Practical Cardiovascular
Medicine

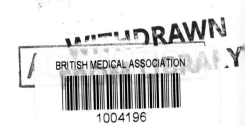

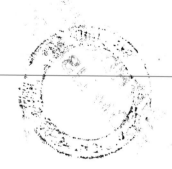

Practical Cardiovascular Medicine

Elias B. Hanna, MD
Associate Professor of Medicine
Associate Program Director of Cardiovascular Disease Fellowship
Associate Program Director of Interventional Cardiology Fellowship
Louisiana State University School of Medicine
University Medical Center
New Orleans, Louisiana, USA

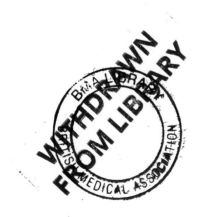

WILEY Blackwell

This edition first published 2017
© 2017 by John Wiley & Sons Ltd

Registered Office
John Wiley & Sons Ltd, The Atrium, Southern Gate, Chichester, West Sussex, PO19 8SQ, UK

Editorial Offices
9600 Garsington Road, Oxford, OX4 2DQ, UK
The Atrium, Southern Gate, Chichester, West Sussex, PO19 8SQ, UK
111 River Street, Hoboken, NJ 07030-5774, USA

For details of our global editorial offices, for customer services and for information about how to apply for permission to reuse the copyright material in this book please see our website at www.wiley.com/wiley-blackwell.

The right of Elias B. Hanna to be identified as the author of this work has been asserted in accordance with the UK Copyright, Designs and Patents Act 1988.

Library of Congress Cataloging-in-Publication Data

Names: Hanna, Elias B., author.
Title: Practical cardiovascular medicine / Elias B. Hanna.
Description: Chichester, West Sussex ; Hoboken, NJ : John Wiley & Sons Inc., 2017. |
   Includes bibliographical references and index.
Identifiers: LCCN 2016055802| ISBN 9781119233367 (pbk.) | ISBN 9781119233497 (epub)
Subjects: | MESH: Cardiovascular Diseases
Classification: LCC RC667 | NLM WG 120 | DDC 616.1–dc23
LC record available at https://lccn.loc.gov/2016055802

A catalog record for this book is available from the British Library.

Wiley also publishes its books in a variety of electronic formats. Some content that appears in print may not be available in electronic books.

Cover image: Science Photo Library - PIXOLOGICSTUDIO/Gettyimages
Cover design: Wiley

Set in 8.5/10.5pt Frutiger Light by SPi Global, Pondicherry, India

Printed in Singapore by C.O.S. Printers Pte Ltd

10 9 8 7 6 5 4 3 2 1

To my mother Marie, my sister Eliana, and my beautiful niece Clara and nephew Marc-Elias, the constant light in my life

To my mentors and my fellows, and to all those who share my love for cardiology

Contents

Preface

You should learn solely in order to create. For willing is creating.

Friedrich Nietzsche, Thus Spoke Zarathustra

Work without ceasing. If you remember in the night, "I have not done what I ought to have done," rise up at once and do it. Believe to the end, even if all men went astray and you were left the only one faithful.

Fyodor Dostoevsky, The Brothers Karamazov

Practical Cardiovascular Medicine is a comprehensive yet practical review of *all* fields of cardiovascular medicine. It addresses various cardiac diseases and presentations using both pathophysiology and clinical evidence, and expands from basic concepts to advanced ones. It should therefore prove useful to experienced physicians as well as trainees. In fact, there is a particular emphasis on the knowledge gaps of cardiologists and cardiology fellows. Organizing fellowship conferences and working with cardiology and interventional cardiology fellows has helped me perceive common deficiencies and focus on them.

Colleagues who read the book will find that it provides them with an in-depth understanding that translates into better patient management. My aim has also been to improve on pre-existing knowledge of pathophysiology and clinical trials. The book follows a comprehensive yet easy, practical, and illustrated flow. To facilitate learning, bottom-line approaches are consistently provided throughout the 38 chapters. There is an extra emphasis on concepts that are frequently misunderstood by practitioners.

Throughout, I have tried to answer daily, practical questions that may not be addressed in any other book. Even classic topics, such as ST-segment elevation myocardial infarction, heart failure, arrhythmias, atrial fibrillation, cardiac catheterization, or electrocardiography are discussed from a different, fresh, and contemporary viewpoint. The book is comprehensive, and many of its chapters could even stand alone as separate books.

In order to consolidate the understanding of complex topics, review questions with detailed answers are provided at the end of clinical chapters, mainly in a clinical vignette format (approximately 400 questions overall). The book will serve cardiologists and cardiology fellows, but will also be valuable to internists, internal medicine residents, and all professionals caring for patients with cardiovascular disease. I have written this book in an effort to embrace the magic and evolving depths of cardiovascular diseases. It is written with love, and with the hope of improving patients' outcomes.

Elias B. Hanna
August 2016

Abbreviations

3D	three-dimensional
AAD	antiarrhythmic drug
AAA	abdominal aortic aneurysm
ABI	ankle–brachial index
ACC	American College of Cardiology
ACCP	American College of Chest Physicians
ACE-I	angiotensin converting enzyme inhibitor
ACS	acute coronary syndrome
ACT	activated clotting time
ADHF	acutely decompensated heart failure
ADP	adenosine diphosphate
AF	atrial fibrillation
Aflutter	atrial flutter
AHA	American Heart Association
AI	aortic insufficiency
AIVR	accelerated idioventricular rhythm
AM	acute marginal
ANA	antinuclear antibodies
Ao	aorta
AoV	aortic valve
AP	accessory pathway
AP	anteroposterior view
ARB	angiotensin-II receptor blocker
ARDS	acute respiratory distress syndrome
ARVC	arrhythmogenic right ventricular cardiomyopathy
ARVD	arrhythmogenic right ventricular dysplasia
AS	aortic stenosis
ASD	atrial septal defect
AT	anterior tibial artery
AT	atrial tachycardia
AT1 receptor	type receptor of angiotensin 2
AT2 receptor	type 2 receptor of angiotensin 2
AT III	antithrombin IIII
AV	atrioventricular
AV block	atrioventricular block
AVA	aortic valve area
AVNRT	atrioventricular nodal reentrant tachycardia
AVR	aortic valve replacement
AVRT	atrioventricular reciprocating tachycardia
BBB	bundle branch block
BiPAP	bilevel positive airway pressure
BiV	biventricular
biVAD	biventricular assist device
BMS	bare-metal stent
BNP	brain natriuretic peptide
BP	blood pressure
bpm	beats per minutes
BSA	body surface area
BUN	blood urea nitrogen
Ca	calcium
CABG	coronary artery bypass grafting
CAD	coronary artery disease
CBC	complete blood count
CCB	calcium channel blockers
CEA	carotid endarterectomy
CIA	common iliac artery

CK	creatine kinase
CK-MB	creatine kinase MB
CKD	chronic kidney disease
CHF	congestive heart failure
CO	cardiac output
COPD	chronic obstructive pulmonary disease
CPAP	continuous positive airway pressure
CRP	C-reactive protein test
CRT	cardiac resynchronization therapy
CT	computed tomography
CTA	computed tomography angiography
CTI	cavotricuspid isthmus
CTO	chronic total occlusion
CTPH	chronic thromboembolic pulmonary hypertension
CVP	central venous pressure
CW	continuous wave Doppler
CYP 450	cytochrome P450
CXR	chest X-ray
DAD	delayed afterdepolarization
DBP	diastolic blood pressure
DC cardioversion	R-wave synchronized direct-current cardioversion
DCM	dilated cardiomyopathy
DES	drug-eluting stent
DHP	dihydropyridine (calcium channel blocker)
dP/dt	delta pressure/delta time (sharpness of rise in pressure over time)
DTI	direct thrombin inhibitor
DTS	Duke treadmill score
DVT	deep vein thrombosis
EAD	early afterdepolarization
ECG	electrocardiogram
echo	echocardiogram
ECMO	extracorporeal membrane oxygenation
ED	emergency department
EF	ejection fraction
EIA	external iliac artery
EP	electrophysiological
ERO	effective regurgitant orifice
ESC	European Society of Cardiology
ESR	erythrocyte sedimentation rate
ESRD	end-stage renal disease
FFR	fractional flow reserve
FiO_2	fraction of inspired oxygen
FMD	fibromuscular dysplasia
GFR	glomerular filtration rate
GI	gastrointestinal
GPI	glycoprotein IIb–IIIa inhibitor
Hb	hemoglobin
HbA1c	glycosylated hemoglobin
HCM	hypertrophic cardiomyopathy
HCTZ	hydrochlorothiazide
HDL	high-density lipoprotein
HF	heart failure
HFpEF	heart failure with preserved ejection fraction
HFrEF	heart failure with reduced ejection fraction
HIT	heparin-induced thrombocytopenia
HIV	Human immunodeficiency virus
HOCM	hypertrophic obstructive cardiomyopathy
HR	heart rate
hs-CRP	high sensitivity C-reactive protein test
HTN	hypertension
IABP	intra-aortic balloon pump
ICD	implantable cardioverter defibrillator
ICU	intensive care unit

INR	international normalized ratio
IV	intravenous or intravenously
IVC	inferior vena cava
IVC-	isovolumic contraction
IVCT	isovolumic contraction time
IVR	isovolumic relaxation
IVRT	isovolumic relaxation time
IVUS	intravascular ultrasound
JVD	jugular venous distension
JVP	jugular venous pressure
K	potassium
LA	left atrium
LAA	left atrial appendage
LAFB	left anterior fascicular block
LAD	left anterior descending artery
LAO	left anterior oblique
LBBB	left bundle branch block
LCx	left circumflex coronary artery
LDL	low-density lipoprotein
LHC	left heart catheterization and coronary angiogram
LIMA	left internal mammary artery
LLSB	left lower sternal border
LM	left main
LMWH	low-molecular-weight heparin
LPFB	left posterior fascicular blockLUSB left upper sternal border
LV	left ventricle or left ventricular
LVAD	left ventricular assist device
LVEDD	left ventricular end-diastolic diameter
LVEDP	left ventricular end-diastolic pressure
LVEF	left ventricular ejection fraction
LVESD	left ventricular end-systolic diameter
LVH	left ventricular hypertrophy
LVOT	left ventricular outflow tract
MAP	mean arterial pressure
MAT	multifocal atrial tachycardia
MET	metabolic equivalent of task
mph	miles per hour
MI	myocardial infarction
MR	mitral regurgitation
MRA	magnetic resonance angiography
MRI	magnetic resonance imaging
MS	mitral stenosis
MV	mitral valve
MV O_2	mixed venous oxygen saturation
MVA	mitral valve area
MVP	mitral valve prolapse
MVR	mitral valve replacement
Na	sodium
NO	nitric oxide
NSAID	non-steroidal anti-inflammatory drug
NSTEMI	non-ST-segment elevation myocardial infarction
NSVT	non-sustained ventricular tachycardia
NT pro-BNP	amino-terminal pro-brain natriuretic peptide
NTG	nitroglycerin
NYHA	New York Heart Association
OCT	optical coherence tomography
OM	obtuse marginal branch of the left circumflex
P	pressure
PA	pulmonary arterial or pulmonary artery
PA O_2	pulmonary arterial oxygen saturation
PAC	premature atrial complex
PaCO$_2$	partial pressure of carbon dioxide in arterial blood
PAD	peripheral arterial disease

PAH	pulmonary arterial hypertension
PAI	plasminogen activator inhibitor
PaO_2	arterial oxygen pressure
PaO_2	alveolar oxygen pressure
PCI	percutaneous coronary intervention
PCSK9	Proprotein convertase subtilisin/kexin type 9
PCWP	pulmonary capillary wedge pressure
PDA	patent ductus arteriosus
PDA	posterior descending artery branch of the right coronary artery or left circumflex
PE	pulmonary embolism
PEA	pulseless electrical activity
PET	positron emission tomography
PFO	patent foramen ovale
PFT	pulmonary function testing
PH	pulmonary hypertension
PHT	pressure half-time
PISA	proximal isovelocity surface area
PJRT	permanent junctional reciprocating tachycardia
PLB	posterolateral ventricular branches of the right coronary artery or left circumflex
PM	pacemaker
PMBV	percutaneous mitral balloon valvuloplasty
PMT	pacemaker-mediated tachycardia
PND	paroxysmal nocturnal dyspnea
POTS	postural orthostatic tachycardia syndrome
PPD	purified protein derivative for *Mycobacterium tuberculosis*
PPI	proton pump inhibitor
PPM	patient/prosthesis mismatch
PR	pulmonic regurgitation
PS	pulmonic stenosis
PT	posterior tibial artery
PTT	partial thromboplastin time
PV loop	pressure–volume loop
$PV O_2$	pulmonary venous oxygen saturation
PVARP	post-ventricular atrial refractory period
PVC	premature ventricular complex
PVR	pulmonary vascular resistance
PW	pulsed wave Doppler
Qp	pulmonary blood flow
Qs	systemic blood flow
QTc	corrected QT interval
RA	right atrium
RAAS	renin-angiotensin-aldosterone system
RAO	right anterior oblique
RAS	renal artery stenosis
RBBB	right bundle branch block
RCA	right coronary artery RHC right heart catheterization
RIMA	right internal mammary artery
rPA	reteplase
rpm	revolutions per minute
r-tPA	recombinant tissue plasminogen activator
RUSB	right upper sternal border
RV	right ventricle/ventricular
RVAD	right ventricular assist device
RVEDP	right ventricular end-diastolic pressure
RVH	right ventricular hypertrophy
RVOT	right ventricular outflow tract
SA	sinoatrial
$SA O_2$	systemic arterial oxygen saturation
SAM	systolic anterior motion
SaO_2	arterial oxygen saturation
SBE	subacute bacterial endocarditis
SBP	systolic blood pressure
SCD	sudden cardiac death

SIRS	systemic inflammatory response syndrome
SFA	superficial femoral artery
SNRT	sinus node reentrant tachycardia
SPECT	single photon emission computed tomography (nuclear imaging)
SQ	subcutaneously
STEMI	ST-segment elevation myocardial infarction
STS	Society of Thoracic Surgeons
SV	stroke volume
SVC	superior vena cava
SVG	saphenous venous graft
SvO_2	mixed venous oxygen saturation
SVR	systemic vascular resistance
SVT	supraventricular tachycardia
TAA	thoracic aortic aneurysm
TdP	torsades de pointes
TEE	transesophageal echocardiogram
TGA	transposition of great arteries
TIA	transient ischemic attack
TID	transient ischemic dilatation
TR	tricuspid regurgitation
TSH	thyroid stimulating hormone
TTE	transthoracic echocardiogram
UA	unstable angina
UFH	unfractionated heparin
VAD	ventricular assist device
V/Q scan	lung ventilation/perfusion scan
VF	ventricular fibrillation
VLDL	very-low-density lipoprotein
Vp	velocity of propagation
VSD	ventricular septal defect
VSR	ventricular septal rupture
VT	ventricular tachycardia
VTI	velocity-time integral
WPW	Wolff–Parkinson–White

Part 1   CORONARY ARTERY DISEASE

1   Non-ST-Segment Elevation Acute Coronary Syndrome

I. Types of acute coronary syndrome (ACS)

A. Unstable angina

Unstable angina is defined as any of the following clinical presentations, with or without ECG evidence of ischemia and with a normal troponin:

- Crescendo angina: angina that increases in frequency, intensity, or duration, often requiring a more frequent use of nitroglycerin
- New-onset (<2 months) severe angina, occurring during normal activities performed at a normal pace
- Rest angina
- Angina occurring within 2 weeks after a myocardial infarction (post-infarction angina)

B. Non-ST-segment elevation myocardial infarction (NSTEMI)

A rise in troponin, per se, is diagnostic of myocardial necrosis but is not sufficient to define myocardial infarction (MI), which is myocardial necrosis secondary to myocardial ischemia. Additional clinical, ECG, or echocardiographic evidence of ischemia is needed to define MI.

In fact, **MI** is defined as a *troponin elevation* above the 99th percentile of the reference limit (~0.03 ng/ml, depending on the assay) *with a rise and/or fall pattern, along with any one of the following four features*: (i) angina; (ii) ST-T abnormalities, new LBBB, or new Q waves on ECG; (iii) new wall motion abnormality on imaging; (iv) intracoronary thrombus on angiography.[1] **NSTEMI** is defined as MI without persistent (>20 min) ST-segment elevation.

Isolated myocardial necrosis is common in critically ill patients and manifests as a troponin rise, sometimes with a rise and fall pattern, but frequently no other MI features. Also, troponin I usually remains <1 ng/ml in the absence of underlying CAD.[2,3]

Practical Cardiovascular Medicine, First Edition. Elias B. Hanna.
© 2017 John Wiley & Sons Ltd. Published 2017 by John Wiley & Sons Ltd.

A rise or fall in troponin is necessary to define MI. A fluctuating troponin or a mild, chronically elevated but stable troponin may be seen in chronic heart failure, myocarditis, severe left ventricular hypertrophy, or advanced kidney disease. While having a prognostic value, this stable troponin rise is not diagnostic of MI. Different cutoffs have been used to define a relevant troponin change, but, in general, a troponin that rises above the 99th percentile with a rise or fall of >50–80% is characteristic of MI (ACC guidelines use a less specific cutoff of 20%; 50–80% cutoff is more applicable to low troponin levels <0.1 ng/ml).[4]

C. ST-segment elevation myocardial infarction (STEMI)

STEMI is defined as a combination of ischemic symptoms and persistent, ischemic ST-segment elevation.[1,5] For practical purposes, ischemic symptoms with ongoing ST-segment elevation of any duration are considered STEMI and treated as such. The diagnosis may be retrospectively changed to NSTEMI if ST elevation quickly resolves without reperfusion therapy, in <20 minutes.

> Unstable angina and NSTEMI are grouped together as non-ST-segment elevation ACS (NSTE-ACS). However, *it must be noted that unstable angina has a much better prognosis than NSTEMI,* and particularly that many patients labeled as unstable angina do not actually have ACS.[6] **In fact, in the current era of highly sensitive troponin assays, a true ACS is often accompanied by a troponin rise. Unstable angina is, thus, a "vanishing" entity.**[7]

II. Mechanisms of ACS

A. True ACS is usually due to plaque rupture or erosion that promotes platelet aggregation (spontaneous or type 1 MI). This is followed by thrombus formation and microembolization of platelet aggregates. In NSTEMI, the thrombus is most often a platelet-rich non-occlusive thrombus. This contrasts with STEMI, which is due to an occlusive thrombus rich in platelets and fibrin. Also, NSTEMI usually has greater collateral flow to the infarct zone than STEMI.

As a result of the diffuse inflammation and alteration of platelet aggregability, multiple plaque ruptures are seen in ~30–80% of ACS cases, although only one is usually considered the culprit in ACS.[8] This shows the importance of medical therapy to "cool down" the diffuse process, and explains the high risk of ACS recurrence within the following year even if the culprit plaque is stented.[8]

Occasionally, a ruptured plaque or, more commonly, an eroded plaque may lead to microembolization of platelets and thrombi and impaired coronary flow without any residual, angiographically significant lesion or thrombus.

B. Secondary unstable angina and NSTEMI (type 2 MI). In this case, ischemia is related to severely increased O_2 demands (demand/supply mismatch). The patient may have underlying CAD but the coronary plaques are stable without acute rupture or thrombosis. Conversely, the patient may not have any underlying CAD, in which case troponin I usually remains <0.5–1 ng/ml.[2,3] *Acute antithrombotic therapy is not warranted.*

> In the absence of clinical or ECG features of MI, the troponin rise is not even called MI.

Cardiac causes of secondary unstable angina/NSTEMI include: severe hypertension, acute HF, aortic stenosis/hypertrophic cardiomyopathy, tachyarrhythmias. Non-cardiac causes of secondary unstable angina/NSTEMI include: gastrointestinal bleed, severe anemia, hypoxia, sepsis.

While acute HF often leads to troponin elevation, ACS with severe diffuse ischemia may lead to acute HF, and in fact 30% of acute HF presentations are triggered by ACS.[9] HF presentation associated with *crescendo angina, ischemic ST changes,* or *severe troponin rise* (>0.5–1 ng/ml) should be considered ACS until CAD is addressed with a coronary angiogram.

> *Acute bleed, severe anemia, or tachyarrhythmia destabilizes a stable angina.* Treating the anemia or the arrhythmia is a first priority in these patients, taking precedence over treating CAD.

> While acute, malignant hypertension may lead to secondary ACS and troponin rise, ACS with severe angina may lead to hypertension (catecholamine surge). In ACS, hypertension drastically improves with angina relief and nitroglycerin, whereas in malignant hypertension, hypertension is persistent and difficult to control despite multiple antihypertensive therapies, nitroglycerin only having a minor effect. Nitroglycerin has a mild and transient antihypertensive effect, and thus a sustained drop in BP with nitroglycerin often implies that hypertension was secondary to ACS.

C. Coronary vasospasm

It was initially hypothesized by Prinzmetal and then demonstrated in a large series that vasospasm and vasospastic angina (Prinzmetal) often occur in patients with significant CAD at the site of a significant atherosclerotic obstruction.[10,11] In one series, 90% of patients with vasospastic angina had significant, single- or multivessel CAD. Most frequently, CAD was not only significant but unstable.[12] In fact, a ruptured plaque is frequently accompanied by vasospasm, as the activated platelets and leukocytes release vasoconstrictors. About 20% of these patients with underlying CAD go on to develop a large MI, while >25% develop severe ventricular arrhythmias or paroxysmal AV block with syncope.

Vasospasm may also occur chronically without plaque rupture, and, sometimes, without any significant atherosclerotic stenosis, and may lead to chronic vasospastic angina. Vasospasm is frequently the underlying disease process in patients with a typical angina or ACS yet no significant CAD (isolated vasospasm).[13,14] The diagnosis is definitely made when: (i) vasospasm is angiographically reproduced with provocative testing, *along with* (ii) symptoms *and* (iii) ST changes during testing. Vasospasm may also occur at the microvascular level (endothelial dysfunction with diffuse microvascular constriction).

III. ECG, cardiac biomarkers, and echocardiography in ACS

A. ECG

The following ECG findings are diagnostic of non-ST elevation ischemia:

- ST depression ≥0.5 mm, especially if transient, dynamic, not secondary to LVH, and occurring during the episode of chest pain.
- Deep T-wave inversion ≥3 mm (T inversion <3 mm is non-specific).
- Transient ST elevation (lasting <20 minutes). This corresponds to a thrombus that occludes the lumen off and on, an unstable plaque with vasospasm, or, less commonly, a stable plaque with vasospasm.

Only 50% of patients with non-ST elevation ACS have an ischemic ECG.[15] In particular, in the cases of NSTEMI and unstable angina, 20% and 37%, respectively, have an absolutely normal ECG.[16] Also, many patients have LVH or bundle branch blocks that make the ECG less interpretable and non-specific for ischemia. Of patients with a normal ECG, 2% end up having MI, mostly NSTEMI, and 2–4% end up having unstable angina.[17]

ECG performed during active chest pain has a higher sensitivity and specificity for detection of ischemia. However, even when performed during active ischemia, the ECG may not be diagnostic, particularly in left circumflex ischemia. In fact, up to 40% of acute LCx total occlusions and 10% of LAD or RCA occlusions are not associated with significant ST-T abnormalities, for various reasons: (i) the vessel may occlude progressively, allowing the development of robust collaterals that prevent ST elevation or even ST depression upon coronary occlusion; (ii) the ischemic area may not be well seen on the standard leads (especially posterior or lateral area); (iii) underlying LVH or bundle branch blocks may obscure new findings; a comparison with old ECGs is valuable. *In general, ~15–20% of NSTEMIs are due to acute coronary occlusion, frequently LCx occlusion, and are, pathophysiologically, STEMI-equivalents missed by the ECG and potentially evolving into Q waves.*[18] NSTEMI patients with acute coronary occlusion have a higher 30-day mortality than patients without an occluded culprit artery, probably related to delayed revascularization of a STEMI-equivalent.[19]

To improve the diagnostic yield of the ECG:

- In a patient with persistent typical angina and non-diagnostic ECG, record the ECG in leads V_7–V_9. ST elevation is seen in those leads in >80% of LCx occlusions, many of which are missed on the 12-lead ECG.
- Repeat the ECG at 10–30-minute intervals in a patient with persistent typical angina.
- Perform urgent coronary angiography in a patient with persistent distress and a high suspicion of ACS, even if ECG is non-diagnostic and troponin has not risen yet.
- *ECG should be repeated during each recurrence of pain, when the diagnostic yield is highest. ECG should also be repeated a few hours after pain resolution* (e.g., 3–9 hours) and next day, looking for post-ischemic T-wave abnormalities and Q waves, even if the initial ECG is non-diagnostic. The post-ischemic T waves may appear a few hours after chest pain resolution.

B. Cardiac biomarkers: troponin I or T, CK-MB

These markers start to rise 3–12 hours after an episode of ischemia lasting >30–60 minutes (they may take up to 12 hours to rise).

Troponin is highly specific for a myocardial injury. However, this myocardial injury may be secondary not to a coronary event but to other insults (e.g., critical illness, HF, hypoxia, hypotension), without additional clinical, ECG, or echocardiographic features of MI.

Kidney disease may be associated, per se, with a chronic mild elevation of troponin I. This is not related to reduced renal clearance of troponin, a marginal effect at best. It is rather due to the underlying myocardial hypertrophy, chronic CAD, and BP swings. This leads to a chronic ischemic imbalance, and, as a result, a chronic myocardial damage.

Any degree of troponin rise, even if very mild (e.g., 0.04 ng/ml), in a patient with angina and without a context of secondary ischemia indicates a high-risk ACS. The higher the troponin rises (meaning >1 ng/ml or, worse, >5 ng/ml), the worse the prognosis.[20] Also, an elevated troponin associated with elevated CK-MB signifies a larger MI and a worse short-term prognosis than an isolated rise in troponin.

CK-MB and troponin peak at ~12–24 hours and 24 hours, respectively. CK and CK-MB elevations last 2–3 days. Troponin elevation lasts 7–10 days; minor troponin elevation, however, usually resolves within 2–3 days. In acutely reperfused infarcts (STEMI or NSTEMI), those markers peak earlier (e.g., 12–18 hours) and sometimes peak to higher values than if not reperfused, but decline faster. Hence, the total amount of biomarkers released, meaning the area under the curve, is much smaller, and the troponin elevation resolves more quickly (e.g., 4–5 days). The area under the curve, rather than the actual biomarker peak, correlates with the infarct size.

Troponin I or T is much more sensitive and specific than CK-MB. Frequently, NSTEMI is characterized by an elevated troponin and a normal CK-MB, and typically CK-MB only rises when troponin exceeds 0.5 ng/ml. To be considered cardiac-specific, an elevated CK-MB must be accompanied by an elevated troponin; the ratio CK-MB/CK is typically >2.5% in MI, but even this ratio is not specific for MI. When increased, CK-MB usually rises earlier than troponin, and thus an elevated CK-MB with a normal troponin and normal CK may imply an early MI (as long as troponin eventually rises). Overall, CK-MB testing is not recommended on a routine basis but has two potential values: (i) in patients with marked troponin elevation and subacute symptom onset, CK-MB helps diagnose the age of the infarct (a normal CK-MB implies that MI is several days old); (ii) CK-MB elevation implies a larger MI.

Cardiac biomarkers, if negative, are repeated at least once 3–6 hours after admission or pain onset. If positive, they may be repeated every 8 hours until they trend down, to assess the area under the curve/infarct size.*

---

* A new generation of high-sensitivity troponin assays (hs-troponin) has a much lower detection cutoff (*detection cutoff* = 0.003 ng/ml vs. 0.01 ng/ml for the older generation; *MI cutoff* = 0.03 ng/ml for both generations). If hs-troponin is lower than the detection cutoff on presentation or lower than the MI cutoff 3 hours later, MI can be ruled out with a very high negative predictive value >99.4%.[4] The positive predictive value of these low values, however, is 75% at best, and is improved by seeking a significant rise or fall pattern.

In patients with a recent infarction (a few days earlier), the diagnosis of *reinfarction* relies on:

- CK or CK-MB elevation, as they normalize faster than troponin, or
- Change in the downward trend of troponin (reincrease >20% beyond the nadir)[1]

In the *post-PCI context*, MI is diagnosed by a troponin elevation >5× normal, *along with* prolonged chest pain >20 min, ischemic ST changes or Q waves, new wall motion abnormality, or angiographic evidence of procedural complications.[1] In patients with elevated baseline cardiac markers that are stable or falling, post-PCI MI is diagnosed by ≥50% reincrease of the downward trending troponin (rather than 20% for spontaneous reinfarction). Note that spontaneous NSTEMI carries a much stronger prognostic value than post-PCI NSTEMI, despite the often mild biomarker elevation in the former (threefold higher mortality). In fact, in spontaneous NSTEMI, the adverse outcome is related not just to the minor myocardial injury but to the ruptured plaques that carry a high future risk of large infarctions. This is not the case in the controlled post-PCI MI.[21,22] Along with data suggesting that only marked CK-MB elevation carries a prognostic value after PCI, an expert document has proposed the use of CK-MB ≥10× normal to define post-PCI MI, rather than the mild troponin rise.[22]

   In the *post-CABG context*, MI is diagnosed by a troponin or CK-MB elevation >10× normal, associated with new Q wave or LBBB, or new wall motion abnormality.[1]

   In randomized trials recruiting patients with high-risk non-ST-segment elevation ACS, only ~60–70% of patients had a positive troponin; the remaining patients had unstable angina. However, with the current generation of high-sensitivity troponin, unstable angina is becoming a rare entity. *In fact, in patients with a serially negative troponin, ACS is unlikely.*[7] **This is particularly true in cases of serially undetectable troponin (<0.003–0.01 ng/ml), where ACS is very unlikely and the 30-day risk of coronary events is <0.5%.**[4,23]

When ischemic imbalance occurs without underlying CAD, troponin I usually remains <0.5–1 ng/ml.[2,3] However, when ischemic imbalance occurs on top of underlying stable CAD, troponin I may rise to levels >0.5–1 ng/ml. Therefore, **a troponin I level >0.5–1 ng/ml suggests obstructive CAD, whether the primary insult is coronary (thrombotic, type 1 MI) or non-coronary (type 2 MI)**; the positive predictive value for CAD is very high and approaches 90%, less so if renal dysfunction is present.[2]

   Conversely, any degree of troponin rise, even if very mild (e.g., 0.04 ng/ml), in a patient with angina and without a context of secondary ischemia indicates a high-risk ACS.

C. Echocardiography: acute resting nuclear scan

The absence of wall motion abnormalities *during active chest pain* argues strongly against ischemia. For optimal sensitivity, the patient must have active ischemia while the test is performed. Wall motion abnormalities may persist after pain resolution in case of stunning or subendocardial necrosis involving >20% of the inner myocardial thickness (<20% subendocardial necrosis or mild troponin rise may not lead to any discernible contractile abnormality).[24]

   On the other hand, wall motion abnormalities, when present, are not very specific for ongoing ischemia and may reflect an old infarct. However, the patient is already in a high-risk category.

   Acute resting nuclear scan, with the nuclear injection performed during active chest pain or within ~3 hours of the last chest pain episode, has an even higher sensitivity than echo in detecting ischemia. An abnormal resting scan, however, is not specific, as the defect may be an old infarct or an artifact.

IV. Approach to chest pain, likelihood of ACS, risk stratification of ACS

Only 25% of patients presenting with chest pain are eventually diagnosed with ACS. On the other hand, ~5% of patients discharged home with a presumed non-cardiac chest pain are eventually diagnosed with ACS, and the ECG is normal in 20–37% of patients with ACS.[17]

   Consider the following approach in patients presenting with acute or recent chest pain.

A. Assess the likelihood of ACS (Table 1.1)

- The relief of chest pain with sublingual nitroglycerin does not reliably predict ACS. Similarly, the relief of chest pain with a "GI cocktail" does not predict the absence of ACS.[25]
- Chest pain lasting over 30–60 minutes with consistently negative markers usually implies a low ACS likelihood. A prolonged pain is usually one of two extremes, an infarct or a non-cardiac pain.

B. Assess for other serious causes of chest pain at least clinically, by chest X-ray and by ECG (always think of pulmonary embolism, aortic dissection, and pericarditis).

C. The patient with a probable ACS should be risk stratified into a high- or low-risk category

   1. High-risk ACS. Any of the following features implies a high risk of major adverse coronary events (mortality, MI, or need for urgent revascularization within 30 days), and justifies early coronary angiography and a more aggressive antithrombotic strategy. *These high-risk features should only be sought after establishing that ACS is highly probable:*[25]

Table 1.1 ACS likelihood.

High likelihood

Elevated troponin or ST-T abnormalities that are definitely ischemic

Prior history of CAD or MI with typical angina or symptoms similar to prior MI

S3, new MR murmur[a]

Chest pain with signs of new HF (and without malignant HTN that could account for both pain and HF)

Typical angina is reproduced or worsened by exertion. In vasospasm, angina may occur only at rest or at night without an exertional component

Severe distress, deep fatigue, diaphoresis, or severe nausea during pain is concerning for angina (the latter symptoms may occur without pain and are called "angina equivalents"). Jaw radiation is concerning for angina

Intermediate likelihood

PAD, age >70, diabetes[b]

In the absence of the above features, the following suggests a low ACS likelihood (the 3 Ps)

Chest pain that is **P**ositional or reproduced with certain chest/arm movements

Pleuritic pain (↑ with inspiration or cough: suggests pleural or pericardial pain, or costochondritis)

Palpable pain localized at a fingertip area and fully reproduced with palpation[c]

Pain >30–60 min with consistently negative markers.

Very brief pain <15 s

---

[a] A new MR murmur in a patient with chest pain is considered ischemic MR until proven otherwise.

[b] **Traditional risk factors are only weakly predictive of the likelihood of ACS.**[25] Once ACS is otherwise diagnosed, diabetes and PAD do predict a higher ACS risk.

[c] True angina and PE pain may seem reproducible with palpation, as the chest wall is hypersensitive in those conditions. **A combination of multiple low-likelihood features** (e.g., reproducible pain that is also positional and sharp), rather than a sole reliance on pain reproducibility, better defines the low-likelihood group.[26,27]

- Elevated troponin (NSTEMI). Any troponin elevation (e.g., 0.05 ng/ml) in a patient with chest pain and no other obvious cardiac or systemic insult (HF, critical illness) implies high-risk ACS.
- Ischemic ECG changes (especially new, dynamic ST depression ≥0.5 mm or transient ST elevation)
- Hemodynamic instability, electrical instability (VT), or HF (S3, pulmonary edema, ischemic MR)
- Angina at rest or minimal exertion that is *persistent/refractory*, or *recurrent* despite the initial antithrombotic and anti-ischemic therapies. In patients with negative ECG/troponin, clinical features are used to decide whether the persistent chest pain is a true angina or not.
- EF <40%
- Prior PCI <6–12 months (time frame of restenosis), or prior CABG
- TIMI risk score ≥3*

While diabetes is associated with a higher risk of adverse outcomes in ACS, it does not, per se, dictate early coronary angiography. Coronary angiography is rather dictated by the above features. As stated in the 2014 ACC guidelines: "decisions to perform stress testing, angiography, and revascularization should be similar in patients with and without diabetes mellitus (class I)."[25]

> The TIMI risk score is used in ACS once the diagnosis of ACS is established or is highly likely. ***The score should not be used for the diagnosis of ACS; it has a prognostic rather than a diagnostic value.*** Also, this score is one risk stratifier out of many. An elevated troponin may be associated with a TIMI risk score of only 1, yet still implies a high-risk ACS. In the right setting, even a mild troponin rise (e.g., 0.05 ng/ml) implies a high-risk ACS.

2. Low-risk ACS and low-likelihood ACS. Low-risk ACS must be differentiated from low-likelihood ACS. The patient may have typical angina or may be older than 70 years with diabetes, which makes ACS probable, yet he has no rest angina, no recurrence of angina at low level of activity, and no recent coronary history with a TIMI risk score that is 1 or 2 (low risk).

Despite being different, those two entities are approached similarly from the standpoint of early conservative vs. early invasive management. They are initially managed conservatively with early stress testing. Patients in this group are characterized by:

- Negative troponin and ECG 3–6 hours after symptom onset
- *AND* no typical angina at rest or minimal exertion; no signs of HF
- *AND* no recent coronary history/MI

Outside a recent PCI or CABG, a prior coronary history places the patient at an intermediate rather than a high risk of coronary events, and stress testing may still be performed.

The patient with persistent atypical chest pain and negative troponin has a low likelihood of ACS and may undergo stress testing while having the atypical pain.

---

* TIMI risk score: 1, Age ≥65 yr; 2, ≥3 risk factors; 3, History of coronary stenosis ≥50%; 4, ≥2 episodes of pain in the last 24 h; 5, Use of aspirin in the prior 7 d (implying aspirin resistance); 6, Elevated troponin; 7, ST deviation ≥0.5 mm. A score of 3 or 4 is intermediate risk; 5–7 is high risk. Early invasive strategy improves outcomes in patients with TIMI risk score ≥3, and thus a score of 3–7 qualifies for an early invasive strategy and full ACS therapy. Risk of mortality/MI/urgent revascularization at 14 days: 13% if score = 3; 20% if score = 4; 26% if score = 5; 40% if score = 6/7.

V. Management of high-risk NSTE-ACS

There are four lines of therapy for high-risk NSTE-ACS:

- Initial invasive strategy
- Antiplatelet therapy:
  1. Aspirin
  2. Platelet ADP receptor antagonists (clopidogrel, prasugrel, ticagrelor)
  3. Glycoprotein IIb/IIIa antagonists
- Anticoagulants
- Anti-ischemic and other therapies
- No thrombolytics. Thrombolytics are only useful for STEMI. In NSTE-ACS, the thrombus is non-occlusive and thrombolytics may promote distal embolization, overall worsening the myocardial perfusion.[28] Also, thrombolytics activate platelets, which may lead to more platelet-rich thrombi in NSTE-ACS.

A. Initial invasive strategy

An initial invasive strategy implies that diagnostic coronary angiography and *possible* revascularization are performed within 72 hours of presentation, and within 12–24 hours in the highest risk subgroup. ***An initial or early invasive strategy does not equate with early PCI. It rather equates with risk stratification by early coronary angiography and subsequent management by PCI, CABG, or medical therapy according to the angiographic findings. It is an early* intent *to revascularize.*** In various clinical trials that managed ACS invasively, ~55–60% of patients received PCI, ~15% received CABG, and 25% received medical therapy only.[29–31] The initial invasive strategy is contrasted with the initial conservative/selective invasive strategy, in which the patient is treated medically and risk-stratified with stress testing, then invasively managed in case of recurrent true angina or high-risk stress test result.

The invasive strategy needs to be performed "*early*" rather than urgently, but becomes "*urgent*" in the following cases:

- ST elevation develops, which indicates the importance of repeating the ECG during each pain recurrence or during persistent pain.
- Refractory or recurrent true angina even if ECG is normal and troponin is initially negative (troponin may be negative up to 12 hours after pain onset).
- Hemodynamic instability or sustained VT attributed to ischemia.

Three major trials (FRISC II, TACTICS-TIMI 18, RITA 3) established the benefit of an initial invasive strategy and showed that in high-risk ACS patients this strategy reduces the combined endpoint of death and MI in comparison to an initial conservative strategy, particularly in patients with positive troponin, ST-segment changes, or TIMI risk score ≥3 (50% reduction in death/MI in those subgroups in all three trials, with an absolute risk reduction of ~5% at 30 days and 1 year).[32–34] The mortality was reduced at 1-year follow-up in the overall FRISC II trial (by ~40%, more so in the highest risk groups), and at 5-year follow-up in the overall RITA 3 trial. Those beneficial results were seen despite the narrow difference in revascularization rates between the initial invasive and initial conservative strategy. For example, in TACTICS, 60% of patients in the initial invasive strategy vs. 35% of patients in the initial conservative strategy received revascularization at 30 days, this difference becoming narrower over the course of 6–12 months. ***These trials did not address revascularization vs. no revascularization in high-risk ACS patients who clinically and angiographically qualify for revascularization, in which case revascularization is expected to show more striking benefits.*** These trials rather addressed the early intent to revascularize vs. the early intent to not revascularize. In trials where the difference in revascularization between groups was narrower, such as the ICTUS trial, the early invasive strategy could not show a benefit over the early conservative strategy (at 1 year, the revascularization rates were 79% vs. 54%).[35] The results of the ICTUS trial do not imply a lack a benefit from revascularization, but rather that an initial conservative strategy with a later invasive strategy if needed, sometimes weeks later, *may be* appropriate in initially stabilized patients who are free of angina, particularly if they have multiple comorbidities and are not ideal candidates for revascularization (class IIb in ACC guidelines; not recommended in ESC guidelines).

The exact timing of the initial invasive strategy has been addressed in the TIMACS trial, where an "early" invasive strategy at <24 hours was compared to a "delayed early" invasive strategy at 36 hours to 5 days (mainly 48–72 hours).[31] The early invasive strategy did not reduce the rate of death/MI in the overall group but reduced it in the highest-risk group, with GRACE risk score >140; beside troponin and ST changes, the GRACE risk score takes into account increasing age, history of HF, tachycardia, hypotension, and renal function. Thus, an "early" invasive strategy <24 hours is reasonable in patients with a GRACE risk score >140, but also in all patients with elevated troponin or dynamic ST changes, per ACC guidelines (class IIa recommendation).[36]

B. Antiplatelet therapy (Figure 1.1, Table 1.2) (see Appendix 4 for a detailed discussion)

Typically, aspirin and one ADP receptor antagonist (ticagrelor, clopidogrel) should be started upon admission, upstream of catheterization.[36] Upstream IIb/IIIa inhibitor therapy is not beneficial and is not an alternative to upstream ADP receptor antagonist therapy.[30,36–38]

C. Anticoagulant therapy (see Appendix 4 for a detailed discussion)

Four anticoagulants are considered in NSTE-ACS: (i) *unfractionated heparin (UFH)*, (ii) *enoxaparin*, (iii) *bivalirudin*, and (iv) *fondaparinux. Upon admission*, anticoagulation with any one of these four drugs should be initiated (class I recommendation). *During PCI*, either UFH or bivalirudin is used (Figures 1.2, 1.3; Table 1.2).

- In high-risk ACS patients, the anticoagulant should not be withheld before the catheterization procedure.
- The dose of UFH used in ACS is lower than the dose used in PE, with a PTT goal of 46–70 seconds. As cornerstone antiplatelet therapy is administered, ***moderate rather than high-level anticoagulation is appropriate for ischemic reduction in ACS*** and minimizes bleeding, which is a powerful prognostic marker in ACS.

- Anticoagulants are typically stopped after the performance of PCI. If PCI is not performed, anticoagulants are typically administered for at least 48 hours, and preferably longer, for the duration of hospitalization (up to 8 days). Longer therapy reduces rebound ischemia, which mainly occurs with heparin.
- In patients undergoing catheterization, upstream enoxaparin therapy is associated with a higher bleeding risk than UFH. Moreover, *the switch between enoxaparin and UFH increases the bleeding risk and should be avoided*. If the patient is going for an invasive strategy and the operator prefers not to use enoxaparin during PCI, the patient should receive UFH or fondaparinux on admission, not enoxaparin.
- A switch from UFH to bivalirudin, or from fondaparinux to other anticoagulants, during PCI has not shown harm.

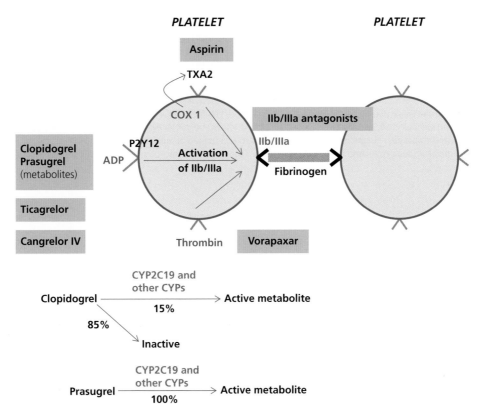

Figure 1.1 Platelet receptors and antiplatelet mechanisms of action.

Cyclooxygenase 1 (COX-1) allows the synthesis of thromboxane A2 (TXA2), which acts on its platelet receptor, eventually activating the IIb/IIIa receptor. Aspirin irreversibly acetylates COX-1. While the pharmacokinetic half-life of aspirin is only ~20 min – 2 h, the pharmacodynamic effect of aspirin lasts the lifespan of the platelet (5–7 days).

The platelet ADP receptor eventually leads to conformational activation of the IIb/IIIa receptors. *Clopidogrel and prasugrel* (thienopyridines) are prodrugs that get metabolized into an active metabolite. This active metabolite irreversibly binds to the P2Y12 ADP receptor, extending the pharmacodynamic effect of these drugs to 5–7 days despite a half-life of 8 h. The prodrugs are metabolized by cytochromes (CYP), particularly CYP2C19; only 15% of clopidogrel vs. 100% of prasugrel is actively metabolized. This explains why prasugrel is a much more potent inhibitor of platelet aggregation (~75% vs. ~35% inhibition of platelet aggregation).

Some patients have a CYP2C19 mutation that slows clopidogrel metabolism and preferentially increases its inactivation by esterases, translating into a poor or no response to clopidogrel. Prasugrel, on the other hand, has only one metabolic pathway, and will be metabolized by cytochromes regardless of how slow the metabolism is.

Ticagrelor directly binds to the P2Y12 ADP receptor and reversibly inhibits it (the effect clears as the drug clears from plasma). Despite being a reversible ADP antagonist, the very potent ADP blockade and the long half-life translates into an antiplatelet effect that lasts 3–4 days (half-life ~15 h). Since it directly acts on its receptor, the response to ticagrelor is consistent and potent (~75% platelet inhibition), including in clopidogrel non-responders.

Cangrelor is an intravenous ADP receptor antagonist that directly and reversibly binds to the ADP receptor. It inhibits 90% of the platelet aggregation. In contrast to ticagrelor, it has a short half-life of 5 min, which, in addition to the reversible receptor binding, leads to a very quick onset and offset of action. Thrombin is also a potent activator of platelet aggregation. *Vorapaxar* blocks the thrombin receptor.

Cyclic AMP, promoted by cilostazol, inhibits platelet aggregation.

The *IIb/IIIa receptor* is the final common pathway of platelet aggregation, and allows linking of the platelets through fibrinogen molecules.

D. Anti-ischemic therapy and other therapies

1. β-Blocker, such as oral metoprolol, is administered at a dose of 25 mg Q8–12 h, and titrated to 50 mg Q8–12 h if tolerated. In the COMMIT-CCS trial, the initiation of β-blockers on the first day of ACS (mainly STEMI) was associated with an increased risk of cardiogenic shock during that first day, the benefit from β-blockers on reinfarction and VF emerging gradually beyond the second day.[39] Overall, β-blockers significantly

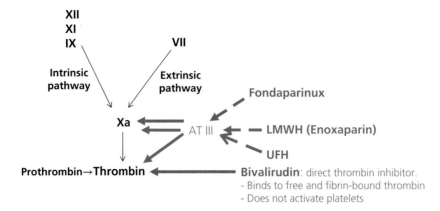

Figure 1.2 Specific effects of the four anticoagulants.

A heparin derivative induces a conformational change in antithrombin III (AT III), which, according to the size of the heparin–AT III complex, predominantly inactivates Xa or the active thrombin. UFH inactivates thrombin preferentially, while low-molecular-weight heparin (LMWH) inactivates Xa preferentially. The smaller fondaparinux molecule inactivates Xa exclusively. The inactivation of Xa eventually inhibits thrombin generation rather than thrombin activity. Heparin activates platelets directly by binding to them, which also triggers antiplatelet antibodies (HIT).

The oral direct thrombin inhibitor (dabigatran) and the oral Xa antagonists (apixaban, rivaroxaban) are used to treat AF, not ACS.

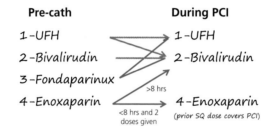

Figure 1.3 Summary of anticoagulant use in NSTE-ACS, before catheterization and during PCI.

Operators who are not comfortable with performing PCI solely under the coverage of a prior subcutaneous dose of enoxaparin should avoid starting enoxaparin on admission and should use any of the other three agents upfront.

Table 1.2 Summary of antithrombotic therapy in ACS.

Antiplatelet therapy
1. Aspirin 325 mg on admission to all, then 81 mg daily (after a 325 mg first dose)
2. Clopidogrel 300 mg or ticagrelor 180 mg on admission of all NSTE-ACS patients
   May withhold in a subgroup of patients with a high probability of needing CABG
3. Upstream GPI *is not indicated*, even if an ADP receptor antagonist is not started on admission
4. After coronary angiography, if PCI is to be performed:
   Add 300 mg of clopidogrel if 300 mg has already been given
   or load with 600 mg of clopidogrel in the lab if no clopidogrel has been given
   or load with prasugrel 60 mg (even if clopidogrel has been given)
   or load with ticagrelor 180 mg (even if clopidogrel has been given)
   GPI if troponin (+) *and* no clopidogrel or ticagrelor preload
   or if PCI complications (bailout use of GPI)
   GPI on top of prasugrel or ticagrelor: unclear benefit

Anticoagulant therapy
   UFH pre-catheterization and during PCI
   or UFH pre-catheterization and switch to bivalirudin during PCI
   or Fondaparinux 2.5 mg SQ once daily pre-catheterization, with standard-dose UFH or bivalirudin during PCI
   or Enoxaparin pre-catheterization. If patient received 1 mg/kg SQ within 8 h of PCI and has already received two doses of enoxaparin, no additional anticoagulation is needed during PCI (if enoxaparin was used 8–12 h ago *or* only one SQ dose was given, add 0.3 mg/kg IV during PCI; if enoxaparin was used >12 h ago, give 0.5–0.75 mg/kg IV bolus)

Note: Avoid switching between UFH and enoxaparin. The switch to bivalirudin is, however, appropriate and does not attenuate the bleeding reduction seen with bivalirudin.

reduced the endpoint of death/MI/cardiac arrest between day 2 and day 15, but increased this endpoint in the first day and in unstable patients, making the overall β-blocker effect neutral. Therefore, β-blockers should be avoided on the first day if there are any HF signs or features predictive of cardiogenic shock: SBP <120 mmHg, heart rate >110 bpm, or age >70 years.* Counterintuitively, β-blockers are avoided in sinus tachycardia, which is often a pre-shock state. Moreover, intravenous β-blockers are generally omitted, as this was the formulation used in COMMIT-CCS on the first day, but may still be used in a patient with active ischemia and none of the previous features (IV metoprolol, 5 mg Q10 min up to 3 times).

2. *ACE-Is or ARBs* are definitely recommended in ACS patients with HF, LV dysfunction, HTN, or diabetes (class I indication). They may also be used in ACS patients who do not have these features (class IIa indication). They are avoided in acute renal failure or when SBP is <100 mmHg or 30 mmHg below baseline.

3. *Statin therapy* should be started during ACS hospitalization regardless of the baseline LDL. Statin's benefit is not immediate, but may become evident within 1 month.[40] The high doses used in secondary prevention trials, such as atorvastatin 80 mg in the PROVE-IT trial, are preferred as they further reduce cardiovascular events (including death/MI), possibly through superior stabilization of vulnerable plaques. Note that, for patients receiving chronic statin therapy, the harm from statin withdrawal is immediate, with an early cardiac risk that is higher than that of statin non-users.[41]

4. *Nitroglycerin (NTG)* is administered sublingually for chest pain (as needed, Q5 min up to three times if tolerated). NTG should be avoided if SBP <100 mmHg or 30 mmHg below baseline, or bradycardia <50 bpm. Acutely in ACS, one can give NTG at a lower BP level than one can give β-blockers. Later on, in case of borderline BP, the priority is given to β-blocker administration.

IV NTG is indicated for frequently recurrent angina, ongoing angina, or ischemia associated with HTN or HF. Angina that is not relieved by 400 mcg of sublingual NTG is often not relieved by the smaller infusion dose of IV NTG (10–200 mcg/min); the latter may however be tried, in conjunction with β-blockers and antithrombotic therapy. IV NTG is initiated at 10 mcg/min and increased by 10 mcg/min every 3–5 minutes until symptoms are relieved or a limiting reduction of SBP <100–110 mmHg occurs. Oral or topical nitrates (patch, paste) are acceptable alternatives in the absence of ongoing angina. After stabilization, IV NTG may be converted to an oral or topical nitrate, with a dosing that prevents tolerance and leaves a 12-hour nitrate-free interval (e.g., isosorbide dinitrate 10–40 mg or nitropaste 0.5–2 inches at 8 a.m., 2 p.m. and 8 p.m.).

5. *Morphine* may be given for angina that is refractory to the above after a decision is made as to whether emergent revascularization will be performed or not. **Thus, morphine should not be used to mask "refractory angina," and resolution of a true angina only after morphine administration should not defer the emergent performance of coronary angiography ± PCI.**

6. *Calcium channel blockers.* Dihydropyridines (DHPs) are vasodilators (nifedipine, amlodipine). Non-dihydropyridines are vasodilators that also have negative ino- and chronotropic effects (verapamil, diltiazem). Short-acting DHPs, such as nifedipine, lead to reflex tachycardia and should be avoided in ACS. Long-acting DHPs may be used in ACS in combination with β-blockers. Non-DHPs may be used in ACS if β-blockers are contraindicated and LV systolic function is normal; as opposed to DHPs, they should generally not be combined with β-blockers.

VI. General procedural management after coronary angiography: PCI, CABG, or medical therapy only

After coronary angiography, a decision is made for PCI vs. CABG vs. continuing medical therapy alone, as dictated by the coronary anatomy. If a decision is made to proceed with CABG, hold clopidogrel and ticagrelor for 5 days before surgery, if possible, and hold enoxaparin for 12–24 hours and eptifibatide for 4 hours before surgery.

A. CABG indications
- Left main disease
- Three-vessel CAD or complex two-vessel CAD involving the LAD (especially proximal LAD), particularly in the case of angiographic SYNTAX score ≥23 (SYNTAX trial) or diabetes (FREEDOM trial)[42,43]

B. PCI indications
- One- or two-vessel disease not involving the proximal LAD
- PCI is an alternative to CABG in single-vessel disease involving the proximal LAD
- PCI is an alternative to CABG in three-vessel CAD or complex two-vessel CAD involving the LAD with a SYNTAX score ≤22 and no diabetes. Multivessel PCI (including proximal LAD PCI) compares favorably with CABG if the stenoses' morphology and location are technically amenable to PCI and if full functional revascularization can be achieved with PCI.[44] The presence of a chronic total occlusion, one or more technically difficult or long lesions, or diabetes, should favor CABG, especially because CABG provides a more complete revascularization.

In STEMI, only the culprit artery is acutely treated, but in NSTEMI and in stable CAD, multivessel PCI may be performed in a single setting without evidence of added risk.[45,46] Moreover, when multiple complex lesions are seen in NSTEMI, the culprit artery may not be clearly identified and multivessel intervention is justified.

---

* Also, always avoid β-blockers acutely and chronically in cases of second- or third-degree AV block, PR interval >240 ms, bradycardia <55 bpm, or active bronchospasm. Beyond the first day, SBP below 100 mmHg, rather than 120 mmHg, is the contraindication to β-blockers.

C. Among patients with high-risk ACS managed invasively, ~25–30% do not undergo any revascularization after coronary angiography

There are two types of patients within this group:

i. ~10–15% have normal coronary arteries or insignificant CAD (<50% obstructive).[47–51] Even among patients with elevated troponin, ~10% have insignificant CAD, this prevalence being higher among women and younger patients (15% of women and 7% of men with NSTEMI do not have significant CAD).[48] Patients without significant CAD have good long-term outcomes,[47–49,51] particularly if the coronary arteries are angiographically normal,[47,50] with a 6-month risk of death of <1% and death/MI of ~2%.

The following causes of chest pain and elevated troponin are considered after angiography and/or IVUS have ruled out significant disease:

1. True ACS/MI from:
   a. isolated coronary spasm[13]
   b. plaque erosion/rupture that has embolized distally without leaving any significant stenosis, or thrombosed then recanalized with antithrombotic therapy (or spontaneously)
   c. an apparently non-obstructive plaque that, in reality, is truly obstructive (e.g., 30–50% hazy stenosis with irregular borders may be anatomically significant by IVUS). Intracoronary imaging may need to be performed to assess moderate disease in patients with ACS.
2. Secondary ischemia from anemia, tachyarrhythmia, or unsuspected hyperthyroidism
3. Hypertensive crisis; diastolic dysfunction with elevated LVEDP
4. Myopericarditis
5. Takotsubo cardiomyopathy
6. Pulmonary embolism

In two studies of patients with severely elevated troponin (up to 27 ng/ml, mean 9 ng/ml) and unobstructed coronary arteries, cardiac MRI established the diagnosis in 90% of patients (three main diagnoses: myocarditis 60%, infarction 15%, and takotsubo ~14%). Infarction may have been due to recanalized/stabilized plaque rupture or vasospasm.[52,53] In another study that analyzed patients with normal or only mildly elevated troponin and unobstructed coronary arteries, coronary vasospasm was diagnosed in half of the cases.[13]

ii. ~15% have significant CAD but are not deemed candidates for revascularization. These patients may have limited CAD in a small branch or a distal coronary segment that supplies a small territory, which is therefore not considered an appropriate revascularization target. The majority of these patients, however, have extensive and diffuse CAD, more extensive than patients undergoing PCI, along with more comorbidities (history of CABG, MI, PAD, stroke, CKD, anemia).[51,54] These patients are not considered candidates for PCI or CABG because of the diffuseness of the CAD, the small diameter of the involved vessels (<2 mm), the lack of appropriate distal targets for CABG, or the medical comorbidities. Their mortality is high, 3–4 times higher than the mortality of patients who are candidates for revascularization (~20% at 3–4 years).[51–55]

The determination of LVEDP is critical in patients with ACS and insignificant CAD. Elevated LVEDP from acute diastolic dysfunction or severe HTN is a common cause of mild troponin elevation in patients with normal coronary arteries. Microvascular coronary flow is driven by the gradient between diastolic blood pressure and LVEDP; thus, microvascular flow is impeded by an elevated LVEDP. In fact, a gradient of 40 mmHg between diastolic blood pressure and CVP, or by extrapolation, LV diastolic pressure, is a zero-flow gradient, as at least 40 mmHg is required to overcome the microvascular resistance.[56]

In patients with insignificant CAD whose angiographic or IVUS appearance suggests stabilized plaque rupture, long-term aggressive medical therapy is indicated (including 1 year of clopidogrel or ticagrelor). This also applies to the patients with significant CAD who do not get revascularized.

In a patient with secondary unstable angina/NSTEMI, the primary therapy is directed towards the primary insult (e.g., sepsis, anemia, severe HTN, tachyarrhythmia). In a patient with gastrointestinal (GI) bleed and angina, the primary treatment consists of transfusion and GI therapy, e.g., endoscopic cauterization. Antithrombotic drugs should be avoided for at least few days, and, if possible, weeks. Depending on the ECG, the echo findings, and the severity of anemia, coronary angiography may not be required. For example, a mild troponin rise <0.3 ng/ml without significant ECG abnormalities, occurring with acute and severe anemia, may not require coronary angiography. On the other hand, troponin rise with a nadir hemoglobin of 8–10 mg/dl and with ST changes often requires coronary angiography.

If acute HF is associated with a positive troponin without ST changes, full ACS therapy is not warranted. In fact, troponin elevation is common in acute HF, and may even reach >1 ng/ml in 6% of patients regardless of any underlying CAD.[57] Thus, an elevated troponin, by itself, does not establish the diagnosis of ACS in a patient presenting with HF.[1] If CAD has not been addressed previously, coronary angiography is still warranted to address the underlying etiology of HF, preferably before discharge, with early revascularization if appropriate. Acute HF with *either ST changes or severe troponin rise* is considered a high-risk ACS and treated as such, unless CAD has been ruled out recently.

In acute HF, chest tightness is frequently a description of dyspnea and does not equate with CAD. Progressive chest tightness that precedes HF decompensation is more suggestive of CAD.

VII. Management of low-risk NSTE-ACS and low-probability NSTE-ACS

Both categories of patients should receive initial therapy with aspirin and β-blockers (unless contraindicated). Clopidogrel may be used when ACS is considered probable, even if low-risk, as in the CURE trial. Anticoagulation is not typically indicated.

Echocardiography and stress testing or coronary CT angiography should be performed 6 hours after presentation (troponin must be negative 3–6 hours after chest pain onset). A high-risk result on the stress test dictates coronary angiography, whereas a normal or low-risk result implies that the patient either does not have significant CAD or has limited CAD with a small or mildly ischemic territory, for which medical therapy is appropriate. Medical therapy is tailored to how much the physician believes the chest pain is anginal based on clinical grounds.

ECG stress testing is appropriate in patients who can perform exercise and do not have baseline ST depression >1 mm or LBBB. Otherwise, exercise or pharmacological stress imaging is recommended.

Alternatively, low-risk patients or low-probability patients may be discharged home on aspirin, β-blockers, and sublingual NTG, with plans for stress testing within 72 hours of discharge. Several large registry analyses showed that this early discharge is safe, with ≤0.1% risk of cardiac death and ≤0.3% risk of cardiac events at 1 month, and <0.5–0.8% risk of cardiac death at 6 months.[58–60] This was particularly true if troponin was undetectable. However, up to 8% of patients were readmitted with chest pain or ACS within 1–6 months, which highlights the importance of early follow-up and testing.[58] Some of these registries included patients with a prior history of CAD but low-risk findings on their current presentation; pre-discharge stress testing is generally preferred for these patients, as they inherently have a higher risk of cardiac events.[58,60]

VIII. Discharge medications

A. High-risk NSTE-ACS: antiplatelet and anticoagulant therapy

1. **Aspirin 81 mg/day.** Chronically, the low dose is as effective as higher doses with a lower risk of GI bleed, even in patients who undergo coronary stenting.

2. **ADP receptor antagonist** (clopidogrel 75 mg/day, prasugrel 10 mg/day, or ticagrelor 90 mg BID).

Even if PCI is not performed, prescribe *clopidogrel* or *ticagrelor* for at least 1 month, and preferably 12 months. This applies to patients with significant CAD who are not revascularized, but also patients with insignificant CAD when moderate disease is present or plaque rupture is believed to be the underlying trigger.[37] In addition, clopidogrel is beneficial in patients who undergo CABG in the context of ACS, where clopidogrel may be started a few days after CABG.[61] In the absence of stenting, the ADP receptor antagonist is more readily stopped if needed (bleeding, surgical procedure).

If PCI is performed, prescribe *clopidogrel*, *prasugrel*, or *ticagrelor* for 12 months whether a bare-metal stent (BMS) or a drug-eluting stent (DES) is used.

Does a longer duration of therapy (>12 months) provide extra benefit? According to the DAPT study, which included patients with MI (26%) or stable CAD undergoing DES placement, the continued administration of a thienopyridine between 1 year and 2.5 years drastically reduced the MI risk in half during this time frame (from 4% to 2%). MI was reduced at the stent site (stent thrombosis) but also at distant lesions, where half of the events occur. This benefit was seen despite the short study duration (1.5 years) and despite the exclusion of patients who had a recurrent coronary event in the first year, the latter likely deriving an even larger benefit from continued thienopyridine administration.[62] A benefit of prolonged therapy was also seen in a separate DAPT study addressing BMS patients. Interestingly, even beyond 1 year, and even with BMS, there was a ~1% risk of stent thrombosis after thienopyridine interruption, similar to DES. The pitfall of this prolonged therapy was an increase in bleeding, cancer diagnoses, and deaths related to cancer and bleeding. Thus, continued thienopyridine therapy seems reasonable in patients who have a low bleeding risk (e.g., age <75) and no suspicion of underlying malignancy; it is expected to be particularly beneficial in the high ischemic risk groups, such as recurrent ACS, multiple complex PCIs, combined CAD + PAD, ischemic HF, or ongoing uncontrolled risk factors, such as smoking or diabetes. Another trial, CHARISMA, addressed prolonged dual antiplatelet therapy regardless of stenting and showed that patients with a prior MI, as opposed to stable CAD, benefited from extended dual antiplatelet therapy for up to 28 months, whether PCI was performed or not; the benefit was larger in patients with a prior MI and PAD.[63] Thus, *prolonged therapy is useful for a general coronary purpose in a high-risk patient, not just a stent thrombosis purpose.*

Conversely, is earlier interruption acceptable? The ADP receptor antagonist may be interrupted at 1 month with BMS, at 3 months with second-generation DES in the stable CAD setting,[64–68] and at 6 months with second-generation DES in the ACS setting, if needed (DES registries and PRODIGY trial).[64,65,69] Note, however, that patients with multiple predictors of stent thrombosis continue to have a low but steady rate of stent thrombosis between 6 and 12 months, even when receiving the safer, new-generation DESs (MI population, long and multiple stents, small stents ≤2.5 mm, stenting for in-stent restenosis, multivessel PCI, renal failure).[64,65] For those patients deemed at high risk of stent thrombosis or recurrent MI, the interruption of clopidogrel may be limited to <7–10 days. In fact, the median time from clopidogrel discontinuation to stent thrombosis is 13.5 days, even in the 1–6-month time interval after stent implantation.[70,71] The interruption of clopidogrel before 1 month with either BMS or DES should be absolutely avoided, as interruption may lead to subacute stent thrombosis and massive MI.

3. **Warfarin.** The combination of aspirin and clopidogrel is the standard post-ACS antithrombotic regimen. Warfarin replaces clopidogrel if the patient has AF or LV thrombus. When the latter patient undergoes stent placement, he needs to be placed on a triple combination of aspirin, clopidogrel, and warfarin (or alternative anticoagulant) if the bleeding risk is low. The triple therapy, however, has a 4× higher major bleeding risk than aspirin + warfarin (12% vs. 3–4% yearly bleeding risk).[72] A BMS may be placed in these patients so that the duration of the mandatory triple therapy is limited to 4 weeks. On the other hand, with the newer-generation DES, triple therapy is safely limited to 6 months even after ACS (ESC and ACC guidelines).[65–69,73] Triple therapy may even be limited to 1 month in patients with a high bleeding risk, including in the setting of ACS and DES (ESC, class IIa).[74] Afterward, the patient is placed on dual therapy with an anticoagulant and either aspirin or clopidogrel.

A recent trial suggested that the double combination of clopidogrel and warfarin is as effective as the triple combination for the prevention of stent thrombosis and ischemic events immediately after any stent, with a lower bleeding risk translating into a mortality benefit.[75] The combined inhibition of thrombin generation with warfarin and the ADP pathway with clopidogrel may lessen the importance of cyclooxygenase inhibition with aspirin. Yet this study consisted mainly of stable CAD (~25% ACS), and those results need to be confirmed in other trials.

Note that warfarin, per se, is protective against coronary events, and data show that the long-term use of aspirin and warfarin combination (INR 2.0–2.5) or warfarin monotherapy (INR 2.5–3.5) is superior to aspirin monotherapy for the secondary prevention of coronary events and stroke after MI at the cost of a higher bleeding risk.[76,77] While this use of warfarin is obsolete in the era of dual antiplatelet therapy, these data imply that warfarin is not just useful for AF but provides anti-ischemic protection after one antiplatelet agent is stopped at 1–6 months. Beyond 12 months after a coronary event or PCI, warfarin monotherapy may be sufficient, and may be superior to aspirin or even aspirin + clopidogrel in preventing coronary events.[73,78]

B. High-risk NSTE-ACS: other therapies

1. β-Blocker therapy: in the pre-reperfusion era, high doses of β-blockers improved post-MI mortality.[79] In the reperfusion era, β-blockers have improved post-MI outcomes over the short term; long-term mortality is improved in the HF and low EF settings.[39,80] β-Blocker therapy is titrated slowly if clinical HF has occurred at any time or if EF is ≤40% (e.g., carvedilol is started as 6.25 mg BID and doubled every 3–10 days) (CAPRICORN trial).[80] In the absence of HF or low EF, the long-term benefit of β-blocker therapy is questionable in reperfused patients;[81] β-blocker therapy is still indicated for 1–3 years, low-to-medium doses being acceptable and equally beneficial in this setting (e.g., metoprolol 25–50 mg/d).[82] High doses may lead to severe fatigue or bradycardia and may not be tolerated.

2. ACE-I is particularly indicated in hypertension or LV dysfunction. If EF is normal and SBP is ≤130 mmHg, long-term ACE-I therapy does not definitely improve outcomes, even in patients with prior MI (PEACE trial).[83] Yet, ACE-I therapy is useful for 6 weeks after any MI (ISIS-4 trial). In light of the recent SPRINT trial, the blood pressure goal is preferably ≤120–130 mmHg.[84]

3. High-intensity statin therapy is administered regardless of LDL. The LDL goal after ACS is <60–70 mg/dl.[85] Other agents can be combined with high-intensity statin if needed (e.g., PCSK9 inhibitors, bile acid-binding resins, niacin, ezetimibe).

4. Aldosterone antagonist is administered for an EF <40% associated with any degree of clinical HF or diabetes; creatinine must be <2 mg/dl.[86]

5. Proton pump inhibitors (PPIs) may inhibit CYP2C19 and thus reduce the conversion of clopidogrel to its active metabolite. PPIs were associated with increased cardiovascular events in some retrospective analyses of clopidogrel therapy. The only randomized trial that compared PPI to placebo in patients requiring clopidogrel therapy showed a reduction of GI events with omeprazole without any increase in cardiac events.[87] Thus, patients who definitely need a PPI, such as patients with an established history of peptic ulcer disease, esophagitis, or GI bleed, or patients receiving a triple antithrombotic combination, are appropriately treated with a PPI. Patients with dyspepsia or symptoms of reflux should not receive a PPI. Patients with a history of peptic ulcer disease should be tested for *H. pylori*.

> NSAIDs should be avoided for their known risks of renal failure, fluid retention, HTN, and GI bleed, especially in combination with aspirin and clopidogrel. Acetaminophen, tramadol, or even a short course of narcotics may be tried for osteoarthritic pain. If an NSAID is absolutely necessary, use the lowest possible dose and *administer aspirin 2 hours before the NSAID.*

6. Return to regular activities, including sexual activities, 1–2 weeks after ACS. Patients with a large infarct and new LV dysfunction should avoid strenuous activities for 4 weeks (high arrhythmic risk during this period).

C. Low-risk NSTE-ACS

If the stress test is normal or low-risk but the patient is believed to have had an unstable angina, secondary prevention measures should be applied, such as aspirin, statin, and a β-blocker. Clopidogrel may be provided for 1–12 months, even in a low-risk unstable angina (class I recommendation).*[37]

D. Low-probability NSTE-ACS

Primary prevention measures should be pursued. Clopidogrel is not indicated. Aspirin may be used in select patients.

IX. Prognosis (Table 1.3)

In-hospital mortality of NSTEMI is lower than STEMI.[88] However, short-term (30 days) and long-term mortality of NSTEMI approximates STEMI mortality (~3% at 30 days, ~5% at 1 year).[30,32,37,88] Short-term mortality of unstable angina without positive markers or ST changes is much lower (≤1.7%).[6,88] The risk of death or MI is 5–10% at 30 days and ~10–15% at 1 year.[29,30,32,34] This risk is much lower beyond the first year (~2% per year).[34,35,42,89,90] Half of these events are recurrences at the site of culprit lesions, while the remaining events are related to non-culprit lesions. Adverse IVUS features (thin cap, heavy atheroma with positive remodeling, small luminal area) predict the progression of a non-culprit lesion to ACS, yet the predictive value is low (~20% progression of this lesion over 3 years).[90] Angiographic stenosis >50% in the context of ACS has up to 25% risk of progression in the ensuing 8 months.

The extent of CAD, NSTEMI (as opposed to unstable angina), and comorbidities affect long-term prognosis and the risk of event recurrence.

---

* The CURE trial of clopidogrel in NSTE-ACS included some low-risk patients, as it mandated any one of the following: ECG abnormalities (not necessarily of the ST segment), biomarker rise, or prior CAD history with age >60. Only 25% of patients had NSTEMI and 40% had ST changes.

Table 1.3 Prognosis of NSTE-ACS.

	30 days	1 year	5 years
Death	3%	**4–5%**	10% *(1% per year past the first year)*
Death or MI	5% (early invasive) 10–14% (early conservative)	**10%** (early invasive) 15% (early conservative)	20% *(2% per year past the first year)*
Death, MI, recurrent ACS, or revascularization		15–20%	30% *(3–5% per year past the first year)*

The most important numbers to remember are 5% death and 10% death/MI at 1 year despite PCI and optimal therapy. The rates herein provided are derived from clinical trial data. Real-world patients tend to be older with more comorbidities and more extensive disease, and thus have higher event rates.

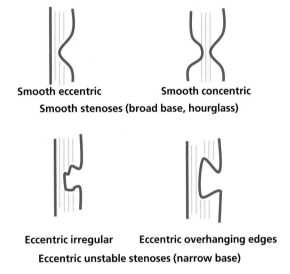

Smooth eccentric   **Smooth concentric**

Smooth stenoses (broad base, hourglass)

Eccentric irregular   **Eccentric overhanging edges**

Eccentric unstable stenoses (narrow base)

Figure 1.4 The concentric and eccentric lesions with smooth borders are predominantly seen in stable CAD, while the lesions with irregular or overhanging borders are predominantly seen in ACS. *Haziness* may be due to an unstable fissured plaque, with contrast faintly seeping through the fissures of the plaque beyond the true lumen; it may also be due to concentric calcium surrounding the lumen and does not necessarily imply instability.

Appendix 1. Complex angiographic disease, moderate disease

A. Complex angiographic plaque

A complex plaque, i.e., a ruptured unstable plaque, is identified angiographically by being ≥50% obstructive (generally), along with one or more of the following features:

i. Thrombus: round intraluminal filling defect *or* contrast stain, i.e., persistence of contrast over a focal area even after it clears from the rest of the vessel. An abrupt thrombotic vessel cutoff may be present.
ii. Plaque ulceration: hazy, usually eccentric plaque with irregular or overhanging margins (Figure 1.4).[91]
iii. Impaired flow from distal microembolization.

Patients with ACS frequently have multiple angiographically complex plaques (~40%). The culprit lesion is identified by seeking these morphological features but also by correlating with the ECG or imaging findings. In NSTE-ACS with multiple complex lesions, a clear single culprit may not be identified, particularly given that the ST depression on the ECG is often not localizing. Multivessel PCI of multiple obstructive stenoses may be performed in one setting without any added risk in NSTE-ACS, and is particularly justified in patients with multiple complex plaques and without one clear culprit.[45,46] Complex ACS lesions that are >50% stenotic have a fast rate of progression.

B. Extent of CAD in patients with NSTE-ACS (Table 1.4)

C. The importance of moderate CAD in patients with NSTE-ACS, recurrent events in NSTE-ACS

If the coronary angiogram shows normal coronaries or minimal disease, the patient is at a very low risk of ischemic events in the ensuing 5 years and the coronary angiogram does not need to be repeated unless there is a strong objective evidence of MI.

The coronary angiogram may show single- or multivessel moderate disease (30–70%), or severe disease (>70%) in a small branch for which PCI is not technically possible or beneficial. The true functional significance of intermediate stenoses (30–70%) is worth assessing using fractional flow reserve (during which the drop in flow across a stenosis is assessed using a pressure wire and maximal hyperemia) (FAMOUS-NSTEMI trial).

Table 1.4 Angiographic findings in NSTE-ACS and rates of revascularization.[29–31]

Angiographic findings	Revascularization
Insignificant disease or normal coronaries ~10%	PCI in ~60–70%
1-vessel CAD ~30%	CABG in ~10–15%
2-vessel CAD ~30%	No revascularization in ~30%
3-vessel CAD ~30%	
Left main disease ~10%	

Intracoronary imaging with OCT or IVUS is also useful to assess moderate ACS lesions (30–50%, and sometimes 50–70%). In fact, in ACS, the question is not only whether the lesion is functionally significant but whether the lesion is anatomically significant and likely to acutely or subacutely progress (e.g., plaque rupture, thrombus). The goal of therapy in ACS is to reduce the high risk of recurrent infarction rather than just improve angina; hence, the assessment of anatomy is more valuable in ACS than in stable CAD. A thrombotic lesion that is not functionally significant at one point in time may still progress within the next hours or days. In addition, the true lumen of a ruptured or ulcerated plaque may be much narrower than its angiographic appearance (contrast seeps through the planes of the ruptured plaque beyond the true lumen, giving the impression of a large lumen that is, nonetheless, hazy). Also, in ACS with serial lesions, anatomical rather than functional features determine which lesion is the culprit.

Even in ACS patients whose symptoms and electrocardiographic ischemia are quickly stabilized with medical therapy, an untreated stenosis of >50% has a 25% chance of progression within 8 months, mostly to a total occlusion, more so when the lesion has a complex appearance; note that this study was performed before the era of widespread statin and ADP receptor antagonist use.[92] Conversely, there is an overall 10% risk of ACS from non-significant, < 50% stenoses in the next 3 years (more so [~20% per lesion] in the presence of complex angiographic or IVUS features).[90,92]

In stable CAD, < 50% stenoses have a slow progression (10% risk of progression at 3 years, with a 2% risk of inducing ACS) (INTACT and COURAGE trials). As in ACS, the risk is higher for stenoses 50–70%, albeit not as high as in ACS (~20% progression, with 10% ACS) (COURAGE trial).[93,94] Also, new moderate lesions frequently appear in these patients during this time frame. FFR further stratifies the risk of progression of *stable* individual lesions.

Appendix 2. Women and ACS, elderly patients and ACS, CKD

A. Women and ACS

In trials of initial invasive vs. initial conservative strategy, low-risk women without elevated troponin, ST changes, or high TIMI risk score had a higher risk of death/MI with an invasive strategy than a conservative strategy (significant in RITA 3, non-significant trend in FRISC II).[34,95] However, high-risk women derive a benefit from an initial invasive strategy (TACTICS, meta-analysis).[32,96] While an initial invasive strategy is not indicated in low-risk men either, a meta-analysis shows that an initial invasive strategy is not harmful to low-risk men but is harmful to low-risk women.[96] This is related to the fact that women have less extensive CAD than men in general, and that in these trials of NSTE-ACS, ~24% of women vs. 8% of men randomized to an invasive strategy had no significant CAD, and even among women with elevated troponin, 15–20% had no significant CAD.[96,97] In fact, women have a *higher burden of macro- or microvascular spasm*. Even among women with CAD, three-vessel or left main disease is less common than among men. In addition, women have a higher bleeding risk, particularly at the vascular access site, which attenuates the benefit from an invasive strategy. Women also have a higher complication rate with CABG.[34]

Despite less extensive CAD, less positive troponin, and less common STEMI vs. NSTE-ACS presentation,[98] the mortality of women with ACS is equal to that of men, and may be higher on unadjusted analyses (GUSTO IIb analysis) or in the specific case of STEMI.[98] Women with ACS are older and have more comorbidities (diabetes, diastolic HF) than men. They have a higher BNP and a higher burden of dynamic ST changes on continuous ECG monitoring than men, indicative of a significant ischemic burden despite less CAD and less troponin rise (MERLIN-TIMI trial).[97] In fact, even among women without obstructive CAD, ~14% have dynamic ST changes on continuous ECG monitoring. Ranolazine may be of particular benefit in women with angina.

B. Elderly patients and ACS

Patients >75 years old with ACS have double the mortality of younger patients. Elderly patients more frequently have atypical presentations with milder ST changes. While associated with a higher major bleeding risk in patients >75 years old, an early invasive strategy drastically reduced the absolute risk of death/MI by 10% at 6 months in those inherently high-risk patients (TACTICS-TIMI-18 trial).[99] This was further confirmed in a trial that randomized octogenarian ACS patients to an invasive vs. conservative strategy (AFTER EIGHTY).[100] However, this benefit may only apply to carefully selected elderly patients with limited comorbidities and bleeding risk, similar to the patients recruited in clinical trials. A careful access (radial) and antithrombotic strategy may maximize the benefit from an invasive strategy, and GPI should be avoided if possible.

C. CKD

Approximately 20–40% of patients presenting with NSTEMI have CKD. Although the bleeding risk is increased in renal failure regardless of the anticoagulant used, bivalirudin (in patients undergoing PCI) and fondaparinux (outside PCI) are associated with less bleeding than UFH or enoxaparin in patients with mild or moderate renal failure.[29] When GFR is <30 ml/min, UFH or dose-adjusted enoxaparin are approved for use; the bleeding risk is, however, higher with enoxaparin at any stage of renal failure and UFH is preferred.[101] A GPI is best avoided in CKD; if used, the bolus and infusion doses of eptifibatide are reduced in half when GFR is <50 ml/min.

CKD patients are inherently high-risk patients. Despite the high prevalence of CKD, large randomized trials that have addressed the benefit of an invasive strategy in ACS have excluded patients with advanced CKD. Subgroup analyses of these trials suggest a benefit of an invasive strategy in patients with mild CKD, and observational data suggest that patients with mild or moderate CKD (GFR 30–60 ml/min) derive a benefit from an invasive strategy, which makes sense, considering the inherently high ischemic risk of these patients.[102,103] This benefit may extend to carefully selected high-risk patients with CKD stages 4 or 5, who, nonetheless, have a higher risk of bleeding and renal and HF complications peri-PCI.[103] CKD stage 3 is a class IIa indication for an initial invasive strategy.

Appendix 3. Bleeding, transfusion, prior warfarin therapy, gastrointestinal bleed

A. The negative impact of bleeding

In the context of ACS or PCI, the occurrence of major bleeding has at least the same prognostic impact as the occurrence of a new MI.[104,105] Compared with patients without bleeding, patients who experience bleeding have a much higher in-hospital but also late mortality (up to 5× higher). In fact, while bleeding is rarely fatal by itself, bleeding strikingly increases the risk of MI, coronary thrombosis, and ischemic events through the following concepts: (i) antithrombotic therapy may need to be temporarily withheld; (ii) bleeding is a very potent activator of the coagulation cascade; (iii) acute anemia may lead to demand ischemia; (iv) blood transfusion, sometimes necessary, leads to untoward proinflammatory and prothrombotic effects. One-half to two-thirds of major bleeding events are femoral access site bleeds, while the remaining events are gastrointestinal or genitourinary bleeds, a drop in hemoglobin without an overt source, or, rarely but fatally, an intracranial bleed.

Radial access drastically reduces bleeding and is associated with improved outcomes when performed by experienced operators. Appropriate antithrombotic therapy, with a limited use of GPI, the avoidance of upstream GPI, and the procedural use of bivalirudin instead of heparin reduce access and non-access bleeding and improve short- but also long-term outcomes.

B. Transfusion in ACS

Anemia may exacerbate myocardial ischemia in patients with CAD or ACS. Yet transfusion, by itself, does not necessarily reverse this ischemia and may be associated with worse clinical outcomes. This is linked to potential prothrombotic (ADP release) and proinflammatory effects of transfusion and to the impaired oxygen-carrying capacity of the transfused red blood cells.[106] In fact, while normal red blood cells transport and dispense nitric oxide to the microvasculature, this function is disrupted in transfused red blood cells, which leads to impaired regional vasodilatation. Two analyses have found that transfusion is associated with increased mortality in ACS patients with a hematocrit >25–27%.[107,108] An analysis from the CRUSADE registry suggested that transfusion in NSTE-ACS was associated with adverse outcomes if the hematocrit was >27%.[108] Other studies have found a strong association between transfusion and adverse outcomes after PCI, performed for ACS or stable CAD, and after CABG.[95] Thus, unless the patient is hemodynamically unstable from bleeding, severely tachycardic, or has refractory angina, transfusion should be withheld when hemoglobin is >8 g/dl or hematocrit is >25% (grade I recommendation, ESC).[109] For patients who continue to exhibit episodes of angina at rest or mild exertion, a higher transfusion cutoff may be used (9–9.5 g/dl). Also, in patients about to undergo PCI, a higher cutoff is generally used (9–9.5 g/dl).[110]

C. Patients on chronic warfarin therapy who present with ACS

Warfarin, per se, is protective against coronary events. There are no data on the management of patients appropriately anticoagulated who present with ACS. If a conservative strategy is selected, it may be reasonable to continue warfarin along with other therapies and withhold from adding any other anticoagulant. There is no reason to believe that combining two anticoagulants reduces ischemic events. In fact, overlapping two anticoagulants worsened the bleeding risk in the SYNERGY trial.

If an invasive strategy is selected, warfarin may be held for a few days before the coronary angiogram and a short-acting anticoagulant used instead of warfarin before and during the procedure. This way, the anticoagulation can be stopped after the procedure, reducing the bleeding complications and allowing for the removal of the arterial sheath. Heparin should be started as soon as the INR starts to trend down (especially below 2). The angiogram may be performed when the INR is ≤1.6. Warfarin is restarted the evening of the procedure, and heparin may be restarted along with warfarin until the INR is ≥2, because an early procoagulant effect occurs upon warfarin reinitiation and may not be tolerated post ACS. Anticoagulation with heparin at a low PTT target (~1.5× normal) may generally be resumed 8–12 hours after sheath removal. Avoid LMWH in those patients with a recent femoral access: LMWH is associated with a higher bleeding risk than controlled-dose heparin (SYNERGY trial), and should a bleeding occur, the prolonged effect of LMWH makes it difficult to control.

Alternatively, warfarin is not withheld, or only one dose is withheld, and the coronary procedure is performed through a radial access with an INR value ≥2. If PCI is performed, heparin is administered and adjusted according to ACT.

D. Gastrointestinal (GI) bleed after a recent stent placement, in patients receiving aspirin and clopidogrel

In case of chronic blood loss and a recently placed stent, dual antiplatelet therapy should probably be continued as mandated, and, if indicated, endoscopic intervention performed while the patient is on dual antiplatelet therapy. PPI is administered and testing for *H. pylori* performed.[111]

In case of a major GI bleed, the cessation of one antiplatelet agent may be judged necessary. Following successful endoscopic therapy of upper GI bleed combined with high-dose PPI therapy, it may be reasonable to reintroduce antiplatelet therapy 3–7 days later in those who remain free of recurrent bleeding. In case of lower GI bleed, one may delay antiplatelet therapy for 7–10 days, depending on the colonic lesion size and the adequacy of endoscopic treatment.[111]

E. Management of elevated troponin in a patient with GI bleed

The elevated troponin often results from the combination of stable CAD and demand ischemia from anemia and tachycardia. Therefore, the treatment of anemia is the first and most important line of therapy. The patients should receive fluid resuscitation ± blood transfusion (particularly in hemodynamic instability, severe tachycardia, persistent angina, or Hb <8 g/dl). PPI therapy is initiated and endoscopy is performed if appropriate, usually before any coronary procedure. A coronary procedure, with the possible ensuing need for anticoagulation and antiplatelet therapy, should only be performed after stabilization and etiologic diagnosis of the GI bleed, typically several days or, if possible in an angina-free patient, weeks later.

Similarly, a patient with stable angina who has chronic anemia should undergo anemia workup before any potential coronary procedure.

A coronary procedure is performed more urgently and potentially before the GI procedure in rare cases: (i) STEMI, (ii) ACS with ongoing angina despite transfusion, or (iii) major ST changes or severe troponin rise occurring with a rather mild or chronic anemia.

Appendix 4. Antiplatelet and anticoagulant therapy

A. Antiplatelet therapy (Table 1.5)

1. Aspirin is given as a 325 mg dose the first day (chewed for rapid absorption and effect), then 81 mg daily. On the second day and beyond, 81 mg is as effective as 325 mg with less bleeding risk, including in patients receiving coronary stents (CURRENT-OASIS trial).[112] In the case of aspirin allergy that consists of asthma or urticaria without anaphylaxis, perform aspirin desensitization, which may be performed urgently over less than 24 hours.

2. Clopidogrel is started as a 300 mg load, followed by 75 mg daily. In the CURE trial of NSTE-ACS patients managed invasively or conservatively, high or low risk, this clopidogrel regimen reduced the combined risk of death/MI by 2% at the cost of an increase in major bleeding risk by 1%; the life-threatening bleeding was not increased, and bleeding was overall attenuated when aspirin 81 mg was used.[33] The benefit was more marked in patients who were eventually managed invasively (~3% risk reduction), even early on (PCI CURE).[113] The benefit was already significant by 24 hours of therapy and maximal within a few days.

Patients who undergo PCI should be loaded with 600 mg of clopidogrel, which has a more potent and faster onset of antiplatelet effect than 300 mg (2 h for 600 mg vs. 6–24 h for 300 mg). If the patient has already received 300 mg, an additional 300 mg is administered during PCI. If the patient requires CABG, clopidogrel is preferably withheld for 5 days to prevent an increase in bleeding risk (absolute risk increase=4%).[37,114] Yet, in the highest-risk patients with critical CAD or ongoing ischemia, CABG may be performed sooner, as clopidogrel cessation for 3 days is often enough.[115,116] In addition, the peri-CABG use of clopidogrel does not adversely affect mortality and actually reduces peri-CABG ischemic events.

Table 1.5 Comparison of the three ADP receptor antagonists.

	Clopidogrel	Prasugrel (60 mg load, 10 mg maintenance)	Ticagrelor (180 mg load, 90 mg BID maintenance)
Inhibition of platelet activation	35–40%	75%	75%
Activation	Prodrug becomes active metabolite Inefficient metabolization by CYP2C19 explains 30% clopidogrel hyporesponsiveness	Prodrug becomes active metabolite ~Always efficiently metabolized by cytochromes	Active drug and active metabolite
Onset of action (i.e., time to 30% platelet inhibition)	600 mg: 2 h 300 mg: 6–24 h	30 min	30 min
Peak effect (hours)	600 mg: 6–8 h	2–4	2–4
Offset of action (days)[a]	5	7	3–4
Population studied and indications	Non-ST elevation or ST elevation ACS managed conservatively or invasively Any PCI (stable or unstable)	Non-ST elevation or ST elevation ACS managed by PCI (not conservatively) Not superior to clopidogrel in stable PCI	Non-ST elevation or ST elevation ACS managed conservatively or invasively
Absolute reduction of death/ MI/stroke in comparison to clopidogrel (at 1 yr)	—	2%	2%
Mortality reduction in comparison to clopidogrel (at 1 yr)	—	None, except in the STEMI subgroup	1%
Stent thrombosis reduction in comparison to clopidogrel	—	1.3%	0.7%
Bleeding	—		
Absolute increase in TIMI major bleeding compared to clopidogrel (non-CABG related)		0.6%	0.6%
Increase in CABG-related bleeding		4 times	No
Increase in fatal bleeding		Yes	No (but increases intracranial bleeding)
High-risk subgroups where it should be avoided	—	Prior stroke/TIA (absolute contraindication) Weight <60 kg Age >75	No specific subgroups

[a] *Note that the duration of effect is related to both the pharmacokinetic half-life and the reversibility of receptor binding.* Aspirin, clopidogrel, and prasugrel have a relatively short half-life yet a very prolonged duration of action, as they irreversibly affect their target. Ticagrelor reversibly binds to ADP receptor but has a combined half-life of ~15 h, which translates into a duration of action of 3–4 days. Cangrelor reversibly binds to ADP receptor and has a very short half-life, translating into a duration of action of 1 hour.

Some institutions prefer to withhold clopidogrel until the coronary angiogram is done, in order to rule out the need for CABG. However, this may deprive patients of the early benefit of clopidogrel therapy. Rather, clopidogrel may be selectively withheld in cases where extensive CAD seems probable, e.g., a man with elevated troponin and PAD, HF, or insulin-dependent diabetes; or a patient with extensive ST segment depressions in >8 leads or ST elevation in aVR.

3. Prasugrel and ticagrelor are more potent than clopidogrel (75% vs. 35% inhibition of platelet aggregation) and have a faster onset of antiplatelet activity (30 min for onset), without the interindividual response variability and the 30% hyporesponsiveness seen with clopidogrel. *These agents have only been studied in ACS (ACS receiving PCI for prasugrel, ACS receiving PCI or medical therapy for ticagrelor).*[117,118] In comparison with clopidogrel, both have shown further reduction of death/MI at the expense of a higher major bleeding risk. Their superiority is particularly marked in the three highest-risk patient groups (STEMI, diabetes, and recurrent ACS).[119,120] On the other hand, three subsets of patients have a marked bleeding risk with prasugrel without any net benefit, and these are contraindications to prasugrel use: (i) history of stroke/TIA, (ii) age >75, (iii) weight <60 kg (the latter two are relative contraindications).

Ticagrelor has several advantages over prasugrel: (i) reversible ADP receptor binding allows reversal of the antiplatelet effect at 3–4 days (vs. 5 days with clopidogrel and 7 days with prasugrel); (ii) reduction in mortality in comparison with clopidogrel (not seen with prasugrel); (iii) ticagrelor increases the release of adenosine, which may improve coronary flow but may also increase the risk of bronchospasm or asymptomatic pauses; (iv) ticagrelor did not increase fatal bleeding and did not specifically harm patients with a prior stroke or patients older than 75, yet both ticagrelor and prasugrel should be used carefully, if at all, in patients deemed at a high bleeding risk; (v) ticagrelor is indicated not only in patients managed with PCI but also in high-risk ACS patients managed conservatively or not deemed appropriate for revascularization. In the latter patients, ticagrelor strikingly reduced death/MI in comparison to clopidogrel; conversely, prasugrel has not shown any benefit in patients not receiving PCI (TRILOGY-ACS trial);[121] (vi) ticagrelor's benefit is early but continues to grow with time; with prasugrel, most of the benefit is early (<30 days).

Moreover, in NSTE-ACS, prasugrel should only be administered after coronary angiography is performed and the need for CABG ruled out (in the event CABG is needed, its performance within 7 days of prasugrel therapy drastically increases the bleeding risk). Clopidogrel or ticagrelor may be administered on admission, upstream of coronary angiography.

A new ADP receptor antagonist, **cangrelor,** is very potent (90% inhibition of platelet aggregation), reversible, and has a very short half-life. It is administered intravenously for the total duration of PCI (and for a total duration of at least 2 hours), and has a very short onset and offset of action (1 hour). It has been studied in patients who have not received clopidogrel upstream of PCI, where it has allowed a quick and potent onset of an ADP antagonist effect during PCI, until the action of the oral ADP antagonist begins.[122] It reduces acute stent thrombosis and intraprocedural complications.

4. Glycoprotein IIb-IIIa inhibitors (GPIs). GPIs are potent IV antiplatelet drugs that block the final common pathway of platelet aggregation (inhibit 95% of platelet aggregation). This comes at the expense of an absolute 2–4% increase in major bleeding risk.[38] In particular, GPI therapy upstream of coronary angiography was associated with an increase in bleeding without a significant reduction in ischemic events, even in patients not receiving clopidogrel, for whom GPI therapy used to be considered appropriate (EARLY ACS trial).[30] Thus, those drugs are typically used *during* PCI in *some* patients with elevated troponin, particularly those who were not pretreated with clopidogrel or ticagrelor (class I).[36,123]

As opposed to GPI, upstream clopidogrel or ticagrelor has proven beneficial in ACS and is the preferred upstream antiplatelet therapy. The bleeding risk associated with GPI drastically increases in patients older than 70, women, and patients with CKD, in which cases GPI, particularly prolonged upstream therapy with GPI, should generally be avoided. Upstream triple therapy with aspirin, clopidogrel, and GPI is rarely justified. The benefit of GPI on top of ticagrelor or prasugrel has not been studied and is likely marginal.

The upstream ADP receptor antagonist therapy theoretically serves to: (i) reduce ischemic events pre-PCI (CURE trial), (ii) optimize PCI outcomes and reduce thrombotic complications during PCI and early afterwards, (iii) obviate the need for any GPI therapy, even during PCI. However, a recent trial has shown that this upstream initiation may not be superior to peri-PCI initiation when a potent and fast ADP receptor antagonist is used, and when catheterization is performed within a few hours of presentation. Note that patients in that trial did not receive GPI, and thus, aspirin and an anticoagulant appeared to be enough therapy before a timely PCI.[124]

B. Clopidogrel resistance is seen in ~30% of patients

Clopidogrel resistance is defined as <30% inhibition of ADP-induced platelet aggregation; or as an absolute platelet reactivity to ADP of <208–230 platelet reactivity units (using a quick point-of-care assay, VerifyNow assay). Clopidogrel resistance is related to impaired clopidogrel activation and is at least partly genetic, determined by mutations of the cytochrome genes (particularly CYP2C19). Other factors, such as ACS presentation, obesity, and CKD may contribute.

Poor clopidogrel response is associated with an increased risk of coronary events and stent thrombosis. However, in hyporesponsive patients undergoing PCI for stable CAD, the tailored use of prasugrel or a higher clopidogrel maintenance (150 mg) did not translate into a clinical benefit.[125,126] In fact, stable CAD PCI is associated with a low risk of stent thrombosis and adverse outcomes even in poor clopidogrel responders, reducing the benefit of more potent antiplatelet strategies.

While it does not have a clear role in stable CAD, platelet reactivity testing may have a role in ACS. Poor clopidogrel response is particularly predictive of poor outcomes in ACS and may be an additional incentive for ticagrelor/prasugrel use and for GPI use during PCI (post-hoc analysis of ISAR-REACT 4 trial).[127] Yet, one may argue that ticagrelor and prasugrel are superior therapies that should be considered in ACS regardless of clopidogrel response.

C. Anticoagulant therapy (Table 1.6)

IV UFH has been shown to reduce early ischemic events and MI in patients with intermediate- or high-risk NSTE-ACS.[128] The starting bolus (60 U/kg) and drip (12 U/kg/h) used in ACS are lower than what is used in pulmonary embolism, with a conservative PTT goal of 46–70 seconds or 1.5–2× normal. **Moderate rather than high-level anticoagulation is appropriate for ischemic reduction in ACS and minimizes the dreaded bleeding.**

SQ Enoxaparin. In NSTE-ACS managed medically, a therapeutic dose of SQ enoxaparin reduces ischemic events compared to UFH at a similar rate of major bleeding (1 mg/kg SQ twice daily, or once daily if GFR <30).[129,130] In patients managed invasively, however, the SYNERGY trial failed to show any superiority of SQ enoxaparin over UFH, and there was a higher major bleeding risk with enoxaparin, particularly in patients who had crossover between heparin and enoxaparin.[131] A similar increase in bleeding risk with enoxaparin was seen in invasively treated patients in the A-to-Z trial.[132] Importantly, pharmacological studies have shown that the effect of SQ enoxaparin does not peak until a second dose is administered.[133] Thus, when two doses have already been administered, PCI may be performed within 8 hours of SQ enoxaparin without additional anticoagulation. However, when PCI is performed within a few hours of presentation, a single subcutaneous dose of enoxaparin does not provide appropriate anticoagulation for PCI and requires supplementation with 0.3 mg/kg of intravenous enoxaparin. The administration of a single SQ dose of enoxaparin is best avoided when PCI is planned in the next few hours; another anticoagulant strategy is preferred in this case.

IV UFH half-life increases with the dose used and is usually ~1.0–1.5 hours. SQ enoxaparin effect peaks at ~3–5 hours and is accelerated by the IV administration of enoxaparin 30 mg one-time dose in medically treated patients or 0.3 mg/kg in PCI. Its half-life is 4.5–7.0 hours, longer in renal failure. The short half-life of UFH may contribute to the "heparin rebound" phenomenon, wherein the abrupt cessation of UFH leads to a rebound increase in ischemia in the following 48 hours in medically treated patients (not PCI). Enoxaparin's antithrombotic effect wanes much more slowly than that of UFH, and enoxaparin inhibits thrombin generation in addition to thrombin action, which attenuates the heparin rebound effect and explains some of the anti-ischemic benefits of enoxaparin in medically treated patients (but not PCI).

SQ Fondaparinux (2.5 mg SQ daily, half-life ~20 hours). This low dose of fondaparinux, equivalent to a DVT prophylaxis dose, has proven to be as effective as a standard dose of enoxaparin (1 mg/kg twice daily) in reducing MI/ischemic events in NSTE-ACS, with a large reduction in major and fatal bleeding risk translating into a mortality reduction (OASIS 5 trial, where 40% of patients underwent PCI).[134] This again corroborates the concept that only moderate-level anticoagulation is required in ACS, less than that required in pulmonary embolism (except during PCI). Patients who are managed invasively after receiving fondaparinux should receive full anticoagulation with heparin or bivalirudin during PCI, as the small fondaparinux dose does not provide the level of anticoagulation required during PCI. In contrast to the harmful enoxaparin–UFH switch, the switch from fondaparinux to UFH during PCI does not attenuate the benefit of fondaparinux on bleeding.[135]

Table 1.6 Comparison of anticoagulants.

	Unfractionated heparin	Enoxaparin	Bivalirudin	Fondaparinux
Action	Binds to AT III in a way that inhibits thrombin >Xa	Is a small heparin derivative. Binds to AT III in a way that inhibits Xa >thrombin. Inhibits thrombin generation	Direct thrombin inhibitor. Inhibits both circulating and clot-bound thrombin[a]	Is a small heparin derivative. Binds to AT III in a way that inhibits Xa only
Effect on platelets	Potential activation	± Activation	Neutral	Neutral
Elimination	Reticulo-endothelial system	Renal	Renal	Renal
Half-life	1–1.5 h	4–7 h. Increases if renal failure	25 min. Increases to 1 hour if GFR <30 ml/min	17–21 h. Increases if renal failure
Time to peak effect	Immediate after IV bolus; few hours after infusion without bolus	3–5 h after SQ dose	Immediate	2–3 h after SQ dose
Dose	ACS: 60 U/kg bolus then 12 U/kg/h IV drip. DVT/PE: 80 U/kg bolus then 15–18 U/kg/h. PTT goal in ACS: 46–70 s (less than PE)	ACS and PE: 1 mg/kg SQ BID[b]	During PCI: 0.75 mg/kg IV bolus then 1.75 mg/kg/h. If started before PCI: 0.2 mg/kg/h	ACS: 2.5 mg SQ QD. DVT/PE: 5–10 mg SQ QD (depending on weight)
Effect of renal failure on dosage	None	Change from 1 mg/kg BID to 1 mg/kg QD if GFR <30 ml/min	Caution if GFR <30 ml/min[a]	Avoid if GFR <30 ml/min

[a] Only bivalirudin inhibits fibrin-bound thrombin. Heparin and fondaparinux cannot act on fibrin-bound thrombin. Bivalirudin has not been studied in advanced renal failure (in ACUITY trial) but is not absolutely contraindicated.
[b] If only one SQ dose was provided before PCI, give additional 0.3 mg/kg IV during PCI. SQ enoxaparin is not well studied in patients >150 kg, where the 1 mg/kg dose is associated with a marked increase in bleeding risk compared to patients with a normal body weight.
AT III, antithrombin III.

IV Bivalirudin. As opposed to UFH, bivalirudin does not activate platelets and inhibits both free and clot-bound thrombin; thus, the effective anticoagulant dose needed with bivalirudin is relatively smaller than the effective anticoagulant dose of UFH, which may explain the lower bleeding with bivalirudin. In addition, bivalirudin is short-acting (half-life 25 min), which is both an advantage (bleeding reduction) but also an ischemic risk, particularly in patients who have not received timely clopidogrel. Bivalirudin is associated with less major bleeding than UFH, whether GPI is additionally used or not (MATRIX and BRIGHT trials).[136] Some studies have shown a higher risk of acute stent thrombosis with bivalirudin vs. UFH, which may be offset by extending the bivalirudin infusion 3–4 hours after PCI. **Being an anticoagulant, bivalirudin is best compared to UFH, not the combination UFH+GPI. In fact, contrary to the design of older trials, the decision to add GPI should not be based on the anticoagulant used.**[29]

Bivalirudin is administered as an intravenous infusion during PCI. On admission and prior to PCI, patients may receive a prolonged bivalirudin infusion, or, alternatively, may receive UFH or fondaparinux with a switch to bivalirudin during PCI. The switch to bivalirudin is safe and still associated with bleeding reduction in comparison to heparin.[137]

Appendix 5. Differences between plaque rupture, plaque erosion, and spontaneous coronary dissection

A vulnerable plaque is characterized by a lipid-rich necrotic core that is surrounded by a thin fibrous cap and infiltrated by inflammatory cells, especially metalloproteinase-rich macrophages (called thin-cap fibroatheroma). The thin cap ruptures, especially at the shoulders/margins of the plaque where the stress is highest, and leads to thrombus formation. *Plaque rupture is, thus, characterized by a ruptured cap and a thrombus in continuity with a necrotic core*. The ruptured cap is identified as a flap on IVUS or OCT. Most plaque ruptures are non-occlusive and silent, contributing to a stair-step progression of coronary stenosis. On IVUS, heavy atherosclerosis and positive remodeling often correlate with instability, as they indicate prior episodes of plaque rupture.

Plaque erosion, on the other hand, is characterized by thrombus formation over a thick cap that has not ruptured (no communication with the necrotic core), or over a fibrointimal plaque rich in smooth muscle cells without a necrotic core (fibrotic plaque).[138–140] Plaque erosion is responsible for ~25% of MIs, more so in women, especially young female smokers (<50 years old). Compared with plaque rupture, plaque erosion occurs, on average, on less stenotic lesions.[138–140]

Plaque rupture leads to the complex eccentric morphology and overhanging borders on angiography. Plaque erosion has an uncomplicated morphology with smooth borders on angiography.

Spontaneous coronary artery dissection may mimic the smooth appearance of vasospasm or plaque erosion. It most frequently involves the *media*, leading to a long smooth stenosis >20–30 mm (average 46 mm) without a flap or stain (intramural hematoma). Less frequently, it involves the *intima* (30–50%), in which case a flap or stain is seen angiographically. The latter being absent in >50% of patients, spontaneous coronary dissection is suspected in a woman with a smooth, long lesion non-responsive to NTG and non-calcified, mimicking a "long refractory vasospasm"; IVUS or OCT may be used, if needed, to confirm the diagnosis by showing the two lumens.[129] It typically involves the mid-to-distal coronary segments, most commonly the LAD, and may involve multiple coronary arteries (~20%). It occurs almost exclusively in women (95%), mainly young and middle-age women (like coronary erosion), and is highly associated with coronary tortuosity, including corkscrew coronary arteries, and peripheral fibromuscular dysplasia. Spontaneous coronary dissection has a relatively high complication rate during PCI, which results from wiring the false lumen or hematoma propagation; in fact, PCI failure is seen in up to 50% of the cases![141,142] Even coronary engagement and contrast injections are associated with a risk of ostial dissection. As opposed to plaque rupture or erosion, the overwhelming majority of spontaneous coronary dissections spontaneously heal on follow-up angiography (≥1 month), justifying conservative management in patients without active ischemia and with non-critical obstruction/TIMI 3 flow (antiplatelet therapy, β-blockade, and 4–7 days of inpatient monitoring).[141,142]

Appendix 6. Harmful effects of NSAIDs and cyclooxygenase-2 inhibitors in CAD

There are two types of cyclooxygenases (COX): COX-1 and COX-2. COX-1, found in the normal epithelium and in platelets, is responsible for the homeostatic prostaglandins but also for the generation of thromboxane A2 and platelet activation. Conversely, COX-2, found in inflammatory cells, generates inflammatory prostanoids but also the protective prostacyclin (vasodilatory and antiplatelet effects). The low aspirin dose predominantly inhibits COX-1 with less effect on COX-2.

NSAIDs are harmful in several ways: (i) NSAIDs bind to COX-1, the site of action of aspirin, yet, as opposed to aspirin, they bind in a reversible manner and do not have a significant antiplatelet effect; (ii) NSAIDs inhibit COX-2 and thus, prostacyclin production. Selective COX-2 inhibitors are potentially worse from a platelet standpoint, as they block prostacyclin without any reduction of COX-1's thromboxane, and are more detrimental to the prostacyclin–thromboxane balance.

Moreover, if aspirin is administered after NSAID, the COX-1 site will be blocked by the NSAID, which prevents aspirin from binding; since the plasma half-life of aspirin is only 20 minutes, aspirin will be eliminated before it gets an opportunity to act.

QUESTIONS AND ANSWERS

Question 1. A 72-year-old man is admitted with fever, severe bilateral pneumonia, and sepsis. His exam does not suggest volume overload. During his first hospitalization day, his ECG shows transient ST depression in the lateral leads. His troponin I peaks at 1.2 ng/ml, with a rise and fall pattern; BNP=65. He has acute renal failure with creatinine of 1.7 mg/dl. He does not complain of chest pain. His echo shows a hyperdynamic LV. What is the next step?
A. His troponin rise is due to ischemic imbalance. He does not fulfill the definition of MI. No need for further cardiac workup
B. His troponin is partly due to ischemic imbalance. He fulfills the definition of MI. Perform stress testing before discharge
C. His troponin is partly due to ischemic imbalance. He fulfills the definition of MI. Perform coronary angiography after stabilization of infectious state and renal function

Question 2. A 72-year-old man is admitted with fever, severe bilateral pneumonia, and sepsis. His exam does not suggest volume overload. His ECG shows mild lateral T inversion. His troponin I peaks at 0.25 ng/ml, with a rise and fall pattern; BNP=65. He has acute renal failure with creatinine of 1.7 mg/dl. He does not complain of chest pain. His echo shows a hyperdynamic LV. What is the next step?

A. His troponin rise is due to ischemic imbalance. He does not fulfill the definition of MI. No need for further cardiac workup at this point

B. His troponin is partly due to ischemic imbalance. He fulfills the definition of MI. Perform stress testing before discharge

C. His troponin is partly due to ischemic imbalance. He fulfills the definition of MI. Perform coronary angiography after stabilization of his infectious state and renal function

Question 3. A 72-year-old man is admitted with melena and severe anemia (hemoglobin 6.5 g/dl). He is tachycardic but not in shock. His ECG shows diffuse 1.5 mm ST depression that has resolved after transfusion. His troponin I peaks at 3 ng/ml, with a rise and fall pattern. He does not complain of chest pain. His echo shows severe anterior hypokinesis. What is the next step?

A. Transfuse and treat with proton pump inhibitors (PPI). No need for coronary angiography. Perform outpatient stress testing

B. Transfuse and treat with PPI. No need for any cardiac workup unless angina occurs despite hemoglobin stabilization

C. Transfuse, treat with PPI, and perform gastroscopy. Perform coronary angiography once bleeding has stabilized for 1–2 weeks

D. Transfuse, treat with PPI, and perform gastroscopy. Administer β-blockers and nitrates. Perform coronary angiography once bleeding has stabilized for 1–2 weeks

Question 4. A 62-year-old man has a history of heart failure with LVEF of 25%. Coronary angiography performed a year previously showed mild, non-obstructive plaques. He presents with acutely decompensated HF, volume overload, and chest tightness. His troponin I peaks at 0.22 ng/ml with a rise and fall pattern (his baseline troponin is 0.05 ng/ml). His ECG shows LVH with a strain pattern; no Q waves are seen. What is the next step?

A. Diuresis and vasodilator therapy. Initiate antithrombotic therapy. Once proper diuresis is achieved, perform coronary angiography.

B. Diuresis and vasodilator therapy. No need to repeat coronary angiography.

Question 5. A 62-year-old man presents with progressive dyspnea and chest tightness for the last week. Exam and X-ray are diagnostic of pulmonary edema and severe HF. Echo shows LVEF 25% with global hypokinesis. Troponin I peaks at 0.22 ng/ml with a rise and fall pattern. ECG shows LVH with strain. Creatinine is 1.7 mg/dl. What is the next step?

A. Diuresis, vasodilator therapy, and antithrombotic therapy. Once proper diuresis is achieved, perform coronary angiography during this hospitalization

B. Diuresis and vasodilator therapy. Once proper diuresis is achieved, perform coronary angiography during this hospitalization

C. Diuresis and vasodilator therapy. Once proper diuresis is achieved, perform stress testing for ischemic evaluation

D. Diuresis and vasodilator therapy. Perform elective coronary angiography in the outpatient setting

Question 6. A 62-year-old man presents with progressive dyspnea and chest tightness for the last week. Exam and X-ray are diagnostic of pulmonary edema and severe HF. Echo shows LVEF 25% with global hypokinesis and inferior akinesis. Troponin I peaks at 0.22 ng/ml with a rise and fall pattern. ECG shows diffuse ST depression and inferior Q waves. Creatinine is 1.7 mg/dl. What is the next step?

A. Diuresis, vasodilator therapy, and antithrombotic therapy. Once proper diuresis is achieved, perform coronary angiography during this hospitalization

B. Diuresis and vasodilator therapy. Once proper diuresis is achieved, perform coronary angiography during this hospitalization

C. Diuresis and vasodilator therapy. Once proper diuresis is achieved, perform stress testing for ischemic evaluation

D. Diuresis and vasodilator therapy. Perform elective coronary angiography in the outpatient setting

Question 7. A 56-year-old man, with no cardiac history, presents with one severe episode of chest pain that started after pushing some furniture. The pain lasted 20 minutes and did not recur. His admission BP is 160/95 mmHg, and no murmur or rub is heard. His ECG is normal. His initial troponin I is 0.02 ng/ml, and peaks at 0.05 ng/ml (99th percentile <0.04 ng/ml). Renal function is normal. What is the next step?

A. Initiate antithrombotic therapy. Coronary angiography within 24 hours.

B. Initiate antithrombotic therapy. Coronary angiography within 72 hours.

C. Stress testing before discharge for risk stratification (troponin I being minimally increased).

Question 8. A 47-year-old man, smoker, diabetic, presents to the emergency department with sharp chest pain that has been occurring intermittently at rest for the last 2 days. It does not prevent him from performing his daily activities. On exam, his BP is 145/92 mmHg, heart rate 85 bpm. He has no HF or murmur. ECG shows inferior T-wave inversion of 1 mm, and the troponin I is undetectable serially (<0.01 ng/ml). What is the next step?

A. Perform inpatient stress testing. Home discharge followed by outpatient stress testing is not acceptable

B. Perform inpatient stress testing. Home discharge followed by outpatient stress testing (within 72 hours) is acceptable

C. Perform coronary angiography

D. Discharge home on aspirin, β-blocker and arrange for clinic follow-up within a week. Further workup depends on progression of symptoms

Question 9. A 56-year-old woman has a history of RCA PCI 2 years previously. She presents with one episode of chest pain that felt similar to her prior angina. It occurred once at rest, 2 days ago, lasted 20 minutes and did not recur. ECG shows LVH with strain and inferior Q waves. Serial troponin levels are <0.04 ng/ml. Creatinine is normal. What is the next step?

A. Coronary angiography within 72 hours

B. Coronary angiography within 24 hours

C. Stress testing 6–12 hours after presentation

Question 10. In comparison with men, women with ACS (multiple answers)

A. Have a higher in-hospital mortality

B. Are less likely to benefit from an early invasive strategy

C. Have fewer underlying comorbidities

D. Have a higher proportion of non-obstructive CAD and less extensive CAD

E. Have a higher bleeding risk

F. Have a higher ischemic burden despite a lower prevalence and extent of CAD

Question 11. A 56-year-old woman presents with severe chest pressure that lasted 2 hours. Her ECG shows deep T-wave inversion across the precordial leads. BP was 190/105 mmHg on presentation. Troponin rises to 2.5 ng/ml. A coronary angiography is performed and only shows minimal plaques <25%. What is the differential diagnosis at this point (multiple answers)?

A. Stabilized plaque rupture

B. Coronary vasospasm

C. Takotsubo cardiomyopathy

D. Myopericarditis

E. Pulmonary embolism

F. Hypertensive crisis with elevated LVEDP and ischemic imbalance

G. Demand/supply mismatch from anemia or tachyarrhythmia

Question 12. For the patient in Question 11, what additional testing best helps establish a diagnosis?

A. Cardiac MRI

B. IVUS

C. Echo

Question 13. A 62-year-old man presents with angina and a troponin of 0.12 ng/ml. ECG shows 1 mm dynamic lateral ST depression. He is started on antithrombotic therapy. Coronary angiography is performed and reveals a 40% hazy lesion in the mid RCA with TIMI grade 3 flow. It is eccentric with overhanging edges (Figure 1.4, Appendix 1). There is minimal disease otherwise. What is the next step?

A. PCI of the hazy lesion

B. FFR of the RCA

C. IVUS of the RCA

D. Medical therapy since lesion is <50%

Question 14. A 66-year-old woman presents with severe chest pain that started 2 hours ago. The pain is ongoing, unrelieved with NTG, with severe distress, diaphoresis, and severe nausea. BP = 165/90, heart rate 90 bpm, O_2 saturation 100% on ambient air. Exam does not reveal signs of HF. No rub is heard and BP is equal in both arms. The abdomen is soft and non-tender. ECG is normal. Troponin I is negative on admission. What is the next step?

A. The pain is unlikely cardiac, as ECG is normal during ongoing pain. ACS likelihood is low. Obtain serial troponin levels then perform stress testing

B. The pain is likely cardiac by clinical features. Give morphine, metoprolol, and anticoagulation, then perform coronary angiography within 24 hours

C. The pain is likely cardiac by clinical features, especially the severe distress. Perform chest X-ray. Perform urgent coronary angiography

Question 15. A 70-year-old man presents with chest pain and inferior ST-segment depression (dynamic). His troponin I is 0.55 ng/ml. He is currently chest pain free, but is tachycardic (sinus tachycardia 105 bpm) with BP of 110/75 mmHg. What is the appropriate therapy?

A. On admission: aspirin, clopidogrel load, UFH and metoprolol. Perform coronary angiography within 24 hours

B. On admission: aspirin, clopidogrel load, and enoxaparin. Perform coronary angiography within 24 hours

C. On admission: aspirin, ticagrelor load, and UFH. Perform coronary angiography within 24 hours

D. On admission: aspirin, ticagrelor load, and UFH. Perform coronary angiography within 72 hours

Question 16. A 70-year-old man who has insulin-dependent diabetes presents with chest pain and inferior ST-segment depression (dynamic). His troponin I is 0.55 ng/ml. He is currently chest pain free. What is the appropriate therapy?

A. On admission: aspirin, clopidogrel load, GPI, and UFH. Perform coronary angiography within 72 hours.

B. On admission: aspirin, GPI, and UFH. Clopidogrel is withheld because the presentation suggests the patient may require CABG. Perform coronary angiography within 72 hours

C. On admission: aspirin, clopidogrel load, and UFH. Perform coronary angiography within 72 hours

Question 17. A 70-year-old woman presents with NSTEMI. Her coronary angiogram shows multiple moderate lesions (30–50%) in the LAD and RCA. The physician decided to treat her medically. What is the best long-term antiplatelet regimen?

A. Aspirin only, as no PCI was performed

B. Aspirin and clopidogrel for 1 year

C. Aspirin and ticagrelor for 1 year

D. Aspirin and prasugrel for 1 year

Question 18. A 52-year-old woman presents with chest pain and is found to have 2 mm T inversion in the lateral leads and troponin I of 0.14 ng/ml. She is given 300 mg of plavix, aspirin 325 mg, heparin 4000 units and drip on admission. She undergoes coronary angiography next day and is found to have 95% mid RCA stenosis. What PCI pharmacotherapy is associated with the best outcomes during and after PCI?

A. Heparin and GPI

B. Bivalirudin

C. Bivalirudin and GPI

D. Bivalirudin and start ticagrelor instead of clopidogrel

Question 19.
 (i) Should the patient in Question 17 receive anticoagulation after coronary angiography? Yes/No
(ii) Should the patient in Question 18 receive anticoagulation after PCI? Yes/No

Question 20. In comparison with clopidogrel (multiple answers):
A. Ticagrelor reduces mortality in invasively and non-invasively managed ACS
B. Ticagrelor may be administered before coronary angiography
C. Ticagrelor is a reversible ADP receptor antagonist, but because of a 15-hour half-life, its effect lasts ~3–4 days
D. Ticagrelor has a higher non-CABG bleeding risk than clopidogrel, but this bleeding hazard is not particularly accentuated in older patients or those with prior stroke. Prasugrel showed excessive hazard in the latter groups
E. Ticagrelor benefit continues to grow with time
F. Prasugrel is only used in patients managed with PCI, and is loaded after coronary angiography (may be loaded before angiography in STEMI)
G. Prasugrel reduces MI but does not reduce mortality, except in STEMI patients (also, a mortality reduction trend is seen in diabetics)

Question 21. Concerning prasugrel and ticagrelor:
A. Ticagrelor and prasugrel are preferred over clopidogrel in all ACS patients (all ACS for ticagrelor, ACS managed with PCI for prasugrel) (class IIa recommendation)
B. Prasugrel and ticagrelor are particularly beneficial in high-risk conditions (STEMI, diabetes, recurrent events, and complex PCI)
C. Consider the bleeding risk, particularly age >75 and prior stroke with both agents, especially prasugrel
D. Even in the absence of the high-risk conditions (STEMI, diabetes, recurrent events), prasugrel and ticagrelor are warranted in ACS. Clopidogrel hyporesponsiveness may be an additional push for the use of these agents

Question 22. A 56-year-old man has NSTEMI and undergoes BMS placement in the mid-RCA. He does not have any prior bleeding history. His EF is normal. Beside lifelong aspirin, which antiplatelet and β-blocker therapies should he receive?
A. Clopidogrel for 1 month
B. Clopidogrel, prasugrel, or ticagrelor for 1 year
C. Clopidogrel, prasugrel or ticagrelor for 1 year. Consider chronic clopidogrel therapy beyond 1 year if he is deemed a low bleeding risk patient
D. Lifelong metoprolol
E. 1–3 years of metoprolol (medium doses if tolerated)

Question 23. A 42-year-old woman with a smoking history presents with a severe episode of resting angina. ECG shows diffuse T inversion. Troponin I peaks at 2 ng/ml. Coronary angiography shows a long (~35 mm), smooth, non-calcified 70% stenosis of the mid-RCA. What is the likely mechanism?
A. Vasospasm
B. Plaque rupture
C. Plaque erosion
D. Spontaneous coronary artery dissection
E. A or C
F. A, C, or D

Question 24. What is the next step for the patient of Question 23?
A. Direct stenting
B. NTG followed by direct stenting
C. NTG, followed by OCT then direct stenting

Question 25. A 55-year-old man has a history of untreated HTN. He presents with chest pain and dyspnea. He has severe HTN upon presentation, 220/120 mmHg. His pain and HTN do not improve with NTG and he requires a 24- hour intravenous drip of nicardipine and multiple agents to control HTN. ECG shows LVH with a strain pattern. Initial troponin I is 0.08 and it peaks at 0.25 ng/ml. Creatinine is 1.5 mg/dl. Echo shows LVH with mild LV systolic dysfunction and elevated LA pressure. What is the diagnosis and the next step?
A. Type 1 MI from plaque rupture. Must perform early invasive strategy
B. Type 2 MI from severe HTN. HTN control is the initial measure. Perform ischemic workup, possibly stress testing, once HTN is controlled and chest pain resolves

Question 26. A 55-year-old man has a history of untreated HTN. He presents with chest pain and dyspnea. He has severe HTN upon presentation, 190/110 mmHg. After the administration of two NTG tablets, chest pain resolves and BP becomes 145/85 mmHg. Troponin I is 0.04 ng/ml and peaks at 0.10 ng/ml. What is the diagnosis and the next step?
A. Type 1 MI from plaque rupture. Must perform early invasive strategy
B. Type 2 MI from severe HTN. HTN control is the initial measure. Perform ischemic workup, possibly stress testing, once HTN is controlled and chest pain resolves

Answer 1. C. He fulfills the MI definition as he has an elevated troponin with a rise and fall pattern, *along with* ST changes. The degree of troponin rise (>0.5–1 ng/ml) as well as the ST changes are concerning for underlying CAD, whether type 1 MI (plaque rupture initiated by the infectious status) or severe ischemic imbalance on top of underlying CAD. In the absence of contraindication, antithrombotic therapy may be initiated and coronary angiography may be performed after his infection and renal function stabilize.

Answer 2. A. He does not fulfill the MI definition as he has an elevated troponin with a rise and fall pattern, but *without associated chest pain, ST changes, or wall motion abnormality*. The severe non-cardiac illness along with the mild degree of troponin rise (<0.5–1 ng/ml) is consistent with ischemic imbalance, and does not necessarily imply underlying CAD. There is no definite need for antithrombotic therapy, and a later, elective evaluation with stress testing may be performed.

Answer 3. C. The patient has NSTEMI. He has a rise and fall in troponin along with ST changes and wall motion abnormality. This is a type 2 MI, related to ischemic imbalance in the context of severe, acute anemia. However, the extensive ST changes, the severity of troponin rise (>0.5–1 ng/ml), and the wall motion abnormality are concerning for severe underlying CAD, which was probably stable and was unveiled by the stress of anemia/tachycardia. CAD needs to be addressed. Stress testing is unlikely to provide additional information, as the patient already shows severe myocardial ischemia and ST depression with the stress of anemia. Coronary angiography, followed by possible revascularization (PCI or CABG), is warranted. However, in a patient with active or recent bleeding, PCI is not advised, as peri-PCI antico-agulation and dual antiplatelet therapy may not be tolerated. Wait 1–2 weeks (at least) after hemoglobin has stabilized and proper gastro-intestinal therapy is performed (PPI, endoscopic cauterization). This allows a safer performance of revascularization if needed. β-Blockers should not be administered acutely, as the patient is in a pre-shock state and tachycardia is compensatory; they may be administered 24–48 hours later.

Answer 4. B. The mild rise in troponin is secondary to the ischemic imbalance of HF (LV dilatation increases wall stress/afterload; LVEDP elevation reduces coronary flow). Similarly, the chest tightness that occurs in decompensated HF is commonly secondary to ischemic imbal-ance. In fact, troponin rise in HF is a prognostic marker that correlates more with the severity of HF decompensation than the coronary status and does not necessarily imply ACS. The fact that a coronary angiography performed in the last 2–3 years did not reveal obstructive CAD strongly argues against ACS.

Answer 5. B. The mild troponin rise is at least partly secondary to the ischemic imbalance of HF. Yet, any HF, particularly acute or systolic HF, warrants evaluation for an underlying ischemic etiology (chronic CAD) using coronary angiography. Antithrombotic therapy does not appear warranted, as the ECG does not suggest acute ischemia. Elevated troponin alone does not establish the diagnosis of ACS in a patient presenting with HF. While the underlying CAD is often stable, ischemic evaluation is preferably performed before discharge. CAD, if present, is likely extensive with an increased risk of recurrent HF or MI. In one analysis, patients with acute HF and CAD who did not undergo revascularization before discharge had a significantly increased mortality in the ensuing 60–90 days; this excess in mortality was attenuated with revascularization.

Answer 6. A. The Q waves suggest an ischemic etiology of HF. The Q-wave infarct may be recent, coinciding with his onset of symptoms. Moreover, global ischemia is suggested by the extensive ST depression and the wall motion abnormality that extends beyond the infarcted territory. Thus, in this particular case, ECG implies that HF is secondary to a recent infarction and acute ischemia. He should be treated as type 1 MI with antithrombotic therapy and he should undergo coronary angiography once he has received proper diuresis. In acute HF, in the absence of acute ST elevation, angiography and PCI are not warranted urgently, as supine positioning and contrast loading are likely to aggravate HF and myocardial ischemia. His Q-wave MI is >24 hours old (by history), without persistent ST elevation.

Answer 7. B. Any increase in troponin above the 99th percentile with a rise and fall pattern, in the context of angina presentation, and in the absence of severe non-cardiac illness (sepsis, anemia, HF, tachyarrhythmia) is diagnostic of primary NSTEMI (ACS). This patient is man-aged with antithrombotic therapy and an initial invasive strategy rather than stress testing. His risk is high but not exceedingly high, as his GRACE risk score is <140 (age <70, no ST depression, HF, hypotension, tachycardia, or renal failure); thus, coronary angiography may be performed at 24–72 hours.

Answer 8. B. Traditional risk factors, like smoking and diabetes, increase the general probability of CAD but only weakly increase the likeli-hood of ACS in a patient with acute chest pain syndrome. Other factors, such as pain timing/duration, troponin, and ECG should be taken into account: (1) the undetectable troponin makes ACS very unlikely; (2) T-wave inversion <3 mm is non-diagnostic and does not signifi-cantly increase the likelihood of ACS or worsen its prognosis; (3) chest pain occurrence and timing are atypical. In this patient with unlikely ACS, early stress testing at 6–12 hours after admission is the best strategy. An early discharge followed by stress testing within 72 hours of discharge is also appropriate. While ACS is unlikely, the acute presentation still warrants stress testing at one point (Answer D is false).

Answer 9. C. A history of PCI dictates an initial invasive strategy in case of recurrence of typical pain within 6–12 months of PCI. Her PCI is >1 year old and while the pain is concerning, it does not have a typical exertional pattern. Considering her troponin and non-specific ECG, the ACS likelihood is not high. In women with negative troponin, no ST changes, and low TIMI risk score, an initial invasive strategy is associ-ated with increased risk of death/MI, and thus initial stress testing is preferably performed.

Answer 10. A, B, D, E, F.

Answer 11. A, B, C, D (see explication under Answer 12).

Answer 12. A. About 10–15% of patients with NSTEMI, particularly women, are not found to have any significant CAD. In those cases, reasons A through G can explain the troponin rise. Demand/supply mismatch without underlying CAD usually causes a troponin rise <0.5–1 ng/ml, and thus is not likely to explain the patient's troponin (causes F and G). Similarly, in pulmonary embolism, troponin does not usually rise beyond 1 ng/ml.

In the absence of obstructive CAD, a myocardial process, such as myocarditis or takotsubo cardiomyopathy, has to be considered. Transient severe myocardial ischemia is also possible (vasospasm or stabilized plaque rupture). The deep T inversion is consistent with takotsubo cardiomyopathy, but also myocarditis and a post-ischemic state. In all those cases, the distribution of the echocardiographic wall motion abnormality helps establish a diagnosis. MRI is most helpful: late gadolinium enhancement rules out takotsubo cardiomyopathy, and is only seen with infarction or myocarditis. The distribution of late gadolinium enhancement distinguishes myocarditis from an ischemic pattern:[52]

- Distribution not consistent with an arterial territory + subepicardial or mid-wall predominance → myocarditis
- Distribution consistent with an arterial territory + subendocardial or transmural predominance → infarction

In all three cases (myocarditis, infarction, takotsubo), edema may be seen on T2-weighed images if the process is acute. The distribution of edema also distinguishes myocarditis from infarction. IVUS may be done when a moderate lesion appears suspicious angiographically (not the case here).

Answer 13. C. In ACS, it is important to ascertain that a seemingly non-obstructive plaque is truly non-obstructive. For example, a 30–50% hazy stenosis with irregular or overhanging borders is possibly unstable and may be anatomically significant by IVUS (more obstructive and ulcerated than the angiography suggests).

Answer 14. C. About 40–45% of acute LCx occlusions do not show any significant ST-T abnormality. **In fact, ~20% of NSTEMIs have acute coronary occlusion, mostly LCx or RCA, and are STEMI-equivalents that lack ST elevation and sometimes ST depression. LCx and RCA occlusions represent 2/3 of these "occluded" NSTEMIs.** Beside the unremarkable ECG, the first troponin may be negative in these patients, which explains the diagnostic delay. Hints to a true ACS: (i) ongoing, unexplained severe distress/pain (rule out clinically and by X-ray aortic dissection, perforated peptic ulcer, and abdominal catastrophe); (ii) posterior-lead ECG; (iii) ECG abnormality may emerge when ECG is repeated every 10 min. Even if the posterior-lead ECG is normal, treat the patient as acute coronary occlusion and perform urgent catheterization. Perform chest X-ray to rule out pneumothorax and any suggestion of aortic dissection or perforated peptic ulcer (subdiaphragmatic air). Morphine should not be used, as it masks an ongoing angina and provides false reassurance.

Answer 15. C. The patient has tachycardia and SBP <120 mmHg, he is in a pre-shock state and should not receive metoprolol in the first 24 hours of ACS. Upstream aspirin, clopidogrel or ticagrelor, and anticoagulation should be provided. The patient has a very high-risk ACS, with a high GRACE score >140 (in light of the age ≥70, tachycardia, SBP <120, and both troponin rise and ST changes). An early invasive strategy <24 hours is preferred. Since coronary angiography will be performed in less than 12–24 hours, heparin is preferred over enoxaparin.

Answer 16. C. Upstream GPI (before PCI) is not justified, whether upstream clopidogrel is administered or not. On admission, the patient should receive dual antiplatelet therapy with aspirin and clopidogrel or ticagrelor. GPI is not an appropriate alternative for clopidogrel. If CABG seems highly likely, one may choose to administer only aspirin and anticoagulation (no clopidogrel or GPI), then perform coronary angiography within 24 hours. In the latter situation, a potent oral ADP receptor antagonist is administered in the catheterization lab if PCI is to be performed (as in the ACCOAST trial).

Answer 17. C (B is also an acceptable option). The patient likely had plaque rupture of one of her moderate lesions, leading to thrombus and microembolization. Her plaques stabilized with antithrombotic therapy. Clopidogrel (CURE trial) and ticagrelor (PLATO) are therapies that have shown benefit in medically treated ACS patients, ticagrelor being the superior agent (ticagrelor showed mortality and MI reductions in this subgroup of medically treated patients). Prasugrel is only studied in ACS patients treated with PCI.

Answer 18. D. The downstream use of GPI (during PCI) is not beneficial in patients who have received proper clopidogrel preload. Ticagrelor provides more reduction of ischemic events and mortality than clopidogrel after ACS.

Answer 19. (i) yes, (ii) no. Anticoagulation for at least 48 hours is warranted in NSTEMI patients managed without PCI. Low-dose UFH may be started 8–12 hours after coronary angiography and continued for a total of 48 hours. Fondaparinux may be used for 2–8 days. Enoxaparin may also be used, but is associated with a higher bleeding risk after catheterization. In patients who undergo PCI, the anticoagulant is stopped after PCI. Only bivalirudin may be infused for 1–4 hours after PCI. In patients who receive GPI during PCI, GPI may be continued for up to 24 hours.

Answer 20. All are correct.

Answer 21. All are correct.

Answer 22. C and E. Regardless of the stent type, true ACS patients should receive 1 year of ADP receptor antagonist. Beyond one year, the recent DAPT trial suggests a benefit of dual antiplatelet therapy in patients who have not bled in the first year, especially the MI subset. If EF is normal, β-blocker does not have a clear benefit beyond 1 year after MI.

Answer 23. F. The smooth angiographic appearance and the age and sex of the patient suggest vasospasm, plaque erosion, or spontaneous coronary dissection. The length of the stenosis is concerning for dissection. A tortuous or corkscrew coronary artery would further support spontaneous coronary dissection.

Answer 24. C. OCT helps show features of plaque erosion. Plaque erosion is characterized by thrombus with an intact intimal cap or a fibrointimal plaque. It may also show spontaneous coronary dissection, in which case conservative management is an alternative.

Answer 25. B. Patients with true ACS/type 1 MI may have HTN secondary to the distress of angina. However, in the case presented here, the persistence of HTN and its requirement for multiple agents implies that malignant HTN is the primary process responsible for the patient's pain and troponin rise. The severe LVH, seen on echo, accentuates ischemic demands and is a marker of uncontrolled HTN. The degree of troponin rise (<0.5 ng/ml) is consistent with ischemic imbalance.

Answer 26. A. Compare this case to Question 25. The quick resolution of HTN with NTG implies that HTN was secondary to myocardial ischemia (catecholamine surge), rather than a cause of ischemia. Even the milder troponin rise, in context, is worrisome for a true ACS and plaque rupture.

References

1. Thygesen K, Alpert JS, Jaffe AS, et al. Third universal definition of myocardial infarction. ESC/ACCF/AHA/WHF expert consensus. Circulation 2012; 126: 220–35.
2. Alcalai R, Planer D, Culhaoglu A, et al. Acute coronary syndrome versus nonspecific troponin elevation. Arch Intern Med 2007; 167: 276–81.
3. Tehrani DM, Seto AH. Third universal definition of myocardial infarction: update, caveats, differential diagnosis. Cleve Clin J Med 2013; 80: 777–86.
4. Keller T, Zeller T, Ojeda F, et al. Serial changes in highly sensitive troponin I assay and early diagnosis of myocardial infarction. JAMA 2011; 306: 2684–93.
5. Hamm CW, Bassand J, Agewall S, et al. ESC Guidelines for the management of acute coronary syndromes in patients presenting without persistent ST-segment elevation. Eur Heart J 2011; 32: 2999–3054.
6. Fox KA, Dabbous OH, Goldberg RJ, et al. Prediction of risk of death and myocardial infarction in the six months after presentation with acute coronary syndrome: prospective multinational observational study (GRACE). BMJ 2006; 333: 1091.
7. Braunwald E, Morrow DA. Unstable angina: is it time for a requiem? Circulation 2013; 127: 2452–7.
8. Goldstein JA, Demetriou D, Grines CL, et al. Multiple complex coronary plaques in patients with acute myocardial infarction. N Engl J Med 2000; 343: 915–22.
9. Niemen MS, Brutsaert D, Dickstein K, et al. EuroHeart Failure Survey II (EHFS II): a survey on hospitalized acute heart failure patients: Description of population. Eur Heart J 2006; 27: 2725–36.
10. Prinzmetal M, Kennamer R, Merliss R, et al. Angina pectoris. 1. A variant form of angina pectoris. Am J Med 1959; 27: 375–88.
11. Prinzmetal M, Ekemecki A, Kennamer R, et al. Variant form of angina pectoris: previously undelineated syndrome. JAMA 1960; 174: 1791–800.
12. Maseri A, Severi S, de Nes M, et al. "Variant" angina: one aspect of a continuous spectrum of vasospastic myocardial ischemia: pathogenetic mechanisms, estimated incidence and clinical and coronary arteriographic findings in 138 patients. Am J Cardiol 1978; 42: 1019–35.
13. Ong P, Athanasiadis A, Hill S, et al. Coronary artery spasm as a frequent cause of acute coronary syndrome: the CASPAR (Coronary Artery Spasm in Patients with Acute Coronary Syndrome) study. J Am Coll Cardiol 2008; 52: 523–7.
14. Ong P, Athanasiadis A, Borgulya G, et al. High prevalence of a pathological response to acetylcholine testing in patients with stable angina pectoris and unobstructed coronary arteries: the ACOVA study (Abnormal COronary VAsomotion in patients with stable angina and unobstructed coronary arteries). J Am Coll Cardiol 2012; 59: 655–62.
15. Fesmire FM, Percy RF, Bardoner JB, et al. Usefulness of automated serial 12-lead ECG monitoring during the initial emergency department evaluation of patients with chest pain. Ann Emerg Med 1998; 31: 3.
16. Pope JH, Ruthazer R, Beshansky JR, et al. Clinical features of emergency department patients presenting with symptoms suggestive of acute cardiac ischemia: a multicenter study. J Thromb Thrombolysis 1998; 6: 63.
17. Pope JH, Aufderheide TP, Ruthazer R, et al. Missed diagnoses of acute cardiac ischemia in the emergency department. N Engl J Med 2000; 342: 1163–70. *Among patients considered normal or non-specific ECG, 2% are eventually diagnosed with MI within 30 d (~75% of which are non-Q MI) and 2% UA (mainly on 1–3 d follow-up visit; prospective analysis). Troponin was not used, just ECG and CK-MB.*
18. Krishnaswamy A, Lincoff AM, Menon V. Magnitude and consequences of missing the acute infarct-related circumflex artery. Am Heart J 2009; 158: 706–12.
19. Gibson C, Pride YB, Mohanavelu S, et al. Angiographic and clinical outcomes among patients with acute coronary syndrome presenting with isolated anterior ST-segment depressions. Circulation 2008; 118: S-654. Abstract 1999.
20. Antman EM, Tanasijevic MJ, Thompson B, et al. Cardiac-specific troponin I levels to predict the risk of mortality in patients with acute coronary syndromes. N Engl J Med 1996; 201: 335: 1342–9.
21. Prasad A, Gersh BJ, Bertrand ME, et al. Prognostic significance of periprocedural versus spontaneously occurring myocardial infarction after percutaneous coronary intervention in patients with acute coronary syndromes. An analysis from the ACUITY trial. J Am Coll Cardiol 2009; 54: 477–86.
22. Moussa ID, Klein LW, Shah B, et al. Consideration of a new definition of clinically relevant myocardial infarction after coronary revascularization. J Am Coll Cardiol 2013; 62: 1563–70.
23. Than M, Cullen L, Aldous S, et al. 2-Hour accelerated diagnostic protocol to assess patients with chest pain symptoms using contemporary troponins as the only biomarker: the ADAPT trial. J Am Coll Cardiol 2012; 59: 2091–8. *With current-generation troponin assay, an undetectable troponin level <0.01 ng/ml is associated with a very low risk of events at 30 days.*
24. Ioannidis JPA, Salem D, Chew PW, et al. Accuracy of imaging technologies in the diagnosis of acute cardiac ischemia in the emergency department: a meta- analysis. Ann Emerg Med 2001; 37: 471–7.
25. Amsterdam EA, Wenger NK, Brindis RG, et al. 2014 AHA/ACC guideline for the management of patients with non-ST-elevation acute coronary syndromes. J Am Coll Cardiol 2014; 64: e139–228. *Note, also, that 2007 AHA/ACC guidelines are relevant: J Am Coll Cardiol 2007; 50: 1–157.*
26. Lee TH, Cook F, Weisberg M, et al. Acute chest pain in the emergency room. Identification and examination of low-risk patients. Arch Intern Med 1985; 145: 65.
27. Swap CJ, Nagurney JT. Value and limitations of chest pain history in the evaluation of patients with suspected acute coronary syndromes. JAMA 2005; 294: 2623–9.
28. Topol EJ, Yadav JS. Recognition of the importance of embolization in atherosclerotic vascular disease. Circulation 2000; 101: 570–80.
29. Stone GW, McLaurin BT, Cox DA, et al. Bivalirudin for patients with acute coronary syndromes. N Engl J Med 2006; 355: 2203–16. *ACUITY trial.*
30. Giugliano RP, White JA, Boden C, et al. Early versus delayed, provisional eptifibatide in acute coronary syndromes. N Engl J Med 2009; 360: 2176–90. *EARLY ACS trial.*
31. Mehta SR, Granger CB, Boden WE, et al. Early versus delayed invasive intervention in acute coronary syndromes. N Engl J Med 2009; 360: 2165–75. *TIMACS trial.*

Invasive strategy > conservative strategy

32. Cannon CP, Weintraub WS, Demopoulos LA, et al. Comparison of early invasive and conservative strategies in patients with unstable coronary syndromes treated with the glycoprotein IIb/IIIa inhibitor tirofiban (TACTICS-TIMI 18 trial). N Engl J Med 2001; 344: 1879–87.
33. Fox KA, Poole-Wilson P, Clayton TC, et al. 5-year outcome of an interventional strategy in non-ST-elevation acute coronary syndrome: the British Heart Foundation RITA 3 randomised trial. Lancet 2005; 366: 914–20.

34. Wallentin L, Lagerqvist B, Husted S, et al. Outcome at 1 year after an invasive compared with a non-invasive strategy in unstable coronary-artery disease: the FRISC II invasive randomised trial. FRISC II Investigators. Lancet 2000; 356: 9–16.

35. de Winter RJ, Windhausen F, Cornel JH, et al. Early invasive versus selectively invasive management for acute coronary syndromes. N Engl J Med 2005; 353: 1095–104. *ICTUS trial*.

36. Amsterdam EA, Wenger NK, Brindis RG, et al. 2014 AHA/ACC guideline for the management of patients with non-ST-elevation acute coronary syndrome. J Am Coll Cardiol 2014; 64: e139–228.

37. Yusuf S, Zhao F, Mehta SR, et al. Effects of clopidogrel in addition to aspirin in patients with acute coronary syndromes without ST-segment elevation. N Engl J Med 2001; 345: 494–502. *CURE trial*.

38. Hanna EB, Rao SV, Manoukian SV, Saucedo JF. The evolving role of glycoprotein IIb-IIIa inhibitors in the setting of percuteneeous coronary intervention. Strategies to minimize bleeding and improve outcomes. J Am Coll Cardiol 2010; 3: 1209–19.

39. Chen ZM, Pan HC, Chen YP, et al. Early intravenous then oral metoprolol in 45,852 patients with acute myocardial infarction: randomised placebo-controlled trial. Lancet 2005; 366: 1622–32. *COMMIT-CCS trial*.

40. Cannon CP, Braunwald E, McCabe CH, et al. Intensive versus moderate lipid lowering with statins after acute coronary syndromes. N Engl J Med 350: 1495, 2004.

41. Heeschen C, Hamm CW, Laufs U, et al. Withdrawal of statins increases event rates in patients with acute coronary syndromes. Circulation 2002; 105: 1446–52.

CABG vs PCI

42. Mohr FW, Morice MC, Kappetein AP, et al. Coronary artery bypass graft surgery versus percutaneous coronary intervention in patients with three-vessel disease and left main coronary disease: 5-year follow-up of the randomised, clinical SYNTAX trial. Lancet 2013; 381: 629.

43. Farkouh ME, Domanski M, Sleeper LA, et al. Strategies for multivessel revascularization in patients with diabetes. N Engl J Med 2012; 367: 2375–84. *FREEDOM trial*.

44. Bravata DM, Gienger AL, McDonald KM, et al. Systematic review: the comparative effectiveness of percutaneous coronary interventions and coronary artery bypass graft surgery. Ann Intern Med 2007; 147: 703–16.

Multivessel PCI

45. Hannan EL, Samadashvili Z, Walford G, et al. Staged versus one-time complete revascularization with percutaneous coronary intervention for multivessel coronary artery disease patients without ST-elevation myocardial infarction. Circ Cardiovasc Interv 2013; 6: 12–20.

46. Brener SJ, Milford-Beland S, Roe MT, et al. Culprit-only or multivessel revascularization in patients with acute coronary syndromes: an American College of Cardiology National Cardiovascular Database Registry report. Am Heart J 2008; 155: 140–6.

ACS without significant CAD

47. Roe MT, Harrington RA, Prosper DM, et al. Clinical and therapeutic profile of patients presenting with acute coronary syndromes who do not have significant coronary artery disease. Circulation 2000; 102: 1101–6.

48. Gehrie ER, Reynolds HR, Chen AY, et al. Characterization and outcomes of women and men with non-ST-segment elevation myocardial infarction and nonobstructive coronary artery disease: results from CRUSADE. Am Heart J 2009; 158: 688–94.

49. Patel MR, Chen AY, Peterson ED, et al. Prevalence, predictors, and outcomes of patients with non-ST-segment elevation myocardial infarction and insignificant coronary artery disease. Am Heart J 2006; 152: 641–7.

50. Rossini R, Capodanno D, Lettieri C, et al. Long-term outcomes of patients with acute coronary syndrome and nonobstructive coronary artery disease. Am J Cardiol 2013; 112: 150–5.

51. Hirsch A, Windhausen F, Tijssen JGP, et al Diverging associations of an intended early invasive strategy compared with actual revascularization, and outcome in patients with non-ST-segment elevation acute coronary syndrome: the problem of treatment selection bias. Eur Heart J 2009; 30, 645–54.

MRI diagnosis in patients with a large troponin rise and normal coronary arteries

52. Leurent G, Langella B, Fougerou C, et al. Diagnostic contributions of cardiac magnetic resolution imaging in patients presenting with elevated troponin, acute chest pain syndrome, and unobstructed coronary arteries. Arch Cardiovasc Dis 2011; 104: 161–70.

53. Assomull RG, Lyne JC, Keenan N, et al. The role of cardiovascular magnetic resonance in patients presenting with chest pain, raised troponin, and unobstructed coronary arteries. Eur Heart J 2007; 28: 1242–9.

Bad outcomes of patients with significant CAD who are not revascularized (in addition to reference 51)

54. Hanna EB, Chen AY, Roe MT, Saucedo JF. Characteristics and in-hospital outcomes of patients presenting with non-ST-segment elevation myocardial infarction found to have significant coronary artery disease on coronary angiography and managed medically: stratification according to renal function. Am Heart J 2012; 164: 52–7.

55. James SK, Roe MT, Cannon CP, et al. Ticagrelor versus clopidogrel in patients with acute coronary syndromes intended for non-invasive management: substudy from prospective randomised PLATelet inhibition and patient Outcomes (PLATO) trial. BMJ 2011; 342: d3527.

56. Spaan JAE, Piek JJ, Hoffman JIE, Siebes M. Physiological basis of clinically used coronary hemodynamic indices. Circulation 2006; 113: 446–55.

57. Peacock WF, De Marco E, Fonarow GC, et al. Cardiac troponin and outcome in acute heart failure. N Engl J Med 2008; 258: 2117–26.

Low-risk and low-probability ACS

58. Koukkunen H, Pyorala K, Halinen MO. Low-risk patients with chest pain and without evidence of myocardial infarction may be safely discharged from emergency department. Eur Heart J 2004; 25: 329–35. *This study had the higher event rate as it included patients with prior CAD: mortality at 6 months 0.8%, readmission 8%.*

59. Conti A, Paladini B, Toccafondi S, et al. Effectiveness of a multidisciplinary chest pain unit for the assessment of coronary syndromes and risk stratification in the Florence area. Am Heart J 2002; 144: 630–5.

60. Smith SW, Tibbles CD, Apple FS, et al. Outcome of low-risk patients discharged home after a normal cardiac troponin I. J Emerg Med 2004; 26: 401–6.

Discharge medications

61. Fox KA, Mehta SR, Peters R. Benefits and risks of the combination of clopidogrel and aspirin in patients undergoing surgical revascularization for non-ST-elevation acute coronary syndrome: the Clopidogrel in Unstable Angina to Prevent Recurrent Ischemic Events (CURE) trial. Circulation 2004; 110: 1202–18.

Duration of dual antiplatelet therapy after ACS or DES

62. Mauri L, Kereiakes DJ, Yeh RW, et al.; DAPT Study Investigators. Twelve or 30 months of dual antiplatelet therapy after drug-eluting stents. N Engl J Med 2014; 371: 2155–66.
63. Bhatt DL, Flather MD, Hacke W, et al. Patients with prior myocardial infarction, stroke, or symptomatic peripheral arterial disease in the CHARISMA trial. J Am Coll Cardiol 2007; 49: 1982–8.
64. Krucoff MW, Rutledge DR, Gruberg L, et al. A new era of prospective real-world safety evaluation primary report of XIENCE V USA (XIENCE V Everolimus Eluting Coronary Stent System condition-of-approval post-market study). JACC Cardiovasc Interv 2011; 4: 1298–309.
65. Naidu SS, Krucoff MW, Rutledge DR, et al. Contemporary incidence and predictors of stent thrombosis and other major adverse cardiac events in the year after Xience V implantation. JACC Cardiovasc Interv 2012; 5: 626–35.
66. Colombo A, Chieffo A, Frasheri A, et al. Second generation drug-eluting stent implantation followed by 6- versus 12- month dual antiplatelet therapy. J Am Coll Cardiol 2014; 64: 2086–97. *SECURITY trial, stable CAD. Similar results were seen in the OPTIMIZE trial (3- versus 12-month of dual antiplatelet therapy).*
67. Palmerini T, Biondi-Zoccai G, Della Riva D. Stent thrombosis with drug-eluting and bare-metal stents: evidence from a comprehensive network meta-analysis. Lancet 2012; 379: 1393–402. *Everolimus-eluting stent is associated with an even lower risk of stent thrombosis than BMS and any other DES.*
68. Palmerini T, Sangiorgi D, Valgimigli M, et al. Short- versus long-term dual antiplatelet therapy after drug-eluting stent implantation: an individual patient data pairwise and network meta-analysis. J Am Coll Cardiol 2015; 65: 1092–102.
69. Valgimigli M, Campo G, Monti M, et al. Short- versus long-term duration of dual antiplatelet therapy after coronary stenting: a randomized multicenter trial. Circulation 2012; 125: 2015–26. *PRODIGY trial, 56% MI.*
70. Airoldi F, Colombo A, Morici N. Incidence and predictors of drug-eluting stent thrombosis during and after discontinuation of thienopyridine treatment. Circulation 2007; 116: 745–54.
71. Schulz S, Schuster T, Mehilli J, et al. Stent thrombosis after drug-eluting stent implantation: incidence, timing, and relation to discontinuation of clopidogrel therapy over a 4-year period. Eur Heart J 2009; 30: 2714–21.

Dual antiplatelet therapy and warfarin

72. Sorensen R, Hansen ML, Abildstrom SZ, et al. Risk of bleeding in patients with acute myocardial infarction treated with different combinations of aspirin, clopidogrel, and vitamin K antagonists in Denmark: a retrospective analysis of nationwide registry data. Lancet 2009; 374: 1967–74.
73. Camm AJ, Kirchhof P, Lip GYH, et al. ESC Guidelines for the management of atrial fibrillation. Eur Heart J 2010; 31: 2369–429.
74. Windecker S, Koth P, Alfonso F, et al. 2014 ESC/EACTS guidelines on myocardial revascularization. Eur Hear J 2014; 35: 2541–619.
75. Dewilde WJ, Oirbans T, Verheugt FW, et al. Use of clopidogrel with or without aspirin in patients taking oral anticoagulant therapy and undergoing percutaneous coronary intervention: an open-label, randomised, controlled trial. Lancet 2013; 30; 381: 1107–15. *WOEST trial.*
76. Hurlen M, Abdelnoor M, Smith P, Erikssen J, Arnesen H. Warfarin, aspirin, or both after myocardial infarction. N Engl J Med 2002; 347: 969–74. *WARIS 2.*
77. Van ES, Jonker JJ, Verheugt FWA, et al. Aspirin and Coumadin after acute coronary syndromes (the ASPECT-2 study). Lancet 2002; 360: 109–11.
78. Lamberts M, Gislason GM, Lip GYH, et al. Antiplatelet therapy for stable coronary artery disease in atrial fibrillation patients on oral anticoagulant: a nationwide cohort study. Circulation 2014; 129: 1577–85.

79. Hjalmarson Å, Herlitz J, Målek L, et al. Effect on mortality of metoprolol in acute myocardial infarction. Lancet 1981; ii: 823–7.
80. CAPRICORN Investigators. Effect of carvedilol on outcome after myocardial infarction in patients with left ventricular dysfunction: the CAPRICORN randomised trial. Lancet 2001; 357: 1385–90.
81. Bangalore S, Steg G, Deedwania P, et al. β-Blocker use and clinical outcomes in stable outpatients with and without coronary artery disease. JAMA 2012; 308: 1340–9. *REACH registry.*
82. Goldberger JJ, Bonow RO, Cuffe M, et al. Effect of beta-blocker dose on survival after acute myocardial infarction. J Am Col Cardiol 2015; 66: 1431–41.
83. PEACE Trial Investigators. Angiotensin-converting-enzyme inhibition in stable coronary artery disease. N Engl J Med 2004; 351: 2058–68. *In CAD patients with normal EF and SBP 130–140 mmHg, the addition of ACE-I did not improve outcomes furthermore (55% had prior MI).*
84. SPRINT Research Group. A randomized trial of intensive versus standard blood pressure control. N Engl J Med 2015; 373: 2103–16.
85. Wiviott SD, Cannon CP, Morrow DA, et al. Can low-density lipoprotein be too low? The safety and efficacy of achieving very low low-density lipoprotein with intensive statin therapy: a PROVE IT-TIMI 22 substudy. J Am Coll Cardiol 2005; 46: 1411–16.
86. Pitt B, Remme W, Zannad F, et al. Eplerenone, a selective aldosterone blocker, in patients with left ventricular dysfunction after myocardial infarction. N Engl J Med 2003; 348: 1309–21.
87. Bhatt DL, Cryer BL, Contant CF, et al. Clopidogrel with or without omeprazole in coronary artery disease. N Engl J Med 2010; 363: 1909–17.

Prognosis

88. Savonitto S, Ardissino D, Granger CB, et al. Prognostic value of the admission electrocardiogram in acute coronary syndromes. JAMA 1999; 281: 707. *From GUSTO 2b.*
89. Lagerqvist B, Husted S, Kontny F, et al. 5-year outcomes in the FRISC-II randomised trial of an invasive versus a non-invasive strategy in non-ST-elevation acute coronary syndrome: a follow-up study. Lancet 2006; 368: 998–1004. *FRISC II, 5-year follow-up.*
90. Stone GW, Maehara A, Lansky AJ, et al. A prospective natural-history study of coronary atherosclerosis. N Engl J Med 2011; 364: 226–35.

Complex plaques and CAD progression

91. Ambrose JA, Winters SL, Stern A, et al. Angiographic morphology and the pathogenesis of unstable angina pectoris. J Am Coll Cardiol 1985; 5: 609–16.
92. Chen M, Chester MR, Redwood S, et al. Angiographic stenosis progression and coronary events in patients with "stabilized" unstable angina. Circulation 1995; 91: 2319–24.

93. Lichtlen PR, Nikutta P, Jost S et al. Anatomical progression of coronary artery disease in humans as seen by prospective, repeated, quantitated coronary angiography. Relation to clinical events and risk factors. The INTACT Study Group. Circulation 1992; 86: 828–38. *Ten percent progression of stenoses at 3 years, but 30–40% of patients develop new moderate stenoses.*

94. Mancini GBJ, Hartigan PM, Bates ER, et al. Angiographic disease progression and residual risk of cardiovascular events while on optimal medical therapy: observations from the COURAGE Trial. Circ Cardiovasc Interv 2011; 4: 545–52.

Women and ACS

95. Clayton TC, Pocock SJ, Henderson RA, et al. Do men benefit more than women from an interventional strategy in patients with unstable angina or non-ST-elevation myocardial infarction? the impact of gender in the RITA 3 trial. Eur Heart J 2004; 25: 1641–50. *RITA 3: increased mortality with an invasive strategy in women.*

96. O'Donoghue M, Boden WE, Braunwald E, et al. Early invasive vs conservative treatment strategies in women and men with unstable angina and non-ST-segment elevation myocardial infarction: : a meta-analysis. JAMA 2008; 300: 71–80.

97. Mega JL, Hochman JS, Scirica BM, et al. Clinical features and outcomes of women with unstable ischemic heart disease: observations from metabolic efficiency with ranolazine for less ischemia in non-ST-elevation acute coronary syndromes-thrombolysis in myocardial infarction 36 (MERLIN-TIMI 36). Circulation 2010; 121: 1809–17.

98. Hochman JS, Tamis JE, Thompson TD, et al. Sex, clinical presentation, and outcome in patients with acute coronary syndromes. Global Use of Strategies to Open Occluded Coronary Arteries in Acute Coronary Syndromes IIb Investigators. N Engl J Med 1999; 341: 226–32.

Elderly and ACS

99. Bach RG, Cannon CP, Weintraub WS, et al. The effect of routine, early invasive management on outcome for elderly patients with non-ST-segment elevation acute coronary syndromes. Ann Intern Med 2004; 141: 186–95.

100. Tegn N, Abdelnoor M, Aaberge L, et al. Invasive versus conservative strategy in patients aged 80 years or older with non-ST-elevation myocardial infarction or unstable angina pectoris (After Eighty study): an open-label randomised controlled trial. Lancet 2016; 387: 1057–65.

CKD

101. Fox KA, Antman EM, Montalescot G, et al. The impact of renal dysfunction on outcomes in the ExTRACT-TIMI 25 trial. J Am Coll Cardiol 2007; 49: 2249–55.

102. Januzzi JL, Cannon CP, DiBattiste PM; TACTICS-TIMI 18 Investigators. Effects of renal insufficiency on early invasive management in patients with acute coronary syndromes (the TACTICS-TIMI 18 Trial). Am J Cardiol 90 2002: 1246–9.

103. Hanna EB, Chen AY, Roe MT, et al. Characteristics and in-hospital outcomes of patients with non-ST-segment elevation myocardial infarction and chronic kidney disease undergoing percutaneous coronary intervention. JACC Cardiovasc Interv 2011; 4: 1002–8.

Bleeding

104. Mehran R, Pocock S, Nikolsky E, et al. Impact of bleeding on mortality after percutaneous coronary intervention. Results from a patient pooled analysis of the REPLACE-2, ACUITY, and HORIZONS-AMI trials. J Am Coll Cardiol 2011; 4: 654–64.

105. Manoukian SV, Feit F, Mehran R. Impact of major bleeding on 30-day mortality and clinical outcomes in patients with acute coronary syndromes: an analysis from the ACUITY trial. J Am Coll Cardiol 2007; 47: 1362–8.

Transfusion in ACS

106. Doyle BJ, Rihal CS, Gastineau DA, Holmes DR. Bleeding, blood transfusion, and increased mortality after percutaneous coronary intervention: implications for contemporary practice. J Am Coll Cardiol 2009; 53: 2019–27.

107. Rao SV, Jollis JG, Harrington RA, et al. Relationship of blood transfusion and clinical outcomes in patients with acute coronary syndromes. JAMA 2004; 292: 1555–62.

108. Alexander KP, Chen AY, Wang TY, et al. Transfusion practice and outcomes in non-ST-segment elevation acute coronary syndromes. Am Heart J 2008; 155: 1047–53.

109. Steg PG, Hubert K, Andreotti F, et al. Bleeding in acute coronary syndromes and percutaneous coronary interventions: position paper by the Working Group on Thrombosis of the European Society of Cardiology. Eur Heart J 2011; 32: 1854–64.

110. Hanna EB, Alexander KP, Chen AY, et al. Characteristics and in-hospital outcomes of patients with non-ST-segment elevation myocardial infarction undergoing an invasive strategy according to hemoglobin levels. Am J Cardiol 2013; 111(8): 1099–103.

GI bleed

111. Bhatt DL, Scheiman J, Abraham NS, et al. ACCF/ACG/AHA 2008 expert consensus document on reducing the gastrointestinal risks of antiplatelet therapy and NSAID use: a report of the American College of Cardiology Foundation Task Force on Clinical Expert Consensus Documents. J Am Coll Cardiol 2008; 52: 1502–17.

Antiplatelet and anticoagulant therapies in ACS

112. Mehta SR, Bassand JP, Chrolavicius S, et al. CURRENT-OASIS 7 Investigators. Dose comparisons of clopidogrel and aspirin in acute coronary syndromes. N Engl J Med 2010; 363: 930–42.

113. Mehta SR, Yusuf S, Peters RJ, et al. Effects of pretreatment with clopidogrel and aspirin followed by long-term therapy in patients undergoing percutaneous coronary intervention: the PCI-CURE study. Lancet 2001; 358: 527–33.

114. Berger JS, Frye CB, Harshaw Q, et al. Impact of clopidogrel in patients with acute coronary syndromes requiring coronary artery bypass surgery: a multicenter analysis. J Am Coll Cardiol 2008; 52: 1693–701.

115. Ebrahimi R, Dyke C, Mehran R, et al. Outcomes following pre-operative clopidogrel administration in patients with acute coronary syndromes undergoing coronary artery bypass surgery: the ACUITY trial. J Am Coll Cardiol 2009; 53: 1965–1972.

116. Firanescu CE, Martens EJ, Schönberger JP, et al. Postoperative blood loss in patients undergoing coronary artery bypass surgery after preoperative treatment with clopidogrel: a prospective randomised controlled study. Eur J Cardiothorac Surg 2009; 36: 856–62.

117. Wiviott SD, Braunwald E, McCabe CH, et al. Prasugrel versus clopidogrel in patients with acute coronary syndromes. N Engl J Med 2007; 357: 2001–15.

118. Wallentin L, Becker RC, Budaj A, et al. Ticagrelor versus clopidogrel in patients with acute coronary syndromes. N Engl J Med 2009; 361: 1045–57. *PLATO trial.*

119. Wiviott SD, Braunwald E, Angiolillo DJ, et al. Greater clinical benefit of more intensive oral antiplatelet therapy with prasugrel in patients with diabetes mellitus in the trial to assess improvement in therapeutic outcomes by optimizing platelet inhibition with prasugrel-thrombolysis in myocardial infarction 38. Circulation 2008; 118: 1626–36.

120. Montalescot G, Wiviott SD, Braunwald E, et al. Prasugrel compared with clopidogrel in patients undergoing percutaneous coronary intervention for ST-elevation myocardial infarction (TRITON-TIMI 38): double-blind, randomised controlled trial. Lancet 2009; 373: 723–31.

121. Roe MT, Armstrong PW, Fox KA, et al. Prasugrel versus clopidogrel for acute coronary syndromes without revascularization. N Engl J Med 2012; 367: 1297–309.

122. Bhatt DL, Stone GW, Mahaffey KW, et al. Effect of platelet inhibition with cangrelor during PCI on ischemic events. N Engl J Med 2013; 368: 1303–13.

123. Kastrati A, Mehilli J, Neumann FJ, et al. ISAR-REACT 2 Trial Investigators Abciximab in patients with acute coronary syndromes undergoing percutaneous coronary intervention after clopidogrel pretreatment: the ISAR-REACT 2 randomized trial. JAMA 295 2006: 1531–8.

124. Montalescot G, Bolognese L, Dudek D, et al. Pretreatment with prasugrel in non-ST segment elevation myocardial infarction. N Engl J Med 2013; 369: 999–1010. *ACCOAST trial.*

125. Price MJ, Berger PB, Teirstein PS, et al. Standard- vs high-dose clopidogrel based on platelet function testing after percutaneous coronary intervention: the GRAVITAS randomized trial. JAMA 2011; 305: 1097–105.

126. Trenk D, Stone GW, Gawaz M, et al. A randomized trial of prasugrel versus clopidogrel in patients with high platelet reactivity on clopidogrel after elective percutaneous coronary intervention with implantation of drug-eluting stents: results of the TRIGGER-PCI study. J Am Coll Cardiol 2012; 59: 2159–64.

127. Sibbing D, Bernlochner I, Schulz S, et al. Prognostic value of a high on-clopidogrel treatment platelet reactivity in bivalirudin versus abciximab treated non-ST-segment elevation myocardial infarction patients. ISAR-REACT 4 platelet substudy. J Am Coll Cardiol 2012; 60: 369–77.

128. Oler A, Whooley MA, Oler J, Grady D. Adding heparin to aspirin reduces the incidence of myocardial infarction and death in patients with unstable angina. A meta-analysis. JAMA 1996; 276: 811–15.

129. Antman EM, McCabe CH, Gurfinkel EP, et al. Enoxaparin prevents death and cardiac ischemic events in unstable angina/non-Q wave myocardial infarction: results of the Thrombolysis In Myocardial Infarction (TIMI) 11B trial. Circulation 1999; 100: 1593–601.

130. Cohen M, Demers C, Gurfinkel EP, et al. A comparison of low molecular-weight heparin with unfractionated heparin for unstable coronary artery disease. Efficacy and safety of subcutaneous enoxaparin in non-Q-wave coronary events study group. N Engl J Med 1997; 337: 447–52.

131. SYNERGY Trial Investigators. Enoxaparin vs unfractionated heparin in high-risk patients with non-ST-segment elevation acute coronary syndromes managed with an intended early invasive strategy: primary results of the SYNERGY randomized trial. JAMA 2004; 292: 45–54.

132. Blazing MA, de Lemos JA, White HD, et al. Safety and efficacy of enoxaparin vs unfractionated heparin in patients with non-ST-segment elevation acute coronary syndromes who receive tirofiban and aspirin: a randomized controlled trial. JAMA 2004; 292: 55–64. *A-to-Z trial.*

133. Levine GN, Ferrando T. Degree of anticoagulation after one subcutaneous and one subsequent intravenous booster dose of enoxaparin: implications for patients with acute coronary syndromes undergoing early percutaneous coronary intervention. J Thromb Thrombolysis 2004; 17: 167–71.

134. Yusuf S, Mehta SR, Chrolavicius S, et al. Comparison of fondaparinux and enoxaparin in acute coronary syndromes. N Engl J Med 2006; 354: 1464–76. *OASIS 5 trial.*

135. Mehta SR, Boden WE, Eikelboom JW, et al. Antithrombotic therapy with fondaparinux in relation to interventional management strategy in patients with ST- and non-ST-segment elevation acute coronary syndromes: an individual patient-level combined analysis of the fifth and sixth organization to assess strategies in ischemic syndromes (OASIS 5 and 6) randomized trials. Circulation 2008; 118: 2038–46.

136. Han Y, Guo J, Zheng Y, et al. Bivalirudin vs heparin with or without tirofiban during primary percutaneous coronary intervention in acute myocardial infarction: the BRIGHT randomized clinical trial. JAMA 2015; 313: 1336–46.

137. White HD, Chew DP, Hoekstra JW, et al. Safety and efficacy of switching from either unfractionated heparin or enoxaparin to bivalirudin in patients with non-ST-segment elevation acute coronary syndromes managed with an invasive strategy: results from the ACUITY trial. J Am Coll Cardiol 2008; 51: 1734–41.

Plaque erosion and spontaneous coronary artery dissection

138. Arbustini E, Dal Bello B, Morbini P, et al. Plaque erosion is a major substrate for coronary thrombosis in acute myocardial infarction. *Heart* 1999; 82: 269–72.

139. Virmani R, Burke AP, Farb A. Plaque rupture and plaque erosion. Thromb Haemost 1999; 82 Suppl 1: 1–3.

140. Braunwald E. Coronary plaque erosion: recognition and management. JACC Cardiovasc Imaging 2013; 6: 288–9.

141. Saw J, Aymong E, Sedlak T, et al. Spontaneous coronary artery dissection. Association with predisposing arteriopathies and precipitating stressors and cardiovascular outcomes. Circ Cardiovasc Interv 2014; 7: 645–55.

142. Tweet MS, Eleid MF, Best PJM, et al. Spontaneous coronary artery dissection. Revascularization versus conservative therapy. Circ Cardiovasc Interv 2014; 7: 777–86.

2 ST-Segment Elevation Myocardial Infarction

1. DEFINITION, REPERFUSION, AND GENERAL MANAGEMENT

I. Definition

STEMI is a clinical syndrome of angina or angina equivalent along with:[1–3]

- ST-segment elevation ≥2 mm in men or ≥1.5 mm in women in leads V_2–V_3, or ≥1 mm in two other contiguous chest or limb leads, *with a shape consistent with ischemic ST elevation*. The shape must be distinguished from early repolarization, pericarditis, or ST-segment elevation secondary to LVH or LBBB; emergent echo or coronary angiography may be performed in case of doubt.

or:

- Isolated or most prominent ST-segment depression in leads V_1–V_3, which is reciprocal to posterior ST elevation in leads V_7-V_9 (true posterior STEMI). In leads V_7–V_9, the ST-segment elevation cutoff is only 0.5 mm, as the distant location of these leads behind the heart minimizes ST-segment elevation.

ST-segment elevation below these cut-points may still imply myocardial injury when the clinical setting or the ST-segment morphology suggests ischemia. Emergent reperfusion may still be indicated in these patients, generally with PCI (thrombolysis is not an established therapy for mild degrees of ST elevation, <1 mm).

Conversely, ST-segment elevation that exceeds these cut-points may not represent STEMI. Careful attention to the morphology of the ST segment and the associated features (Q wave, inverted or ample T wave) is critical.

STEMI usually evolves into electrocardiographic Q waves (Q-wave MI) and is usually a transmural and large MI. NSTEMI usually evolves into a non-Q-wave MI and is usually a subendocardial, smaller MI. However, there is some overlap: STEMI may not generate Q waves while NSTEMI may generate Q waves.

Since it takes 3–12 hours for cardiac biomarkers to rise after the onset of infarction, they should not be relied upon for the diagnosis or initiation of emergent therapies.

Approximately 12.5% of MIs are totally silent and ~12.5% have a mild, atypical presentation (e.g., nausea, dyspnea, malaise).[4] These cases go unrecognized, and patients may present with HF days or months after acute MI. This presentation is more common in female, diabetic, and elderly patients.

II. Timing of reperfusion

a. Emergent reperfusion with PCI or fibrinolytics is indicated in patients who present *within 12 (24) hours of symptom onset* and who have *persistent* ST elevation in two or more contiguous leads or ST depression that is isolated or most prominent in V_1–V_3 (class I recommendation for PCI or fibrinolytics at ≤12 h, class IIa for PCI at 12–24 h).[1] This applies even if ischemic symptoms have resolved, as long as ST elevation is persistent and the onset of ischemic symptoms is ≤24 hours.

PCI is the preferred strategy, and it should be performed with a door-to-balloon time (DTB) of ≤90 min in patients presenting to PCI-capable hospitals, and ≤120 min in patients transferred from non-PCI-capable to PCI-capable hospitals. If PCI cannot be performed with a DTB of ≤120 min, fibrinolytics should be given to patients presenting within 12 hours of symptom onset.*

b. Patients presenting *>24 hours after symptom onset* generally do not have an indication for emergent PCI. *Emergent PCI (not fibrinolysis) is selectively indicated* in some of these patients, such as patients with persistent ischemic symptoms, cardiogenic shock, acute severe HF with massive pulmonary edema, or when the onset of STEMI is not clearly >24 hours.

Otherwise, *non-urgent coronary angiography* and PCI are indicated in patients with recurrent chest pain at rest or mild exertion or severe ischemia on stress testing.

While a timely primary PCI is favored over fibrinolysis in all STEMI patients, it is more heavily favored in the following circumstances, where the efficacy of fibrinolysis is reduced:

- Cardiogenic shock or severe HF attributed to STEMI should undergo emergent PCI regardless of the delay to presentation (even if >24 hours). Fibrinolytics should not be a standalone therapy for cardiogenic shock, but may be used en route to PCI in early presenters, when delays are expected.
- Late presenters, 3–12 hours.
- Age >75 years.
- History of CABG with suspicion of SVG thrombosis. Both PCI and fibrinolytics have reduced efficacy in this high-risk subset, but PCI remains more effective than fibrinolytics. PCI re-establishes TIMI 3 flow in 50–70% of SVG MIs, vs. 25–50% with fibrinolytics.
- ECG is not definite for STEMI (e.g., LBBB without ST concordance) or time of onset of symptoms is unclear (may be >12 hours).

Myocardial effect of reperfusion therapy:

- In the first 2–3 hours, reperfusion prevents myocardial necrosis.
- Between 3 (or 6) and 12 hours, reperfusion may not prevent further necrosis, but treats peri-infarct ischemia, prevents deleterious remodeling, improves scar turgor, and decreases mortality (absolute mortality reduction >2%).

---

* DTB is defined as the time from first medical contact to first establishment of reperfusion with an interventional device. In studies, the door time has been defined as the time of arrival to the hospital, but is ideally defined by the on-scene arrival of emergency medical service. First establishment of reperfusion corresponds to the first thrombectomy or balloon inflation that successfully re-establishes coronary flow.

III. ECG phases of STEMI (Figure 2.1)

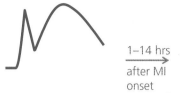
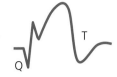

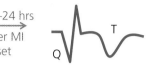
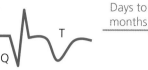
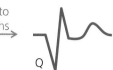

1–14 hrs after MI onset

12–24 hrs after MI onset

Days to months

Phase 1:
ST elevation
Hyperacute wide/large T

Phase 2:
ST elevation persists
Q starts to develop
T starts to invert

Phase 3:
ST elevation subsides
Q becomes deeper
T inversion becomes deeper
QT prolongs

Acute STEMI
→Emergent reperfusion if persistent chest pain or last chest pain within 12 (24) hrs

Recent or subacute STEMI
→Reperfusion with PCI may be indicated for persistent/recurrent chest pain, but is not emergent from the ECG standpoint. Fibrinolytics are not indicated.

This pattern may also be seen after less prolonged, transient ischemia without extensive infarction (e.g, 1–2 hrs), where PCI is beneficial

Old MI

Figure 2.1 Phases of STEMI.

Phase 3 does not imply that MI has already been too prolonged to benefit from PCI; some patients with phase 3 morphology have had only a brief period of ischemia.

ST elevation may persist for days, weeks, or chronically >3 weeks in patients with a dyskinetic or aneurysmal myocardium. In this case, the age of the infarct is implied clinically. Let's take the case of a patient who had chest discomfort several days previously and currently has HF without angina; if his ECG shows Q waves and ST elevation his STEMI is likely >24 hours old and the persistent ST elevation likely reflects dyskinesia. An echocardiogram showing a dilated LV with thin aneurysmal wall confirms this suspicion.

The inverted T waves may persist for days, weeks, months, or even years. Patients with LV dyskinesia and persistent ST-segment elevation may have chronic T-wave inversion as well.

IV. STEMI diagnostic tips and clinical vignettes

1. A patient presents with one episode of chest pain that lasted 10 minutes. He does not have any pain currently. He reports a prior history of a large MI 2 years previously. His ECG shows 1.5 mm ST elevation in the anterior leads with Q waves and T-wave inversion. Should he undergo emergent reperfusion?

Emergent reperfusion is probably not warranted. It is important to seek old ECGs and urgently obtain an echocardiogram. In fact, ST elevation may represent an old STEMI with a chronic dyskinetic myocardium and a chronic, persistent ST elevation with Q waves; T waves may be inverted or upright, but not ample. A history of an old MI, an old ECG (if available), or a quick bedside echocardiogram may allow the diagnosis. Echocardiography shows a thin, bright (scarred) and possibly an aneurysmal myocardium in case of an old infarct, whereas in acute STEMI the myocardium is neither thin nor scarred yet. *If the patient does not report a history of MI, if T wave is ample, or if the patient had a typical angina within the last 24 hours, ST elevation is generally considered acute STEMI.*

2. A patient presents with ongoing chest pain for the last 8 hours. His ECG shows inferior ST elevation of 1 mm with deep Q waves. Should he undergo emergent reperfusion?

Q waves often develop at 1–14 hours after STEMI onset, while the ST segment is still elevated. The appearance of abnormal and deep Q waves does not lessen the benefit from reperfusion therapy and the potential reduction of the infarct size, and does not necessarily mean that the infarct is old, as long as ST elevation is persistent and the presentation is within the reperfusion window (<24 hours). Q waves are not synonymous with irreversible myocardial damage.[5]

3. A patient presents with intermittent chest pain for the last 3 days. He had an episode of pain 2 hours previously, but is currently free of any pain. His ECG shows anterolateral ST elevation. Should he undergo emergent reperfusion?

Some patients have episodes of unstable angina for hours or days before STEMI. Presume that the onset of STEMI is the onset of the last episode of prolonged chest pain. Thus, this patient qualifies for emergent reperfusion.

4. A patient presents with chest pain that started 4 hours previously and inferior ST elevation. His pain has just resolved with aspirin and nitroglycerin, but ST elevation is persistent. Should he undergo emergent reperfusion?

Some patients have resolution of chest pain with nitroglycerin or antithrombotic therapies *but ST elevation persists*. These patients should still undergo emergent reperfusion therapy, as long as they present within 24 hours of pain onset.

5. A patient presents with chest pain that started 4 hours previously and inferior ST elevation. Both his pain and ST elevation resolve after aspirin and nitroglycerin administration. Should he undergo emergent reperfusion?

Chest pain and ST elevation *may both resolve spontaneously* or with the acute therapies. This often indicates spontaneous thrombolysis and occurs in ~15% of STEMIs, leading to a much lower mortality and a smaller infarct size.[6] Occasionally, this may represent resolution of

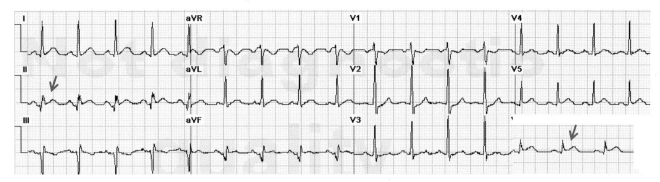

Figure 2.2 The patient presents with chest discomfort that has lasted 3 hours and resolved 2 hours ago. Subtle ST elevation is seen in leads II and aVF, and in leads V$_5$ and V$_6$, with subtle ST depression in V$_1$–V$_2$. Three features suggest that this mild ST elevation is actually STEMI: (i) Q waves; (ii) ST depression in reciprocal leads (V$_1$–V$_2$); (iii) wide T-wave morphology and fused ST-T segments in leads I, II, V$_5$, and V$_6$ (*arrows*). This patient qualifies for emergent catheterization since his discomfort occurred in the last 24 hours. He is found to have an acutely occluded large obtuse marginal branch.

a coronary spasm. Coronary angiography is preferably performed emergently, but this is no longer mandatory. Full ACS therapy and early coronary angiography, within the next day, are indicated.

6. A patient presents with chest pain that lasted 2–3 hours earlier today and has now resolved. His ECG shows subtle ST elevation (<1 mm) in leads II, aVF, V$_5$, and V$_6$ (Figure 2.2). Should he undergo emergent reperfusion?

Yes, he should. This patient has mild ST elevation (<1 mm) with a morphology that is, nonetheless, consistent with STEMI. Q waves are also present. STEMI may be over 12–24 hours old, at a stage where ST elevation is resolving but has not fully resolved yet (close to phase 3). Alternatively, STEMI may be more recent with ongoing or resolving ischemia. This patient does not qualify for fibrinolytics, as ST elevation is <1 mm and the occlusion duration is questionable, but qualifies for emergent PCI if the discomfort is ongoing or if the discomfort occurred within the last 24 hours, even if it is not ongoing.

7. A patient presents with chest pain that has lasted 2–3 hours earlier today and has now resolved. His ECG shows inferior Q waves and T-wave inversion, without any significant ST elevation. Should he undergo emergent reperfusion?

PCI is preferably, but not necessarily, performed emergently. Resolution of ST elevation with appearance of Q waves (phase 3) often implies a late presentation, >12–24 hours, but may also occur after a brief ischemia, e.g., 1–2 hours, as in this case. This patient does not qualify for fibrinolysis (no residual ST elevation). He still qualifies for PCI, not necessarily on an emergent basis, if the discomfort is recurrent or ongoing or if the discomfort occurred within the last 24 hours.

> In general, a patient qualifies for emergent PCI with either of the following two conditions: (i) persistent ST elevation with a presentation less than 24 hours after pain onset (even if pain is not persistent); (ii) persistent pain, even if the patient presents later than 24 hours after pain onset and even if ST elevation has resolved.

V. Specific case of new or presumably new LBBB

Normally, LBBB is associated with ST-segment deviation that is discordant to QRS, i.e., directed opposite to QRS. If a patient has an ischemic presentation and LBBB on the ECG, one cannot tell whether this ST elevation is purely secondary to LBBB, if an ischemic injury is partially contributing to the ST elevation, or if there is ST depression masked by the ST elevation. STEMI is definite if ST abnormality is concordant to QRS, but STEMI or non-ST elevation ischemia is still possible if ST changes are discordant to QRS. This would be the case of a patient with a true anterior injury in V$_1$–V$_4$ or inferior injury, where QRS is negative and where ischemic ST elevation would inherently appear discordant. RBBB, on the other hand, is not associated with significant ST abnormality, and thus ST changes in a patient with RBBB are diagnostic of ischemia. Early thrombolytic trials and their meta-analysis have shown a striking benefit from thrombolytic therapy in patients with any bundle branch block, particularly that a new bundle branch block in STEMI indicates a high-risk STEMI.[7] Both types of bundle branch blocks, if secondary to STEMI, represent high-risk categories, but since only LBBB poses a diagnostic challenge, a new or presumably new LBBB has been considered a STEMI equivalent in previous ACC guidelines, in order not to miss a high-risk STEMI.

However, STEMI rarely causes left bundle branch infarction, because the left bundle is supplied by both the LAD and RCA and is only affected in extensive infarction. In the GUSTO-1 trial, only ~1% of STEMIs had LBBB on presentation. In fact, a **new LBBB often results from a chronic cardiomyopathy, ischemic or non-ischemic, with a dilated or hypertrophied myocardium, rather than an extensive acute infarction.**[8] A new LBBB may also be rate-related and may have been unveiled by an increase in heart rate.

Evidence has shown that only ~10% of patients with an ischemic presentation and a new LBBB have a STEMI-equivalent (acute coronary occlusion on angiography), and <40% have any MI, most commonly NSTEMI.[9–12] *STEMI is even far less likely when all comers with new LBBB, both atypical or typical presentations, are included (<5%).*[11] Therefore, in order to make the diagnosis of STEMI, an ischemic presentation is required (ongoing angina, flash pulmonary edema) along with additional ECG features:

- Concordant ST-segment depression or elevation of ≥1 mm is >95% specific for the diagnosis of STEMI, but has a limited sensitivity of 20% (Sgarbossa's concordance). If present, STEMI diagnosis is definite, and emergent reperfusion with fibrinolytics or PCI should be achieved.
- Concordant negative T wave or biphasic T wave in multiple leads increases the likelihood of STEMI.
- Extreme discordance increases the likelihood of STEMI, but has a reduced specificity: discordant ST elevation that exceeds 25% of the QRS height; or upright T wave that exceeds 50% of the QRS height. This discordance ratio is more sensitive and specific than an absolute ST discordance >5 mm, but may still be seen in 9% of control patients without MI.[13]

In the absence of these features, particularly Sgarbossa's concordance, and in the absence of ongoing typical angina, it is reasonable to urgently perform bedside echocardiography. The presence of a segmental wall motion abnormality without severe thinning, aneurysm, or severe LV dilatation suggests acute ischemia and warrants early angiography; fibrinolytics are preferably avoided since many of these patients have NSTEMI rather than STEMI, and transfer for angiography is preferred even if delays are expected to exceed 120 minutes.[9] Abnormal septal motion is universal with LBBB but the anterior and apical contraction is preserved; therefore, anterior and apical akinesis implies ischemia. Global hypokinesis may imply ischemic or non-ischemic cardiomyopathy, such as hypertensive cardiomyopathy, rather than acute ischemia;[8] early, usually non-urgent angiography may be needed.

Thus, the 2013 STEMI guidelines state that **"new or presumably new LBBB should not be considered diagnostic of acute myocardial infarction (MI) in isolation."**[1]

VI. Reperfusion strategies: fibrinolytics, primary PCI, and combined fibrinolytics–PCI

A. Fibrinolytics (also called thrombolytics): mortality benefit

In the GISSI-1 and ISIS-2 trials and a large meta-analysis, fibrinolytics (mainly streptokinase) have shown:[7,14–16]

- A striking 6.5% absolute mortality reduction and 50% relative mortality reduction in the first hour after STEMI onset, called the golden hour
- A 4% absolute mortality reduction in the second hour
- A plateau 3% mortality reduction between 3 and 6 hours (relative mortality reduction ~25%)
- Absolute mortality reduction of ~2% between 6 and 12 hours. Beyond that, between 12 and 24 hours, the benefit is marginal and questionable.

This time-dependent benefit is due to the fact that very early reperfusion of the occluded coronary artery may lead to full recovery of the ischemic tissue and thus prevent necrosis. In addition, fibrinolytic therapy in the first 2–3 hours is highly efficacious in lysing a fresh thrombus.

The benefit is more striking in high-risk subgroups, such as anterior STEMI, STEMI with bundle branch block, or high STEMI risk score (tachycardia, hypotension). *The elderly subgroup is the only high-risk subgroup that, paradoxically, only derives a marginal benefit from fibrinolysis;* this is partly because of the high bleeding risk but also because of the more extensive CAD that makes it less likely for fibrinolysis to re-establish perfusion.

The mortality benefit is also more striking with the fibrin-specific fibrinolytics (~1% additional mortality reduction).

B. Fibrinolytics: limitations, contraindications, definition of successful response, and definition of TIMI flow (Table 2.1)[1,7,17,18]

In addition to the classic contraindications, fibrinolysis is contraindicated in a patient with an expected intracranial bleeding risk of >4% (e.g., an elderly [>75] small woman with HTN).[17]

Table 2.1 Limitations and contraindications of fibrinolysis.

Limitations

- Patency of the infarct-related artery (TIMI 2 or 3 flow) is achieved in ~75–80%. TIMI 3 flow is achieved in 55–60%[a]
- Intracranial hemorrhage: 0.5–1.5%
- Major bleeding: ~5%
- Early recurrent ischemia or MI: 10–20% (within hours or days)

Most important absolute contraindications

- Any prior intracranial hemorrhage
- Ischemic stroke <3 months. Ischemic stroke >3 months is a relative contraindication
- Severe acute hypertension unresponsive to acute therapy
- Active bleeding (except menses)
- Cranial or spinal surgery <2 months
- Closed head or facial trauma <3 months, even without a documented bleed (e.g., recent fall with head trauma)

Most important relative contraindications

- Ischemic stroke >3 months
- Severe acute HTN (SBP >180 or DBP >110) responsive to acute therapy
- Chronic severe hypertension
- Recent major surgery or internal bleed <2–4 weeks. Proliferative retinopathy is not a contraindication
- Oral anticoagulant therapy, including warfarin with INR >2 (strong relative contraindication)

[a] Full patency with <50% residual disease is achieved in only 15–20%.

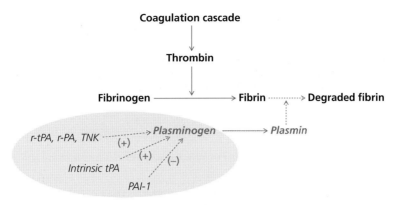

Figure 2.3 Fibrinolysis cascade and mechanism of action of fibrinolytics. Fibrinolytics activate plasminogen into plasmin, which degrades fibrin. PAI-1, plasminogen activator inhibitor (~ tPA inhibitor); r-PA, reteplase; r-tPA, alteplase; TNK, tenecteplase; tPA, tissue plasminogen activator.

Consider fibrinolytic therapy successful if: chest pain resolves *and* initial ST-segment elevation decreases by more than 50% (preferably 70%) at 60–90 minutes after therapy initiation, in the lead showing the worst ST-segment elevation. Also, the occurrence of an accelerated idioventricular rhythm (AIVR) *in conjunction* with the preceding features is highly specific for reperfusion. In the absence of a response (persistent ischemic symptoms, ST elevation, or both), plan for emergent *rescue PCI*. It is best to start transferring the patient to a PCI-capable hospital as soon as fibrinolytic therapy is started, so that, if no response is seen at 60 minutes, cardiac catheterization is readily available.

A successful fibrinolysis correlates with TIMI 3 flow on coronary angiography. *TIMI grade 0 flow* implies the absence of any flow. *TIMI 1* flow implies the presence of some flow beyond the obstruction but without full distal perfusion. *TIMI 2* flow means that the vessel is fully perfused but the flow is slow compared with a normal artery and/or the contrast material clears more slowly than in a normal artery; TIMI 2 flow is related to a residual mechanical obstruction or to microvascular obstruction from microvascular emboli. *TIMI 3* flow means full perfusion of the vessel with normal flow. In fibrinolytic trials, TIMI 3 flow has been shown to be associated with the lowest mortality. TIMI 2 flow is associated with an intermediate mortality, while TIMI 0–1 flow is associated with the highest mortality.[19,20] The outcome is improved in patients whose TIMI 2 flow eventually improves to TIMI 3 flow within a few days (this happens two-thirds of the times).[21] In a patent artery, TIMI 2 and 3 flow patterns are associated with divergent outcomes and should not be grouped together.

Following PCI and in the absence of any residual mechanical obstruction, the flow may still be TIMI 0–2 flow because of microvascular embolization, spasm, or edema; this is called *no reflow*, i.e., TIMI 0–2 flow without any residual epicardial stenosis. *The term "no reflow" is used only with PCI, not with fibrinolysis.*

C. Fibrinolytics: various agents

Fibrinolytics bind to the clot-bound plasminogen and convert it to plasmin, which promotes the degradation of fibrin (Figure 2.3). The old fibrinolytic *streptokinase* also binds to free plasminogen; thus, in addition to lysing fibrin, it depletes systemic, free fibrinogen and affects systemic coagulation for 12–24 hours.

Alteplase (recombinant tissue plasminogen activator [r-tPA]) binds to the plasminogen entrapped in a thrombus and thus mainly degrades fibrin of a thrombus, rather than systemic fibrinogen (fibrin-specific fibrinolytic). Being more concentrated at the thrombus level, it is a more effective lytic than streptokinase. It generally does not affect the systemic fibrinogen and has a short half-life of only 6 minutes; thus, after the infusion is discontinued and the drug eliminated (~30 min), there is no significant residual effect on systemic coagulation. Therefore, the performance of PCI soon after r-tPA administration is not necessarily associated with a significant increase in bleeding. On the other hand, this short half-life and the lack of residual effect on the systemic coagulation explain the high risk of recurrent thrombosis and the need to *start heparin infusion immediately* at the end of r-tPA infusion in MI.

In the GUSTO trial of r-tPA vs. streptokinase, r-tPA further reduced mortality by 1% and reduced major bleeding in general, but increased intracranial hemorrhage by 0.25% in comparison with streptokinase.[18]

Reteplase (r-PA) is a mutation variant of r-tPA. It is slightly less fibrin-specific than r-tPA and has a longer half-life (~15 min), allowing its administration in two boluses rather than an infusion. It has the same mortality benefit and bleeding risk as r-tPA.

Tenecteplase (TNK) is also a mutation variant of r-tPA that is 14 times more fibrin-specific than r-tPA and less likely to be degraded by tPA inhibitors. Thus, TNK is slightly more effective, which explains the higher TIMI 3 flow rate achieved with TNK vs. r-tPA (~65% vs. 60%). It also has a longer half-life than r-tPA, with a duration of effect of ~120 minutes. In the ASSENT-2 trial, TNK was associated with the same overall mortality as r-tPA, but a reduction in major non-cerebral bleeding and a reduction in mortality of patients presenting >4 hours after symptom onset.[22]

D. Primary PCI is superior to fibrinolytic therapy; importance of time of presentation, door-to-balloon time, and PCI delay

In comparison with fibrinolytic therapy, primary PCI is more effective in re-establishing TIMI 3 flow (95%), and thus reduces 30-day mortality by 2% (7% vs. 9%), recurrent MI by 4% (3% vs. 7%), and stroke by 1%.[23–25] However, this superiority of PCI depends on a DTB <120 minutes and PCI-related delay <60 minutes (delay between the expected time of fibrinolytic therapy and the expected time of balloon inflation). *The "90-minute" and "120-minute" cutoffs of DTB have actually been established in terms of PCI delays beyond which PCI loses its advantage over fibrinolysis (those times correspond to equipoise between PCI and fibrinolysis).*

DTB is particularly important if the patient presents early, <3 hours after symptom onset, *or* if the patient is high-risk (anterior MI, tachycardia, SBP <100 mmHg, Killip class ≥II, age ≥65), as those patients derive the greatest benefit from fibrinolytics and are most harmed by reperfusion delays. In CAPTIM, PRAGUE-2, and more recently the STREAM trial, fibrinolytic therapy (+ rescue PCI if needed) resulted in the same mortality reduction as primary PCI in patients presenting <2–3 hours after symptom onset.[26–28] Conversely, in low-risk patients presenting late, DTB is less important and, in a large MI registry, PCI-related delays of 100 minutes did not negate the survival advantage of primary PCI over fibrinolytic therapy in those patients.[29] In fact, the superiority of PCI over fibrinolysis widens as the presentation is more delayed; while the benefit from fibrinolysis strikingly drops beyond 3 hours, PCI has a less pronounced drop in benefit.[30] In two other retrospective analyses, DTB >90–120 minutes did not impair outcomes in low-risk patients presenting late.[31,32] Yet in all patients, systems should strive for as small a DTB as possible. In high-risk patients presenting early, any DTB delay, even within the 90-minute window, is associated with increased mortality compared to a shorter DTB (mortality difference of 0.5–1% for every 30 min DTB delay, e.g., between DTB of 30 min and 60 min).[33]

Elderly patients (age >75) – In the fibrinolytic trials, the benefit from fibrinolytic therapy was much less striking in the elderly than in the young.[7,34] Conversely, primary PCI remains effective in elderly people, with more absolute mortality reduction in the elderly subgroup than in young patients. This makes fibrinolytic therapy, whether standalone or combined with PCI, a less attractive alternative to primary PCI in the elderly. Studies of combined fibrinolytic therapy and PCI included very few patients over the age 75.[35]

E. Combination of PCI and fibrinolytic therapy

Three different combinations of PCI and fibrinolytics have been studied in STEMI (Figure 2.4):[35]

- **Facilitated PCI** is a strategy of emergent PCI with a planned door-to-balloon time of <120 minutes. Fibrinolytic therapy is administered "on the way" to a timely PCI.[36,37]
- **Pharmacoinvasive therapy** means that fibrinolytic therapy is administered at a non-PCI facility, then the patient is promptly and systematically transferred to a PCI facility, where PCI is performed 2–3 to 24 hours after the start of fibrinolytic therapy, regardless of whether fibrinolysis results in successful reperfusion. Thus, the time to PCI is longer than with facilitated PCI. *Facilitated PCI addresses patients primarily treated with a timely PCI*, and looks at the value of pre-treatment with fibrinolytics or glycoprotein IIb/IIIa inhibitors (GPI), whereas *pharmacoinvasive therapy addresses patients who are primarily treated with fibrinolytics*, as they cannot undergo a timely PCI, and looks at the value of routine early PCI after fibrinolysis.[38–40]
- **Rescue PCI** refers to PCI that is performed urgently *if* fibrinolysis fails, failure being defined as persistent hemodynamic or electrical instability, persistent ischemic symptoms, or failure to achieve at least a 50–70% resolution of the maximal ST-segment elevation 90 minutes after fibrinolysis is started.[41] Approximately 35% of patients treated with fibrinolysis require rescue PCI.[27,38,39]

Facilitated PCI has been associated with worse outcomes than primary PCI, probably because the administration of fibrinolytics before a timely PCI cannot offer any ischemic advantage yet increases the bleeding risk. Also, fibrinoytics expose clot-bound thrombin, a potent platelet activator, which heightens platelet activation and aggregation. PCI facilitated with fibrinolytics is associated with increased mortality, ischemic complications, HF, and bleeding (ASSENT-4 trial). Even PCI facilitation with a brief upstream GPI therapy leads to increased bleeding without any ischemic benefit (FINESSE trial).[36,37] Conversely, *pharmacoinvasive therapy*, also called *routine early PCI 3–24 hours after fibrinolytics*, has been shown to improve outcomes, mainly recurrent MI and recurrent ischemia in high-risk STEMI, without increasing the bleeding risk (despite the use of femoral access in the trials). Patients who achieve successful reperfusion with fibrinolytics are actually left with severe residual disease in ~85% of the cases, and benefit from early PCI.

F. Putting it all together: management of patients presenting to non-PCI-capable hospitals

1. If there is a pre-established transfer system with a predicted DTB <120 minutes, a transfer for primary PCI is the best strategy and is superior to fibrinolysis (DANAMI and PRAGUE trials).[24] This usually implies a distance <60 miles, often with a helicopter transfer, a door-in door-out time <30 minutes, direct activation of the outside PCI team through a central pager, and direct transfer to the outside cath lab.[42]

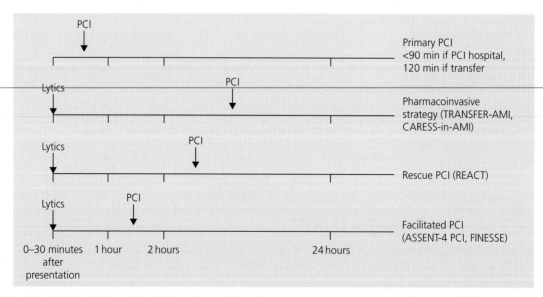

Figure 2.4 The timing of PCI in relation to thrombolysis in the pharmacoinvasive strategy, rescue PCI strategy, and facilitated PCI strategy, with the clinical trials that addressed and defined these strategies.

2. When DTB is expected to be >120 minutes, administer primary fibrinolytic therapy and immediately transfer the patient to allow the performance of *routine early PCI* 3–24 hours later, or to allow immediate rescue PCI in the absence of a response to fibrinolysis. Several registries suggest that timely fibrinolysis followed by semiurgent transfer for PCI offers a benefit similar to that seen in patients presenting to a PCI hospital and undergoing a timely primary PCI.[42,43]

Beside fibrinolytics, the patient should receive aspirin, heparin bolus and infusion, and 300 mg of clopidogrel. Prasugrel, ticagrelor, or 600 mg of clopidogrel have not been studied in the first 24 hours of fibrinolytic therapy and may only be used if PCI is performed >24 hours later. Subcutaneous enoxaparin is not appropriate in patients undergoing early PCI. Glycoprotein IIb/IIa inhibitors may be used during PCI (rather than upstream of PCI).[38]

3. When DTB is expected to be >120 minutes but the patient is presenting >3–4 hours after symptom onset and has a non-anterior MI with low-risk clinical features (Killip class I, heart rate <100 bpm, SBP >100 mmHg), a transfer for primary PCI without preceding fibrinolytic therapy may be reasonable in individual cases, although not clearly expressed in the guidelines.

4. If fibrinolytic therapy is contraindicated, immediately transfer for primary PCI regardless of the expected DTB.

5. For cardiogenic shock or acute severe HF (Killip class III or IV), administer fibrinolytic therapy if DTB is expected to be >120 minutes, and immediately transfer for PCI.

6. Prehospital fibrinolytic therapy delivered by paramedics and followed by early transfer to a PCI facility has been associated with further reduction in mortality rates compared with in-hospital fibrinolytic therapy (as in the Swedish registry), and a mortality reduction comparable to that of primary PCI in patients presenting early (CAPTIM trial).[27,44] This is an adequate strategy in regions where such a system can be implemented.[43]

VII. Coronary angiography and PCI later than 24 hours after presentation: role of stress testing

In the OAT trial, patients with MI older than 24 hours (1–28 days old specifically, mainly STEMI/Q-wave MI), who were selected based on the following features did not benefit from PCI and had a trend towards more frequent reinfarctions:[45]

- Totally occluded infarct-related artery (TIMI 0 or 1 flow)
- Akinetic or dyskinetic infarcted wall
- One- or two-vessel CAD
- No recurrent rest or low-threshold angina
- No severe ischemia on stress testing
- No shock and no persistent functional class III–IV HF

Further analysis showed that PCI was not beneficial even among patients enrolled 1–3 days after MI onset.[46] Thus, late PCI of an occluded infarct artery is only indicated in patients with persistent ischemic symptoms, persistent severe HF, or severe ischemia on stress testing.

On the other hand, data suggest that an infarct artery *that is not totally occluded* (TIMI 2–3 flow) may benefit from late revascularization (>24 h) to the same extent that it may benefit from early revascularization, as a patent infarct artery with good collaterals is associated with a more limited MI size and a significant amount of viable myocardium that can be salvaged with revascularization.[47–49] Approximately 35% of totally occluded infarct-related arteries spontaneously recanalize in the first 24 hours and may qualify for late revascularization.

Therefore, patients who did not receive emergent reperfusion (late presenters >24 hours) or patients who received fibrinolytics, with or without response, but did not undergo angiography in the first 24 hours after symptom onset may still undergo angiography later than 24 hours (class II):

- A non-occluded infarct-related artery may be treated with PCI (class IIb).
- Left main disease or three-vessel CAD that largely extends beyond the occluded artery should receive revascularization, typically surgical revascularization, after a post-MI waiting period of at least 3–7 days (in stable patients).
- A totally occluded artery should not be treated with PCI unless the patient has a low-threshold angina, severe ischemia on stress testing (class I), persistent HF after initial therapy (high-risk case with stress test contraindication), or a corresponding myocardial wall that is not akinetic. If not performed before angiography, the stress test may be performed afterwards and the patient brought back for PCI once severe ischemia is documented.
- If one is unsure that the MI is >24 hours old, PCI may still be performed. While not beneficial, late PCI in the OAT trial was not significantly harmful either, which may justify its use when timing is unclear.

Table 2.2 summarizes the PCI timelines. Questions 2 and 9–11 at the end of this chapter illustrate these concepts.

As a preferred alternative to coronary angiography, patients who have not been managed invasively in the first 24 hours of STEMI and who are stable, without persistent HF and angina, may *undergo stress testing rather than angiography* (class I). In those stable patients, a submaximal stress test (modified Bruce protocol) may be performed 4 days after STEMI onset, and a maximal stress test (symptom-limited Bruce protocol) may be performed 5–14 days later. Severe ischemia or angina on stress testing dictates coronary angiography and revascularization. If no significant residual ischemia is detected, only medical therapy is provided.

As opposed to NSTEMI, where stress testing is avoided even in patients who become free of angina, stress testing is indicated in stable post-STEMI patients free of angina. In NSTEMI, the amount of myocardial necrosis is usually minor and revascularization is needed to salvage a large area of ischemic but non-infarcted myocardium. In non-reperfused STEMI, the myocardium is already largely infarcted and unlikely to benefit from revascularization, unless residual angina or ischemia is shown.

Table 2.2 Revascularization timelines in STEMI.

<12 h after STEMI onset: Emergent primary PCI or fibrinolytic therapy (class I, level of evidence A)
12–24 h: Emergent primary PCI if persistent angina or persistent ST elevation (class IIa)
>24 h: Delayed, non-emergent PCI for: (i) recurrent angina, (ii) severe ischemia on stress testing (class I), (iii) persistent HF

After fibrinolytic therapy
- Delayed routine PCI 3–24 h later (class IIa)
- Rescue PCI for fibrinolytic failure (class IIa, should be class I)

If PCI was not performed in the first 24 h, whether the patient received fibrinolytic therapy, with or without success, or did not receive fibrinolytic therapy
In the absence of angina recurrence, stress testing is preferred to coronary angiography. Coronary angiography is a less favored alternative, with the following recommendations:
- Coronary angiography >24 h after STEMI onset: class IIb
- PCI of a stenotic but not totally occluded artery: class IIb
- Avoid PCI of a totally occluded artery (OAT trial, class III), except in cases of *recurrent angina, high-risk stress test (class I), persistent HF with severe functional limitation, or uncertain timing*
- CABG if left main or three-vessel CAD

Cardiogenic shock *or* acute severe HF (massive pulmonary edema = Killip III): emergent PCI regardless of time (class I)

> **Note that ischemia and viability are two different entities, ischemia being the one most definitely improved with revascularization,** with a potentially striking reduction in the long-term risk of cardiac death and MI (SWISSI-2 trial). *Viability* implies that at rest, the infarcted territory can uptake significant nuclear agent. Conversely, *ischemia* implies that at stress, the nuclear defect in the infarcted or peri-infarct territory is significantly more intense or more extensive than at rest; or significant/ extensive ST-segment deviations occur. **An ischemic territory is viable; conversely, a territory may be viable but non-ischemic**, in which case the benefit of revascularization and the functional recovery are less clear. In a substudy of OAT patients who received viability testing, viability did not predict a benefit from late PCI.[50] Conversely, in the SWISSI-2 trial, asymptomatic patients who had a STEMI or a NSTEMI within the preceding 3 months, documented ischemia on stress testing, and one- or two-vessel CAD derived a 70% reduction of cardiovascular events, including cardiac death, with PCI.[51]

The OAT trial does not apply to a coronary chronic total occlusion (CTO) that has not led to a large transmural infarct, in which case the myocardial contractility is fairly preserved because of the collateral network. A progressive occlusion that allows for an adequate collateral network to develop may not present as MI. It typically presents as chronic angina or a small NSTEMI, not STEMI. Opening a CTO has a beneficial effect on symptoms and LV function.

VIII. Angiographic findings, PCI, and cellular reperfusion; multivessel disease in STEMI

A. PCI: microvascular and cellular reperfusion

Approximately 15% of occluded arteries acutely recanalize before the PCI procedure, in the first 4 hours, and achieve TIMI 2 or 3 flow (from spontaneous or antithrombotic-induced lysis). If recanalization occurs and biomarkers rise only mildly (CK <2× normal), the STEMI is called "aborted STEMI." Residual stenosis usually persists.[52–54]

During PCI, the lesion is dilated with balloon angioplasty then stented. In comparison with standalone balloon angioplasty, stenting reduces the early risk of reocclusion/reinfarction by 50% (to <2%) and the late risk of restenosis, without affecting mortality.[53] Drug-eluting stents may be used, as they have shown similar safety to bare-metal stents in STEMI, without any increase in the hazard of late stent thrombosis, and with the known late benefit on restenosis.[54] A routine initial use of aspiration thrombectomy has not shown superiority to balloon angioplasty in two large trials.[55]

Following primary PCI, ~95% of patients achieve TIMI 3 flow, while 5% achieve TIMI 0–2 flow despite wide macrovascular patency, also called "no reflow." *The term "no reflow" implies poor microvascular flow and is only used after treating all significant epicardial stenoses.* TIMI flow <3 is a predictor of poor outcomes, but TIMI 3 flow does not necessarily imply appropriate microvascular flow. In fact, only ~60% of patients with TIMI 3 flow achieve significant ST-segment resolution (= cellular reperfusion), and only 70% achieve appropriate myocardial blush (= microvascular reperfusion).[55,56] "Appropriate myocardial blush," also called "myocardial blush grade 2 or 3," is used to describe brisk contrast staining of the myocardium followed by contrast clearance and no residual myocardial stain by the next injection. Impaired coronary flow, impaired myocardial blush, or the lack of ST resolution implies: (i) distal microembolization, (ii) microvascular spasm, or (iii) myocyte injury and swelling from ischemia or reperfusion injury, especially late reperfusion, sometimes irreversible. The best long-term outcomes (survival and LV function) are seen in patients with ST-segment resolution and good myocardial blush, while intermediate outcomes are seen in patients with discordant findings.[57]

> Persistent ST-segment elevation after successful primary or rescue PCI implies microvascular obstruction or cellular injury, and thus worse long-term prognosis. The patient may have mild persistent chest pain. As opposed to persistent ST elevation after thrombolysis, persistent ST elevation after a successful PCI does not dictate any further procedure, unless the patient has severe recurrence of pain.
> **Patients with no-reflow and ongoing myocardial ischemia, chest pain, or ventricular arrhythmia are generally treated with IABP.** After treatment of the epicardial stenosis, IABP improves coronary flow and relieves ongoing ischemia.

When angiography is performed in patients who have been successfully reperfused with fibrinolytics, data from the pharmacoinvasive trials suggests that ~15–20% of the infarct-related arteries have a residual stenosis <50% that does not require PCI.[27,37,58,59] Many of those lesions represent plaque erosion rather than plaque rupture, the latter being more likely to occur on a severe stenosis.

B. Multivessel disease in STEMI

Approximately 50–60% of patients presenting with STEMI have multivessel CAD, and up to 40% have multiple complex plaques.[39,53,60] In the absence of cardiogenic shock, only the culprit artery is usually treated with PCI. In order to achieve a good flow across the culprit artery, allow myocardial healing, and reduce the risk of stent thrombosis, multiple lesions may need to be treated within the culprit artery. Conversely, PCI of non-culprit arteries is prone to complications in the strong prothrombotic and proinflammatory milieu of STEMI, and distal embolization or side branch compromise may diminish flow in those stable, non-infarct arteries. These complications will be less tolerated in a patient who has already lost or stunned part of the myocardium, and therefore PCI of non-culprit arteries is generally performed at a later setting rather than acutely.[61,62] Conversely, in cardiogenic shock, PCI of all critical lesions is performed, as shock, per se, induces ischemia in all territories with obstructive CAD; ischemia of non-culprit territories contributes to the downhill course.

CABG is rarely required acutely in STEMI (~1%; 0.2% in TAPAS trial),[54,55,63] but may be more frequently required in patients with cardiogenic shock and severe left main or three-vessel disease. In fact, in the SHOCK trial, 37% of invasively managed patients were emergently revascularized with CABG (a median of 2.7 hours after randomization, 19 hours after MI).[64] Acute CABG may also be required after a failed PCI.

In hemodynamically stable patients with multivessel disease, culprit artery PCI is performed acutely. If CABG is required for full revascularization of non-culprit arteries after a large MI, it is preferred to wait at least 24 hours, and preferably 3–7 days. CABG mortality is increased in the first 3 days after a large MI.[65] In patients who developed RV infarct and were not successfully reperfused in the first 6 hours, it is better to delay CABG 4 weeks to let the RV heal (otherwise, there may be severe, intractable RV dilatation upon opening the pericardium during CABG). For example, in a patient with left main or three-vessel disease and RCA-related MI, the RCA is treated with bare-metal stent and CABG performed 1 month later. If CAD is critical (e.g., >75% left main stenosis), one may recanalize the RCA with balloon angioplasty and perform CABG sooner, a few days later.

If staged multivessel PCI rather than staged CABG is deemed appropriate, the non-culprit PCI is preferably performed before hospital discharge, a few days later. It may also be performed a few weeks later (within 2 months). Staged multivessel PCI, even if the patient is free of angina, is superior to culprit-only PCI according to one meta-analysis and two trials (CvLPRIT and DANAMI-3 trials, before discharge), probably because significant lesions progress more readily in the setting of ACS than in stable CAD.[61,62] While pre-discharge PCI is favored in all patients, it is particularly indicated in patients with recurrent low-level angina (class I) or critical stenosis >90%. Less severe lesions may alternatively be assessed within 8 weeks either by stress testing (at 3–6 weeks) or repeat angiography (± FFR if needed), then treated if appropriate.

> While it is appropriate to revascularize non-culprit lesions, and while these lesions may progress and lead to events, one should also note that many of these stenoses paradoxically improve on repeat angiography by a mean absolute value of 10%, with 21% of angiographically significant stenoses becoming non-significant. Vasospasm that occurs in the setting of MI likely exaggerates the severity of lesions.[66] Thus, reassessment of non-culprit lesions with either angiography or stress imaging is reasonable before non-culprit PCI.

IX. Antithrombotic therapies in STEMI

A. Antithrombotic therapies in conjunction with primary PCI

1. *Aspirin* 325 mg upon presentation.

2. *Clopidogrel* 600 mg is preferably administered in the emergency room before transport to the cath lab.[67,68] As opposed to non-ST-elevation ACS, urgent CABG is rarely required in STEMI, except STEMI with cardiogenic shock.

Alternatively, *ticagrelor* 180 mg load or *prasugrel* 60 mg load may be used as they further reduce ischemic events in comparison with clopidogrel, particularly in STEMI. Prasugrel is contraindicated in patients with a prior stroke or TIA. As opposed to NSTE-ACS, prasugrel may be loaded before coronary angiography in STEMI.

3. *Upstream therapy with glycoprotein IIb/IIIa inhibitors (GPI) in the emergency room, pre-catheterization, is not indicated*. While it increases the rate of pre-PCI TIMI 3 flow, it increases bleeding without improving any ischemic outcome (FINESSE trial).[37]

4. *Upstream unfractionated heparin* (UFH) in the ED (60 units/kg, up to a maximum dose of 4000 units).

5. *During PCI*:

- ***UFH***. In patients appropriately preloaded with 600 mg of clopidogrel in the emergency room, the routine addition of GPI to UFH may not be beneficial (BRAVE-3 trial).[68]
- ***Bivalirudin monotherapy*** is associated with bleeding reduction and 0.6% mortality reduction in comparison to UFH monotherapy (MATRIX trial), and may thus be the preferred antithrombotic strategy even if the patient received UFH in the emergency room. However, bivalirudin is associated with a higher risk of acute stent thrombosis than UFH, which can be reduced by providing a UFH bolus in the emergency department and early clopidogrel preload. Providing several hours of high-dose bivalirudin post-PCI may offset this risk.[69]

  Except for this optional brief infusion of bivalirudin, anticoagulants are stopped after PCI.

- ***Downstream use of GPI*** during PCI, in conjunction with either UFH or bivalirudin, may be reserved for patients who are inadequately preloaded with ADP-receptor antagonist *or* who have a large thrombus burden (class IIa). Intracoronary GPI, more specifically abciximab delivered onto the occlusive thrombus through a weeping balloon (same dose as the standard bolus dose of abciximab), may reduce infarct size and translate into improved 1-year clinical outcomes. The latter may be the preferred administration route of GPI in patients who need it.[70] In contemporary trials, ~15% of STEMI patients require the use of GPI.

B. Antithrombotic therapies in patients treated with fibrinolytics (started upon presentation)

1. *Aspirin* 325 mg.

2. *Clopidogrel* 300 mg load if patient is <75 years old, or 75 mg if >75 years old (300 mg rather than 600 mg is the dose studied with fibrinolytics, even in pharmacoinvasive trials; 75 mg is the only dose studied with fibrinolytics in elderly patients).[71,72]

3. *UFH* IV bolus 60 units/kg (not more than 4000 units), followed *immediately* by heparin drip 12 units/kg/h, adjusted Q6h to keep the PTT 1.5–2.0× the control.

If the patient is going to have fibrinolytic reperfusion rather than PCI reperfusion, and if PCI is not expected in the next 24 hours, **enoxaparin** SQ or **fondaparinux** SQ may be used instead of UFH. In the patient receiving primary fibrinolytic reperfusion, enoxaparin or fondaparinux has a more favorable effect on reinfarction risk than UFH, with less major bleeding with fondaparinux, vs. more major bleeding with enoxaparin.[73,74] Patients undergoing fibrinolytic therapy should receive anticoagulants for at least 48 hours and preferably for the duration of the hospitalization. Regimens other than UFH are preferred if anticoagulation is used for >48 hours, because UFH therapy is of no proven benefit beyond 48 hours.

- Dosage of enoxaparin: initial 30 mg IV dose, followed 15 minutes later by 1 mg/kg SQ Q12h
  - For patients >75 years old, avoid IV dose and administer 0.75 mg/kg Q12h
  - If GFR <30 ml/min, administer 1 mg/kg SQ Q24h
- Dosage of fondaparinux: 2.5 mg IV initially, then 2.5 mg SQ Qday. Avoid if GFR <30 ml/min.

> Clopidogrel 600 mg load, prasugrel, and ticagrelor have not been studied within 24 hours of fibrinolytics, and thus should be avoided during this time frame. Conversely, if delayed PCI is performed >24 hours after fibrinolysis, one of these regimens should be used.

X. Other acute therapies

1. *β-Blockers* (e.g., metoprolol orally 25 mg Q8–12h, titrated to 50 mg Q8–12h). A meta-analysis of old trials addressing β-blockers in acute MI has shown that β-blockers reduce mortality after MI, whether HF is present or not.[75] In the COMMIT-CCS trial, the use of β-blockers beyond the first 24–48 hours after MI was beneficial and significantly reduced the risk of recurrent MI and VF at 15 days.[76] However, the earlier administration of β-blockers, especially IV β-blockers, increased the risk of cardiogenic shock overall, particularly in high-risk subgroups, where a net adverse effect was seen. Thus, β-blockers should be acutely avoided in these subgroups:

- Killip class ≥ II (any degree of HF); age >70 years.
- Sinus tachycardia >110 bpm: The more tachycardic the patient, the less likely he is to acutely benefit from β-blockers. In general, tachycardia reflects a large MI and compensates for a reduced stroke volume (pre-shock state). Slowing the heart rate will trigger a shock.
- Sinus bradycardia <60 bpm.
- SBP <120 mmHg or 30 mmHg lower than baseline, or evidence of low output. However, beyond the first 24–48 hours, SBP <90–100 mmHg, rather than 120 mmHg, is the contraindication to β-blocker use.
- Also, avoid β-blockers in other classic contraindications: PR >0.24 s, any second- or third-degree AV block, history of severe asthma, or active bronchospasm.

β-Blockers are generally titrated to the maximal tolerated dose before hospital discharge and are expected to have a short- and long-term benefit. In patients with LVEF <40% or patients who developed HF but are now stable, β-blockers are started slowly, later than 24 hours, then titrated in the outpatient setting (e.g., carvedilol is started as 6.25 mg BID in the hospital, 3 days after MI, and uptitrated every 3–10 days, as in the CAPRICORN trial; this regimen reduced late mortality in patients with low EF, with or without HF).[77]

2. *Oral ACE-Is (or ARBs if cough or angioedema occurs with ACE-I).* Wait a few hours before starting an ACE-I to ensure the patient is stable and not evolving into cardiogenic shock. Try to start an ACE-I early, in the first 24 hours. In landmark trials of ACE-inhibition in acute MI, ACE-I was initiated in the first 24 hours of all types of MI, whether anterior or inferior, accompanied by HF or not, and improved early mortality (survival curves start to diverge at day 1 and become significant at 1 week and 6 weeks).[78,79] ACE-I therapy is particularly beneficial in patients with LV dysfunction, anterior MI or HF (SAVE trial). The benefit is less marked when ACE-I is used unselectively in all MI patients, including those with inferior MI and without HF, but ACE-I is still reasonable for a duration of 6 weeks, as in those trials. ACE-I is avoided in acute renal failure or when SBP <100 mmHg or 30 mmHg below baseline; intravenous ACE-I is avoided in all patients because of the risk of hypotension. A low-dose, short-acting ACE-I may be used in the acute setting in order to verify tolerability. Examples:

- Captopril 6.25 mg TID, to be doubled with each subsequent dosage, until 50 mg TID
- *or* Lisinopril 5 mg Qday, to be increased to 20–40 mg Qday

3. *Nitroglycerin.* Administer 0.4 mg of sublingual NTG up to three times during active angina, then start IV drip if tolerated hemodynamically. NTG is useful for chest pain, HTN, or HF concomitant to MI. It may lead to hypotension or vagal shock and should be avoided if SBP <100 mmHg, bradycardia <50 bpm, tachycardia >100 bpm, or if RV infarct is suspected with inferior MI (even if RV infarct is clinically silent).

4. *Morphine.* Administer morphine if the pain is severe and uncontrolled despite NTG, provided that additional therapy is used to manage the underlying ischemia.

5. *High statin dose* (atorvastatin 80 mg, rosuvastatin 20 mg)

6. *Glucose control.* In hyperglycemia, with or without prior diabetes, insulin (IV or SQ) is administered to maintain blood glucose ≤180 mg/dl during acute MI/ACS. Afterwards, when the patient is less ill, try to achieve normoglycemia.[80]

7. *Monitoring.* The patient is monitored in a coronary care unit for 12–24 hours, then transferred to a step-down unit in the absence of complications. In general, an uncomplicated STEMI is safely discharged after 72 hours of hospitalization (PAMI-II trial), or even 48 hours according to recent data.[81–83] Patients qualify for early discharge if they undergo a successful reperfusion with primary PCI, have one- or two-vessel CAD, are younger than 70 years of age without major comorbidities, and have no arrhythmias or pump failure.

8. *Echo.* Echo should be performed before hospital discharge in all patients, and should be performed or repeated urgently in a patient with shock or suspected mechanical complication.

XI. Risk stratification

A. Killip classification uses clinical features upon *presentation* to assess STEMI prognosis.
- Class I: no HF (30-day mortality = 3%)[84]
- Class II: crackles up to one-third of the lung fields or S3 (= HF, mortality = 13%)
- Class III: pulmonary edema (mortality = 27%)
- Class IV: cardiogenic shock (mortality = 50–60%)

Note that Killip classification is only applied at presentation. It also has a prognostic value in NSTE-ACS.

B. TIMI risk score for STEMI
Depending on the STEMI TIMI risk score (Table 2.3), the 30-day mortality of fibrinolytic-treated STEMI patients ranges from 1% to 35%.[85] The benefit of reperfusion is highest in the higher risk groups.

C. Troponin I peaks at a level of 50–300 ng/ml (at ~24 h), CK typically peaks at 2500–5000 units/l (at 18–24 h). Reperfusion therapy makes these biomarkers peak earlier and often at higher levels; however, the total volume of CK or troponin released is smaller, i.e., the distribution curves over time are narrower and the decline is faster (3–4 days for troponin I). The CK or troponin mass, but not the CK or troponin peak, correlates with the infarct size and the prognosis. Aborted STEMI, whether aborted spontaneously or with very early reperfusion, is characterized by a biomarker rise that is only mild (total CK <2× normal).

XII. LV remodeling and infarct expansion after MI (see Figure 2.5)

XIII. Discharge, EF improvement, ICD

A. Discharge medications
See Chapter 1, Section VIII.

B. EF improves 1–3 months after discharge and justifies follow-up echocardiography for risk assessment. There are two explanations for EF improvement:

- LV dysfunction that occurs immediately after MI is partly due to post-ischemic stunning rather than necrosis. When an artery occludes transiently, necrosis occurs in part of the myocardium, while dysfunction without necrosis, called stunning, occurs in other parts. The stunned myocardium recovers over the course of days to weeks after arterial recanalization.
- ACE-Is, β-blockers, and aldosterone antagonists reduce LV remodeling and LV size, allowing an increase in EF for the same amount of necrotic myocardium (Figure 2.5). Each one of these drugs allows an EF improvement of up to 5%.

C. ICD
The risk of sudden death is highest in the first 30 days after MI (1.2%) and increases with HF and severe LV dysfunction (~3%).[86] However, placing an ICD in the first 40 days after MI has not been shown to reduce the overall mortality; it reduces sudden-death mortality by 50%, but the patients prone to early sudden death are typically high-risk patients also prone to dying from pump failure or recurrent MI.[87,88] Early ICD placement only changes the mode of death of these patients, from sudden death to pump-failure death (conversion hypothesis). Also, early LV dysfunction/stunning may improve and some patients may turn out to be at a lower long-term risk than expected, and thus would not require an ICD. *Therefore, ICD is indicated for primary prevention of VT/VF if EF is ≤35% at 40 days post-MI.*

On the other hand, ICD is indicated early on, before hospital discharge, for the patient who develops sustained VT or VF anytime beyond the first 2 days after MI.

Table 2.3 STEMI TIMI risk score.

Variable	Score
Age ≥65 yr/≥75 yr	2 for ≥65; 3 for ≥75
SBP <100 mmHg	3
Sinus tachycardia >100 bpm	2
Killip class ≥ II	2
Anterior location of MI or LBBB	1
Prior history of diabetes, HTN, or angina	1
Time to treatment >4 h after symptom onset	1
Weight <67 kg (higher bleeding with fibrinolytics)	1

30-day mortality according to the score: score ≤2 → <2.2%; score 3–4 → 4–7%; score ≥5→ >12%.

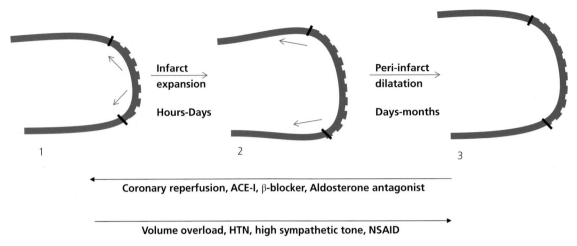

Figure 2.5 Stages of negative LV remodeling post-MI, also called infarct expansion.

For the same amount of necrosis, the dashed infarcted area thins and stretches out *(from 1 to 2).* Then, this stretched infarcted area increases tension at its edges *(arrows),* which eventually leads to progressive dilatation of the normal, non-necrotic myocardium *(from 2 to 3).* The dilatation occurs as a compensatory attempt to increase stroke volume, albeit counterproductive and maladaptive. The LV loses its normal elliptical shape and becomes a sphere, which further increases wall stress and reduces the efficiency of the non-infarcted myocardium.

Thus, *for the same amount of tissue necrosis,* the infarcted area and the EF vary largely, depending on:

(a) Loading conditions.

(b) Opening of the occluded artery, even at a time when necrosis has already occurred (e.g., 3–24 h). Reperfusion accelerates myocardial scar formation and turgor and reduces the thinning of the necrotic area, even if it does not salvage myocardium beyond 3–6 hours.

(c) Medical therapy: ACE-Is reduce afterload and exert a direct myocardial effect that reduces LV dilatation and reduces fibrosis in peri-infarct areas. Aldosterone antagonists also exert a direct myocardial effect that reduces LV dilatation and fibrosis. β-Blockers reduce the high wall stress induced by the sympathetic tone. Diuretics reduce preload and afterload.

2. STEMI COMPLICATIONS

I. Cardiogenic shock

A. Differential diagnosis (see Table 2.4)

Clinically, RV-related shock leads to a high JVP and clear lungs, whereas LV-related shock leads to a high JVP with pulmonary edema. PCWP is frequently increased in RV shock, with a mean PCWP of 23 mmHg, because of concomitant LV failure and RV/LV interdependence.[89]

When a patient with inferior MI develops cardiogenic shock, consider the following:

- RV shock
- Mechanical complication
- Relative sinus bradycardia or AV block
- Prior MI or LV dysfunction
- Superdominant RCA with apical, posterior, or lateral involvement

In the SHOCK trial and registry, ~60% of patients with LV shock had anterior MI, while 34% had inferior MI without any acute anterior involvement.[64,90] Concerning the latter 34% of patients, 14% had prior MI and 11% had concomitant apical, posterior or lateral involvement, while only 9% had isolated, new inferior MI.[90]

B. Pathophysiology of LV-related cardiogenic shock and failure in acute MI

In the SHOCK trial, LVEF was ~30 ± 12%, implying that at least half the patients only had a moderate LV insult and a moderate reduction of LV systolic function.[64] Also, ~40% of patients had non-anterior MI, mainly inferior MI.[64,90] Thus, an EF that is well tolerated in chronic HF may be associated with cardiogenic shock in acute MI. In a way, this is similar to tolerating chronic MR or AI vs. developing shock with acute MR or AI. Beside systolic dysfunction, several mechanisms explain cardiogenic shock in acute MI:

- While the progressive LV dilatation that occurs chronically raises afterload and is maladaptive, some early degree of LV dilatation is adaptive and increases stroke volume at a given LV contractility. Also, some degree of LA dilatation is adaptive and lessens the rise in

Table 2.4 Differential diagnosis of a shock.

---

1. **LV-related cardiogenic shock**: anterior MI, MI with a prior history of MI or LV dysfunction, or MI in a patient with severe multivessel CAD. Cardiogenic shock occurs in 4–7% of STEMI (vs. 2.5% of NSTEMI). It is occasionally present on admission, and more typically develops soon after admission, at a median of 5.5 hours after MI onset (vs. a later shock development, at ~3 days, in NSTEMI with three-vessel disease).

2. **RV infarct:** RV-related shock should be considered **whenever hypotension occurs in inferior MI**. RV infarct occurs in 30% of inferior MIs, mainly with proximal RCA occlusion. Only one-half of RV infarcts produce clinical RV failure.

3. **Mechanical complications** (mitral regurgitation, ventricular septal rupture, free wall rupture) or **tamponade**.

4. **Arrhythmias** (inappropriate bradycardia, advanced AV block, VT).

5. **Vagal stimulation and vagal shock** in inferior MI. It manifests as bradycardia with clear lungs and low JVP. It is treated with atropine and fluid administration.

6. **Hypovolemic hypotension**: hypotension with clear lungs, low JVP, and no bradycardia. May attempt small fluid challenge in this situation.

During or after PCI, shock may develop from the use of sedative and vasodilatory drugs in a patient with limited cardiac output reserve, or from myocardial reperfusion injury that aggravates myocardial depression. Coronary reocclusion, coronary perforation with tamponade, and bleeding complications may also be considered.

backward pressure. This is similar to the chronic LV adaptation to MR or AI. In fact, half of patients with cardiogenic shock have a small or normal-size LV, which represents failure of the mechanism of acute LV dilatation.[91,92]

- For a given LV contractility, the more severe impairment of LV compliance in acute MI leads to a more severe rise of LV filling pressure, which further reduces coronary perfusion pressure.

- Transient hypotension (drugs, arrhythmia, sedation) in an initially stable patient may transiently reduce coronary blood flow and thus initiate a vicious circle of progressive myocardial ischemia that sustains the hypotension. Furthermore, since the pulmonary edema of MI results from volume redistribution rather than florid volume overload, aggressive diuresis may precipitate shock in MI. *Also, β-blockers, ACE-Is, and other vasodilators, including sedatives administered during PCI or during intubation, may precipitate shock in a pre-shock patient who depends on the compensatory vasoconstriction and tachycardia.* This partly explains why cardiogenic shock often develops after hospital admission.

While hypotension unloads the LV and may be tolerated in chronic LV failure, it is not well tolerated in a patient with acute ischemia and unstable CAD or in a patient with RV failure.

- In over 25% of MI-associated cardiogenic shock, SVR is inappropriately low or normal rather than elevated, despite the use of vasopressors (SVR ≤1000 dyn.s.cm^{-5}).[93] *This mismatch between myocardial depression and inappropriate vasodilatation (or lack of compensatory vasoconstriction) may result in cardiogenic shock.* Also, 18% of patients, mainly those with a low initial SVR, go on to develop a clinical picture of sepsis with fever or leukocytosis 2–4 days later, mostly with positive bacterial cultures. Thus, inappropriate vasodilatation is initiated by a systemic inflammatory response syndrome (SIRS) secondary to MI early on, then a septic process later on, and contributes to shock in a substantial proportion of patients. This implies a role for vasopressors in this subset of patients. High levels of cytokines and *inducible* nitric oxide synthase, beyond the healthy levels of *endothelial* nitric oxide synthase, precipitate vasodilatation and further myocardial depression. The initial vasodilatation, per se, is associated with an increased risk of later sepsis (bacterial translocation?).[93]

Some patients with a pre-shock state before PCI develop a full-blown shock after PCI. PCI may initiate a reperfusion injury with further activation of inducible nitric oxide synthase, and thus vasodilatation and myocardial depression. This is a temporary phenomenon, as the benefit from PCI eventually takes over. Also, the use of sedatives may precipitate shock during PCI.

C. Management of LV-related cardiogenic shock

A shock is defined as sustained SBP <90 mmHg for at least 30 minutes, *with* signs of low perfusion (oliguria <30 ml/h, cold/clammy extremities, impaired mentation, increased lactate >2 mmol/l).[64] LV-related cardiogenic shock is characterized by additional features suggestive of increased left-sided filling pressure, such as clinical or radiographic pulmonary edema. Supportive hemodynamic features consist of a cardiac index ≤2.2 l/min and PCWP ≥15 mmHg, but right heart catheterization was not absolutely required in the SHOCK trial when pulmonary congestion was evident in a patient with anterior MI. Echo may be used to assess left-sided filling pressures and confirm the diagnosis, in addition to ruling out mechanical complications.

In the SHOCK trial, patients with cardiogenic shock and STEMI or Q-wave MI of less than 36 hours' duration were randomized to emergent revascularization vs. medical therapy. The median time from the onset of MI to shock was 5.6 hours, from MI to PCI 11 hours, and from MI to CABG 19 hours. Approximately 65% of patients had three-vessel disease and ~20% had left main disease. Revascularization with PCI or CABG, as appropriate, reduced the absolute 6-month mortality by a drastic 13% (30-day mortality 46% vs. 56%, with a lower mortality of 38% if successful PCI was performed; 6-month mortality 50% vs. 63%). Patients who survive the acute phase of cardiogenic shock have a good long-term survival, with two-thirds being alive at 6 years.[94,95]

Notably, fibrinolytics were administered to 63% of the SHOCK trial patients managed medically and were associated with a marked and significant 40% mortality reduction in comparison to no fibrinolytic therapy.[96] In addition, fibrinolytics were administered to ~50% of patients managed with revascularization, as half of SHOCK trial patients presented to non-PCI-capable hospitals; the mortality benefit of fibrinolytics in this subgroup was less clear. In the SHOCK registry, the use of fibrinolytic therapy was associated with a mortality reduction even in those who eventually underwent revascularization.[97] The impaired systemic perfusion may impede the lytic delivery to its target; fibrinolysis remains, nonetheless, effective, particularly if IABP is used.

In the SHOCK trial, 37% of patients received emergent CABG rather than PCI, and CABG was performed briskly, at a median of 2.7 hours after randomization. CABG was associated with the same survival as PCI, despite the higher prevalence of extensive CAD.[98] However, this quick CABG is not feasible at many institutions and the CABG rate in the community is lower.

IABP was recommended in all SHOCK trial patients, including medically treated patients and those initially presenting to a non-PCI hospital, and was used in 86% of patients. In the SHOCK registry, IABP was associated with a reduced mortality.[97] However, randomized trials failed to show a benefit of IABP in STEMI patients with LV failure,[99] and lately, the IABP-SHOCK II trial failed to show a benefit of IABP even in MI patients with cardiogenic shock.[100] The failure of the IABP-SHOCK II trial may be due to the heterogeneity of cardiogenic shock and the inclusion of patients whose shock was not purely related to LV dysfunction (median EF was 35%, 33% of patients had NSTEMI, and 45% had post-cardiac arrest shock); and to the fact that IABP was placed after rather than before PCI. In patients with true LV shock, it is reasonable to place the IABP before PCI as an early measure to stabilize the patient, reduce O$_2$ demands, and perform a safer PCI with a potential for less reperfusion injury. Unloading the LV before primary PCI, in carefully selected patients with true LV shock, may prove beneficial. Also, outside shock, IABP is useful in patients with a large STEMI who have persistent ischemia/slow coronary flow after primary PCI.

In sum, the following strategy is recommended in cardiogenic shock:

a. *Emergent revascularization* of the infarct-related artery *and* all critical stenoses of other major arteries, irrespective of the time of presentation (even >24 hours after MI onset). *Ongoing* ischemia and necrosis are typical of the vicious cycle that characterizes shock, even late shock. *As opposed to non-shock patients, full revascularization is recommended in cardiogenic shock.*

b. In patients presenting to non-PCI-capable hospitals within 6 hours of MI onset, administer **fibrinolytics** whenever transfer delays are expected. Also, IABP may be placed before transfer. Augmentation of blood pressure with IABP or vasopressors may increase coronary flow and facilitate fibrinolysis.

c. *In patients with multivessel CAD* on angiography:
- Severe three-vessel CAD (>90%) or critical left main disease dictates immediate CABG if possible. Alternatively, PCI of the infarct-related artery is performed then followed by PCI of the remaining critical stenoses if the patient's hemodynamics do not improve. Balloon angioplasty of the culprit artery followed by early CABG is another alternative.
- Significant but non-critical three-vessel CAD dictates PCI of the infarct artery, followed by PCI of the remaining arteries if the patient's hemodynamics do not improve.

d. *IABP* may be placed during or before the revascularization procedure.

e. *Mechanical ventilation* is often necessary to reduce the respiratory work, improve oxygenation, and reduce LV preload and afterload.

f. *Inotropic support:* dobutamine or dopamine is used in patients whose SBP is >70 mmHg, while norepinephrine is required in patients with SBP <70 mmHg or inappropriately low or normal SVR. While vasoconstriction may be harmful, the maintenance of an appropriate systemic perfusion pressure, including coronary perfusion pressure, is a priority and justifies the use of norepinephrine in severely hypotensive patients. Also, norepinephrine stimulates the myocardial release of local coronary vasodilators which counteract its direct α$_1$ constrictive effect. Patients whose shock has been precipitated by vasodilators or sedation may also be temporarily treated with vasopressors, until the effect of the drugs wears off.

g. *Temporary pacing,* usually at a rate over 80–100 bpm, is required if the heart rate is inappropriately low or even "normal" (60–70 bpm).

h. *PA catheter* may be placed to support the diagnosis and guide management, but is not necessary unless the patient does not improve with revascularization; the finding of a low SVR may dictate the use of vasopressors.

    Echo should be done to rule out mechanical complications and to assess left-sided filling pressures.

    Alternatively, *LV pressure measurement and LV angiography* are performed during the emergent cardiac catheterization.

i. *LV assist device*, such as percutaneous Impella or TandemHeart, may be considered in patients with refractory shock as it provides better hemodynamic support than IABP. The survival benefit in patients with irreversible stage of shock and multiple organ failure is, however, uncertain.

E. Management of severe acute left heart failure without shock

In acute MI, pulmonary edema results from volume redistribution to the lungs without overt volume overload and sometimes without LV dilatation. Treatment consists of small doses of furosemide (e.g., 20–40 mg IV), along with a low dose of intravenous NTG to reduce preload. *Excessive preload or afterload reduction may, however, precipitate shock.*

Severe HF (Killip class III), i.e., massive pulmonary edema with hypoxemia that frequently requires mechanical ventilation, is an indication for primary PCI irrespective of the delay to presentation (approach similar to cardiogenic shock). Multivessel PCI of non-infarct arteries may not be necessary in the absence of shock.

> Conversely, *less severe HF with late presentation (>24 hours) and no residual angina does not dictate urgent PCI.* Coronary angiography and PCI may be performed on a non-urgent basis if HF, i.e., severe functional limitation, persists after initial diuresis; otherwise, stress testing may be performed first to assess for residual ischemia.

F. RV-related cardiogenic shock: characteristics and management

If the patient survives the acute phase of RV MI, RV function usually improves spontaneously within 1 month, as RV ischemia is usually reversible and does not lead to chronic RV failure, even if the RV is not reperfused.[101] In fact, the long-term survival is excellent in survivors of the acute phase. RV is thin (less oxygen demands), easily recruits collaterals because of its lower coronary microvascular resistance, and has a capacity to derive oxygen from the RV cavity through the deep trabeculations; thus, RV usually recovers most of its contractile function. Acutely, however, RV shock is associated with a very high mortality, almost similar to LV shock (~50%), despite a younger age, a higher

⬡BMA

BMA Library

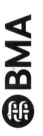

Freepost RTKJ-RKSZ-JGHG
British Medical Association
PO Box 291
LONDON
WC1H 9TG

FREE RETURN POSTAGE FOR STUDENTS, FY DOCTORS & REFUGEE DOCTORS

Use this label for the **FREE** return of books to the BMA Library

LVEF, and a much lower likelihood of three-vessel CAD.[89] Similarly to LV shock, RV shock benefits from emergent reperfusion with PCI or CABG. In fact, reperfusion promptly improves RV function within 1 hour and normalizes it within 3–5 days, dramatically and quickly improving the survival and the clinical status.[101] Non-reperfused patients continue to have a poor RV function and poor hemodynamics at 3–5 days; RV function eventually normalizes at 1 month, which may be too late.

In the SHOCK registry, PCWP was equally elevated in RV shock as in LV shock (23 ± 11 mmHg), and was equalized with RA pressure.[89] This is mainly related to the RV–LV interdependence. The dilated RV pushes the septum, forcing the LV diastolic pressure to equalize with the RV diastolic pressure and reducing LV output. RV is thin, intolerant to the increased afterload, and thus intolerant to RV dilatation which begets more dilatation. The LV is underfilled, yet LA and LV diastolic pressures are elevated.

The usual culprit of RV shock is RCA in 96% of the cases, usually proximal RCA affecting flow to the acute marginal branches (RV free wall) and the PDA (inferior septum). The left coronary is responsible for RV infarction in 4% of the cases; this occurs when the left coronary supplies collaterals to a chronically occluded RCA, when the septal infarction affects the septal contribution to RV function, but also when RV MI leads to ST elevation beyond V_1 and V_2, falsely creating an ECG impression of anterior MI.

Treatment of RV shock (beside emergent reperfusion):

a. *Fluid administration.* In patients without significant pulmonary hypertension, one may increase the RA pressure to passively force flow through the PA and therefore increase the cardiac output. However, this is only effective as long as the RV does not dilate. Once the RV dilates, fluid administration worsens ventricular interdependence, further reduces LV output, and increases TR. Thus, 500 ml fluid boluses are provided while carefully assessing the hemodynamic response to each bolus, and preferably while checking RV size on echo. Boluses are stopped if RV is significantly dilated *or* if no improvement in SBP and pulse pressure is noted.
While RA pressure may not correlate with volume responsiveness of the stiff RV, a study has suggested that in RV MI, the best stroke volume is seen when RA pressure is 10–14 mmHg, beyond which the stroke volume declines.[102]

b. *Inotropes/vasopressors.* After RV preload has been optimized, the patient with persistent hypotension is treated with inotropes/vasopressors. Since at least half of the RV coronary flow occurs in systole, RV coronary flow depends on the driving gradient between SBP and RV systolic pressure. Thus, the RV is very sensitive to decreased SBP, more so than the LV, which may thrive with a slightly reduced SBP. Inotropes used in RV MI should be able to increase SBP, and thus norepinephrine is often the agent of choice.[103]

c. *Maintenance of AV synchrony* is critical in acute RV failure, as the RV but also the underfilled LV are dependent on the extra-filling provided by the atrial contraction, *more so than a failing, overfilled LV.*[104] AF may need to be DC cardioverted. Patients with AV block or AV dissociation from an accelerated junctional rhythm need to have atrial and ventricular sequential pacing. Transvenous atrial and ventricular leads are placed through separate venous accesses (e.g., bilateral femoral accesses).
As in any shock, a "normal" heart rate of 60–70 bpm is inappropriate and dictates pacing to a rate >80 bpm.

d. *Hypoxemia* should be aggressively treated with mechanical ventilation if necessary, as hypoxemia increases pulmonary vascular resistance and RV afterload.

e. *IABP* may be useful to increase flow across the reperfused RCA. It is more definitely indicated when concomitant LV failure is present (pulmonary edema).

f. *Inhaled NO* may be used in refractory RV shock and has been shown to reduce RA pressure and pulmonary vascular resistance, and increase stroke volume, in RV MI.[105]

Beware of two processes that may mimic RV infarct: pulmonary embolism and tamponade.

II. Mechanical complications
Mechanical complications occur within the first 14 days of STEMI, and have two peaks (24 hours and 3–5 days). They are responsible for 12% of cases of cardiogenic shock (severe mitral regurgitation, 7%; ventricular septal rupture, 3.9%).[90] Myocardial rupture usually results from the shear stress at the border between the live and the infarcted area. In the reperfusion era, myocardial rupture is most frequently seen in the first 24 hours (SHOCK registry).[106,107] It may occur at 3–5 days, particularly in non-reperfused patients, when the forming scar thins, expands, and exerts excessive tension at the border. In the second week, the rupture may involve the thin necrotic area itself.

A. Severe mitral regurgitation (MR)
- *Posterior leaflet tethering* – A degree of ischemic MR is seen in ~30% of acute MI. *Inferior MI* with localized inferior/posterior akinesis pulls the posterior papillary muscle posterolaterally, with subsequent tethering of the posterior mitral leaflet (predominantly). This tethering may lead to severe MR, a dynamic form of MR that may be mild at rest and severe with increased ventricular loading. *Tethering may also occur with anterior MI and is usually a posterior tethering as well.* In anterior MI, posterior tethering is secondary to global LV dilatation.
- *Papillary muscle rupture* – Severe MR may also result from rupture of a papillary muscle head, usually the posterior papillary muscle in the context of an *inferior or posterior MI* (two-thirds of severe MR cases in the SHOCK registry).[106] The posterior papillary muscle is supplied by one artery, the PDA (from a dominant RCA or LCx), whereas the anterolateral muscle has a dual blood supply from the LAD (usually first diagonal) and the LCx. Papillary muscle rupture occurs in ~1% of MIs, and, unlike ventricular septal rupture, the infarct is relatively small in 50% of the cases. Each papillary muscle extends chordae to both leaflets, and therefore flailing of *either or both leaflets* may occur with rupture of *either papillary muscle.*

Echo distinguishes papillary muscle rupture (treated surgically) from leaflet tethering (initially treated with revascularization and supportive measures). In the former, the leaflet(s) are flail, prolapsed, with flailing of chordae and flailing of an echogenic piece of papillary muscle; in the latter, the posterior leaflet is restricted and the jet is usually posterior.

B. Ventricular septal rupture (VSR) occurs in ~1% of MIs (only 0.2% of reperfused MIs). Anterior MI (LAD) and inferior MI (mainly RCA) were equally common causes of VSR in the SHOCK registry, while other registries suggest that anterior MI is slightly more common.[107] Patients with a wrap-around LAD have less septal collaterals and are at a higher risk of septal rupture with anterior MI. The location is apical septal in anterior MI and basal inferior in inferior MI. VSR leads to a severe left-to-right shunting with severe hypotension and LV volume overload.

C. Free wall rupture occurs in ~2% of MIs and is the most common and most underdiagnosed mechanical complication (≤1.5% of patients treated with PCI, 3% of patients treated with thrombolysis, 6% of patients not reperfused).[108,109] The most common location is anterior MI (LAD culprit); the second most common location is lateral MI (LCx culprit).[110]

Free wall rupture often leads to tamponade and a bradycardic pulseless electrical activity. It commonly has one of the following prodromes: chest pain, re-elevation of ST segments, bradycardia, or syncope from a vagal shock.[109] In ~30% of the cases, it is preceded by a concealed rupture and a moderate pericardial effusion, where the pericardium temporarily seals the rupture.[109]

> Risk factors for VSR and free wall rupture: female sex, older age, first MI, absence of collaterals, history of HTN, anterior MI. Also, the use of NSAIDs or steroids increases the risk of rupture. Anticoagulants do not clearly increase the risk of rupture.
>
> Reperfusion with thrombolysis or PCI reduces the incidence of all mechanical complications. While early thrombolysis reduces the risk of free wall rupture, late thrombolysis >12 hours, particularly in elderly patients, may increase the risk of free wall rupture according to a meta-analysis of thrombolytic trials.[111,112]
>
> The majority of patients with VSR have multivessel disease, while patients with papillary muscle or free wall rupture usually have a single-vessel disease with good LV function.

D. Clinical manifestations

Patients with either MR or VSR present with cardiogenic shock and pulmonary edema.

- Pulmonary edema is less marked with VSR than with MR. Patients with VSR can typically lie supine, which is not the case with MR.
- The murmur may be faint or absent with acute MR, because of the near-equalization of LV and LA pressures. The murmur is usually loud in VSR and is associated with a thrill at the left lower sternal border.

E. Diagnosis

a. *Transthoracic echo* (TTE) is the initial test. TTE shows a left-to-right shunt in VSR. It may miss severe acute MR because of the narrowing of the pressure difference between the LV and the LA, leading to attenuation of the regurgitant color flow. TTE may show a pericardial effusion with layered echodensities, corresponding to blood, in free wall rupture; however, it may miss a concealed rupture (an effusion is not seen in 25% of concealed ruptures).[110]

b. If the severity/mechanism of MR is unclear on TTE in a patient with shock, perform ***transesophageal echocardiography***.

c. *MRI* is needed when a concealed free wall rupture is suspected but not well delineated by echo.

d. *Right heart catheterization* may also be useful to diagnose VSR and MR:

- In VSR, there is O_2 saturation step-up ≥7% between RA and RV.
- In MR, PCWP tracing has a giant V wave; however, a large V wave may also occur with VSR or severe LV failure. In both MR and VSR, PCWP is higher than LVEDP.

e. *Left ventriculography* may be performed during PCI in a patient with cardiogenic shock. It allows the diagnosis of severe MR, VSR, or free wall rupture.

F. Treatment

All mechanical complications are treated by emergent surgical repair and coronary revascularization. Surgery reduces mortality from 90–100% to ~20–50%.

a. *MR* – Papillary muscle rupture dictates emergent valvular surgery + CABG. Place IABP preoperatively and administer IV vasodilators (nitroprusside) as in all cases of acute severe MR. Mitral valve replacement is most often performed as it is more expeditious than repair, but repair may be performed in some cases. The operative mortality is 20–40%.[106]

When severe acute MR is secondary to acute mitral leaflet tethering, the patient may be treated with percutaneous revascularization, vasodilators and temporary IABP support. It is expected that leaflet tethering improves once the function of the reperfused territory improves.[113–115] This is not the case in chronic leaflet tethering seen with chronic infarction. Surgery should be considered a second-line therapy for those patients who do not improve with medical therapy.

b. *VSR* – The operative mortality is ~50% and is higher in basal-inferior VSR, because the latter is more serpiginous and often associated with RV infarct. Prepare the patient with IABP/nitroprusside/inotropes.

> The long-term survival of patients who survive any of the three mechanical complications is good.

G. Another mechanical complication: dynamic left ventricular outflow tract obstruction

This complication occurs in 1–2% of MIs and up to 12% of anterior MIs in women. It is due to anteroapical akinesis associated with a compensatory hyperkinesis of the LV base. This narrows the LVOT and leads to drawing of the mitral valve to the septum and systolic anterior motion (SAM) of the mitral valve, similar to HOCM (Figure 2.6).[116]

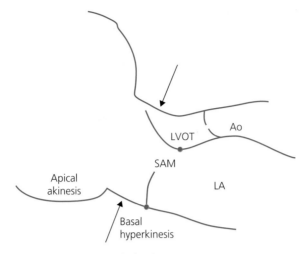

Figure 2.6 Dynamic left ventricular outflow tract obstruction in apical infarction.

Hypotension and pulmonary edema may subsequently occur. Clinically, a new, dynamic systolic murmur, similar to HOCM murmur, is heard. MR murmur (SAM) may also be heard.

As opposed to the treatment of cardiogenic shock, inotropes, diuretics, and IABP should be avoided, as they worsen the basal hyperkinesis and LVOT narrowing. β-Blockers are used to reduce the LVOT hyperkinesis. α-Agonists may be used in case of hypotension.

III. Recurrent infarction and ischemia

Within 30 days, recurrent infarction or ischemia occurs in ~10–15% of patients treated with fibrinolytic therapy, vs. <4% of patients treated with PCI (less so with stenting, ~2%).[23,38,39] Recurrent infarction is usually due to reocclusion and is also called "infarct extension," which is different from "infarct expansion" (LV remodeling).

It is diagnosed based on clinical grounds, ECG, and a reincrease of a downtrending troponin by >20%.

Treatment – Escalate β-blockers, NTG, and readminister anticoagulants. Emergent PCI is indicated in STEMI, refractory angina, or hemodynamic instability. Otherwise, a non-urgent coronary angiogram is usually performed. For recurrent ST elevation, the fibrin-specific fibrinolytics may be (re-)administered if PCI cannot be performed in a timely fashion.

IV. Tachyarrhythmias

A. Ventricular tachyarrhythmias: VF and sudden death

Improvements in reperfusion therapy have reduced the 30-day mortality of a STEMI patient presenting to the hospital from 15% to 5–6%. Yet, out-of-hospital mortality remains very high, and is responsible for most MI fatalities, mainly in the first hour after MI onset. In fact, the risk of out-of-hospital cardiac arrest in STEMI is ~30%,[117,118] mainly in the first hour after STEMI onset, when over half of all VF episodes occur (risk of VF during the first hour ≥12%);[119] and between hours 1 and 4, where most of the remaining VF events occur.

Conversely, for patients who make it to the hospital without cardiac arrest, the risk of primary VF within 48 hours is ~4%, mostly in the first 4 hours after symptom onset, and the risk of VT and/or VF is ~10%.[120]

B. Ventricular tachyarrhythmias: VF

In the reperfusion era, sustained VF occurs in 4% of patients hospitalized with acute STEMI. There are three types of VF, mostly characterized in fibrinolytic trials:

• *Primary VF* is defined as VF occurring in the first 48 hours after MI without an associated shock or severe HF (Killip class I). It occurs because of rapid potassium fluxes with increased automaticity and dispersion of repolarization, or increased sympathetic or vagal tone. It mostly occurs in the first 4 hours. Primary VF, whether in the first 4 hours or at 4–48 hours, is associated with a 2–4 times increased in-hospital mortality, from the VF episode itself, VF recurrence, or the larger ischemic burden. However, VF does not affect long-term mortality in survivors, even on unadjusted analyses.[120–122] *In fact, primary VF correlates with the extent of initial ischemia and is much more commonly seen in STEMI than NSTEMI, but does not correlate with the eventual infarct size and is at least as frequently seen in inferior as in anterior MI* (GISSI-2, Apex-AMI analyses). Sinus bradycardia or pauses may precipitate VF in patients with inferior MI.

Even after primary PCI, a small but significant proportion of patients have VT/VF at 24–48 hours (~1.5% of patients).[123,124] This post-PCI VT/VF carries an increase in short-term,[124] but not long-term, mortality.

Post-PCI VF may reflect stent thrombosis, and warrants thorough clinical and ECG investigation.

- *Secondary VF* is defined as VF occurring in association with HF or shock (<48 h or >48 h) and portends a poor early and long-term survival, mainly from a downhill HF course.[121,122]
- *Late VF* is defined as VF occurring after 48 hours without an associated HF or shock. It is secondary to the myocardial scar and correlates with pump failure, extensive myocardial damage, and increased long-term mortality.[120]

C. Ventricular tachyarrhythmias: sustained VT
There are two types of VT:

- *Polymorphic VT* is usually an ischemic rhythm that occurs in the first 48 hours of MI or during ischemic recurrences.[125] In contrast to torsades de pointes, this polymorphic VT is usually associated with a normal or a minimally prolonged QT interval. Similar to primary VF, it is associated with increased short-term but not long-term mortality.[126]
- *Monomorphic VT*, whether occurring early (in the first 48 hours) or late (>48 hours), is a sign of extensive myocardial damage and portends a strikingly increased in-hospital but also long-term mortality, even when it is not accompanied by HF or shock (GUSTO-1 data).[120,127,128] It is rarely seen, in ~2% of MI.

Polymorphic VT usually corresponds to active ischemia, many times without underlying anatomic substrate/scar or with less underlying anatomic substrate and higher EF than monomorphic VT.[129] Monomorphic VT, on the other hand, usually reflects the presence of an often large substrate in the border zone between viable and infarcted tissue.[120]

D. Ventricular tachyarrhythmias: non-sustained VT (NSVT)
Early NSVT (<48 hours) is not associated with any impairment of short- or long-term survival.[126] Late NSVT (≥4 beats) is associated with impaired long-term survival.[130] NSVT does not require any specific therapy; provide general MI therapy and, more specifically, a β-blocker if possible.

E. Accelerated idioventricular rhythm = slow VT = slow wide ventricular rhythm at a rate of 60–100 (120) bpm. Its incidence is 20% in the first 48 hours, mostly after successful reperfusion. Its occurrence immediately after fibrinolytic therapy may signal reperfusion; however, since it frequently occurs without reperfusion, it cannot be used as a standalone reperfusion marker. In any case, it is benign and resolves spontaneously; no specific treatment is required.

F. Acute therapy of sustained VT/VF
- DC cardioversion and IV amiodarone (first choice), procainamide, or lidocaine for 6–24 hours. Use procainamide cautiously in HF, as it has a negative inotropic effect.
- Revascularization
- β-Blockers if possible
- Keep K levels >4.0–4.5 mEq/l and Mg >2 mg/dl
- Consider repeating the coronary angiogram in case of recurrent VT or VF despite earlier reperfusion therapy
- Primary VT prophylaxis with antiarrhythmic drugs (e.g., lidocaine) is not indicated and does not improve outcomes

G. Atrial fibrillation, atrial flutter
In the reperfusion era, the incidence of new AF or atrial flutter in acute MI, usually paroxysmal AF/atrial flutter, is ~10%. This incidence is increased in patients with HF, large MI (including RV MI), pericarditis, or older age. AF is associated with an increased in-hospital as well as long-term mortality, which is partly related to the associated pump failure and the late VT/VF.[131] Post-MI AF has been associated with a striking increase in the risk of in-hospital but also long-term stroke across multiple studies, even when AF is only transient.[131] In the GUSTO-1 trial, the in-hospital stroke risk was 3.1% with AF vs. 1.3 % without AF.[132] Another study addressed patients with inferior MI and preserved EF who had transient AF, i.e., AF that spontaneously reverted to sinus rhythm before hospital discharge; these patients had a much higher risk of AF at 1 year than patients without transient AF (22% vs. 1.3%) and a high risk of stroke under aspirin therapy (~10% vs. 2%), despite a normal EF. This suggests that AF occurring during MI is not a transient phenomenon, but rather a chronic process with a high stroke risk.[133]

This high risk of stroke supports anticoagulation for peri-MI AF and is further supported by one registry analysis.[134] However, in the era of PCI and routine dual antiplatelet therapy, the role of anticoagulation for transient, peri-MI AF is unclear. The in-hospital use of unfractionated heparin is encouraged to reduce the in-hospital stroke risk, and long-term triple therapy with warfarin, aspirin, and clopidogrel may be considered in patients with a low bleeding risk, provided that aspirin or clopidogrel therapy is kept short if possible (e.g., 1–6 months).

β-Blockers are used for rate control, but are not appropriate in patients with acute HF. In ill patients with acute HF, some degree of tachycardia may be tolerated to prevent a shock state (e.g., heart rate of 100–110 bpm). Anticongestive measures and afterload reduction improve the AF rate; if needed, digoxin and IV amiodarone may be added for rate control.

H. Accelerated junctional rhythm (also called non-paroxysmal junctional tachycardia)
The accelerated junctional rhythm is an automatic rhythm originating from the AV node at a rate of 70–130 bpm, often ~80 bpm. The junctional rhythm is faster than the sinus rhythm, which leads to AV dissociation. Sometimes, the junctional and sinus rhythms compete at close rates, leading to isorhythmic AV dissociation, i.e., some beats may be sinus beats preceded by sinus P waves, while the other beats may be junctional beats dissociated from P waves and showing up at any deceleration of the sinus P rate (see Chapter 13, Figure 13.9). The QRS is narrow, except in patients with a baseline bundle branch block. This rhythm may occur with inferior MI, is benign and transient, and does not generally require any specific therapy unless the patient is in shock. In shock, atrial pacing at a rate faster than the junctional rhythm may be performed to promote AV synchrony and a more appropriate rate for shock.

Persistent sinus tachycardia is a strong negative prognostic marker; it often signifies pump failure from a large MI. Do not necessarily attempt to slow it down, and avoid β-blockers in the first 24 hours if the heart rate exceeds 110 bpm. One may attempt to slow it down in young patients with hyperdynamic circulation and limited-size MI. Sinus tachycardia may improve with anticongestive measures and afterload reduction.

V. Bradyarrhythmias, bundle branch blocks, fascicular blocks

A. Inferior MI

The sinus nodal artery originates from the proximal RCA (60%) or the LCx (40%). The AV nodal artery originates from the AV groove continuation of a dominant RCA (90%) or a dominant LCx (10%).

In inferior MI, sinus bradycardia and AV blocks may develop in the first 24 hours, at which time they are usually brief and result from the increased vagal tone that accompanies inferior MI. Beyond 24 hours, the AV block is due to ischemia and edema of the AV node and is more persistent, but eventually resolves within a few days (<1 week). The AV node is resistant to ischemia, and therefore it almost never infarcts. When AV block is seen along with a fast P-wave rate, the block is due to nodal ischemia or edema, rather than a high vagal tone.

The AV block being at the nodal level, it may manifest as first-degree AV block, second-degree type I AV block, or complete AV block with a junctional rhythm (rate 40–100). Those blocks are usually well tolerated, develop gradually (first-degree to second-degree then third-degree AV block), and resolve gradually. Complete AV block is seen in ~11% of inferior MIs, mostly on the first day.

Complete AV block is associated with a larger MI, more RV MI, and a higher in-hospital mortality. Patients who survive to hospital discharge, however, do not have an increase in long-term mortality in some,[135] but not all studies.[136]

Treatment – AV block that occurs in the first 24 hours responds to atropine, which should be used in case of hemodynamic instability. Since it is not driven by a high vagal tone, later AV block (>24 hours) does not typically respond to atropine; being usually well tolerated with a good escape, it only requires temporary transvenous ventricular pacing in case of shock, HF, symptoms of weakness/dizziness, or complete AV block with a rate <40 bpm.

Symptomatic sinus bradycardia or pauses are initially treated with up to 2 mg of atropine. Transcutaneous or transvenous pacing may be used if symptomatic bradycardia persists.

B. Anterior MI

The bundle branches and fascicles are, at least partially, supplied by the LAD. Anterior MI may lead to bundle branch blocks and AV block. The AV block is Hisian or infra-Hisian and is usually preceded by bundle branch blocks. A second- or third-degree AV block is seen in ~3.5% of anterior MIs and portends a very high mortality related to pump failure (3–4 times increase in mortality; mortality was >50% in the pre-reperfusion era).[136,137] The anterior MI's AV block often resolves but may recur in a minority of patients.[137]

Transvenous pacing, while indicated for any high-grade second- or third-degree AV block occurring with anterior MI, even if asymptomatic, does not improve the grim overall prognosis that is dictated by the pump function. Permanent pacing is indicated for persistent, infranodal second- or third-degree AV block.

C. Bundle branch and fascicular blocks

Approximately 2–8% of STEMI patients develop some form of new intraventricular block, LAFB being the most common block. Note the following arterial supply:[138]

- The right bundle mainly has a single arterial supply from the LAD (first septal branch).
- The left anterior fascicle has a single arterial supply from the LAD (first septal branch).
- The His bundle, the main left bundle, and the posterior fascicle have a dual supply from the LAD septal branches and the AV nodal artery. Thus, the composite of the anterior and posterior fascicles, the branching left bundle, usually has a dual supply. This explains why it is difficult to infarct the left bundle and why most new LBBBs are non-ischemic in nature.

RBBB or LAFB are most commonly seen in anterior MI,[139] but may also be seen in inferior MI if the LAD has severe disease and is dependent on the RCA for collaterals. LBBB may result from either anterior or inferior MI, and is more likely seen when both RCA and LAD are compromised, with one acutely occluded and the other chronically obstructed (in the GUSTO trial, LBBB was associated with an RCA culprit at least as much as an LAD culprit).[7,140]

The conduction system is more resistant to ischemia than the myocardium, as the myocardial cells require much more O_2 for their continuous mechanical work than the electrical cells, which also frequently receive dual or collateral supply. This explains why conduction blocks are frequently due to edema or ischemia rather than necrosis and are usually reversible (75% of the cases).[139] If not reversible, and if secondary to MI rather than degenerative disease, the myocardial injury is usually quite extensive (e.g., persistent RBBB or LBBB).

While a chronic bundle branch block (BBB) has a very low risk of progression to complete AV block, 20% of acute BBBs progress to complete AV block, and 25–40% of acute bifascicular blocks progress to complete AV block.

Beside the risk of progressing to complete AV block, *a new BBB is independently associated with a two- to sixfold increase in in-hospital mortality, HF, and VF, particularly because it correlates with a more extensive infarction* (mortality 18% vs. 11% in GUSTO trial; 35–50% in the pre-reperfusion era).[140] Approximately 75% of these blocks are transient, and transient blocks do not portend any increase in mortality.[139,140] Old BBBs do not portend any increase in mortality either. *Both RBBB and LBBB are associated with the same increase in mortality.*[139,140]

A standby temporary transcutaneous or transvenous pacemaker is indicated for a new BBB or bifascicular block occurring in anterior MI.

VI. LV aneurysm and LV pseudoaneurysm

A. LV aneurysm

Dyskinesis signifies that a non-contractile myocardial segment moves out during myocardial contraction and moves in during relaxation (paradoxical motion). **LV aneurysm** is an extreme form of dyskinesis and consists of a *thin* area of infarcted, dyskinetic myocardium that forms a myocardial pocket. Dyskinesis without an aneurysm implies that the myocardium protrudes only during systole, whereas an *aneurysm protrudes in both systole and diastole, forming a separate chamber, and always has thin walls*. LV aneurysm usually reflects the presence of extensive transmural necrosis; contrarily, dyskinesis may be seen with acute reversible ischemia, post-ischemic stunning, or takotsubo cardiomyopahty without any necrosis, in which case the myocardial wall is not thin (it may appear thin in systole from the lack of thickening, but it is not thin in diastole). Dyskinesis without an aneurysm is much more common than a true aneurysm.

LV aneurysm is a form of adverse LV remodeling and dilatation of the necrotic area. ~50% develop acutely in the first 48 hours, from early dilatation of the necrotic, expansile myocardium, and the remainder usually appear within 2 weeks.[141] The mature, thick scar appears several weeks later, followed by calcifications. The early use of ACE-I, β-blocker, and aggressive blood pressure control prevents LV aneurysm from appearing or expanding.

An aneurysm leads to increased preload and afterload, and a double mortality for the same EF.[142] LV aneurysm occurs in 5% of STEMI cases, mainly anteroapical STEMI (80% of LV aneurysms are anteroapical; the rest are inferoposterior). LV aneurysm may initiate or worsen: (i) HF, (ii) angina (from the adverse loading conditions), (iii) VT, and (iv) mural thrombosis.

The diagnosis is made by echo. ST elevation that persists >3 weeks suggests LV aneurysm, but may also be seen with a dyskinetic, often non-viable wall.

Treatment consists of HF therapy to reverse LV remodeling. Aneurysmectomy is indicated for refractory HF or refractory VT, mainly in conjunction with CABG. Operative mortality is <10%.

B. LV pseudoaneurysm

Pseudoaneurysm is a myocardial rupture that has been concealed by pericardium, organized thrombus and fibrosis. Unlike a true LV aneurysm, the LV pseudoaneurysmal wall does not contain any myocardium. Note that thrombus is layered inside both the LV aneurysm and LV pseudoaneurysm. A pseudoaneurysm may also be seen after trauma or cardiac surgery (especially mitral surgery, at the posterobasal level) (Figure 2.7).

A pseudoaneurysm has a 40–50% risk of progressing to a full rupture, and thus warrants urgent surgical suturing. Rupture often occurs in the first week,[143] but rupture of chronic pseudoaneurysms, even small pseudoaneurysms, has been described.[144] Conversely, a true aneurysm does not rupture (it may, rarely, rupture in the first 2 weeks of MI, but does not rupture later on, once it is fully fibrosed).

The distinction between a true LV aneurysm and a pseudoaneurysm is made by echo: a pseudoaneurysm has a narrow neck with a neck-to-internal diameter ratio <0.5,[145] although occasionally, it can be 0.5–1.[143] Doppler may also support the diagnosis of pseudoaneurysm

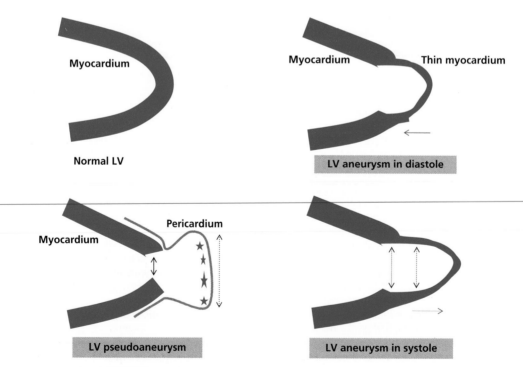

Figure 2.7 LV aneurysm and LV pseudoaneurysm.

In comparison with the normal LV, note the bulging pocket seen in LV aneurysm and LV pseudoaneurysm. The aneurysmal wall consists of thin scarred myocardium ± clot, whereas the pseudoaneurysmal wall consists of adherent pericardium and clot (*stars*). The neck of the LV pseudoaneurysm is narrow; the neck/internal diameter ratio is <0.5 in pseudoaneurysm vs. >0.5, usually 0.8–1, in aneurysm (ratio of *double arrows*). The dyskinetic motion of the aneurysm is indicated by the *horizontal arrows*.

by showing a to-and-fro turbulent flow through the narrow neck, which corresponds to a murmur on exam. However, echo-Doppler does not always allow this distinction. MRI may be used in equivocal cases and shows loss of epicardial fat across the pseudoaneurysm.

Left ventriculography is also highly accurate in distinguishing an aneurysm from a pseudoaneurysm.[143] In case of a pseudoaneurysm, it shows a pocket with a contrast stain that persists over multiple beats. Moreover, in contrast with a true aneurysm, the coronary arteries do not extend over the pseudoaneurysmal wall.

VII. Pericardial complications

A. Acute post-infarction pericarditis
In the reperfusion era, inflammatory pericarditis occurs in ~5% of STEMIs, usually large or anterior STEMIs (it was more common in the pre-reperfusion era, ~10–20%). Less commonly, it may occur in large NSTEMIs. The incidence may be higher if only pericarditic chest pain is used to define post-infarction pericarditis, without mandating a rub.[146] On the other hand, asymptomatic rubs are also common in the first 48 hours of MI. Pericarditis, including asymptomatic rub, correlates with a larger MI size, and thus carries a worse prognosis despite being innocuous per se.

A minimal or small pericardial effusion is seen in up to a third of patients with MI.[147] *Pericarditis and pericardial effusion do not necessarily coincide.* Over half of pericarditis cases are not associated with any effusion; similarly, half of pericardial effusions are not inflammatory (no rub), and rather result from pump failure and transudation.[147]

1. *Diagnosis* – Pericarditis develops in the first few days of MI, most commonly the first or second day, and usually lasts a few days only. The pain is typically pleuritic, and radiation to the trapezius is characteristic. A fleeting rub may be heard. On ECG, a pattern of diffuse pericarditis with diffuse ST elevation is rare (<20%);[146] rather, pericarditis is localized to the infarcted area with ECG findings of localized ST elevation. The latter may simulate reinfarction or may be overshadowed by the pre-existing ST elevation. *The persistence of upright T waves or the reversal from inverted T waves to upright T waves very early after MI* is 100% sensitive for the diagnosis of pericarditis, but may also be seen with ischemia (normally, inverted T waves are seen a few hours after MI onset, and persist several days at least).[148]

2. *Treatment* – NSAIDs should not be used post-MI because of the risk of adverse LV remodeling and free wall rupture. High-dose aspirin (325–650 mg Q 6–8 h) may be used; alternatively, acetaminophen or colchicine may be used for this transient process.

The risk of hemorrhagic transformation of acute post-MI pericarditis is theoretical and very rarely reported. Thus, pericarditis should not alter the antiplatelet regimen and anticoagulation may be continued in patients who need it, with close monitoring. However, in the presence of a moderate or large effusion, anticoagulants should be discontinued (antiplatelet agents are usually continued).

B. Pericardial effusion
Small pericardial effusions (5–9 mm) are seen in 5% of STEMIs, usually appearing during the first 5 days and slowly resolving over several weeks.[149,150] A small pericardial effusion may be secondary to pericarditis or to pump failure and may be associated with an increase in long-term mortality. It is not usually associated with a free wall rupture unless it progresses to a moderate effusion, which happens in a minority of patients.[150] Echo surveillance is warranted for a small effusion.

Moderate or large pericardial effusions (≥10 mm) were seen in 5% of STEMIs before the reperfusion era, and are probably less common in the PCI era. A moderate pericardial effusion, even asymptomatic, is associated with an 8% risk of death from free wall rupture, which tends to occur over a week late. While it may result from pump failure or pericarditis in some patients, a moderate pericardial effusion represents a sealed, subacute myocardial rupture with self-limited bleeding in a substantial proportion of patients. A large effusion with tamponade or pulseless electrical activity is usually due to free wall rupture and warrants emergent surgical repair. A moderate effusion, if diagnosed on a pre-discharge echo or in a symptomatic patient, warrants at least a more prolonged monitoring, close echo surveillance, and potentially a cardiac MRI to diagnose impending rupture. Anticoagulation should be discontinued.

C. Dressler syndrome or post-cardiac injury syndrome
This nowadays rare syndrome is an inflammatory and likely autoimmune process related to anticardiac antibodies. It occurs 1–8 weeks after MI, and leads to fever, pericarditis, but also pericardial and pleural effusions. It is treated similarly to early post-MI pericarditis.

VIII. LV thrombus and thromboembolic complications
LV thrombus is most common in patients with anteroapical MI, with a 30–40% incidence in the pre-reperfusion era, down to 10% in the thrombolytic era and 5–10% in the PCI era.[151,152] It usually forms in the first week after MI, with at least 25% of thrombi forming in the first 24 hours;[152,153] however, a few thrombi form 1–3 months later. In addition to akinesis, the hypercoagulable state of STEMI promotes the formation of LV thrombi, particularly early LV thrombi. Severe global LV dysfunction is not a prerequisite for LV thrombus formation. LV thrombus may rarely form over a large inferoposterior MI.

In the absence of anticoagulation, LV thrombus is associated with a ~10–15% embolization risk (contrast this risk with the 1% stroke risk in patients without AF or LV thrombus).[154] In one study, all embolic events occurred within 3–4 months of MI. Beyond this period, the thrombus becomes organized and unlikely to embolize.[155] Some studies suggest that a mobile or a pedunculated thrombus bulging in the LV has a higher risk of embolization than a laminated, mural thrombus. More importantly than the pedunculated morphology, AF, severe HF, severe LV dysfunction, and older age are associated with higher embolization rates.[151]

Echo is usually used for diagnosis. However, echo may give a false positive diagnosis because of side lobe artifacts or reverberations from the ribs. On the other hand, MRI studies have shown that echo frequently misses apical thrombi, in up to 50% of the cases, particularly when the thrombus is laminated/flat or when the echo plane does not cut through the true apex. Delayed-enhancement MRI allows an accurate diagnosis and allows the distinction between thrombus and the underlying myocardial scar.[156]

Treatment – Warfarin anticoagulation almost abolishes the embolization risk.[152,154,155] In addition, warfarin allows intrinsic lysis of the thrombus or, at least, organization and endothelialization. In fact, ~50% of LV thrombi resolve within 6–12 months of anticoagulation, while the rest organize and become laminated. It is believed that an organized thrombus actually has beneficial effects, as it adheres to the dyskinetic apex preventing further infarct expansion and reducing the paradoxical myocardial motion by a plugging effect.

Thus, ACC guidelines recommend the use of warfarin for at least 3 months in patients with LV thrombus (class IIa), as most emboli occur within 3–4 months of MI. Warfarin may be continued longer than 3 months in patients who continue to have a low bleeding risk and a high embolic risk, such as: (i) history of embolization with persistent akinesis, (ii) severe HF or severe LV dilatation, (iii) persistently pedunculated thrombus. In the era of dual antiplatelet therapy, the benefit of warfarin on top of antiplatelet therapy is unclear, but warfarin remains justified in patients with LV thrombus and a low bleeding risk, particularly for the first 3 months.

IX. Early and late mortality after STEMI

The short-term mortality (30 days) is, on average, 4–5% for patients treated with primary PCI, 6–7% for patients treated with fibrinolytics, and ~11–12% for patients not treated with reperfusion therapy. This varies according to the risk criteria listed in Section 1.XI (Killip class and TIMI risk score), the ST-segment response to reperfusion therapy, and the coronary microvascular perfusion achieved with reperfusion therapy.

Afterward, the yearly mortality is 2–6% depending on the degree of LV dysfunction, the presence of HF, and the presence and extent of residual ischemia and residual severe CAD.

The risk of sudden death is highest in the first 30 days after MI (1.2%), followed by a 1.2% sudden death risk per year.[86] The risk is higher in patients with HF or severe LV dysfunction (2.5–3%).

Note that NSTEMI and ACS with ST-segment depression have the same short- and long-term mortality as STEMI (but lower in-hospital mortality).[157]

Appendix 1. Out-of-hospital cardiac arrest: role of early coronary angiography and therapeutic hypothermia

Of 100 patients suffering out-of-hospital cardiac arrest (OHCA), ~30–40 are successfully resuscitated in the field with return of spontaneous circulation and reach the hospital. Of those 30–40, ~5–10 survive to hospital discharge (5–10% overall survival).[158] A better survival is seen in patients whose initial rhythm is VF/VT (22% survival to discharge). In patients with VF, the survival decreases by 7–10% for each minute of delay to defibrillation.

A. Role of immediate coronary angiography

Several French investigators performed immediate coronary angiography in cardiac arrest patients without any obvious extracardiac cause of arrest (such as severe sepsis, major bleed, previous respiratory failure, or metabolic abnormalities). Regardless of ECG findings, 50% of patients were found to have an acute coronary occlusion and an additional 20% were found to have significant CAD with complex angiographic features.[159] This translated into an overall CAD prevalence of 70%. The initial arrest rhythm was mostly VT/VF, but PEA and asystole were also included (93% VF, 7% PEA/asystole in one study; 68% VF, 32% PEA/asystole in the PROCAT study).[160] In patients with CAD but no apparent acute occlusion, the cardiac arrest may have resulted from a recanalized coronary thrombosis, coronary spasm, or ischemia without coronary thrombosis.

Patients with CAD who underwent successful PCI of the culprit artery derived a striking survival benefit in comparison with patients who either did not have CAD or did not get revascularized (50–70% survival if revascularized, vs. <30% if not revascularized).

Importantly, in these studies, over 80–90% of survivors had a favorable neurological recovery. Thus, the initial neurological status should not preclude urgent catheterization. In fact, while the survival to hospital discharge is >90% in patients who regain consciousness early on or who display a minimal response, ~50% of patients who are initially unresponsive survive with good neurological recovery.[161,162]

While PCI may not improve neurological outcomes per se, it improves the hemodynamic status and reduces cardiac complications of survivors, as it would in any STEMI or hemodynamically unstable ACS (reduces shock, HF, electrical instability, and mechanical complications). The better outcomes associated with PCI are partly related to PCI itself, but also to the fact that PCI-treated patients have a reversible, cardiac cause of arrest, as opposed to advanced cardiomyopathy or severe non-cardiac comorbidity.

Note that coronary angiography is typically performed in patients who are successfully resuscitated and whose systemic pressure is maintained on reasonable and stable doses of vasopressors. The performance of PCI in patients actively receiving chest compressions, using an external compression device, did not improve the grim mortality in one study and was not recommended in an expert viewpoint.[158,163]

B. Role of post-resuscitation ECG and echocardiography

ST elevation is seen on one-third of post-resuscitation ECGs. However, in the PROCAT study, only 43% of patients with significant CAD (stenosis or occlusion) had ST elevation, <80% of patients with acute coronary occlusion had ST elevation,[159] and 58% of patients without ST elevation had CAD.[160]

Also, 4% (PROCAT) to 20% of patients with ST elevation do not have CAD.[159,162] In those cases, ST elevation is related to a myocardial injury from the cardiac arrest itself, hyperkalemia, PE, or intracranial hemorrhage.

In addition, no difference in survival or favorable neurological function was seen among survivors with or without ST elevation.[158]

Thus, overall, the ECG has a relatively poor predictive value for coronary occlusion. Patients with OHCA and without a clear non-cardiac explanation should undergo immediate coronary angiography regardless of the ECG findings.

Echo findings are not specific. Echo often shows LV dysfunction that is non-specific, as it may be secondary to acute ischemia but also post-cardiac arrest myocardial stunning or chronic cardiomyopathy.

C. No role for thrombolysis during the resuscitation of cardiac arrest

In patients undergoing cardiopulmonary resuscitation for an arrest of presumed cardiac origin, the administration of tenecteplase during resuscitation did not improve the 30-day survival, the return of spontaneous circulation, or the neurological outcome, and increased intracranial hemorrhage. During cardiac arrest, the poor systemic perfusion may preclude the delivery of the lytic agent to its target, explaining the lack of efficacy. Also, bleeding, including intracranial hemorrhage, may be a cause of arrest in a small proportion of patients and is aggravated by thrombolysis.[164] However, after the return of spontaneous circulation in a patient with STEMI, thrombolysis may be appropriate, as suggested by a small analysis.[165]

D. Mild therapeutic hypothermia

Two randomized trials of resuscitated post-cardiac arrest patients have shown that mild therapeutic hypothermia drastically improves survival with appropriate neurological recovery (49% vs. 26% in one trial, 55% vs. 39% in the other trial).[166,167] Based on the inclusion criteria of these trials, patients with the following features have a class I recommendation for hypothermia:

- Patients with VF/VT arrest who had return of spontaneous circulation within 60 minutes of cardiac arrest. Hypothermia may be used in patients with asystole or PEA (less evidence and generally poorer outcomes in comparison to VT/VF).
- Persistent coma with Glasgow Coma scale <8.
- Cardiac arrest is not due to trauma or drug overdose.

Exclusion criteria:

- Persistent hypotension (mean pressure <60 mmHg) despite the use of one vasopressor. The requirement for IABP is not a contraindication.
- Uncontrolled active bleeding or intracranial hemorrhage ± severely abnormal coagulation studies or platelets <50 × 10^9/l.

Patients in the hypothermia protocol should have hypothermia induced as soon as possible after arrival to the emergency department, with a *temperature goal of 32–36 °C within 6 hours after return of spontaneous circulation.* The temperature is reduced by 0.5–1 °C per hour. In one of the trials, hypothermia was initiated as late as several hours after restoration of circulation, and the goal temperature was achieved at a mean of 8 hours (interquartile range, 4–16 hours).[167] However, hypothermia should not be initiated later than 6 hours, as there is probably no benefit beyond this point.

Hypothermia is achieved using ice packs, cold intravenous saline, or a cooling blanket with adjustable settings. The patient is given paralytic agents to prevent the counterproductive shivering during induction of hypothermia. Paralytic agents are not usually necessary once the goal temperature is reached. Sedation is also administered.

Hypothermia is maintained for 24 hours, then the patient is rewarmed very slowly, at a rate no faster than 0.5 °C per hour. Since the patient is sedated, the neurologic prognosis of cardiac arrest patients undergoing hypothermia may not be properly assessed until 72 hours after rewarming.

In the control group of the two major hypothermia trials, the post-arrest temperature was close to 38 °C. A recent study suggested that the mere prevention of this post-arrest hyperthermia with a low normal temperature of 36 °C is as effective as a temperature goal of 33 °C, which was used in the two early trials.[168]

During hypothermia, the patient is monitored for the following side effects:[169]

- Metabolic: hypokalemia (resulting from intracellular K shift), hyperglycemia, mild reduction of GFR, cold-induced diuresis. Hypokalemia should not be aggressively replaced, as severe hyperkalemia may occur during rewarming.
- Bradyarrhythmia, VT.
- Bleeding (coagulation factors are less effective during hypothermia).
- Increased infectious risk; seizures.
- Hypotension is multifactorial in these patients but may be worsened by hypothermia. Hypothermia reduces cardiac output and increases systemic vascular resistance.

> The early initiation of hypothermia does not preclude the early performance of coronary angiography and PCI. The induction of hypothermia prior to or on arrival to the catheterization laboratory has been shown to be safe in several studies.[158] In fact, PCI should be performed urgently, and hypothermia started as soon as possible, preferably before the initiation of PCI (international consensus recommendation).[170] Antithrombotic therapies may also be used and have not significantly increased bleeding risk in hypothermic patients, but the patient should still be carefully monitored for bleeding.[169]

E. Hemodynamic status post cardiac arrest

Hemodynamic instability after a cardiac arrest may be secondary to myocardial infarction, myocardial stunning that results from the arrest itself, or post-cardiac arrest syndrome, which is a form of systemic inflammatory response syndrome (SIRS) with systemic vasodilatation similar to sepsis. Post-cardiac arrest syndrome is managed similarly to sepsis with an early goal-directed therapy. The SBP goal is usually >90 mmHg; one study has shown that a mean blood pressure >70 mmHg in the first 6 hours is associated with better neurological outcomes.[171] 1–2 liters of normal saline is initially administered, followed by dopamine or norepinephrine.

QUESTIONS AND ANSWERS

Question 1. A 52-year-old man presents to a non-PCI hospital with 2 hours of chest pain. His ECG shows anterior ST-segment elevation. His blood pressure is 109/67 and his heart rate is 105. He has no known contraindication to thrombolysis. The closest PCI hospital is 90 miles away and no community transfer system is in place. The best reperfusion strategy for this patient is:
A. No administration of thrombolysis. Transfer for primary PCI
B. Immediate thrombolysis and immediate transfer to a PCI hospital for consideration of routine early PCI within 24 hours of presentation or for rescue PCI if thrombolysis fails
C. Immediate thrombolysis. Transfer to the PCI center only if thrombolysis fails at 90 min after starting therapy
D. Administer aspirin, heparin and clopidogrel 300 mg before transfer
E. B and D
F. C and D

Question 2. A 49-year-old man presents with progressive dyspnea over the last week. He recalls having 2 hours of mild chest discomfort and nausea 10 days ago. No chest pain is currently reported. His ECG shows anterior Q waves with 1 mm ST elevation and T inversion. The exam and X-ray suggest pulmonary edema. The echo shows anteroapical akinesis and thinning. Beside diuresis and medical therapy, what is the appropriate management?
A. Coronary angiography emergently
B. Coronary angiography is not urgent but should be performed before discharge. Attempt to open an occluded LAD
C. Perform stress SPECT before discharge, then perform coronary angiography only if there is evidence of severe ischemia
D. Test for viability of anterior wall. If viable, perform coronary angiography and attempt to open an occluded LAD

Question 3. A 76-year-old female presents with 2 hours of chest pain to a non-PCI hospital. The closest PCI hospital is 100 miles away. ECG shows anterior ST-segment elevation. BP = 170/85, weight 62 kg. She has not had any recent bleed, surgery, fall, or history of stroke. A recent hemoglobin is 12 g/dl. What is the next step?
A. Administer fibrinolytics then transfer for routine early PCI
B. Do not administer fibrinolytics, transfer for primary PCI

Question 4. A 72-year-old man presents with 3–4 hours of chest pain and respiratory distress. BP = 80/60, heart rate = 120. He is intubated by paramedics and transferred to a non-PCI-capable hospital. ECG shows 5 mm ST elevation anterior leads. The closest cath lab is 3 hours away. What is the next step?
A. Emergent transfer for PCI; thrombolysis is not helpful in cardiogenic shock
B. Thrombolysis and emergent transfer for PCI
C. IABP and emergent transfer
D. Thrombolysis, IABP, and emergent transfer for PCI

Question 5. The patient in Question 4 arrives to the cath lab. He still has ST elevation and is in shock. He is found to have thrombotic 100% proximal LAD, CTO of mid RCA, and 80% stenosis of mid LCx. What is the next step?
A. PCI of LAD only
B. PCI of LAD and LCx
C. PCI of LAD initially. If no hemodynamic improvement, proceed with PCI of LCx
D. Emergent CABG

Question 6. A 68-year-old man presents with inferior and lateral STEMI. He undergoes primary PCI of a large, thrombotic, codominant proximal LCx. While he has been doing well, he suddenly becomes near-syncopal on day 2. BP 70/40, pulse 35, and no murmur is heard. ECG shows sinus bradycardia with re-elevation of ST segments in the inferior leads. What is the most important next step?
A. Immediate coronary angiography ± PCI
B. Immediate echocardiography
C. Immediate placement of a transvenous pacemaker

Question 7. A 57-year-old man presented with anterior STEMI and received primary PCI of the proximal LAD at 16 hours after pain onset. At day 3, the patient is doing well, ambulating without angina and no HF on exam. He had an asymptomatic 14-beat run of NSVT. At day 4, a pre-discharge echo is performed and shows a large area of anterior akinesis with LVEF 25%, mild MR, and moderate size (1 cm) pericardial effusion. What is the next step?
A. Discharge home on ACE-I, carvedilol, spironolactone, statin, aspirin/plavix, and check echo in 40 days. If EF <35% → ICD
B. Discharge home on ACE-I, carvedilol, statin, aspirin and plavix, and check echo in 40 days. If EF <35% → ICD
C. Monitor the patient in the hospital for a longer period of time, repeat echo next day and obtain cardiac MRI.
D. Discharge home on ACE-I, carvedilol, statin, aspirin/plavix. Place a lifevest and then ICD at 40 days if EF <35%

Question 8. A 64-year-old man presents with anterior STEMI, BP 105/75, pulse 110, and bibasilar crackles. He is found to have occluded LAD and mid RCA 80%. What is the next step?
A. Perform multivessel PCI at the time of primary PCI
B. Perform culprit PCI only. Plan for elective PCI of RCA only if the patient has residual angina
C. Perform LAD PCI, then plan for elective RCA PCI before home discharge, regardless of symptoms
D. Perform LAD PCI, then plan for elective RCA angiography before home discharge, then RCA PCI if appropriate, regardless of symptoms

Question 9. A 70-year old female had chest pain 3 days previously. The chest pain resolved after 8 hours. She has syncope on the day of presentation and is currently dizzy and dyspneic. BP 80/60, pulse 30 bpm. ECG shows complete AV block with ventricular escape rhythm, and ST elevation concordant with the wide QRS in the anterolateral leads suggestive of STEMI (even though the rhythm is a ventricular rhythm). She has bibasilar crackles and is hypoxic. What is the 30-day mortality of this patient?

A. <10%

B. 20%

C. 50%

Question 10. For the patient in Question 9, what is the next step?

A. Place a temporary pacemaker and take emergently to the catheterization laboratory for PCI of LAD

B. Place a temporary pacemaker. Take to the catheterization laboratory if shock persists

C. Place a temporary pacemaker. Do not take to the catheterization laboratory as PCI later than 24 hours after an infarct is not beneficial

Question 11. For the patient in Question 9, a temporary pacemaker is placed. Her BP improves to 110/70, and she is not dizzy anymore. She is dyspneic at rest with bibasilar crackles on exam. What is the next step, beside starting diuretics?

A. Take urgently to the cath lab for PCI of LAD

B. Perform coronary angiography after HF improves

C. Perform stress testing after HF improves, to assess for residual ischemia

Question 12. A 66-year-old man presents with chest pain that has lasted 3 hours earlier today and has now resolved. His ECG shows subtle ST elevation (<1 mm) in leads II, aVF and in leads V_5 and V_6 (Figure 2.2). Should he undergo emergent reperfusion?

A. No emergent reperfusion

B. Emergent reperfusion with PCI

C. Emergent reperfusion with thrombolysis

D. B or C

Question 13. A 50-year-old woman presents with a persistent, mild chest pain for the last 6 hours. Chest pain fully resolves after nitroglycerin administration. The ECG performed after pain resolution is shown (Figure 2.8). What is the next step?

A. Perform coronary angiography/PCI next day (not urgent anymore)

B. Perform emergent reperfusion, whether with thrombolysis or PCI

C. Obtain serial troponin levels, as the ECG is not definite for MI

Question 14. A 72-year-old man presents with waxing and waning episodes of resting chest pain for the last 10 hours. Chest pain is reproducible with palpation and the patient does not appear to be in distress. He is not actively having chest pain. The first troponin is 0.03 ng/ml. ECG is shown (Figure 2.9). What is the next step?

A. Emergent reperfusion with PCI

B. Emergent reperfusion with thrombolysis

C. Follow serial cardiac markers (ECG non-diagnostic)

D. Initiate antiplatelet therapy, heparin, and NTG and perform non-urgent coronary angiography (next day)

Question 15. A 66-year-old woman presents with anterior STEMI. She receives thrombolysis at a non-PCI hospital, with resolution of chest pain and >50% resolution of ST elevation. She had a mild degree of pulmonary edema on admission, which quickly responded to diuresis. Echo shows severe anterior hypokinesis with LVEF of 35%. Three days later, she is able to ambulate without chest pain and with a mild degree of dyspnea. What is the next step?

A. Coronary angiography

B. Treadmill nuclear imaging (modified Bruce protocol)

C. Pharmacological nuclear imaging

D. Continue medical therapy without any further intervention

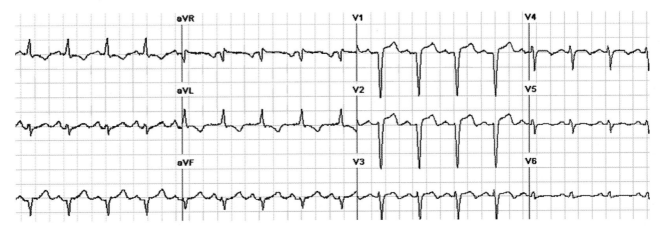

Figure 2.8

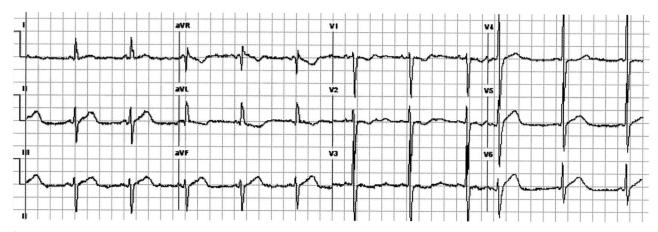

Figure 2.9

Question 16. A 67-year-old man presents with chest pain that started 45 minutes ago. His ECG shows 5 mm anterior ST elevation with ample T waves and no Q waves. His BP is 130/75, pulse is 105 bpm. He can be transferred for PCI with a DTB <90 minutes. Which reperfusion strategy achieves the lowest mortality?
A. Primary PCI
B. Thrombolysis
C. Thrombolysis followed by routine PCI 3–24 hours later
D. Any of the above

Question 17. A patient presents with chest pain. ECG shows a new LBBB, severe discordant ST elevation in the anterior leads (>25% of S wave) and concordant ST elevation in the lateral leads. Which statement is incorrect?
A. The left bundle receives dual arterial supply, hence LBBB rarely occurs in STEMI
B. LBBB implies a high-risk STEMI with extensive infarction and extensive CAD
C. LBBB is associated with 3–4 times higher mortality and a more drastic benefit from reperfusion
D. LBBB is associated with increased mortality only when persistent
E. A new LBBB is associated with a higher mortality than a new RBBB
F. A new RBBB is usually seen with LAD-related infarct

Question 18. Which statement is incorrect?
A. LV pseudoaneurysm has a neck to internal diameter ratio <0.5 (vs. >0.5 in LV aneurysm)
B. LV pseudoaneurysm may be characterized by to-and-fro flow on Doppler and a murmur on exam (not present with aneurysm)
C. MRI may help differentiate pseudoaneurysm from aneurysm in equivocal cases
D. Left ventriculogram does not help differentiate pseudoaneurysm from aneurysm
E. Post-MI pericarditis often occurs in the 1st or 2nd day and implies a large MI
F. A persistently upright T wave (lack of T inversion) or a reversal of T wave from an inverted to an upright position is 100% sensitive for post-MI pericarditis

Question 19. A 68-year-old man presents with chest pain. He is dizzy and weak. Blood pressure is 80/55 and pulse is 55 bpm. JVP is 5 cmH$_2$O and lungs are clear. ECG shows sinus rhythm with 2:1 AV block and a ventricular rate of 55 bpm, along with inferior ST elevation. What is the immediate next step?
A. IV fluids
B. IV fluids + dopamine
C. IV fluids + atropine
D. Atropine + transvenous pacing + IV fluids
E. Primary PCI
F. IABP followed by primary PCI

Question 20. The patient in Question 19 receives atropine and a fluid bolus. AV conduction improves and heart rate is 100 bpm. He remains hypotensive and dizzy. Peripheral O$_2$ saturation is 94% on ambient air. No murmur or thrill is present. What is the most likely diagnosis?
A. RV MI shock
B. Mechanical complication (papillary muscle rupture or ventricular septal rupture)
C. LV shock from an isolated inferior MI
D. LV shock from inferior MI extending to the lateral wall or inferior MI associated with an old anterior MI

Question 21. The patient in Question 19 now has a JVP of 12 cmH$_2$O. What is the next step?
A. Administer another 500 ml IV fluid bolus. If he remains hypotensive, add dopamine
B. Administer another 500 ml IV fluid bolus. If he remains hypotensive, add norepinephrine

C. Primary PCI

D. IABP followed by primary PCI

E. B + C

F. B + D

Question 22. With the administration of more fluids, the patient in Question 19 now develops arterial desaturation (85%), which is minimally responsive to supplemental O_2. His lungs are still clear and no murmur is heard. What is the most likely cause?

A. Ventricular septal rupture

B. Patent foramen ovale

C. Severe MR

D. LV failure

Question 23. A 67-year-old woman had severe nausea 2 days ago. This was followed by dyspnea and cough. On presentation, she is hypotensive (90/45 mmHg) and has respiratory distress with lung crackles and orthopnea. A holosystolic mumur is heard with S3 and without a thrill. ECG shows lateral ST elevation of 1 mm in leads I and aVL. She later develops fever. What is the most likely diagnosis?

A. Cardiogenic shock from extensive infarction

B. RV shock

C. Posterior papillary muscle rupture

D. Anterior papillary muscle rupture

E. Septic shock

F. C + E

G. D + E

Answer 1. E (Section 1.VI.F).

Answer 2. C (Section 1.VII). This is a patient presenting with Q-wave MI >24 hours after MI onset without residual angina. Stress test may be performed and angiography ± revascularization performed only in the presence of severe residual ischemia in the infarcted territory. Alternatively, angiography may be performed first (class II): (i) if left main or three-vessel CAD is found, CABG may be considered on a non-urgent basis (>3–7 days after MI); (ii) if the culprit is not totally occluded, PCI may be performed (class IIb); (iii) if the culprit is totally occluded, PCI should not be immediately performed. Stress testing should be performed and the patient brought back for PCI if severe ischemia is present. Viability is different from ischemia. It is important to document that the wall is ischemic with stress, not just viable. A moderate viability without documented ischemia is not a clear indication to revascularize. Ischemia is documented clinically (angina), by ECG (ST depression), or by reduction of nuclear uptake at stress.

Answer 3. B (Section 1.VI.B). This patient has a combination of four features (elderly small woman with HTN). The combination predicts >4% risk of intracranial hemorrhage with fibrinolytics.

Answer 4. D (Section 2.I.C). Thrombolysis improved survival in the medically treated arm of the SHOCK trial and in all arms of the SHOCK registry. The insertion of IABP was part of the protocol of the SHOCK trial and was associated with better outcomes in the SHOCK registry (although recent data question its benefit).

Answer 5. D (Section 2.I.C). Full revascularization should be attempted in a patient with cardiogenic shock, rather than PCI of the culprit only. Answer C is reasonable at institutions where emergent CABG cannot be promptly performed, which is commonly the case.

Answer 6. B. The presentation is consistent with free wall rupture. Stent thrombosis is a second possibility. Echocardiography is immediately followed by pericardiocentesis and surgical correction if the diagnosis of myocardial rupture/tamponade is confirmed.

Answer 7. C. A moderate pericardial effusion is concerning for a sealed cardiac rupture (in at least 8% of the cases) and warrants further observation and MRI if possible. Late NSVT, while carrying a worse prognosis, does not, per se, change management and does not dictate earlier ICD or Lifevest placement.

Answer 8. D (Section 1.VIII.B). Non-culprit lesions are generally revascularized electively, even in the absence of angina. They are preferably revascularized before discharge, even more so in the presence of critical disease or low level of angina. Non-critical lesions may improve on subsequent angiograms; thus, before elective revascularization of these lesions in asymptomatic patients, the lesion is reassessed on repeat angiography and non-culprit FFR performed. LAD PCI followed by elective stress testing would also be an appropriate answer to this question.

Answer 9. C. AV block in anterior MI indicates extensive anterior infarction. The patient likely has multivessel disease preventing collateral supply to the left bundle. In the pre-reperfusion era, the mortality of complete AV block in anterior MI was ≥50%. Also, a shock that persists with pacing (Killip IV) portends a mortality of ≥50%.

Answer 10. B. She may be in shock because of bradyarrhythmia. Cardiogenic shock qualifies for emergent reperfusion regardless of the time of presentation, as long as it is not purely secondary to the bradyarrhythmia (a purely bradycardic shock was excluded from the SHOCK trial).

Answer 11. B (Section 1.VII). Since the patient does not have cardiogenic shock or massive HF, there is no indication for emergent PCI >24 hours after the infarct. Massive HF is defined as Killip class III, i.e., massive pulmonary edema frequently requiring mechanical ventilation. **A persistent severe HF, however, prevents the patient from receiving stress testing and was an exclusion criterion in the OAT trial, the trial wherein late post-STEMI PCI was not beneficial.** A patient with persistent severe HF qualifies for coronary angiography after diuresis and stabilization (non-urgently, e.g., after 24 hours of diuresis), and may benefit from late revascularization. A patient who stabilizes and becomes ambulatory without severe HF qualifies for risk stratification with stress testing, in which case angiography and PCI are only performed if severe ischemia is documented.

Answer 12. B. STEMI may be over 12–24 hours old, at a stage where ST-segment elevation is resolving but has not fully resolved yet (close to phase 3). Alternatively, STEMI may be more recent with ongoing or resolving ischemia. This patient does not qualify for fibrinolytics, as ST elevation is <1 mm and the occlusion duration is questionable, but qualifies for primary PCI if the discomfort is ongoing, or if the discomfort occurred within the last 24 hours, even if it is not ongoing.

Answer 13. B. The ECG shows persistent ST elevation in leads V_1–V_4. ST elevation is barely 2 mm, but the morphology is typical of STEMI (terminal T inversion, reciprocal ST depression in I–aVL, and lack of alternative explanation of the mild ST elevation in V_1–V_3, i.e., no LVH/LBBB). Even if chest pain resolves, a persistent ST elevation along with a presentation <12 hours qualifies the patient for primary PCI or thrombolysis.

Answer 14. A. The ECG shows subtle signs of inferior, lateral, and posterior ST elevation injury. In fact, the isolated ST depression in leads V_1–V_3 implies posterior ST elevation. The ST segment is minimally elevated in the inferior leads and in leads V_5 and V_6 (~0.5 mm), but has a strikingly convex morphology with a wide hyperacute T wave, particularly evident on the aberrant beat. Also, reciprocal ST depression is seen in lead aVL. All this confirms that the ECG, while subtle, is definitely consistent with ST elevation injury. Being <1 mm, thrombolysis is not justified. Emergent PCI is warranted even if pain resolved (presentation within 24 hours). In reality, this patient was not emergently reperfused, his troponin ended up peaking at 76 ng/ml, and he was found to have subtotal OM occlusion.

Answer 15. B. The patient would have best been treated with early coronary angiography and PCI at 3–24 hours after thrombolysis. Beyond 24 hours, coronary angiography has a weak recommendation (class IIb) in the absence of recurrent pain or persistent HF (the patient only had transient HF on admission). Coronary angiography may be performed; however, stress testing has a higher recommendation. Exercise testing is preferred as the patient is able to ambulate.

Answer 16. D. In the first 3 hours of STEMI, especially the first hour, and in the absence of shock, the mortality reduction with thrombolysis is likely equivalent to that of primary PCI, provided that rescue PCI is performed if needed (CAPTIM, PRAGUE [<3 hours subgroup], STREAM trials). If thrombolysis is used as a primary revascularization strategy, outcomes are improved when thrombolysis is followed by routine early PCI (further reduction of recurrent MI in comparison to thrombolysis alone).

Answer 17. E. Both new LBBB and RBBB are associated with a similarly increased mortality. A transient LBBB or RBBB is not associated with increased mortality.

Answer 18. D.

Answer 19. C. The patient is in shock, which is aggravated by the inappropriate heart rate. In shock, compensatory tachycardia is expected, but the 2:1 AV block is cutting the patient's ventricular rate in half. In the first 24 hours of inferior MI, AV block is responsive to atropine. In the context of inferior MI, hypotension with clear lungs suggests hypovolemia or RV shock, so fluid administration is appropriate. Those simple measures are performed while PCI is being arranged.

Answer 20. A. The patient has shock with clear lungs and no hypoxia, which suggests RV shock. Inferior MI does not usually lead to LV shock, unless a mechanical complication occurs or the inferior MI is associated with posterolateral extension or an old anterior MI. The exam does not suggest LV failure or mechanical complication.

Answer 21. E. The most definitive therapy of RV shock is primary PCI. Simultaneously, IV fluids are administered. In acute RV failure, the RV is small and non-compliant, in a way that JVP of 10–15 cmH$_2$O does not preclude fluid challenge; many of the latter patients with elevated JVP may be fluid-responsive. If JVP is elevated and the patient is unresponsive to a fluid challenge, norepinephrine therapy is appropriate (preferred to dopamine). In RV shock, IABP is warranted if high-dose pressors are required despite reperfusion or if LV failure is concomitantly present.

Answer 22. B. Clinically, the patient does not appear to have pulmonary edema. His hypoxemia is likely due to an underlying, previously innocent PFO. With RV failure and fluid resuscitation, the RA pressure rises and causes exaggerated flow through the PFO and a right-to-left shunt with hypoxemia refractory to O$_2$.

Answer 23. G. The patient's nausea represents the true onset of MI (angina-equivalent). Her shock 2 days later is due to a papillary muscle rupture. It is likely that the anterior papillary muscle is ruptured in this patient with non-inferior MI (likely LCx-related MI). The anterior papillary muscle is supplied by both the LCx and the LAD (usually first diagonal); an LCx-related MI may lead to papillary muscle rupture if the LAD also has an underlying stenosis. The infarct associated with papillary muscle rupture may be small, as in this case. The wide pulse pressure and the fever suggest an associated vasodilatory or septic shock, which is seen in 25% of post-MI cardiogenic shock. In this patient, echo is subsequently performed and shows rupture of the anterolateral papillary muscle (echodense mass attached to the leaflets) with flailing of both leaflets and both a central and a posterior jet. SVR is low (~600–700) and cardiac index relatively high, despite MR (~4 l/min/m²), confirming an associated vasodilatory/septic shock.

References

1. O'Gara PT, Kushner FG, Ascheim DD, et al. 2013 ACCF/AHA guideline for the management of ST-elevation myocardial infarction: a report of the American College of Cardiology Foundation/American Heart Association Task Force on Practice Guidelines. J Am Coll Cardiol 2013; 61: e78–140.
2. Steg PG, James SK, Atar D, et al. ESC Guidelines for the management of acute myocardial infarction in patients presenting with ST-segment elevation. Eur Heart J 2012; 33: 2569–619.
3. Thygesen K, Alpert JS, Jaffe AS, et al. Third universal definition of myocardial infarction. ESC/ACCF/AHA/WHF expert consensus. Circulation 2012; 126: 220–35.
4. Kannel WB, Abbott RD. Incidence and prognosis of unrecognized myocardial infarction: an update on the Framingham study. N Engl J Med 1984; 311: 1144–7.
5. Delewi R, Ijff G, van de Hoef TP, et al. Pathological Q waves in myocardial infarction in patients treated by primary PCI. JACC Cardiovasc Imaging 2013; 6: 324–31.
6. Fefer F, Hod H, Hammerman H, et al. Relation of clinically defined spontaneous reperfusion to outcome in ST-elevation myocardial infarction. Am J Cardiol 2009; 103: 149–53. *Also, an analysis of patients with spontaneous ECG reperfusion from ASSENT-4 PCI is concordant with this finding (spontaneous ECG reperfusion defined as ST resolution >70%).*
7. Fibrinolytic Therapy Trialists' (FTT) Collaborative Group. Indications for fibrinolytic therapy in suspected acute myocardial infarction: collaborative overview of early mortality and major morbidity results from all randomised trials of more than 1000 patients. Lancet 1994; 343: 311–22.
8. Strauss DG, Loring Z, Selvester RH, et al. Right, but not left, bundle branch block is associated with large anteroseptal scar. J Am Coll Cardiol 2013; 62: 959–67.
9. Neeland IJ, Kontos MC, de Lemos JA. Evolving considerations in the management of patients with left bundle branch block and suspected myocardial infarction. J Am Coll Cardiol 2012; 60: 96–105.
10. Jain S, Ting HT, Bell M, et al. Utility of left bundle branch block as a diagnostic criterion for acute myocardial infarction. Am J Cardiol 2011; 107: 1111–16.
11. Chang AM, Shofer FS, Tabas JA, Magid DJ, McCusker CM, Hollander JE. Lack of association between left bundle-branch block and acute myocardial infarction in symptomatic ED patients. Am J Emerg Med 2009; 27: 916–21.
12. Rokos IV, Farkouh ME, Reiffel J, et al. Correlation between index electrocardiographic patterns and pre-intervention angiographic findings: Insights from the HORIZONS-AMI trial. Cath Cardiovasc Interv 2012; 79: 1092–8.
13. Smith SW, Dodd KW, Henry TD, et al. Diagnosis of ST-elevation myocardial infarction in the presence of left bundle branch block with the ST-elevation to S-wave ratio in a modified Sgarbossa rule. Ann Emerg Med 2012; 60: 766–76.
14. Boersma E, Maas AC, Deckers JW, Simoons ML. Early thrombolytic treatment in acute myocardial infarction: reappraisal of the golden hour. Lancet 1996; 348: 771–5.
15. Gruppo Italiano per lo Studio della Streptochinasi nell'Infarto Miocardico (GISSI). Effectiveness of intravenous thrombolytic treatment in acute myocardial infarction. Lancet 1986; 1: 397–402.
16. ISIS-2 (Second International Study of Infarct Survival) Collaborative Group. Randomised trial of intravenous streptokinase, oral aspirin, both, or neither among 17,187 cases of suspected acute myocardial infarction: ISIS-2. Lancet 1988; 2: 349–60.
17. Antman EM, Anbe ET, Armstrong PW, et al. ACC/AHA guidelines for the management of patients with ST elevation myocardial infarction. J Am Coll Cardiol 2004; 44: 671–719.
18. GUSTO-I Investigators. An international randomized trial comparing four thrombolytic strategies for acute myocardial infarction. N Engl J Med 1993; 329: 673–82.
19. Ross AM, Coyne KS, Moreyra E, et al. Extended mortality benefit of early postinfarction reperfusion. GUSTO-I Angiographic Investigators. Global Utilization of Streptokinase and Tissue Plasminogen Activator for Occluded Coronary Arteries Trial. Circulation 1998; 97: 1549. *Outcomes of TIMI 2 flow intermediate between TIMI 0/1 and TIMI 3, but closer to TIMI 0/1.*
20. Lincoff AM, Topol EJ, Califf RM, et al. Significance of a coronary artery with thrombolysis in myocardial infarction grade 2 flow 'patency' (outcome in the Thrombolysis and Angioplasty in Myocardial Infarction trials). Am J Cardiol 1995; 75: 871–6. *Intermediate outcomes for TIMI 2 flow (between TIMI 0/1 and TIMI 3).*
21. Reiner JS, Lundergan CF, Fung A, et al. Evolution of early TIMI 2 flow after thrombolysis for acute myocardial infarction. Circulation 1996; 94: 2441–6. *If TIMI 2 flow persists, LV function/wall motion is as poor as TIMI 0–1 flow. IF TIMI 2 flow improves to TIMI 3 flow at 5–7 days, LV function improves, slightly less than TIMI 3 flow.*
22. Assessment of the Safety and Efficacy of a New Thrombolytic (ASSENT-2) Investigators. Single-bolus tenecteplase compared with front-loaded alteplase in acute myocardial infarction: the ASSENT-2 double-blind randomised trial. Lancet 1999; 354: 716–22.

PCI vs. thrombolysis, DTB time

23. Keeley EC, Boura JA, Grines CL. Primary angioplasty versus intravenous thrombolytic therapy for acute myocardial infarction: a quantitative review of 23 randomised trials. Lancet 2003; 361: 13–20.
24. Andersen HR, Nielsen TT, Rasmussen K, et al. A comparison of coronary angioplasty with fibrinolytic therapy in acute myocardial infarction. N Engl J Med 2003; 349: 733–42. *DANAMI-2 trial.*
25. Grines CL, Browne KF, Marco J, et al. A comparison of immediate angioplasty with thrombolytic therapy for acute myocardial infarction. The Primary Angioplasty in Myocardial Infarction Study Group. N Engl J Med 1993; 328: 673–9. *PAMI trial.*
26. Widimský P, Budesínský T, Vorác D, et al. Long distance transport for primary angioplasty vs immediate thrombolysis in acute myocardial infarction. Final results of the randomized national multicentre trial: PRAGUE-2. Eur Heart J 2003; 24: 94–104.
27. Steg PG, Bonnefoy E, Chabaud S, et al. Comparison of Angioplasty and Prehospital Thrombolysis in Acute Myocardial infarction (CAPTIM) Investigators. Impact of time to treatment on mortality after prehospital fibrinolysis or primary angioplasty: data from the CAPTIM randomized clinical trial. Circulation 2003; 108: 2851–6.
28. Armstrong PW, Gershlick AH, Goldstein P, et al. Fibrinolysis or primary PCI in ST-segment elevation myocardial infarction. N Engl J Med 2013; 368: 1379–87. *STREAM trial: PCI vs. TNK in patients presenting <3 h, with expected DTB >60 min (appears though that the mean PCI delay was ~78 min, i.e., not severely delayed, DTB close to 90 min). PCI and TNK were equivalent, trend toward less HF and shock with TNK, more bleeding in TNK (mainly if age >75). By design, most patients were randomized in the ambulance and transferred to PCI-capable hospital. Routine early PCI was performed in all TNK patients, at a median of 17 h.*

29. Pinto DS, Kirtane AJ, Nallamothu BK, et al. Hospital delays in reperfusion for ST-elevation myocardial infarction: implications when selecting a reperfusion strategy. Circulation 2006; 114: 2019–25.

30. Boersma E. Primary Coronary Angioplasty vs Thrombolysis Group. Does time matter? A pooled analysis of randomized clinical trials comparing primary percutaneous coronary intervention and in-hospital fibrinolysis in acute myocardial infarction patients. Eur Heart J 2006; 27: 779–88.

31. Brodie BR, Gersh BJ, Stuckey TD, et al. When is door-to-balloon time critical? Analysis From the HORIZONS-AMI (Harmonizing Outcomes with Revascularization and Stents in Acute Myocardial Infarction) and CADILLAC (Controlled Abciximab and Device Investigation to Lower Late Angioplasty Complications) trials. J Am Coll Cardiol 2010; 56: 407–13.

32. Brodie BR, Hansen C, Stuckey TD, et al. Door-to-balloon time with primary percutaneous coronary intervention for acute myocardial infarction impacts late cardiac mortality in high-risk patients and patients presenting early after the onset of symptoms J Am Coll Cardiol 2006; 47: 289–95.

33. Rathore SS, Curtis JP, Chen J, et al. Association of door-to-balloon time and mortality in patients admitted to hospital with ST elevation myocardial infarction: national cohort study. BMJ 2009; 338: b1807.

34. Thiemann DR, Coresh J, Schulman SP, et al. Lack of benefit for intravenous thrombolysis in patients with myocardial infarction who are older than 75 years. Circulation 2000; 101: 2239–46.

Combined PCI–thrombolysis. Management in non-PCI hospitals with expected PCI delays

35. Hanna EB, Hennebry TA, Abu-fadel MS. Combined reperfusion strategies in patients with ST-segment elevation myocardial infarction: Rationale and current role. Clev Clin J Med 2010; 77: 629–39.

36. Assessment of the Safety and Efficacy of a New Treatment Strategy with Percutaneous Coronary Intervention (ASSENT-4 PCI) investigators. Primary versus tenecteplase-facilitated percutaneous coronary intervention in patients with ST-segment elevation acute myocardial infarction (ASSENT-4 PCI): randomised trial. Lancet 2006; 367: 569–78.

37. Ellis SG, Tendera M, de Belder MA, et al; FINESSE Investigators. Facilitated PCI in patients with ST-elevation myocardial infarction. N Engl J Med 2008; 358: 2205–17.

38. Cantor WJ, Fitchett D, Borgundvaag B, et al; TRANSFER-AMI Trial Investigators. Routine early angioplasty after fibrinolysis for acute myocardial infarction. N Engl J Med 2009; 360: 2705–18.

39. Di Mario C, Dudek D, Piscione F, et al; CARESS-in-AMI Investigators. Immediate angioplasty versus standard therapy with rescue angioplasty after thrombolysis in the Combined Abciximab REteplase Stent Study in Acute Myocardial Infarction (CARESS-in-AMI): an open, prospective, randomised, multicentre trial. Lancet 2008; 371: 559–68.

40. Bøhmer E, Hoffmann P, Abdelnoor M, Arnesen H, Halvorsen S. Efficacy and safety of immediate angioplasty versus ischemia-guided management after thrombolysis in acute myocardial infarction in areas with very long transfer distances results of the NORDISTEMI. J Am Coll Cardiol 2010; 55: 102–10.

41. Carver A, Rafelt S, Gershlick AH, et al. Longer-term follow-up of patients recruited to the REACT (Rescue Angioplasty Versus Conservative Treatment or Repeat Thrombolysis) trial. J Am Coll Cardiol 2009; 54: 118–26.

42. Henry TD, Sharkey SW, Burke MN, et al. A regional system to provide timely access to percutaneous coronary intervention for ST-elevation infarction. Circulation 2007; 116: 721–8.

43. Danchin N, Coste P, Ferrières J, et al. FAST-MI Investigators. Comparison of thrombolysis followed by broad use of percutaneous coronary intervention with primary percutaneous coronary intervention for ST-segment-elevation acute myocardial infarction: data from the French registry on Acute ST-elevation Myocardial Infarction (FAST-MI). Circulation 2008; 118: 268–76.

44. Björklund E, Stenestrand U, Lindbäck J, et al. Pre-hospital thrombolysis delivered by paramedics is associated with reduced time delay and mortality in ambulance-transported real-life patients with ST-elevation myocardial infarction. Eur Heart J 2006; 27: 1146–52.

OAT and late presenters

45. Hochman JS, Lamas GA, Buller CE, et al. Coronary intervention for persistent occlusion after myocardial infarction. N Engl J Med 2006; 355: 2395–407. *OAT trial.*

46. Menon V, Pearte CA, Buller CE, et al. Lack of benefit from percutaneous intervention of persistently occluded infarct arteries after the acute phase of myocardial infarction is time dependent: insights from Occluded Artery Trial. Eur Heart J 2009; 30: 183–91.

47. Schdmig A, Mehilli J, Antoniucci D, et al.; Beyond 12 hours Reperfusion AlternatiVe Evaluation (BRAVE-2) Trial Investigators. Mechanical reperfusion in patients with acute myocardial infarction presenting more than 12 hours from symptom onset: a randomized controlled trial. JAMA 2005; 293: 2865–72. *In this study, late reperfusion 12–48 h improved LV infarct size. ~50% of these patients had subtotal occlusion, mostly with TIMI 2–3 flow.*

48. Busk M, Kaltoft A, Nielsen SS, et al. Infarct size and myocardial salvage after primary angioplasty in patients presenting with symptoms for <12 h vs. 12–72 h. Eur Heart J 2009; 30: 1322–30. *When the infarct artery is patent (TIMI 1–3), late presenters >12 h derive the same percent salvage of the infracted territory as early presenters <12 h.*

49. Sim DS, Jeong MH, Ahn Y, et al. Benefit of percutaneous coronary intervention in early latecomers with acute ST-segment elevation myocardial infarction. Am J Cardiol 2012; 110: 1275–81.

50. Udelson JE, Pearte CA, Kimmelstiel CD, et al. The occluded artery trial (OAT) viability ancillary study (OAT-NUC): impact of infarct zone viability on left ventricular remodeling after percutaneous coronary intervention versus optimal medical therapy alone. Am Heart J 2011; 161: 611–21.

51. Erne P, Schoenenberger AW, Burchkardt D, et al. Effects of percutaneous coronary interventions in silent ischemia after myocardial infarction. The SWISSI 2 randomized controlled trial. JAMA 2007; 297: 1985–91.

PCI flow

52. Montalescot G, Barragan P, Wittenberg O; ADMIRAL Investigators. Platelet glycoprotein IIb/IIIa inhibition with coronary stenting for acute myocardial infarction. N Engl J Med 2001; 344: 1895–903.

53. Stone G.W., Grines C.L., Cox D.A.; CADILLAC Investigators. Comparison of angioplasty with stenting, with or without abciximab, in acute myocardial infarction. N Engl J Med 2002; 346: 957–66.

54. Stone GW, Witzenbichler B., Guagliumi G., et al.; HORIZONS-AMI Trial Investigators Paclitaxel-eluting stents versus bare-metal stents in acute myocardial infarction. N Engl J Med 2009: 360: 1946–59.

55. Jolly SS, Cairns JA, Yusuf S, et al. Randomized trial of primary PCI with or without routine manual thrombectomy. N Engl J Med 2015; 372: 1389–98. *TOTAL trial. In contrast to the TAPAS trial, the TASTE and TOTAL trials did not show any clinical benefit of the routine use of thrombectomy.*

56. Gibson CM, Cannon CP, Murphy SA, et al.; TIMI Study Group. Relationship of the TIMI myocardial perfusion grades, flow grades, frame count, and percutaneous coronary intervention to long-term outcomes after thrombolytic administration in acute myocardial infarction. Circulation 2002; 105: 1909–13.

57. Sorajja P, Gersh BJ, Costantini C, et al. Combined prognostic utility of ST-segment recovery and myocardial blush after primary percutaneous coronary intervention in acute myocardial infarction. Eur Heart J 2005; 26: 667–74.

58. Marshall JC, Waxman HL, Sauerwein A. Frequency of low-grade residual coronary stenosis after thrombolysis during acute myocardial infarction. Am J Cardiol 1990; 66: 773–8.

59. Holmes D, Lerman A, Moreno PR, et al. Diagnosis and management of STEMI arising from plaque erosion. JACC Cardiovasc Imaging 2013; 6: 290–6.

Multivessel CAD, PCI, and CABG in STEMI

60. Goldstein JA, Demetriou D, Grines CL, et al. Multiple complex coronary plaques in patients with acute myocardial infarction. N Engl J Med 2000; 343: 915–22.

61. Vlaar PJ, Mahmoud KD, Holmes DR, et al. Culprit vessel only versus multivessel and staged percutaneous coronary intervention for multivessel disease in patients presenting with ST-segment elevation myocardial infarction. J Am Coll Cardiol 2011; 58: 692–703. *Meta-analysis of staged PCI for non-culprit arteries after STEMI, non-culprit PCI was performed anywhere between index admission and 2 months.*

62. Hannan EL, Samadashvili Z, Walford G. Culprit vessel percutaneous coronary intervention versus multivessel and staged percutaneous coronary intervention for ST-segment elevation myocardial infarction patients with multivessel disease. JACC Cardiovasc Interv 2010; 3: 22–31.

63. Wiviott SD, Braunwald E, McCabe CH, et al. Prasugrel versus clopidogrel in patients with acute coronary syndromes. N Engl J Med 2007; 357: 2001–15.

64. Hochman JS, Sleeper LA, Webb JG, et al.; Should We Emergently Revascularize Occluded Coronaries for Cardiogenic Shock (SHOCK) Investigators. Early revascularization in acute myocardial infarction complicated by cardiogenic shock. N Engl J Med 1999; 341: 625–34. *SHOCK trial.*

65. Crossman AW, D'Agostino HJ, Geraci SA. Timing of coronary artery bypass graft surgery following acute myocardial infarction: a critical literature review. Clin Cardiol 2002; 25: 406–10.

66. Hanratty CG, Koyama Y, Rasmussen HH, et al. Exaggeration of nonculprit stenosis severity during acute myocardial infarction: implications for immediate multivessel revascularization. J Am Coll Cardiol 2002; 40: 911–16.

Antithrombotics

67. Dangas G, Mehran R, Guagliumi G, et al. Role of clopidogrel loading dose in patients with ST-segment elevation myocardial infarction undergoing primary angioplasty: results from the HORIZONS-AMI trial. J Am Coll Cardiol 2009; 54: 1438–46.

68. Mehilli J, Kastrati A, Schulz S; BRAVE-3 Study Investigators. Abciximab in patients with acute ST-segment-elevation myocardial infarction undergoing primary percutaneous coronary intervention after clopidogrel loading: a randomized double-blind trial. Circulation 2009; 119: 1933–40.

69. Valgimigli M, Frigoli E, Leonardi S, et al. Bivalirudin or unfractionated heparin in acute coronary syncromes. N Engl J Med 2015; 373: 997–1009. *MATRIX trial.*

70. Stone GW, Witzenbichler B, Godlewski J, et al. Intralesional abciximab and thrombus aspiration in patients with large anterior myocardial infarction: one-year results from the INFUSE-AMI trial. Circ Cardiovasc Interv 2013; 6: 527–34.

71. COMMIT collaborative group. Addition of clopidogrel to ASA in 45,852 patients with acute myocardial infarction: randomized placebo controlled trial. COMMIT. Lancet 2005; 366: 1607–21.

72. Sabatine MS, Cannon CP, Gibson CM, et al, for the CLARITY-TIMI 28 Investigators. Addition of clopidogrel to aspirin and fibrinolytic therapy for myocardial infarction with ST-segment elevation. N Engl J Med 2005; 352: 1179–89.

73. Yusuf S, Mehta SR, Chrolavicius S, et al. Effects of fondaparinux on mortality and reinfarction in patients with acute ST-segment elevation myocardial infarction: the OASIS-6 randomized trial. JAMA 2006; 295: 1519–30.

74. Antman EM, Morrow DA, McCabe CH, et al. Enoxaparin versus unfractionated heparin with fibrinolysis for ST-elevation myocardial infarction. N Engl J Med 2006; 354: 1477–88.

Other acute therapies

75. Freemantle N, Cleland J, Young P, Mason J, Harrison J. Beta blockade after myocardial infarction: systematic review and meta regression analysis. BMJ 1999; 318: 1730–7. *β-Blockers reduce mortality 23% over long-term (6–24 months), not short-term follow-up.*

76. Chen ZM, Pan HC, Chen YP, et al. Early intravenous then oral metoprolol in 45,852 patients with acute myocardial infarction: randomised placebo-controlled trial. Lancet 2005; 366: 1622–32. *COMMIT-CCS trial.*

77. CAPRICORN Investigators. Effect of carvedilol on outcome after myocardial infarction in patients with left ventricular dysfunction: the CAPRICORN randomised trial. Lancet 2001; 357: 1385–90.

78. ISIS-4 Collaborative Group. ISIS-4: A randomised factorial trial assessing early oral captopril, oral mononitrate, and intravenous magnesium sulphate in 58050 patients with suspected acute myocardial infarction. Lancet 1995; 345: 669–85.

79. Gruppo Italiano per lo Studio della Sopravvivenza nell'Infarto Miocardico. GISSI-3: effects of lisinopril and transdermal glyceryl trinitrate singly and together on 6-week mortality and ventricular function after acute myocardial infarction. Lancet 1994; 343: 1115–22. *GISSI-3 and ISIS-4 proved a mortality reduction with early initiation of ACE-I in all STEMI patients. Another trial, SAVE trial, proved a more drastic mortaltiy reduction with captopril in MI patients with LV dysfunction.*

80. Deedwania P, Kosiborod M, Barrett E, et al. Hyperglycemia and acute coronary syndrome: a scientific statement from the American Heart Association Diabetes Committee of the Council on Nutrition, Physical Activity, and Metabolism. Circulation 2008; 117: 1610–19.

Early discharge

81. Grines CL, Marsalese DL, Brodie B, et al. Safety and cost-effectiveness of early discharge after primary angioplasty in low risk patients with acute myocardial infarction. PAMI-II Investigators. Primary Angioplasty in Myocardial Infarction. J Am Coll Cardiol 1998; 31: 967–72.

82. Noman A, Zaman AG, Schechter C, et al. Early discharge after primary percutaneous coronary intervention for ST-elevation myocardial infarction. Eur Heart J Acute Cardiovasc Care 2013; 2: 262–9.

83. Jones DA, Rathod KS, Howard JP, et al. Safety and feasibility of hospital discharge 2 days following primary percutaneous intervention for ST-segment elevation myocardial infarction. Heart 2012; 98: 1722–7.

Prognosis

84. Papp A, Bueno H, Gierlotka M, et al. Value of Killip classification first described in 1967 for risk stratification of STEMI and NSTE-ACS in the new millennium. Lessons from the Euro Heart Survey ACS registry. J Am Coll Cardiol 2011; 57: 14: E1062.

85. Morrow DA, Antman EM, Chrlesworth A, et al. TIMI risk score for ST-segment elevation myocardial infarction: A convenient bedside, clinical score for risk assessment at presentation. Circulation 2000; 102: 2031.

ICD

86. Solomon SD, Zelenkofske F, McMurray JJV, et al. Sudden death in patients with myocardial infarction and left ventricular dysfunction, heart failure, or both. N Engl J Med 2005; 352: 2581–8. *Analysis from VALIANT trial; similar results reported by: Adabag AS, Therneau TM, Gersh BJ, et al. Sudden death after myocardial infarction. JAMA 2008; 300: 2022–9.*

87. Hohnloser SH, Kuck KH, Dorian P, et al. Prophylactic use of an implantable cardioverter defibrillator after acute myocardial infarction. N Engl J Med 2004; 351: 2481–8.

88. Steinbeck G, Andresen D, Seidl K, et al. Defibrillator implantation early after myocardial infarction. N Engl J Med 2009; 361: 1427–36. *IRIS trial.*

Shock (+ SHOCK trial, reference 64)

89. Jacobs AK, Leopold JA, Bates E, et al. Cardiogenic shock caused by right ventricular infarction: a report from the SHOCK registry. J Am Coll Cardiol 2003; 41: 1273–9.

90. Hochman JS, Buller CE, Sleeper LA, et al. Cardiogenic shock complicating acute myocardial infarction: etiologies, management and outcome: a report from the SHOCK Trial Registry. J Am Coll Cardiol 2000; 36 (3 Suppl A): 1063–70.

91. Reynolds HR, Hochman JS. Cardiogenic shock: current concepts and improving outcomes. Circulation 2008; 117: 686–97.

92. Yehudai L, Reynolds HR, Schwarz SA, et al. Serial echocardiograms in patients with cardiogenic shock: analysis of the SHOCK Trial. J Am Coll Cardiol 2006; 47 (suppl A): 111A.

93. Kohsaka S, Menon V, Lowe AM, Lange M, Dzavik V, Sleeper LA, Hochman JS. Systemic inflammatory response syndrome after acute myocardial infarction complicated by cardiogenic shock. Arch Intern Med 2005; 165: 1643–50.

94. Hochman JS, Sleeper LA, Webb JG, Dzavik V, Buller CE, Aylward P, Col J, White HD. Early revascularization and long-term survival in cardiogenic shock complicating acute myocardial infarction. JAMA 2006; 295: 2511–15.

95. Singh M, White J, Hasdai D, Hodgson PK, Berger PB, Topol EJ, Califf RM, Holmes DR. Long-term outcome and its predictors among patients with ST-elevation myocardial infarction complicated by shock: insights from the GUSTO-I trial. J Am Coll Cardiol 2007; 50: 1752–8.

96. French JK, Feldman HA, Assmann SF, et al.Influence of thrombolytic therapy, with or without intra-aortic balloon counterpulsation, on 12-month survival in the SHOCK trial. Am Heart J 2003; 146: 804–10.

97. Sanborn TA, Sleeper LA, Bates ER, et al. Impact of thrombolysis, intra-aortic balloon pump counterpulsation, and their combination in cardiogenic shock complicating acute myocardial infarction: a report from the SHOCK Trial Registry. J Am Coll Cardiol 2000; 36: 1123–9.

98. White HD, Assmann SF, Sanborn TA, at al. Comparison of percutaneous coronary intervention and coronary artery bypass grafting after acute myocardial infarction complicated by cardiogenic shock: results from the SHOCK trial. Circulation 2005; 112: 1992–2001.

99. Patel MR, Smalling RW, Thiele H, et al. Intra-aortic balloon counterpulsation and infarct size in patients with acute anterior myocardial infarction without shock: the CRISP AMI randomized trial. JAMA. 2011; 306: 1329–1337. *Trend towards lower mortality with IABP at 6 months (1.9% vs 5.2%, p = 0.12) and significant reduction in death/shock/HF. IABP was placed before PCI. A substudy showed improvement of survival in the small subgroup of patients with severe baseline ST elevation≥15 mm in total and persistent ischemia/ST elevation. Another study, PAMI II trial, showed a lack of benefit of IABP in STEMI with HF but no shock.*

100. Thiele H, Zeymer U, Neumann FJ, et al. Intraaortic balloon support for myocardial infarction with cardiogenic shock. N Engl J Med 2012; 367: 1287–96.

RV shock (+ reference 89 above)

101. Bowers TR, O'Neill WW, Grines C, et al. Effect of reperfusion on biventricular function and survival after right ventricular infarction. N Engl J Med 1998; 338: 933–40.

102. Berisha S, Kastrati A, Goda A, Popa Y. Optimal value of filling pressure in the right side of the heart in acute right ventricular infarction. Br Heart J 1990; 63: 98–102.

103. Price LC, Wort SJ, Finney SJ, et al. Pulmonary vascular and right ventricular dysfunction in adult critical care: current and emerging options for management: a systematic literature review. Crit Care 2010; 14: R169.

104. Haddad F, Doyle R, Murphy D, et al. Right ventricular dysfunction in cardiovascular disease, part II. Pathophysiology, clinical importance and management of right ventricular failure. Circulation 2008; 117: 1717–31.

105. Inglessis I, Shin JT, Lepore JT, et al. Hemodynamic effects of inhaled nitric oxide in right ventricular myocardial infarction and cardiogenic shock. J Am Coll Cardiol 2004; 44: 793–8.

Mechanical complications

106. Thompson CR, Buller CE, Sleeper LA, et al. Cardiogenic shock due to acute severe mitral regurgitation complicating acute myocardial infarction: a report from the SHOCK Trial Registry. J Am Coll Cardiol 2000; 36 (3 Suppl A): 1104–9. *Problem: this registry does not distinguish severe MR due to tethering from severe MR due to papillary muscle rupture.*

107. Menon V, Webb JG, Hillis LD, et al. Outcome and profile of ventricular septal rupture with cardiogenic shock after myocardial infarction: a report from the SHOCK trial registry. J Am Coll Cardiol 2000; 36: 1110–16.

108. Moreno R, Lopez-Sendon J, Garcia E, et al. Primary angioplasty reduces the risk of left ventricular free wall rupture compared with thrombolysis in patients with acute myocardial infarction. J Am Coll Cardiol 2002; 39: 598–603.

109. Lopez-Sendon J, Gonzalez A, Lopez de Sa E, et al. Diagnosis of subacute ventricular wall rupture after acute myocardial infarction (sensitivity and specificity of clinical, hemodynamic and echocardiographic criteria). J Am Coll Cardiol 1992; 19: 1145–53.

110. Slater J, Brown RJ, Antonelli TA, et al. Cardiogenic shock due to cardiac free-wall rupture or tamponade after acute myocardial infarction: a report from the SHOCK Trial Registry. J Am Coll Cardiol 2000; 36: 1117–22.

111. Honan MB, Harrell FE, Reimer KA, et al. Cardiac rupture, mortality and the timing of thrombolytic therapy: a meta-analysis. J Am Coll Cardiol 1990; 16: 359–67. *Early thrombolysis reduces cardiac rupture, late thrombolysis increases it.*

112. Bueno H, Martínez-Sellés M, Pérez-David E, López-Palop R. Effect of thrombolytic therapy on the risk of cardiac rupture and mortality in older patients with first acute myocardial infarction. Eur Heart J 2005; 26: 1705–11. *Thrombolysis increases cardiac rupture in the elderly.*

113. Heuser RR, Maddoux GL, Goss JE, et al.; Coronary angioplasty for acute mitral regurgitation due to myocardial infarction. A nonsurgical treatment preserving mitral valve integrity. Ann Intern Med 1987; 107: 852–5. *Three cases of acute ischemic dynamic MR that resolved with angioplasty.*

114. Shawl F.A, Forman M.B, Punja S, Goldbaum T.S; Emergent coronary angioplasty in the treatment of acute ischemic mitral regurgitation. long- term results in five cases. J Am Coll Cardiol 1989; 14: 986–91.

115. Le Feuvre C, Metzger J.P, Lachurie M.L, Georges J.L, Baubion N, Vacheron A; Treatment of severe mitral regurgitation caused by ischemic papillary muscle dysfunction. indications for coronary angioplasty. Am Heart J 1992; 123: 860–5.

116. Chockalingam A, Tejwani L, Aggarwal K, Dellsperger KC. Dynamic left ventricular outflow tract obstruction in acute myocardial infarction with shock: cause, effect, and coincidence. Circulation 2007; 116: e110–13.

Arrhythmias
VF

117. Tunstall-Pedoe H, KuulasmaaK, Amouyel P, et al. Myocardial infarction and coronary deaths in the World Health Organization MONICA registration project: registration procedures, event rates and case fatality rates in 30 populations from 21 countries in 4 continents. Circulation 1994; 90: 583–612.

118. Norris RM, on behalf of the United Kingdom Heart Attack Study Collaborative Group. Fatality outside hospital from acute coronary events in three British health districts. BMJ 1998; 316: 1065–70.

119. Sayer JW, Archbold RA, Wilkinson P, et al. Prognostic implications of ventricular fibrillation in acute myocardial infarction: new strategies required for further mortality reduction. Heart 2000; 84: 258–61.

120. Newby KH, Thompson T, Stebbins A, et al. Sustained ventricular arrhythmias in patients receiving thrombolytic therapy: incidence and outcomes. Circulation 1998; 98: 2567–73. *Data from GUSTO-1.*

121. Volpi A, Cavalli A, Santoro L, Negri E. Incidence and prognosis of early primary ventricular fibrillation in acute myocardial infarction--results of the GISSI-2 database. Am J Cardiol 1998; 82: 265–71.

122. Tofler GH, Stone PH, Muller JE, et al. Prognosis after cardiac arrest due to ventricular tachycardia or ventricular fibrillation associated with acute myocardial infarction (the MILIS study). Am J Cardiol 1987; 60: 755–61.

123. Mehta RH, Yu J, Piccini JP, et al. Prognostic significance of postprocedural sustained ventricular tachycardia or fibrillation in patients undergoing primary percutaneous coronary intervention (from the HORIZONS-AMI trial). Am J Cardiol 2012; 109: 805–12.

124. Mehta RH, Starr AZ, Lopes RD, et al.; APEX AMI Investigators. Incidence of and outcomes associated with ventricular tachycardia or fibrillation in patients undergoing primary percutaneous coronary intervention. JAMA 2009; 301: 1779–89. *VT/VF post-PCI: VT/VF that occurs during or after primary PCI is not associated with any long-term increase in mortality (APEX, HORIZONS), but increase in short-term mortality (APEX).*

VT

125. Wolfe CL, Nibley C, Bhandari A, et al. Polymorphous ventricular tachycardia associated with acute myocardial infarction. Circulation 1991; 84: 1543–51.

126. Eldar M, Sievner Z, Goldbourt U, et al. Primary ventricular tachycardia in acute myocardial infarction: clinical characteristics and mortality. Ann Intern Med 1992; 117: 31–6.

127. Mont L, Cinca J, Blanch P, et al. Predisposing factors and prognostic value of sustained monomorphic ventricular tachycardia in the early phase of acute myocardial infarction. J Am Coll Cardiol 1996; 28: 1670–6.

128. Hatzinikolaou-Kotsakou E, Tziakas D, Hotidis A, et al. Could sustained monomorphic ventricular tachycardia in the early phase of a prime acute myocardial infarction affect patient outcome? J Electrocardiol 2007; 40: 72–7.

129. Vaitkus PT, Kindwall KE, Marchlinski FE, et al. Differences in electrophysiological substrate in patients with coronary artery disease and cardiac arrest or ventricular tachycardia. Insights from endocardial mapping and signal-averaged electrocardiography. Circulation 1991; 84: 672–8.

130. Scirica BM, Braunwald E, Belardinelli L, et al. Relationship between nonsustained ventricular tachycardia after non-ST-elevation acute coronary syndrome and sudden cardiac death: observations from MERLIN-TIMI 36 randomized controlled trial. Circulation 2010; 122: 455–62.

AF

131. Atrial fibrillation in acute myocardial infarction: a systematic review of the incidence, clinical features and prognostic implications. Eur Heart J 2009; 30: 1038–45.

132. Crenshaw BS, Ward SR, Granger CB, et al. Atrial fibrillation in the setting of acute myocardial infarction: the GUSTO-I experience. Global Utilization of Streptokinase and TPA for Occluded Coronary Arteries. J Am Coll Cardiol 1997; 30: 406–13.

133. Siu CW, Jim MH, Ho HH, et al. Transient atrial fibrillation complicating acute inferior myocardial infarction: implications for future risk of ischemic stroke. Chest 2007; 132: 44–9.

134. Stenestrand U, Lindback J, Wallentin L. Anticoagulation therapy in atrial fibrillation in combination with acute myocardial infarction influences long-term outcome: a prospective cohort study from the Register of Information and Knowledge About Swedish Heart Intensive Care Admissions (RIKS-HIA). Circulation 2005; 112: 3225–31.

AV block

135. Nicod P, Gilpin E. Dittrich H, et al. Long-term outcome in patients with inferior myocardial infarction and complete atrioventricular block. J Am Coll Cardiol 1988; 12: 589–94.

136. Meine TJ, Al-Khatib SM, Alexander JH, et al. Incidence, predictors, and outcomes of high-degree atrioventricular block complicating acute myocardial infarction treated with thrombolytic therapy. Am Heart J 2005; 149: 670–4.

137. Ginks WR, Sutton R, Oh W, Leatham W. Long-term prognosis after acute anterior infarction with atrioventricular block. Br Heart J 1977; 39, 186–9.

138. Engel TR, Wolf NM. Left bundle branch block does not mean left coronary artery block. J Am Coll Cardiol 2013; 62: 968–9.

139. Newby KH, Pisano E, Krucoff MW, et al. Incidence and clinical relevance of the occurrence of bundle branch block in patients treated with thrombolytic therapy. Circulation 1996; 94: 2424–8. *Data from GUSTO-1 and TAMI, continuous ECG monitoring. 75% of BBB are transient, mortality higher for LBBB.*

140. Sgarbossa EB, Pinski SL, Topol EJ, et al. Acute myocardial infarction and complete bundle branch block at hospital admission: clinical characteristics and outcome in the thrombolytic era. J Am Coll Cardiol 1998; 105–10. *Data from GUSTO 1. 25% of BBB are transient; LBBB more RCA than LAD; mortality higher for RBBB.*

Aneurysm and pseudo-aneurysm

141. Ba'albaki HA, Clements SD. Left ventricular aneurysm: a review. Clin Cardiol 1989; 12: 5–13.
142. Heras M, Sanz G, Betriu A, et al. Does left ventricular aneurysm influence survival after acute myocardial infarction? Eur Heart J 1990; 11 (5): 441–6.
143. Frances C, Romero A, Grady D. Left ventricular pseudoaneurysm. J Am Coll Cardiol 1998; 32: 557–61.
144. Vlodaver Z, Coe JI, Edwards JE. True and false left ventricular aneurysms. Propensity for the altter to rupture. Circulation 1975; 51: 567–72.
145. Gatewood RP, Nanada NC. Differentiation of left ventricular pseudoaneurysm from true aneurysm with two dimensional echocardiography. Am J Cardiol 1980 46: 869–78.

Post-MI pericarditis

146. Oliva PB, Hammill SC, Edwards WD. Electrocardiographic diagnosis of postinfarction regional pericarditis: ancillary observations regarding the effect of reperfusion on the rapidity and amplitude of T wave inversion after acute myocardial infarction. Circulation 1993; 88: 896–904.
147. Sugiura T, Iwasaka T, Takayama Y, et al. Factors associated with pericardial effusion in acute Q wave myocardial infarction. Circulation 1990; 81: 477–81.
148. Oliva PB, Hammill SC, Talano JV. Effect of definition on incidence of postinfarction pericarditis. It is time to redefine postinfarction pericarditis? Circulation 1994; 90: 1537–41.
149. Widimský P, Gregor P. Pericardial involvement during the course of myocardial infarction. A long-term clinical and echocardiographic study. Chest 1995; 108: 89–93.
150. Figueras J, Barrabes JA, Serra V, et al. Hospital outcome of moderate to severe pericardial effusion complicating ST-elevation acute myocardial infarction. Circulation 2010; 122: 1902–9.

LV thrombus

151. Delewi R,Zijlstra F, Piek JJ. Left ventricular thrombus formation after acute myocardial infarction. Heart 2012; 98: 1743–9.
152. Shacham Y, Leshem-Rubinow E, Ben Ass E, et al. Frequency and correlates of early left ventricular thrombus formation following anterior wall acute myocardial infarction treated with primary percutaneous coronary intervention. Am J Cardiol 2013; 111: 667–70.
153. Asinger RW, Mikell FL, Elsperger J, et al. Incidence of left ventricular thrombosis after acute transmural myocardial infarction. Serial evaluation by two-dimensional echocardiography. N Engl J Med 1981; 305: 297–302.
154. Vaitkus PT, Barnathan ES. Embolic potential, prevention and management of mural thrombus complicating anterior myocardial infarction: a meta-analysis. J Am Coll Cardiol 1993; 22: 1004–9.
155. Meltzer RS, Visser CA, Fuster V. Intracardiac thrombi and systemic embolization. Ann Intern Med 1986; 104: 689–98.
156. Mollet NR, Dymarkowski S, Volders W, et al. Visualization of ventricular thrombi with contrast-enhanced magnetic resonance imaging in patients with ischemic heart disease. Circulation 2002; 106: 2873–6.

Prognosis

157. Savonitto S, Ardissino D, Granger CB, et al. Prognostic value of the admission electrocardiogram in acute coronary syndromes. JAMA 1999; 281: 707–13.

Cardiac arrest

158. Kern KB. Optimal treatment of patients surviving out-of-hospital cardiac arrest. JACC Cardiovasc Interv 2012; 5: 597–605.
159. Spaulding CM, Joly LM, Rosenberg A. Immediate coronary angiography in survivors of out-of-hospital cardiac arrest. N Engl J Med 336 1997: 1629–33.
160. Dumas F., Cariou A., Manzo-Silberman S. Immediate percutaneous coronary intervention is associated with better survival after out-of-hospital cardiac arrest: insights from the PROCAT (Parisian Region Out of hospital Cardiac ArresT) registry. Circ Cardiovasc Interv 2010; 3: 200–7.
161. Gorjup V, Radsel P, Kocjancic ST, et al. Acute ST-elevation myocardial infarction after successful cardiopulmonary resuscitation. Resuscitation 2007; 72: 379–85.
162. Hosmane VR, Mustafa NG, Reddy VK. Survival and neurologic recovery in patients with ST-segment elevation myocardial infarction resuscitated from cardiac arrest. J Am Coll Cardiol 2009; 53: 409–15.
163. Larsen AI, Hjørnevik AS, Ellingsen CL, Nilsen DW. Cardiac arrest with continuous mechanical chest compression during percutaneous coronary intervention. A report on the use of the LUCAS device. Resuscitation 2007; 75: 454–9.
164. Bottiger BW, Arntz H, Chamberlain DA, et al. Thrombolysis during resuscitation for out-of-hospital cardiac arrest. N Engl J Med 2008; 359: 2651–62.
165. Arntz HR, Wenzel V, Dissmann R, et al. Out-of-hospital thrombolysis during cardiopulmonary resuscitation in patients with high likelihood of ST-elevation myocardial infarction. Resuscitation 2008; 76: 180–4.
166. Bernard SA, Gray TW, Buist MD, et al. Treatment of comatose survivors of out-of-hospital cardiac arrest with induced hypothermia. N Engl J Med 2002; 346: 557–63.
167. Hypothermia after Cardiac Arrest Study Group. Mild therapeutic hypothermia to improve the neurologic outcome after cardiac arrest. N Engl J Med 2002; 346: 549–56.
168. Nielsen N, Wetterslev J, Cronberg T, et al. Targeted temperature management at 33 °C versus 36 °C after cardiac arrest. N Engl J Med 2013; 369: 2197–206.
169. Oomen SS, Menon V. Hypothermia after cardiac arrest: beneficial, but slow to be adopted. Clev Clin J Med 2011; 78: 441–8.
170. O'Connor RE, Bossaert L, Arntz HR, et al. Part 9: Acute coronary syndromes: 2010 International Consensus on Cardiopulmonary Resuscitation and Emergency Cardiovascular Care Science With Treatment Recommendations. Circulation 2010; 122 (Suppl 2): S422–5.
171. Kilgannon JH, Robert BW, Jones AE, et al. Arterial blood pressure and neurologic outcome after resuscitation from cardiac arrest. Crit Care Med 2014; 42: 2083–91.

3   Stable CAD and Approach to Chronic Chest Pain

I. Causes of angina; pathophysiology of coronary flow

A. Angina caused by fixed coronary obstruction

Coronary blood flow constitutes ~5% of the total cardiac output and may increase up to 5 times with exercise. Normally, the coronary microcirculatory resistance constitutes the only resistance to myocardial flow; the epicardial vessels are just conductance vessels that offer no resistance to myocardial flow. In the presence of a functionally significant stenosis, classically a 70% diameter stenosis, the trans-stenotic flow drops during exertion; at a 90% diameter stenosis, the trans-stenotic flow drops at rest. During exercise or adenosine infusion, extensive microvascular dilatation occurs, requiring an extensive increase in flow to fill the dilated circulation; since the flow cannot increase across a flow-limiting stenosis, ischemia occurs.[1]

Supply ischemia is typically caused by ≥50% diameter stenosis of the left main coronary artery or ≥70% diameter stenosis of the major epicardial vessels. However, a 40–70% stenosis may be functionally significant, i.e., may impede maximal coronary flow during stress. The functional significance of a fixed lesion depends not only on the luminal narrowing, but also on:[1]

- The size of the territory supplied by the vessel: a 50% proximal LAD stenosis is often significant, whereas a 50% diagonal or distal LAD stenosis may not be. A larger flow across a stenosis translates into a larger percentage of flow drop across the stenosis.
- Lesion length, as resistance across a stenosis correlates with (viscosity × length)/radius⁴ (Poiseuille law).
- Amount of viable myocardium.

Therefore, stress imaging may be useful to assess the functional significance of a borderline lesion. Also, in the cath lab, fractional flow reserve (FFR), i.e., the relative drop in flow across a lesion, may be invasively measured. FFR implies the assessment of pressure drop across a lesion using a coronary pressure wire; this pressure drop corresponds to a flow drop in patients with maximal microcirculatory hyperemia that exhausts autoregulation (flow=pressure/microvascular resistance). A flow drop ≥20%, i.e., FFR flow ratio ≤0.80, implies functional significance. In the FAME trial of multivessel PCI, 35% of lesions that were 50–70% stenotic, 80% of lesions that were 70–90% stenotic, and almost all lesions >90% stenotic were functionally significant (FFR ≤0.80).[2] This highlights the limitations of angiography even for stenoses of 70–90%.

B. Vasospastic angina (Prinzmetal angina) or dynamic coronary obstruction

It was initially hypothesized by Prinzmetal and then demonstrated in a large series that vasospasm and vasospastic angina often occur **at the site of a significant atherosclerotic obstruction in patients with significant CAD**;[3,4] in two series, 60–90% of patients with vasospastic angina had significant single- or multivessel CAD. CAD was not only significant but frequently unstable.[4] Later reports suggest that **vasospasm is also a common diagnosis in patients with angina and no significant CAD**, particularly women.[5] Even in patients with normal or near-normal coronary arteries, atherosclerosis is documented at the site of vasospasm, and, in fact, vasospasm correlates with the atherosclerotic burden at this site.[6,7] Vasospasm may be related to vasoconstrictors released by platelets and leukocytes at the atherosclerotic site, or endothelial dysfunction and abnormal vasomotor response induced by atherosclerosis.[6] Paradoxical vasoconstriction may occur during exercise, adrenergic stimulation (stress), or cold exposure. Approximately 60% of patients only have symptoms at rest or mild activity without exertional limitation, sometimes in a cyclic nocturnal pattern; in those patients, angina only occurs when the dynamic component exacerbates the fixed obstruction.[4] On the other hand, many patients have exertional angina, whether from the CAD itself or from the exertional vasospasm, and some patients only have exertional angina.[5] Vasospastic angina is classically more severe than fixed-threshold angina, as the episodic obstruction is totally or subtotally occlusive, with more frequent arrhythmia, high-grade AV block, or syncope during the episodes. While characteristically more common in women, the vasospasm occurring on top of CAD was more common in men in one series (see Appendix 2 for more details).[4]

C. Angina secondary to severely increased demands

This is seen with severe LV hypertrophy, severe HTN, valvular heart disease, HF, marked tachycardia, or metabolic disorders (anemia or hyperthyroidism). Some of these patients have underlying significant CAD, but many do not, angina being completely explained by the severely increased demands.

Note on coronary flow physiology

Because of systolic compression of the microcirculation, the LV receives blood mainly during diastole (>80% of the left coronary flow occurs in diastole). Tachycardia, in addition to increasing O_2 demands, reduces myocardial O_2 supply by reducing diastolic time.

As opposed to the LV, the RV is thin, which explains why its microcirculation is not as affected by systole as the LV's microcirculation. Approximately 50% of the right coronary-to-RV flow occurs in systole.

The LV coronary blood flow is directly related to the pressure gradient between DBP and LVEDP (coronary perfusion pressure) and inversely related to the microvascular resistance; the latter depends on myocardial stiffness, and, thus, on LVEDP as well (flow=delta pressure/microvascular resistance). A reduction of DBP or an increase in LVEDP reduces coronary flow, even in the absence of a coronary stenosis.

Since the RV receives significant flow during systole, the coronary blood flow of the RV is partly related to the gradient between SBP and RV systolic pressure, not just DBP and RVEDP.

II. Diagnostic approach
A. Clinical features of typical angina

Typical angina is characterized by three features:

1. Retrosternal or epigastric discomfort; neck/jaw/arm pain; or angina equivalent (dyspnea, fatigue, dizziness).
2. Occurrence with stress or exertion.
3. Quick relief by rest or nitroglycerin (within 30 s – 5 min). A prolonged pain (>20 min), or a delay to relief with rest or nitroglycerin (>5 min) usually implies one of two extremes: acute MI or non-cardiac pain.

Angina is precipitated by walking uphill, in the cold, or after a meal.* Nausea or diaphoresis during pain increases the likelihood of angina. *Postprandial angina* is often a marker of severe, sometimes multivessel CAD. As opposed to biliary colic or peptic ulcer disease, angina occurs immediately after the meal and is *exacerbated by postprandial physical activity*. *Nocturnal angina* may imply severe CAD or vasospasm on top of fixed CAD; the increased venous return in the recumbent position increases O_2 demands and triggers ischemia in patients with critical, sometimes multivessel, CAD. *Rest angina* without an exertional component may be seen in patients with significant CAD whose angina is mainly triggered by a vasospastic reduction of O_2 supply (although many of the latter patients also have exertional angina). *Dyspnea* may be an angina equivalent and may indicate extensive CAD with secondary increase in ventricular stiffness and LVEDP. *"Warm-up" angina* is angina that starts with the onset of activity and improves with further exertion (e.g., in the morning); it suggests a very severe stenosis, with collaterals that get recruited during exertion and a myocardium that adapts to ischemia (ischemic preconditioning).

---

*Cold leads to vasoconstriction (afterload increase) and shivering, increasing O_2 demands. The severity of angina is classified using the Canadian Cardiovascular Society grading (CCS). CCS IV is angina with minimal activities, CCS III is angina at a low level of activity, such as walking one flight of stairs or 1–2 flat blocks at a normal pace, CCS II is angina with walking more or at a faster pace, and does not usually occur on a daily level, and CCS I is angina with strenuous lifting or running.

B. Pre-test clinical probability of significant CAD

The presence of all three features defines typical (definite) angina, while two features define possible angina, and chest pain without any additional feature defines non-anginal chest pain. The combination of (1) angina features, (2) age and sex, and (3) risk factors establishes the probability of CAD (Forrester and Duke classifications, combined in Figure 3.1).[8–10]

In addition, primary ST-T changes or Q waves on the resting ECG imply a higher probability of CAD and a higher-risk CAD, even outside unstable angina.[10]

Only 50% of women with classic angina have CAD (as opposed to ~90% of men). The WISE registry shows that ~40% of women undergoing coronary angiography for suspected myocardial ischemia have CAD; the remaining patients likely have macro- or microvascular spasm without obstructive CAD. While fewer women have obstructive CAD than men, women without obstructive CAD who continue to have chest pain have a worrisome ~9% risk of death/MI at 4 years (WISE).[11]

C. Pre-test probability of high-risk CAD (multivessel, extensive CAD)

Hubbard et al. identified five clinical parameters that predict severe (three-vessel or left main) CAD, beside age: male sex, typical angina, diabetes, insulin dependency, prior MI by history or ECG.[12] A 40-year-old patient with four or more of these parameters, or a 60-year-old patient with three or more of these parameters, has a probability of severe CAD of over 40% (e.g., a 60-year-old diabetic man with typical angina). *Such patients are appropriately referred directly to coronary angiography without stress testing,* as it is highly unlikely that the latter will be normal and, if normal, it may represent a false negative test.[13]

Other clinical features are predictive of severe CAD and may justify direct referral to angiography (class I for severe angina, class IIa for the rest):[10,14]

- High-probability angina that is severe or frequent. A severe angina is likely to require revascularization for symptom control regardless of stress test results or extent of CAD, as standalone medical therapy is less effective than PCI for symptom control of class III or IV angina.
- PAD (doubles the risk of severe CAD).
- HF that is likely ischemic (HF with angina, flash pulmonary edema, or older age/combination of risk factors).
- Q waves or primary ST-T abnormalities on the baseline ECG, or regional wall motion abnormalities on echo.

D. Indications for testing (diagnostic and prognostic purposes):

In a patient with suspected CAD, two questions are initially addressed: (i) clinical probability of CAD; (ii) clinical risk of CAD (probability of severe, left main or three-vessel CAD). The patient is managed accordingly:[12]

- *High pre-test probability:*
  - Stress testing is not useful for *diagnostic* purposes, as the likelihood of CAD remains high even with a negative test. Stress testing is, however, performed for *risk stratification* if the clinical risk does not appear high (class I).
  - Coronary angiography is performed if the clinical risk is high.
- *Intermediate pre-test probability:* stress testing is performed for diagnosis and prognosis (class I). CTA may be performed (class II). CTA is also indicated in patients with an intermediate or inconclusive stress test result or a negative stress test yet persistent symptoms.
- *Low pre-test probability* (young patient with atypical angina): stress testing may not need to be performed. Even if the stress test is positive, the probability of CAD will increase from <10% up to 20%, i.e., the stress test is likely to be falsely positive in this context. However, if judged necessary, ECG or echo stress testing may be performed (class IIa).

E. Risk stratification with stress testing

Treadmill stress ECG, more specifically the Duke Treadmill Score (DTS), is a powerful risk stratifier. A high-risk DTS implies an increased cardiac mortality and a 75% probability of left main or three-vessel CAD, regardless of imaging results. A low-risk DTS often implies a low mortality; however, ~10% of patients with a low-risk DTS have severe three-vessel or left main disease with a high mortality, and another 10% have two-vessel or proximal LAD disease, and overall, 20% of symptomatic patients with normal stress ECG have significant, high-risk CAD.[15] These patients are likely to be picked up by stress imaging.[16,17] *In fact, a high-risk result on nuclear or echo stress imaging overrules*

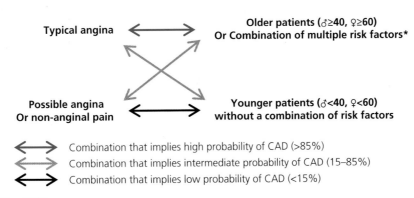

Figure 3.1 Clinical probability of CAD.

*Combination of diabetes, smoking, or hyperlipidemia (LDL >160–190 mg/dl), especially when all three are present.[10]

a low- or intermediate-risk result on stress ECG.[16,17] Thus, stress imaging is preferred to stress ECG in patients with a high probability of CAD or with prior coronary revascularization (class IIa), while stress ECG is enough in patients with an intermediate or low CAD probability who are able to walk and have an interpretable baseline ECG (Table 3.1).[18]

A high-risk DTS, on the other hand, implies a high risk regardless of imaging results, with a 75% probability of left main or three-vessel CAD and >99% probability of any significant CAD.[15] Because of balanced ischemia, some patients with extensive disease have normal or mildly abnormal perfusion imaging but are picked up by ECG variables, DTS, severe angina during testing, and post-stress LV dysfunction.

Table 3.2 stratifies the risk according to stress testing.

F. Putting it together: diagnostic approach and management of chronic chest pain (Figure 3.2)

G. Additional clinical scenarios

If the coronary angiogram is not done because of a low-risk stress test, or if it is done but PCI is not performed (medical therapy selected for a lesion supplying a moderate area of myocardium or for a technically difficult lesion), yet the patient continues to have refractory typical angina, especially angina at mild exertion despite medical therapy, perform a coronary angiogram and consider or reconsider PCI.

If a patient with a prior revascularization (PCI or CABG) presents with chest pain, assess the probability of angina based on the three clinical features and on the similarity with the prior angina that was relieved with revascularization. Perform stress imaging, or repeat the coronary angiogram if a typical angina occurs on mild exertion.

In patients who have undergone PCI, the coronary angiogram is more readily repeated if: (i) angina recurs in the first 12 months after PCI, which is the time frame of restenosis, or (ii) untreated, significant coronary stenoses are known to be present. Chest pain relief followed by recurrence months later is typical of in-stent restenosis, or, less often, progression of moderate disease outside the stented area (especially in patients who initially presented with ACS). A persistent chest pain without a pattern of relief and recurrence suggests either non-cardiac pain or residual, non-revascularized disease.

Warranty periods

When should stress testing be repeated in patients with prior negative studies who present with chest pain? Stress tests have "warranty periods" during which the risk of cardiovascular events is low (<1% per year) and during which there is no need to perform a coronary angiogram unless the patient has objective evidence of new CAD, such as ACS with positive cardiac markers or new, severe ischemia on the ECG.

This "warranty period" of a stress test varies according to the context:[20]
- History of CAD: 1 year.
- Diabetes: 2 years; shorter for women.
- Elderly (>70–80 years old) undergoing pharmacological stress testing: 1 year
- The combination of these factors or the use of pharmacological imaging, as opposed to treadmill testing, further limits the warranty periods.
- Outside of these contexts, in the absence of a history of CAD or diabetes, the warranty period of a low-risk stress test result is 2–3 years.

When a coronary angiogram shows normal coronary arteries or minimal disease, the risk of coronary events is very low for 5 years, and unless there is evidence of MI, the angiogram is not usually repeated within the next 5 years. As per the CASS registry, the 7-year survival is 96% for patients with normal EF and normal coronaries and 92% for patients with mild coronary disease <50% (much better prognosis than obstructive CAD).[21]

How about patients who had a coronary angiogram showing single- or multivessel moderate disease (30–70%), or showing severe disease (>70%) in a small branch where PCI is not technically possible or beneficial? If they present with recurrent or persistent chest pain a few months or 1–2 years later, the coronary angiogram may not need to be repeated unless there is an ischemic ST abnormality, a positive troponin, or a dramatic change in the severity of a typical, exertional angina. *Also, the true functional significance of intermediate stenoses (50–70%) is worth assessing with stress imaging or FFR.*

Note that CAD progresses faster in patients whose initial presentation was ACS: the risk of ACS from nonsignificant lesions is 10% at 3 years, and up to 20% from each lesion that has high-risk features on intracoronary imaging.

These "warranty periods" are used for guidance; ultimately, decisions are based on clinical judgment.

III. Silent myocardial ischemia

A totally silent myocardial ischemia is uncommon. The more common form of silent myocardial ischemia consists of silent ischemia interspersed with episodes of symptomatic ischemia, such as angina or prior MI. Even if asymptomatic, ischemia is a strong predictor of cardiac events and mortality and probably has the same prognostic significance as symptomatic ischemia.[22] Therapy in this case is guided by the resolution of objective ischemia on stress testing. Silent ischemia 6 months after PCI, if severe, is associated with a high risk of clinical events.[23]

Table 3.1 Indications for stress imaging, as opposed to plain treadmill stress ECG.

Treadmill stress imaging (nuclear or echo) >Treadmill stress ECG
- Baseline ST depression >1 mm[a]
- High pre-test probability of CAD
- Prior coronary revascularization (stress imaging allows localization of ischemia and has a higher sensitivity in detecting single-vessel ischemia)
- Prior stress ECG with intermediate result

Pharmacological stress imaging (nuclear or echo)
- Unable to walk
- Able to walk but baseline ECG has LBBB or ventricular paced rhythm (classically, pharmacological nuclear imaging is performed, but exercise or dobutamine echo has shown an appropriate yield as well)[b] [19]

[a]LVH without ST depression is appropriately tested with stress ECG.
[b]Exercise and dobutamine exaggerate the septal motion abnormality and septal defect present in LBBB, falsely suggesting ischemia.

Table 3.2 Risk stratification with stress testing.

High risk: yearly cardiac mortality >3%, yearly cardiac events >5%
- DTS ≤–11[a]
- Reversible, large *or* severe perfusion defect (summed stress score >+8, corresponding to ischemia involving >10% of the myocardium)
- Fixed, large *or* severe perfusion defect with LV dilatation/low EF
- Rest- or stress-induced LV dysfunction with EF ≤35%, even if the defect is mild or moderate
- On stress echo: ischemia of ≥3 segments (out of 17), or >one coronary distribution, especially if it occurs at a low rate <120 bpm or a low dose of dobutamine (≤10 mcg/kg/min)

Intermediate risk: yearly cardiac mortality 1–3%, cardiac events 1–5%
- DTS –10 to +4
- Summed stress score 4–8

Low risk: yearly cardiac mortality and cardiac events <1% (~0.5% with stress imaging)
- DTS ≥+5 (≥ +8 is very low risk)
- No perfusion defect or small perfusion defect with a summed stress score <4

[a]Duke Treadmill Score (DTS) = prognostic score for treadmill stress testing
= Exercise time on Bruce protocol – 5 × (the deepest ST depression on ECG) – 4 × (angina score)
(Angina score: 0 = no angina, 1 = non-limiting angina, 2 = exercise-limiting angina)

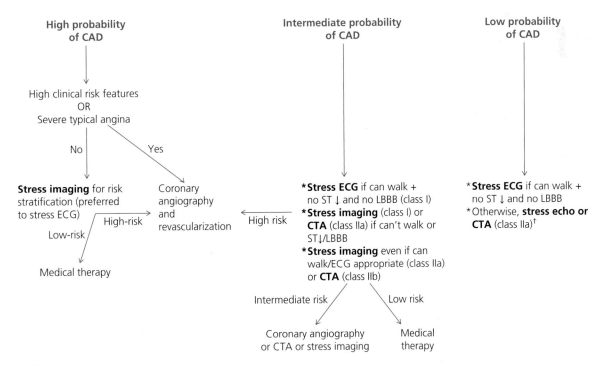

Figure 3.2 Diagnostic approach to chronic chest pain.
[†]Avoid nuclear stress testing in low-probability patients, as nuclear imaging has a high rate of false positives in a low-probability population.

However, screening asymptomatic patients based solely on risk factors is not indicated, nor is screening of post-PCI patients indicated. In the DIAD study, asymptomatic diabetic patients, who constitute a relatively high-risk population, were screened for CAD with nuclear stress imaging. These asymptomatic patients actually had a low risk of cardiac events (0.6% per year), and while this risk was higher in the small subgroup of patients with moderate or severe ischemia (2.5% per year), 70% of events eventually occurred in patients with normal testing. In fact, a 0.6% event rate in 90% of the population leads to more total events than a 2.5% event rate in 10% of the population. Even if revascularization reduces the risk of late MI in this small subgroup, the benefit is compounded by the periprocedural risk of MI and by the risk of unnecessary diagnostic angiograms in patients with false positive stress tests. This explains why the event rate was similar in the screened and non-screened diabetic populations. Thus, stress testing is not generally useful in asymptomatic patients, even those at seemingly high risk, particularly if risk factors and hemoglobin A1c are well controlled (as in the DIAD study).[24] These findings were corroborated by another study, wherein asymptomatic diabetic patients were randomized to coronary CTA screening vs. routine care. Coronary CTA found significant CAD (>70% stenosis) in 11% of patients and resulted in a 6% revascularization rate, which did not translate into any reduction of death, MI, or unstable angina (FACTOR-64 study).[25]

If stress testing is done in asymptomatic patients, the detection of severe ischemia would lead to coronary angiography and revascularization of extensive CAD (similarly to symptomatic patients). In comparison with medical therapy, revascularization with CABG or PCI reduced mortality and MI in patients with asymptomatic ischemia or medically controlled ischemic symptoms in the ACIP trial.[26] CABG reduced mortality in patients with asymptomatic left main or three-vessel CAD in the CABG trials.[27]

IV. Medical therapy: antiplatelet therapy to prevent cardiovascular events

While the combination of aspirin and clopidogrel is beneficial for up to 1 year after ACS or stent placement, this combination has not shown superiority to aspirin monotherapy in stable CAD and peripheral vascular disease (CHARISMA trial).[28] However, in a substudy of CHARISMA, stable patients with prior MI appeared to derive a benefit from prolonged combination therapy for up to 28 months, especially if they had disease in multiple vascular locations (e.g., MI and PAD).[29] Clopidogrel is an alternative to aspirin and may be slightly superior in reducing coronary and cerebrovascular events with a slightly lower risk of GI bleed.[30]

Patients with CAD who also have an indication for anticoagulation (AF or a history of DVT) may receive the combination of aspirin and warfarin (INR goal, 2.0–2.5). Warfarin may be administered alone beyond 1 year of MI or coronary stenting (INR goal, 2.0–3.0). Warfarin, per se, effectively reduces coronary events. In fact, warfarin monotherapy or warfarin–aspirin combination is more effective than aspirin in preventing coronary events, at the cost of a higher bleeding risk.[31]

V. Medical therapy: antianginal therapy

Myocardial oxygen demands are related to the following four factors: inotropism, chronotropism, afterload, and preload. Each antianginal agent targets some of these factors. Nitrates and vasodilatory calcium channel blockers reduce ischemia by reducing preload and afterload, and, except in vasopastic angina, the coronary vasodilatory effect is a less important effect.

A. β-Blockers

a. In patients with established CAD and angina, β-blockers are titrated to achieve a resting heart rate of 55–60 bpm. This tight rate control has not been associated with improved outcomes in HTN and is not pursued when β-blockers are used solely for HTN control.[32]
Because they have been shown to reduce mortality after MI, β-blockers are the first-line therapy for angina (class I). However, in stable CAD without prior MI or HF, there is no evidence of mortality reduction and the main benefit is angina relief.[33] In the absence of angina, prior MI, or HF, the recommendation for β-blocker therapy is weak (class IIb).

b. Myocardial β_1-receptors have a positive inotropic and chronotropic effect, thus increasing myocardial O_2 demands. β_2-Receptors mainly have a vasodilatory and bronchodilatory effect, with a limited inotropic and chronotropic effect at baseline. However, the latter effect is exaggerated when β_1-receptors are blocked. Thus, β_2-blockade may be useful in patients requiring a comprehensive blockade of all myocardial adrenergic receptors, such as HF (carvedilol), but may induce a harmful vasoconstrictive and bronchospastic effect.

c. Four types of β-blockers:
  i. Non-selective β_1- and β_2-blockers (e.g., propranolol).
  ii. Selective β_1-blockers (e.g., metoprolol, atenolol, bisoprolol). Selectivity is lost at high doses.
  iii. β-Blockers with intrinsic sympathomimetic activity – β-blockade mainly occurs during catecholamine surges; these agents do not decrease mortality and are preferably avoided.
  iv. β-Blockers with combined α- and non-selective β-blocker activity (carvedilol, labetalol) have a vasodilatory effect and, thus, a more pronounced antihypertensive effect. However, the α-blocking effect gets attenuated with time, in particular with labetalol.[34]

d. Contraindications
  i. Bradycardia <55 bpm or symptomatic bradycardia.
  ii. PR interval >0.24 s, any second- or third-degree AV block.
  iii. Decompensated HF (start β-blockers once HF is compensated).
  iv. History of clinically severe asthma, even if the patient is currently stable, or actively decompensated COPD with wheezes. A low or moderate dose of a selective β-blocker, such as metoprolol 100 mg/day, may be used in stable, mild/moderate asthma.
  v. Use caution in diabetic patients with hypoglycemic episodes.

e. Doses:
  • Metoprolol tartrate 25 mg BID, titrated every 3–7 days to a target dose of 50–100 mg BID if tolerated (maximum 200 mg BID). Metoprolol succinate (Toprol XL): the once-daily dose of Toprol XL is almost equivalent to the total daily dose of metoprolol tartrate.
  • Atenolol 12.5–25 mg BID (or Qday in advanced renal failure), titrated up to 50 mg BID.
  • Carvedilol: 3.125–25 mg BID; labetalol 100–400 mg BID.

Notes

Severe PAD was considered a relative contraindication to non-selective β-blockers, because of an initial β$_2$-blocker vasoconstrictive effect. However, this is no longer a contraindication to β-blockers, as they proved safe in patients with PAD.[35] Also, PAD patients often die of CAD, and thus, β-blockers are valuable in the PAD setting. However, individual responses may vary, and be aware of a potential worsening of severe rest symptoms.

In diabetic patients, metoprolol appears to slightly worsen diabetes control (HbA1c). This is not the case with carvedilol and nebivolol, which should be the preferred β-blockers in diabetic patients (GEMINI trial).[36]

B. Nitrates

a. Nitrates are venodilators and thus reduce ischemia primarily by reducing preload. They also improve coronary flow by reducing intramyocardial diastolic tension, i.e., LVEDP. They are also, to a lesser extent, arterial vasodilators and thus reduce afterload.

The dilatation of epicardial coronary arteries is a less important anti-ischemic mechanism than preload reduction, but dilatation of collaterals may be particularly useful. Vasodilators, in general, may worsen myocardial ischemia in critical CAD as they increase flow through the normal coronary arteries at the expense of the abnormal artery that cannot dilate, creating a coronary steal phenomenon through collaterals (e.g., adenosine). This, however, does not usually happen with nitrates as they do not drastically affect the microvascular tone, and thus do not drastically increase coronary flow to the normal myocardium.

b. While sublingual nitroglycerin (NTG) is used as needed (during angina or before exertion) and has a short effect <5 min, long-acting formulations are used as adjunct to background β-blocker or calcium channel blocker therapy:
- Isosorbide dinitrate (ISDN) 10–40 mg TID, isosorbide mononitrate (ISMN) 30–240 mg Qday, NTG paste 0.5–2 inches TID, NTG patch 0.2–0.6 mg/h Q24h.

c. Tolerance to nitrates develops quickly, within 24 hours of therapy. It is minimized by providing nitrate-free intervals (e.g., administer ISDN at 8 a.m., 2 p.m., and 8 p.m., with 10–14 hours free interval; administer ISMN once daily; or place NTG patch for 12 out of 24 hours every day). However, rebound ischemia may occur during the nitrate-free intervals.

d. Nitrates are metabolized into NO by the endothelium of large arteries. NO promotes the release of cGMP, a smooth muscle relaxant. ***In contrast to large arteries, arterioles cannot metabolize nitrates into NO.***

Nitrate tolerance occurs as the beneficial NO eventually gets metabolized into reactive oxygen species, which reduce NO generation and NO effect and increase the vascular sensitivity to vasoconstrictors; nitrates may, in fact, impair endothelial function.[37] Neurohormonal activation may also contribute to nitrate tolerance. The same phenomenon leads to vasoconstriction and rebound ischemia in the first 4 hours after nitrate withdrawal. Several studies have shown that statin, ACE-I (and possibly ARB), hydralazine, and carvedilol reduce nitrate tolerance as they reduce the production of reactive oxygen species and counteract the neurohormonal activation.[37–40] Thus, with the contemporary drug regimens, nitrate tolerance and rebound are minimized.

C. Calcium channel blockers (CCBs)

a. Non-dihydropyridines (non-DHPs) decrease cardiac inotropism and chronotropism and have a vasodilatory effect (afterload reduction). Also, they dilate the coronary arteries.
- **i.** Examples: diltiazem and verapamil. Verapamil has more negative inotropic effect, slightly more AV and SA nodal depressant effect, and stronger vasodilatory effect than diltiazem.
- **ii.** Non-DHPs are contraindicated in bradycardia or systolic HF. Avoid non-DHPs, particularly verapamil, in combination with a β-blocker. Diltiazem may be combined with a β-blocker in rate-uncontrolled AF.
- **iii.** Doses: diltiazem 30–90 mg TID–QID, diltiazem CD 120–480 mg Qday; verapamil 80–120 mg TID–QID, verapamil SR 180–480 mg/d.

b. Dihydropyridines (DHPs) are vasodilators that reduce afterload and vasodilate the coronary arteries.
- **i.** Only the long-acting formulations are used. Short-acting DHPs may cause reflex tachycardia, which leads to ischemia.
- **ii.** Except for nifedipine, DHPs are not contraindicated in bradycardia or HF. Nifedipine has some negative inotropic effects and should not be used in HF; other DHPs have minimal to no negative inotropic effects.
- **iii.** In contrast to non-DHPs, DHPs are preferably combined with a β-blocker to counteract any potential reflex tachycardia.
- **iv.** DHPs are the first-choice antianginal therapy in patients with bradycardia or AV block, and are the second choice in patients already on β-blockers.
- **v.** Examples are amlodipine, felodipine, and nifedipine XL.
- **vi.** Doses: amlodipine 2.5–10 mg Qday (same for felodipine); nifedipine XL 30–90 mg Qday.

D. Choice of antianginal drugs

β-Blockers are first-line agents. If β-blockers are contraindicated because of bronchospasm, use a non-DHP; if β-blockers are contraindicated because of bradycardia, use a DHP. A long-acting nitrate is used as a second- or third-line agent.

If one agent does not greatly relieve the angina, use a combination of a first-, second-, or third-line agent:

- β-blocker + DHP, nitrate, or ranolazine.
- β-blocker + DHP + nitrate or ranolazine triple combination.
- Non-DHP + nitrate if severe bronchospastic disease contraindicates β-blockers.
- DHP, nitrate, or ranolazine if bradycardia contraindicates β-blockers. The combination DHP + nitrates may be used but is less favored, as both agents are vasodilators.

In HF patients with angina, β-blockers are started slowly. Nitrates may be added for angina or the combination of nitrates + hydralazine may be used for HF. DHP or ranolazine may be added if needed (amlodipine or felodipine may be slowly added, only if HF is compensated).

E. Ranolazine

Ranolazine blocks the late current of the inward sodium channel (I_{Na}, phase 0), a channel that is particularly active in ischemia or HF. This reduces intracellular sodium and, subsequently, intracellular calcium through the sodium–calcium sarcoplasmic exchange (*opposite to digoxin effect*). The main effect of ranolazine is the reduction of diastolic calcium overload, which reduces O_2 consumption and improves LV relaxation. Moreover, the improvement of LV relaxation reduces LVEDP and the coronary compression, which improves microvascular function and coronary flow.

Ranolazine has been shown to reduce angina burden, increase exercise duration, and reduce ischemic burden on nuclear imaging, particularly in patients with the most severe or frequent angina, whether used in monotherapy or in combination with other antianginal drugs.[41,42]

In the MERLIN-TIMI 36 trial of NSTE-ACS patients, ranolazine added to standard therapy reduced the endpoint of recurrent ischemia or worsening angina. The benefit was most striking in *women* and in patients with *elevated BNP* (in the latter group, ranolazine also reduced the composite endpoint of MI/recurrent ischemia).[43–45] Ranolazine has not shown any effect on mortality.

Ranolazine only slightly prolongs QT from I_K blockade (by 2–6 ms) and does not increase the risk of arrhythmia. The blockade of I_{Na} serves to shorten the action potential, similarly to the effect of lidocaine, and counteracts the I_K blockade. In fact, in the MERLIN trial, ranolazine significantly reduced the risk of VT, SVT, and AF. *In addition, ranolazine appeared to reduce the risk of sudden death in patients with VT lasting over 8 beats, in the setting of NSTE-ACS.*[46] However, ranolazine should only be used cautiously in patients with prolonged QT or patients receiving QT-prolonging drugs.

Thus, ranolazine has the advantages of:

• Reduction of ischemia *without affecting the systemic pressure or heart rate*. It is particularly valuable when systemic pressure or heart rate limits the use of other antianginal agents.
• Improvement of LV diastolic function.
• Reduction of arrhythmias.
• Reduction of HbA1c of ~1% in patients with HbA1c ≥8% (MERLIN analysis).

Ranolazine may be used as *initial therapy* in patients who do not tolerate β-blockers (alternative to CCB and nitrates), or as *additional therapy* in patients with persistent angina despite standard therapy.

VI. Medical therapy: treatment of risk factors

1. Statin, regardless of LDL. If needed, ezetimibe, niacin, or a bile acid sequestrant may be added to achieve LDL <100 or 70 mg/dl.
2. HTN is controlled to ≤140/90 mmHg, with a preferable SBP goal ≤130 mmHg (SPRINT trial).[47]
3. ACE-Is are beneficial in CAD patients (HOPE and EUROPA trials),[48] more so in cases of EF <50%, HTN, diabetes, or CKD. In CAD patients with SBP 130–140 mmHg and normal EF, ACE-I did not show any benefit (PEACE trial).[49] In the post-CABG setting with normal EF, ACE-I did not improve outcomes and was associated with more adverse events in the first 3 months postoperatively (IMAGINE trial).[50]
4. Control of diabetes to a Hb A1c ≤7%.
5. Smoking cessation leads to a 50% reduction of the excessive risk of MI and stroke within 1 year (mostly within 2 months). At 3–5 years, the risk approaches that of never-smokers.

VII. Indications for revascularization

The first step is to determine if the patient requires coronary angiography (Figure 3.2). The *second step* is to determine if the patient requires revascularization. The *third step* is to determine whether CABG or PCI is appropriate. The need for coronary angiography does not imply a need for revascularization once CAD is found. In fact, medical therapy is frequently appropriate in a patient with significant, but not extensive CAD (no left main or three-vessel CAD). *Coronary angiography serves as a risk stratification tool that helps determine whether medical therapy alone is appropriate.*

In order to revascularize, one of the following two features must be present: (i) severe or refractory angina, *or* (ii) severe ischemia on stress testing. The appropriate indications for revascularization are as follows (ACC appropriateness criteria 2012) (Table 3.3):[51]

a. *Angina that is severe (class III–IV) and refractory,* even if the stress test is low-risk. Refractory angina is defined as angina that persists despite the use of at least two antianginal medications (or less in case of intolerance or a baseline low BP and heart rate).
b. *High-risk stress test suggesting that a large myocardial territory is at risk, or low FFR of a major epicardial vessel supplying a large territory,* along with any degree of angina, even if antianginal therapy has not been initiated.
c. *In asymptomatic patients,* revascularization is indicated if the stress test is high-risk despite maximal medical therapy, or high-risk along with proximal LAD, left main, or three-vessel CAD.

Table 3.3 Indications for revascularization and modality (PCI vs. CABG).

---

1. *Severe (class III–IV) **and** refractory angina,* even if the stress test is mildly positive
2. *High-risk stress test along with any degree of angina,* even if medical therapy is not yet initiated or maximized[a]
3. *Asymptomatic* but stress test is high-risk despite maximal medical therapy, OR *high-risk along with proximal LAD, left main, or three-vessel CAD*
4. *If one vessel CTO* (not proximal LAD), revascularize *only if* high-risk stress test + severe *or* refractory angina

PCI	CABG
One- or two-vessel CAD not involving the proximal LAD	Left main disease
Alternative to CABG in one- or two-vessel CAD involving the proximal LAD, or three-vessel CAD, if SYNTAX score ≤22 and no diabetes	Three-vessel CAD, or one- or two-vessel CAD involving the proximal LAD

[a] *Moderate-risk stress test* requires more angina (severe, or mild but refractory), or multivessel disease with proximal LAD involvement to qualify for revascularization.

d. *In single-vessel disease with chronic total occlusion (CTO)*, PCI is only indicated if the patient has a high-risk stress test *and* severe *or* refractory angina. This also depends on angiographic features that make PCI favorable (short CTO, non-calcified, no branches at the proximal cap). CTO is almost always associated with ischemia of the subtended territory, unless it is already largely infarcted. The degree of ischemia depends on the size of the supplied territory and the appropriateness of collaterals, and thus ischemia may only be mild. CTO PCI is technically challenging, but may be associated with improved survival, particularly in patients with LAD CTO and severe ischemia.[52,53]

Evidence supporting the use of ischemia to guide revascularization: In one large retrospective analysis, revascularization in the setting of extensive ischemia involving ≥10% of the myocardium (summed stress score of ≥8) was associated with a reduction of mortality (half of the patients received CABG, the other half received PCI).[54] This mortality reduction is definitely established in the subset of patients with extensive disease undergoing CABG.[27] PCI of major epicardial vessels subtending a large territory reduced coronary events, mainly ACS presentation and the need for urgent revascularization, when FFR was ≤0.80 (FAME 2 trial, in which 65% of patients had proximal or mid-LAD disease).[55] In the ACIP trial, revascularization with either CABG or PCI markedly reduced mortality and MI in patients with asymptomatic or medically controlled ischemia (especially if proximal LAD disease or multivessel CAD was present).[26]

> Note that the results of coronary angiography have, per se, strong prognostic value independent of stress test results. In fact, some studies suggest that the anatomic burden of disease is a better predictor of outcomes than ischemia.[56] *Significant left main disease, three-vessel CAD, or proximal LAD disease implies high-risk CAD and qualifies for revascularization according to a meta-analysis of CABG vs. medical therapy (definitely required in left main disease).*[27] However, when the stress test is negative or low-risk in patients with multivessel CAD, the significance of CAD needs to be proven by FFR, IVUS, or a clinically severe angina. The negative stress test may be a false negative (balanced ischemia),[57] or a true negative in a patient with non-hemodynamically significant, moderate three-vessel CAD, who would not benefit from revascularization.[2,27]
>
> In chronic stable CAD, revascularization of a non-proximal, single-vessel lesion mainly has a symptomatic value, particularly in patients with refractory angina, with no clear effect on survival or MI prevention.

VIII. CABG

CABG is the only revascularization modality shown to improve survival in the high-risk subsets of stable CAD. In a meta-analysis that included the three classic trials of CABG vs. medical therapy, the Coronary Artery Surgery Study (CASS), the European Coronary Surgery Study (ECSS), and the VA study, CABG reduced mortality by 40–50% in the following groups:[27]

- Left main disease (mortality reduction of ~75%).
- Three-vessel CAD, or one- or two-vessel CAD involving the proximal LAD. CABG is beneficial in these patients irrespective of LV function, but more so in the case of mild LV dysfunction with EF 35–50% or evidence of moderate/severe ischemia on stress testing (i.e., make sure CAD is functionally significant).

CABG is superior to PCI in three-vessel CAD or complex two-vessel CAD involving the LAD (especially proximal LAD) with SYNTAX score >22 or diabetes.

CABG was beneficial in the classic trials despite a 25% crossover to CABG in the medical therapy arm at 5 years, implying that the absolute CABG benefit is even higher. This CABG benefit was seen irrespective of symptom status, and extended to asymptomatic patients. *Note that the survival benefit in stable CAD does not emerge until 2 years after CABG, partly because of the early surgical hazard;* thus, CABG is an appropriate therapy in patients who are otherwise likely to have a good longevity. CABG is expected to be beneficial sooner in patients with unstable CAD. Those trials were done in the 1970s, at a time when CABG technique was suboptimal (LIMA was not routinely used, which explains why the survival advantage of CABG gradually narrowed beyond 10 years). But in those trials medical therapy was also suboptimal (mainly consisting of β-blockers, with very limited use of aspirin and no statin). In fact, in the CABG stratum of the modern BARI 2D trial, initial CABG did not reduce the mortality of diabetic patients with multivessel, non-left main disease (vs. initial medical therapy).

The above trials excluded patients with severe LV dysfunction (EF <35%). In patients with severe ischemic LV dysfunction (EF <35%), no or mild angina, and no severe HF, CABG improved the secondary endpoints of cardiovascular death and cardiovascular hospitalizations at 5 years in the STICH trial.[58] The benefit was, however, less marked than the benefit seen in mild LV dysfunction in the above trials (~20% reduction of cardiovascular death). *Once again, the benefit did not emerge until 2 years after CABG. This benefit was irrespective of viability testing.*

CABG may also be performed for single- or two-vessel CAD not involving the LAD, if PCI is not technically feasible and the patient has refractory, severe angina. The value of a single- or two-vessel CABG to a non-LAD vessel is mainly symptomatic.

The well-known benefit of CABG in diabetic patients is seen in CABG vs. PCI trials, rather than in the above trials of CABG vs. medical therapy.

IX. PCI

Consider the following three settings:

- PCI is a first-line therapy for one- or two-vessel CAD not involving the proximal LAD, along with an indication for revascularization (severe ischemia or severe angina).
- PCI is an alternative to CABG in three-vessel CAD, or one- or two-vessel CAD involving the proximal LAD, with an angiographic SYNTAX score ≤22 and no diabetes.

Table 3.4 Reasons for superiority of CABG vs. PCI.

---

i. CABG success is much less affected by the anatomical complexity (e.g., CTO) and the diffuseness of CAD

ii. While PCI treats focal disease, a graft improves flow to the whole coronary territory, including segments with moderate diffuse disease, and protects from MI resulting from occlusion of the proximal 6–8 cm coronary segment

iii. Very long longevity of LIMA graft

iv. More complete revascularization with CABG (vessels with CTO are sometimes left untreated in a multivessel PCI strategy)

- In three-vessel CAD, or complex two-vessel disease involving the LAD (especially proximal LAD), with *either diabetes or SYNTAX score >22*, CABG significantly improves survival in comparison with PCI (SYNTAX and FREEDOM trials).[18]

PCI is flawed by a risk of restenosis of 15–20% with BMS, which is reduced to <10% with DES. At the 5-year follow-up of PCI populations without extensive CAD and with a low prevalence of multivessel CAD, 25% of patients had recurrent events, mainly recurrent symptoms with a need for revascularization. Approximately 50–60% of these events occur in the target vessel, mainly the target stented lesion, while 40–50% occur in remote vessels (non-culprit disease progression).[59,60] Those events would be more common in patients with diffuse and complex CAD, who not only have a higher risk of restenosis but also a higher risk of progression of non-target lesions/vessels, as PCI only addresses the focal disease. CABG outcome is less dependent on the complexity and diffuseness of lesions than PCI, and when a graft is placed, the whole proximal 6–8 cm of the coronary artery is protected from MI induced by plaque rupture (Table 3.4). Hence, CABG is consistently associated with a lower risk of MI and angina recurrence than PCI. Even when MI occurs after CABG, it is less likely to be fatal and more likely a small MI, as compared with patients receiving medical therapy or PCI (CASS, BARI).

While a significant stenosis has a much higher individual risk of plaque rupture and ACS or MI (5–10% per year) than a non-significant plaque (<0.5–1%) (COURAGE, FAME, FAME 2 trials),[57,61–63] non-significant plaques are much more common throughout the coronary vasculature than significant plaques; therefore, MI or ACS often occurs over a lesion that is <50% stenotic (those lesions were responsible for 1/3 and 2/3 of ACS events upon long-term follow-up in COURAGE and PROSPECT trials, respectively).[60,61] The individual risk of a functionally significant lesion is reduced from 5–10% to 3% per year with stenting (3% is the combined risk of MI from periprocedural injury, stent thrombosis, and severe restenosis). Thus, in carefully selected stable CAD patients, PCI guided by functional significance (stress testing or FFR) may reduce the risk of future events, mainly ACS. However, a significant number of events continues to arise from non-culprit lesions or from the stented areas, which underscores the role of aggressive medical therapy.

X. PCI vs. medical therapy

The **COURAGE trial** evaluated patients with stable, rather mild angina, normal EF, and a good functional status (mean stress test exercise time = 7 min).[64] It included a large population of patients with multivessel CAD (~70%, including 30% three-vessel CAD) and patients with proximal LAD disease (~35%), although the stenoses' functional significance was unclear and only a third of patients undergoing nuclear stress testing had severe ischemia. *Initial* PCI did not improve death or MI outcomes as compared to *initial* medical therapy ± delayed PCI (PCI was eventually performed in 31% of patients in the medical therapy arm). COURAGE results, however, do not dismiss the value of PCI in highly symptomatic patients with frequent anginal episodes (i.e., daily), those with severely limiting angina, or those with persistent angina despite medical therapy, patients in whom PCI has strong effects on quality of life and functional status, according to the COURAGE quality-of-life substudy.[65] Also, as unveiled by the COURAGE nuclear substudy, PCI may still improve cardiovascular outcomes in the highest risk category of stable angina patients, with objective evidence of moderate to large myocardial ischemia on stress imaging. *PCI was far more effective than medical therapy in reducing ischemia on nuclear imaging.*[66]

Similar results were replicated in the **BARI 2D trial**.[67] In diabetic patients with mild angina, *initial* revascularization did not reduce death or MI in comparison to *initial* medical therapy, although 40% of patients eventually crossed over from medical therapy to revascularization over 5 years. More specifically, in patients with one- or two-vessel CAD, initial revascularization with PCI did not reduce death or MI in comparison with medical therapy (PCI stratum). In patients with extensive CAD randomized to initial CABG vs. medical therapy (CABG stratum), initial CABG reduced MI (14.6% vs. 7.4% at 5 years) but not death in comparison with medical therapy.

Those studies were flawed by the fact that PCI was performed in patients with mild symptoms, no objective evidence of severe ischemia, probably non-critical stenoses (COURAGE nuclear substudy), and no extensive CAD.

The **FAME 2 trial** randomized patients who mainly had one- or two-vessel CAD (65% proximal/mid-LAD) to FFR-guided PCI vs. medical therapy. PCI strikingly reduced the risk of urgent revascularization within 8 months (1.6% vs. 11%), including the risk of revascularization for MI or high-risk ACS (0.9% vs. 5.2%), despite the fact that most patients had mild angina (class I–II) and some patients only had asymptomatic ischemia (~15%). While PCI reduced the risk of late *spontaneous* MI, which occurred in 3% of patients in the medical therapy arm, it was associated with a small risk of periprocedural MI and stent thrombosis, which negated the overall benefit on MI at 8 months. A spontaneous MI is associated with a much larger increase in long-term mortality than periprocedural MI, and thus the reduction of spontaneous MI with PCI is a valuable finding.[68] The FAME-2 trial is, in a way a "COURAGE 2" trial of PCI vs. medical therapy, differing from the COURAGE trial mainly in the use of FFR guidance, since only lesions that are functionally significant have a high individual risk of evolving into ACS/MI or progressing symptomatically. PCI was more strikingly beneficial in lesions with FFR ≤0.65.

In the FAME 2 trial, patients who had >50% stenoses without a significant FFR had a low risk of coronary events with medical therapy, a risk lower than that of patients with significant CAD receiving PCI. While the individual risk of MI for every lesion with FFR >0.80 is 0.2% at 2 years, the overall risk of MI in these patients was ~2% at 8 months (risk summation of all non-significant plaques). This implies that patients with non-significant disease have a low but not a negligible risk of MI, a risk that does not result from one particular lesion but rather from the diffuse process, which warrants aggressive medical therapy.

In stable CAD, ischemia appears to be the greatest driver of outcomes; PCI is much more effective than medical therapy in reducing severe ischemia *and* severe angina. ***Overall, the COURAGE and BARI 2D trials support* initial *medical therapy in patients with no or mild angina, no severe functional limitation, and no severe ischemia on stress testing. PCI is superior for angina relief*** and is particularly helpful in patients with severe functional limitation, and in patients with angina and a combination of low heart rate/low blood pressure, whose myocardial demands are inherently low (low rate-pressure product) and whose angina is mainly driven by the severe stenosis rather than hemodynamic variables. ***PCI is far superior for the* relief of the ischemic burden *in patients*** with severe baseline ischemia on nuclear imaging (>10% of the myocardium).[66,69] Moreover, PCI improves coronary outcomes, mainly future ACS and the need for urgent revascularizations, in lesions with documented severe ischemia or FFR ≤0.80 (especially ≤0.65), regardless of the severity of angina. Yet even for those lesions, initial medical therapy did not translate into increased mortality or overall MI risk in the FAME 2 trial, and thus *initial* medical therapy is appropriate in selected cases. Also, up to half of patients with severe ischemia achieve >5% absolute reduction of ischemia with medical therapy (vs. 78% of patients treated with PCI).[66,69]

Furthermore, it is unclear if PCI improves survival in patients with left main or extensive multivessel disease who would derive a survival benefit from CABG, but who are not candidates for CABG or whose SYNTAX score is ≤22. By extrapolation from the results of CABG vs. PCI trials, PCI is presumed to improve survival in those patients (PCI and CABG are associated with equivalent survival in select patients with multivessel or left main CAD).

XI. PCI vs. CABG in multivessel disease

BARI and ARTS trials – In the balloon angioplasty era, the *BARI trial* randomized very select patients with focal multivessel CAD to CABG vs. PCI. In comparison with PCI, CABG dramatically reduced mortality in diabetic patients by an absolute 16% at 5 years, and dramatically reduced repeat revascularizations in all patients.[70] The benefit on repeat revascularizations was shown in the BMS era as well (*ARTS trial*).[71] The superiority of CABG was seen despite the very careful selection of patients with non-extensive CAD amenable to PCI (<10% of screened patients were randomized to CABG vs. PCI).

Isolated proximal LAD disease – A meta-analysis of randomized trials of CABG vs. PCI for isolated proximal LAD disease suggests the lack of mortality difference, although repeat revascularizations were much lower with CABG (pre-DES era).[72]

SYNTAX trial – In the DES era, the *SYNTAX trial* randomized patients with three-vessel and/or left main disease to CABG vs. PCI with DES. This trial included patients with extensive, complex CAD, and graded the angiographic severity of CAD using the SYNTAX score. In the overall trial, at 5 years of follow-up, CABG was associated with a significant reduction in MI (~10% vs. 4%), a marked reduction in the need for repeat revascularizations (26% vs. 14%), and a strong trend towards mortality reduction (14% vs. 11%, significant at 4 years). CABG significantly improved all of these outcomes in patients with intermediate SYNTAX scores (23–32) and high SYNTAX scores (>32), with 8% absolute mortality reduction in the latter group.[73,74] Patients with a low SYNTAX score (≤22) had similar death and MI rates with CABG and PCI, whether they had three-vessel or left main disease, yet even in this subgroup repeat revascularization rates were lower with CABG. Interestingly, *CABG outcomes were not affected by SYNTAX score, meaning that CABG success and post-CABG survival is not affected by angiographic complexity, in contradistinction with PCI.* The only pitfall of CABG was the higher early risk of stroke in all subgroups (2.2% vs. 0.6% at 1 year).

The SYNTAX score assigns a number for the location of each stenosis (e.g., left main 5, proximal LAD 3.5, RCA 1), and multiplies this number by 2 in case of a 50–99% stenosis, and 5 in case of a CTO. Additional points are added at every lesion for tri- or bifurcation, long disease, calcium, and CTO complexity. Overall, the score emphasizes proximal stenoses (especially LAD) and angiographic complexity, especially CTO.

FREEDOM trial – Diabetic patients with two- or three-vessel CAD involving the LAD were randomized to CABG vs. PCI with DES.[75] At 5-year follow-up, CABG significantly reduced mortality vs. PCI, more dramatically than in the overall SYNTAX trial and almost as much as in the high SYNTAX group (16.3% vs. 10.9%). It reduced MI (~14% vs. 6%) at the price of an increase in postoperative stroke and a higher early postoperative mortality. The benefit in these diabetic patients was consistent across all SYNTAX score groups, including the low SYNTAX group.

Overall, both SYNTAX and FREEDOM trials support the use of CABG in multivessel CAD with LAD involvement. PCI is an option in patients with a low SYNTAX score ≤22 and no diabetes, although repeat revascularizations are higher with PCI even in this group.

PCI is also a viable option for patients with left main disease, high surgical risk >5%, and favorable PCI features: left main disease with SYNTAX score ≤22, or ostial or mid-shaft left main disease (where PCI would not involve the bifurcation).

Note some of the features of the SYNTAX and FREEDOM trials:

- LVEF was normal or >40% in almost all patients. Very few patients had HF (4% in SYNTAX trial).
- Patients with acute MI, including large acute NSTEMI, were excluded. The superiority of CABG is extrapolated to those patients whose event rates are higher than stable CAD.

- While the CABG benefit on repeat revascularization emerges early within the first year, the survival and MI benefit only starts to emerge beyond 2 years of follow-up, after an early perioperative hazard (in both trials). This benefit appeared sooner in the high SYNTAX score group in SYNTAX trial. Overall, this implies that CABG mainly applies to patients who are expected to have a long longevity (e.g., > 3–4 years).
- Consistent increase in the risk of stroke with CABG (by an absolute ~2%).
- Patients with prior stroke were essentially excluded from both trials. In fact, very few patients had carotid disease. Yet, despite this, CABG led to a higher risk of stroke than PCI, which is expected to be even higher in patients with prior stroke or carotid disease.
- Randomized patients were relatively young (median age ~65).

Thus, these trials do not necessarily prove the superiority of CABG in a sicker population: older patients, higher prevalence of stroke, lower expected longevity, severe LV dysfunction or HF. Age, by itself, may not increase the risk of CABG. A meta-analysis of CABG vs. PCI trials has shown that old patients (>65) derive more mortality benefit from CABG than younger patients, which is consistent with an analysis of Medicare beneficiaries;[76] a New York registry analysis has shown that CABG is associated with a lower mortality than PCI in carefully selected octogenarians.[77] However, when an older but also sicker population was randomized to CABG vs. PCI in the VA-AWESOME trial, the 6-month survival was better with PCI, and the 5-year survival was equivalent with both strategies.[78] In the VA-AWESOME trial, patients had at least one of the following: age >70 (50%), MI <7 days (33%), EF ≤35% (20%), prior CABG (33%). Thus, PCI still has a role in ill patients with multivessel CAD and comorbidities who are deemed at a high surgical risk.

XII. High-surgical-risk patients

In a patient with multivessel disease where CABG or PCI is considered, two risk scores are used: (i) SYNTAX score to determine PCI outcomes, and (ii) STS score or EuroSCORE to assess surgical mortality (Table 3.5).[79,80] The average CABG mortality is 3% (1–5%), but increases to >5% with the combination of several risk factors, especially combined CABG and valve surgery, redo CABG, age >80, prior disabling stroke, severe lung disease, or acute or critical coronary status. Patients who are at a high surgical risk, much higher than the 2% seen in randomized trials (e.g., > 5%), may be better served with multivessel PCI. *Thus, in the era of an aging population with comorbidities, multivessel complex PCI still has a role.* A heart team discussion is warranted for these patients.

In addition to the high surgical risk patients, patients with small vessels and diffuse distal disease that is severe or calcified may not have appropriate distal targets for CABG and may not be candidates for CABG, especially when the LAD cannot be grafted. They may undergo PCI of focal, critical, proximal disease. A third reason that may preclude CABG is the lack of conduits, in particular venous conduits in patients with large varicose veins and venous insufficiency.

The use of LIMA necessitates surgical entry into the pleural cavity, with a high risk of pleural effusion and deterioration of pulmonary function in patients with severe lung disease.

XIII. Role of complete functional revascularization

Complete revascularization is defined as revascularization of all functionally significant stenoses in vessels ≥1.5 mm supplying viable territories. However, this has been defined differently across studies, and some based it on angiographic disease >50–70% rather than on functionally significant disease, or on achieving revascularization of the three major epicardial vessels (as opposed to all branches).[81] CABG generally achieves more complete revascularization than PCI, as it is less affected by lesion complexity (e.g., CTO) (67% vs. 53% in SYNTAX patients).[82] *In most registries and post-hoc analyses, only incomplete revascularization with PCI was associated with impaired outcomes* (New York and ARTS registries).[83,84] This adverse outcome may be related to the residual disease itself or to the fact that residual disease is a marker of more extensive and aggressive atherosclerosis even across the revascularized arteries, which explains why incomplete revascularization is more unfavorable after PCI than CABG. In fact, the intense pursuit of complete revascularization may not, by itself, improve outcomes. In two analyses of CABG patients, incomplete revascularization of a small/poor target RCA or LCx in patients receiving LIMA-to-LAD graft did not adversely affect long-term outcomes; in fact, too aggressive revascularization of >1 non-LAD vessel may be associated with worse outcomes.[85,86] This is called "reasonable" incomplete revascularization. This *reasonable revascularization* concept fits with the *functional revascularization* concept where *only large and ischemic* territories are revascularized. Incomplete revascularization usually has a worse connotation with PCI than with CABG, as (i) PCI is a suboptimal therapy for extensive disease, and (ii) PCI more frequently omits large, otherwise graftable vessels because of technical challenge, such as CTO.

Table 3.5 Variables analyzed in surgical risk scores (STS and EuroSCORE).

1. Underlying patient-related factors and comorbidities
(i) age (the risk doubles with every 10 yr >60); (ii) women (~50% higher risk than men); (iii) moderate or severe COPD; (iv) severe CKD; (v) prior disabling stroke or neurological illness; (vi) carotid disease, PAD

2. Underlying EF–HF
(i) EF (<50%: mild score; < 30%: severe score); (ii) HF functional class IV

3. Prior cardiac surgery, especially redo CABG

4. Isolated CABG <isolated valve surgery <CABG+valve surgery

5. Current cardiac status
(i) recent MI; (ii) unstable vs. stable angina; (iii) hemodynamic or electrical instability and requirements for IABP and/or inotropes

XIV. Hybrid CABG–PCI

The superiority of CABG mainly results from the longevity of the LIMA-to-LAD graft. DES stenting of non-LAD vessels, when feasible (e.g., no CTO, no diffuse calcified disease), is likely associated with equal or superior results to placement of venous grafts, ~25% of which occlude by the first year. The so-called hybrid strategy consists of performing LIMA–LAD using off-pump (beating heart) CABG, followed by DES PCI of the remaining stenoses during the same hospitalization (hours or days later, with clopidogrel loading after CABG). Occasionally, in patients with critical non-LAD disease, non-LAD disease is stented first, followed by performance of off-pump CABG under clopidogrel therapy.

The off-pump LIMA-to-LAD surgery offers the advantage of avoiding aortic manipulation, which is necessary during on-pump CABG or during SVG grafting (whether off- or on-pump). Also, the shorter surgical time, the lower blood loss, and the avoidance of cardioplegia and cardiopulmonary bypass are advantages.

Currently, the hybrid approach is particularly applicable to: (i) patients with heavily calcified, porcelain aorta in whom aortic manipulation needs to be avoided; and (ii) patients with good LAD target but poor LCx and RCA targets that, nonetheless, have severe proximal disease amenable to PCI.

XV. Enhanced external counterpulsation (EECP)

This therapy consists of inflating cuffs around the lower extremities during diastole, and deflating them in systole, creating an effect similar to IABP. The systolic cuff depression reduces LV afterload and O_2 demands. It may also have a sustained effect on endothelial function, collateral function, and oxidative stress, explaining the sustained benefit. EECP consists of 35 one-hour sessions. Non-randomized and limited randomized data suggest a reduction of angina and a reduction of ECG and nuclear ischemia with this therapy (class IIb for refractory angina).[18]

XVI. Mortality in CAD (Table 3.6)

Note on left main disease – Medical therapy has not been addressed as a standalone therapy for left main disease in any contemporary trial. Old studies such as the VA-CABG trial and the CASS registry have shown that the mortality of medically treated left main disease, whether symptomatic or asymptomatic, is ~10% per year, with a dramatic reduction of mortality to 2% per year after CABG, the largest mortality benefit of CABG in any subgroup of patients.[89,90]

Appendix 1. Note on outcomes with various surgical grafts

A. SVG

1. General SVG outcomes

SVG grafts occlude at the following rates: ~10% in the first month, 15–25% in the first year, and 2–4% per year beyond the first year. Thus, the fastest occlusion rate occurs in the first year, and at 10 years, 50% of SVGs are occluded while 20% are significantly stenotic (Table 3.7). In addition, 20–40% of patients have native disease progression in non-grafted vessels or in grafted vessels distal to the anastomoses at 5–10 years of follow-up.

CABG patients who present with ACS often have an SVG culprit. However, < 50% of SVG occlusions lead to MI (STEMI or NSTEMI), the remaining being either silent or leading to stable angina;[73] this is related to the status of the native vessel and the presence of collaterals. Overall, additional revascularization is required in ~15–20% of patients at 5 years, and MI occurs at a rate of ~1–2% per year (CASS, SYNTAX trials).[74]

2. Factors determining SVG patency

Early and late SVG patency is dependent on a good flow through the graft and requires: (i) good distal runoff and good size of the recipient artery (>1.5–2.0 mm) without distal disease; (ii) significant proximal disease in the recipient artery (otherwise, the flow through the recipient artery prevents appropriate flow through the graft); (iii) well-matched size of the graft and recipient artery.[91–93] This dependency on size and flow explains that SVG graft to LAD has higher patency than SVG to RCA or LCx, and that SVG to a diagonal or to a small vessel has the lowest patency.

Table 3.6 CAD mortality.

Older data of medically treated CAD patients (CASS registry)[87,88]

One- or two-vessel CAD: 1.5–2% mortality per yr
Three-vessel CAD with normal EF: 4.5% mortality per yr
Multivessel CAD with EF <35%: 10% morality per yr

Contemporary data in non-extensive single or multivessel CAD, treated with PCI or medical therapy (COURAGE, BARI 2D PCI group)

1.5% mortality per yr
20–25% event rate at 5yr

Contemporary data in patients with multivessel CAD and normal EF undergoing CABG (SYNTAX, FREEDOM, BARI 2D CABG group)

2–3% mortality per yr (after a higher 1st-yr mortality of 3.5%)
1.5% repeat revascularization per yr (after a higher 1st-yr repeat revascularization rate of 6%)
1% MI per yr (3.5% MI in 1st yr, with 3.5% symptomatic graft occlusion in 1st yr)
27% overall death or cardiovascular event rate at 5yr (12.5% in first yr) vs. 37% event rate with PCI

Contemporary data in multivessel CAD with EF <35% but no or mild HF (STICH)

6.5% mortality per yr with CABG, 8% mortality per yr with medical therapy (mortality would be higher with worse HF status)

Mortality is higher in patients with ACS, low EF, symptomatic HF, or comorbidities.

Table 3.7 Causes and histology of SVG failure.

< 1 month
Graft thrombosis, often before hospital discharge, sometimes related to distal native disease past the anastomosis or to technical issues (anastomotic stenosis from the suture, SVG kinking or stretching)

1 month to 1–3 years
Fibrointimal hyperplasia leads to peri-anastomotic or mid-graft stenosis (exposure of the vein to the arterial pressure leads to endothelial injury with formation of a hard neointima, called fibrointimal hyperplasia)

>1–3 years
Atherosclerosis starts to develop at >1–3 years, with similar risk factors to native atherosclerosis
As compared with native atherosclerosis, SVG atherosclerosis is more extensive, friable, with more foam cells and no fibrous cap, and may be mixed with thrombi. Aggressive lipid lowering slows down this process

3. Treatment of SVG failure

In the first 30 days, ST elevation is often the result of venous graft thrombosis with distal embolization, which worsens the perfusion of a previously stable territory subtended by a stenotic artery or by collaterals. Since the main issue is distal embolization, routine PCI for any post-CABG ST elevation may not be helpful. If there is a clinical, electrical, or hemodynamic manifestation of ischemia, the patient often needs to be revascularized. Reoperation may need to be performed the first day after CABG; beyond the first day, angiography may be performed to identify the problem and potentially treat anastomotic SVG disease or native distal disease with PCI. If a thrombotic SVG occlusion is found, PCI of the native artery may be attempted if possible. A review of the preoperative anatomy is critical: e.g., an expected occlusion of a graft supplying a small distal RCA may not have any revascularization option when the native RCA has a CTO. ST elevation may also result from arterial graft spasm.

Beyond the first 30 days, when SVG disease develops, it is best to treat the native artery if possible, as long-term patency of a percutaneously treated SVG is low. If the native artery is not amenable to PCI (CTO), SVG PCI is performed, unless the SVG is also chronically occluded, in which case medical therapy is the best option. *Location and timing* of the disease determine long-term success. Distal SVG stenosis has the best long-term success rate with PCI, especially when it occurs in the first year, or even up to 5 years after CABG, in which case it is due to intimal hyperplasia without atherosclerosis (20% restenosis after plain angioplasty). Mid-shaft disease has intermediate long-term success rate, while proximal disease has the lowest success rate.

Disease occurring at <1–3 years without significant atherosclerosis has the best long-term success.[94,95] In fact, the extent of atherosclerosis >1–3 years after CABG is a major determinant of long-term success. Treating the focal lesion, particularly a proximal lesion, does not prevent the eventual progression of the diffuse atherosclerotic disease and the eventual ~50% occlusion rate at 2 years. While DES may prevent the focal restenosis, it does not eliminate this aggressive disease progression outside the stented area and the long-term occlusion risk in diffusely diseased grafts. Degenerated SVGs with diffuse atherosclerosis have a high adverse event rate at 2 years (up to 45%), even if SVG stenosis is only moderate.[96]

Patients with multiple failing SVGs and no patent graft to the LAD have an indication for redo CABG, unless the operative risk is prohibitively high.

B. LIMA

LIMA graft is usually used as an in-situ graft: the distal part of the LIMA is connected directly to the LAD, while the proximal LIMA is not touched and remains connected to the subclavian artery. LIMA atherosclerosis is extremely uncommon, thus the excellent long-term patency of 90% at 10 years; *a LIMA that is patent beyond the first few months post-CABG usually remains patent for life*. LIMA has an intact internal elastic membrane that prevents smooth muscle migration and atherosclerosis. Early LIMA failure is possible, however, and is related to anastomotic fibrointimal hyperplasia or to poor LIMA development. LIMA may not develop or may regress because of a subclavian stenosis, poor distal LAD flow, or insignificant LAD stenosis proximal to the anastomosis. Significant native proximal disease is necessary to allow SVG and, more particularly, LIMA and radial grafts to remain patent; a good native flow may impede LIMA or SVG flow, leading to thrombosis of the SVG or spasm of an arterial graft. In fact, bypassing a LAD that has <50–60% stenosis leads to disuse atrophy of the LIMA or "string sign" in up to 80% of patients.

Always attempt to use LIMA to the LAD, except in emergent cases with hemodynamic instability, where SVG-to-LAD may be preferred, because SVG has a higher and more expeditious flow initially.[92] Also, LIMA is occasionally avoided in patients with severe lung disease in order to avoid pleural dissection and the subsequent left pleural effusion.

While LIMA does not develop atherosclerotic disease, ischemia of the LIMA territory may be caused by:
1. Subclavian stenosis (this is the most common cause of LIMA ischemia). The assessment of BP in both arms is critically important in CABG patients presenting with angina.
2. Atresia of the LIMA graft related to insignificant proximal LAD disease, poor distal LAD runoff, or subclavian stenosis. It is usually seen early after CABG.
3. Stenosis of the LIMA-to-LAD anastomosis, which often occurs in the first 3–6 months and results from intimal hyperplasia. Since it is not due to an atherosclerotic process, plain angioplasty provides good long-term patency (as good as BMS). Stenting may be reserved for a suboptimal result but is more systematically used in the DES era.
4. Progression of native LAD disease distal to the anastomosis.
5. If the LIMA's intercostal branches are not clipped, the flow may be directed away from the LAD (steal phenomenon). However, this is an unlikely phenomenon, as the coronary flow is mainly diastolic, while the flow into the intercostal branches is mainly systolic.

C. Other arterial grafts

Radial grafts have similar 1-year patency to SVG, but very low attrition rate beyond the first year and better long-term patency (85% at 5 years).[97,98] Radial grafts are very prone to spasm and more prone than any other graft to early failure if the underlying native stenosis is not severe or the target artery is not large. They are probably best used when stenosis is >90% and the recipient artery is very large.[98] Moreover, radial grafts are more susceptible to atherosclerosis than mammary arteries.

RIMA may also be used, as in-situ or free graft, mainly for RCA or LCx arteries. It is used as a free rather than in-situ graft to the distal RCA and sometimes LCx branches, because RIMA may be too short to reach these branches. RIMA has a better patency than radial and SVG grafts, but may be technically more challenging with a risk of sternal wound infection, especially in patients with diabetes.[99] The gastroepiploic artery may be used as a free or in-situ graft.

A classical CABG surgery involves grafting a LIMA to the LAD, one or several SVGs to diagonal(s), obtuse marginal branch(es), and distal RCA (or its PDA or PLB branch). Instead of SVGs, radial or free RIMA grafts may be used.

In distal left main disease, both the LAD and one of the obtuse marginal branches are bypassed.

D. Grafts with multiple distal anastomoses (see Chapter 34, Figure 34.41)

Some grafts connect to two or multiple distal targets. A **sequential graft** (or jump graft) connects to one branch, e.g. OM1, in a side-to-side anastomosis, then continues and connects to another branch, e.g., OM2, in an end-to-side anastomosis. A **split graft** (or Y graft) consists of a graft A that connects to one branch and a second graft B that is anastomosed to graft A and that separately connects to another branch. Sequential and split grafts reduce the number of aortic anastomoses and may improve patency in light of the higher flow across the graft. However, when the runoff is good, grafts with single targets have a higher patency than sequential grafts.[92,93] Sequential grafting is useful in patients with poor runoff or patients with limited venous conduits (e.g., varicose veins). The best sequential graft patency is obtained by placing the last distal anastomosis onto the coronary branch with the greatest runoff, while the smaller coronary branch is anastomosed more proximally in a side-to-side fashion (e.g., graft to diagonal and LAD, LAD being the last anastomosis); this allows an increase in flow throughout the whole graft.[93]

E. Off-pump CABG

During on-pump CABG, cardioplegia is induced, the aorta is cannulated and cross-clamped, and a cardiopulmonary bypass (heart–lung pump) is used between the venae cavae and the aorta. The pulmonary ventilation is then turned off. *Off-pump CABG* is performed on a beating heart without cannulation of the aorta, although partial aortic cross-clamping is still needed if SVG anastomoses are performed.

Off-pump CABG has the advantage of less bleeding/less requirement for transfusion, less renal failure, less respiratory complications, and probably less stroke as aortic manipulation is limited.[100,101] In fact, in patients with heavy aortic calcifications or atherosclerosis, off-pump CABG with only LIMA or LIMA and RIMA grafting is particularly valuable, as it avoids aortic manipulation. Off-pump CABG is, however, associated with less complete revascularization and a higher risk of early ischemia and graft failure.[100] MIDCAB (minimally invasive direct CABG) is a form of off-pump CABG performed through a mini-thoracotomy between two ribs, and mainly consists of single-vessel grafting of the LIMA to the LAD. Off-pump LIMA–LAD may be used as part of a hybrid strategy, where non-LAD disease is treated with PCI.

Appendix 2. Coronary vasospasm (variant angina, Prinzmetal angina)

A. Underlying CAD: patterns of vasospasm

While Prinzmetal angina was initially described in patients who had underlying obstructive CAD, sometimes unstable CAD,[3,4,102,103] later reports suggest that vasospasm is also commonly diagnosed in patients with typical angina and no obstructive CAD.[5] Even when the coronary arteries appear angiographically normal, IVUS imaging demonstrates that the sites of vasospasm exhibit underlying atherosclerosis. Atherosclerosis induces endothelial dysfunction and dysregulation of nitric oxide production, which leads to local vascular hyperreactivity.[6]

Vasospasm may be **epicardial and focal**, i.e., involving one coronary segment, or **epicardial and diffuse**, involving two or more coronary segments. It may also occur solely at the **microvascular level**.

Additional features of vasospasm:

- Epicardial vasospasm often involves one site and *recurs at the same atherosclerotic site*; less commonly, it may involve multiple sites, sometimes two separate coronaries, or occur at separate sites at different times (~15% of cases).[104]
- The LAD and RCA are most commonly involved. The proximal and distal segments have been variously involved in different reports.
- In the absence of CAD, spontaneous remissions within 6–12 months of follow-up or remissions with CCBs are common (up to 82% of patients). Yet up to a third of these patients may experience recurrences.[103–105]
- Vasospasm that occurs without significant CAD is more commonly seen in women,[5] although some series suggest it is more common in men.[102,103,106] It is generally described in patients >40 years of age, with a mean age of 55–65. Smoking and chronic alcohol or cocaine use increase the risk of vasospasm.

B. ECG, arrhythmias, and clinical manifestations

Vasospasm usually leads to a more severe ischemia than fixed stenosis and is occlusive or subtotally occlusive, particularly when it occurs on top of obstructive, fixed stenosis. It typically leads to transient ST elevation, reflecting transmural ischemia, but it may also lead to ST-segment depression when the spasm is not totally occlusive. Post-ischemic T-wave inversion may be seen. Since ischemia may be severe, serious arrhythmias (VT, VF, AV block), syncope, sudden death, or MI may be seen. The latter complications are particularly common (~20%) when vasospasm occurs on top of a significant stenosis;[3,4] otherwise, spontaneous remissions are common and the course is often, but not always, benign.[103–105]

Angina is most commonly a rest angina without exertional limitation, even in patients with CAD (angina manifests when the dynamic component exaggerates the fixed stenosis).[4,104,105] It may also be a mixed rest/exertional angina, or, less commonly, a purely exertional angina.[5,106] The rest angina typically has a cyclic, often nocturnal pattern, and is more prolonged and more severe than classic angina.

Exercise ECG testing is frequently positive in these patients (50–70%),[4,5] partly from the underlying CAD, and partly from exercise-induced vasospasm.

C. Diagnosis of vasospasm

Epicardial (macrovascular) vasospasm is definitely diagnosed on coronary angiography when the following three features occur, spontaneously or with provocation:[5]

- Focal or diffuse vasospasm leading to ≥75% dynamic luminal reduction
- ST-segment elevation or depression
- Reproduction of the patient's symptoms

Microvascular vasospasm is diagnosed when ST-segment changes and symptoms occur with provocation, without any visualized spasm.[5] An additional feature of microvascular spasm is a slow coronary flow (delayed TIMI frame count) without epicardial obstruction.

When present spontaneously, vasospasm is frequently confused with a true fixed obstruction; the diagnosis of vasospasm is made when the stenosis improves to <50% with intracoronary NTG administration. High doses of NTG are sometimes required to yield severe vasospasm (800 mcg). While it is reasonable to administer NTG whenever any coronary stenosis is seen (to rule out a dynamic component before any PCI), vasospasm is particularly suspected when the stenosis is concentric with smooth borders. *Conversely, ostial spasm occurring at the catheter tip does not have a diagnostic value.*

Vasospasm may be provoked with intracoronary ergonovine, intracoronary acetylcholine, hyperventilation for 6 minutes, or hand immersion in ice water for 2 minutes (the latter two have low sensitivity). Angiographic vasospasm without symptoms or ECG changes is suspicious but not diagnostic of vasospastic angina.

Although safe, pharmacological provocation is rarely performed because of reported cases of refractory vasospasm. Thus, the diagnosis is often presumptive in a patient with either one of the following:

i. Typical *rest angina* and documentation of transient ST elevation or ST depression on stress ECG or ambulatory ECG (with or without significant CAD)
ii. *Effort angina* with ST changes on stress ECG but *no significant CAD.*

This is how the diagnosis of variant angina has historically been made.[4,102,106]

In vessels with normal endothelial function, acetylcholine induces the synthesis of NO and coronary vasodilatation. In vessels with endothelial dysfunction, the endothelium cannot generate NO and acetylcholine directly acts as a vasoconstrictor.

D. Frequency of vasospasm in patients with exertional chest pain and no significant CAD

One study assessed patients (age 63±10) with typical exertional chest pain and unobstructed coronary arteries (<20%) on angiography. Among patients who underwent a stress ECG before angiography, half had ischemic ECG changes while the other half did not. Upon provocative testing with acetylcholine, 62% of these patients developed macrovascular or microvascular spasm (28% macrovascular, 34% microvascular). Macrovascular spasm was often diffuse and distal.[7] Most of these patients were women.

Thus, variant angina is not only a cause of rest angina, but is also a very common cause of exertional angina in patients without CAD. The stimulation of adrenergic α-receptors may induce epicardial coronary spasm. Alternatively, the epicardial or microvascular spasm induced by acetylcholine testing may be a marker of abnormal coronary vascular tone that prevents appropriate micro- and macrovascular dilatation with exercise.

E. Treatment and prognosis of vasospasm

An underlying significant CAD is treated with PCI or CABG as appropriate. Beware that, sometimes, the lesion is only moderate and not hemodynamically significant, but becomes significant when vasospasm aggravates it; in those cases, revascularization is not indicated and good results are obtained with CCBs.

In the absence of severe CAD, CCBs are first-line therapy. CCBs are very effective (control of symptoms in 83% of patients),[107] and spontaneous remission is also very common.[103–105] Nitrates may also be used, but are less effective (31%).[107] β-Blockers may exaggerate vasospasm through blocking the β_2-receptor, but may be beneficial in patients with a fixed stenosis and exertional symptoms. In comparison with CCB monotherapy, the combination of CCB and statin has been shown to dramatically reduce vasospasm in one trial.[108]

The prognosis is usually benign and is related to the extent of underlying CAD. Patients with underlying CAD have a high risk of MI (~20%) or serious arrhythmias (20–30%) in the short-term follow-up (<30 days).[3,4] In five series, patients without CAD had a lower, but still significant, risk of MI (up to 15%),[4,102,105–107] VT (25%),[4,105,107] syncope from arrhythmia (20%), and particularly cardiac arrest (2.5%)[102,106] at several years of follow-up; these patients, for the most part, were not receiving CCB. In fact, vasospasm has been well documented as a cause of cardiac arrest in five patients without significant CAD; CCB prevented ergonovine-induced spasm and arrhythmias in these patients.[109] The severity of spasm, as evidenced by the severity and extent of ST elevation, correlates with adverse events and ventricular arrhythmias regardless of the underlying CAD.[102,106] Similarly, prior MI or cardiac arrest are strong predictors of future events.[106]

Patients receiving CCBs have a much more benign course with much less angina, much less unstable angina (6% at 3 years), and 10× lower risk of MI and cardiac death (<1% at 3 years), which suggests the great efficacy of CCBs.[102,104,106] However, in patients who have already had a cardiac arrest, CCB therapy does not fully eliminate the risk of VF, and ICD may be justified (in one series, 15% of patients receiving ICD had appropriate shocks despite CCB therapy; in another series, > 50% had VT/VF or ICD shock despite CCB therapy).[106,110] Abstinence from smoking and alcohol is also associated with a reduction of events.

F. Microvascular endothelial dysfunction or syndrome X

Microvascular dysfunction has two forms, both reflective of endothelial dysfunction:

i. Microvascular spasm, which is part of the spectrum of coronary vasospasm
ii. Impaired capacity to vasodilate the microcirculation and increase flow during exercise

It is diagnosed by provocative coronary testing with acetylcholine, seeking ST-segment and chest pain response, or by demonstration of impaired coronary flow reserve after acetylcholine or adenosine (<2.5× increase in coronary flow, measured with a coronary flow wire).[5,111–113] In the absence of CAD, a slow angiographic flow also suggests microvascular dysfunction ("coronary slow flow phenomenon"). Impaired coronary flow may elevate LVEDP or may be due to an elevated LVEDP. In fact, microvascular dysfunction may be associated with left ventricular hypertrophy.[113]

The diagnosis of vasospasm or microvascular dysfunction is often made presumptively in a patient with chest pain, documented ST changes or convincing ischemia on stress testing, and no significant CAD. Echo stress imaging is not very sensitive in these patients; nuclear SPECT or, better, stress imaging with PET or MRI is preferred to detect abnormal vasodilatory reserve. *While the stress test is sometimes considered falsely positive (e.g., artifact), patients with convincing angina and ischemic ECG or imaging defects most likely have microvascular dysfunction, or, less frequently, macrovascular spasm.* One study has found a correlation between impaired coronary response to acetylcholine and ischemic defects on nuclear testing.[112] As opposed to nuclear SPECT imaging, nuclear PET is able to quantify the absolute myocardial flow, both at rest and after stress.

CCBs, nitrates, statins, and ACE-Is have been used for this syndrome with a variable success rate. Nitrates are not microvascular dilators, but lessen ischemia through preload reduction. Ranolazine appears to be particularly effective in reducing angina and improving myocardial flow.[114] In one study of microvascular dysfunction, L-arginine significantly improved myocardial flow.[111,115] L-arginine is available as an over-the-counter supplement.

Appendix 3. Women with chest pain and normal coronary arteries

While women with CAD frequently have atypical angina, including prolonged pain sometimes unrelated to exertion, women with typical angina frequently (~50%) do not have any significant CAD and their angina is explained by microvascular dysfunction. In fact, in the WISE study, ~60% of women with chest pain undergoing coronary angiography (median age, 58) did not have any significant CAD, despite an abnormal stress test in the majority of them.[116] Half of the women without CAD continued to have chest pain for over a year, likely those with macrovascular or microvascular spasm/dysfunction.[117,118] Despite the lack of CAD, women with persistent chest pain (>1 year) had a significant risk of MI (5.5%), HF (7.5%), stroke, and combined cardiovascular events (20%) at 6-year follow-up, much higher than patients without persistent chest pain, albeit far lower than patients with CAD.[116] Another analysis of the WISE study showed *that among women with chest pain and no obstructive CAD, half had microvascular dysfunction (as assessed by coronary flow reserve), more so if ischemia was present on stress testing.*[117] Yet, microvascular dysfunction may be present without stress test abnormality.[117] Perfusion stress PET or MRI is a better diagnostic modality.

The high rate of events on follow-up may be directly related to the following:

- Ischemic events/MI triggered by coronary vasospasm.
- Endothelial dysfunction and abnormal response to acetylcholine predicts the future development of obstructive CAD,[118] and a 14% risk of cardiac events, including progressive CAD, at 3 years.[119]
- Since patients with spasm and endothelial dysfunction have underlying atherosclerosis, erosion of non-obstructive plaque is another potential mechanism of MI. A dysfunctional endothelium may contribute to plaque destabilization and erosion because of its reduced antioxidative potential.

> Note that diastolic dysfunction with elevated LVEDP may be the cause or consequence of microvascular dysfunction. This partly explains HF events in these patients.

> In sum, abnormalities of coronary flow may be due to obstructive CAD, coronary epicardial spasm, or microvascular spasm/dysfunction. While obstructive CAD is associated with the highest risk of events, abnormal vasomotion is associated with an intermediate risk of events, including MI, arrhythmias, and progressive CAD, much higher than in patients with no CAD and normal vasomotion.

Appendix 4. Myocardial bridging

The coronary arteries normally take an epicardial course over the surface of the heart, but they occasionally have an intramyocardial segment that may get compressed in systole and cause symptomatic ischemia. This is called "myocardial bridging," and it is characterized by angiographic off-and-on narrowing of the intramyocardial segment by >70%, only *during systole*. This phasic obstruction distinguishes bridging from spasm, which is present throughout the cardiac cycle. Bridging is seen in 2% of coronary angiograms and is almost always limited to the LAD. Intramyocardial coronary segments are even more commonly diagnosed on coronary CT, with a frequency of up to 25%.[120]

Since over 80% of the left coronary blood flow occurs during diastole, bridging does not usually cause ischemia and often does not explain chest pain.[121] During tachycardia, systolic coronary flow gains more importance as systole occupies a larger part of the cardiac cycle, while stronger inotropism leads to a stronger squeeze of the bridged LAD with a spillover into diastole, which may lead to exertional ischemia. This explains that up to 20% of patients with bridging may have ischemia on stress testing.[122] The combination of exertional angina, ischemia on stress testing, and bridging on angiography without obstructive CAD suggests the diagnosis of symptomatic myocardial bridging. Ischemia correlates with the severity of the narrowing and the intramyocardial depth of the bridge.

Even when symptomatic, myocardial bridging is a very benign condition with a very low risk of MI or arrhythmia.[123] Nitrates and diuretics aggravate bridging as they may lead to reflex tachycardia and increased inotropism; the patient may improve enough upon their withdrawal. **In fact, NTG administration is a useful diagnostic test during angiography, as it unveils the severity of bridging (opposite effect on vasospasm)**. β-Blockers are the mainstay of therapy.

Appendix 5. Coronary collaterals, chronic total occlusion

In a patient with a coronary total occlusion, the presence of coronary collaterals does not imply that the occlusion is chronic. Underdeveloped intercoronary channels often pre-exist in normal individuals before the occurrence of the coronary occlusion; coronary occlusion or severe stenosis leads to widening of these channels within the first 24 hours, followed by progressive enlargement and maturation of the collateral wall. Mature collaterals that approximate 1 mm in diameter with grade 3 filling of the recipient artery require >1 day to form, typically 1–6 weeks.[124]

Basic collateral filling may be seen in acute MI. In fact, half of patients with acute MI develop collateral flow in the first 6 hours, while all patients develop collaterals within 24 hours.[124] More mature collaterals may be seen early in MI if it was preceded by a chronic, severe coronary stenosis (e.g., ≥90% chronic stenosis). Grade 3 intercoronary collaterals suggest an occlusion that is at least several weeks old, but do not rule out the possibility of acute occlusion on top of a chronic, subtotally occlusive stenosis. Intercoronary collaterals are angiographically graded as follows: grade 1 = side branch filling of the recipient occluded artery, without visualization of the body of the recipient artery; grade 2 = partial, faint filling of the body of the recipient artery; and grade 3 (mature collaterals) = complete filling of the recipient artery. Nitric oxide promotes collateral growth; traditional risk factors, *particularly diabetes*, may impede the development of collaterals.

Mature collateral flow may provide up to 50% of the native antegrade flow, and thus drastically reduce ischemia.[125] Chronic total occlusions (CTOs) most often develop slowly, allowing collaterals to develop and allowing normal function of the subtended myocardium at rest. While a CTO is almost always associated with stress-induced ischemia, the degree of ischemia depends on the size of the territory and the maturity of collaterals.[126]

CTO is defined as a total occlusion that is >3 months old without any antegrade filling (*true CTO*), or with faint antegrade filling through microchannels (*functional CTO*). CTO is distinguished from an acute or recent occlusion by the clinical presentation and the ECG (stable angina in CTO, recent ACS or MI in recent occlusion). The duration of the occlusion is gauged by the date of onset or sudden worsening of angina or the date of MI.[125] *Bridging collaterals*, which are fine collateral vessels that form a caput medusae around the CTO, usually imply an old occlusion >3 months old and a low PCI success rate. This fine bridging network is sometimes confused with intra-CTO microchannels (functional CTO), yet the two entities have radically opposite implications: the former implies a low PCI success rate, while the latter implies a high PCI success rate.

> After successful PCI of a CTO, a considerable fraction (50%) of the collateral function is immediately reduced through spasm and is non-recruitable should acute reocclusion occur.[125] The patient may have a stable CTO for years; however, if a CTO is recanalized with PCI then acutely reoccludes, an acute MI will ensue, even if reocclusion occurs as early as a few hours or days after recanalization. This is due to: (i) early loss of collateral flow (spasm early on, anatomic involution later on), (ii) distal embolization from the upstream thrombosis, which occludes the microcirculation and any patent collaterals (similar to early SVG thrombosis). Yet sometimes, when reocclusion occurs early, collateral flow may be quickly recruited and may limit MI size.

Appendix 6. Hibernation, stunning, ischemic preconditioning

Hibernation is chronic impairment of the myocardial function that results from a severe, **persistent** coronary stenosis; the myocardium downregulates its function and its metabolism to survive and remains viable. Chronic ischemia may, however, lead to irreversible fibrosis. The myocardial segment has reduced nuclear uptake at rest and with stress, but preserved metabolic uptake on PET study.

Stunning is transient myocardial dysfunction occurring after a severe, **transient** episode of ischemia. Ischemia resolves and leaves a viable myocardium that will recover in time. This is the case of an acutely occluded artery that is opened with PCI or fibrinolytics (acute MI), exertional ischemia that occurs at stress and resolves at rest, or ischemia induced by cardiac surgery or PCI. Some myocardium is necrotic already, some is stunned; only time will show. As opposed to hibernation, the artery is now open and there is no persistent ischemia, hence the stunned myocardium does not remain dysfunctional. In the post-MI and post-cardiac surgery cases, temporary support with inotropes or IABP is sometimes needed until the myocardium recovers, provided there is no ongoing ischemia. Unlike hibernation, the nuclear uptake is usually normal at rest. Repetitive stunning (exertional ischemia) can lead to persistent dysfunction and hibernation.

Recovery of function occurs 1–6 months after revascularization (faster with stunning, days to 1 month). See Chapter 4 for viability evaluation.

> In a patient with active chest pain and severe CAD, the myocardial dysfunction is usually an actively ischemic dysfunction, rather than hibernation or stunning.

Ischemic preconditioning is the phenomenon whereby brief exposure to ischemia preconditions the heart and makes it more resilient to a later, prolonged and severe ischemia. In fact, ischemia stimulates protective myocyte receptors, such as adenosine receptors and G-protein receptors (protein kinase C). There are two windows of protection: the first starts within a few minutes of the brief ischemia and lasts a few hours; the second occurs at 24 hours and lasts 96 hours. This is partly why patients with pre-infarct angina suffer from smaller infarcts and have better outcomes. Also, patients with severe pre-existing disease have already formed mature collaterals, which attenuate the infarct size.

QUESTIONS AND ANSWERS

Question 1. A 67-year-old man with a history of HTN and diabetes presents with exertional chest pain CCS III for 3–4 months. Chest pain is relieved with rest and with his wife's NTG. He has left lower extremity claudication. On exam, distal left lower extremity pulses are not palpable. ECG shows LVH with 0.5 mm ST-segment depression. What is the most appropriate next step?
A. Coronary angiography
B. Exercise stress ECG
C. Exercise stress SPECT
D. Adenosine SPECT

Question 2. A 67-year-old man with a history of LAD stent placed 2 years ago presents with mild angina on heavy exertion (CCS I). He is on atenolol, amlodipine, aspirin, and atorvastatin. BP 110/65, pulse 58 bpm. Exercise stress test result: 8 min on a Bruce protocol, mild angina occurred, DTS score +4. Nuclear perfusion shows a small area of apical–lateral ischemia, with a summed stress score of +3. Coronary angiography shows 80% proximal LCx stenosis, 30% mid-LAD, 40% mid-RCA. What is the next step?
A. PCI of LCx. No need for FFR since the lesion is angiographically significant
B. PCI of LCx. No need for FFR since the stress test is positive
C. FFR of LCx. Stent if FFR <0.80
D. Continue medical therapy, no PCI

Question 3. A 76-year-old man presents with chest pain on heavy activity. His home medications consist of aspirin and a statin. A nuclear stress test shows mild/moderate anterior ischemia, and coronary angiography shows 80% mid-LAD stenosis. What is the next step?
A. Medical therapy. There is no mortality difference between CABG, PCI, and medical therapy for this lesion
B. PCI
C. CABG, since it provides mortality benefit compared to PCI or medical therapy

Question 4. Same scenario as Question 3, except the patient has 80% proximal LAD stenosis.
A. Medical therapy.
B. PCI
C. CABG, since it provides mortality benefit compared to PCI or medical therapy

Question 5. A 76-year-old man presents with chest pain on heavy activity (walking >2 blocks). He receives aspirin and a statin. A nuclear stress test shows moderate anterior ischemia, and coronary angiography shows 80% proximal LAD stenosis and 75% mid-RCA and mid-LCx stenoses. What is the next step?
A. Medical therapy
B. PCI
C. CABG

Question 6. A 76-year-old man presents with chest pain on heavy activity (walking >2 blocks). He receives aspirin and a statin. A nuclear stress test shows severe anterior ischemia with summed stress score of +8, and coronary angiography shows 80% proximal LAD stenosis. What is the next step?
A. Medical therapy
B. PCI
C. CABG
D. B or C

Question 7. A 47-year-old executive man, asymptomatic, is starting an exercise program at the gym. He is asymptomatic during daily activities. A stress test is ordered by his family physician. He exercises for 5 minutes and develops 1.5 mm ST depression without chest pain. Nuclear images show a large anterior and anterolateral reversible defect, with a normal EF and no TID.
A. Because he is asymptomatic, there is no need for coronary angiography since there is no need for revascularization. Just initiate medical therapy
B. Perform coronary angiography, but only revascularize if left main or three-vessel CAD is present
C. Perform coronary angiography, but only revascularize if left main, three-vessel CAD, or one- or two-vessel CAD involving the proximal LAD is found. If isolated mid-LAD stenosis is found, start intense medical therapy and repeat stress test before going for PCI
D. Perform coronary angiography, but only revascularize if left main, three-vessel CAD, or one- or two-vessel CAD involving the proximal LAD is found. Do not revascularize if isolated mid-LAD stenosis is found

Question 8. A 56-year-old man presents with angina walking up one flight of stairs or less (= CCS III). He is not receiving any antianginal therapy. His nuclear stress test shows severe inferior ischemia. His angiogram shows CTO of the RCA with features that make it favorable for PCI (non-calcified, ~2 cm long).
True or false: PCI is not appropriate, as the patient is not receiving maximal antianginal therapy

Question 9. A 46-year-old diabetic woman, smoker, who also has dyslipidemia and whose diabetes is not insulin-dependent, presents with a typical exertional angina CCS III. ECG shows LVH without ST changes. She has no arterial bruits and peripheral pulses are normal. What is the most appropriate next step?

A. Coronary angiography
B. Exercise stress ECG
C. Exercise stress SPECT, as the patient cannot receive stress ECG with the baseline LVH
D. Exercise stress SPECT, because it is more appropriate for this patient's presentation
E. Adenosine SPECT

Question 10. A 50-year-old female, smoker, presents with chest pain that occurs with exertion, but not consistently, and sometimes occurs at rest. Each episode lasts ~45 minutes. BP = 160/95, HR = 78. She undergoes a treadmill nuclear stress testing. She walks for 5 minutes, does not report any chest pain, and no ST abnormality is seen. Her nuclear images show a large reversible anterior defect with a summed stress score of +10. The patient prefers to try medical therapy first if deemed appropriate by the physician. What is her Duke Treadmill Score? What is the most appropriate next step?
A. Start aspirin, statin, β-blockers and amlodipine. Coronary angiography is not indicated, as her risk of cardiac events is <1% per year
B. Start aspirin, statin, β-blockers and amlodipine and proceed with coronary angiography, as her risk of cardiac events is >5% per year
C. Start amlodipine, since the likely diagnosis is vasospasm

Question 11. A 65-year-old diabetic patient is planning to undergo elective cholecystectomy. He has mild dyspnea on exertion (>4 METs) but no angina. He undergoes preoperative testing with a nuclear SPECT, which shows severe inferior ischemia and preserved EF. Coronary angiography shows CTO of the RCA with angiographic features favorable for PCI. What is the next step?
A. Aggressive medical regimen. Revascularization is not indicated. His surgical risk is intermediate but revascularization will not improve this
B. Aggressive medical regimen. Revascularization is not indicated. His surgical risk is low
C. Aggressive medical regimen and PCI of the RCA with BMS
D. Aggressive medical regimen and PCI of the RCA with DES

Question 12. A 58-year-old woman has exertional chest pain (and some episodes of pain with mental stress). While undergoing treadmill stress ECG, she develops severe chest pain, inferior ST-segment elevation, and multiple runs of non-sustained VT. The pain and ST elevation resolve at 5 minutes of recovery. Coronary angiography is performed and shows a smooth 80% stenosis of the mid-RCA, which improves to a mild, 25% stenosis with NTG. What is the prognosis and what is the treatment?
A. Even in the absence of obstructive CAD, her risk of unstable angina/MI/VT is ~20% at several years of follow-up. She must be placed on amlodipine and statin
B. In the absence of obstructive CAD, her risk of unstable angina/MI/VT is low (<5%) at several years of follow-up. Provide CCB for symptomatic relief
C. Vasospasm frequently occurs on top of obstructive CAD. Perform IVUS to ensure that the residual stenosis is not a more severe stenosis or a ruptured plaque.

Question 13. A 55-year-old woman, smoker, presents with exertional chest pain. A nuclear stress test shows a reversible anterior defect. Coronary angiography is performed and does not show any obstructive CAD. Moderate bridging of the mid-LAD (50% obstructive) is seen. What is the diagnosis?
A. Myocardial bridging
B. Coronary epicardial vasospasm
C. Microvascular dysfunction
D. All of the above

Question 14. What diagnostic testing could help establish the diagnosis in the patient of Question 13?
A. Stress echo
B. Stress MRI
C. Intracoronary acetylcholine testing
D. Intracoronary or intravenous adenosine testing
E. Administer NTG during coronary angiography, even if no spasm is seen
F. B, C, D, and E
G. All of the above

Question 15. A 50-year-old man presents with resting chest pain and ST-segment elevation in the inferior leads. His coronary angiography shows a smooth 90% mid-RCA stenosis that is relieved with NTG. Which statement is *incorrect*?
A. Prinzmetal angina often occurs in patients without underlying CAD
B. Without CCB therapy, recurrent MI occurs in a substantial proportion of patients with Prinzmetal angina (~20%), even in the absence of underlying CAD
C. The definite diagnosis requires a concomitant documentation of the following three features: vasospasm on angiography, chest pain, and ST-segment changes
D. Among patients with exertional chest pain, abnormal stress testing, yet unobstructed coronary arteries, the incidence of coronary vasospasm on provocative testing is up to 50% (macrovascular or microvascular)

Question 16. A 69-year-old man has chronic exertional angina, CCS III. He undergoes coronary angiography and is found to have 90% proximal RCA stenosis. Which statement is correct?
A. Initial PCI, as opposed to initial medical therapy only, reduces his risk of MI
B. Initial PCI reduces his cardiovascular mortality
C. Initial PCI reduces angina
D. Single-vessel CABG reduces his risk of death or MI

Question 17. A 59-year-old woman has occasional, atypical, non-exertional chest pain. She undergoes stress testing, which shows a large anterior defect. Coronary angiography shows 80% proximal LAD stenosis. Which statement is correct (multiple possible answers)?

A. Initial PCI reduces her risk of MI

B. Initial PCI reduces her cardiovascular mortality

C. Initial PCI reduces angina

D. If the patient is undergoing non-cardiac surgery, PCI of LAD reduces her risk of perioperative MI

E. Single-vessel CABG may reduce her risk of death or MI

Question 18. After undergoing coronary revascularization, which statement is *incorrect*?

A. After one- or two-vessel PCI, the risk of repeat revascularization is ~20% at 5 years

B. After multivessel revascularization, the risk of repeat revascularization is 15% with CABG and ~30% with PCI at 5 years

C. After high-risk PCI (e.g., complex proximal LAD PCI), stress testing is indicated routinely at 6–12 months

Question 19. A 70-year-old man has undergone PCI of the mid-LAD with one DES 1 year ago. He presents with recurrent mild angina. Coronary angiography shows 90% in-stent restenosis of the LAD. What is the next step?

A. Medical therapy

B. PCI

C. CABG

D. PCI or CABG

Question 20. A 51-year-old woman presents with exertional angina. She undergoes a standard treadmill ECG testing, where she exercises for 7 minutes and exhibits her typical angina without any ST change. What is the next step?

A. Risk factor modification, aspirin, statin, and antianginal therapy

B. Refer to coronary angiography

Question 21. The patient of Question 20 continues to have angina. A coronary angiography is performed and does not reveal any significant CAD. What is the next step?

A. Reassure the patient that her pain is not of a cardiac origin. Consider gastroesophageal reflux therapy.

B. The patient likely has coronary vasospasm. Prescribe amlodipine.

C. Perform adenosine PET perfusion imaging or adenosine MRI perfusion imaging. If the diagnosis is confirmed, consider adding ranolazine or L-arginine.

Question 22. A 50-year-old diabetic man has exertional angina (2 flights of stairs, 4 blocks). On stress echo, he walks 7 minutes on Bruce protocol, develops mild pain, 2 mm of ST depression in leads V_4–V_6, and inferior hypokinesis. Coronary angiography shows 80% proximal RCA stenosis, with no disease in the LAD or LCx. What is the next step?

A. Optimize medical therapy

B. Perform RCA PCI

C. Perform RCA FFR, then PCI if appropriate

Question 23. In the diabetic patient of Question 22, which of the following is *incorrect*:

A. β-Blockers reduce mortality in patients with stable CAD and without prior MI

B. Metoprolol worsens HbA1c, while carvedilol does not affect HbA1c and actually improves insulin resistance

C. The higher the HbA1c, the more effective ranolazine is in reducing angina of diabetic patients

D. Ranolazine improves HbA1c by up to 1%

Question 24. A 60-year-old diabetic man has dyspnea on exertion and occasional episodes of rest chest discomfort. A resting ECG shows borderline inferior Q waves. On stress echo, he walked 8 minutes and had 1 mm of ST segment depression in V_4–V_6, with dyspnea and no chest pain. His inferior wall is akinetic with EF 35–40% at rest and without worsening during exercise. Coronary angiography shows a totally occluded RCA in its mid-segment, and moderate, 50% disease in the proximal LAD. What is the next step?

A. Aggressive statin and antianginal therapy. No revascularization of RCA CTO

B. Revascularize RCA CTO (beside medical therapy)

C. Perform FFR of LAD. If significant, refer to CABG (LAD and RCA). If insignificant, perform PCI of RCA

D. Perform FFR of LAD. If significant, refer to CABG. If insignificant, perform medical therapy only

E. Perform FFR of LAD. If significant, perform LAD PCI, and continue medical therapy for RCA. If insignificant, perform medical therapy only

Question 25. In stable CAD, which three features guide the decision to revascularize?

Answer 1. A (Section II.C). According to Hubbard et al., the patient has >40% risk of severe CAD (age, sex, diabetes, typical angina).[13] Also, PAD predicts severe CAD. He has not only a high probability of CAD, but a high probability of severe CAD. The severity of his angina is another indicator of the need for invasive angiography with possible revascularization.

Answer 2. D. This is a typical COURAGE patient with mild angina, good functional capacity, and low-risk stress test. For this patient, medical therapy is as good as PCI + medical therapy. If the stress test is high-risk (≥10% ischemia), or angina is severe despite medical therapy, COURAGE nuclear and functional substudies would support PCI (PCI would be superior to medical therapy for reduction of angina and reduction of ischemic burden). Also, a large retrospective analysis suggested improved survival when revascularization is performed for high-risk ischemia on nuclear imaging.[16] FFR is not necessary, since ischemia has already been proven by nuclear imaging.

Answer 3. A. A patient with mild angina and mild/moderate ischemia is appropriately treated with medical therapy only. The MASS trial showed that for isolated LAD disease >80%, there was no difference in mortality between CABG vs. angioplasty vs. medical therapy, although angina was reduced with angioplasty and more so with CABG. The LAD disease addressed in the MASS trial was proximal LAD disease.

Answer 4. A. Again, a patient with mild angina, mild/moderate ischemia and no severe functional limitation is appropriately treated with medical therapy only (typical COURAGE patient). A proximal LAD with mild/moderate rather than severe ischemia may be initially treated conservatively according to the ACC appropriateness criteria. While revascularization with either CABG or PCI may be performed, the value of this strategy in patients with no severe ischemia, no severe or refractory angina, and isolated proximal LAD disease (no two- or three-vessel CAD) is questionable. The appropriateness criteria puts it in an "uncertain" category. If the mild angina persists despite two antianginal drugs, revascularization becomes appropriate.

Answer 5. C. As opposed to Questions 3 and 4, the patient has three-vessel CAD (>70%). According to the ACC appropriateness criteria, even if angina is mild and only moderate ischemia is induced on non-invasive testing, revascularization is justified for three-vessel CAD or two-vessel CAD with proximal LAD involvement, particularly because the stress test may underestimate the true severity of ischemia. Nuclear defects being comparative to the best segment, the LCx and RCA may appear to be normally perfused when, in fact, they are ischemic but less ischemic than the LAD. FFR may be warranted in the absence of a high-risk stress test result, and will allow adequate assessment of RCA and LCx.

Answer 6. D. A patient with severely positive stress test is appropriate for revascularization even if angina is mild and antianginal therapy has not been initiated. A meta-analysis of early trials of CABG vs. medical therapy suggests that survival with CABG is superior to medical therapy in proximal LAD disease, even single-vessel LAD (as long as LAD stenosis is definitely significant, typically with high-risk ischemia). A meta-analysis of randomized data of CABG vs. PCI suggests no mortality difference in isolated proximal LAD disease. Thus, revascularization with CABG or PCI, if technically feasible, is appropriate for this patient.

Answer 7. C. Asymptomatic patients qualify for revascularization if the stress test is high-risk despite maximal medical therapy, *or* high-risk along with proximal LAD, left main, or three-vessel CAD. This is supported by data from the ACIP trial (trial of revascularization of asymptomatic patients with ischemia) and old CABG vs. medical therapy trials.

Answer 8. False. PCI of CTO is appropriate as long as stress test is high-risk and angina is either severe or refractory. He qualifies for PCI by the fact that his angina is severe and the CTO has favorable PCI features, even if he is not on maximal antianginal therapy. Being appropriate does not mean it is necessary, and one may alternatively maximize antianginal therapy and proceed with PCI only if angina persists.

Answer 9. D. Despite being a young woman <60 years of age, the patient has a high pre-test probability of CAD based on the fact that she has typical angina and multiple risk factors. Her pre-test clinical risk, however, is not high based on Hubbard et al.'s risk estimation (age <60 and only two of the five factors: typical angina, male sex, diabetes, insulin dependency, prior MI).[13] Thus, stress testing is appropriate for her risk stratification, before proceeding with angiography. LVH without ST changes does not preclude the use of stress ECG; however, in a patient with a high pre-test probability, stress imaging is preferred to stress ECG for risk stratification.

Answer 10. B. The patient has low-risk DTS of +5. A low-risk stress ECG/low risk DTS does not necessarily rule out high-risk CAD. In fact, 10% of patients with low-risk DTS have left main or three-vessel CAD. A high-risk stress imaging result overrules a low or intermediate DTS. This patient has a high-risk stress imaging result, and thus should undergo coronary angiography. Any degree of angina along with severe ischemia qualifies for revascularization. Atypical symptoms are common in women.

Answer 11. A. The patient does not have a clear angina. Revascularization of a CTO is only indicated if symptoms are severe or refractory, along with a high-risk stress test. The inferior ischemia implies that the patient has an increased surgical risk, including a risk of functional ischemia/infarction of the RCA territory during surgery. However, except for left main disease or extensive three-vessel CAD, preoperative revascularization does not change postoperative cardiac complications. If surgery is necessary, medical therapy with a statin and a β-blocker, initiated more than a week before surgery, and careful perioperative monitoring are the strategies that improve outcomes.

Answer 12. A. Even in the absence of CAD, vasospastic angina is associated with a significant risk of cardiac events (~20% within a few years), especially when extensive or severe ST changes or arrhythmias have been demonstrated. With CCB, this risk is reduced to <1% (unstable angina may occur at a higher rate). Statin has additional benefit on top of CCB. IVUS is reasonable if the lesion is ≥50% obstructive on angiography or has worrisome angiographic features (overhanging borders, eccentric, hazy).

Answer 13. D. Even if coronary angiography does not show any obstruction, a convincing chest pain history along with a perfusion abnormality suggest that the chest discomfort is a true angina. *Half of women whose symptoms are worrisome enough to warrant coronary angiography but who are not found to have significant coronary obstruction have, in fact, microvascular dysfunction. This is particularly the case of patients with typical angina features and abnormal stress testing.* Myocardial bridging is usually incidental, even when severe; however, it may be considered the culprit in a patient with typical angina and anterior ischemia.

Answer 14. F. Stress MRI is the best non-invasive modality for the diagnosis of microvascular dysfunction, followed by nuclear imaging (which has the pitfall of a high false-positive rate in women). Stress echo and stress ECG have a lower yield. Invasively, there are two aspects of microvascular dysfunction: (i) microvascular spasm, unveiled by acetylcholine, (ii) inability to vasodilate and increase coronary flow, unveiled by adenosine infusion. For diagnostic purposes, coronary flow reserve is checked after adenosine infusion or intracoronary acetylcholine. Concerning myocardial bridging, NTG administration may worsen it and further suggest it as a culprit.

Answer 15. A. In the majority of patients with variant angina, significant coronary obstruction of at least one vessel is present. Vasospasm occurs at the site of obstruction or within 1 cm.

Answer 16. C. In stable CAD, PCI only improves angina control. There is no demonstrated effect on MI or mortality, even if the lesion appears angiographically critical. It may improve unstable angina presentations (FAME II trial), but not MI. PCI is appropriate in a patient with severe angina, especially if it persists despite antianginal therapy. In the stable CAD setting, revascularization with CABG improves mortality of patients with left main disease and likely that of patients with three-vessel disease or two-vessel disease with proximal LAD (in multivessel disease without left main involvement, CABG may only reduce MI risk, not mortality, as per BARI 2D trial).

Answer 17. C and E. In stable CAD, PCI has not demonstrated a reduction of mortality or MI in comparison with medical therapy, even when the proximal LAD is treated (COURAGE, MASS, MASS II trials). CABG may reduce mortality in single-vessel proximal LAD according to a meta-analysis of old CABG vs. medical therapy trials, but not according to more recent trials (MASS, BARI 2D). Preoperative revascularization has not demonstrated an improvement of postoperative outcomes, except, possibly, in the case of left main or three-vessel CAD.

Answer 18. C. Even when asymptomatic, recurrent ischemia from restenosis has a negative prognostic value. However, there is no evidence that PCI for recurrent, asymptomatic ischemia improves outcomes, and thus routine testing is not indicated. Concerning choice B, note that, after CABG, ~15% of patients require repeat revascularization at 5 years, yet each SVG has a 25% risk of occlusion in the first year (most SVG occlusions are asymptomatic).

Answer 19. D. Angina is mild, but the ischemic territory is presumably large, so revascularization is appropriate. DES restenosis is often treated with repeat PCI: intracoronary imaging is performed to check for stent expansion, as stent underexpansion accounts for at least 50% of DES restenosis and is treated with high-pressure balloon inflation. If restenosis is mainly due to neointimal hyperplasia or if it is diffuse or extending outside the stent, repeated DES stenting is performed (stent inside a stent). CABG is an alternative therapy for LAD in-stent restenosis.

Answer 20. A. The stress test does not reveal high-risk findings and proves a good functional capacity. Thus, medical therapy for low-risk CAD may be initiated. CTA or stress imaging may be performed for further risk stratification, but is not necessary.

Answer 21. C. Half of women with typical angina have no significant CAD. The most likely cause of angina in this case is endothelial dysfunction, with inability of the microvasculature to dilate during stress. Macrovascular vasospasm is less likely. The diagnosis is made non-invasively by comparing the rest and post-adenosine myocardial perfusion using PET or MRI.

Answer 22. A. The patient has mild angina (CCS I), mild functional limitation, and intermediate-risk stress test (not high risk by Duke Treadmill Score and echo). This is a typical COURAGE trial patient, where PCI does not improve survival or MI rates. To qualify for revascularization, his angina needs to be severe or persistent despite two antianginal drugs, his ischemia needs to be severe, or his CAD needs to be more extensive.

Answer 23. A.

Answer 24. D. The patient does not clearly have angina, although dyspnea may be an angina equivalent (exertional dyspnea is commonly multifactorial and is not as specific as chest pain for CAD). His stress test is intermediate in risk by both DTS and echo features. If he has single-vessel CAD (RCA), revascularization would not be appropriate in the absence of severe angina. The key is, thus, to demonstrate the significance of LAD disease. If it is significant, the patient has moderate-risk stress test result and multivessel CAD involving the LAD, which qualifies him for revascularization, preferably CABG in the context of diabetes.

Answer 25. Severity of angina, severity of ischemia on non-invasive testing, and extent of CAD on coronary angiography (especially whether left main, extensive three-vessel CAD, or proximal LAD disease is present).

References

1. Hanna EB, Glancy DL. Coronary hemodynamics: fractional flow reserve concepts, pitfalls, and special applications. In: Hanna EB, Glancy DL, Practical Cardiovascular Hemodynamics. New York: Demos Medical, 2012, pp. 193–210.
2. Tonino PAL, Fearon WF, De Bruyne B, et al. Angiographic versus functional severity of coronary artery stenoses in the FAME study, fractional flow reserve versus angiography in multivessel evaluation. J Am Coll Cardiol 2010; 55: 2816–21.
3. Prinzmetal M, Ekemecki A, Kennamer R, et al. Variant form of angina pectoris: previously undelineated syndrome. JAMA 1960; 174: 1791–800.
4. Maseri A, Severi S, de Nes M, et al. "Variant" angina: one aspect of a continuous spectrum of vasospastic myocardial ischemia: pathogenetic mechanisms, estimated incidence and clinical and coronary arteriographic findings in 138 patients. Am J Cardiol 1978; 42: 1019–35.
5. Ong P, Athanasiadis A, Borgulya G, et al. High prevalence of a pathological response to acetylcholine testing in patients with stable angina pectoris and unobstructed coronary arteries: the ACOVA study (Abnormal COronary VAsomotion in patients with stable angina and unobstructed coronary arteries). J Am Coll Cardiol 2012; 59: 655–62.
6. Yamagishi M, Miyatake K, Tamai J, et al. Intravascular ultrasound detection of atherosclerosis at the site of focal vasospasm in angiographically normal or minimally narrowed coronary segments. J Am Coll Cardiol 1994; 23: 352–7.
7. Zeiher AM, Schächlinger V, Hohnloser SH, Saurbier B, Just H. Coronary atherosclerotic wall thickening and vascular reactivity in humans. Elevated high-density lipoprotein levels ameliorate abnormal vasoconstriction in early atherosclerosis. Circulation 1994; 89: 2525–32.
8. Diamond GA, Forrester JS. Analysis of probability as an aid in the clinical diagnosis of coronary-artery disease. N Engl J Med 1979; 300: 1350–8.
9. Chaitman BR, Bourassa MG, Davis K, et al. Angiographic prevalence of high-risk coronary artery disease in patient subsets (CASS). Circulation 1981; 64: 360–7.
10. Pryor DB, Shaw L, McCants CB, et al. Value of the history and physical in identifying patients at increased risk for coronary artery disease. Ann Intern Med 1993; 118: 81–90.
11. Johnson BD, Shaw LJ, Pepine CJ, et al. Persistent chest pain predicts cardiovascular events in women without obstructive coronary artery disease: results from the NIH-NHLBI-sponsored Women's Ischemia Syndrome Evaluation (WISE) study. Eur Heart J 2006; 27: 1408–15.
12. Hubbard BL, Gibbons RJ, Lapeyre AC, et al. Identification of severe coronary artery disease using simple clinical parameters. Arch Intern Med 1992; 152: 309–12.

13. Gibbons R, Chatterjee K, Daley J, et al. ACC/AHA 1999 guidelines for the management of patients with chronic stable angina: a report of the American College of Cardiology/American Heart Association Task Force on Practice Guidelines (Committee on the Management of Patients With Chronic Stable Angina). J Am Coll Cardiol 1999; 33: 2092–197.

14. Pryor DB, Shaw L, Harrell FE, et al. Estimating the likelihood of severe coronary artery disease. Am J Med 1991; 90: 553–62.

15. Shaw LJ, Peterson ED, Shaw LK, et al. Use of a prognostic treadmill score in identifying diagnostic coronary disease subgroups. Circulation. 1998; 98: 1622–30.

16. Hachamovitch R, Berman DS, Kiat H, et al. Exercise myocardial perfusion SPECT in patients without known coronary artery disease: incremental prognostic value and use in risk stratification. Circulation 1996; 93: 905–14.

17. Bouzas-Mosquera A, Peteiro J, Álvarez-García N. Prediction of mortality and major cardiac events by exercise echocardiography in patients with normal exercise electrocardiographic testing. J Am Coll Cardiol 2009; 53: 1981–90.

18. Fihn SD, Gardin JM, Abrams J, et al. 2012 ACCF/AHA/ACP/AATS/PCNA/SCAI/STS Guideline for the diagnosis and management of patients with ischemic heart disease. J Am Coll Cardiol 2012; 60: e44–164 (+2014 update).

19. Bouzas-Mosquera A, Peteiro J, Alvarez-Garcia N, et al. Prognostic value of exercise echocardiography in patients with left bundle branch block. JACC Cardiovasc Imaging 2009; 2: 251–9.

20. Hachamovitch R, Hayes S, Friedman JD, et al. Determinants of risk and its temporal variation in patients with normal stress myocardial perfusion scans. What is the warranty period of a normal scan? JAm Coll Cardiol 2003; 41: 1329–40.

21. Kemp HG, Kronmal RA, Vlietstra RA, Frye RL. Seven year survival of patients with normal or near normal coronary arteriograms: a CASS registry study. J Am Coll Cardiol 1986; 7: 479–83.

22. Geh AK, Ali S, Na B, et al. Inducible ischemia and the risk of recurrent cardiovascular events in outpatients with stable coronary heart disease: the heart and soul study. Arch Intern Med 2008; 168: 1423–8.

23. Zellweger MJ, Weinbacher M, Zutter AW. Long-term outcome of patients with silent versus symptomatic ischemia six months after percutaneous coronary intervention and stenting. J Am Coll Cardiol 2003; 42: 33–40.

24. Young LH, Wackers FJT, Chyun DA, et al. Cardiac outcomes after screening for asymptomatic coronary artery disease in patients with type 2 diabetes. JAMA 2009; 301: 1547–55.

25. Muhlestein JB, Lappe DL, Lima JA, et al. Effect of screening for coronary artery disease using CT angiography on mortality and cardiac events in high-risk patients with diabetes. The Factor-64 randomized clinical trial. JAMA 2014; 312: 2234–43.

26. Davies RF, Goldberg AD, Forman S, et al. Asymptomatic Cardiac Ischemia Pilot (ACIP) Study two-year follow-up. Outcomes of patients randomized to initial strategies of medical therapy versus revascularization. Circulation 1997; 95: 2037–43.

27. Yusuf S, Zucker D, Peduzzi P, et al. Effect of coronary artery bypass surgery on survival: Overview of 10-year results from randomized trials by the Coronary Artery Bypass Surgery Trialists Collaboration. Lancet 1994; 344: 563. *In this CABG vs. PCI meta-analysis, patients with normal stress test did not derive a clear benefit from CABG.*

28. Bhatt DL, Fox KA, Hacke W, et al. Clopidogrel and aspirin versus aspirin alone for the prevention of atherothrombotic events. N Engl J Med 2006; 354: 1706–17.

29. Bhatt DL, Flather MD, Hacke W, et al. Patients with prior myocardial infarction, stroke, or symptomatic peripheral arterial disease in the CHARISMA trial. J Am Coll Cardiol 2007; 49: 1982–8.

30. A randomised, blinded, trial of clopidogrel versus aspirin in patients at risk of ischaemic events (CAPRIE) CAPRIE Steering Committee. Lancet 1996; 348: 1329–39.

31. Hurlen M, Abdelnoor M, Smith P, et al. Warfarin, aspirin, or both after myocardial infarction. N Engl J Med 2002; 347: 969–74. *WARIS 2.*

32. Bangalore S, Sawhney S, Messerli FH. Relation of beta-blocker-induced heart rate lowering and cardioprotection in hypertension. J Am Coll Cardiol 2008; 52: 1482–9.

33. Bangalore S, Steg PHG, Deedwania P, et al. Beta blocker use and clinical outcomes in stable outpatients with and without coronary artery disease. JAMA 2012; 308: 1340–9. *REACH registry.*

34. Giannattasio C, Cattaneo BM, Seravalle G, et al. Alpha 1-blocking properties of carvedilol during acute and chronic administration. J Cardiovasc Pharmacol 1992; 19 Suppl 1: S18–22.

35. Narins CR, Zareba W, Moss AJ, et al. Relationship between intermittent claudication, inflammation, thrombosis, and recurrent cardiac events among survivors of myocardial infarction. Arch Intern Med 2004; 164: 440–6.

36. Bakris GL, Fonseca V, Katholi RE, et al. Metabolic effects of carvedilol vs. metoprolol in patients with type 2 diabetes mellitus and hypertension: a randomized controlled trial. JAMA 2004; 292: 2227–36.

37. Munzel T, Daiber A, Gori T. Nitrate therapy: new aspects concerning molecular action and tolerance. Circulation 2011; 123: 2132–44.

38. Liuni A, Luca MC, Di Stoffo G, et al. Coadministration of atorvastatin prevents nitroglycerin-induced endothelial dysfunction and nitrate tolerance in healthy humans. J Am Coll Cardiol 2011; 57: 93–8.

39. Katz RJ, Levy WS, Buff L, et al. Prevention of nitrate tolerance with angiotensin converting enzyme inhibitors. Circulation 1991; 83: 1271–7.

40. Watanabe, H, Kahihana, M, Ohtsuka, S, et al. Randomized, double-blind, placebo-controlled study of carvedilol on the prevention of nitrate tolerance in patients with chronic heart failure. J Am Coll Cardiol 1998; 32: 1194–200.

41. Chaitman BR, Skettino SL, Parker JO, et al. Anti-ischemic effects and long-term survival during ranolazine monotherapy in patients with chronic severe angina. J Am Coll Cardiol 2004; 43: 1375–82.

42. Chaitman BR, Pepine CJ, Parker JO, et al. Effects of ranolazine with atenolol, amlodipine, or diltiazem on exercise tolerance and angina frequency in patients with severe chronic angina. JAMA 2004; 291: 309–16.

43. Morrow DA, Scirica BM, Karwatowska-Prokopczuk E, for the MERLIN-TIMI 36 Trial Investigators. Effects of ranolazine on recurrent cardiovascular events in patients with non-ST-elevation acute coronary syndromes: the MERLIN-TIMI 36 randomized trial. JAMA 2007; 297: 1775–83.

44. Mega JL, Hochman JS, Scirica BM, et al. Clinical features and outcomes of women with unstable ischemic heart disease: observations from metabolic efficiency with ranolazine for less ischemia in non-ST-elevation acute coronary syndromes-thrombolysis in myocardial infarction 36 (MERLIN-TIMI 36). Circulation 2010; 121: 1809–17.

45. Morrow DA, Scirica BM, Sabatine MS, et al. B-type natriuretic peptide and the effect of ranolazine in patients with non-ST-segment elevation acute coronary syndromes: observations from the MERLIN–TIMI 36 trial. J Am Coll Cardiol 2010; 55: 1189–96.

46. Scirica BM, Braunwald E, Belardinelli L, et al. Relationship between nonsustained ventricular tachycardia after non-ST-elevation acute coronary syndrome and sudden cardiac death: observations from MERLIN-TIMI 36 randomized controlled trial. Circulation 2010; 122: 455–62.

47. SPRINT Research Group. A randomized trial of intensive versus standard blood pressure control. N Engl J Med 2015; 373: 2103–16.

48. HOPE Study Investigators. Effects of an angiotensin-converting-enzyme inhibitor, ramipril, on cardiovascular events in high-risk patients. N Engl J Med 2000; 342: 145–53. *HOPE study.*

49. PEACE Trial Investigators. Angiotensin-converting-enzyme inhibition in stable coronary artery disease. N Engl J Med 2004; 351: 2058–68.

50. Rouleau J, Warnica WJ, Baillot R, et al. Effects of angiotensin-converting enzyme inhibition in low-risk patients early after coronary artery bypass surgery. Circulation 2008; 117: 24–31.

Revascularization

51. Patel MR, Dehmer GJ, Hirshfeld JW, et al. ACCF/SCAI/STS/AATS/AHA/ASNC/HFSA/SCCT 2012 Appropriate use criteria for coronary revascularization focused update. J Am Coll Cardiol 2012; 59: 857–81.

52. Olivari Z, Rubartelli P, Piscione F, et al. Immediate results and one-year clinical outcome after percutaneous coronary interventions in chronic total occlusions: data from a multicenter, prospective, observational study (TOAST-GISE). J Am Coll Cardiol 2003; 41: 1672–8.

53. Safley DM, House JA, Marso SP, et al. Improvement in survival following successful percutaneous coronary intervention of coronary chronic total occlusions: variability by target vessel. JACC Cardiovasc Interv 2008; 1: 295–302.

54. Hachamovitch R, Hayes SW, Friedman JD, et al. Comparison of the short-term survival benefit associated with revascularization compared with medical therapy in patients with no prior coronary artery disease undergoing stress myocardial perfusion single photon emission computed tomography. Circulation 2003; 107: 2900–6.

55. De Bruyne B, Pijls N, Kalesan B, et al. Fractional flow reserve-guided PCI versus medical therapy in stable coronary disease. N Engl J Med 2012; 367: 991–1001.

56. Mancini GB, Hartigan PM, Shaw LJ, et al. Predicting outcomes in the COURAGE trial: coronary anatomy versus ischemia. JACC Cardiovasc Interv 2014; 7: 195–201.

57. Melikian N, De Bondt P, Tonino O, et al. Fractional flow reserve and myocardial perfusion imaging in patients with angiographic multivessel coronary artery disease. JACC Cardiovasc Interv 2011; 3: 307–14.

58. Velazquez EJ, Lee KL, Deja MA, et al.; STICH Investigators. Coronary-artery bypass surgery in patients with left ventricular dysfunction, N Engl J Med 2011; 364: 1607–16.

59. Zellweger MJ, Kaiser C, Jeger R, et al.Coronary artery disease progression late after stent implantation. J Am Coll Cardiol 2012; 59: 793–9.

60. Stone G.W., Maehara A., Lansky A.J., et al. PROSPECT Investigators A prospective natural-history study of coronary atherosclerosis. N Engl J Med 2011; 364: 226–35.

PCI vs. medical therapy

61. Mancini GB, Hartigan PM, Bates ER, et al. Angiographic disease progression and residual risk of cardiovascular events while on optimal medical therapy. Observations from the COURAGE Trial. Circ Cardiovasc Interv 2011; 4: 545–52.

62. Pijls NH, Fearon WF, Tonino PA, et al. Fractional flow reserve versus angiography for guiding percutaneous coronary intervention in patients with multivessel coronary artery disease: 2-year follow-up of the FAME study. J Am Coll Cardiol 2010; 56: 177–84.

63. Pijls NHJ, Sels JEM. Functional measurement of coronary stenosis. J Am Coll Cardiol 2012; 59: 1045–57.

64. Boden WE, O'Rourke RA, Teo KK, et al. Optimal medical therapy with or without PCI for stable coronary disease. N Engl J Med 2007; 356: 1503–1516. *COURAGE trial.*

65. Weintraub WS, Spertus JA, Kolm P, et al. Effect of PCI on quality of life in patients with stable coronary disease. N Engl J Med 2008; 359: 677–87.

66. Shaw LJ, Berman DS, Maron DJ, et al. Optimal medical therapy with or without percutaneous coronary intervention to reduce ischemic burden: results from the Clinical Outcomes Utilizing Revascularization and Aggressive Drug Evaluation (COURAGE) trial nuclear substudy. Circulation 2008; 117: 1283–91.

67. Frye RL, August P, Brooks MM, et al.; BARI 2D Study Group. A randomized trial of therapies for type 2 diabetes and coronary artery disease. N Engl J Med 2009; 360: 2503–15.

68. Prasad A, Gersh BJ, Bertrand ME, et al. Prognostic significance of periprocedural versus spontaneously occurring myocardial infarction after percutaneous coronary intervention in patients with acute coronary syndromes. An analysis from the ACUITY trial. J Am Coll Cardiol 2009; 54: 477–86.

69. Berman DS, Kang X, Schisterman EF, et al. Serial changes on quantitative myocardial perfusion SPECT in patients undergoing revascularization or conservative therapy. J Nucl Cardiol 2001; 8: 428–37.

CABG vs. PCI

70. The Bypass Angioplasty Revascularization Investigation (BARI) Investigators. Comparison of coronary bypass surgery with angioplasty in patients with multivessel disease. N Engl J Med 1996; 335: 217–25.

71. Abizaid A, Costa MA, Centemero M, et al. Arterial Revascularization Therapy Study Group. Clinical and economic impact of diabetes mellitus on percutaneous and surgical treatment of multivessel coronary disease patients: insights from the Arterial Revascularization Therapy Study (ARTS) trial. Circulation 2001; 104: 533–8.

72. Kapoor JR, Gienger AL, Ardehali R, et al. Isolated disease of the proximal left anterior descending artery comparing the effectiveness of percutaneous coronary interventions and coronary artery bypass surgery. JACC Cardiovasc Interv 2008; 1: 483–91.

73. Serruys PW, Morice MC, Kappetein AP, et al. Percutaneous coronary intervention versus coronary-artery bypass grafting for severe coronary artery disease. N Engl J Med 2009; 360: 961–72. *SYNTAX one year follow-up.*

74. Mohr FW, Morice M, Kappetein AP, et al. Coronary artery bypass graft surgery versus percutaneous coronary intervention in patients with three-vessel disease and left main coronary disease: 5-year follow-up of the randomised, clinical SYNTAX trial. Lancet 2013; 381: 629–38.

75. Farkouh ME, Domanski M, Sleeper LA, et al. Strategies for multivessel revascularization in patients with diabetes. N Engl J Med 2012; 367: 2375–84. *FREEDOM trial.*

76. Hlatky MA, Boothroyd DB, Bravata DM, et al. Coronary artery bypass surgery compared with percutaneous coronary interventions for multivessel disease: a collaborative analysis of individual patient data from ten randomised trials. Lancet 2009; 373: 1190–7.

77. Hannan EL, Wu C, Walford G, et al. Drug-eluting stents vs. coronary-artery bypass grafting in multivessel coronary disease. N Engl J Med 2008; 358: 331–41.

78. Morrison DA, Sethi G, Sacks J, et al. Percutaneous coronary intervention versus coronary artery bypass graft surgery for patients with medically refractory myocardial ischemia and risk factors for adverse outcomes with bypass: a multicenter, randomized trial. J Am Coll Cardiol 2001; 38: 143–9. *AWESOME trial.*

79. Nashef SA, Rogues F, Michel P, et al. European system for cardiac operative risk evaluation (EuroSCORE). Eur J Cardiothorac Surg 1999; 16: 9–13.
80. Society of Thoracic Surgeons. STS risk calculator: http://riskcalc.sts.org/STSWebRiskCalc273.

Complete vs. incomplete revascularization

81. Dauerman HL. Reasonable incomplete revascularization. Circulation 2011; 123: 2337–40.
82. Farooq V, Serruys PW, Garcia-Garcia HM, et al. The negative impact of incomplete angiographic revascularization on clinical outcomes and its association with total occlusions: the SYNTAX trial. J Am Coll Cardiol 2013; 61: 282–94. *Incomplete revascularization, whether with CABG or PCI, was associated with impaired long-term outcomes in SYNTAX trial (≠ references 80, 81).*
83. Hannan EL, Wu C, Walford G, *et al.* Incomplete revascularization in the era of drug-eluting stents: impact on adverse outcomes. JACC Cardiovasc Interv 2009; 2: 17–25.
84. van den Brand MJ, Rensing BJ, Morel MA, et al. The effect of completeness of revascularization on event-free survival at one year in the ARTS trial. J Am Coll Cardiol. 2002; 39: 559–564
85. Rastan AJ, Walther T, Falk V et al. Does reasonable incomplete surgical revascularization affect early or long-term survival in patients with multivessel coronary artery disease receiving left internal mammary artery bypass to left anterior descending artery? Circulation 2009; 120: S70–7.
86. Vander Salm TJ, Kip KE, Jones RH, et al. What constitutes optimal surgical revascularization? Answers from the Bypass Angioplasty Revascularization Investigation (BARI). J Am Coll Cardiol 2002; 39: 565–72.

Mortality

87. Mock MB, Ringqvist I, Fisher LD, et al. Survival of medically treated patients in the coronary artery surgery study (CASS) registry. Circulation 1982; 66: 562–8.
88. Emond M, Mock MB, Davis KB, et al. Long-term survival of medically treated patients in the Coronary Artery Surgery Study (CASS) Registry. Circulation 1994; 90: 2645–57.

Left main

89. Detre K, Murphy ML, Hultgren H. Effect of coronary bypass surgery on longevity in high and low risk patients. Report from the V.A. Cooperative Coronary Surgery Study. Lancet 1977; 2: 1243–5.
90. Taylor HA, Deumite NJ, Chaitman BR, et al. Asymptomatic left main coronary artery disease in the Coronary Artery Surgery Study (CASS) registry. Circulation 1989; 79: 1171–9.

Bypass grafts

91. Motwani JG, Topol EJ. Aortocoronary saphenous vein graft disease: pathogenesis, predisposition, and prevention. Circulation 1998; 97: 916–31.
92. Nwasokwa ON. Coronary artery bypass graft disease. Ann Intern Med 1995; 123: 528–33.
93. Sabik JF. Understanding saphenous vein graft patency. Circulation 2011; 124: 273–5.
94. Douglas JS, Weintraub WS, Lieberman HA, et al. Update of saphenous graft (SVG) angioplasty: restenosis and long-term outcome. Circulation 1991; 84 (Suppl II): II-249.
95. de Feyter PJ, van Suylen RJ, de Jaegere PP, Topol EJ, Serruys PW. Balloon angioplasty for the treatment of lesions in saphenous vein bypass grafts. J Am Coll Cardiol 1993; 21: 1539–49.
96. Ellis SG, Brener SJ, DeLuca S, et al. Late myocardial ischemic events after saphenous vein graft intervention: importance of initially "nonsignificant" vein graft lesions. Am J Cardiol 1997; 79: 1460–4.
97. Posatti G, Gaudino M, Pratti F, et al. Long-term results of radial artery use for myocardial revascularization. Circulation 2003; 108: 1350–4.
98. Barner HB. Radial artery patency. Eur J Cardiothorac Surg 2012; 41: 92–3.
99. Ruttmann E, Fischler N, Sakic A, et al. Second internal thoracic artery versus radial artery in coronary artery bypass grafting. A long-term, propensity score-matched follow-up study. *Circulation* 2011; 124: 1321–9
100. Lamy A, Devereaux PJ, Prabhakaran D, et al. Off-pump or on-pump coronary-artery bypass grafting at 30 days. N Engl J Med 2012; 366: 1489–97.
101. Hannan EL, Wu C, Smith CR, et al. Off-pump versus on-pump coronary artery bypass graft surgery: differences in long-term outcomes and in long-term mortality and need for subsequent revascularization. Circulation 2007; 116: 1145–52.

Coronary spasm

102. Yasue H, Takizawa A, Nagao M, et al. Long-term prognosis for patients with variant angina and influential factors. Circulation 1988; 78: 1–9. *60% had CAD; CAD not particularly predictor of events.*
103. Waters DD, Bouchard A, Theroux P. Spontaneous remission is a frequent outcome of variant angina. J Am Coll Cardiol 1983; 2: 195–9. *Excluded those who developed MI, CABG.*
104. Ozaki Y, Takatsu F, Osuqi J, et al. Long-term study of recurrent vasospastic angina using coronary angiograms during ergonovine provocation tests. Am Heart J 1992; 123: 1191–8. *This study only took patients without CAD; only 38% had recurrence, often (84%) consistent location and ECG.*
105. Cipriano PR, Koch FH, Rosenthal SJ, Schroeder JS. Clinical course of patients following the demonstration of coronary artery spasm by angiography. Am Heart J 1981; 101: 127–34. *Bad outcome in those with CAD, good if no CAD or receive CABG, but still 3/11 patients without CAD had VT, 1/11 had MI.*
106. Takagi Y, Yasuda S, Tsunoda R, et al. Clinical characteristics and long-term prognosis of vasospastic angina patients who survived out-of-hospital cardiac arrest: multicenter registry study of the Japanese Coronary Spasm Association. Circ Arrhythm Electrophysiol 2011; 4: 295–302. *14% had CAD.*
107. Bott-Silverman C, Heupler FA. Natural history of pure coronary artery spasm in patients treated medically. J Am Coll Cardiol 1983; 2: 200–5.
108. Yasue H, Mizuno Y, Harada E, et al. Effects of a 3-hydroxy-3-methylglutaryl coenzyme A reductase inhibitor, fluvastatin, on coronary spasm after withdrawal of calcium-channel blockers. J Am Coll Cardiol. 2008; 51: 1742–8.
109. Myerburg RJ, Kessler KM, Mallon SM, et al. Life-threatening ventricular arrhythmias in patients with silent myocardial ischemia due to coronary-artery spasm. N Engl J Med 1992; 326: 1451–5.
110. Meisel SR, Mazur A, Chetboun I, et al. Usefulness of implantable cardioverter-defibrillators in refractory variant angina pectoris complicated by ventricular fibrillation in patients with angiographically normal coronary arteries. Am J Cardiol 2002; 89: 1114–16.

Microvascular dysfunction

111. Cannon RO. Microvascular angina and the continuing dilemma of chest pain with normal coronary angiograms. J Am Coll Cardiol 2009; 54: 877–85.

112. Hasdai D, Gibbons RJ, Holmes DR, et al. Coronary endothelial dysfunction in humans is associated with myocardial perfusion defects. Circulation 1997; 96: 3390–5.

113. Hamasaki S, Al Suwaidi J, Higano ST, et al. Attenuated coronary flow reserve and vascular remodeling in patients with hypertension and left ventricular hypertrophy. J Am Coll Cardiol 2000; 35: 1654–60.

114. Mehta PJ, Goykhman P, Thomson LE, et al. Ranolazine improves angina in women with evidence of myocardial ischemia but no obstructive coronary artery disease. JACC Cardiovasc Imaging 2011; 4: 514–22.

115. Lerman A, Burnett JC, Higano ST, et al. Long-term L-arginine supplementation improves small-vessel coronary endothelial function in humans. Circulation 1998; 97: 2123–8.

Women

116. Johnson BD, Shaw LJ, Pepine CJ, et al. Persistent chest pain predicts cardiovascular events in women without obstructive coronary artery disease: results from the NIH-NHLBI-sponsored Women's Ischaemia Syndrome Evaluation (WISE) study. Eur Heart J 2006; 27: 1408–15.

117. Reis SE, Holubkov R, Smith AJC, et al. Coronary microvascular dysfunction is highly prevalent in women with chest pain in the absence of coronary artery disease: results from the NHLBI WISE study. The WISE investigators. Am Heart J 2001; 141: 735–41.

118. Bugiardini R, Manfrini O, Pizzi C, et al. Endothelial function predicts future development of coronary artery disease: a study of women with chest pain and normal coronary angiograms. Circulation 2004; 109: 2518–23.

119. Al Suwaidi J, Hamasaki S, Higano ST, et al. Long-term follow-up of patients with mild coronary artery disease and endothelial dysfunction. Circulation 2000; 101: 948–54.

Myocardial bridging

120. Mohlenkamp S, Hort W, Ge J, Erbel R. Update on myocardial bridging. Circulation 2002; 106: 2616–22.

121. Greenspan M, Iskandrian AS, Catherwood E, et al. Myocardial bridging of the LAD: evaluation using exercise thallium-201 myocardial scintigraphy. Cathet Cardiovasc Diagn. 1980; 6: 173–80.

122. Tang K, Wang L, Shi R, et al. The role of myocardial perfusion imaging in evaluating patients with myocardial bridging. J Nucl Cardiol 2011; 18: 117–22.

123. Juillière Y, Berder V, Suty-Selton C, et al. Isolated myocardial bridges with angiographic milking of left anterior descending coronary artery: a long-term follow-up study. Am Heart J 1995; 129: 663–5.

Collaterals

124. Schwartz H, Leiboff R, Bren G, et al. Temporal evolution of the human coronary collateral circulation after myocardial infarction. J Am Coll Cardiol 1984; 4: 1088–93.

125. Werner GS, Richartz BM, Gatmann O, et al. Immediate changes of collateral function after successful recanalization of chronic total coronary occlusions. Circulation 2000; 102: 2959–65.

126. Aboul-Enein F, Kar S, Hayes SW, et al. Influence of angiographic collateral circulation on myocardial perfusion in patients with chronic total occlusion of a single coronary artery and no prior myocardial infarction. J Nucl Med 2004; 45: 950–5.

Part 2 HEART FAILURE (CHRONIC AND ACUTE HEART FAILURE, SPECIFIC CARDIOMYOPATHIES, AND PATHOPHYSIOLOGY)

4   Heart Failure

DEFINITION, TYPES, CAUSES, AND DIAGNOSIS OF HEART FAILURE

1. DEFINITION AND TYPES OF HEART FAILURE

I. Heart failure is diagnosed clinically, not by echocardiography

It is a combination of congestive findings and low output findings.

A. Congestive findings

- *Orthopnea and paroxysmal nocturnal dyspnea (PND)*, both relatively specific for HF. They result from the increase in venous return during recumbency and the subsequent increase in pulmonary capillary pressure. Many patients present with nocturnal cough or wheezes rather than nocturnal dyspnea; a dry cough may be a dyspnea equivalent and should suggest HF. Wheezes result from congestion of the bronchial mucosa and from the interstitial edema that narrows the small airways.

  Orthopnea can be tested by asking the patient to lie supine for 2 minutes. Beside HF, orthopnea may be seen in obese patients or those with advanced lung disease and flattened diaphragm. Beside HF, PND may be seen in lung disease; whereas HF-related PND is relieved by upright posture, COPD-related PND results from mucus hypersecretion and is relieved by cough and albuterol, and asthma-related PND results from nocturnal bronchospasm and is relieved by albuterol.

- *Exertional dyspnea*. This may be a manifestation of a rise in pulmonary capillary pressure during exertion, even without overt pulmonary edema and without significant hypoxemia. The pulmonary venous engorgement stiffens the lungs and reduces vital capacity, leading to dyspnea. Dyspnea may also be a manifestation of an inappropriate rise in cardiac output during exertion, with a subsequent peripheral and respiratory muscle fatigue and reduced pulmonary perfusion (increased pulmonary dead space). *Thus, outside florid edema, diuretics do not necessarily improve exertional dyspnea.* Dyspnea is frequently described as "chest pressure" and therefore, in HF, especially decompensated HF, chest pressure is not necessarily secondary to CAD.

- *Quick weight gain* or quick weight loss in response to treatment implies volume overload.

- *Crackles/pulmonary edema/pleural effusions*. Note that crackles are frequently (80%) absent in patients with decompensated chronic HF, even when pulmonary capillary pressure is severely elevated. The increased lymphatic drainage of alveolar fluid prevents alveolar pulmonary edema.[1]

- *Increased JVP ≥ 8 cmH₂O*. JVP exam assesses the height of the *internal,* or sometimes external, jugular vein pulsations. In patients with a normal JVP, a hepatojugular reflux maneuver may be performed to unveil HF: a positive result is defined as a *sustained* rise of JVP of ≥4 cmH₂O following > 10 seconds of pressure on the right upper quadrant during normal breathing (no Valsalva), or a fall of JVP of 4 cmH₂O upon release of pressure.[2–4]

  JVD means distension of the *external* jugular vein, which is the visible jugular vein, and usually implies an elevated JVP. When JVD is present, JVP may be assessed on the external jugular vein.

- *S_3*: in patients > 40 years old, S_3 is highly specific (~90%) for an elevated pulmonary capillary wedge pressure (PCWP) (but insensitive).[5] *A loud P_2* implies significant pulmonary hypertension, suggestive of HF in the right context. Normally, P_2 is soft and is only heard at the left upper sternal border, where S_2 is split; *a loud P_2 translates into an S_2 split that is loud and more diffusely heard* over the lower sternum or apex. S_4 is less specific for an elevated PCWP and may be seen with compensated LV dysfunction.

- *Peripheral edema ± ascites; congestive and sometimes painful hepatomegaly (pulsatile hepatomegaly if severe TR); and rarely, congestive splenomegaly in prolonged failure*. Over 4 liters of volume overload are required to see peripheral edema. Therefore, peripheral edema is an insensitive finding and may be absent in 60% of patients with elevated PCWP; moreover, in many cases, pulmonary edema results from volume redistribution to the lungs rather than florid volume overload.[2,6] Edema is, however, specific for HF in a dyspneic patient.

As opposed to HF and constrictive pericarditis, the liver is atrophic in cirrhotic ascites.

- *Congestion on X-ray*: similarly to the limitations of the pulmonary exam in chronic HF, the increased lymphatic drainage prevents the appearance of alveolar or even interstitial pulmonary edema in the majority of patients with chronically elevated PCWP. Pulmonary vascular cephalization, pleural effusion, and perivascular haziness are the most sensitive findings, but overall, X-ray may not show any congestive finding in ~40% of patients with elevated PCWP.[1,2] CT scan is more helpful: *interlobular septal thickening* is a marker of interstitial pulmonary edema and is highly sensitive and specific for elevated PCWP.

In general *one to two congestive signs* along with at least *one congestive symptom* are required for the clinical diagnosis of HF. The most reliable congestive findings are orthopnea, elevated JVP, S_3, and a recent, quick weight gain. In particular, elevated JVP at rest or with hepatojugular reflux is the most sensitive and specific finding (>80%) for the diagnosis of elevated right- but also left-sided filling pressures (PCWP).[2-4]

B. Low-output findings (also known as "cold" signs) correlate with a more advanced HF stage:

- Severe fatigue.
- Since **the pulse pressure corresponds to stroke volume**, a narrow pulse pressure (<25% SBP) or a borderline systolic blood pressure implies a low stroke volume. In fact, *a narrow pulse pressure is the physical finding that most reliably predicts a low cardiac output* (>85% sensitivity and specificity).[1] Occasionally, severe arterial noncompliance prevents pulse pressure from narrowing.
- Pulsus alternans, which refers to an *every-other-beat variation in pulse intensity.* This is different from pulsus paradoxus, seen in tamponade.
- Cold, clammy extremities.
- Compensatory tachycardia.
- Renal failure, hyponatremia, poor response to diuretics.
- At an advanced stage: impaired mentation, drowsiness, central hypoventilation with Cheyne–Stokes pattern (hyperpnea alternating with hypopnea/apnea).
- Abdominal pain may result from functional bowel ischemia or from liver distension.

The functional capacity of HF patients is classified into four classes (NYHA class I: no limitation, can jog or carry > 24 lb up a flight of stairs; class II: can walk more than a flight of stairs or a block without symptoms, but symptoms occur with heavy weight carrying or walking two blocks; IIIA: symptoms with walking one block; IIIB symptoms with mild activities, such as dressing, showering, short walking; IV: symptoms at rest). *This functional classification applies to patients at their most stable cardiac status, outside of HF exacerbations.* Frequent HF hospitalizations, however, usually imply a worse functional class and a poor prognosis.

II. After HF is defined clinically, echocardiography is used to differentiate the three major types of HF

A. HF secondary to LV systolic dysfunction, where EF is reduced (≤40%)
In order to improve the stroke volume, the LV cavity dilates, but may be of normal size in acute systolic HF (acute MI, acute valvular regurgitation, acute myocarditis).

B. HF secondary to LV diastolic dysfunction, where EF is normal (≥50%), sometimes supranormal, and LV is generally of normal size, sometimes small
Diastolic HF is also called HF with normal or preserved EF (HFpEF), and this constitutes 40–50% of all HF presentations. In order to make a diagnosis of HFpEF, two other diagnoses have to be ruled out:

1. Transient, ischemic LV systolic dysfunction. HFpEF is best defined when the echo is performed within 72 hours of HF presentation and ACS is ruled out.
2. Dynamic ischemic MR in patients with off/on or persistent inferior wall dysfunction.

HFpEF is diagnosed when the following three features are present (ESC) (Figure 4.1):[7]

1. Clinical HF
2. Normal EF and normal or only mildly increased LV volume
3. Invasive, echocardiographic, or BNP evidence of elevated LVEDP or LA pressure, or diastolic dysfunction

The following mechanisms are incriminated (see detailed discussion in Chapter 5):

1. Abnormal diastolic function: (i) LV does not relax well (reduced active relaxation or tau index), and (ii) LV is not "elastic" enough to further distend after relaxation and accept the diastolic filling (increased diastolic stiffness or beta index). This limited LV filling results in a *backward* rise of PCWP despite a normal LV volume, and a *forward* drop of stroke volume.
2. Other mechanisms are found in many patients with HFpEF. Thus, **HFpEF does not always equate with diastolic HF:**

- Impaired contractility. A normal EF does not necessarily imply normal contractility. EF being equal to stroke volume divided by end-diastolic volume, EF is affected by contractility but also by changes in loading conditions. For the same contractility, a reduction in preload reduces the EF denominator and thus improves EF; a reduction in afterload increases stroke volume and thus improves EF.
- Increased arterial stiffness, which leads to exaggerated exertional hypertension.
- Pulmonary vascular stiffness with a rise in PA pressure disproportionate to LA pressure.
- Very small and stiff LV cavity that cannot distend in diastole, sometimes with cavity obliteration in systole and LVOT obstruction.
- Volume overload conditions, with a stretch of a normal LV, or only mildly abnormal LV, beyond its compliance point (e.g., end-stage renal disease).
- Chronotropic incompetence, seen in ~50% of patients, may be secondary to HF but may also be a contributor to exercise intolerance.

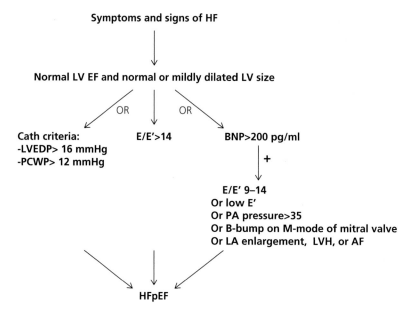

Figure 4.1 Diagnosis of HFpEF by catheterization, echo, or BNP features, according to ESC criteria.[7] A normal or mildly dilated LV is defined as LV end-diastolic volume $<75\,ml/m^2$ or $96\,ml/m^2$, respectively.

Patients with LV systolic dysfunction usually have a variable degree of impairment of diastolic filling and diastolic properties. LV systolic dysfunction is, in fact, a combined systolic and diastolic dysfunction. However, by definition, to use the term *diastolic HF*, EF should be preserved.

Patients with HF and EF 40–50% constitute a specific group wherein the LV pressure–volume relationship may be as steep as in diastolic failure, and wherein the diastolic function is more severely impaired than systolic function. **HF with EF 40–50% is a form of systolic dysfunction with predominant diastolic failure and is generally considered HFpEF or called** HF with midrange EF.

C. HF due to severe valvular disease, in which the ventricular function is initially normal. Ultimately, with most valvular disorders except MS, left ventricular systolic and diastolic dysfunction results.

> Whether HF is due to systolic or to diastolic dysfunction, the same congestive and low-output manifestations are seen. Advanced low-output failure is mainly seen with severe LV systolic dysfunction but may be seen with severe restrictive cardiomyopathy (such as amyloidosis).

III. Two additional types of HF
A. High-output heart failure
See Chapter 5, Section 3.IX.

B. Predominant or isolated right heart failure
Left HF is often (~55–80%) associated with a secondary right systolic or diastolic failure, manifested as increased RA pressure. In fact, left HF is the most common cause of right HF; back-up pressure overload from the left side and loss of the septal contribution to RV contraction lead to biventricular failure. Therefore, an elevated JVP or an abnormal hepatojugular reflux suggests not only right but also left HF, and predicts an elevated PCWP with a sensitivity of 55–80% and a positive predictive value of 85–95%.[1–4]

In some patients, the right HF becomes clinically more prominent than left HF as the lungs become underfilled, attenuating the pulmonary edema. Also, in non-ischemic cardiomyopathy, the RV may be directly involved by the myocardial process and may, in some cases, be more affected than the LV.

> Note that an overlooked LV diastolic failure is one of the most common and missed causes of what appears to be a predominant RV failure. In fact, RV failure/dilatation is present in ~20–30% of cases of HFpEF.

A truly isolated RV failure may be seen with ASD shunt, lung disease, or pulmonary vascular disease. It is clinically characterized by peripheral edema and elevated JVP yet clear lungs, and invasively, *an elevated RA pressure with either a normal PCWP or a mildly increased PCWP that is equalized to the RA pressure*. Pleural effusions may be seen with isolated right HF as the parietal pleura drains in the venae cavae (visceral pleura drains in the pulmonary veins).

2. CAUSES OF HEART FAILURE

I. Systolic HF (or HF with reduced EF)

A. CAD

CAD is the most common cause of systolic HF. Systolic HF that is secondary to CAD is called "ischemic cardiomyopathy." Two ischemic processes may explain LV dysfunction:

1. Large transmural Q-wave MI.

2. Hibernating myocardium. Severe coronary artery stenosis with chronic ischemia at rest or recurrent exertional ischemia may cause the myocardium to "shut down," i.e., hibernate without dying. Hibernation can be reversed with revascularization because the tissue usually remains viable.

LV dysfunction associated with single-vessel angiographic CAD, not involving the left main or the proximal LAD and without evidence of prior infarction, is disproportionate to the severity of CAD and implies a mortality that is similar to non-ischemic cardiomyopathy; this LV dysfunction is better classified as non-ischemic cardiomyopathy.[8] Ischemic cardiomyopathy, which has ~1.5-fold higher mortality than non-ischemic mortality, requires one of the following: (1) history of a large MI; (2) ≥ two-vessel CAD; or (3) single-vessel CAD that involves the left main or the proximal LAD. More extensive CAD is associated with further increase in mortality.[8] Some patients have mixed cardiomyopathies (e.g., LV dysfunction secondary to two-vessel CAD and exaggerated by HTN).

> An ischemic etiology is often suspected by history (history of MI, coronary revascularization, or angina/acute coronary syndrome). Occasionally, HF is the first manifestation of CAD: among patients with unexplained cardiomyopathy and unsuspected ischemic etiology, 7% are classified as ischemic cardiomyopathy after coronary angiography.[9]

B. Hypertension

Hypertension is the second most common cause of systolic HF. Chronic, severe hypertension leads to diastolic dysfunction initially, followed by systolic dysfunction. Without underlying myocardial disease or a chronic hypertensive cardiomyopathy, acute blood pressure rise does not usually cause acute LV systolic dysfunction, as a normal LV can tolerate acute pressure overload. This acute blood pressure rise more readily causes pulmonary edema through acute diastolic dysfunction.[10]

C. Advanced valvular heart disease (MR, AI, AS)

D. Dilated cardiomyopathy (DCM)

1. DCM is characterized by LV ± RV systolic dysfunction that is not due to ischemia, uncontrolled HTN, or valvular disease. The LV dysfunction is often global, but segmental wall motion abnormalities may be seen and do not necessarily imply ischemic cardiomyopathy.

2. Causes (see Chapter 5, Section 1):
- *Viral myocarditis.* There are several forms of myocarditis: (i) subclinical myocarditis, usually self-limited, although a minority of these cases progress to chronic cardiomyopathy; (ii) mild clinical myocarditis with EF 45–50%, usually recovers within weeks or months; (iii) severe myocarditis, i.e., myocarditis manifesting as HF or significant LV dysfunction, fully reverses in one-third of the cases, improves in another 40%, but may rapidly progress in a minority.[11]
- *Idiopathic.* Viral and idiopathic DCMs are the most common forms of DCM.
- *Toxic:* long-standing alcohol abuse with or without thiamine deficiency (reversible); cocaine use; radiation therapy; certain chemotherapy agents, such as doxorubicin (irreversible), cyclophosphamide and trastuzumab (reversible).
- *Genetic inheritance* in 30% of patients, mainly autosomal dominant.
- *HIV cardiomyopathy.*
- *Metabolic:* hyper- or hypothyroidism.
- *Infiltrative:* sarcoidosis, hemochromatosis.
- *Tachycardia-mediated cardiomyopathy.*
- *Peripartum cardiomyopathy* develops in the last month of pregnancy or within 5 months of delivery, without any identifiable cause, and without pre-existing heart disease. 50–60% of the cases are reversible within 6 months.
- *Takotsubo cardiomyopathy.*

The worst prognosis is seen with the following three cardiomyopathies: HIV cardiomyopathy, amyloidosis, and doxorubicin-associated cardiomyopathy.[9]

3. Some DCMs may be reversible:
- Myocarditis.
- Alcoholic cardiomyopathy reverses if the alcohol abuse is stopped at an early stage ± thiamine supplemented.
- Hypertensive cardiomyopathy.
- Peripartum cardiomyopathy.
- Tachycardia-mediated cardiomyopathy.
- Takotsubo cardiomyopathy.
- Other stress-related cardiomyopathies: sepsis or critical illness-associated cardiomyopathy, and neurogenic cardiomyopathy (following hemorrhagic or ischemic stroke).
- Cardiomyopathy related to thyroid disorders.

On average, ~35% of recent-onset DCMs (<6 months) that are idiopathic or secondary to myocarditis resolve spontaneously or with medical therapy within 6 months (*HF-recovered EF*), while another 40% have a significant improvement of EF.[11] This rate is higher for hypertensive cardiomyopathy and lower for genetic cardiomyopathy. Until they recover, these patients have an increased risk of arrhythmias and sudden death, well described with severe myocarditis. HF medical therapy should probably be continued over the long term, even after LV function normalizes.

Patients with *HF-recovered EF* of any etiology, including ischemic, have a good long-term prognosis, much better than HF-reduced EF and HFpEF, but continue to have a 1–2% cardiac mortality per year, > 5% risk of HF hospitalization per year, and a frequent BNP abnormality.[12]

II. HF with preserved EF

A. Hypertension with or without LV hypertrophy

Hypertension is the most common risk factor for diastolic HF. LV hypertrophy is common in diastolic HF; however, LV mass is normal in up to 50% of patients, and LV thickness is normal in up to 25% of patients.[13] Diastolic dysfunction may precede LV hypertrophy and is more prevalent than LV hypertrophy.

Arterial, ventricular, and atrial stiffness are increased as a result of increasing collagen, cytoskeletal proteins, and abnormal calcium homeostasis. This stiffness makes the LV filling pressure, LA pressure, and systolic blood pressure markedly increase with relatively minor volume overload. The arterial stiffness explains a very striking rise in SBP with exercise, which is an important component of diastolic HF in many patients.

Other risk factors for diastolic HF include age (>65 years), diabetes (30–50% of diastolic HF patients have diabetes), obesity (30–50%), female sex, renal failure, and AF.

B. CAD (ischemia without infarction)

Relaxation being an active process, CAD may contribute to diastolic dysfunction. In fact, in patients with CAD, a rise in LVEDP (diastolic stiffening) is an early hemodynamic manifestation of angina induced by pacing or exercise.[14]

As importantly, CAD may lead to transient LV systolic failure or dynamic ischemic MR that is mislabeled as diastolic failure, and thus, CAD needs to be considered in all heart failure cases that are labeled diastolic failure.

Overall, CAD is a less common etiology of HFpEF than HF with reduced EF, but is still considered the underlying etiology of HFpEF in 25–45% of patients in large HFpEF trials.[15,16] As with systolic HF, significant, usually multivessel CAD must be present to be considered the underlying mechanism of HFpEF.

C. Hypertrophic cardiomyopathy

D. Restrictive cardiomyopathy (RCM)

RCM is characterized by:[17,18]

a. *LV is small and stiff with severe diastolic failure*. Unlike in dilated cardiomyopathy, the LV cavity is small. Systolic function is relatively preserved and becomes progressively impaired at an advanced stage, yet the LV remains small. The RV may also be stiff and small or may be dilated; *RV dilatation/RV systolic dysfunction is common* at an advanced stage and is a poor prognostic sign.[19]
b. As in any decompensated ventricular failure, *LA and RA are markedly dilated* and functional TR and MR, sometimes severe, may be seen.
c. The *myocardial thickness is normal or near-normal* in idiopathic restrictive cardiomyopathy but is *increased* in infiltrative restrictive cardiomyopathies, particularly amyloidosis, where it may reach levels seen with hypertrophic cardiomyopathy (>20 mm) and may occasionally be asymmetric.[18] As opposed to hypertrophic or hypertensive cardiomyopathy, the increase in thickness is due to myocardial infiltration rather than myocardial hypertrophy, explaining the discrepancy between the low voltage on the ECG on the one hand and the thick myocardium on echocardiography on the other hand. As opposed to hypertensive cardiomyopathy, *the thickening frequently involves both ventricles, not just the LV.*

Moreover, amyloidosis has the following echo characteristics: a small pericardial effusion, valvular thickening, and a granular, "sparkling" myocardial texture. The sparkles are bright echo spots corresponding to amyloid deposits; note that the heterogeneous texture of HCM may simulate the sparkled texture of amyloidosis.[20]
d. On ECG, two findings are common with the thick amyloid cardiomyopathy, corresponding to replacement of the myocardium by the amyloid material: pseudo-Q waves and low QRS voltage, or at least a QRS voltage that is disproportionate to the thickness of the myocardium. LVH voltage criteria are never seen in the limb leads in amyloidosis.

Hypertensive cardiomyopathy may have the same echocardiographic features and severely restrictive filling as RCM, especially in the elderly. Hypertensive cardiomyopathy is sometimes labeled restrictive cardiomyopathy, but is better labeled "*restrictive process*" ("*restrictive process*" accounts for the pathophysiology, regardless of the underlying etiology).

In a patient with a thick myocardium and severely restrictive filling/HF, three diagnoses are considered: (i) hypertensive cardiomyopathy, (ii) hypertrophic cardiomyopathy, (iii) infiltrative cardiomyopathy. ECG and MRI help with the differential diagnosis.

In addition to echocardiography, right and left heart catheterization may be performed in a patient with suspected RCM to confirm the severe elevation of filling pressures and differentiate it from constrictive pericarditis. MRI and endomyocardial biopsy may be needed to diagnose the etiology of infiltrative cardiomyopathy.

Causes of RCM:

- Idiopathic, primary RCM (rarely familial). ~50% of RCMs are idiopathic.
- Infiltrative disease, most commonly amyloidosis, but also hemochromatosis, sarcoidosis, and hypereosinophilic syndrome.
- Scleroderma.
- Radiation heart disease, which leads to a combination of RCM, constrictive pericarditis, valvular heart disease (AS/AI, MR, TR), CAD, and pulmonary fibrosis. All these develop 5–30 years after radiation exposure.

E. Constrictive pericarditis
Constrictive pericarditis mimics the presentation of RCM and RV failure.

Obstructive sleep apnea not only worsens right HF but also left HF. The deep negative intrathoracic pressure increases the LV transmural pressure (= LV pressure minus surrounding pressure), and thus increases the LV wall tension (= afterload), an opposite effect to positive-pressure mechanical ventilation. Venous return is also increased, which distends the RV and creates RV–LV ventricular interdependence, further reducing LV flow. In addition, the episodes of hypoxia lead to sympathetic activation and systemic and pulmonary vasoconstriction, and thus both left and right HF and ischemia.[21] *While a normal individual may recover from these effects quickly upon apnea termination, recovery is delayed in patients with underlying HF.* LV filling pressure, LV diastolic function, but also LVEF and myocardial ischemia are affected by sleep apnea.

Tachycardia decompensates any compensated LV failure, whether systolic or diastolic, by reducing the diastolic time provided for the slow LV filling. On Doppler, an impaired relaxation pattern with a reversed E/A ratio and a slow E flow at rest becomes a high E/A ratio with a narrow and brief E flow during tachycardia (Figure 4.2). Once LV failure is decompensated, tachycardia should not be immediately reversed; at this point, the diastolic filling (E wave) is brief and impeded by the quick rise of LV diastolic pressure. Prolonging diastole will not increase diastolic filling; it is rather tachycardia that improves cardiac output and LV filling by providing more cardiac cycles. Only in compensated failure, a controlled heart rate (60–80 bpm) may allow better diastolic filling.

A newly diagnosed tachyarrhythmia at a rate > 105–110 bpm, coinciding with a new HF diagnosis, suggests the possibility of tachycardia-mediated cardiomyopathy. This is the case in 25–50% of new-onset atrial arrhythmias associated with a new-onset HF and warrants aggressive rate and possibly rhythm control, after treating HF decompensation.[22–24]

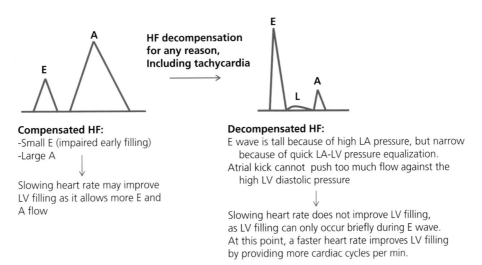

Figure 4.2 Change of LV filling pattern between compensated and decompensated HF.
The E and A waves correspond to the transmitral flow in diastole. The L wave is a marker of elevated LA pressure which attempts to push flow throughout diastole.

III. Right HF

Left HF is the most common cause of right HF. Overall, there are three mechanisms of RV failure, including isolated RV failure:

a. *Pressure overload:* pulmonary hypertension secondary to left heart disease, lung disease, PE, or pulmonary vascular disease.

b. *Volume overload:* ASD, tricuspid or pulmonic regurgitation. TR is often functional and secondary to RV failure but exaggerates its progression through the extra volume load. Conversely, primary TR may be a cause of an otherwise unexplained RV failure. In the absence of severe pulmonary hypertension, TR and especially PR are usually well tolerated for years before leading to RV failure. The adult RV is more tolerant of volume overload than pressure overload.

c. *Intrinsic RV dysfunction:* ARVD or RV infarct. Acute myocarditis, tachycardia-mediated cardiomyopathy, and idiopathic, HIV, or alcoholic cardiomyopathy usually lead to RV and LV involvement, but one may be more predominantly involved than the other.

> In any patient presenting with right heart failure, do not overlook the possibility of *pericardial processes, the great mimickers of right heart failure*. Tamponade mimics acute right heart failure, while constrictive pericarditis mimics chronic right heart failure.
>
> Moreover, restrictive cardiomyopathy, a form of biventricular failure, frequently presents clinically as a predominant right heart failure.

3. DIAGNOSTIC TESTS

I. Echocardiography

As mentioned under *Definition*, HF is a clinical diagnosis. The severity of HF is assessed using the NYHA functional classification. **Echocardiography is done to differentiate the three major categories of HF based on the assessment of EF, valvular function, diastolic dysfunction (low E'), and LA pressure (elevated E/E'):**

> A normal EF suggests diastolic dysfunction or transient systolic dysfunction (as in ischemia). One should look for specific signs of diastolic dysfunction such as reduced mitral tissue Doppler E' (E' corresponds to myocardial recoil in diastole). A normal E' is very unusual in diastolic or systolic HF.[13] Patients with diastolic HF usually have signs of elevated LA pressure if they are in active HF (elevated E/E' ratio > 14), or signs of stage 1, compensated diastolic dysfunction if they are not in HF (low E' < 8 cm/s with normal E/E' ratio and reversed E/A ratio).
>
> The septum is thickened in most but not all patients with HFpEF (mean septal thickness 1.18 cm in one study).[13]
>
> Also, typically and almost uniformly, LA is enlarged if the patient is in decompensated HF (whether systolic or diastolic HF). Regardless of decompensation, LA volume and/or diameter is enlarged in 80% of HFpEF (LA volume is enlarged in 46%, LA diameter is enlarged in 64%).[13]
>
> In the absence of *diastolic dysfunction or LA enlargement* on echo, reconsider the diagnosis of diastolic HF and consider other causes of dyspnea.[13]

- Echo estimates left atrial pressure and pulmonary arterial pressure, which, if high, are signs of decompensation and of some degree of pulmonary congestion. Pulmonary hypertension, per se, may persist after resolution of the pulmonary congestion. In fact, a chronic increase in pulmonary pressure may lead to a reactive pulmonary hypertension that may be slow to resolve after normalization of left-sided filling pressures.
- Echo can suggest a cause, such as ischemia in the case of focal wall motion abnormalities (albeit not very specific), or hypertensive cardiomyopathy in the case of a thickened septum.
- Echo assesses for other forms of HF:
  ○ Isolated RV failure with its various causes (pulmonary arterial hypertension, ASD).
  ○ HF mimickers: constrictive pericarditis, tamponade.

II. BNP

BNP is useful in acute dyspneic presentation. BNP is a peptide synthesized in response to cardiomyocyte stretch. Atrial or ventricular wall stress, especially *LV wall stress* from volume or pressure overload, is the primary driver of BNP secretion, but ischemia and neurohormones may also directly stimulate BNP gene expression. RV and/or atrial stretch may increase BNP to lesser degrees than LV stretch, as RV and the atria have a smaller mass. Pro-BNP is the precursor of BNP; it is cleaved into BNP and NT-pro-BNP.

A. BNP > 400–500 pg/ml (or NT-pro-BNP > 1200 pg/ml) is highly suggestive of acute left HF in a patient with acute dyspnea. It correlates with increased LVEDP; however, the exact BNP value does not correlate with the exact degree of LVEDP rise. For a given filling pressure, dilated ventricles secrete more peptide because of the greater wall stress/stretch and chamber mass. This explains why BNP is higher in LV systolic than in LV diastolic failure, and how it may be high despite a normal LVEDP. Also, several factors such as age, sex, and renal failure contribute to the absolute BNP levels.

B. BNP < 100 pg/ml (or NT-pro-BNP < 300 pg/ml) excludes acute left HF as a cause of acute dyspnea. The patient may, however, have asymptomatic LV dysfunction or mildly symptomatic LV dysfunction (exertional symptoms). In fact, patients with diastolic or even severe systolic dysfunction who do not have overt HF frequently have BNP values that overlap with normal individuals' BNP (BNP

<50pg/ml). In one study, most patients with asymptomatic LV systolic dysfunction, even severe LV dysfunction, had BNP levels<50pg/ml.[25] In another study that focused on LV diastolic dysfunction, a significant proportion (~25%) of patients with echocardiographic diastolic dysfunction had BNP<50, but this was very uncommon in patients with a history of HF, current clinical HF, or severe diastolic abnormalities on echo (the mean BNP in these patients was>300).[26] *A cutoff of 35pg/ml is a better cutoff to exclude chronic HF as a cause of chronic exertional symptoms (ESC).*

C. In the acute setting, BNP levels of 100–500pg/ml are in the intermediate range. Dyspnea may be due to acute left HF but also to acute pulmonary or pulmonary vascular illness (with RA/RV stretch), or sepsis. BNP may also be increased because of RV failure, renal failure, or myocardial ischemia.

In the chronic setting, BNP levels of 35–200pg/ml are in the intermediate range. Chronic dyspnea may be due to HF or non-cardiac disease.

D. Evolution and follow-up of BNP levels. In most patients with acute HF, BNP decreases with diuresis and the reduction of LV filling pressure but may not return to normal, as the LV remains dilated even after LVEDP is normalized (BNP may be as high as several hundred pg/ml, but is not usually higher than 1000pg/ml). This residual BNP correlates with the degree of underlying LV and RV remodeling.[27,28] Even when euvolemia is achieved and LVEDP normalized, a dilated LV will continue to generate an elevated BNP (called residual, *dry BNP*). Also, the reduction in BNP may be delayed because of reduced clearance, especially in renal failure. Thus, daily BNP measurements are not warranted; when clinical euvolemia is established, a *pre-discharge BNP level* may be determined and used in follow-up.[28] A persistently elevated BNP upon discharge is a predictor of HF readmission and has a negative prognostic value. In one analysis, a 30–50% BNP or NT-pro-BNP reduction during the hospital stay strongly predicted a reduction in hospitalizations, beyond clinical variables, suggesting that BNP may be used as a target before HF discharge.[29]

BNP levels may be followed in stable outpatients to detect early congestion, but this has pitfalls, because BNP has an intra-individual biological variability of up to 25–50% unrelated to the development of symptoms.[28] Conversely, a rise in BNP of over 25–50% may herald a clinical decompensation and suggests drug titration. Several studies and a meta-analysis have shown the utility of a BNP-guided outpatient drug titration in patients<75years old with systolic HF (ACE-I, β-blocker, aldosterone antagonist, and diuretic titration to a BNP<100–300). This strategy reduced HF hospitalizations and improved survival in the meta-analysis (class IIa recommendation).[30,31] In those studies, BNP was checked every 1–3 months. ACE-I, β-blocker, and aldosterone antagonist titration may be prioritized over diuretics if the patient is not clinically congested. The utility of BNP-guided therapy in older patients and in patients with diastolic dysfunction is unclear; overzealous therapy to reduce BNP in these patients may be associated with more side effects (dizziness, fatigue).

> BNP tends to be higher in the elderly, in women, in renal failure, and in cirrhosis. BNP is mostly cleared by tissue peptidase, but is partially cleared renally.
>
> BNP is lower in obese patients because of a higher BNP clearance. In obese patients, a lower BNP cutoff of 50 ng/ml may be used to rule out acute left HF. Also, in comparison with left ventricular HF, HF induced by mitral stenosis and acute mitral regurgitation has a lower BNP (cases where LVEDP is not necessarily increased). BNP takes 1 hour to rise and may be initially normal in hyperacute HF.
>
> In a patient with clinical HF, JVD, and edema yet normal BNP, consider the diagnosis of constrictive pericarditis.

In critically ill patients with severe sepsis or shock, BNP levels do not correlate well with left-sided filling pressures; BNP levels higher than 1000 may be found with normal PCWP and better correlate with renal failure in this setting.[28]

III. ECG
A completely normal ECG almost excludes the diagnosis of HF, particularly systolic HF and acute HF.[32]

Q waves usually point towards ischemic cardiomyopathy. Other abnormalities are non-specific but may have prognostic values: LVH with strain pattern, ST–T abnormalities, RBBB or LBBB, AF and various arrhythmias.

Advanced AV block is more characteristic of myocarditis and infiltrative disease than other cardiomyopathies.

The association of a large QRS voltage in the precordial leads with a low QRS voltage in the limb leads suggests reduced systolic function with dilated LV.

LBBB with QRS>130ms has therapeutic implications (benefit from CRT).

IV. Coronary angiography and other ischemic workup
An ischemic etiology of LV dysfunction should be sought. Coronary angiography is generally indicated in all cases of systolic or diastolic HF (ACC guidelines class IIa), especially if there is any history of angina, CAD, or acute severe presentation.

Alternatively, any one of the following studies is performed (class IIa):

- *Nuclear rest and stress perfusion* scan, looking for segmental defects suggestive of CAD. However, nuclear defects are common in non-ischemic cardiomyopathy (patchy scar tissue). On the other hand, up to 30% of patients with multivessel CAD have balanced ischemia without any apparent defect.[33,34] Therefore, nuclear testing is not very sensitive or specific to diagnose CAD as the underlying cause of cardiomyopathy, *but may be useful to assess for residual ischemia in an infarcted territory in ischemic cardiomyopathy.*
- *Stress echocardiography:* a biphasic response (i.e., an initial increase in contractility at low doses of dobutamine followed by a decrease in contractility at higher levels of stress) suggests that LV is viable and able to increase its contraction, but gets ischemic with high stress. A uniphasic response with a progressive increase in contractility from lower to higher doses suggests non-ischemic cardiomyopathy or ischemic cardiomyopathy related to a coronary stenosis that has been revascularized, but the myocardium has not recovered yet or full recovery is prevented by a severe subendocardial scar. The absence of any increase in contractility suggests the absence of myocardial

reserve: LV dysfunction could be ischemic or non-ischemic and is possibly irreversible (non-viable), but viability and the potential benefit from revascularization should not be ruled out based purely on this finding.

- *Coronary CT angiography* may be used to rule out CAD, mainly when the probability of ischemic HF is low.

V. Diastolic stress testing

Chronic dyspnea that is associated with a normal systolic function on echo and no clinical signs of HF may be falsely considered a dyspnea of non-cardiac origin. These patients may have normal pulmonary capillary pressure and PA pressure at rest. However, exertion and the increase in venous return may increase their left-sided filling pressures; also, exertion may markedly increase their blood pressure. This is a masked form of LV diastolic dysfunction that is unveiled with exercise. Thus, ***"diastolic stress testing"*** is valuable in patients with chronic unexplained dyspnea, ***especially if they have borderline BNP or echo findings at rest*** (e.g., low E', LA enlargement, or LVH but normal E/E' ratio). It consists of reassessing PA pressure and LA pressure (E/E' ratio) after exercise testing. In addition, stress testing allows the assessment of ischemia, transient ischemic MR, and the objective functional limitation.[35]

Some patients with diastolic dysfunction but normal left-sided filling pressure at rest truly have a non-cardiac cause of exertional dyspnea. Diastolic stress testing helps sort out whether dyspnea is due to diastolic dysfunction or to a non-cardiac cause.

Diastolic stress testing may also be performed invasively, using a Swan catheter and a supine bicycle. As an alternative to exercise, passive leg raising may be used as a diastolic stress test.

VI. Endomyocardial biopsy

Endomyocardial biopsy is indicated when severe, progressive myocarditis is suspected, in which case ***fulminant myocarditis*** (reversible) and ***hypersensitivity eosinophilic myocarditis*** (treatable and reversible) need to be distinguished from the downhill progressive ***giant-cell myocarditis***.[36] Fulminant myocarditis recovers in a few weeks but requires aggressive early support, while giant-cell myocarditis dictates cardiac transplantation with immunosuppressive therapy and LV assist device in the interim period. Thus, a biopsy is indicated in the case of unexplained, non-ischemic, new-onset HF (<3 months) with hemodynamic compromise, failure to adequately respond to 1–2 weeks of usual care, or intractable ventricular arrhythmias or advanced AV block. It is also indicated, less strongly, in unexplained HF of >3 months duration unresponsive to 1–2 weeks of usual care; and when drug reaction is suspected but HF is not quickly improving after drug withdrawal (biopsy establishes the diagnosis of eosinophilic myocarditis and allows steroid therapy).

In addition, a biopsy is indicated when infiltrative disease is suspected: (i) amyloidosis is suspected but an abdominal fat pad biopsy and serum/urinary immunofixation are inconclusive; (ii) sarcoidosis is suspected without a typical pulmonary involvement; (iii) thick myocardial walls with suspicion of amyloidosis vs. HCM.

VII. Cardiac MRI

Normally, gadolinium does not penetrate the myocardial cells and briefly and mildly penetrates the myocardial circulation during first-pass MRI perfusion imaging (myocardial cells are tightly packed with no significant interstitium). Late gadolinium enhancement (LGE) on T1 usually implies necrotic or fibrotic tissue, to which gadolinium has a high affinity. Cardiac MRI has four major applications in HF: (i) assessment of LGE patterns that are specific for some cardiomyopathies (subendocardial or transmural LGE implies ischemic cardiomyopathy, subepicardial or midwall LGE or LGE in a non-coronary distribution implies non-ischemic cardiomyopathy); (ii) diagnosis of myocarditis in unexplained cardiomyopathy or unexplained, large troponin elevation; (iii) diagnosis of infiltrative cardiomyopathy vs. hypertrophic cardiomyopathy in a patient with thick myocardium (*global* subendocardial LGE suggests amyloidosis, patchy midwall enhancement suggests HCM); (iv) viability assessment in ischemic cardiomyopathy.

CHRONIC TREATMENT OF HEART FAILURE

1. TREATMENT OF SYSTOLIC HEART FAILURE

I. Treat the underlying etiology

Valvular surgery should be performed in severe valvular disease. HTN should be treated to a goal ≤ 140/90 mmHg. In systolic HF, HTN may get "normalized" or reduced as a result of the low cardiac output; HF drugs are provided regardless of blood pressure, as long as clinically tolerated. Revascularization with CABG or PCI should be considered in patients with ischemic cardiomyopathy, i.e., CAD extensive enough to explain the cardiomyopathy, rather than incidental single-vessel CAD (as explained under *Causes of heart failure*). Revascularization should also be considered in patients with diastolic HF and extensive CAD.

II. Value of revascularization in ischemic cardiomyopathy: STICH trial

The STICH trial randomized patients with ischemic cardiomyopathy and EF < 35% to revascularization with CABG vs. medical therapy.[37] Most of these patients had three-vessel CAD, often with proximal LAD disease, and a prior history of MI; patients were not excluded based on viability testing. The trial excluded patients with significant (CCS 3 or 4) angina and patients with class IV HF, and consisted mainly of patients with LV dysfunction, no angina, and mild HF (class I–II for the most part). At 5 years, CABG was associated with a strong trend towards mortality reduction (~8% per year vs. 6.5% per year, p=0.12), and a significant reduction of each of the following endpoints: cardiovascular mortality and hospitalization for HF or cardiovascular causes. In addition, the early hazard with CABG was relatively low in the trial (3.6 % mortality at 30 days).

Thus, overall, this trial supports CABG in ischemic cardiomyopathy. Furthermore, the benefit is higher in the as-treated analysis that takes into account the 17% crossover rate to CABG in the medical therapy group. The benefit is also potentially higher in the sicker, real-world patients with angina or more advanced HF, although the immediate surgical risk is expected to be higher.

Yet the benefit from CABG in these stable patients did not appear until 2 years of follow-up and the benefit was not dramatic, which implies that CABG is not urgent in patients with ischemic cardiomyopathy who are stabilized with medical therapy.

III. Subsets of patients who are likely to benefit from revascularization: role of viability testing and ischemic testing

In the STICH trial, ~50% of patients underwent viability testing (with echo or SPECT) and were randomized to CABG vs. medical therapy regardless of the result. CABG was beneficial regardless of viability, and viability did not provide any discriminatory effect.[38] This suggests that in the chronic ischemic setting, revascularization for ischemic LV dysfunction is likely beneficial regardless of viability testing.

A. Definition of global and regional viability; viability tests

Viability implies that a dysfunctional myocardium is still metabolically active, but is hibernating from persistent severe ischemia; or stunned after a transient episode of severe ischemia, even if perfusion is re-established. Those processes are called *hibernation* and *stunning*, respectively. A dysfunctional myocardial area is considered viable if:[39-43]

- The regional dysfunction significantly improves after revascularization by at least one point (from akinesis to hypokinesis, or from hypokinesis to normal). This is called **regional viability.**
  or:
- The overall EF significantly improves (>5%). This is called **global viability**.

Thus, viability can only be confirmed in retrospect, after revascularization is performed. In general, 60–70% of patients with chronic ischemic LV dysfunction have significant improvement in LV function after revascularization. Four imaging modalities have been used to assess viability:

- *Thallium myocardial uptake* at rest and at 4 hours and 24 hours post-rest injection (rest-redistribution imaging). Also, *technetium uptake* at rest (or after nitrates administration) may be used to assess viability. An uptake ≥50% at rest or after thallium redistribution implies that the regional myocardium is viable.[44] Also, an absolute change of 12% during redistribution implies regional viability even if the uptake remains <50%.[38,45]
- *Low-dose dobutamine echocardiography* evaluates for an improvement of myocardial contraction in response to low doses of dobutamine (<10 mcg/kg/min): from dyskinesis to hypokinesis, akinesis to hypokinesis, or hypokinesis to normal contraction (a change from dyskinesis to akinesis is not considered improvement). This is called myocardial contractile reserve. A decline in myocardial contraction at subsequent higher doses reflects ischemia; this biphasic response is highly predictive of myocardial recovery and viability. Conversely, a uniphasic response (progressive improvement of contractility at high doses of dobutamine) does not always indicate viability as it may be seen with subendocardial scarring, where the myocardial segment responds to dobutamine because of augmentation of the subepicardium but does not always recover its function. The absence of any response may imply non-viability; 25–30% of viable segments, however, do not augment with dobutamine. This is why nuclear studies are more sensitive for the detection of viability, albeit less specific.
- *PET scan* assesses metabolic uptake of a glucose analog tracer (metabolic viability). It can also assess perfusion with N^{13} tracer. A mismatch between a low perfusion and a high metabolic uptake implies viability. A reduction in both perfusion and metabolic uptake implies irreversible injury. PET has the highest sensitivity (~90%) but the lowest specificity (~58%) for viability assessment.
- *Cardiac MRI:* late myocardial hyperenhancement 10 minutes after gadolinium injection is a sign of scarring and implies non-viability of the myocardial segment when it involves >50% of the transmural myocardial thickness.

Also, several ECG, echocardiographic, and angiographic features are helpful, to a limited extent, in assessing viability:

i. *The lack of Q waves* implies less scar and necrosis and strongly predicts recovery.[46,47] However, Q waves may be seen with a hibernating myocardium, and thus *the presence of Q waves* does not rule out viability.[46]

ii. *As compared to akinesis, hypokinesis does not* necessarily imply a higher likelihood of recovery with revascularization. After revascularization, akinesis and dyskinesis frequently improve, while occasionally hypokinesis does not improve. The hypokinetic wall may be tethered by adjacent akinetic walls or there may be extensive subendocardial necrosis and scarring.[48] Yet, hypokinesis implies the presence of viable tissue, and thus revascularization of a hypokinetic wall may prevent further deterioration of LV function and is more readily performed.

iii. *A thin and bright myocardium* ≤5.5 mm on echo may imply a scarred, non-viable myocardium. Yet, if it is not extensive, it does not preclude a revascularization benefit to the surrounding walls. Also, a recent study has shown that 18% of thin myocardial regions have a limited scar burden by MRI and recover myocardial thickness and contractility with revascularization, with Q-wave disappearance; thus, a thin myocardium does not preclude revascularization.[49]

iv. Severe LV dilatation (end-diastolic volume ≥twice normal, which often corresponds to a diastolic diameter ≥70 mm) usually implies extensive scarring and negative remodeling that would not be reversed with revascularization and predicts a poor prognosis after revascularization.[50]

v. When a dysfunctional segment is supplied by an occluded artery, *good collateral flow* predicts myocardial recovery.[51] In one study, the presence of grade 2 or 3 collaterals on coronary angiography, i.e., good collaterals that reconstitute partially or fully the epicardial vessel, predicted regional and global myocardial recovery in 81% of the cases.[52]

B. Variations in the definition of global viability

For revascularization to be useful, the percentage of the LV that must be viable is a matter of debate. In patients with multivessel disease considered for multivessel revascularization, several studies have focused on the assessment of global LV viability rather than regional viability. Global LV viability has been defined as viability of ≥65% of all myocardial segments (11 out of 17 segments), counting both dysfunctional segments and segments with normal contractility.[38,53,54]

Conversely, most studies have defined global viability with a focus on the dysfunctional segments. When the viable dysfunctional segments constitute ≥25% of the LV, global viability is considered present and a global improvement of EF is expected (e.g., ≥ **4 of the dysfunctional myocardial segments are viable**).[39-43,45,55]

C. Limitations of viability testing

Viability testing has the following limitations:

- Viability tests have positive and negative predictive values of ~75–80%, for both regional and global viability. This is particularly the case in thallium or technetium nuclear viability testing (sensitivity ~80%, specificity ~60%) and dobutamine echocardiography testing (sensitivity 65%, specificity 85%), which were used in the STICH trial.[39,56] The assessment of the extent of transmural scarring by MRI is more valid (sensitivity ~80%, specificity ~80%).
- The definition is not uniform. Studies have variably defined viability as regional viability versus global LV viability.[39,45] Global LV viability may be the most valuable way of assessing viability before considering surgical revascularization (adopted in the STICH viability study), but has been defined differently across studies. Some have considered viability present when ≥65% of the overall LV is viable (STICH),[38,54] while most studies have defined viability to be present when the dysfunctional but viable segments constitute ≥25 % of the LV.[40] For example, in a patient with anteroapical infarction, regional viability addresses the viability of the anteroapical segments to decide whether LAD revascularization is beneficial; conversely, global viability addresses what percentage of the overall LV is represented by the dysfunctional yet viable LAD territory (<25% vs. ≥ 25%), or how much of the overall LV is viable (if ≥65% of the LV is viable, full revascularization of all territories, including LAD, is performed, as suggested in the STICH viability study protocol).
- Even without any viability and any contractile and EF improvement, revascularization may improve symptom status, HF, and mortality.[57] Revascularization may improve LV remodeling, prevent further MI and further deterioration of LV function, preserve infarct border zone integrity, and reduce arrhythmogenesis.
- The benefit from CABG may be higher in the sickest patients, such as those with limited viability.[38]

D. Role of ischemic testing; difference between ischemia and viability

The concepts of ischemia and viability are different, and the presence of ischemia is a much stronger marker of prognosis and functional myocardial recovery than the mere presence of viability.[58–61] On nuclear imaging, *viability* implies that at rest, the dysfunctional territory uptakes significant nuclear agent. *Ischemia* implies that at stress, the nuclear defect in the infarcted or peri-infarct territory is significantly more intense or more extensive than at rest; or significant/extensive ST-segment deviations occur. *An ischemic territory is viable; conversely, a viable territory may not be ischemic,* in which case the benefit of revascularization and the functional recovery are less clear.[62] A territory may have a center that is non-ischemic, but a surrounding area that is ischemic, in which case revascularization is beneficial. This is one of the main applications of nuclear stress testing in cardiomyopathy (Figures 4.3, 4.4).

Ischemia of the infarcted territory may also be documented by invasive FFR testing, which correlates with the potential benefit from revascularization.[62]

Nonetheless, while valuable, the assessment of ischemia in patients with LV dysfunction and significant baseline nuclear defects is cumbersome, as fixed defects on nuclear imaging or fixed wall motion abnormality on echo may very well represent severe ischemia with hibernation, particularly when the nuclear uptake is ≥50%; up to 75% of these defects reverse with revascularization.[63,64] This lessens the predictive value of ischemic testing in LV dysfunction (STICH stress substudy).[65] **The fixed defect likely represents ischemia if the nuclear uptake is ≥50%, or if the patient has angina, ST deviation or no Q wave.**

E. Proposed algorithm to guide revascularization of patients with ischemic LV dysfunction

Based on the STICH trial, revascularization may be useful in chronic ischemic cardiomyopathy regardless of viability. On the other hand, regardless of viability, revascularization may not be beneficial in patients with a recent large clinical infarct that is 1–28 days old and responsible for the low EF (those patients were excluded from the STICH trial). As shown in the OAT trial, patients with acute MI who do not receive culprit artery reperfusion in the first 24 hours of presentation, and have an akinetic wall, a totally occluded culprit artery, and no residual angina or peri-infarct ischemia, do not benefit from revascularization.[66]

In sum, the following features may be used to guide revascularization of patients with ischemic LV dysfunction (Figure 4.5):

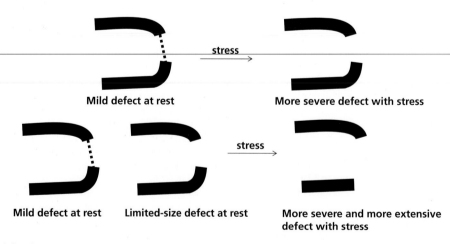

Mild defect at rest → stress → More severe defect with stress

Mild defect at rest / Limited-size defect at rest → stress → More severe and more extensive defect with stress

Figure 4.3 Peri-infarct ischemia.

In a patient with a clinical history of MI or Q waves on ECG, the worsening of a resting defect is indicative of peri-infarct ischemia (extension of the defect area *or* severity).

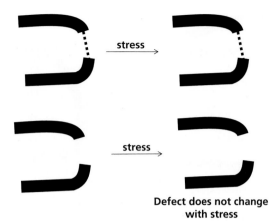

**Defect does not change
with stress**

Figure 4.4 Fixed defect.

In a patient with a clinical history of MI or Q waves on ECG, the fixed defect indicates the lack of significant ischemia in the viable area (if any viable area exists).

Conversely, if the patient has angina and no Q waves, or if the nuclear uptake is ≥ 50%, this fixed defect may indicate hibernation and ischemia.

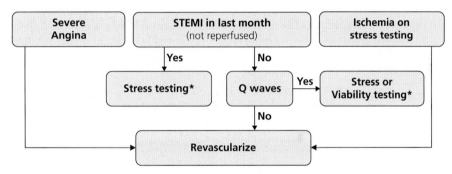

Figure 4.5 Proposed algorithm to guide revascularization in patients with ischemic LV dysfunction.

*Also, consider myocardial wall thickness (≤5 mm is less likely to derive a benefit from revascularization), and wall motion (hypokinesis vs. akinesis).

1. Angina, particularly severe angina, is an indication of ischemia and often dictates revascularization, even if a significant amount of myocardium appears non-viable.

2. Stress testing showing significant stress-induced ischemia in or around the infarcted territory favors revascularization.

3. i. Clinical history of a large STEMI that was not acutely reperfused, *particularly recent STEMI in the last month*, argues against revascularization.

   ii. Q waves: the lack of Q waves strongly predicts recovery, while their presence does not rule it out.

   • If neither (i) nor (ii) is present, the territory is likely viable and revascularization is likely appropriate.

   • If (i) or (ii) is present, consider stress testing to look for residual ischemia. Viability testing may be considered for (ii). Also, take into account the thickness of the myocardial wall (≤5 mm is less likely to benefit), and hypokinesis vs. akinesis.

IV. Drugs that affect survival

Three compensatory mechanisms occur in HF and are ultimately harmful.

1. LV remodeling is the process of LV dilatation, LV change in geometry, and LV eccentric hypertrophy that attempt to increase the stroke volume of a hypocontractile myocardium. This process may be useful to a certain degree early on. Over time, however, as the LV undergoes progressive remodeling, it becomes less elliptical and more spherical, progressively more dilated, thin, and fibrotic, with increased wall stress (afterload); all this ultimately decreases the stroke volume.

LV end-systolic volume is the best measurement of LV remodeling. *EF, often considered a contractility index, is affected by preload and afterload and is, in fact, more a remodeling index than a contractility index (Figure 4.6).*

2. Increased activity of the sympathetic system increases cardiac contractility but ultimately exhausts the myocardium, makes it less responsive to catecholamines, and promotes apoptosis.

3. Increased activity of the renin–angiotensin–aldosterone system (RAAS) elicits vasoconstriction and increases blood volume. This aims to maintain the blood pressure and the kidney perfusion, but is deleterious to the LV. In addition, angiotensin II directly acts on harmful myocardial AT1 receptors that promote cellular growth, LV dilatation, and LV fibrosis and increase the release of myocardial norepinephrine.

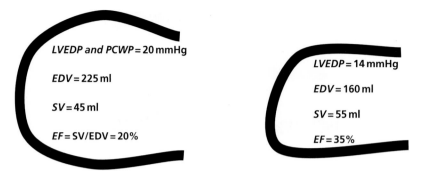

Figure 4.6 Case of chronic HF with LV dilatation and mild increase in PCWP.

Left figure corresponds to LV volume/pressure before diuresis and before drug therapy. After diuresis, RAAS blockade, and β-blockade (*right figure*), LV volume decreases and LV morphology changes from a sphere to an ellipse. Stroke volume increases because of reduced afterload (smaller LV), reduced functional MR, and reduced RV–LV interdependence. Diuresis is beneficial, although PCWP is only mildly elevated at baseline.

Note that afterload correlates with LV size and is not simply equivalent to aortic pressure (afterload=wall stress=LV radius x LV pressure/2x LV thickness).

EDV, end-diastolic volume; SV, stroke volume.

Four main treatments improve mortality and are directed against the sympathetic system and RAAS activity. They reduce LV remodeling, promote reverse remodeling, and, eventually, *increase EF even if myocardial contractility is unchanged*:

1. Angiotensin-converting-enzyme inhibitors (ACE-Is) or angiotensin receptor blockers (ARBs). ACE-Is and ARBs improve HF outcomes not only through afterload reduction but also through blocking the harmful RAAS effect on volume status and on the AT1 myocardial receptor. In fact, afterload reduction with amlodipine or with α-blockers does not improve HF outcomes.

2. β-Blockers blunt the high sympathetic tone of HF.

3. Aldosterone antagonists.

4. Neprilysin inhibitor combined with ARB.

5. A fifth treatment, hydralazine and nitrate combination. This vasodilator combination reduces mortality and symptoms in black patients and reduces symptoms in white patients.

V. Specifics of drugs that affect survival

ACE-Is/ARBs and β-blockers are indicated in all patients with systolic LV dysfunction, including asymptomatic patients.

A. ACE-I or ARB*

1. ACE-Is and ARBs increase cardiac output, reduce LV remodeling, and improve EF. They reduce mortality by ~20% and reduce HF hospitalizations by ~30%.[67–70]

2. ARB is an alternative to ACE-I when cough or angioedema occurs with ACE-I. There is a small cross-risk of angioedema with ARB (<5%), and thus extreme caution is advised when substituting ARB for ACE-I in a patient who had angioedema with ACE-I; this is not a contraindication to ARB (CHARM-Alternative). The main ARBs studied in HF are candesartan and valsartan.[71–73] When used as an alternative to ACE-I therapy, ARB therapy reduces mortality in systolic HF (CHARM alternative trial and ValHeFT substudy).

3. Avoid or be cautious in cases of:

- Hypotension with SBP<80mmHg or with symptoms of low output (dizzy, obtunded, oliguric). A low SBP of 80–90mmHg may be well tolerated in HF because it helps unload the LV; ACE-I is started slowly and the diuretic is reduced if possible.

- Elevation of creatinine of over 50% within 1–2 weeks of ACE-I/ARB initiation. In advanced HF, the worsening of renal function may be related to the low output/low BP/low kidney perfusion state aggravated by ACE-I initiation, which impairs renal autoregulation. It may also be due to volume depletion. A rise in creatinine of over 25% and/or over 0.3mg/dl early after initiation of ACE-I is not associated with a loss of benefit with continued ACE-I therapy, and renal function largely recovers on follow-up; in fact, in one study, patients with early worsening of renal function appeared to derive the largest benefit from ACE-I.[74] If creatinine rises ≥50% or ≥0.5mg/dl, reduce other BP-lowering drugs, make sure the patient is not using NSAIDs, assess for excessive diuresis and consider reducing the dose of the diuretic in the absence of hypervolemia. Along with reducing other drugs and the diuretic if possible, hold the ACE-I for a few days to allow renal recovery then restart half the initial dose. Bilateral renal artery stenosis may need to be ruled out.

  Avoid starting ACE-I in clinically decompensated HF or acute renal failure, because ACE-I may acutely worsen kidney perfusion and the diuretic response. However, if the patient was already on an ACE-I before HF decompensation, the ACE-I is usually continued unless severe, acute renal failure is present.

- Hyperkalemia (>5mEq/l). If hyperkalemia occurs upon ACE-I initiation without a severe rise in creatinine, discontinue potassium supplements, then, if needed, reduce the dose of the aldosterone antagonist and the ACE-I.

---

*ACE-Is inhibit the conversion of angiotensin I to angiotensin II and increase kinin (and nitric oxide) availability; some angiotensin II is, however, still produced by myocardial chymase. ARBs block the harmful AT1 angiotensin II receptor, without affecting the potentially useful AT2 receptor, but ARBs do not increase the beneficial kinin. Despite this difference, the clinical effects of ACE-Is and ARBs are grossly the same, and the risks are the same, except for cough and angioedema with ACE-I (related to kinin).

Note that ACE-I therapy is beneficial even in patients with advanced baseline renal dysfunction and cardiorenal syndrome (up to a creatinine of 3.4 mg/dl in the CONSENSUS trial),[67] and in patients with mild degree of renal deterioration upon ACE-I initiation. Thus, an ACE-I or ARB should be given in these contexts.

4. Attempt titration every 5 days to the optimal dose used in randomized trials, which is approximately one-half of the maximal dose. In comparison with the low dose, the intermediate or high dose further reduces HF hospitalizations by 24% but does not significantly improve mortality and symptoms (ATLAS trial, where lisinopril 2.5–5 mg was compared with 30–40 mg). Thus, even if a high dose is not reached, it is expected that the low dose will lead to similar benefit on mortality and symptoms.[75]
Examples of doses:

- Lisinopril (ACE-I): start 5 mg Qday and try to reach 20–40 mg Qday. It is renally eliminated and the effect is doubled in patients with renal failure, wherein the starting dose may be 2.5 mg Qday.
- Enalapril (ACE-I): start 2.5 mg BID and reach 10 mg BID (also renally eliminated).
- Candesartan (ARB): 4 mg Qday; goal, 32 mg Qday.
- Valsartan (ARB): 40 mg BID; goal, 160 mg BID.

5. Significant, sometimes drastic, improvement of exercise duration (20–50%) and functional class is seen with ACE-I.[71] Symptomatic improvement may occur within 48 hours of ACE-I initiation, but is generally delayed weeks to months. Abrupt withdrawal of ACE-I can lead to clinical deterioration and should be avoided, except in decompensated HF with low output and hypotension, or severe deterioration of renal function.

6. In one trial, the addition of ARB (candesartan) to ACE-I in class II–III HF already receiving a β-blocker reduced both HF hospitalizations and cardiovascular death in comparison to ACE-I alone, without an effect on total mortality (CHARM-Added trial).[72] Yet in patients receiving ACE-I, preference should be given to adding an aldosterone antagonist rather than ARB, as an aldosterone antagonist is associated with a larger reduction of HF hospitalizations and cardiovascular death, and a striking reduction of total mortality. Because the triple combination ACE-I/ARB/aldosterone antagonist is contraindicated (risk of hyperkalemia), the role of the ARB/ACE-I combination is limited in HF.

B. β-Blockers

1. β-Blockers used to be contraindicated in HF, and in fact they may worsen HF initially, especially in the first 2–3 months after therapy initiation and/or up-titration. This is due to their initial negative inotropic effect. But when used over the long term, β-blockers:
- Improve contractility, EF (by 5–15%), and HF symptoms, and reduce mortality by 35–60% and HF hospitalizations by 40%.[76–78]
- Reverse the deleterious and apoptotic effects of catecholamines on the heart. The reduction in energy demands reduces apoptosis.
- Reverse remodeling and reduce cardiac chamber size by reducing LV wall stress.
- Prevent arrhythmias.

2. The three agents that have been shown to improve survival and outcomes in HF are:
- **a.** Long-acting metoprolol (metoprolol XL): metoprolol is a selective $β_1$-blocker, but loses selectivity with high doses > 100 mg. Long-acting metoprolol has a more sustained effect than regular metoprolol; this limits the daily fluctuations of the β-blocker effect and the β-blocker withdrawal effect that occurs between the doses of regular metoprolol.
  - Dose: Start 12.5 or 25 mg Qday and titrate to 200 mg Qday
- **b.** Carvedilol: carvedilol is a non-selective $β_1$-blocker, $β_2$-blocker, and $α_1$-blocker (vasodilatory effect), with additional antioxidant properties. Despite its α-blocker effect, it is as well tolerated as metoprolol in patients with borderline BP. The non-selective blockade of adrenergic receptors is advantageous. While metoprolol upregulates β-receptor density towards normal levels, carvedilol maintains a low density of these receptors. Moreover, selective $β_1$-blockade with metoprolol may enhance the ino- and chronotropic response to $β_2$-adrenergic stimulation, an untoward effect.[79] Thus, carvedilol is a more potent antiadrenergic agent than metoprolol, as manifested by the more significant blunting of heart rate response.[80] With its more comprehensive blockade of all adrenergic receptors, carvedilol improves myocardial function, EF, and cardiac hemodynamics such as stroke volume, PA pressure, and PCWP, more than other β-blockers and reverses remodeling more effectively.[79,80] Because of the α-blocking effect, carvedilol acts as a moderate vasodilator acutely, but with long-term treatment the vasodilator activity is no longer prominent, as tolerance to the α-blocking effect occurs. This transient α-blocker effect is useful, as it allows an early improvement in stroke volume and LV remodeling before the long-term effect of β-blockade kicks in.[81]
  - Dose: start 3.125 mg BID; titrate to the goal of 25 mg BID if patient's weight < 85 kg, 50 mg BID if weight > 85 kg.
  - A long-acting formulation of carvedilol, Coreg CR, is available. It is given once daily. Coreg CR 10 mg is equivalent to carvedilol 3.125 mg BID. Start Coreg CR 10 mg Qday and titrate up to 80 mg Qday.
- **c.** Bisoprolol, a selective $β_1$-blocker. Start 1.25 mg Qday; goal, 10 mg Qday.

3. Keys to β-blocker therapy:
- **a.** Start "low and slow." Patients have to be euvolemic and stable. During hospitalization for HF, low-dose β-blockade can be started before discharge, after the patient has stabilized.
- **b.** Contraindications: overt HF, SBP < 80 mmHg or symptomatic hypotension, bradyarrhythmia (bradycardia < 55 bpm, any second- or third-degree AV block, PR > 0.24 s), bronchospasm.
- **c.** *Double the dose every 2 weeks* and monitor for worsening of dyspnea, edema, weight gain, bradycardia, and hypotension. If the patient is off the β-blocker for over 1 week for any reason, or after an episode of cardiogenic shock, restart at the lowest dose and retitrate.

d. If *edema* increases or HF develops within a week of titration, increase the diuretic dose; if this is not effective, decrease the β-blocker dose and titrate more slowly.

In case of *severe fatigue*, decrease the dose of β-blocker (and sometimes the diuretic) or titrate more slowly. Most often, fatigue resolves spontaneously in a few weeks.

In case of *bradycardia* (symptomatic bradycardia < 55 bpm, asymptomatic bradycardia < 50 bpm, or AV block), try to decrease the dosage of digoxin and amiodarone first, then, if needed, reduce the β-blocker.

> Patients with severe systolic HF can tolerate SBP of 80–90 mmHg, and doses of medications should not be decreased unless the patient is symptomatic (dizzy, severe fatigue) or has signs of low perfusion, in which case the medications should be started at lower doses and titrated slowly, hypovolemia corrected (↑ BUN), the timing of ACE-I and β-blocker staggered, and the diuretic dose reduced if possible. A spontaneously low SBP (<100 mmHg) is, per se, an adverse prognostic factor; however, it does not limit the benefit and tolerability of β-blockers, ACE-Is/ARBs, or hydralazine–nitrate.[82–84] A substudy of the COPERNICUS trial showed that HF patients with chronic SBP < 95 mmHg derived the same benefit from carvedilol as patients with higher SBP, and did not have a significant drop of SBP with carvedilol; in fact, SBP increased over time above baseline, as a result of the increased cardiac output.[84] A similar phenomenon was seen with candesartan in CHARM, valsartan in ValHeft, and hydralazine–nitrate in A-Heft. *In fact, those drugs reduce BP in patients with HTN, but increase BP in patients with severe HF and low BP.*

e. It is not necessary to reach an optimal dose of an ACE-I before starting a β-blocker. In fact, it is preferred to start low doses of both and titrate up in an alternating fashion. The combination of a low β-blocker dose and a low ACE-I dose produces a greater symptomatic improvement and mortality reduction than an increase in the ACE-I dose.

Order of therapy: start low-dose ACE-I (lisinopril ~5 mg), then start low-dose β-blocker and titrate β-blocker every 2 weeks. After reaching the maximally tolerated dose of β-blocker, and if it is possible from the blood pressure and renal standpoints, start up-titrating the ACE-I at 1-week intervals.

f. If the patient has been on a β-blocker for more than a few weeks and is hospitalized with HF decompensation, the β-blocker should not generally be withheld. In low-output HF decompensation with borderline BP, the β-blocker dosage may be reduced. In full-blown shock, the β-blocker is withheld. Discontinuation of β-blocker therapy is independently associated with increased short- and long-term mortality and should be avoided if possible.[85] If interrupted, β-blocker is restarted at the lowest dose after the patient stabilizes, before hospital discharge, then retitrated.

> Try to reach the high target doses and the high degrees of β-blockade that are proven to be beneficial. In the only trial comparing various doses of β-blockers in HF, carvedilol showed a survival benefit that started at 6.25 mg BID and further increased at a dose of 25 mg BID.[86] Also, LVEF further improved with the high dose. A post-hoc analysis of a metoprolol XL trial showed that doses of 25–100 mg achieved the same mortality reduction as doses > 100 mg, and a post-hoc analysis of a bisoprolol trial showed similar mortality reduction with low vs. medium or high doses.[87,88]

g. ***Should β-blockers be titrated to achieve a specific target heart rate (HR)?*** The improvement in outcomes with β-blocker therapy is incremental and is related to the following two factors, in order of importance: (1) dose achieved; (2) HR achieved and HR reduction.[89,90] The HR achieved with β-blocker therapy is multifactorial and depends on the overall HF severity and catecholamine level, rather than just the degree of β-blockade. A more severe or decompensated HF is associated with a higher HR. Therefore, β-blockers are not titrated to achieve a specific target HR, although a low HR (~60–70 bpm) is desirable, is associated with a reduced mortality, and implies better HF control through both β-blockade and adjunctive HF therapy. Part of the reason metoprolol XL achieved similar benefit at low and high doses is the similar HR achieved with both doses in the trial (patients in the low-dose group may have been less sick and more readily achieved optimal HR). ***Either a high β-blocker dose or a low HR (<70 bpm) should at least be achieved***. Even if HR remains > 70 bpm, the mortality is low when a high dose of β-blocker is reached.[89]

While a high HR is essentially secondary to HF, it may also, by itself, perpetuate systolic HF through perpetuating myocardial ischemia. A trial of a pure sinus node blocker (ivabradine) showed that pure HR reduction was associated with reduced HF hospitalizations, confirming a direct role of HR in the pathophysiology of systolic HF.[91]

C. Aldosterone receptor antagonists (spironolactone, eplerenone)

1. The high aldosterone levels seen in HF not only induce renal sodium retention but directly act on the myocardial and arterial aldosterone receptors, leading to myocardial and arterial remodeling and fibrosis and baroreceptor dysfunction. In fact, the small doses of aldosterone antagonists studied in HF only have a mild or no diuretic effect (RALES trial).[92] The benefit in HF mainly results from: (i) blockade of the myocardial aldosterone receptors; (ii) increase in potassium (antiarrythmic effect); (iii) reduction of the tubular resistance to loop diuretics.[93] Aldosterone antagonists reduce HF mortality by 30%, HF hospitalization by 30–40%, and improve NYHA functional class (RALES trial).[92,94,95]

Aldosterone acts at the DNA level and induces the genomic synthesis of Na tubular channels and Na/K pumps that absorb sodium and secrete potassium. The aldosterone receptor blockers inhibit this synthesis rather than directly block Na/K pumps, and therefore *have a slow onset of action of 2–3 days and a slow offset (3–4 days), similar to aldosterone and other steroids.*

2. An aldosterone receptor antagonist is indicated in chronic HF with EF≤35% and NYHA classes III–IV.[92] More recently, aldosterone antagonist therapy has reduced mortality in class II systolic HF (EF≤35%) with elevated BNP or recent cardiovascular hospitalization in the last 6 months, and is now recommended for these patients (class I recommendation).[94]

It is also indicated after a recent ACS (within 30 days) when EF is<40% and any degree of clinical HF or diabetes is present.[95]

3. Contraindications: creatinine>2 mg/dl or GFR<30 ml/min; K>5 mEq/l. In the RALES trial, patients with mild renal failure (GFR 30–60 ml/min) had a higher risk of worsening renal function and hyperkalemia with spironolactone in comparison to those with normal renal function, but derived the largest absolute mortality reduction. Thus, patients with mild renal failure are appropriate candidates for this therapy if well monitored.[96]

4. Dosage of spironolactone: 12.5–25.0 mg daily; careful up-titration to 37.5–50.0 mg daily may be tried in patients with refractory HF or persistent hypokalemia. If gynecomastia develops, eplerenone may be used instead of spironolactone. Potassium and creatinine should be checked within 3 days and again at 1 week after therapy initiation, then Q2–4wk for the next 3 months. Typically, all potassium supplements need to be stopped at the initiation of the aldosterone antagonist; a minority of patients will continue to require a potassium supplement, but this is restarted only after blood testing. In real-world registries, hyperkalemia is common with aldosterone antagonists (up to 20%), therefore justifying careful K monitoring. In fact, these agents should be avoided if K monitoring is not possible (compliance issues), and the patient should be instructed about interruption of therapy should diarrhea or dehydration occur (renal failure).

5. RAAS activation leads to a marked elevation of aldosterone levels in both HF and cirrhosis with ascites, exaggerated by the fact that aldosterone catabolism, a hepatic process, is impaired. In cirrhosis, a high dose of spironolactone (100–400 mg), higher than the one studied in HF, has been shown to induce more natriuresis than a loop diuretic. In fact, the avid distal sodium reabsorption induced by hyperaldosteronism makes loop diuretics ineffective in 50% of cirrhotic patients.[97] This high dose has not been largely studied in HF because of the combined therapy with ACE-I, but illustrates the potential value of spironolactone in patients with combined heart and liver failure and the possible role of higher spironolactone doses in patients resistant to loop diuretics.[97]

D. Neprilysin inhibitor combined with ARB (sacubitril–valsartan combination)

Neprilysin is a peptidase that degrades natriuretic peptides, bradykinin, and adromedullin. Neprilysin inhibition increases the level of these substances, counteracting vasoconstriction, sodium retention, and LV remodeling. In fact, natriuretic peptides reduce cellular proliferation in the heart and kidneys. In a trial of patients with systolic HF, NYHA II–IV, and BNP>150 or a prior HF hospitalization in the last year, neprilisyn inhibitor+valsartan (combined in one molecule, not just one pill) reduced the 2-year mortality by ~3% in comparison with ACE-I (relative risk reduction 16%).[98] Hospitalization for HF was also reduced by ~3%. Neprilyin inhibitor+valsartan was associated with less renal dysfunction and hyperkalemia than ACE-I, but more symptomatic hypotension. This benefit was seen despite a background therapy that included β-blockers and aldosterone antagonists (PARADIGM-HF trial). Most patients had class II symptoms, and the benefit was seen in stable and relatively low-risk patients, which argues that *even early-stage HF patients who are stable on ACE-I are better switched to this therapy*; the indication is more compelling in patients with recent HF hospitalization or elevated BNP. In order to prevent angioedema, the recommended washout period between an ACE inhibitor and sacubitril–valsartan is 36 hours. A prior history of angioedema with ACE-I contraindicates the use of sacubristil–valsartan, but a prior history of cough is not a contraindication.

Of note, neprilysin inhibitor is the only HF therapy that increases BNP, a consequence of its direct effect. This affects the diagnostic value of BNP, at least during therapy initiation, but BNP remains useful for monitoring in respect to the new baseline. Conversely, NT-pro-BNP is not directly affected.

E. Hydralazine–nitrate combination

In the *V-HeFT-I trial*, the hydralazine–nitrate combination reduced mortality by 34% in comparison to placebo or α-blocker therapy; this was the first trial ever to show a mortality reduction with vasodilator therapy in HF.[99] The mortality reduction was mainly driven by the benefit in black patients. In the *V-HeFT-II trial* of hydralazine–nitrate vs. ACE-I, the hydralazine–nitrate combination reduced mortality as much as ACE-I in black patients, and was superior to enalapril in terms of exercise tolerance and EF improvement.[100–102] The hydralazine–nitrate combination was also beneficial in white patients, in whom it was superior to enalapril in terms of exercise tolerance and EF improvement, although the mortality was lower with enalapril. The reduction in hospitalization with hydralazine–nitrate was similar to enalapril and similar between white and black patients.[102] In the *A-HeFT trial* of class III–IV black patients already receiving ACE-I and β-blocker therapy, the hydralazine–nitrate combination therapy strikingly reduced mortality by an additional 43% and reduced HF hospitalizations by 40%.[103]

Therefore, the combination is indicated as an additional therapy to ACE-I/ARB and β-blocker in black patients with a functional class III–IV (class I recommendation). It may be considered in non-black patients with persistent symptoms or persistent HTN (>140/90 mmHg); nitrates, per se, may be used for decongestion and symptom relief in all races (CHAMPION trial algorithm). The combination may also be used *instead* of ACE-I or ARB in case of intolerance to ACE-I/ARB, i.e., renal failure occurs with ACE-I/ARB and does not improve by reducing the dose of furosemide, or hyperkalemia occurs with ACE-I/ARB and does not improve with potassium restriction (class IIa recommendation regardless of race).

The benefit is partly related to the afterload and preload reduction. More importantly, nitrates increase the local production of nitric oxide (NO), while hydralazine prevents the oxidation of NO through its antioxidant properties, allowing to maintain the NO effect. ACE-I also prevents NO oxidation and may be beneficial in combination with nitrates. NO promotes endothelial and vascular homeostasis and appropriate myocardial remodeling and contractility, which improves EF by up to 5%. Hydralazine–nitrate combination may also directly reduce pulmonary vascular resistance in patients with left HF-associated pulmonary hypertension. Black patients frequently have a defective genetic variant of NO synthase that may explain the particular benefit; many white patients also have this variant, and thus pharmacogenomics rather than race may guide hydralazine–nitrate therapy in the future.

Dosing: start hydralazine 12.5 mg TID, increase it to 25 mg TID in 2–4 days, then increase by 25 mg/dose Qweek. Target is ~50–75 mg TID (may reduce to BID in renal failure). Start isosorbide dinitrate 20 mg TID and titrate up to 40 mg TID.

BiDil is a pill that combines 37.5 mg of hydralazine and 20 mg of isosorbide dinitrate (ISDN); BiDil may be started at one-half pill TID and titrated up to two pills TID.

VI. Drugs that improve symptoms and morbidity
A. Diuretics

- *Overview and effect of disease states.* Thiazide diuretics are weak diuretics that work on the distal tubule, where ~3–5% of sodium is reabsorbed, and are mainly used in chronic HTN rather than HF. Loop diuretics (furosemide, bumetanide, torsemide) work on the ascending loop of Henle, where ~25% of sodium is reabsorbed, and are often the mainstay diuretic therapy in HF. Both loop and thiazide diuretics are secreted by the proximal tubule into the lumen and work from the luminal side of the nephron.

  In HF and renal failure with reduced renal blood flow, less diuretic reaches the kidneys and gets secreted into the lumen, implying the need for *higher doses*. Moreover, the reduced amount of renally filtered sodium reduces the total amount of sodium that can be eliminated with every single diuretic dose, implying the need for more *frequent administration*.[104]

  All diuretics are highly bound to albumin, which traps them and delivers them to the secretory site of the nephron. In very low albumin states (<2 g/dl), some of the diuretic is lost in the extravascular space, and in nephrotic syndrome, even the diuretic that gets to the nephron's lumen is bound to the urinary albumin, preventing it from acting on the sodium pump.

- *Renal failure and diuretics (especially thiazide).* In patients with GFR < 30 ml/min, less sodium is filtered overall. Thus, less sodium can be eliminated by any diuretic (especially a thiazide diuretic), particularly because each of the remaining nephrons is already maximizing its sodium elimination. Hence, thiazide diuretics are less effective in patients with advanced renal failure, but, contrary to common belief, remain effective after cumulative dosing or in combination with a loop diuretic that increases the salt delivery to the distal tubule.[105,106] Metolazone, a thiazide-like diuretic that also works on the proximal tubule, maintains its efficacy in advanced renal failure; it also has a prolonged duration of action (~1 week). All thiazide diuretics are renally eliminated and have a long half-life, and thus cumulate in renal failure (not just metolazone), which further potentiates their effect after multiple dosing. Some data suggest that thiazide monotherapy is effective in hypertensive patients with advanced CKD after multiple dosing.[105,106]

- *Diuretic threshold.* A diuretic dose is only effective if it exceeds the required threshold at the tubular level. This threshold varies between individuals and diseases. Once the threshold is exceeded, there is a point at which maximal natriuresis is achieved, and beyond which no further natriuresis is gained with higher doses.[104]

For a normal patient, the threshold IV dose of furosemide may be 10 mg, while the maximum effective dose is 40 mg. For a patient with HF, where both the diuretic delivery is reduced (reduced renal flow) and nephron responsiveness is reduced, the IV threshold may be 20–40 mg, and the oral threshold 40 mg. In the latter scenario, the administration of 20 mg BID does not achieve any diuresis in comparison to 40 mg Qday. On the other hand, if 40 mg Qday is effective (i.e., urination > 500 ml after the dose) but does not maintain euvolemia, 40 mg BID is a better strategy than 80 mg Qday. Patients with *HF have a reduced maximal response to any single dose*, and therefore, once the threshold is identified, they are best managed by giving this threshold dose more frequently rather than giving larger doses, allowing a larger and more sustained diuresis (Figure 4.7). With IV furosemide, urine output is assessed 30–60 minutes after dose administration; with oral furosemide, the effect is seen 1–2 hours later (slower with severe edema).

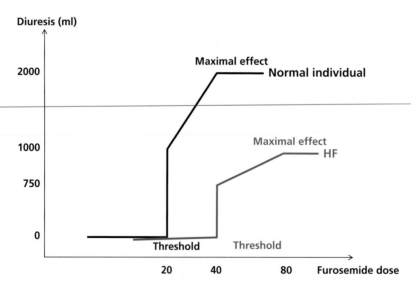

Figure 4.7 Diuretic response in a normal individual and in HF. Note that no diuretic response occurs before achieving the threshold dose. The threshold is higher in HF and the diuresis achieved with the threshold dose is lower in HF than in normal individuals. Also, the difference between the threshold and the maximal effect is narrow in HF, suggesting the value of frequent dosing, rather than higher dosing, to increase the overall efficacy. *Figure inspired by reference 104.*

- *Pharmacokinetics of loop diuretics.*[104] Approximately 50% of oral furosemide is absorbed, with a high intra- and inter-individual variation (10–90%). Thus, in general, the effective oral dose of furosemide is numerically twice the intravenous dose. Bumetanide and torsemide are more consistently and thoroughly absorbed (80–100%). With all these agents, the absorption may be slowed and reduced by the intestinal edema or the poor intestinal flow, requiring higher doses or an intravenous course of therapy before oral dosing is effective again.

  The duration of action is short (~4–6 h) and the nephron may avidly retain sodium between doses, which shows the importance of splitting the dose when a high total daily dose is required. Torsemide is 2–3 times longer acting (~12 hours), has better oral bioavailability than furosemide, has a hepatic metabolism, and is given once daily. It may be considered in patients with erratic diuretic effect or those with refractory fluid retention. While torsemide and bumetanide are metabolized by the liver, furosemide is partly inactivated by renal metabolism; thus, in renal failure, the elimination of furosemide is delayed, which prolongs its action and narrows its dose equivalence to the other two agents.

  Bumetanide dose equivalent: 1 mg = 40 mg of furosemide (or 20 mg in advanced renal failure); torsemide dose equivalent: 20 mg = 40 mg furosemide.

- Practical use of oral loop diuretics:
  - Use the lowest chronic oral dose to maintain euvolemia: furosemide 20 mg once daily, up to 40–80 mg 2–3 times daily. If the patient has a diuretic response to 40 mg of furosemide and is requiring a total of 80 mg per day, it is better to give 40 mg BID than 80 mg Qday to provide a more sustained diuretic effect and less metabolic perturbations.
  - The patient needs to take extra dose(s) if weight increases > 3–4 lb in < 5 days. He needs to continue taking an extra dose of diuretic daily until the weight returns to baseline. If in 1–2 days, the weight continues to rise, a clinic visit is immediately warranted.
  - Patients with mild HF receiving a small dose of furosemide may be switched to chlorthalidone. On the other hand, patients with severe HF requiring high chronic doses of furosemide (>200 mg/d) may be supplemented with a biweekly or triweekly dose of chlorthalidone or metolazone.
  - Oral potassium (~20–40 mEq per day) may need to be supplemented, particularly if the patient is not receiving an aldosterone antagonist. K goal in HF is ≥ 4 mEq/l. *Patients requiring high doses of potassium are often magnesium-deficient and should receive magnesium supplementation.*

> *In acutely decompensated HF, a rise in BUN and creatinine with diuretic therapy is often related to worsening HF and does not imply over-diuresis*, as most of these patients remain volume overloaded; diuresis should be maintained until euvolemia is achieved. *However, in the chronic, stable setting, a rise in BUN and creatinine usually implies excessive volume contraction*, and a reduction of the diuretic dose is often needed, unless signs of fluid retention are present.[107] Chronic high doses of furosemide (>160 mg/day) may be needed in advanced HF and may even be associated with a mortality reduction on adjusted analysis, as long as BUN is not increased.[107] In fact, one study of stable HF suggests that diuretic therapy favorably affects markers of tubular function.[108]

B. Digoxin

Digoxin has the unique property of combining a mildly positive inotropic action with a negative chronotropic action, making it the only positive inotrope that does not increase mortality. Digoxin inhibits the sarcolemmal Na/K-ATPase, which increases intracellular Na and subsequently increases the intracellular Ca through the Ca/Na sarcoplasmic passive exchange, leading to an inotropic effect. Digoxin also increases the vagal tone, which counteracts some of the catecholaminergic hyperactivity in HF, reduces HR, increases HR variability, and achieves some vasodilatation. This *neurohormonal modulation* is achieved at low levels of digoxin and actually explains most of the digoxin's benefits in HF and the rate control in AF.[109,110] EF improves with digoxin, including low-dose digoxin (up to 5%).[110]

The inotropic action of digoxin becomes stronger and begins to offset the therapeutic benefits provided by neurohormonal modulation at moderate and high serum digoxin levels, possibly explaining the increased mortality with higher levels.[109] Higher doses may further improve EF and contractility parameters without further symptomatic or rate improvement.[111] In addition, some believe that high digoxin levels have fewer neurohormonal effects than low levels.

Digoxin is indicated in HF that is still symptomatic despite all of the above medications (class IIa indication). In the DIG trial of patients with HF and sinus rhythm, the addition of digoxin to standard therapy reduced pump failure death but was offset by an increased risk of arrhythmic death, making it neutral on mortality. Digoxin was overall beneficial and reduced HF hospitalizations by ~30%, particularly in the more severe cases (EF < 25%, class III or IV).[112] Women had more hazard with digoxin, probably because of higher serum digoxin levels.

In a patient with *HF and AF*, digoxin is added as a second-line agent when β-blockers do not achieve appropriate rate control.

Once a patient is on digoxin, the withdrawal of digoxin worsens HF and increases HF hospitalizations. Therefore, once digoxin is started, it should not be withdrawn unless toxicity occurs.[113]

Dosing: 0.125 mg daily in the majority of patients, particularly small patients, women, old patients > 70, and patients with renal failure. Digoxin level monitoring should be performed in the latter patients, and every-other-day dosing considered. A dose of 0.25 mg daily may be used in young, large men with normal renal function. Loading doses are not necessary; loading is used for supraventricular arrhythmias rather than HF.

Digoxin level monitoring is encouraged in all patients, once steady state is achieved (~2 weeks after digoxin initiation). This is even more important in cases of renal failure, female sex, drug interactions, or suspicion of toxicity. The goal trough level is ≤ 0.8 ng/ml (serum level is checked at least 6 hours after the last dose). *Trough levels of 0.5–0.8 ng/ml were associated with a lower mortality than placebo in the DIG trial;* trough levels > 1.1 ng/ml were associated with a higher mortality than placebo.[109] In addition, a dosing study has shown that all of the hemodynamic, EF, and autonomic improvement with digoxin is seen at the lower dose (0.125 mg/day) and lower concentrations, without further improvement with higher doses.[110] *This reflects the importance of neurohormonal modulation over further inotropic activity.*

Signs of toxicity:

- Bradyarrhythmias, tachyarrhythmias (atrial tachycardia with block, non-paroxysmal junctional tachycardia, and VT, including the characteristic bidirectional VT)
- Nausea and vomiting, visual scotomas or halos, neurologic changes

Digoxin toxicity is usually seen with levels > 1.5–1.8 ng/ml, but may be seen at lower levels, particularly over the long term or when hypokalemia coexists. Digoxin half-life is ~36 hours, so digoxin effects are expected to last ~4 days after discontinuation. Digoxin Fab antibodies (DigiFab) are indicated for bradyarrhythmias or tachyarrhythmias associated with hemodynamic instability.*

C. Ivabradine

Ivabradine is a pure heart rate reducer (sinus node inhibitor). In the SHIFT trial of patients with class II–IV systolic HF (EF ≤ 35%), prior HF hospitalization in the last year, and sinus rate ≥ 70 bpm despite maximally tolerated dose of β-blockers, ivabradine reduced HF hospitalizations and HF death by 26%.[91] This benefit is consistent among patients with severe class IV HF. Being a sinus node blocker, this drug has no role in patients with AF. See discussion under *Chronic treatment of heart failure*, Section 1.V.B, last paragraph.

VII. Devices

A. ICD

Fifty percent of patients with HF die of VT or VF. The remaining 50% of patients die of end-stage, low-output HF. Late MI contributes to 30–50% of both types of mortality in ischemic HF.[114] Sudden death is less common in absolute value, but more common in relative value, in mild class II HF than severe class IV HF.

An ICD is indicated as a secondary prevention measure if the patient has a history of sustained VT. It is indicated as a primary prevention measure in ischemic or non-ischemic cardiomyopathy with a low EF (≤ 35%) that is persistent over time despite optimal medical therapy, a functional class of II or III, and an expected survival of over 1 year. Patients with functional class I qualify for ICD in ischemic cardiomyopathy with EF < 30%:[115]

- Wait > 40 days after an MI.
- Wait > 3 months after revascularization for chronic ischemia.
- Wait 3–6 months in non-ischemic cardiomyopathy, to ensure that it is not reversible and that it persists after a few months of medical therapy and BP control. Three to six months of waiting are reasonable but are not necessary according to the ACC guidelines.

Patients with functional class IV do not have an indication for ICD because of their high mortality. While they have a higher risk of VT/VF than other functional classes, they also have a much higher risk of death from pump failure; ICD simply converts their mode of death from VT to pump failure. If class IV patients are ambulatory and have an indication for BiV pacemaker, the combo BiV/ICD is indicated and improves their mortality as well as their quality of life.

B. Biventricular (BiV) pacemaker = cardiac resynchronization therapy (CRT)

Approximately 20–30% of HF patients have QRS > 120 ms, mostly LBBB (80%). This leads to dyssynchronous contraction of the LV, which means that different LV segments contract at different times (intraventricular dyssynchrony), and the LV and RV contract at different times (interventricular dyssynchrony), leading to an ineffective ventricular effort and dyssynchronous mitral leaflets movement (→ MR). A prolonged QRS independently correlates with increased mortality and symptoms. CRT paces LV and RV at approximately the same time, and restores the delayed lateral LV contraction.

BiV is indicated in patients with EF ≤ 35% + QRS ≥ 150 ms (mainly LBBB morphology or RV-paced rhythm) + functional class II, III, or ambulatory IV despite an adequate medical regimen, whether they are in sinus rhythm or AF. These same patients have an indication for a BiV/ICD combined device. Patients with LBBB but a QRS 130–150 ms, or RBBB with a QRS > 150 ms, have a class IIa indication for BiV.

Thirty percent of patients do not respond to CRT, i.e., do not achieve reverse remodeling on echo, for the following reasons:

- Wide QRS does not always mean dyssynchrony. The wider the QRS (i.e., QRS > 150 ms), the more likely a response is seen. Echocardiographic dyssynchrony features help select patients whose QRS is 130–150 ms, according to the CARE HF trial.[116]
- Ischemic cardiomyopathy with large infarcts is poorly responsive to CRT. Irreversible scars respond less well to CRT than non-ischemic cardiomyopathy.
- LV lead placement may not be optimal (apex rather than the basal lateral wall).
- Patients with a pure RBBB are less likely to respond to CRT, especially if the RV is the main side that is dyssynchronous and delayed. RBBB, per se, is associated with at least the same negative prognosis as LBBB, but is less responsive to CRT;[117] this partly explains why, in CRT registries, RBBB is associated with a higher mortality than LBBB. Patients who, in addition to RBBB, have LV dyssynchrony and slow left bundle conduction may respond to CRT (RBBB would be wider than 150 ms, or echocardiographic features of LV dyssynchrony would be present).

---

*Dose of DigiFab in chronic toxicity: number of vials = digoxin level (ng/mL) × weight (kg)/100 (e.g., a 50 kg patient with a digoxin level of 3 ng/ml would be given 1.5 vials). DigiFab binds to digoxin and then is slowly excreted by the kidneys (half-life 15–20 hours, more prolonged with renal failure). After DigiFab administration, the serum digoxin level remains high or higher for several days and is no longer meaningful. Monitor for hypokalemia with DigiFab treatment.

- Echocardiographic evaluation of dyssynchrony is likely helpful in selecting patients with QRS 130–150 ms and those with RBBB. Conversely, it is not helpful for QRS <130 ms. Approximately 30% of HF patients with QRS <130 ms have dyssynchrony on echo; however, CRT is not beneficial in these patients.[118]

CRT improves survival, symptoms, and EF. It decreases LV systolic size (= reverse remodeling) and reduces functional MR (the two leaflets coapt at the same time when all segments contract simultaneously). CRT improves diastolic function as it reduces systolic time, thus increasing the diastolic filling time. It leads to immediate improvement of symptoms, then reverse remodeling within months.

BiV pacing is mainly validated in patients who are in sinus rhythm. Data show that AF patients with EF≤35% and wide QRS benefit from BiV pacing to the same extent as patients in sinus rhythm. However, patients with AF need to have aggressive rate control to guarantee continuous BiV pacing instead of spontaneous QRS conduction (this may include, if necessary, AV nodal ablation followed by BiV pacing).[119]

Approximately 5–10% of patients with HF and low EF (≤35%) develop bradyarrhythmias that mandate PM placement for rhythm rather than heart failure purposes. In the case of AV block requiring frequent ventricular pacing, the implantation of a BiV PM rather than a RV PM is the best option,[119] and is given a class IIa recommendation in the guidelines regardless of the functional class.
   Both ICD and BiV devices improve survival.

VIII. Other therapeutic measures

A. Salt restriction (<2–3 g/day). Fluid restriction to 1.5–2 liters/day is necessary in advanced HF, decompensated HF, or hyponatremia.[36]

B. Exercise training in stable HF. Exercise training improves vascular function, muscular O_2 extraction, and symptoms.

C. Avoidance of harmful medications such as NSAIDs, non-dihydropyridines (negative inotropic effect), glitazones, and anti-TNF-α drugs. Dihydropyridines are not indicated for HF per se, but are not contraindicated either, with the exception of nifedipine, which has a mild negative inotropic effect; they have been shown to be safe in HF (amlodipine, felodipine) and may be used in combination with ACE-I/β-blocker for HTN or angina control, if needed.

D. Warfarin is indicated for patients with AF, LV thrombus, or a history of stroke or transient ischemic attack in the context of severe LV dysfunction. Aspirin is indicated for ischemic cardiomyopathy. Aspirin's benefit is uncertain in HF patients without CAD, and it may counteract some of the benefit of ACE-Is.
   Two trials have addressed the use of aspirin vs. warfarin in patients with severe ischemic or non-ischemic LV dysfunction and sinus rhythm (EF<35%) (WATCH and WARCEF trials).[120,121] In both trials, the yearly risk of ischemic stroke on aspirin therapy was low (~1.3%), and while it was significantly reduced in half with warfarin, intracranial and major hemorrhage increased. As a result, the overall risk of death/MI/stroke was not different between groups. This lack of benefit of warfarin is mainly due to the low stroke risk of stable HF patients who are in sinus rhythm.

E. Omega-3 fatty acids. Omega-3 fatty acids, at a small dose of 1 g/day, have been shown to slightly reduce mortality in class II–IV HF with any EF, in the GISSI-HF trial (class IIa recommendation).[122]

F. 25% of HF patients have obstructive sleep apnea. Treatment with CPAP and nocturnal oxygen improves LVEF (by 8% in one study). It also improves LV diastolic function, RV function, and functional capacity.[123]

   Up to 35% of HF patients, especially patients with more advanced HF, have central sleep apnea (Cheyne-Stokes). It is treated with nocturnal O_2, which leads to symptomatic improvement.

G. Iron therapy. Iron deficiency is highly prevalent in HF, affecting ~40% of patients, including ~30% of patients without anemia. Iron deficiency impairs myocardial and musculoskeletal metabolism, even in the absence of anemia. In HF, higher cutoffs of ferritin are used to define iron deficiency, as some iron is misused and blocked in the reticuloendothelial system (ferritin<100, or 100–300 with iron saturation<20%). In two HF trials, intravenous iron therapy improved walking distance and NYHA class and reduced HF hospitalizations (CONFIRM-HF trial). Conversely, erythropoietin therapy did not provide any benefit.

IX. Prognosis

The average yearly mortality of patients with class II or III HF is ~6–10%. Half of deaths are sudden deaths, the other half are pump failure deaths. MI contributes to 30–50% of each death modality in ischemic HF. The sudden death is less common in absolute value, but more common in relative value, in class II HF than class IV HF. Several factors negatively affect prognosis in HF patients:[124]

- Severely decreased EF (<30%).
- Refractory functional class III.B or IV: 1-year mortality 30–50%.
- Hospitalization for decompensated HF is associated with a high mortality, especially in the first few months after hospitalization (4- to 10-fold higher mortality). The risk progressively decreases throughout the ensuing 12 months, but does not reach the level of risk of the patient without HF hospitalization. The risk further increases with the number of HF hospitalizations in the last year (up to 10-fold).[125]
- Low-output profile, i.e., renal failure, poor response to diuretics, hypotension, resting tachycardia, cachexia, hyponatremia<133 mmol/l, anemia of HF with Hb<12 g/dl.
- Borderline BP<100 mmHg with inability to tolerate ACE-I and/or β-blocker therapy, or a need to discontinue them in hypotensive, low-output states with frequent episodes of renal deterioration.

- Low peak oxygen consumption on exercise testing (<14 ml/min/kg).
- Mortality of ischemic HF is approximately 1.5–2 times that of non-ischemic HF.[8,9]
- Right ventricular failure in addition to left ventricular failure.
- Enlarged LV size/volume is a powerful negative prognostic indicator and a reflection of negative LV remodeling and HF decompensation. Current therapies (ACE-I, β-blockers, spironolactone, BiV pacing) decrease LV size and remodeling.
- Severe functional MR and AF.
- Baseline renal failure (including cardiorenal syndrome, as described under *Acute heart failure*, Section IV) and renal failure upon hospital discharge are strong mortality predictors.

2. TREATMENT OF HFPEF

HFpEF is epidemiologically characterized by an older age, less underlying CAD, and more HTN, AF, and female sex than systolic HF. While two epidemiologic studies have suggested that the long-term mortality of HFpEF approximates that of systolic HF,[126,127] a recent meta-analysis has shown that the yearly mortality of HFpEF is lower than the mortality of systolic HF (~30% lower), particularly cardiovascular mortality.[16] Overall, however, the mortality in HFpEF is high, and this is partly explained by the old age and the non-cardiac comorbidities of HFpEF, which lead to a relatively high non-cardiac mortality. Furthermore, in contrast to systolic HF, no specific therapy improves survival in HFpEF.

In fact, in HFpEF, the mode of death is cardiovascular in 60% of patients.[128] Only 15% of deaths are due to HF, while 27% are sudden deaths and 5% are MI deaths. This is in contrast to systolic HF, where cardiac death (sudden or HF) accounts for 85% of the deaths. Patients with HFpEF may develop ischemia secondary to increased LVEDP, LVH, and demand/supply mismatch, as well as the underlying CAD, which explains arrhythmia and sudden death. Sudden death may also be related to the scattered increase in collagen and myocardial fibrosis seen with HFpEF. Thus, patients with HFpEF are at increased risk of sudden death, albeit less than patients with systolic HF (the more prevalent CAD, myocardial distension, and scarring contribute to the higher rate of arrhythmias in systolic HF).[128] Currently, there is no indication for ICD therapy in HFpEF per se.

Both types of HF are associated with the same yearly risk of rehospitalization for HF.[126]

> Unlike systolic HF, no drug has been shown to improve survival in HFpEF per se, and thus no drug is specifically indicated to improve survival in HFpEF. The only treatment that improves outcomes is the aggressive treatment of the underlying disease (HTN, CAD).

A. Treatment of HTN to ≤ 140/90 (ESC HTN guidelines)

Afterload reduction has lusitropic effects and improves the LV pressure–volume relationship. In addition, vasodilator therapy with ACE-I or CCB improves arterial compliance, the impairment of which being a cornerstone of HFpEF and exertional HTN.[129]

Afterload reduction also improves stroke volume. However, excessive afterload reduction may not be as well tolerated in diastolic HF as in systolic HF. ***Vasodilators are less likely to increase stroke volume and more likely to reduce BP in patients with diastolic HF than systolic HF, and thus vasodilators may not be tolerated in diastolic HF with normal or low-normal BP.***[130] A borderline BP (e.g., SBP 100 mmHg) is less tolerated in diastolic HF than systolic HF (see Chapter 5, Section 3).

B. Decongestion and diuretics

Patients with decompensated HFpEF and peripheral edema usually tolerate high doses of diuretics. However, in light of the steep pressure–volume relationship, a high PCWP may be seen despite a normal LV volume, i.e., an LV volume that is necessary to maintain cardiac output. This is the preload dependency of severe diastolic failure. Therefore, diuretics are more likely to reduce cardiac output in these patients than in systolic HF, and chronically, only a small diuretic dose is advised.

Long-acting nitrate may also be considered as an additional decongestive measure, particularly in patients who appear euvolemic on exam. Yet, in a recent trial, nitrate did not improve exercise capacity in stable patients with HFpEF, most of whom had normal NT-pro-BNP.

> HFpEF requires afterload reduction to improve relaxation and cardiac output, and preload reduction to reduce congestion, but the therapeutic window is narrower than in systolic HF

C. Rate or rhythm control of tachyarrhythmias, especially in the chronic setting

A rhythm-control strategy may be considered chronically when the patient remains symptomatic from the arrhythmia or from HFpEF despite rate control, provided that long-term maintenance of sinus rhythm can be expected.

D. Revascularization of CAD that is extensive enough to contribute to HF

In HFpEF, revascularization has been associated with mortality reduction and prevention of EF deterioration.[131]

E. β-Blockers or non-DHP calcium channel blockers

Acute use – As explained in Figure 4.2, slowing the heart rate does not improve diastolic filling in decompensated HF, where the diastolic filling is brief and limited and cannot be improved by prolonging diastole. Therefore, these drugs are not helpful in the acute setting. However, as opposed to acute systolic HF, these drugs can be used when a fast tachyarrhythmia (>110–120 bpm) dictates acute rate control. They can also be used acutely in patients with hyperdynamic LV and LVOT obstruction.

Chronically, once LV filling pressures are reduced, these drugs may be used to prolong and improve diastolic filling, especially in patients whose heart rate is > 80 bpm. However, it is unclear whether this theoretical mechanism translates into any symptomatic relief in HFpEF. To the contrary, β-blockers may worsen symptoms in the subset of patients with chronotropic incompetence (~50% of HFpEF), or patients with a small and stiff cavity and limited preload reserve, whose cardiac output totally depends on heart rate. In fact, *pure heart rate slowing with ivabradine worsens exercise capacity in HFpEF* (Circulation 2015; 132:1719), and most data suggest that β-blockers do not improve outcomes in HFpEF.

Only a cardioselective β-blocker with vasodilatory effect, nebivolol, has been shown to reduce the composite of mortality and cardiovascular hospitalization in all types of HF in the elderly, including HFpEF.[132]

F. ACE-I or ARB

Beyond their use for HTN and beyond having the greatest LVH reverting effect, the role of ACE-I or ARB in HFpEF is questionable. Candesartan significantly reduced HF hospitalizations in the CHARM-Preserved trial (by an absolute value of only 2% at 3 years);[133] other trials, like I-PRESERVE, failed to show a benefit from ARB.[15] In both trials, HTN was well controlled at baseline with SBP of ~135 mmHg. These trials have been flawed by the inclusion of dyspneic patients who may have been mislabeled as HFpEF without solid echo or BNP features of diastolic dysfunction.

In addition, while early worsening of renal function after ACE-I/ARB initiation does not affect the long-term benefit from this therapy in systolic HF, early worsening of renal function after ACE-I/ARB initiation is associated with worsening of cardiovascular outcomes and mortality in HFpEF (worsening renal function defined as a creatinine rise ≥ 0.3 mg/dl and ≥ 25%, or GFR decline ≥ 20%).[134]

G. Spironolactone

In one trial of patients with HFpEF, mostly stable functional class II patients with controlled HTN, spironolactone improved diastolic parameters (E/E' ratio), LV mass, and NT-pro-BNP, but did not affect symptoms or exercise performance (AldoHF trial).[135] In the TOPCAT trial, patients with HFpEF, current class II or III, and elevated BNP or prior hospitalization for HF were randomized to spironolactone vs. placebo. For patients recruited from American countries, spironolactone was associated with a 26% reduction of cardiovascular mortality (from ~5% to 3.5% per year) and a 20% reduction of hospitalization for HF (from 10% to 8% per year).[136] Benefit is expected to be higher in sicker patients, as long as objective evidence of HF is present (high BNP).

ACUTE HEART FAILURE AND ACUTELY DECOMPENSATED HEART FAILURE

Acute HF presentation encompasses three syndromes:[137]

1. Deterioration of a chronic compensated HF, called **acutely decompensated HF** (ADHF). ADHF is the most common form of acute HF presentation (~70%), and is sometimes the first presentation of a chronic progressive HF. The underlying causes are the same as chronic HF, with additional decompensating triggers.

2. *De novo acute HF*, due to acute ischemia/MI, acute valvular regurgitation (acute AI or MR), hypertensive crisis, or acute fulminant myocarditis. The LV is not as dilated in these cases as it is in chronic HF and ADHF. The accompanying pulmonary edema is called *flash pulmonary edema*. Approximately 25% of acute HF presentations are de novo, acute HF.

De novo HF, but also many cases of ADHF, develop abruptly and only have mild volume overload: there is volume redistribution more than volume overload.[6,137]

3. A small proportion of acute HF presentations (~5%) are secondary to a chronic severe systolic HF with a relentless and progressive deterioration of a low-output state.

Overall, ~50–60% of patients who present with acute HF have systolic HF; the rest have HFpEF.

While volume overload is evident clinically in most patients (*clinical congestion*), a subgroup of patients, particularly those with abrupt onset of symptoms, only have a mild degree of volume overload yet a severe rise in LV filling pressure (*hemodynamic congestion, fluid redistribution*). In general, though, even in the latter patients, the rise in LV filling pressure precedes the clinical presentation by several days or weeks and, in contrast to the abruptness of symptoms and the limited weight gain, the hemodynamic change is generally progressive over weeks (Figure 4.8).[138]

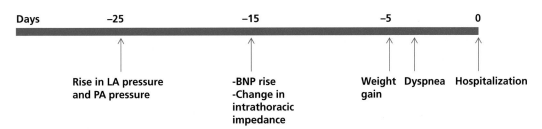

Figure 4.8 Hemodynamic decompensation starts several weeks before clinical decompensation, even when the presentation seems abrupt and the weight gain is only mild, and even in HFpEF. Modified from Zile et al. (2008).[138]

I. Triggers of acute decompensation
A. Non-compliance with medical therapy, salt and fluid restriction, or NSAID use

B. Acute HTN. Vascular dysfunction is characterized by abnormal arterial compliance, arterial vasoconstriction, and venoconstriction, and is currently viewed as a central abnormality in many cases of acute heart failure. The abnormal vascular compliance leads to marked blood pressure lability with relatively minor changes in the intravascular volume; this causes a precipitous increase in afterload and decompensates LV failure. *Bilateral renal artery stenosis* is underlying a few of these cases, particularly unexplained recurrent ADHF. 50% of ADHF patients have HTN on presentation; 70% of patients have HTN at baseline.[137,139]

Note, however, that acute HTN may at least partly be the result of the acute pulmonary edema and the accompanying sympathetic surge. This explains the precipitous blood pressure fall commonly seen with initiation of diuresis. Besides which, the impaired vascular compliance leads not only to a sudden blood pressure rise with a slight volume change but also to a sudden blood pressure fall.

While vasodilatation increases stroke volume of the failing heart, excessive vasodilatation, seen sometimes in patients who get intubated and sedated, may not be matched by enough rise in cardiac output, as the cardiac reserve is limited, which leads to precipitous hypotension. Thus, the aggressive initiation of vasodilators or multiple antihypertensive drugs on admission should be avoided until diuresis has been started.

C. Acute ischemia/ACS. ACS is responsible for up to 30% of acute HF presentations, especially de novo HF; CAD without ACS is documented in another ~30% of patients with acute HF.[139] Diffuse ischemia may lead to acute diastolic dysfunction, systolic dysfunction, or ischemic MR.

In an autopsy study, acute MI was responsible for ~54% of sudden deaths in patients with ischemic HF, and 30% of pump failure deaths.[114] Acute MI occurred on top of underlying CAD, sometimes with a thrombotic or ruptured plaque. Acute MI is a far less likely mode of death in patients without CAD. This highlights the importance of detection and treatment of CAD in HF patients, especially ADHF (high-risk group).

D. Arrhythmias, such as *AF* with a rapid ventricular rate. Approximately 30–40% of patients with ADHF have AF.[137,139] The occurrence or the acceleration of AF can be secondary to HF rather than the cause of HF.

A patient with decompensated HF typically has an elevated rate (80–110bpm). *AV block or sinus bradycardia,* even at a rate of 50–60bpm, is inappropriate and signifies that the bradyarrhythmia is a factor underlying HF decompensation (bradycardia further reduces cardiac output).

E. Any systemic infection; anemia. Normally, during infectious states and chronic anemia, both preload and inotropism increase, allowing cardiac output to increase and match the high metabolic demands. This is similar to the physiology of exercise. In systolic or diastolic dysfunction, three untoward effects occur: (i) LV is unable to accommodate the increased preload and fails, leading to an increase in filling pressures; (ii) the stroke volume cannot increase enough to match the dilated circulation, which reduces tissue perfusion; (iii) the incumbent tachycardia may decompensate HF.

F. Acute valvular insufficiency, including acute ischemic MR.

G. Notes
On admission, 30–64% of acute HF patients have moderate or severe renal failure. This may be either a cause of HF (acute tubular necrosis, intrinsic renal disease) or, more often, a result of HF. It is not usually related to over-diuresis. Either way, renal failure worsens the volume overload and leads to further neurohormonal activation, increasing the susceptibility to dietary indiscretions and ultimately worsening HF, which leads to a vicious circle of mutual HF-renal damage.

PE may exacerbate RV failure. It does not usually lead to pulmonary edema.

40–50% of acute heart failure episodes have no known precipitant.[140]

II. Profiles of acute HF: congestion without low cardiac output, congestion with low cardiac output
A. Always assess for:
1. Congestion, also known as "wet" picture[141]
- Orthopnea (90% sensitive), crackles (uncommon), peripheral edema, pleural effusions, ascites
- Elevated JVP, S_3, loud P_2 that is heard at the lower left sternum or apex (usually with split S_2).
- Also, the lack of a 30% decrease of the systolic and pulse pressure during the strain phase of Valsalva's maneuver is a highly sensitive and specific (~90%) sign of volume overload*[141–143]

---

*This is done using continuous non-invasive pressure monitoring and a 10–15s strain; alternatively, using a BP cuff inflated at systolic pressure or slightly above it, Korotkoff sounds remain heard throughout the strain phase of Valsalva and do not overshoot after the release.

2. Peripheral perfusion. Low-output signs are referred to as "cold" signs and portend a worse prognosis, with a *mortality that is twice as high as "warm" HF.*[141] Cold signs are:

- Borderline or low SBP (<90–100 mmHg), narrow pulse pressure (pulse pressure < 25% SBP, reflecting a reduced stroke volume), or pulsus alternans. *A narrow pulse pressure is the most sensitive and specific finding in low stroke volume.*
- Cool and/or cyanotic extremities.
- Severe fatigue, drowsiness, Cheyne–Stokes respiration.
- Severe worsening of renal failure.
- Hyponatremia.
- Poor or no response to diuretics.

B. Then classify the acute HF into the following hemodynamic profiles:
1. Wet and warm: pulmonary/peripheral edema without signs of low cardiac output. This is the most common ADHF profile (~2/3 of the cases).
2. Wet and cold: pulmonary/peripheral edema with signs of low cardiac output (~30% of the cases). Hypotension is present in only 2% of acute HF.[137,139]
3. Dry and cold: low output is present without edema. This may be due to hypovolemia, or to a euvolemic severe HF (~5% of acute HF), in which case it portends the worst ADHF prognosis.

Note: While cardiogenic shock is classically described in patients with acute large MI, it may also be seen in patients with chronic severe cardiomyopathy and decompensating factors (acute infection, arrhythmia, excessive vasodilators or sedation, cases where the limited cardiac output reserve cannot match the dilated circulation). In addition, volume overload, by itself, increases ventricular filling pressures and reduces myocardial perfusion and cardiac output.

III. Treatment of acute HF: diagnosis and treatment of triggers
A. Ischemia must be ruled out and treated.
If ACS is diagnosed by *dynamic ST-segment abnormalities or a marked troponin rise > 1 ng/ml*, antiplatelet and anticoagulant therapies are initiated with a plan for an early invasive strategy. Revascularization is emergent in case of ST elevation or cardiogenic shock considered secondary to ACS. Even when ACS is not suspected, a coronary angiogram needs to be performed as part of acute or severe HF workup, unless previously done; it is preferably performed during the index HF hospitalization before discharge, after appropriate diuresis. In one analysis, patients with acute HF and CAD who did not undergo revascularization before discharge had a significantly higher 60-to-90-day mortality than patients without CAD, whether EF was low or preserved; this excess in mortality was abolished with revascularization performed before or during hospitalization (OPTIMIZE-HF registry).[144]

B. HTN treatment

C. AF.
While a rate of 100–120 bpm may trigger HF decompensation, this rate is appropriate once the patient is in decompensated HF and allows an increase in cardiac output and left atrial emptying (Figure 4.2). *Aggressive acute rate control (<80 bpm) may be harmful as it may reduce cardiac output,* and should only be attempted later on, once HF has been diuresed and stabilized. AF may convert or slow down spontaneously with HF therapy and with reduction of left atrial pressure. Along with diuresis, digoxin may be started for rate control, followed by β-blocker therapy after initial stabilization. *β-Blocker is slowly titrated in systolic HF, but may be started and titrated more quickly in patients with uncontrolled AF rate, after initiating diuresis and relieving dyspnea.*

Beside rate control, consider *elective* rhythm control and DC cardioversion for persistent AF that is believed to be a major contributor to the HF exacerbation, even if the rate is appropriate, as reinstitution of atrial systole may help a subgroup of HF patients. Also, a new HF coinciding with a newly diagnosed atrial tachyarrhythmia is a tachycardia-mediated cardiomyopathy 25–50% of the time, justifying aggressive rate control or elective rhythm control in this setting. The AF-CHF trial does not support AF cardioversion in stable class II HF, but does not preclude a benefit in patients who had a recent decompensation.[145]

D. Echocardiography.
Echocardiography should be obtained to assess for systolic and diastolic dysfunction, acute valvular disease, and acute segmental wall motion abnormalities suggestive of ischemia.

E. Look for anemia, any infection, renal failure, and hyponatremia.
Hyponatremia usually signifies advanced low-output HF or hemodilution from hypervolemia. *Outpatient hypernatremia signals dehydration* and is very unusual in acute HF.

F. Consider endomyocardial biopsy when acute/fulminant myocarditis is suspected.

Note that with acute HF, the LV end-diastolic pressure increases, leading to microcirculatory coronary compression and reduction of the pressure gradient between the aortic pressure and LVEDP, i.e., the pressure gradient that drives coronary microcirculatory flow. This explains the common mild troponin increase in ADHF, unrelated to any thrombotic coronary event. In 6% of ADHF, troponin rose to striking levels > 1 ng/ml, regardless of the presence of coronary disease.[146] Troponin is a marker of increased mortality in acute HF independent of coronary disease.

In decompensated HF, dyspnea is frequently described as chest tightness; thus, acutely, chest tightness does not equate with angina and is not a specific marker of CAD.

IV. Treatment of acute HF: diuretics, cardiorenal syndrome, aggressive decongestion, ultrafiltration
A. Diuretics
Loop diuretics are the mainstay of acute HF therapy. Furosemide dosing:

- Intravenous 40–80 mg bolus.
- Intravenous 20 mg may be effective in patients who are not receiving chronic treatment with furosemide. Doses larger than 80 mg may be needed in renal failure (up to 200 mg single dose).
- A 40 mg intravenous dose of furosemide is approximately equivalent to 80 mg of oral furosemide.
- Acutely, intestinal edema and low intestinal perfusion may be present and may prevent any response to oral furosemide.

Immediate relief is due to venodilatation and is followed by a diuretic effect that peaks at 30–60 minutes and lasts ~4–6 hours. When the patient is euvolemic, switch to oral, lower maintenance dose of furosemide.

The lack of response to dose "X" in ~30–60 minutes (<500 ml of urine within 30–60 minutes) means that "X" is below a patient-specific threshold dose. Twice the dose "X" should be administered in 30–60 minutes. In HF without renal failure, the furosemide IV threshold is usually 40–80 mg; in renal failure, higher single doses may be needed (up to 200 mg IV dose given over 30 minutes).[104] After a dose is determined to be effective, the frequency of administration is tailored to achieve the 24-hour goal (e.g., 4 liters of urine output).

Administer multiple daily doses of furosemide in acute HF, such as Q6–12h. Once the threshold is defined, not much is gained by providing higher single doses, as the maximal response to a single dose is reduced in HF. Frequent dosing of the threshold provides a more effective diuresis and prevents the post-diuretic sodium reabsorption that occurs during the diuretic-free intervals. For someone whose diuretic threshold is 40 mg IV, the administration of 40 mg Q6h is likely better than 80 mg Q12h. Alternatively, furosemide may be administered as IV drip when more than 250 mg of IV furosemide is required per day (drip of 10–40 mg of furosemide per hour). *A drip may only be started after an effective bolus dose initiates a diuretic response*, and each time the drip is up-titrated, the bolus dose is typically administered again.

In a patient receiving chronic loop diuretic therapy, *the total daily dose of IV diuretic that should be used is ~2.5 times the total daily oral dose*, with the bolus dose being numerically equal or superior to the single oral dose (this regimen proved beneficial in two trials).[147,148] For a patient chronically using 80 mg of oral furosemide Q12h, an appropriate initial regimen in ADHF may be 80 mg IV Q6h or 120 mg IV Q8h. **This dose is tailored according to: (i) the response to the first dose, and (ii) the 24-hour diuresis goal (3–5 liters of urine).**

If there is **no response** *to the maximal single dose of furosemide*, two diagnoses should be considered: (1) very low renal flow resulting from an inappropriate cardiac output at the renal level or inappropriate BP (e.g., 90–100 mmHg); (2) acute, intrinsic kidney injury unresponsive to the diuretic (e.g., acute tubular necrosis). Inotropic therapy is administered and often initiates diuresis in the case of low renal flow.

If there is a **moderate response** *to the maximal single dose of furosemide* (e.g., 500 ml of urine output over several hours after a 160–200 mg dose), a thiazide diuretic may be added to boost the overall, 24-hour urine output.

Examples of thiazide diuretics include oral metolazone 2.5–20 mg Qday, oral hydrochlorothiazide 25–50 mg Qday, or IV chlorothiazide 500–1000 mg Qday. Thiazide diuretics attenuate the distal tubular escape from the loop diuretic effect; thus, *they increase the total diuresis but do not initiate diuresis in unresponsive patients*. Note that metolazone is a thiazide-like drug that works on both the proximal and distal tubules and remains effective in advanced renal failure. Other thiazide diuretics also remain effective in advanced renal failure, particularly when combined with loop diuretics. Thiazide is probably best administered ≥ 1 hour before the loop diuretic, to prevent the distal tubular reabsorption of the sodium released by the loop diuretic. Spironolactone may also be added early on (ESC) and may potentiate diuresis in HF, which is a high aldosterone state, but it has a slow onset of action of 2–3 days.[149]

Goal of diuresis:

- *2–3 liters of net negative fluid balance per day, which corresponds to 3–5 liters of urine/day*. The goal is lower in patients who meet both of the following conditions: no significant peripheral edema (abrupt HF) *and* no LV dilatation (steep pressure–volume relationship). It is also lower in isolated right heart failure (~1 l/day) and when the predominant manifestation is ascites.*

Laboratory monitoring is necessary to detect adverse metabolic effects:

- Worsening of renal function.
- Hypokalemia, hypomagnesemia, hypocalcemia.

---

*The volume clearance across the peritoneal membrane cannot exceed 500 ml/day; in patients with predominant ascites, a diuresis of 2 liters per day comes at the expense of the intravascular volume.

- Hypernatremia (the urine induced by loop diuretics is half-tonic, similar to 0.45% half-saline); or hyponatremia from neurohormonal activation. The loop diuretic–thiazide combination is associated with marked hypokalemia and more frequent hyponatremia.
- Contraction metabolic alkalosis signals chloride depletion and the need to slow the diuresis or replete the potassium deficit. Diuresis needs to be continued in patients with persistent volume overload, possibly at a slower rate with aggressive potassium replacement.

Moderate renal failure is present in 30–64% of acute HF patients on hospital admission. Furthermore, worsening of renal function occurs in ~30% of patients hospitalized with ADHF (worsening = ↑ creatinine by ≥ 0.3 mg/dl).[150]

> If the patient is still clinically or radiographically congested, continue diuresis even if creatinine rises. In this case, the rise in creatinine is due to the low output or the venous congestion per se (cardiorenal syndrome) rather than "overdiuresis," or to a necessary drop of the preload in patients with acute or diastolic HF. In fact, in most patients, the filling pressures are high at the time of worsening of renal function.[150-152]

B. Acute cardiorenal syndrome

Acute cardiorenal syndrome (type 1) refers to worsening renal function and progressive volume overload in a patient with acute HF.[148] This syndrome may reduce diuretic response. While it may be related to a low-output cold HF, the ESCAPE trial suggests a poor correlation between cardiac index and baseline or worsening renal function.[150] In fact, **cardiac output may be normal at the central level but the local renal flow is reduced**. Cardiorenal syndrome is most often related to the following mechanisms:

- Volume overload itself, which increases the **renal venous afterload** and consequently impedes the forward renal flow.[150,153] In fact, renal flow is driven by the gradient between mean arterial pressure and renal venous pressure. This gradient should be high enough to overcome the renal arteriolar resistance. According to one analysis, the admission and post-therapy RA pressure was the most important factor driving renal deterioration in acute HF.[151]
- A reduction of arterial pressure with therapy. Multiple analyses showed that renal deterioration in ADHF strongly correlates with SBP reduction during therapy (e.g., >10 mmHg reduction from a baseline SBP of ~115 mmHg).[154]
- Slow plasma refill time. The plasma refill time is the time required for the extracellular edema to refill the intravascular volume that is being diuresed. At the plasma refill rate, the intravascular volume only marginally decreases with diuresis, whereas the interstitial volume markedly decreases. However, a patient with 20 liters of volume overload may not tolerate 5 liters of negative balance per day if his plasma refill time is 3 l/day.
- A diuretic bolus induces a pulse diuresis (e.g., 1.5 l within 2 h) that may be faster than the plasma refill time, which creates transient effective hypovolemia, activates the renin–angiotensin and sympathetic systems, and reduces GFR, even if central cardiac output is eventually preserved.
- Increased intra-abdominal pressure, secondary to ascites and visceral edema, leads to an abdominal compartment syndrome with increased renal venous pressure and reduced renal perfusion, regardless of the central venous pressure.[153]

This pathophysiology explains why many cases of cardiorenal syndrome (up to 50%) occur in patients with EF > 40%. This syndrome may potentially worsen with diuresis, but more often improves with diuresis. In fact, although ~30% of acute HF patients have worsening of renal function during therapy,[150] slightly over 50% of HF patients have an improvement in renal function with adequate diuresis, even more so when creatinine is assessed at 30–60 days after hospitalization.[147,148] This is related to:

- Reduction of renal venous pressure and renal venodilatation with loop diuretics and vasodilators (↓ renal "afterload")
- Reduction of intra-abdominal pressure
- Reduction of right and left ventricular volumes, and, as a result, improvement of cardiac output (Table 4.1)

> ***Thus, congestion is at the center of acute HF syndromes. Aggressive decongestion greatly improves renal and myocardial flow and ventricular loading conditions.*** This allows renal function to improve enough to sustain diuresis with lower diuretic doses. This also allows the patient to tolerate lower systemic pressure without compromise of myocardial or renal perfusion.

Prior underlying kidney disease, diabetes, hypertension, NSAID use, or repeated episodes of subclinical acute kidney injury predispose to the cardiorenal syndrome.[150,155]

Table 4.1 Reduction of ventricular volume improves cardiac output through four mechanisms.

1. Reduction of ventricular wall tension, which is afterload (↓ afterload → ↑ cardiac output)
2. Reduction of functional MR and TR
3. Reduction of RV–LV interdependence
4. Reduction of LVEDP and RVEDP, which improves myocardial perfusion

While cardiorenal syndrome is the most common form of progressive renal dysfunction encountered in acute HF, *intrinsic acute renal failure may occur as well*, and should be suspected in patients who are oliguric and diuretic-resistant. Acute tubular necrosis may occur as a result of the sustained ischemic injury and may persist for 7–10 days, requiring hemodialysis in the interim. On the other hand, post-renal obstruction, NSAID injury, glomerulonephritis, or acute interstitial nephritis may be present and make renal failure the cause rather than the result of acute HF. Urinalysis and urinary microscopic exam are thus warranted, and can exclude parenchymal disease.

The combination of two particular factors predicts a poor renal tolerance of acute diuresis: (i) *no or minimal peripheral edema*, and (ii) *non-dilated LV and RV with steep pressure–volume relationship* (e.g., de novo acute HF, diastolic HF). Patients with severe edema usually tolerate aggressive diuresis, especially if they have a good plasma refill time. Conversely, in patients without severe peripheral edema *and* with poorly compliant, normal-size ventricles, the preload volume is not dramatically increased, but the preload pressure (LVEDP) is. Hence, these patients have pulmonary edema despite being "preload volume-dependent." Diuresis may be poorly tolerated in the absence of peripheral edema, leading to a reduction in cardiac output, and, as a result, renal failure. However, *mild and careful diuresis, in conjunction with vasodilator therapy, is usually well tolerated and may be the best option in this case (e.g., negative fluid balance 1–1.5 l/day).*

Note: Other types of cardiorenal syndrome:[155] (i) type 2 or chronic cardiorenal syndrome: renal dysfunction results from chronic HF and has similar mechanisms to type 1 syndrome, except that these mechanisms are more persistent; (ii) type 3 or acute renocardiac syndrome: acute kidney injury leads to HF decompensation; (iii) type 4 or chronic renocardiac syndrome; (iv) type 5: systemic illnesses, such as diabetes, HTN, vasculitis, or separate disease processes cause combined cardiac and renal dysfunction.

C. Importance of aggressive decongestion, even in the face of a rising creatinine

One analysis has shown that aggressive decongestion with hemoconcentration (rise in hematocrit and albumin) is associated with a profound 70% reduction in mortality at 6 months, despite a strong association with creatinine rise.[156] In fact, in this and other analyses, the incomplete relief of congestion during acute heart failure, rather than the worsening of creatinine levels, strongly contributed to HF progression and worsening survival.[156,157] Therefore, the increase in creatinine does not portend a negative prognosis *if* decongestion is achieved. Besides, the rise in creatinine does not necessarily imply a worsening of renal function; it may simply reflect hemoconcentration, a desired effect.

Other data corroborate that baseline renal function has a prognostic value, but not the in-hospital worsening of renal function.[150] In addition, in the DOSE trial, a high dose of diuretic was associated with more worsening of renal function at 72 hours but better clinical outcomes. The creatinine level eventually trended down at 60 days in patients receiving the high diuretic dose, while it progressively trended up at 60 days in patients who did not achieve appropriate decongestion. Although creatinine may fluctuate initially, it generally becomes lower than baseline at 30–60 days in patients appropriately decongested.[147]

D. Continuous loop diuretic drip vs. intermittent boluses: role of ultrafiltration

The bolus diuretic dose induces pulse diuresis (e.g., 1 liter in 1 hour) that may be faster than the plasma refill time, potentially leading to a transient effective hypovolemia with subsequent RAAS and sympathetic activation and avid post-diuretic sodium reabsorption. This is how, in theory, diuretics may increase mortality, but, as shown below, this did not prove to be true.

The use of a continuous infusion of furosemide, rather than bolus doses, may allow a steady-state fluid removal at the plasma refill rate. In the DOSE trial, a continuous diuretic infusion was associated with similar renal and clinical outcomes as bolus administration. Conversely, the use of a high diuretic dose, as opposed to a low dose, achieved more net fluid loss and weight loss, superior decongestion, more dyspnea reduction, and a trend towards lower hospitalizations despite a transient worsening of renal function.[147]

Continuous ultrafiltration constitutes a non-pharmacological modality of fluid removal. One device, Aquadex, is simpler than renal replacement devices and uses a smaller central or peripheral venous catheter with a lower venous flow (10–40 ml/min) and a small blood volume outside the body (40 ml) that is more tolerated hemodynamically. It removes fluid at a rate of 100–250 ml/h (≤6 l/day). In theory, the intravascular volume remains unchanged as fluid shifts from the extracellular space to the intravascular space at the plasma refill rate, with potentially less harmful neurohormonal activation. Also, ultrafiltration removes isotonic fluid, as opposed to the half-tonic diuresis induced by diuretics; thus, for a similar amount of fluid removed, ultrafiltration removes more sodium than diuretics. Yet, in the CARRESS-HF trial of patients with acute HF and cardiorenal syndrome, ultrafiltration at a rate of 200 ml/h was not more effective than high-dose diuretics in achieving decongestion, weight loss, or clinical improvement, and led to significantly more creatinine rise that persisted at 60 days.[148] Ultrafiltration probably failed because of catheter-related complications and a frequent need to interrupt therapy (e.g., catheter clotting). It is also possible that diuretics have protective renal effects through blocking the ATP pump at the loop of Henle and reducing medullary O_2 consumption.[108]

Those two trials illustrate that the principal goal of acute HF therapy is aggressive decongestion, achieved through a high-volume diuresis and a high diuretic dose if needed (urine output 3–5 liters/day), even in the face of transient/mild increase in creatinine. *Beware that patients with abrupt acute HF without significant peripheral edema and with a non-dilated LV may not tolerate this high-volume diuresis.*

E. Diuretic resistance

Diuretic resistance is defined as reduced diuresis and natriuresis despite intermediate or high diuretic doses, precluding the resolution of congestion (e.g., net negative fluid balance < 1 liter/day despite a daily dose of intravenous furosemide > 160–240 mg). It is seen in up to 25% of ADHF cases. Several mechanisms are implicated:

- Reduced renal flow, partly related to a high renal afterload and a renal compartment syndrome (high outflow pressure), and partly related to a low local cardiac output and a low systemic pressure (low inflow pressure).
- Intrinsic renal failure.
- Activation of the renin–angiotensin–aldosterone system.
- Hyperfunction of the Henle loop with repeated loop diuretic administration after a first dose (braking phenomenon).
- Post-diuretic rebound effect, i.e., tubular reabsorption of sodium in between doses.
- Hypertrophy of the distal tubules after chronic loop diuretic administration (thiazide benefit), and hyperaldosteronism with exaggeration of the distal sodium retention (spironolactone benefit).

As mentioned earlier, it is treated by increasing loop diuretic doses and frequency of administration, and by combining them with thiazide diuretics, if needed, and spironolactone.

> Patients who do not achieve appropriate diuresis with a high diuretic dose generally have a very low renal flow; inotropic therapy and/or ultrafiltration may be considered for these patients. If no response is achieved with inotropic therapy, acute tubular necrosis is suspected and hemodialysis may be required.

After 24–48 hours of inotropic therapy or ultrafiltration, diuretic responsiveness is often restored, as cardiac output improves with the reduction of afterload, RV–LV interdependence, and functional MR, while renal perfusion improves with the reduction of renal venous afterload.
In patients with severe intrinsic renal dysfunction, full hemodialysis rather than ultrafiltration should be used, as ultrafiltration worsens outcomes in advanced renal failure.

V. Treatment of acute HF: vasodilators

Vasodilators decrease afterload and improve cardiac output; they also have a venodilatory effect that reduces preload, relieves pulmonary edema, and reduces renal afterload. They counteract the vasoconstrictive effect of loop diuretics. However, even *transient hypotension* impairs renal function and outcomes. **Vasodilators are definitely avoided if SBP < 100 mmHg, and should often be avoided if SBP < 110 mmHg.**[32] *Vasodilators are only started after ensuring that SBP is stable at > 110 mmHg, rather than maintained by the high catecholamine state of HF* (in which case BP may precipitously drop with the relief of dyspnea). When properly used, a small vasodilator dose increases cardiac output, thereby counteracting any direct hypotensive effect. Vasodilators are indicated in "warm-wet" HF, particularly the fluid redistribution type (in which HTN and vascular dysfunction are primary targets), and in patients whose symptoms do not quickly improve with diuresis.[32,158,159] Data from the ADHERE registry, the Cleveland Clinic, and a randomized trial of nitroglycerin suggest a benefit from acute vasodilator use.[158–160]

Patients with *diastolic HF* are more vasodilator-sensitive than those with systolic HF, and may have a precipitous BP drop with vasodilators, even if they are hypertensive on presentation. Patients with *low-output, cold HF* have a limited cardiac output reserve which may prevent them from filling a dilated circulation: BP and tissue perfusion may precipitously drop with vasodilators. **In general, initiate diuresis and ensure BP is stable before initiating vasodilators.**

A. Intravenous nitroglycerin (NTG). Nitroglycerin is a venodilator that acts as a mixed venous and arterial vasodilator at medium doses. NTG has arterial vasodilatory effects, particularly in the context of severely increased systemic vascular resistance or high-dose diuresis (diuretics activate the RAAS and may lead to vasoconstriction). Nitrate tolerance develops after several hours of NTG therapy and appears to be improved by the combination with hydralazine or ACE-I. Start with 20 mcg/min, then titrate by 10–20 mcg/min every 5 min, up to 200 mcg/min, as long as SBP ≥ 110 mmHg.

B. Intravenous nitroprusside. Nitroprusside has arterial, venous, and pulmonary vasodilatory properties. Classically, an arterial line is needed to monitor BP during nitroprusside therapy, but this is not always necessary. One study suggested improved outcomes and mortality with the acute use of nitroprusside in acute HF.[158]

C. Switch to oral vasodilators when stable, such as ACE-Is and/or the combination of hydralazine and oral nitrates, mainly in case of LV systolic dysfunction.

- A patient who is receiving chronic ACE-I therapy should continue to receive it even if there is some worsening of renal function during the hospital stay, because holding ACE-I may impair outcomes. However, ACE-I should be held and avoided acutely in hypotensive, cold HF or severe acute kidney injury.
- If the patient was not on an ACE-I chronically, avoid starting ACE-I acutely, in the first few hours, before making sure the patient is hemodynamically stable and is not developing a cardiogenic shock. In addition, ACE-I may reduce kidney perfusion and the response to diuretics acutely.
- The combination of hydralazine and nitrates can be started acutely in HF, with some evidence suggesting benefit.[158]

D. Nesiritide. Nesiritide is a recombinant form of BNP that is administered intravenously. It is a potent venous and arterial vasodilator with a mild direct diuretic effect.

The duration of action of nesiritide is 3 hours, i.e., longer than NTG and nitroprusside, the effect of which lasts only minutes. If hypotension occurs, this prolonged effect increases the chances of renal failure and mortality. This hypotension is potentially more harmful than the hypotension seen with other IV vasodilators. There is evidence suggesting that nesiritide at effective doses increases the risk of renal dysfunction and mortality in acute HF.[161] In one randomized trial, lower doses of nesiritide appeared safe but did not provide any clinical benefit on top of standard therapy.[162]

Thus, nesiritide has an unclear role and should be avoided if SBP < 110 mmHg.[32] Loop diuretics and other vasodilators are first-line agents.

E. Serelaxin (investigational): Serelaxin, an intravenous vasodilator, is a recombinant form of relaxin, the natural hormone that promotes vasodilatation in pregnancy. In the RELAX-HF trial of ADHF patients with SBP > 125 mmHg, the use of serelaxin for 2 days on top of diuretic therapy was associated with improved dyspnea, improved mortality at 60 days, and an early improvement of biomarkers (troponin, renal function, BNP).

VI. Treatment of acute HF: IV inotropic agents (dobutamine, milrinone, dopamine)

IV inotropic agents may worsen survival over the long term even when used temporarily; therefore, they should be avoided if possible.[160] In the OPTIME-HF trial, the short-term use of milrinone increased in-hospital death and the 60-day risk of death or rehospitalization in ischemic HF, and increased arrhythmias in all HF.[163–165] Exogenous cardiac stimulation, at a time when the myocardium is significantly energy-depleted, may result in further ischemic and apoptotic damage and lead to the poor outcomes associated with these agents, despite immediate short-term hemodynamic improvement. Note that OPTIME-HF did not include cases where inotropic therapy was considered essential. ***An inotrope, typically dobutamine, is still indicated temporarily in: (i) wet and cold HF* with SBP < 85–90 mmHg, *or (ii) wet and cold HF not responding to diuresis.***[32]

A. Dobutamine (β_1- and β_2-agonist) and milrinone (phosphodiesterase-5 inhibitor) have inotropic and vasodilatory effects

Milrinone is a phosphodiesterase-5 inhibitor that increases intracellular cAMP along the β-receptor pathway. It has more marked vasodilatory and hypotensive effects and a more prolonged effect than dobutamine, with a 2.5-hour half-life, more so in renal failure. Milrinone should be avoided if SBP < 80 mmHg, and the dose should be reduced by 50% in renal failure. Also, the bolus dose of milrinone is particularly hypotensive and is better avoided. Start a small drip of milrinone (0.2 mcg/kg/min) and titrate it very slowly every few hours, allowing the increase in cardiac output to catch the vasodilatory effect, therefore preventing hypotension. Milrinone has significant pulmonary vasodilatory potential and may be the preferred inotrope in patients with pulmonary hypertension.

Dobutamine has a marked β_1-agonist effect, and a less marked β_2- and α_1-agonist effect. The β_2- and α_1-receptors have counter effects on the vasculature (vasodilatation and vasoconstriction, respectively), which explains that the vasodilatory and hypotensive effects of dobutamine are usually mild, and in fact BP often improves with the increase in cardiac output. Only in critical patients with severe vasoconstriction and occupancy of all α-receptors, dobutamine may have a predominant β_2 and vasodilatory effect. A low dose of dobutamine (2–5 mcg/kg/min) usually provides the desired effect. Higher doses (up to 10 mcg/kg/min) may be required in patients previously receiving β-blockers.

The most common arrhythmia with milrinone is AF (up to 25%), while the most common arrhythmia with dobutamine is sinus tachycardia. Asymptomatic PVCs are common with both, more so dobutamine, but VT is rare.

> Note that chronic β-blocker therapy with carvedilol and, to a lesser extent, metoprolol, may lessen the hemodynamic effects of dobutamine, mandating higher dobutamine doses.[166,167] On the other hand, chronic β-blocker therapy seems to enhance the effects of milrinone. Milrinone increases cAMP downstream of the β-receptor pathway, uninhibited by blockade of the β-receptor.

B. Dopamine and norepinephrine have inotropic and vasoconstrictive effects.

These agents are used in severe hypotension (SBP < 70–80 mmHg). For a similar increase in cardiac output, dopamine produces greater elevation in heart rate and more arrhythmias than dobutamine and norepinephrine.

Inotropes can often be weaned off within a few days. Inotropes initiate diuresis and reduce ventricular volumes, and thus improve ventricular afterload, functional MR/TR, and myocardial perfusion in a sustained fashion. This allows the patient to tolerate inotrope discontinuation and tolerate lower systemic pressures without compromise of myocardial perfusion. Also, renal function improves enough to allow the sustainment of diuresis. In patients with less severe HF, aggressive diuresis achieves a similar sustained benefit to inotropes (Figure 4.9).

VII. In-hospital and pre-discharge use of ACE-Is and β-blockers

ACE-I and β-blockers should be continued in the majority of acute HF cases, except in shock (discontinuation of both), or severe azotemia (discontinuation of ACE-I). In low-output HF with borderline BP, the β-blocker and ACE-I dosages may be reduced.

If ACE-Is and/or β-blockers were discontinued or never started, they should be initiated or reinitiated ≥ 24 hours before discharge. β-blockers are initiated after successful discontinuation of inotropes. Pre-discharge initiation of carvedilol reduces the 60-day mortality by 54%.

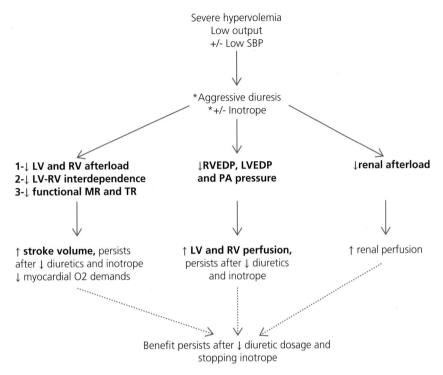

Figure 4.9 Mechanisms through which diuresis and inotropes initiate a benefit that is sustained over time.
LV perfusion is mainly diastolic and depends on the gradient between aortic DBP and LVEDP. RV perfusion is diastolic and systolic and depends on the gradient between aortic DBP and RVEDP, as well as the gradient between aortic SBP and RV systolic pressure. A reduction in LVEDP improves LV perfusion, while a reduction in RVEDP and RV systolic pressure, i.e., PA pressure, improves RV perfusion.

If the patient has required inotropic support, he should be monitored for one or more additional days after β-blocker initiation; the same applies to the initiation of ACE-I in a patient who has developed azotemia.

VIII. Treatment of acute HF: O₂, non-invasive ventilatory support (CPAP, BiPAP), intubation

CPAP or BiPAP may be acutely used in severe respiratory distress as a bridge until pulmonary edema is relieved with diuretics. CPAP or BiPAP should only be tried in a patient with appropriate level of wakefulness who is not severely hypoxic or acidotic (pH > 7.2), and not hypotensive, and should be quickly removed within < 30 minutes if it proves ineffective. Its prolonged ineffective use may paradoxically increase and prolong respiratory work, gastric distension and aspiration, and delay a salutary intubation. Intubation is required in patients with severe respiratory distress if CPAP/BiPAP and furosemide have not been effective quickly.

Intubation with positive-pressure ventilation reduces both preload and afterload, creating optimal loading conditions and an immediate reduction of pulmonary edema. Intracavitary LV pressure is not the only pressure affecting afterload; a positive pressure surrounding the myocardium negates some of the intracavitary pressure and reduces the tension against the inner myocardial wall. In fact, afterload correlates with the transmural pressure (LV pressure minus pericardial pressure) and is reduced with positive-pressure ventilation. Conversely, extubation may be poorly tolerated in HF patients or patients with critical CAD, as it drastically increases both preload and afterload.

IX. Summary: keys to the treatment of acute HF (Table 4.2)

- "Wet and warm" state: treat with diuretics + vasodilators.
- "Cold" state (low perfusion): treat with diuretics. Vasodilators may be carefully added if SBP is stable at ≥ 110 mmHg (vasodilators are only used after ensuring that SBP is stable).
- "Cold" state not achieving diuresis despite high doses of diuretics: add inotropic support to diuretic therapy, and consider ultrafiltration.
- "Cold" state associated with SBP < 90 mmHg: use inotropic support and diuretics (typically high diuretic dose).

The clinical assessment of "wet" and "cold" signs is usually enough to guide initial therapy. The routine use of a Swan–Ganz catheter (PA catheter) in acute HF does not improve outcomes.[168] It is used selectively to monitor RA pressure, pulmonary capillary pressure, and cardiac output, if:

- The patient's BP or respiratory status does not improve after initiation of medical treatment and the volume status is unclear. This includes some cases of diuretic resistance.

Table 4.2 Acute HF therapy according to volume status and peripheral perfusion status.

| Perfusion signs | Overload/congestive signs | |
	Wet	*Dry*
Warm	Diuresis + vasodilators	Not HF
Cold	Diuresis ± vasodilators If no response or if SBP < 90 mmHg: inotropes	Could be hypovolemia → hold diuretics and give volume gradually (oral rather than IV replacement) Consider the possibility of overdosage with medical therapy (especially if hypotension)[a] Consider inotropes if still hypoperfused

[a] Swan–Ganz catheter may be of use to guide therapy in this patient goup.

- There is progressive renal failure with diuretic resistance.
- A mixed shock is suspected (cardiogenic and septic).
- There is uncertainty about the diagnosis of cardiogenic shock, especially in the "cold" and "dry" subgroup.

X. Discharge

Patients need to achieve near optimal volume before discharge. They should be able to ambulate without dizziness and with minimal dyspnea. Transition from intravenous to oral diuretic needs to be completed and stable for 12–24 hours before discharge. Oral diuretic dose should maintain a slightly negative input/output balance. If the patient was receiving 60 mg IV Q8h, the patient is placed on a maintenance dose of 40–60 mg of oral furosemide, twice a day (i.e., a total oral furosemide dose that is numerically 0.5–0.75 the intravenous dose used, taking into account how well decongested the patient is). This oral dose is far lower than the intravenous dose, but is usually effective enough at the compensated stage in a patient who is almost euvolemic with improved renal perfusion. Appropriate diuresis should be ensured within a few hours of the oral dose. **Early clinical and creatinine/K/BNP checkup should be performed within a week of discharge, and the oral dose of furosemide up- or down-titrated during this visit.**

The in-hospital mortality of acutely decompensated heart failure, whether systolic or diastolic, is ~4%. There are four major prognostic risk factors: [146,169] ↑ BUN or creatinine on admission, SBP < 115 mmHg, "cold" low-output HF, positive troponin (especially > 1 ng/ml, regardless of the presence of ischemia). Mortality can go up to 10–20% with one or more of these factors and down to 2% with no factors. The mortality and rehospitalization rates at 60–90 days are 8–10% and 30%, respectively.[144] The mortality and rehospitalization rates at 1 year are 30% and 50%, respectively, much higher than MI mortality.[125,170]

XI. Inability of severe HF to tolerate vasodilatation or hemodialysis

In patients with severely *limited cardiac output reserve*, vasodilatation may not be matched by enough rise in cardiac output to fill the dilated circulation, which leads to precipitous hypotension.

While decongestion improves cardiac output, quick fluid removal during dialysis (2–3 liters in 3 hours) exceeds plasma refill time and creates transient reduction of intravascular volume. In patients with preserved cardiac function, the LV increases its contractility, stroke volume, and EF to fill the empty circulation. This cannot happen in patients with *limited cardiac output reserve*, especially those whose BP is borderline low. BP will precipitously drop during dialysis. Norepinephrine may be used to constrict the empty circulation and maintain BP during dialysis; in patients with hypotension, norepinephrine does not increase afterload untowardly, as it only raises the SBP to 90–100 mmHg.

XII. Outpatient monitoring of HF and prevention of hospitalization

Fluid accumulation in the lungs generally occurs over time, typically 1–3 weeks, and is generally believed to precede episodes of overt decompensation in most patients.[171] Daily monitoring of body weight is the easiest method of monitoring fluid status, with a gain of over 3 lb in less than a week indicating the need for extra doses of diuretics. However, weight gain may not be sensitive enough (~20% sensitivity) to detect HF deterioration, and the weight increase is smaller than considered clinically relevant in > 50% of patients (~2 lb).[172,173] Fluid redistribution with only mild fluid retention might explain this diagnostic gap.[6] Afterload increase, ischemia, AF, infection, may all cause a *sudden deterioration that may not be heralded by weight gain*. In fact, in one study using a PA sensor, changes in the continuously monitored PA diastolic pressure reliably predicted HF hospitalization, while weight minimally changed throughout the decompensation.[138] PA diastolic pressure started to rise ~20 days prior to HF hospitalization, even earlier in systolic HF. Thus, in stable HF outpatients, several monitoring methods have been developed to prevent HF hospitalization:

- BNP monitoring, particularly in patients < 75 years of age with systolic HF.
- Impedance cardiography. The chest bioimpedance or resistance correlates with intrathoracic fluid volume and is measured non-invasively using external electrodes (the higher the fluid volume, the lower the chest resistance). Measuring bioimpedance every 2 weeks allowed the prediction of decompensation, but this is not widely used or validated.[174] Bioimpedance may also be monitored more accurately with implantable devices (ICD, CRT) that perform a daily measurement of electrical impedance between the device box and the right-ventricular

electrode (OptiVol feature). This information may be transmitted daily and wirelessly to a bedside communicator which transmits it to a service center. OptiVol is less subject to external electrode positioning bias and produces an audible alert once the impedance is lower than a certain cutoff. Bioimpedance change has ~60–80% sensitivity and positive predictive value for HF decompensation and warrants at least a clinic visit and a probable up-titration of diuretics, vasodilators, and HTN therapy.[171,175] It correlates with PCWP changes and fluid loss in patients hospitalized with HF.[171] Home monitoring of devices improves clinical outcomes in HF, through impedance monitoring but also through the early detection of atrial and ventricular arrhythmias (IN-TIME trial).[176]

- Invasively implanted hemodynamic monitors, such as CardioMEMS, which is a small, invasively implanted PA sensor that wirelessly transmits PA pressure (checked at least once weekly). In patients with class III HF and prior HF hospitalization in the last year, CardioMEMS-guided therapy reduced the risk of recurrent HF hospitalizations, whether EF was reduced or preserved (CHAMPION trial).[177]

> With the CardioMEMS device, decongestive therapy is titrated to achieve a normal PA pressure. The PA pressure is recorded by the patient every morning and the numbers are telemonitored by the physician at least once weekly. An upward trend over several days is more alarming than daily fluctuations. Beside diuretics, long-acting nitrate may be used for decongestion.

Appendix 1. Management of isolated or predominant RV failure

A. Causes of right HF (see Table 4.3)[178]

Causes of RV failure have been discussed under *Causes of heart failure* (Section 2.III), and are organized in three categories: **(i) pressure overload, (ii) volume overload, and (iii) intrinsic RV disease**.

Acute RV failure is caused by RV infarct, acute PE, or any acute pulmonary hypertension (sepsis, ARDS). It may also result from the decompensation of any of the chronic causes, typically by acute pulmonary hypertension. *Acute pulmonary hypertension is at the center of most cases of acute RV failure.*

B. RV morphological features; echocardiographic features of RV dysfunction

As opposed to the LV, which has an elliptical shape, the RV has the shape of a pyramid connected to an infundibular tube. While the RV diameter is smaller than the LV diameter on the apical four-chamber view, *the three-dimensional RV volume is actually larger than the LV volume, which implies that normally the RV EF is lower than LV EF*, with 40% as the lower limit of normal (EF = stroke volume/ventricular diastolic volume; for the same stroke volume, the ventricular volume is larger on the right). In pathological states, the dilated RV assumes a spherical shape.

On echo, the diagnosis of subtle RV dilatation is difficult because of the complex RV geometry. RV that is larger than LV on the four-chamber view, or RV that is spherical rather than crescentic on the long-axis view, suggests RV dilatation but is not specific. RV septal motion should be analyzed for RV volume overload (septum pushed towards the LV in diastole, with paradoxical motion in systole), and RV pressure overload (septum pushed towards the LV in systole, called D-shaped septum).

Two echo indices are valuable for the assessment of RV systolic function: (i) *TAPSE* (tricuspid annular plane systolic excursion, normal > 16 mm), which is the systolic excursion of the lateral tricuspid annulus toward the apex, measured on M-mode; (ii) *tissue Doppler of the lateral tricuspid annulus* (called S′, normal > 10 cm/s). RV volume and EF are better assessed by MRI or first-pass nuclear scan.

> Unexplained RV dilatation or unexplained pulmonary hypertension often warrants TEE and a bubble study seeking an *overlooked shunt*, particularly ASD (e.g., sinus venosus ASD).

C. Pathophysiology, ventricular interdependence

1. *Afterload sensitivity.* The thin RV poorly tolerates an increase in PA pressure and quickly fails and distends. *As opposed to the normal LV, the RV is very sensitive to acute afterload changes and is more likely to fail from acute pressure overload* (such as pulmonary embolism) *than from volume overload* (such as atrial septal defect, primary tricuspid or pulmonic regurgitation). This is due to the fact that the RV wall is thinner than the LV wall, afterload inversely correlating with myocardial thickness (Laplace law: wall stress or afterload = pressure × radius/ [2 × wall thickness]). Chronic pulmonary hypertension stimulates thickening of the RV wall, which helps reduce wall tension; this is not seen in the acute setting, where RV is intolerant to any rise in afterload.

Table 4.3 Diagnosis of the underlying mechanism of RV failure and tricuspid regurgitation: measurement of PA systolic pressure and PVR (pressure overload vs. volume overload vs. intrinsic RV disease).

PA pressure > 50, or PVR ↑

Pulmonary hypertension, possibly from left HF. PA pressure may be normal if cardiac output is poor (severe RV failure), but PVR unveils the diagnosis of pulmonary hypertension

PA pressure normal or < 50, and PVR normal

Isolated right HF from volume overload (ASD, TR), or intrinsic RV disease (cardiomyopathy, RV MI). A mild pulmonary hypertension with normal PVR may not explain RV failure

---

As the RV severely fails and dilates, progressive RV dilatation leads to progressively more wall stress on the thin walls, which leads to further RV dilatation (vicious circle of RV dilatation). The pericardium is helpful in those cases as it tries to contain the RV; pericardiotomy/cardiac surgery may lead to massive RV dilatation.

2. *Ventricular interdependence.* LV failure leads to RV failure through pulmonary hypertension and through the loss of septal contribution to RV function. In fact, the septum and the RV free wall contribute almost equally to the RV function, and 20–40% of RV systolic pressure and output result from LV contraction.[179] On the other hand, RV failure, particularly when acute, may lead to LV failure. RV dilatation causes pericardial stretching and functional pericardial constriction, which forces the RV to eventually compress the LV in diastole. These changes decrease LV distensibility and preload and may severely reduce cardiac output.

3. *Secondary right-to-left shunt.* Severe RV failure may lead to refractory hypoxemia. The high RA pressure may induce a large right-to-left shunting in patients with PFO.

4. In patients with severe pulmonary hypertension, the PA pressure may decline into the mild/moderate range as RV failure develops. In those patients, a high systolic PA pressure predicts recovery of RV function with therapy and better outcomes than patients with lower systolic PA pressure

---

The Fontan procedure illustrates the concept that, in patients with normal PA pressure, the RV may not be a necessary structure for many years and blood can flow passively from the RA to the PA. Therefore, RV failure is only detrimental if PA pressure is elevated, TR is present (further reducing the forward cardiac output), or severe RV dilatation compresses the LV. The septum maintains its stability and function as long as the RV is not dilated. *In a way, it is better not to have an RV (Fontan) than to have an enlarged, dysfunctional RV.*

As opposed to the adult RV, the thick congenital RV tolerates pressure overload and does not fail (e.g., pulmonic stenosis, Eisenmenger syndrome).

D. Treatment of acute, isolated, or predominant RV failure

- *Respiratory failure with hypoxemia*, often a major culprit of acute RV failure, should be aggressively treated, with mechanical ventilation if needed.
  Underlying causes of RV failure should be treated.
- *Preload management:* In chronic RV failure, mild progressive diuresis (negative balance of 0.5–1.0 liter/day) is very beneficial to reduce RV dilatation, improve RV function, improve functional TR (which is secondary to RV dilatation), and reduce ventricular interdependence, all of which improve cardiac output. High doses of diuretics or a loop–thiazide combination may be needed.[180] Unless left-sided volume overload is also present, aggressive diuresis (>1 liter/day) is avoided, as it may worsen the underfilling of the already small LV cavity.

  In cases of acute RV failure secondary to RV MI or PE, two concepts justify volume loading: (i) a non-dilated RV increases its stroke volume with increasing preload, before reaching the point of ventricular interdependence; (ii) a high CVP does not imply a high preload in acute, de novo, RV failure. The RV compliance curve is shifted leftward, meaning that the CVP increases even if RV volume is normal. Thus, if *RV is not dilated*, give a 500–1000 ml saline load regardless of CVP (even if 12–15 mmHg), as long as pulmonary edema is not present. If there is no hemodynamic response (i.e., increased urine output and BP), or if the RV is dilated along with elevated CVP > 15 mmHg, volume loading should not be continued, as it may lead to further RV dilatation, failure, and hemodynamic compromise.

  At this point, consider inotropes and consider afterload reduction with inhaled nitric oxide. Note that digoxin may also be useful in RV failure.[181]
- *Maintenance of an appropriate systemic systolic blood pressure (SBP) and resistance (SVR)*

As opposed to the failing LV, the failing RV is less tolerant of a low SBP. In LV failure, a low SBP reduces afterload of the exquisitely sensitive LV and may significantly increase cardiac output. The RV, on the other hand, is not favored by a low SBP from an afterload standpoint and, in fact, the RV depends on an adequate SBP for its coronary perfusion. While the LV coronary flow is mostly diastolic, the RV coronary flow is at least 50% systolic, and depends on the gradient between SBP and systolic RV pressure. If the SBP is low in a patient with a high PA pressure, the gradient between SBP and systolic RV pressure is drastically reduced, which reduces RV coronary flow leading to RV ischemia and failure. The ratio of SBP/systolic PA pressure, or SVR/PVR, is an important ratio in RV failure.[182]

Thus, norepinephrine, which increases RV contractility and increases SVR, is often the preferred inotrope in RV failure; it does not have a significant effect on PVR at low/medium doses (<0.5 mcg/kg/min), and thus favorably affects the SVR/PVR ratio.[182]

Systemic vasodilators are poorly tolerated in RV failure because of the reduction of SVR but also because the underfilled LV cannot increase its output to match the vasodilated circulation. Low-dose dobutamine (<10 mcg/kg/min) and milrinone increase RV contractility and reduce PVR; however, they are also systemic vasodilators and thus must be used in conjunction with vasopressors, such as norepinephrine or vasopressin.

- *Afterload reduction (PVR):* Treatment of hypoxemia is key. In addition, inhaled NO, inhaled milrinone, or inhaled epoprostenol may be used. The inhaled forms are less likely to reduce SVR or impair V/Q matching than the systemic forms.
- *Maintain sinus rhythm and AV synchrony:* AF or AV dissociation may have more profound hemodynamic effects in RV failure than LV failure. In RV failure, the LV is small, compressed, and underfilled, which makes it highly dependent on the atrial kick. LA contraction is a major contributor to LV filling and LV output in RV failure (more than in LV failure); also, RA contraction directly raises RV pressure and, thus, flow into the PA. Consider prompt DC cardioversion in AF associated with acute RV shock, even if the rate is reasonably controlled. Also, AV synchronous pacing should be performed in RV shock associated with AV block (temporary atrial and ventricular leads are placed through two separate venous accesses).
  As in decompensated LV failure, an increase in heart rate (80–120 bpm) is often necessary to allow RV filling and emptying through providing more cardiac cycles.
- *Effect of mechanical ventilation:* Mechanical ventilation reduces hypoxia, and thus improves PVR and RV output. However, positive-pressure ventilation with a high pressure or volume compresses the alveolar capillaries and increases PVR, while a very low volume ventilation leads to atelectasis and arterial compression. A strategy of low tidal volume with limited plateau pressure should be implemented.
- *Right-to-left shunting through a PFO* serves to unload the RV, reduce RA pressure, and increase the LV filling and cardiac output. Thus, although this shunt induces hypoxemia (arterial O_2 saturation 80–85%), some degree of shunting improves the cardiac output, the overall oxygen delivery, and the patient's symptoms and functional status and should not be closed. In fact, patients with Eisenmenger syndrome (with inherent R–L shunt) and patients with idiopathic pulmonary hypertension who have a PFO live longer than patients with pulmonary hypertension and no shunt.[183,184] That is why balloon atrial septostomy has been beneficial in cases of refractory right HF.[185] Only excessive shunting, as in patients with very high RA pressure > 20 mmHg and very poor RV function, may drastically reduce pulmonary blood flow and induce severe hypoxemia (overall untoward effect).

QUESTIONS AND ANSWERS

Question 1. A 62-year-old man with a history of HTN, moderate COPD, CKD, and obesity (BMI 37 kg/m²) presents with dyspnea on exertion. Exam does not reveal significant volume overload. Echo shows normal EF, moderate LVH, and LA enlargment. Grade 1 diastolic dysfunction is present with normal LA pressure and PA pressure (E′ is reduced but E/E′ratio is < 8). What is the next step in assessing his dyspnea?
A. BNP
B. Exercise testing or leg raising with echo measurement of E/E′ ratio and PA pressure with exercise
C. Right and left heart catheterization with measurement of PCWP and LVEDP at rest and with leg raising, exercise or adenosine testing
D. Any of the above
E. None of the above. Dyspnea is due to obesity and COPD

Question 2. A 62-year-old man with a history of HTN, moderate COPD, CKD, and obesity (BMI 37 kg/m²) presents with dyspnea on exertion. Exam does not reveal significant volume overload. Echo shows normal LVEF and moderate LVH. LA size is normal. Diastolic function appears normal (normal E′) with normal LA pressure and PA pressure. What is the next step in assessing his dyspnea?
A. BNP
B. Exercise testing or leg raising with echo measurement of E/E′ ratio and PA pressure with exercise
C. Right and left heart catheterization with measurement of PCWP and LVEDP at rest and with leg raising, exercise or adenosine testing
D. Any of the above
E. None of the above. Dyspnea is due to obesity and COPD

Question 3. A 64-year-old man presents with progressive dyspnea on exertion. He has a history of HTN, CKD, and moderate COPD. Cardiac exam reveals a persistently split, loud S_2, heard at the upper but also lower left sternal border; and an early systolic murmur most prominent at the left lower sternal border. He has a left parasternal lift. The left apical impulse is discrete. JVP is elevated at 15 cmH$_2$O, with prominent V waves and Kussmaul's sign. The abdominal exam reveals mild hepatomegaly with a pulsatile liver. Mild peripheral edema is present. Chest X-ray shows enlarged RA and PA, with small pleural effusions but no parenchymal findings. BNP is 400 pg/ml. What is the most likely cause of the patient's presentation?
A. RV failure secondary to primary TR
B. RV failure secondary to pulmonary arterial hypertension
C. RV failure secondary to a shunt
D. Restrictive cardiomyopathy with pulmonary venous hypertension and RV failure
E. Intrinsic RV dysfunction
F. Constrictive pericarditis
G. B, C, or D
H. B or C
I. All of A through F

Question 4. In the patient of Question 3, echo shows enlarged RA and RV with plethoric IVC. PA pressure is 70 mmHg. The LA is enlarged and LV is small and hyperdynamic. No shunt is seen. A chest CT does not show any pulmonary embolus. What is the next step?
A. TEE looking for a left-to-right shunt
B. Pulmonary function testing
C. Sleep study
D. Right and left heart catheterization

Question 5. A 60-year-old man presents with a clinical picture of severe RV failure and anasarca. BP is 85/60, heart rate is 105 bpm, and he has cool extremities with oliguria. On echo, RV is severely dilated, while LV is small with normal EF. Right and left heart catheterization reveals a severely elevated RA pressure ~25 mmHg with a large V wave, and elevated PCWP and LVEDP ~25 mmHg. PA pressure is 75/28 mmHg. Cardiac index is 1.7 l/min/m². During simultaneous RV–LV pressure recording: (i) in diastole, RV and LV end-diastolic pressures are equalized, with LV pressure exceeding RV pressure at times; (ii) in systole, RV and LV peaks are concordant. What is the diagnosis?
A. Restrictive cardiomyopathy with a stiff, failing LV, secondary pulmonary hypertension, and secondary RV failure
B. Constrictive pericarditis
C. Isolated RV failure secondary to pulmonary arterial hypertension. LVEDP is elevated from RV compression

Question 6. How is the patient in Question 5 acutely treated?
A. Diuretic therapy
B. Diuretic and vasodilator therapy
C. Diuretic therapy and inotropic therapy with dobutamine
D. Diuretic therapy and inotropic therapy with norepinephrine
E. Diuretic therapy, inotropic therapy, and pulmonary vasodilators

Question 7. A 56-year-old patient presents with a new diagnosis of HF and LVEF of 20%. His symptoms improve with diuresis and initiation of medical therapy. He has no significant CAD on coronary angiography. What is the likelihood of significant improvement or full recovery of his LVEF in the next 6 months, under proper medical therapy?

Question 8. A 60-year-old with a history of non-ischemic cardiomyopathy (LVEF 25%) presents with ADHF (progressive dyspnea and edema over the last week). He chronically takes furosemide 40 mg BID, carvedilol 6.25 mg BID, and lisinopril. BP is 145/85 mmHg, JVP is 13 cmH₂O. ECG shows AF, rate 125 bpm (newly diagnosed AF). What is the next step?
A. Furosemide 80 mg IV Q8h, digoxin load, and same dose of carvedilol
B. Furosemide 80 mg IV Q8h, digoxin load, and increase carvedilol to 12.5 mg BID
C. Furosemide 80 mg IV Q8h and acute DC cardioversion of AF
D. Furosemide 40 mg IV Q12h and acute DC cardioversion of AF
E. Furosemide 80 mg IV Q12h, digoxin load, and nitroglycerin IV

Question 9. A 60-year-old with a history of non-ischemic cardiomyopathy (LVEF 25%) presents with ADHF (progressive dyspnea and edema over the last week). He chronically takes furosemide 40 mg BID, carvedilol 6.25 mg BID, and lisinopril. BP is 145/85 mmHg, JVP is 13 cmH₂O. ECG shows sinus bradycardia 55 bpm. What is the next step?
A. Furosemide 80 mg IV Q8h, continue same dose of carvedilol
B. Furosemide 80 mg IV Q8h, reduce carvedilol
C. Furosemide 40 mg IV Q12h, reduce carvedilol

Question 10. A 60-year-old with a history of non-ischemic cardiomyopathy (LVEF 25%) presents with ADHF (progressive dyspnea and edema over the last week). He chronically takes furosemide 40 mg BID, carvedilol 6.25 mg BID, and lisinopril 10 mg daily. BP is 98/70 mmHg, heart rate is 85 bpm, JVP is 15 cmH₂O. Creatinine is 2.4 mg/dl (baseline 1.4 mg/dl), and he is drowsy and weak with cool extremities. What is the initial treatment?
A. Furosemide IV and inotropic therapy. Discontinue carvedilol and lisinopril
B. Furosemide IV. Discontinue lisinopril and reduce the dose of carvedilol. Inotropes are initiated in case of poor response to furosemide

Question 11. A 60-year-old with a history of non-ischemic cardiomyopathy (LVEF 25%) presents with ADHF (progressive dyspnea and edema over the last week). He is initiated on a proper dose of diuretic and achieves a proper response (3 liters of urine output). Next day, he is still congested clinically with JVP 12 cmH₂O, but his creatinine rises from 1.5 mg/dl to 1.8 mg/dl. BP is 110/70 mmHg.
A. The patient is over-diuresed. Hold the diuretic therapy.
B. Continue the same diuretic dose
C. Add inotropic therapy

Question 12. A 60-year-old man with ischemic cardiomyopathy and LVEF 20% is started on furosemide 40 mg BID, lisinopril 5 mg, and carvedilol 3.125 mg BID. A week later, he complains of dizziness and fatigue. His JVP is normal with no peripheral edema. His BP is 120/75 mmHg, with significant orthostatic drop. His creatinine rises from a baseline of 1.3 mg/dl to 1.8 mg/dl, BUN rises from 24 mg/dl to 50 mg/dl, and K rises to 5.5 mEq/l. What is the next step?
A. Discontinue lisinopril
B. Reduce the dose of furosemide to 40 mg Qday
C. Reduce furosemide and discontinue lisinopril
D. Hold furosemide then resume it at a lower dose, hold lisinopril for 4 days, then start lisinopril 2.5 mg Qday

Question 13. A 60-year-old man with ischemic cardiomyopathy and LVEF 20% is started on furosemide 40 mg BID, lisinopril 5 mg, and carvedilol 3.125 mg BID. A week later, he complains of mild exertional dyspnea but no dizziness. JVP is normal with no peripheral edema. BP is 120/75 mmHg, without orthostatic drop. His creatinine rises from a baseline of 1.3 mg/dl to 1.6 mg/dl, BUN rises from 24 mg/dl to 29 mg/dl. What is the next step?
A. Discontinue lisinopril
B. Reduce the dose of furosemide to 40 mg Qday
C. Reduce furosemide and discontinue lisinopril

D. Reduce furosemide, hold lisinopril for 4 days, then start lisinopril 5 mg Qday

E. Continue the same regimen

Question 14. A 60-year-old man with ischemic cardiomyopathy and LVEF 20% is started on furosemide 40 mg BID, lisinopril 5 mg, and carvedilol 3.125 mg BID. A week later, he complains of dizziness and fatigue. His JVP is still mildly increased (~8–9 cm), with 1+ peripheral edema. His BP is 105/75 mmHg with a significant orthostatic drop, and heart rate is 60 bpm. His creatinine rises from a baseline of 1.3 mg/dl to 1.7 mg/dl, BUN rises from 24 mg/dl to 32 mg/dl. What is the next step?

A. Discontinue lisinopril

B. Reduce the dose of furosemide to 40 mg Qday

C. Reduce furosemide and discontinue carvedilol and lisinopril

D. Reduce furosemide, hold lisinopril for 4 days, then start lisinopril 2.5 mg Qday

E. Continue furosemide, hold carvedilol, hold lisinopril for 4 days, then start lisinopril 2.5 mg Qday

Question 15. A 69-year-old man with no known cardiac history presents with decompensated HF. ECG shows LVH and ST depression (no Q waves). Echo shows anteroapical dyskinesis with LVEF 25%. The myocardial thickness of the anterior wall is 7 mm. Coronary angiography shows a totally occluded LAD with grade 3 collateral flow and severe RCA disease. Exercise stress testing is performed and shows a large, mainly fixed anteroapical defect with 55% uptake, and mild, reversible inferior defect. The patient walked 3 minutes and experienced chest tightness early on. Beside proper medical therapy, what is the best revascularization option?

A. Revascularization does not improve outcomes at this point

B. Revascularize with CABG without further testing

C. Perform viability testing. Perform CABG only if the anterior wall is viable

Question 16. A 69-year-old man with no known cardiac history presents with decompensated HF. He does not have exertional chest pain. ECG shows anterior Q waves. Echo shows anteroapical dyskinesis with EF of 25%. The myocardial thickness of the anterior wall is 7 mm. Coronary angiography shows a totally occluded LAD with grade 3 collateral flow and severe RCA disease. Stress testing is performed and shows a large, mainly fixed anteroapical defect, and inferior reversible defect. The patient only walked 3 minutes and experienced severe dyspnea and dizziness. Beside proper medical therapy, what is the best revascularization option?

A. Revascularization does not improve outcomes at this point

B. Revascularize with CABG without further testing

C. Perform viability testing with MRI. Perform CABG if the anterior wall is viable

D. Perform viability testing with MRI. Perform CABG if four segments of the anterior or apical wall are deemed viable

Question 17. A 37-year-old man presents with severe chest pain and diffuse ST elevation. A rub is heard on exam. Troponin peaks at 20 ng/ml. Echo shows global hypokinesis with inferior akinesis (EF 25%) and no pericadial effusion. A coronary angiography is performed and shows normal coronary arteries. He develops acute pulmonary edema and severe hypoxia requiring mechanical ventilation. He does not improve with diuresis and develops a shock requiring two vasopressors. What is the next step?

A. IABP, endomyocardial biopsy, and LVAD

B. IABP, LVAD, and cardiac transplant

C. IABP and immunosuppressive drugs

Question 18. A 64-year-old hypertensive man with CKD presents with severe dyspnea and lower extremity edema. On exam, BP is 85/72 mmHg, JVP is > 15 cmH$_2$O, ascites is present. S$_2$ is loud and persistently split, with S$_3$ gallop. ECG shows low QRS voltage in the limb leads and no features of LVH; septal Q waves are present. His echo shows severe LV thickening (septum = 18 mm) with small cavity and normal EF, dilated RV, and biatrial enlargement. What workup and treatment should be performed?

A. This is most likely an advanced stage of hypertensive cardiomyopathy. Diurese. Once stable, initiate carvedilol

B. Endomyocardial biopsy, diuretic therapy

C. Serum and urine immunofixation and fat pad biopsy. If negative, perform endomyocardial biopsy. Gently diurese. Avoid digoxin, ACE-I, and β-blocker in this condition

Question 19. A 50-year-old Mexican man presents with dyspnea on exertion and orthopnea. On exam, he has elevated JVP with a deep Y descent, hepatomegaly, ascites, and peripheral edema. Lungs are clear. Echo shows normal LVEF and LV size, and a dilated IVC. Which of the following initial tests is *not* appropriate?

A. Fat pad biopsy

B. Right and left heart catheterization

C. Chest CT

D. Tuberculin skin testing

E. Coronary angiography

F. Iron studies

Question 20. A 54-year-old man with a history of non-ischemic cardiomyopathy (EF 15% for 5 years) had two admissions for ADHF in the last 4 months. He presents with severe dyspnea and fatigue on exertion. On exam, he is cachectic (BMI 20) and lethargic, with BP 90/70 and pulse 100 bpm. JVP is 8–9 cmH$_2$O. Extremities are cool without peripheral edema. He has MR murmur. Korotkoff sounds are heard throughout the strain phase of Valsalva. Creatinine is 1.7 mg/dl. What is the next step?

A. Discontinue carvedilol and lisinopril

B. Administer intravenous furosemide

C. Right heart catheterization

Question 21. The patient in Question 20 undergoes right heart catheterization, which shows RA pressure of 8 mmHg, PCWP of 18 mmHg, PA pressure of 38/20 mmHg, and cardiac index of 1.7 l/min/m². What is the next step?

A. Cardiopulmonary stress testing, inotropic therapy, and referral for LVAD and transplant

B. Hold β-blocker and diuretic therapy and encourage fluid intake

C. Add intravenous vasodilator then increase lisinopril dose to increase cardiac output

Question 22. The patient improves with inotropic therapy but deteriorates 2 weeks later. SBP is 75–80 mmHg. His cardiac index worsens (1.6 l/min/m²) and his PCWP rises to 30 mmHg despite inotropic therapy. LVAD is placed. What is the likelihood of RV failure after LVAD placement?

Question 23. A 28-year-old man presents with chest pain, palpitations lasting 10 seconds, and mildly elevated troponin I (0.09 ng/ml). No HF is present on exam. ECG shows deep, biphasic anterior T waves. Coronary angiography shows normal coronary arteries. Echo shows normal LVEF and no pericardial effusion. CRP is normal but mild leucocytosis is present. What is the diagnosis, and how should it be confirmed?

A. MI resulting from a plaque rupture that has healed. Perform IVUS

B. Coronary vasospasm. Perform intracoronary acetylcholine testing

C. Mild acute myocarditis. Perform cardiac MRI

Question 24. Three weeks later, the patient of Question 23 presents with prolonged palpitations and dyspnea. ECG shows VT, which is successfully cardioverted. His ECG then shows intermittent Mobitz 2 AV block. EF has deteriorated to 25% (global hypokinesis) and the ventricular walls are unusually thickened. BP is 90/70 mmHg after cardioversion. Beside placing a transvenous pacemaker and initiating amiodarone, what is the most important next step?

A. Cardiac MRI

B. Endomyocardial biopsy

C. EP study and consideration for ICD

Question 25. A 38-year-old man presents with HF. He has a history of HTN and end-stage renal disease requiring dialysis for 2 years. HTN has always been well controlled. Echo shows severe biventricular hypertrophy, biatrial enlargement, restrictive LV filling, and a small pericardial effusion. ECG shows normal voltage in the limb leads, prominent voltage in the precordial leads (no definite LVH), and short PR with delta wave. What is the diagnosis?

A. Hypertensive cardiomyopathy

B. Hypertrophic cardiomyopathy

C. Genetic amyloidosis (transthyretin gene deficiency)

D. Fabry disease

E. B, C, or D

Question 26. Had the patient in Question 25 not had renal failure, what would the most likely diagnosis be?

A. Hypertensive cardiomyopathy

B. Hypertrophic cardiomyopathy

C. Genetic amyloidosis (transthyretin gene deficiency)

D. Fabry disease

E. B, C, or D

Question 27. A 41-year-old woman from Guatemala presents with dyspnea, orthopnea, and severe peripheral edema and ascites. She has a history of tuberculosis and a prior history of heavy menometrorrhagia. She had coronary angiography showing normal coronary arteries 3 years ago. On exam, BP is 110/50, pulse is 100 bpm, JVP is 15 cmH₂O, RV lift is present, S₂ is loud, and 3/6 murmur is heard at the left lower sternal border. Echo shows LVEF of ~45% with mild LV dilatation, marked RV dilatation, severe TR, and systolic PA pressure of 70 mmHg. On catheterization, RA and PCWP are severely elevated and equal (~20 mmHg with V wave of ~30 mmHg), and cardiac index is 5 l/min/m². BNP is 650 pg/ml. What is the most likely diagnosis?

A. Constrictive pericarditis (tuberculosis)

B. Restrictive cardiomyopathy

C. Pulmonary arterial hypertension with secondary RV failure and secondary TR

D. RV failure from intrinsic dysfunction, primary TR, or shunt

E. High-output HF

Question 28. A 50-year-old man presents with syncope followed by severe lightheadedness. He is found to have a monomorphic VT. After successful DC cardioversion, echo shows LVEF of ~35% with inferior wall akinesis. Coronary angiography shows normal coronary arteries. The patient continues to experience breakthroughs of VT despite amiodarone therapy. What is the diagnosis and the next step?

A. Ischemic scar related to prior cocaine use or vasospasm. Perform MRI.

B. Sarcoidosis. Perform endomyocardial biopsy, MRI, or chest CT

C. Severe myocarditis, including giant-cell myocarditis. Perform endomyocardial biopsy or MRI

D. ARVD. Perfrom MRI

E. B or C

Question 29. A 70-year-old woman with chronic systolic HF of ischemic origin presents with progressive dyspnea and edema. She receives chronic therapy with lisinopril, carvedilol, furosemide, and digoxin. Intravenous diuresis is initiated. Dyspnea improves, but the patient starts to experience fatigue, nausea, and anorexia on day 2. She notes a yellow vision once. On exam, BP is 120/75, pulse is 65 bpm, edema has resolved, and JVP is normal. Her creatinine has risen from 1.1 to 1.3 mg/dl and BUN has risen to 25 mg/dl. What is the next step?

A. Hold the diuretic

B. Reduce the dose of carvedilol

C. Check digoxin level 6 hours after a dose and consider digoxin interruption

D. Administer a small saline bolus

Question 30. A 58-year-old man with ischemic cardiomyopathy, EF 20% and multiple hospitalizations with low-output HF is placed on chronic inotropic therapy. ACE-I and β-blockers are discontinued because of hypotension. On right heart catheterization, PCWP is 12 mmHg, and RA pressure is 16 mmHg, cardiac index is 2 l/min/m² at rest (on inotrope therapy). He has LBBB with QRS of 150 ms. What is the best device therapy?

A. LVAD

B. LVAD + RVAD

C. CRT

Question 31. A 65-year-old man presents with progressive dyspnea and fatigue. He has a history of well-controlled HTN. ECG shows sinus rhythm with complete LBBB, and echo shows LVEF of 35–40% with global hypokinesis, and severe pulmonary hypertension. Right heart catheterization confirmed severe pulmonary hypertension (PA pressure 75/35 mmHg) that is precapillary/arterial in nature, unrelated to the left heart disease (PCWP is 12 mmHg). Coronary arteries are normal. MRI shows delayed enhancement of the basal and inferolateral walls with inferior LV aneurysm. What is the most likely diagnosis?

A. Cardiac amyloidosis

B. Cardiac sarcoidosis. ICD is indicated

C. Cardiac sarcoidosis. ICD is not indicated yet, endomyocardial biopsy needs to be performed

D. Idiopathic pulmonary arterial hypertension

E. Hypertensive cardiomyopathy

Question 32. A 62-year-old woman with no prior medical problem presents with chest pain and dizziness after an argument with a cow-orker. She is hypotensive (80/55) and tachycardic (110 bpm). She has a loud mid-systolic murmur at the right upper sternal border. ECG shows 1 mm ST elevation in the anterior leads with T inversion. On catheterization, her coronary arteries are normal. Yet on the left ventriculogram she has anterior akinesis with EF of 30%, moderate MR, and a 45 mmHg pressure gradient between the LV and aorta. What is the next step?

A. This is likely a self-aborted STEMI. Place IABP temporarily for support

B. Place IABP and administer inotropic therapy

C. Check echo for AS and consider AVR ± MVR

D. May administer α-agonist therapy for hypotension. IABP should be avoided. After the patient stabilizes, β-blocker therapy may be started and will improve MR

Question 33. A 33-year-old woman without prior medical history presents with fever and shock state requiring norepinephrine. Bedside echo shows small ventricular chambers with severely reduced left and right ventricular function (LVEF ~20%). The patient remains hypotensive despite norepinephrine and dobutamine. A right heart catheterization shows severely elevated RA and LA pressures (20 mmHg and 30 mmHg, respectively), with a cardiac index of 1.8 l/min/m² despite inotropes. Coronary angiography is normal. What is the diagnosis and next diagnostic step?

Question 34. What is the next therapeutic step for the patient of Question 33?

A. Impella

B. LVAD

C. Extracorporeal biventricular VAD (CentriMag)

D. Venoarterial ECMO

E. C or D

Question 35. A 70-year-old man was recently admitted with HFpEF. His creatinine is 1 mg/dl. He is diuresed and his HTN is well controlled, but he still has dyspnea NYHA III. His medications are furosemide 40 mg once daily, lisinopril, and metoprolol. On exam, he has no edema and JVP is normal. Which of the following is appropriate?

A. Add spironolactone to reduce HF hospitalization

B. Implant a CardioMEMS (PA monitor device). If PA pressure is elevated, increase the dose of diuretic or add a nitrate

C. Increase the diuretic dose

D. A and B

Question 36. A 62-year-old man with a history of HTN (on lisinopril and thiazide) presents with progressive dyspnea and peripheral edema. He is hypoxemic, with BP of 190/110 and a heart rate of 105 (sinus). Troponin is 0.15 ng/ml (2nd set 0.18 ng/ml), creatinine is 1.6 mg/dl, BNP is 1000 pg/ml. ECG shows LVH with lateral ST depression. Echo shows normal EF. Which of the following is *incorrect*?

A. Diurese then perform cardiac catheterization

B. This is acutely decompensated, hypertensive HFpEF. Diurese and administer intravenous NTG for persistent HTN. In the first 24 hours, reinstitute oral antihypertensives and add other drugs to control HTN.

C. The troponin rise is not of coronary etiology

D. Obtain pre-discharge BNP and ensure it drops > 30–50% before discharge

E. After discharge, patient should have follow-up with BNP reassessment. Consider CardioMEMS if class III symptoms persist.

Question 37. Review Chapter 36, Case 5 questions. In brief, a 69-year-old hypertensive, obese woman presents with dyspnea on exertion. Echo shows normal EF and grade 1 diastolic dysfunction. Right heart catheterization shows a normal mean PCWP at rest, but severe rise of PCWP and PA pressure with supine cycling. Cardiac output rose, but not enough, and stroke volume index did not significantly rise with exercise. She became hypoxemic with exercise. All of the following can improve her dyspnea, *except* which one?

A. The two most important interventions are weight loss and HTN control, both of which have lusitropic effects

B. Heart rate reduction with β-blocker therapy improves filling and stroke volume

C. O$_2$ therapy with exercise

D. Add a small dose of furosemide (or raise its dose if she already receives it).

E. Add spironolactone

Answer 1. D. The differential diagnosis of dyspnea includes diastolic HF or a combination of COPD, obesity, and deconditioning. LVH, LA enlargement, and the mild diastolic dysfunction suggest the possibility of diastolic HF. To establish the diagnosis of diastolic HF (beyond just diastolic dysfunction), one must prove high left-sided filling pressures at rest, or if normal at rest, high left-sided filling pressures at stress, whether by echo or catheterization. The mere presence of diastolic dysfunction does not prove diastolic HF. Stress may be performed using exercise testing or passive leg raising. Adenosine infusion is another option in the cath lab (increases LV preload). BNP measurement is an alternative testing. An elevated BNP > 200 pg/ml, along with borderline echo abnormalities (LVH, LA enlargement, grade 1 diastolic dysfunction), provides evidence that LVEDP rises at times and is diagnostic of diastolic HF in the chronic setting (ESC). A BNP that ranges between 35 and 200 pg/ml may be consistent with chronic diastolic HF; BNP < 35 may be used to exclude chronic diastolic HF (ESC).

Answer 2. E. HTN and LVH imply that diastolic HF is a possible cause of the patient's dyspnea. However, the combination of normal LA size and normal diastolic function, especially normal E′, makes diastolic HF extremely unlikely.

Answer 3. G. The loud S$_2$ implies pulmonary hypertension, while the persistent S$_2$ split in inspiration and expiration implies RV failure or RBBB (delayed closure of the pulmonic valve). The left parasternal lift implies RV enlargement. The large JVP V waves, and particularly the pulsatile liver, imply severe TR. Kussmaul's sign, wherein JVP further increases with inspiration, may be seen in constrictive pericarditis, or, commonly, severe RV failure. Causes A through F are all causes of RV failure. In this patient, RV failure is associated with pulmonary arterial or venous hypertension, and thus it is not intrinsic RV dysfunction or primary TR. Constrictive pericarditis is a mimic of RV failure, but severe pulmonary hypertension and large V waves make it unlikely. Also, the elevated BNP makes constrictive pericarditis unlikely. While the patient does not have clinical or X-ray signs of left HF, an overlooked left HFpEF is a common cause of RV failure, particularly at his age and with his history of HTN and CKD (lung findings are frequently absent in chronic left HF).

Answer 4. D. Frequently, HFpEF is characterized by a small and stiff LV, which, despite being hyperdynamic, has a limited filling reserve and thus limited stroke volume reserve. In fact, a small LV does not contradict the diagnosis of HFpEF. Cardiac catheterization will be done to: (1) measure PCWP and LVEDP, seeking a diagnosis of left HF – if left HF is absent, the diagnosis of pulmonary arterial hypertension is made; (2) perform oximetry run to diagnose left-to-right shunt. In the absence of left HF, TEE is reasonable to further investigate a left–right shunt. This patient was eventually diagnosed with a sinus venosus ASD, missed by TTE. Oximetry run confirmed a shunt and TEE made the diagnosis. ASD and anomalous pulmonary venous return are forms of left-to-right shunt that may manifest late in life, as LA pressure rises and leads to more shunting.

Answer 5. A. This is restrictive cardiomyopathy with severely elevated right-and left-sided pressures. RV is dilated and RV failure is more prominent clinically and echocardiographically than LV failure, but the LV is failing as well (LVEDP ≥ RVEDP).

Answer 6. D. The patient has a picture of hypotension and low-output state; he is not likely to respond to standalone diuretic therapy. BP < 110 mmHg is a contraindication to acute vasodilator therapy in decompensated HF. While inotropic therapy will not help the LV, which is small with limited filling rather than limited contractile reserve, it will help the severely dysfunctional RV. More importantly, in a patient whose systolic PA pressure matches the systemic pressure, the RV is not perfused (50% of RV perfusion occurs in systole and depends on the gradient between SBP and RV systolic pressure, which is only 10 mmHg in this case). Thus, inotropic therapy, beside improving RV contractility, must raise systemic pressure to improve RV perfusion, hence the preferred therapy with norepinephrine. Once intropic therapy is started, the patient will respond to diuretic therapy. Diuresis will further improve ventricular perfusion by reducing RVEDP and LVEDP, and improve cardiac output by reducing RV–LV interdependence and functional TR.

Answer 7. 70–75%.

Answer 8. A. The new AF is likely the decompensating factor for HF. However, once HF is decompensated, the atrial kick (if restored) would not contribute much to the ventricular filling (see Figure 4.2, and *Acute heart failure and acutely decompensated heart failure*, Section III). In addition, some degree of tachycardia may be compensatory in ADHF. The best strategy is to treat HF with diuretic therapy, which will indirectly slow AF, and initiate digoxin therapy. In the acute setting, a heart rate < 110 bpm is acceptable; if needed, amiodarone may be added temporarily, the first day, for rate control. Eventually, 1 or 2 days later, once HF has improved, β-blocker therapy may be initiated or up-titrated to achieve a better rate. A few days later, AF may be cardioverted after TEE. The total 24-hour dose of intravenous furosemide used in ADHF is ~2.5 times the chronic oral daily dose. The dose is adjusted according to the diuresis goal (negative balance of 2–3 liters/day). IV nitroglycerin may be administered; however, BP may precipitously fall with diuretic therapy after relieving the distress of pulmonary edema. Nitroglycerin is better reserved for the situation where the patient remains hypertensive after the initial diuretic administration.

Answer 9. B. A patient with ADHF is expected to have a compensatory increase in heart rate. A heart rate of 60 bpm or less is inappropriate and implies a loss of chronotropic reserve. This may be a factor contributing to the HF decompensation. While carvedilol is generally continued in ADHF, it may be reduced in this case of inappropriate bradycardia.

Answer 10. B. The patient has ADHF, wet and cold category, with narrow pulse pressure and acute kidney dysfunction. His SBP is > 90 mmHg, and thus inotropic therapy does not absolutely need to be initiated on admission. Yet, in light of the poor cardiac output, the patient may not respond to diuretic therapy, in which case inotropic therapy may be initiated. Lisinopril needs to be discontinued because of the acute azotemia. Carvedilol needs to be reduced because of the severity of ADHF (low-output state with borderline BP). If an inotrope needs to be started, carvedilol is fully interrupted.

Answer 11. B. The patient is still congested, and thus the rise in creatinine is due to the acute cardiorenal syndrome and congestion itself rather than diuresis. With further diuresis, creatinine level improves in most congested patients. In fact, creatinine level correlates with RA pressure and renal venous afterload more than cardiac output.

Answer 12. D. Note that, as compared to Question 11, this patient is a stable outpatient with no volume overload on exam. The rise in BUN and creatinine likely represents hypovolemia from furosemide. This is evidenced by the dizziness, orthostatic hypotension, and the more striking rise of BUN than creatinine. The rise in BUN and creatinine is aggravated by the initiation of ACE-I. The diuretic may be held for 2 days then resumed at a lower dose. While unlikely to be a culprit for this creatinine rise, lisinopril is still held for a few days to allow renal recovery, then restarted at a lower dose (2.5 mg).

Answer 13. E. Note that, as compared to Question 12, the patient is not dizzy and does not appear hypovolemic. Moreover, the rise in creatinine is within the acceptable range (<0.5 mg/dl, < 50%). Such a rise in creatinine may be related to the low output/low BP/low kidney perfusion state aggravated by ACE-I initiation. This early rise in creatinine after ACE-I initiation is not associated with a loss of benefit from continued ACE-I therapy, and renal function largely recovers on follow-up. The patient is not hypovolemic, so furosemide does not need to be reduced; in some instances, one may choose to reduce the furosemide dose for 1 or 2 days to allow better tolerance of ACE-I initiation.

Answer 14. E. The rise in creatinine is not due to hypovolemia, nor a direct effect of lisinopril. It is due to a symptomatic hypotension that was triggered by the combination of all the drugs. Orthostatic hypotension, in this case, is due to the interruption of the autonomic baroreflex by carvedilol and ACE-I, rather than hypovolemia. Since the patient still shows signs of hypervolemia, furosemide should be continued. Both lisinopril and carvedilol are interrupted to allow a BP rise and renal recovery. Afterwards, a lower dose of lisinopril is initiated. A week later, in the absence of dizziness, carvedilol may be re-initiated. The timing of drug intake should be staggered.

Answer 15. B. In the absence of Q waves or a history of a recent large MI, the anterior wall is likely hibernating rather than infarcted and revascularization is likely helpful. Stress testing may help better select these patients. Large reversible defects imply extensive ischemia and a definite benefit from revascularization. Also, a moderate fixed defect (>50% nuclear uptake), or a moderate fixed defect with angina or ST changes or no Q waves, often implies hibernation and ischemia rather than infarction. Thus, CABG is indicated in this patient.

Answer 16. D. This patient has no angina, no anterior ischemia on stress testing, and has Q waves. This is a subgroup of patients where viability testing may still have a value, particularly MRI viability (MRI being a superior modality that was not used in the STICH trial). Global viability has to be present when deciding about CABG. Global viability implies that four of the dysfunctional segments, in this case anterior segments, are viable (four segments correspond to ~25% of the whole LV).

Answer 17. A. The patient has acute myocarditis with manifestations of pericarditis (rub, pain, ST elevation) and severe HF/cardiogenic shock. This myocarditis is very severe. It may be reversible (fulminant myocarditis) or irreversible (giant-cell myocarditis). It may also be a hypersensitivity eosinophilic myocarditis. IABP needs to be immediately placed for support, and endomyocardial biopsy needs to be done. This patient will need LVAD support as a bridge to recovery (fulminant myocarditis) or bridge to transplant (giant-cell myocarditis). Percutaneous LVAD may be used (Impella). Immunosuppressive drugs may be used if the biopsy reveals giant-cell myocarditis; steroids may be used for eosinophilic myocarditis.

Answer 18. C. The clinical picture suggests severe left and right HF. Echo suggests a restrictive process, which may result from either hypertensive or infiltrative disease. Hypertensive cardiomyopathy is unlikely, as the ECG shows a disproportionately low QRS voltage and pseudo-Q waves. The latter suggest that myocardial thickening results from infiltration rather than hypertrophy. Amyloid cardiomyopathy is suspected. The pressure–volume relationship is very steep, and thus LA pressure may be elevated despite a normal or even reduced LV volume; stroke volume is low because of the limited LV filling. Diuresis may further reduce stroke volume and must be gentle.

Answer 19. E. The exam is consistent with RV failure. This may be due to isolated RV failure (from pulmonary arterial hypertension or shunt), restrictive cardiomyopathy, or constrictive pericarditis. Heart catheterization is useful for the diagnosis of all the prior diagnoses. Fat pad biopsy (amyloidosis) and iron studies (hemochromatosis) are useful for the diagnosis of restrictive cardiomyopathy. Chest CT and tuberculin testing are useful for the diagnosis of constrictive pericarditis and pulmonary disease. Coronary angiography is not useful here.

Answer 20. C. The patient has a cold picture without clear congestion on exam (possibly dry and cold). Cardiac output is significantly reduced, as evidenced by the narrow pulse pressure, tachycardia, lethargy/fatigue, cachexia, and rise in creatinine. Right heart catheterization helps confirm the low cardiac output and define his filling pressures (→ need to hold the diuretic if filling pressures are low vs. need for inotropes).

Answer 21. A. The patient's right filling pressure is normal while the left is minimally elevated. His symptoms are due to the reduced cardiac output. In fact, beside the low cardiac output at rest, the cardiac output reserve is severely impaired with inability to augment cardiac output with exertion. Cardiopulmonary stress testing will confirm this inability to increase cardiac output and O_2 consumption, which would remain < 14 ml/kg/min at anaerobic threshold. At this stage, since inotropic therapy is considered, carvedilol may be withheld. The issue is cardiac function rather than hypovolemia, so that holding the diuretic or administering fluid will not help. The lack of BP decline with Valsalva implies that the LV is at the flat portion of the Starling curve and is not fluid-responsive. Vasodilators are unlikely to be tolerated in patients with such limited cardiac output reserve. Vasodilatation without a capacity to raise cardiac output leads to severe hypotension.

Answer 22. RV failure is a common complication after LVAD placement and is predicted by the baseline RV function. In this case, RA pressure is < 0.65 × PCWP, and RV stroke work index, a measure of the overall RV performance, is > 300 (stroke work index = stroke volume index × [mean PA – RA pressure] = 374). Thus, RV failure is not likely.

Answer 23. C. The patient has acute myocarditis presenting as a chest pain syndrome (pericarditis syndrome). It is mild as EF is normal and no HF is present. A and B may explain the patient's presentation, but are less likely in light of the normal coronary arteries. The ECG of myocarditis may show diffuse pericarditic findings, but may also show focal findings and a pseudoinfarction pattern as in this case (Q waves and focal ST elevations may be seen).

Answer 24. B. The severe, rapidly progressive myocarditis with VT and AV block in a young patient is concerning for giant-cell myocarditis. The differential diagnosis also includes cardiac sarcoidosis, necrotizing eosinophilic myocarditis, and fulminant non-giant-cell myocarditis, which are more likely to recover after supportive therapy. The thick walls are consistent with the edema of hyperacute myocarditis. He has a class I indication for endomyocardial biopsy (sensitivity of 85% for giant-cell myocarditis). If giant-cell myocarditis is confirmed, a downhill course is expected, and thus immunosuppressive therapy is initiated and VAD and cardiac transplantation are considered. If lymphocytic myocarditis is found (clinically fulminant form), improvement is expected but the patient may require aggressive hemodynamic support.

Answer 25. D.

Answer 26. E. Ventricular hypertrophy at a young age, without severe HTN, should suggest hypertrophic or infiltrative cardiomyopathy, rather than hypertensive cardiomyopathy, especially when hypertrophy is biventricular. The accessory pathway is further suggestive of a primary cardiomyopathy. The ECG is consistent with hypertrophic cardiomyopathy or Fabry (high voltage) rather than amyloidosis. Renal failure may be seen in systemic amyloidosis and in Fabry disease, but not in genetic amyloidosis.

Answer 27. E. The patient has congestive signs of right HF, which may be seen with any of the cases A through E. However, the wide pulse pressure is only characteristic of a high-output HF. Catheterization shows biventricular failure with equalization of RA and PCWP. This may be seen with constrictive pericarditis or restrictive cardiomyopathy; however, both conditions are characterized by a low cardiac output. Also, constrictive pericarditis is unlikely in the presence of large V waves, severe pulmonary hypertension, and elevated BNP. High-output HF may be due to chronic severe anemia. TSH and thiamine need to be checked, and fistulas should be sought by physical exam, especially at the site of the prior femoral access.

Answer 28. E. The patient has a non-ischemic cardiomyopathy that is prone to frequent recurrences of VT. This is most suggestive of one of the following four entities: hyperacute myocarditis, sarcoidosis, ARVD, or Chagas disease. ARVD is unlikely in the absence of RV involvement. Segmental wall motion abnormalities may be seen with any non-ischemic cardiomyopathy, especially sarcoidosis, myocarditis, or Chagas disease.

Answer 29. C. The patient's fatigue and creatinine rise may be related to excessive diuresis. However, it is more likely that, with diuresis and the rise in creatinine, less digoxin is excreted and the patient is experiencing digoxin toxicity (nausea, visual halos). This should always be considered in a patient receiving chronic digoxin therapy who is admitted with an acute condition. Older women with a small body mass are particularly susceptible to the rise in digoxin level. In fact, digoxin level should have been checked before symptoms of toxicity developed. If digoxin level is > 1.1 ng/ml, one or two doses are held and a lower maintenance dose is initiated.

Answer 30. B. CRT is beneficial in patients with class IV symptoms who are still ambulatory. CRT is not beneficial in an unstable, inotrope-dependent patient. RA pressure is higher than PCWP, implying severe RV failure. This is a contraindication to isolated LVAD therapy, as RV failure will worsen following LVAD placement.

Answer 31. B. LBBB may be seen with any cardiomyopathy. However, the basal delayed enhancement is highly suggestive of cardiac sarcoidosis. In context, the pulmonary arterial hypertension also supports the diagnosis of sarcoidosis. Endomyocardial biopsy is poorly sensitive for sarcoidosis (~25%), as the septal involvement is basal. The most common cause of death is arrhythmia, and ICD is indicated whenever cardiac involvement is evident, even if EF > 35%. Chest CT is indicated to look for noncardiac involvement.

Answer 32. D. The patient has takotsubo cardiomyopathy, with ECG changes mimicking STEMI and a clinical presentation mimicking ACS and cardiogenic shock. The hypercontractile LV base leads to LVOT obstruction and a sucking effect on the anterior mitral leaflet, hence the MR. The murmur and pressure gradient are due to dynamic LVOT obstruction, not AS (the lack of aortic valve calcium and the shape of the LV-aortic tracings help make that distinction). Inotropic therapy and afterload reduction (e.g., IABP) will worsen LVOT obstruction, hypotension, and MR in this case. If needed, α-agonist may be used until the patient stabilizes. These patients typically stabilize quickly.

Answer 33. The patient likely has severe, progressive myocarditis: either lymphocytic fulminant myocarditis (will eventually reverse) or giant-cell myocarditis (will keep progressing). An endomyocardial biopsy is indicated.

Answer 34. E. The patient is in refractory cardiogenic shock with biventricular failure. Impella, a form or percutaneous LVAD, only supports the LV. In this patient, biventricular support is preferred. Temporary devices are preferred to implantable devices, as the condition may be reversible (bridge to recovery or bridge to decision). ECMO may be used for a few days, while CentriMag may be used for weeks. CentriMag requires surgical placement of the cannulae in the cardiac chambers.

Answer 35. D. The TOPCAT trial strongly suggests that spironolactone reduces HF hospitalization in HFpEF. In a patient who appears euvolemic clinically, increasing the diuretic dose should be guided by objective measurement of PA pressure or left-sided filling pressure, or BNP, rather than just symptoms.

Answer 36. A. The patient has acutely decompensated, hypertensive HFpEF. The troponin rises to a mild degree (<0.5–1 ng/ml) without a typical rise-and-fall pattern (<20–50%) and without other features supportive of NSTEMI. The ST depression is consistent with LVH strain pattern. Ischemia is secondary to HF and HTN, rather than the cause of HF.

Answer 37. B. The LV cavity is small and stiff and is unable to dilate and accept the increased venous return (limited preload reserve). It is unable to use the Frank–Starling mechanism, wherein a higher preload would lead to a rise of stroke volume. It does not accept preload, which backs up in the pulmonary circulation. The LV is stiff and is unlikely to increase its preload with β-blocker therapy. Heart rate reduction will likely worsen the patient's symptoms, as the rise of cardiac output is totally dependent on heart rate rather than stroke volume. Diuretic therapy would prevent some of the exertional rise in filling pressures and improve dyspnea. Spironolactone has the additional benefit of improving LV diastolic function (AldoHF). Exertional hypoxemia may be partly related to HF, but is mostly related to a lack of appropriate rise of ventilation during exercise (obesity).

References

1. Stevenson LW, Perloff JK. The limited reliability or physical signs for estimating hemodynamics in chronic heart failure. JAMA 1989: 261: 884–8.
2. Chakko S, Woska D, Martinez H, et al. Clinical, radiographic, and hemodynamic correlations in chronic congestive heart failure: conflicting results may lead to inappropriate care. Am J Med 1991; 90: 353–9.
3. Butman SM, Ewy GA, Standen JR, et al. Bedside cardiovascular examination in patients with severe chronic heart failure: importance of rest or inducible jugular venous distension. J Am Coll Cardiol 1993; 22: 968–74.
4. Drazner MH, Hamilton MA, Fonarow G, et al. Relation between right and left-sided filling pressures in 1000 patients with advanced heart failure. J Heart Lung Transpl 1999; 18: 1126–32.

   Sensitivity (Se) and specificity (Sp) of elevated JVP for predicting elevated PCWP: Chakko: Se 50%, Sp > 90%. Stevenson: Se 55%, Sp 100%. Butman: Se 80%, Sp 80–93%. Drazner: Se 85%, Sp ~94%. Overall, there is 80% correlation between PCWP and RA pressure.

5. Marcus GM, Gerber IL, McKeown BH, et al. Association between phonocardiographic third and fourth heart sounds and objective measures of left ventricular function. JAMA 2005; 293: 2238–44.
6. Cotter G, Felker GM, Adams KF, et al. The pathophysiology of acute heart failure: is it all about fluid accumulation? Am Heart J 2008; 155: 9–18.
7. Paulus WJ, Tschope C, Sanderson JE, et al.; European Society of Cardiology. How to diagnose diastolic heart failure: a consensus statement on the diagnosis of heart failure with normal left ventricular ejection fraction by the Heart Failure and Echocardiography Associations of the European Society of Cardiology. Eur Heart J 2007; 28: 2539–50.
8. Felker GM, Shaw LK, O'Connor CM. A standardized definition of ischemic cardiomyopathy for use in clinical research. J Am Coll Cardiol 2002; 39: 210–18.
9. Felker CM, Thompson RE, Hare JM, et al. Underlying causes and long-term survival in patients with initially unexplained cardiomyopathy. N Engl J Med 2000: 342: 1077–84.
10. Gandhi SK, Powers JC, Nomeir AM, et al. The pathogenesis of acute pulmonary edema associated with hypertension. N Engl J Med 2001; 344: 17–22.
11. McNamara DM, Holubkov R, Starling RC, et al. Controlled trial of intravenous immune globulin in recent-onset dilated cardiomyopathy. Circulation 2001; 103; 2254–9.
12. Basuray A, French B, Ky B, et al. Heart failure with recovered ejection fraction: clinical description, biomarkers, and outcomes. Circulation 2014; 129: 2380–7.
13. Shah AM, Shah SJ, Anand IS, et al. Cardiac structure and function in heart failure with preserved ejection fraction. Circ Heart Fail 2014; 7: 104–15.
14. O'Brien KP, Higgs LM, Glancy DL, Epstein SE. Hemodynamic accompaniments of angina. Circulation 1969; 39: 735–43.
15. Massie BM, Carson PE, McMurray JJ, et al. Irbesartan in patients with heart failure and preserved ejection fraction. N Engl J Med 2008; 359: 2456–67. *CAD is the cause of 25% of HFpEF.*
16. Meta-analysis Global Group in Chronic Heart Failure (MAGGIC). The survival of patients with heart failure with preserved or reduced left ventricular ejection fraction: an individual patient data meta-analysis. Eur Heart J 2012; 33: 1750–7.
17. Richardson P, McKenna W, Bristow M, et al. Report of the 1995 World Health Organization/International Society and Federation of Cardiology Task Force on the Definition and Classification of Cardiomyopathies. Circulation 1996; 93: 841–2.
18. Ammash NM, Seward JB, Bailey KR, et al. Clinical Profile and Outcome of Idiopathic Restrictive Cardiomyopathy. Circulation 2000; 101: 2490–6.
19. Patel AR, Dubrey SW, Mendes LA, et al. Right ventricular dilation in primary amyloidosis: an independent predictor of survival. Am J Cardiol 1997; 80: 486–92.
20. Falk RH. Diagnosis and management of the cardiac amyloidosis. Circulation 2005; 112: 2047–60.
21. Kasai T, Bradley TD. Obstructive sleep apnea and heart failure. Pathophysiologic and therapeutic implications. J Am Coll Cardiol 2011; 57: 119–27.
22. Medi C, Kalman JM, Haqqani H, et al. Tachycardia-mediated cardiomyopathy secondary to focal atrial tachycardia. J Am Coll Cardiol 2009; 53: 1791–7.
23. Redfield MM, Kay GN, Jenkins LS, et al. Tachycardia-related cardiomyopathy: a common cause of ventricular dysfunction in patients with atrial fibrillation referred for atrioventricular ablation. Mayo Clin Proc 2000; 75: 790–5.
24. Simantirakis EN, Koutalas EP, Vardas PE. Arrhythmia-induced cardiomyopathies: the riddle of the chicken and the egg still unanswered? Europace 2012; 14: 466–73.

BNP

25. Vasan RS, Benjamin EJ, Larson MG, et al. Plasma natriuretic peptides for community screening for left ventricular hypertrophy and systolic dysfunction: the Framingham heart study. JAMA 2002; 288: 1252–9.

26. Lubien E, DeMaria A, Krishnaswamy P, et al. Utility of B-natriuretic peptide in detecting diastolic dysfunction: comparison with Doppler velocity recordings. Circulation 2002; 105: 595–601.

27. Dokainish H, Zoghbi WA, Lakkis NM, et al. Optimal noninvasive assessment of left ventricular filling pressures. A comparison of tissue doppler echocardiography and B-type natriuretic peptide in patients with pulmonary artery catheters. Circulation 2004; 109: 2432–9.

28. Maisel A, Mueller C, Adams K Jr, et al. State of the art: using natriuretic peptide levels in clinical practice. Eur J Heart Fail 2008; 10: 824–39.

29. Kociol RD, McNulty SE, Hernandez AF, et al. Markers of decongestion, dyspnea relief, and clinical outcomes among patients hospitalized with acute heart failure. Circ Heart Fail 2013; 6: 240–5.

30. Jourdain P, Jondeau G, Funck F, et al. Plasma brain natriuretic peptide-guided therapy to improve outcome in heart failure: the STARS-BNP Multicenter Study. J Am Coll Cardiol 2007; 49: 1733–9. *Also PROTECT trial, JACC 2011, focus the titration on non-diuretic therapies; TIMES-CHF trial.*

31. Porapakkham P, Porapakkham P, Zimmet H, et al. B-type natriuretic peptide-guided heart failure therapy: a metaanalysis. Arch Intern Med 2010; 170: 507–14.

32. Ponikowski P, Voors AA, Anker SD, et al. 2016 ESC Guidelines for the diagnosis and treatment of acute and chronic heart failure.Eur Heart J 2016 May 20. pii: ehw128. [Epub ahead of print]

33. Lima RSL, Watson DD, Goode AR, et al. Incremental value of combined perfusion and function over perfusion alone by gated SPECT myocardial perfusion imaging for detection of severe three vessel coronary artery disease. J Am Coll Cardiol 2003; 42: 64–70.

34. Melikian N, De Bondt P, Tonino O, et al. Fractional flow reserve and myocardial perfusion imaging in patients with angiographic multivessel coronary artery disease. JACC Cardiovasc Interv 2010; 3: 307–14.

35. Burgess MI, Jenkins C, Sharman JE, Marwick TH. Diastolic stress echocardiography: hemodynamic validation and clinical significance of estimation of ventricular filling pressure with exercise. J Am Coll Cardiol 2006; 47: 1891–900.

36. Yancy CW, Jessup M, Bozkurt B, et al. 2013 ACCF/AHA guideline for the management of heart failure. Circulation 2013; 128: e240–327.

Revascularization in ischemic cardiomyopathy, viability testing

37. Velazquez EJ, Lee KL, Deja MA, et al.; STICH Investigators. Coronary-artery bypass surgery in patients with left ventricular dysfunction, N Engl J Med 2011; 364: 1607–16.

38. Bonow RO, Maurer G, Lee KL, et al.; STICH Investigators. Myocardial viability and survival in ischemic left ventricular dysfunction, N Engl J Med 2011; 364: 1617–25.

Regional vs. global viability

39. Schinkel AFL, Bax JJ, Poldermans D, et al. Hibernating myocardium: diagnosis and patient outcomes. Current Problems in Cardiology 2007; 32: 375–410. *Most important reference.*

40. Hanekom L1, Jenkins C, Jeffries L, et al. Incremental value of strain rate analysis as an adjunct to wall-motion scoring for assessment of myocardial viability by dobutamine echocardiography: a follow-up study after revascularization. Circulation 2005; 112: 3892–900.

41. Haas F, Haehnel CJ, Picker W, et al. Preoperative positron emission tomographic viability assessment and perioperative and postoperative risk in patients with advanced ischemic heart disease. J Am Coll Cardiol 1997; 30: 1693–700.

42. Bax JJ, Poldermans D, Elhendy A, et al.Improvement of left ventricular ejection fraction, heart failure symptoms and prognosis after revascularization in patients with chronic coronary artery disease and viable myocardium detected by dobutamine stress echocardiography. J Am Coll Cardiol 1999; 34: 163–9.

43. Piscione F, De Luca G, Perrone-Filardi P, et al.Relationship between contractile reserve, Tl-201 uptake, and collateral angiographic circulation in collateral-dependent myocardium: implications regarding the evaluation of myocardial viability. J Nucl Cardiol 2003; 10: 17–27.

44. Perrone-Filardi P, Pace L, Prastaro M, et al. Assessment of myocardial viability in patients with chronic coronary artery disease: rest-4-hour-24-hour 201Tl tomography versus dobutamine echocardiography. Circulation 1996; 94: 2712–19.

45. Chareonthaitawee P, Gersh BJ, Araoz PA, Gibbons RJ. Revascularization in severe left ventricular dysfunction: the role of viability testing. J Am Coll Cardiol 2005; 46: 567–74.

46. Jeon H, Shah GA, Diwan A, et al. Lack of pathologic Q waves: a specific marker of viability in myocardial hibernation. Clin Cardiol 2008; 31: 372–7.

47. Delewi R, Ijff G, van de Hoef TP, et al. Pathological Q waves in myocardial infarction in patients treated by primary PCI. JACC Cardiovasc Imaging 2013; 6: 324–31.

48. Chia KKM, Picard MH, Skopicki HA, Hung J. Viability of hypokinetic segments. Influence of tethering from adjacent segments. Echocardiography 2002; 19: 475–82.

49. Shah DJ, Kim HW, James O, et al. Prevalence of regional myocardial thinning and relationship with myocardial scarring in patients with coronary artery disease. JAMA 2013; 309: 909–18.

50. Buckley O, Di Carli M. Predicting benefit from revascularization in patients with ischemic heart failure. Imaging of myocardial ischemia and viability. Circulation 2011; 123: 444–50.

51. Sabia PJ, Powers ER, Ragosta M, et al: An association between collateral blood flow and myocardial viability in patients with recent myocardial infarction. N Engl J Med 1992; 327: 1825–31.

52. Kozman H, Cook JR, Wiseman AH, et al. Presence of angiographic coronary collaterals predicts myocardial recovery after coronary bypass surgery in patients with severe left ventricular dysfunction. Circulation 1998; 98 (19 Suppl): II57–61.

53. Ragosta M, Beller GA, Watson DD, Kaul S, Gimple LW. Quantitative planar rest-redistribution 201Tl imaging in detection of myocardial viability and prediction of improvement in left ventricular function after coronary bypass surgery in patients with severely depressed left ventricular function. Circulation 1993; 87: 1630–41.

54. Pagano D, Bonser RS, Townend JN, et al. Predictive value of dobutamine echocardiography and positron emission tomography in identifying hibernating myocardium in patients with postischaemic heart failure. Heart 1998; 79: 281–8.

55. Chareonthaitawee P, Gersh BJ, Panza JA. Is viability testing still relevant in 2012? JACC Cardiovasc Imaging 2012; 5: 550–8.

56. Marwick TH. Stress echocardiography. Heart 2003; 89: 113–18.

57. Samady H, Elefteriades JA, Abbott BG, et al. Coronary revascularization for ischemic cardiomyopathy is not associated with worse outcomes. Circulation 1999; 100: 1298–304.

58. Weiner DA, Ryan TJ, McCabe CH, et al. The role of exercise testing in identifying patients with improved survival after coronary artery bypass surgery, J Am Coll Cardiol 1986; 8: 741–8.

59. Rogers WJ, Bourassa MG, Andrews TC, et al. The Asymptomatic Cardiac Ischemia Pilot Study (ACIP) study: outcome at one year for patients with asymptomatic cardiac ischemia randomized to medical therapy or revascularization, J Am Coll Cardiol 1995; 26: 594–605.

60. Hachamovitch R, Hayes SW, Friedman JD, Cohen I, Berman DS. Comparison of the short-term survival benefit associated with revascularization compared with medical therapy in patients with no prior coronary artery disease undergoing stress myocardial perfusion single photon emission computed tomography, Circulation 2003; 107: 2900–7.

61. Kitsiou AN, Srinivan G, Quyyumi AA, et al. Stress-induced reversible and mild to moderate irreversible thallium defects: Are they equally accurate for predicting recovery of regional left ventricular function after revascularization? Circulation 1998; 98: 501–8.

62. De Bruyne B, Pijls NH, Bartunek J, et al. Fractional flow reserve in patients with prior myocardial infarction. Circulation 2001; 104: 157–62.

63. Hendel RC. Interpretation of myocardial perfusion imaging. In: Heller GV, Hendel RC. Nuclear Cardiology: Practical Applications. new York: McGraw Hill, 2004.

64. Liu P, Kiess MC, Okada RD, et al. The persistent defect on exercise thallium imaging and its fate after myocardial revascularization: does it represent scar or ischemia? Am Heart J 1985; 110: 996–1001.

65. Panza JA, Holly TA, Asch FM, et al. Inducible myocardial ischemia and outcomes in patients with coronary artery disease and left ventricular dysfunction. J Am Coll Cardiol 2013; 61: 1860–70.

66. Hochman JS, Lamas GA, Buller CE, et al. Coronary intervention for persistent occlusion after myocardial infarction. N Engl J Med 2006; 355: 2395–407.

ACE-I

67. CONSENSUS Trial Study Group. Effects of enalapril on mortality in severe congestive heart failure: results of the Cooperative North Scandinavian Enalapril Survival Study (CONSENSUS). N Engl J Med 1987; 316: 1429–35.

68. SOLVD Investigators. Effect of enalapril on mortality and the development of heart failure in asymptomatic patients with reduced left ventricular ejection fractions. N Engl J Med 1992; 327: 685–91.

69. SOLVD Investigators. Effect of enalapril on survival in patients with reduced left ventricular ejection fractions and congestive heart failure. N Engl J Med 1991; 325: 293–302.

70. Narang R, Swedberg K, Cleland JGF. What is the ideal study design for evaluation of treatment for heart failure? Insights from trials assessing the effect of ACE-inhibitors on exercise capacity Eur Heart J 1996; 17: 120–34. *Improvement of exercise duration with ACE-I.*

ARB and other ACE-I data

71. Granger CB, McMurray JJ, Yusuf S, et al. Effects of candesartan in patients with chronic heart failure and reduced left-ventricular systolic function intolerant to angiotensin-converting-enzyme inhibitors: the CHARM-Alternative trial. Lancet 2003; 362: 772–6.

72. McMurray JJ, Ostergren J, Swedberg K, et al. Effects of candesartan in patients with chronic heart failure and reduced left ventricular systolic function taking angiotensin-converting enzyme inhibitors: the CHARM-Added trial. Lancet 2003; 362: 767–71.

73. Cohn JN, Tognoni G. A randomized trial of the angiotensin-receptor blocker valsartan in chronic heart failure. N Engl J Med 2001; 345: 1667–75. *Val HeFT trial.*

74. Testani JM, Kimmel SE, Dries DL, Coca SG. Prognostic importance of early worsening renal function after initiation of angiotensin-converting enzyme inhibitor therapy in patients with cardiac dysfunction. Circ Heart Fail 2011; 4: 685–91. *Data from SOLVD trial.*

75. Packer M, Poole-Wilson PA, Armstrong PW, et al. Comparative effects of low and high doses of the angiotensin-converting enzyme inhibitor, lisinopril, on morbidity and mortality in chronic heart failure. Circulation 1999; 100: 2312–18. *ATLAS trial: in comparison with 2.5–5 mg of lisinopril, 30–40 mg of lisinopril non-significantly reduced mortality by 8%; it significantly reduced HF hospitalization by 24%.*

β-Blockers

76. Hjalmarson A, Goldstein S, Fagerberg B, et al,. Effects of controlled- release metoprolol on total mortality, hospitalizations, and well-being in patients with heart failure: the Metoprolol CR/XL-Randomized Intervention Trial in congestive heart failure (MERIT-HF). JAMA 2000; 283: 1295–302.

77. Packer M, Coats AJ, Fowler MB, et al. Effect of carvedilol on survival in severe chronic heart failure. N Engl J Med 2001; 344: 1651–8. *COPERNICUS.*

78. The Cardiac Insufficiency Bisoprolol Study II (CIBIS-II): a randomised trial. Lancet 1999; 353: 9–13.

79. Gilbert EM, Abraham WT, Olsen S, et al. Comparative hemodynamic, left ventricular functional, and antiadrenergic effects of chronic treatment with metoprolol versus carvedilol in the failing heart. Circulation 1996; 94: 2817–25.

80. M Metra, R Giubbini, S Nodari, et al. Differential effects of beta-blockers in patients with heart failure: a prospective, randomized, double-blind comparison of the long-term effects of metoprolol versus carvedilol. Circulation 2000; 102: 546–51.

81. Doughty RN, Whalley GA, Walsh HA, et al. Effects of carvedilol on left ventricular remodeling after acute myocardial infarction: the CAPRICORN Echo Substudy. Circulation 2004; 109: 201–6.

82. Anand IS, Tam SW, Rector TS, et al. Influence of blood pressure on the effectiveness of a fixed-dose combination of isosorbide dinitrate and hydralazine in the African-American Heart Failure Trial. J Am Coll Cardiol 2007; 49: 32–9.

83. Meredith PA, Ostergren J, Anand IS, et al. Clinical outcomes according to baseline blood pressure in patients with a low ejection fraction in the CHARM Program. J Am Coll Cardiol 2008; 52: 2000–7.

84. Rouleau JL, Roeker EB, Tendera M, et al. Influence of pretreatment systolic blood pressure on the effect of carvedilol in patients with severe chronic heart failure : The Carvedilol Prospective Randomized Cumulative Survival (COPERNICUS) study. J Am Coll Cardiol 2004; 43: 1423–8.

85. Fonarow GC, Abraham WT, Albert NM, et al. Influence of beta-blocker continuation or withdrawal on outcomes in patients hospitalized with heart failure: findings from the OPTIMIZE-HF program. J Am Coll Cardiol 2008; 52: 190–9.

86. Bristow MR., Gilbert EM, Abraham WT, et al. Carvedilol produces dose-related improvements in left ventricular function and survival in subjects with chronic heart failure. MOCHA Investigators. Circulation 1996; 94: 2807–16.

87. Wikstrand J, Hjalmarson A, Waagstein F, et al. Dose of metoprolol CR/XL and clinical outcomes in patients with heart failure: analysis of the Experience in Metoprolol CR/XL Randomized Intervention Trial in Chronic Heart Failure (MERIT-HF). J Am Coll Cardiol 2002; 40: 491–8.

88. Simon T, Mary-Krause M, Funck-Brentano C, et al. Bisoprolol dose–response relationship in patients with congestive heart failure: a subgroup analysis in the cardiac insufficiency bisoprolol study (CIBIS II). Eur Heart J 2003; 24: 552–9.

89. Fiuzat M, Wojdyla D, Pina I, et al. Heart rate or beta-blocker dose? Association with outcomes in ambulatory heart failure patients with systolic dysfunction: results from the HF-ACTION Trial. JACC Heart Fail 2016; 4: 109–15. *Only β-blocker dose was associated with mortality reduction on adjusted analysis. The combination of low β-blocker dose and high HR is associated with the worst outcomes.*

90. McAlister FA, Wiebe N, Ezekowitz JA, et al. Meta-analysis: beta-blocker dose, heart rate reduction, and death in patients with heart failure. Ann Int Med 2009; 150: 784–94. *β-Blocker benefit correlates with heart rate reduction rather than dose (≠ reference 89).*
91. Swedberg K, Komadja M, Bohm M, et al. Ivabradine and outcomes in chronic heart failure (SHIFT): a randomized, placebo-controlled trial. Lancet 2010; 376: 875–85.

Aldosterone antagonists

92. Pitt B, Zannad F, Remme WJ, et al. The effect of spironolactone on morbidity and mortality in patients with severe heart failure. Randomized Aldactone Evaluation Study Investigators. N Engl J Med 1999; 341: 709–17.
93. van Vliet AA, Donker AJ, Nauta JJ, Verheugt FW. Spironolactone in congestive heart failure refractory to high-dose loop diuretic and low-dose angiotensin-converting enzyme inhibitor. Am J Cardiol 1993; 71: 21A–28A.
94. Zannad F, McMurray JJV, Krum H, et al. Eplerenone in patients with systolic heart failure and mild symptoms. N Engl J Med 2011; 364: 11–21.
95. Pitt B, Remme W, Zannad F, et al. Eplerenone, a selective aldosterone blocker, in patients with left ventricular dysfunction after myocardial infarction. N Engl J Med 2003; 348: 1309–21.
96. Vardeny O, Wu DH, Desai A, et al. Influence of baseline and worsening renal function on efficacy of spironolactone in patients With severe heart failure: insights from RALES (Randomized Aldactone Evaluation Study). J Am Coll Cardiol 2012; 60: 2082–9.
97. Bansal S, Lindenfeld J, Schrier RW. Sodium retention in heart failure and cirrhosis: potential role of natriuretic doses of mineralocorticoid antagonist? Circ Heart Fail 2009; 2: 270–6.

Neprilysin antagonist, ARB

98. McMurray JJV, Packer M, Desai AS, et al. Angiotensin-neprilysin inhibition versus enalapril in heart failure. N Engl J Med 2014; 371; 993–1004.

Hydralazine, nitrates

99. Cohn JN, Archibald DG, Ziesche S, et al. Effect of vasodilator therapy on mortality in chronic congestive heart failure: results of a Veterans Administration cooperative study. N Engl J Med 1986; 314: 1547–52.
100. Cohn JN, Johnson G, Ziesche S, et al. A comparison of enalapril with hydralazine-isosorbide dinitrate in the treatment of chronic congestive heart failure. N Engl J Med 1991; 325: 303–10.
101. Carson P, Ziesche S, Johnson G, Cohn JN. Racial differences in response to therapy for heart failure: analysis of the vasodilator-heart failure trials. J Card Fail 1999; 5: 178–87.
102. Cole RT, Kalogeropoulos AP, Georgiopoulou VV, et al. Hydralazine and isosorbide dinitrate in heart failure: historical perspective, mechanisms, and future directions. Circulation 2011; 123: 2414–22.
103. Taylor AL, Ziesche S, Yancy C, et al. Combination of isosorbide dinitrate and hydralazine in blacks with heart failure. N Engl J Med. 2004; 351: 2049–57.

Diuretics

104. Brater DC. Diuretic therapy. N Engl J Med 1998; 339: 387–95.
105. Dussol B, Moussi-Frances J, Morange S, et al. A randomized trial of furosemide vs hydrochlorothiazide in patients with chronic renal failure and hypertension. Nephrol Dial Transplant 2005) 20: 349–53.
106. Knauf H, Mutschler E. Diuretic effectiveness of hydrochlorothiazide and furosemide alone and in combination in chronic renal failure. J Cardiovasc Pharmacol 1995; 26: 394–400.
107. Testani JM, Cappola TP, Brensinger CM, Shannon RP, Kimmel SE. Interaction between loop diuretic-associated mortality and blood urea nitrogen concentration in chronic heart failure. J Am Coll Cardiol 2011; 58: 375–82.
108. Damman K, Chuen MJN, MacFadyen RJ, et al. Volume status and diuretic therapy in systolic heart failure and the detection of early abnormalities. J Am Coll Cardiol 2011; 57: 2233–41. *Diuretic favorably affects tubular function in stable HF.*

Digoxin

109. Sathore SS, Curtis JP, Wang Y, Bristow MR, Krumholz HM. Association of serum digoxin concentration and outcomes in patients with heart failure. JAMA 2003; 289: 871–8. *DIG trial dose substudy.*
110. Slatton ML, Irani WN, Hall SA. et al. Does digoxin provide additional hemodynamic and autonomic benefit at higher doses in patients with mild to moderate heart failure and normal sinus rhythm? J Am Coll Cardiol 1997; 29: 1206–13.
111. Gheorghiade M, Hall VB, Jacobsen G, et al. Effects of increasing maintenance dose of digoxin on left ventricular function and neurohormones in patients with chronic heart failure treated with diuretics and angiotensin-converting enzyme inhibitors. Circulation 1995; 92: 1801–7.
112. Digitalis Investigation Group. The effect of digoxin on mortality and morbidity in patients with heart failure. N Engl J Med 1997; 336: 525–33.
113. Packer M, Gheorghiade M, Young JB, et al. Withdrawal of digoxin from patients with chronic heart failure treated with angiotensin-converting-enzyme inhibitors. RADIANCE Study. N Engl J Med 1993; 329: 1–7.

Devices

114. Uretsky BF, Thygesen K, Armstrong PW, et al. Acute coronary findings at autopsy in heart failure patients with sudden death: results from the Assessment of Treatment With Lisinopril and Survival (ATLAS) Trial. Circulation 2000; 102: 611–16.
115. Tracy CM, Epstein AE, Darbar D, et al. 2012 ACCF/AHA/HRS focused update incorporated into the ACCF/AHA/HRS 2008 guidelines for device-based therapy of cardiac rhythm abnormalities. J Am Coll Cardiol 2013; 61: e6–75.
116. Cleland JG, Daubert JC, Erdmann E, et al. The effect of cardiac resynchronization on morbidity and mortality in heart failure. N Engl J Med 2005; 352: 1539–49. *CARE HF trial.*
117. Wang NC, Maggioni AP, Konstam MA, et al. Clinical implications of QRS duration in patients hospitalized with worsening heart failure and reduced left ventricular ejection fraction. JAMA 2008; 299: 2656–66.
118. Beshai JF, Grimm RA, Nagueh SF, et al. Cardiac-resynchronization therapy in heart failure with narrow QRS complexes. N Engl J Med 2007; 357: 2461–71. *RETHINQ trial.*
119. Doshi RN, Daoud EG, Fellows C, et al. Left ventricular-based cardiac stimulation post AV nodal ablation evaluation (the PAVE study). J Cardiovasc Electrophysiol 2005; 16: 1160–5.

120. Massie BM, Collins JF, Ammon SE, et al. Randomized trial of warfarin, aspirin, and clopidogrel in patients with chronic heart failure: the Warfarin and Antiplatelet Therapy in Chronic Heart Failure (WATCH) trial. Circulation 2009; 119: 1616–24.
121. Homma S, Thompson JLP, Pullicino PM, et al. Warfarin and aspirin in patients with heart failure and sinus rhythm. N Engl J Med 2012; 366: 1859–69. *WARCEF trial.*
122. Tavazzi L, Maggioni AP, Marchioli R, et al. Effect of n-3 polyunsaturated fatty acids in patients with chronic heart failure (the GISSI-HF trial): a randomised, double-blind, placebo-controlled trial. Lancet 2008; 372: 1223–30.
123. Kaneko Y, Floras JS, Usui K, et al. Cardiovascular effects of continuous positive airway pressure in patients with heart failure and obstructive sleep apnea. N Engl J Med 2003; 348: 1233–41.
124. Russell SD, Miller LW, Pagani FD. Advanced heart failure: a call to action. Congest Heart Fail 2008; 14: 316–21.
125. Solomon SD, Dobson G, Pocock A, et al. Influence of nonfatal hospitalization for heart failure on subsequent mortality in patients with chronic heart failure. Circulation 2007; 116: 1482–7. *Analysis from CHARM.*

HFpEF
126. Owan TE, Hodge DO, Herges RM, et al. Trends in prevalence and outcome of heart failure with preserved ejection fraction. N Engl J Med 2006; 355: 251–9.
127. Bhatia RS, Tu JV, Lee DS, et al. Outcome of heart failure with preserved ejection fraction in a population-based study. N Engl J Med 2006; 355: 260–9. *Also, MAGGIC meta-analysis and I-Preserve trial.*
128. Zile MR, Gaasch WH, Anand IS, et al. Mode of death in patients with heart failure and a preserved ejection fraction: results from the Irbesartan in Heart Failure With Preserved Ejection Fraction Study (I-Preserve) trial. Circulation 2010; 121: 1393–405.
129. Williams B, Lacy PS, Thom SM, et al. Differential impact of blood pressure-lowering drugs on central aortic pressure and clinical outcomes: principal results of the Conduit Artery Function Evaluation (CAFE) study. Circulation 2006; 113: 1213–25.
130. Schwartzenberg S, Redfield MM, From AM, et al. Effects of vasodilation in heart failure with preserved or reduced ejection fraction. J Am Coll Cardiol 2012; 59: 442–51.
131. Hwang SJ, Melenovsky V, Borlaug BA. Implications of coronary artery disease in heart failure with preserved ejection fraction. J Am Coll Cardiol 2014; 63: 2817–27.
132. Flather MD, Shibata MC, Coats AJ, et al. Randomized trial to determine the effect of nebivolol on mortality and cardiovascular hospital admission in elderly patients with heart failure (SENIORS). Eur Heart J 2005; 26: 215–25.
133. Yusuf S, Pfeffer MA, Swedberg K, et al. Effects of candesartan in patients with chronic heart failure and preserved left-ventricular ejection fraction: the CHARM-Preserved Trial. The Lancet. 2003; 362: 777–81.
134. Damman K, Perez AC, Anand IS, et al. Worsening renal function and outcome in heart failure patients with preserved ejection fraction and the impact of angiotensin receptor blocker treatment. J Am Coll Cardiol 2014; 64: 1106–13.
135. Edelman F, Wachter R, Schmidt AG, et al. Effect of spironolactone on diastolic function and exercise capacity in patients with heart failure with preserved ejection fraction: the Aldo-DHF randomized controlled trial. JAMA. 2013; 309: 781–91.
136. Pfeffer MA, Claggett B, Assmann SF, et al. Regional variation in patients and outcomes in the Treatment of Preserved Cardiac Function Heart Failure With an Aldosterone Antagonist (TOPCAT) trial. Circulation 2015; 131: 34–42. *TOPCAT selected HFpEF based on clinical diagnosis of HF with HF hospitalization (~2/3 of patients) or elevated BNP>100. It did not mandate echo parameters of diastolic dysfunction.*

HF has a lower mortality in women, and is less often systolic in women. Women derived more mortality benefit than men from CRT in MADIT-CRTtrial (men had no mortality benefit). Trend towards benefit from ICD in SCD Heft and MADIT II.

ADHF
137. Gheorghiade M, Zannad F, Sopko G, et al. Acute heart failure syndromes. Current state and framework for future research. Circulation 2005; 112: 3958–68.
138. Zile MR, Bennett TD, St John Sutton M, et al. Transition from chronic compensated to acute decompensated heart failure: pathophysiological insights obtained from continuous monitoring of intracardiac pressures. Circulation 2008; 118: 1433–41.
139. Niemen MS, Brutsaert D, Dickstein K, et al. EuroHeart Failure Survey II (EHFS II): a survey on hospitalized acute heart failure patients: Description of population. Eur Heart J 2006; 27: 2725–36. + *Similar and complementary data from: ADHERE scientific advisory committee: Core Module Q1 2006 Final Cumulative National Benchmark Report: Scios, Inc.; July 2006.*
140. Opasich C, Rapezzi C, Luzzi D, et al. Precipitating factors and decision-making processes of short-term worsening heart failure despite "optimal" treatment (from the IN-CHF Registry). Am J Cardiol 2001; 88: 382–7.
141. Nohria A, Tsang SW, Fang JC, et al. Clinical assessment identifies hemodynamic profiles that predict outcomes in patients admitted with heart failure. J Am Coll Cardiol 2003; 41: 1797–804.
142. McIntyre KM, Vita JA, Lambrew CT, Freeman J, Loscalzo J. A noninvasive method of predicting pulmonary-capillary wedge pressure. N Engl J Med 1992; 327: 1715–20.
143. Weilenmann D, Rickli H, Follath F, et al. Noninvasive evaluation of pulmonary capillary wedge pressure by BP response to the Valsalva maneuver. Chest 2002; 122: 140–5.

Revascularization in acute HF
144. Rossi JR, Flaherty JD, Fonarow GC, et al. Influence of coronary artery disease and coronary revascularization status on outcomes in patients with acute heart failure syndromes: a report from OPTIMIZE-HF. Eur J Heart Fail 2008; 10: 1215–23.
145. Roy D, Talajic M, Nattel S, et al. Rhythm control versus rate control for atrial fibrillation and heart failure. N Engl J Med 2008; 358: 2667–77. *AF CHF trial.*
146. Peacock WF, De Marco E, Fonarow GC, et al. Cardiac troponin and outcome in acute heart failure. N Engl J Med 2008; 358: 2117–26.
147. Felker GM, Lee KL, Bull DA, et al. Diuretic strategies in patients with acute decompensated heart failure. N Engl J Med 2011; 364: 797–805. *DOSE trial.*
148. Bart BA, Goldsmith SR, Lee KL, et al. Ultrafiltration in decompensated heart failure with cardiorenal syndrome. N Engl J Med 2012; 367: 2296–304. *CARESS HF trial.*
149. McMurray JJ, Adamopoulos S, Anker SD, et al. ESC Guidelines for the diagnosis and treatment of acute and chronic heart failure 2012: the Task Force for the Diagnosis and Treatment of Acute and Chronic Heart Failure 2012 of the European Society of Cardiology. Eur Heart J 2012; 33: 1787–847.

150. Nohria A, Hasselbad V, Stebbins A, et al. Cardiorenal interactions. Insights from the ESCAPE trial. J Am Coll Cardiol 2008; 51: 1268–74. *Correlation between RA pressure and renal failure (r=0.64), less strong than in Mullens study.*

151. Mullens W, Abrahams Z, Francis GS, et al. Importance of venous congestion for worsening of renal function in advanced decompensated heart failure. J Am Coll Cardiol 2009; 53: 589–96. *Cleveland Clinic registry.*

152. Weinfeld MS, Chertow GM, Stevenson LW. Aggravated renal dysfunction during intensive therapy for advanced chronic heart failure therapy. Am Heart J 1999; 138: 285–90.

153. Mullens W, Abrahams Z, Skouri HN, et al. Elevated intra-abdominal pressure in acutely decompensated heart failure: a potential contributor to worsening renal failure? J Am Coll Cardiol 2008; 51: 300–6.

154. Dupont M, Mullens W, Finucan M, et al. Determinants of dynamic changes in serum creatinine in acute decompensated heart failure: the importance of blood pressure reduction during treatment. Eur J Heart Fail 2013; 15: 433–40.

155. Ronco C, Cicoira M, McCullough PA. Cardiorenal syndrome type 1: pathophysiological crosstalk leading to combined heart and kidney dysfunction in the setting of acutely decompensated heart failure. J Am Coll Cardiol 2012; 60: 1031–42.

156. Testani JM, Chen J, McCauley BD, et al. Potential effects of aggressive decongestion during the treatment of decompensated heart failure on renal function and survival. Circulation 2010; 122: 265–72. *Escape trial analysis.*

157. Metra M, Davison B, Bettari L, et al. Is worsening renal function an ominous prognostic sign in patients with acute heart failure? The role of congestion and its interaction with renal function. Circ Heart Fail 2012; 5: 54–62.

Vasodilators and inotropes in acute heart failure

158. Mullens W, Abrahams Z, Francis GS, et al. Sodium nitroprusside for advanced low-output heart failure. J Am Coll Cardiol 2008; 52: 200–7.

159. Cotter G, Metzkor E, Kaluski E, et al. Randomised trial of high-dose isosorbide dinitrate plus low-dose furosemide versus high-dose furosemide plus low-dose isosorbide dinitrate in severe pulmonary oedema. Lancet 1998; 351: 389–93.

160. Abraham WT, Adams KF, Fonarow GF, et al. In-hospital mortality in patients with acute decompensated heart failure requiring intravenous vasoactive medications: an analysis from the Acute Decompensated Heart Failure National Registry (ADHERE). J Am Coll Cardiol 2005; 46: 57–64.

161. Sackner-Bernstein JD, Kowalski M, Fox M, et al. short-term risk of death after treatment with nesiritide for decompensated heart failure: a pooled analysis of randomized controlled trials. JAMA 2005; 293: 1900–5.

162. O'Connor CM, Starling RC, Hernandez AF, et al. Effect of nesiritide in patients with acute decompensated heart failure. N Engl J Med 2011; 365: 32–43.

163. Cuffe MS, Califf RM, Adams KF, et al. Short-term intravenous milrinone for acute exacerbation of chronic heart failure: a randomized controlled trial. JAMA 2002; 287: 1578–80. *OPTIME-HF.*

164. Felker GM, Benza RL, Chandler AB, et al. Heart failure etiology and response to milrinone in decompensated heart failure: results from the OPTIME-HF study. J Am Coll Cardiol 2003; 41: 997–1003.

165. Packer M, Carver JR, Rodeheffer RJ, et al. Effect of oral milrinone on mortality in severe chronic heart failure. N Engl J Med 1991; 325: 1468–75.

166. Metra M, Nodari S, D'Aloia A, et al. Beta-blocker therapy influences the hemodynamic response to inotropic agents in patients with heart failure. A randomized comparison of dobutamine and enoximone before and after chronic treatment with metoprolol or carvedilol. J Am Coll Cardiol 2002; 40: 1248–58.

167. Lowes BD, Tsvetkova T, Eichhorn EJ, Gilbert EM, Bristow MR. Milrinone versus dobutamine in heart failure subjects treated chronically with carvedilol. Int J Cardiol 2001; 81: 141–9.

168. Binanay C, Califf RM, Hasselblad V, et al. Evaluation study of congestive heart failure and pulmonary artery catheterization effectiveness: the ESCAPE trial. JAMA 2005; 294: 1625–33.

169. Fonarow GC, Adams KF, Abraham WT, Yancy CW, Boscardin WJ; ADHERE Scientific Advisory Committee, Study Group, and Investigators. Risk stratification for in-hospital mortality in acutely decompensated heart failure: classification and regression tree analysis. JAMA 2005; 293: 572–80.

170. Tavazzi L, Maggioni AP, Lucci D, et al. Nationwide survey on acute heart failure in cardiology ward services in Italy. Eur Heart J 2006; 27: 1207–15.

Prevention of HF hospitalizations

171. Yu CM, Wang L, Chau E, et al. Intrathoracic impedance monitoring in patients with heart failure: correlation with fluid status and feasibility of early warning preceding hospitalization. Circulation 2005; 112: 841–8.

172. Zhang J, Goode KM, Cuddihy PE, Cleland JG. Predicting hospitalization due to worsening heart failure using daily weight measurement: analysis of the Trans-European Network-Home-Care Management System (TEN-HMS) study. Eur J Heart Fail 2009; 11: 420–7.

173. Lewin J, Ledwidge M, O'Loughlin C, et al. Clinical deterioration in established heart failure: what is the value of BNP and weight gain in aiding diagnosis? Eur J Heart Fail 2005; 7: 953–7.

174. Packer M, Abraham WT, Mehra MR, et al. Utility of impedance cardiography for the identification of short-term risk of clinical decompensation in stable patients with chronic heart failure. J Am Coll Cardiol 2006; 47: 2245–52.

175. Abraham WT, Compton S, Haas G; FAST investigators. Superior performance of intrathoracic impedance-derived fluid index versus daily weight monitoring in heart failure patients: results of the Fluid Accumulation Status Trial (FAST). J Card Fail 2009; 15: 813.

176. Hindricks G, Taborsky M, Glikson M, et al. Implant-based multiparameter telemonitoring of patients with heart failure (IN-TIME): a randomized controlled trial. Lancet 2014; 384: 583–90.

177. Abraham WT, Adamson PB, Bourge RC, et al. Wireless pulmonary artery haemodynamic monitoring in chronic heart failure: a randomised controlled trial. Lancet 2011; 377: 658–66.

RV failure

178. Ling LF, Marwick TH. Echocardiographic assessment of right ventricular dysfunction: how to account for tricuspid regurgitation and pulmonary hypertension. JACC Cardiovasc Imaging 2012; 5: 747–53.

179. Haddad F, Doyle R, Murphy D, et al. Right ventricular dysfunction in cardiovascular disease. Part II. Pathophysiology, clinical importance and management of right ventricular failure. Circulation 2008; 117: 1717–31.

180. Haddad F, Hunt SA, Rosenthal DN, Murphy DJ. Right ventricular function in cardiovascular disease. Part I. Anatomy, physiology, aging, and functional assessment of the right ventricle. Circulation 2008; 117: 1436–48.

181. Rich S, Seidlitz M, Dodin E, et al. The short-term effects of digoxin in patients with right ventricular dysfunction from pulmonary hypertension. Chest 1998; 114: 787–92.

182. Price LC, Wort SJ, Finney SJ, et al. Pulmonary vascular and right ventricular dysfunction in adult critical care: current and emerging options for management: a systematic literature review. Crit Care 2010; 14: R169.

183. Hopkins WE, Ochoa LL, Richardson GW, Trulock EP. Comparison of the hemodynamics and survival of adults with severe primary pulmonary hypertension or Eisenmenger syndrome. J Heart Lung Transplant 1996; 15: 100–5.

184. Rozkovec A, Montanes P, Oakley CM. Factors that influence the outcome of primary pulmonary hypertension. Br Heart J 1986; 55: 449–58.

185. Sandoval J, Gaspar J, Pulido T, et al. Graded balloon dilation atrial septostomy in severe primary pulmonary hypertension: a therapeutic alternative for patients nonresponsive to vasodilator treatment. J Am Coll Cardiol. 1998; 32: 297–304.

5 Additional Heart Failure Topics

1. SPECIFIC CARDIOMYOPATHIES

I. Specific dilated cardiomyopathies

A. Tachycardia-mediated cardiomyopathy

Severe biventricular dilatation and failure may develop with uncontrolled tachyarrhythmias that persist for over 2 weeks, typically several months. This ventricular failure results from depletion of energy stores. In a way, it is a form of ischemic hibernation. While faster rates increase the risk and speed of its occurrence, this cardiomyopathy may be observed with chronic rates of only 105–110 bpm, rates that are usually well tolerated chronically and do not come to medical attention until the patient develops HF. It is seen with uncontrolled AF, atrial flutter, atrial tachycardia, or the slow and incessant form of AVRT (PJRT).[1] Interestingly, the tachyarrythmia may not be persistent; tachycardia that occurs over 10–15% of the day may cause a cardiomyopathy.[2] Frequent PVCs, with a burden of >10% of the patient's total rhythm on a Holter monitor, may also lead to this cardiomyopathy; up to one-third of patients with frequent PVCs develop cardiomyopathy.[3]

While a tachycardia of 110 bpm in the acute phase of decompensated HF may be secondary to HF and may not be targeted acutely, a newly diagnosed tachyarrhythmia at this rate, coinciding with HF exacerbation, suggests the possibility of tachycardia-mediated cardiomyopathy.[4] This is the case in 25–50% of new-onset AFs or atrial arrhythmias coinciding with a new HF presentation.[2,4,5] *Also, the persistence of the fast heart rate after diuresis and HF improvement suggests this diagnosis.*

After HF is treated (diuresis) and compensated, the tachyarrhythmia is targeted with a heart rate goal <80 bpm. In addition, rhythm control is often attempted (e.g., ablation for atrial flutter and atrial tachycardia, DC cardioversion and antiarrhythmics for AF). This cardiomyopathy usually reverses several months after rate control, typically within 6 months.[1,4] Residual ultrastructural abnormalities persist, explaining *a fast recurrence of LV dysfunction with recurrence of the arrhythmia.*

Practical Cardiovascular Medicine, First Edition. Elias B. Hanna.
© 2017 John Wiley & Sons Ltd. Published 2017 by John Wiley & Sons Ltd.

B. Viral myocarditis

There are several forms of myocarditis:

- **Subclinical myocarditis** signifies asymptomatic myocarditis (no HF). It is usually self-limited, but a minority of patients develop chronic HF and are diagnosed years later with idiopathic dilated cardiomyopathy.
- **Clinical myocarditis** implies myocarditis that manifests clinically with HF or with signs of pericarditis. It can take several forms:

  a. **Mild acute myocarditis** presents with LVEF of 40–50% and sometimes mild HF, along with acute pericarditis signs. It usually recovers, in >90% of the patients, within weeks or months.[6]

  b. **Severe acute or chronic myocarditis** is a myocarditis that manifests as HF or significant LV dysfunction. It reverses in ~35%, significantly improves in ~40%, and progresses to a more severe HF in ~25% of patients.[7,8] The overall 5-year mortality of patients with persistent HF is similar to idiopathic DCM (~50%).[9]

  c. **Very severe acute myocarditis** manifests as severe HF of recent onset (typically 2 weeks) with cardiogenic shock or ventricular arrhythmias, usually with a *normal-size LV* that has not had time to dilate and with severe thickening/edema of the ventricular walls. There are two forms of very severe myocarditis: (i) **fulminant lymphocytic myocarditis**, in which the patient is unstable acutely but eventually fully recovers if appropriately supported with vasopressors or ventricular assist devices, as the process mainly consists of myocardial depression by cytokines rather than necrosis (the long-term prognosis is excellent, with >90% 10-year survival);[10,11] (ii) **giant-cell myocarditis**, in which autoimmune myocardial destruction occurs and the illness continues its aggressive downhill course and intractable ventricular arrhythmias occur. These very severe forms are seen in young patients with aggressive immune systems.

Myocarditis is associated with three types of clinical manifestations:

- *HF*
- *Severe HF or shock*
- *A syndrome of acute pericarditis* or recent viral illness may be seen with any acute or hyperacute myocarditis, along with pericarditic ECG changes, increased CRP, and an inflammatory pericardial effusion. **ECG changes may be diffuse, similar to acute pericarditis, or more localized, mimicking STEMI (local myocarditis with "pseudoinfarction" pattern)**. Coronary angiography frequently needs to be performed to rule out CAD in these patients with ST elevation and troponin rise.

> In a patient presenting with acute HF and no CAD, a large troponin rise, higher than seen with HF, is a hint to myocarditis.
> Ventricular arrhythmias and high-grade AV block are more frequent in giant-cell myocarditis and cardiac sarcoidosis than in lymphocytic myocarditis.

Diagnosis

A definitive diagnosis of myocarditis is made by endomyocardial biopsy: lymphocyte-rich inflammatory infiltrate *and* myocyte necrosis (Dallas criteria); or positive viral genome on molecular analysis. Because of patchy myocardial involvement, the biopsy only has a 35–50% sensitivity. The yield is higher (85%) in giant-cell myocarditis, where the myocardium is more diffusely involved and multinucleate giant cells are seen. Biopsy is only indicated in cases of very severe myocarditis, where an urgent diagnosis of giant-cell myocarditis needs to be made and ventricular assist device and transplant considered; immunosuppressive therapy may temporarily slow the progression of giant cell myocarditis.

In patients acutely presenting with chest pain, troponin rise, and ST abnormality (diffuse or focal), a presumptive diagnosis of perimyocarditis is made after coronary angiography rules out CAD, in the absence of a takotsubo pattern of LV dysfunction.

In patients presenting with HF, a presumptive diagnosis of myocarditis or genetic DCM is made when non-ischemic cardiomyopathy has no clear explanation. Recently, MRI has emerged as a useful modality for the diagnosis of myocarditis: (i) increased T2 signal indicates edema (acute inflammation), and (ii) late gadolinium enhancement (LGE) on T1 indicates cellular death and/or scarring. Both findings may be seen with acute MI; however, as opposed to acute MI, the coronaries are not significantly diseased in myocarditis, the abnormalities are not distributed in a particular coronary territory, and **the pattern of late enhancement is different (subepicardial or mid-wall in myocarditis vs. subendocardial or transmural in MI)**. The subendocardium is usually spared in myocarditis, and transmural enhancement is rare.[8]

C. Eosinophilic hypersensitivity myocarditis

This is a form of myocarditis that occurs as a reaction to drugs (e.g., penicillins, sulfa) and may be accompanied by constitutional symptoms, rash and peripheral eosinophilia. It may be severe but transient and reversible if the drug is withdrawn; corticosteroids may be used. Endomyocardial biopsy, which is indicated in severe progressive cases of uncertain cardiomyopathy, shows eosinophilic infiltration.

D. HIV cardiomyopathy

HIV cardiomyopathy is often related to a direct myocardial HIV infection, but is sometimes related to an autoimmune process triggered by HIV, coinfections (e.g., cytomegalovirus, *Toxoplasma*, Epstein–Barr virus), or selenium deficiency. It should be distinguished from a reversible, acute illness cardiomyopathy sometimes seen in hospitalized HIV patients. HIV cardiomyopathy is typically seen in patients with CD4 counts <400 and develops in ~8% of these patients over a 5-year follow-up;[12] it may present as acute myocarditis. Dilated cardiomyopathy is associated with a high mortality risk of >50% at 2 years that is partly related to the advanced HIV disease.[13,14] Patients with a progressive course should undergo an endomyocardial biopsy to rule out and treat opportunistic coinfections. The effect of highly active antiretroviral therapy on stabilizing HIV cardiomyopathy is unclear. Diastolic dysfunction is common in HIV; in the absence of reduced EF, it may not affect the long-term prognosis.[14]

E. Chagas cardiomyopathy

Chagas disease occurs in endemic Latin American countries. It is due to a parasite (trypanosome) that is transmitted through the bite of a bug. Acute infection leads to a picture of acute myocarditis with HF that is usually reversible. Years later, ~30% develop chronic Chagas disease, which is characterized by a progressive biventricular failure and, frequently, a characteristic large apical aneurysm. Thromboembolic complications, conduction blocks, and arrhythmias are common. Chagas disease, whether acute or chronic, is due to a combination of active and persistent myocardial infestation and a damaging immune response.[15] The diagnosis is confirmed by serology. Beside HF therapy, antiparasitic agents are useful in acute disease and may be useful in slowing the progression of chronic disease, unless severe HF is already present.

F. Sarcoidosis

Sarcoid cardiyomyopathy is characterized by myocardial sarcoid infiltration, with granulomas and edema early on and fibrosis later on. The LV wall may be thickened by granulomas, which leads to LV diastolic dysfunction; or thinned by fibrosis with localized aneurysms, which leads to LV systolic dysfunction. Dilated or restrictive cardiomyopathy may be seen, sometimes with focal akinetic areas.

Sarcoidosis typically involves the basal septum and the lateral LV, leading to localized akinesis or dyskinesis of these segments.[16] This basal septal involvement leads to infra-His AV block, RBBB, or LBBB, as well as pseudo-Q waves. VT is also common. Echo is not very sensitive for detecting the early small granulomas and localized dysfunction, and arrhythmias or conduction blocks may be the earliest manifestation. The RV is not directly involved, but pulmonary hypertension may occur and lead to secondary RV failure.

Approximately 20–30% of patients with sarcoidosis have myocardial involvement, but only 5% have clinical myocardial involvement; it usually occurs in conjunction with pulmonary involvement. Sudden death from ventricular tachyarrhythmias or conduction blocks is the most common cause of death in cardiac sarcoidosis, accounting for 30–65% of deaths.[16] Progressive cardiomyopathy is the second most common cause of death.

> Sarcoidosis should always be considered in a young patient with VT, conduction block, cardiomyopathy with conduction block, and non-ischemic cardiomyopathy with thick walls, segmental dysfunction, or pseudo-Q waves. The diagnosis is suggested by non-cardiac sarcoid involvement and MRI finding of either edema or late gadolinium enhancement at the basal septal and inferolateral walls (subepicardial or mid-wall involvement). RV endomyocardial biopsy has a low sensitivity (~25%) as the septal infiltration is patchy. At an early stage, granulomas, MRI defects, and myocardial contractility improve with steroid therapy; however, AV block and the risk of VT do not reliably improve with steroids.[16] The prognosis of sarcoid cardiomyopathy is similar to idiopathic DCM, and much better than other infiltrative cardiomyopathies (e.g., amyloid).[13] Patients with cardiac manifestations, including high-degree AV block, have a high risk of VT on follow-up (up to 50% at 2–3 years), justifying ICD therapy early on.

G. LV non-compaction

Embryologically, the normal myocardium has subendocardial and subepicardial layers that are initially loose then become packed and thin, i.e., compacted. In LV non-compaction or "spongy myocardium," the subepicardium becomes compacted but the subendocardial meshwork remains loose, leading to prominent trabeculations and deep recesses, particularly in the mid-LV and apex. Doppler flow is seen through the recesses and thus helps define the excessively trabeculated morphology. LV non-compaction has been defined as an end-systolic ratio of the loose inner myocardium to the compacted outer myocardium ≥2, with an impaired or normal LVEF. Occasionally, LV non-compaction may be mistaken for LV thrombus, but echo contrast allows the differentiation. Early reports suggested that non-compaction is frequently associated with severe LV dysfunction and high incidence of arrhythmia and thromboembolic complications.[17] In fact, the deep sluggish recesses allow for thrombus formation. Later reports suggested that non-compaction, per se, may not carry any additional diagnostic or prognostic value beyond that provided by EF and HF status.[18]

Viral and hypertensive cardiomyopathies may lead to prominent trabeculations, that, at times, may fulfill the definition of LV non-compaction (false-positive diagnosis).[19] In the latter cases, the prominent trabeculations are acquired rather than congenital. In fact, in one analysis, ~25% of patients with systolic HF fulfilled the diagnostic criteria of LV non-compaction,[20] including many patients with underlying CAD (CAD was present in 29% of HF with LV non-compaction).[21] In addition, up to 8% of normal individuals, particularly black individuals, have prominent trabeculations that fulfill the diagnosis of LV non-compaction.[20] One analysis has shown that 8% of healthy women develop a non-compaction morphology during pregnancy, which reverses in the few months postpartum without any untoward clinical events or EF deterioration.[22] Also, 8% of athletes have a non-compaction morphology. Thus, LV non-compaction is likely a non-specific phenotype, induced by volume overload, rather than a specific entity.

The prognosis depends on the underlying LVEF and HF functional status, and the impact of the non-compaction morphology, per se, is unclear. Patients with normal EF at baseline have an excellent prognosis, with no increased risk of death or HF and no deterioration of LV function at 9.5 years.[18,21,23]

H. Takotsubo cardiomyopathy (TC, also called "stress-induced cardiomyopathy" or "apical ballooning syndrome")

This is a transient form of cardiomyopathy that occurs after a major stress and typically leads to dyskinesis and "ballooning" of the ventricular apex. Massive catecholamine surge leads to contraction band necrosis, which is actually a form of stunning rather than necrosis, similar to what is seen with cocaine overdose. Multivessel spasm and microvascular spasm have been incriminated as well. Atypical variants of TC have been described, such as the mid-ventricular ballooning and the basal ballooning (inverted TC).

TC typically involves post-menopausal women (~95% of cases), and only 2% of affected patients are <50 years of age. TC uncommonly presents as HF and more typically mimics ACS, particularly STEMI, and presents with chest pain, anterior ST elevation with deep anterior T-wave inversion, and elevated troponin. *ST elevation is seen in >80%* of the cases and involves the *anterior and lateral leads*, with rare inferior extension; isolated inferior ST elevation is not seen. ST elevation evolves into deep anterior T-wave inversion and prolonged QT within 24–48 hours; patients sometimes present at the stage of T-wave inversion without residual ST elevation, *T-wave inversion being the most universal finding.* Transient anterior/lateral Q waves are seen in 30% of the cases. On echo and left ventriculography, the apex is akinetic/dyskinetic while the base is hypercontractile, and the overall EF is ~30% (20–40%). RV is commonly involved (~1/3 of cases). Up to 17% of TCs are mid-cavitary rather than apical.[24,25]

The ECG and echo findings characterize anterior MI as much as TC, and coronary angiography should be performed in all these cases to rule out LAD disease. In TC, no significant CAD is found. Troponin increases to mild degrees (up to 5 ng/ml), much less than in anterior STEMI. As opposed to STEMI and myocarditis, MRI does not show any LGE (while helpful, MRI is not a necessary diagnostic tool).

All cases of TC are reversible within 2 months (half of them resolve within a week). *In fact, the diagnosis can only be made in retrospect, once recovery of LV function is confirmed.* A risk of recurrence of 11% has been described over a 4-year follow-up.[26]

TC has a good prognosis, with ~1% in-hospital mortality. Complications similar to STEMI complications may be seen acutely, but are much less common than in STEMI: HF (17%), shock (4%), VT/VF (1–6%), LV thrombus (2.5%) with a stroke risk of ~1%, usually within 48 hours.

HF and cardiogenic shock may result from the poor LV function but also from the basal hypercontractility that leads to LVOT obstruction, the latter being seen in ~15% of TCs. These two forms of HF or shock need to be differentiated by echo and are treated differently. In LVOT obstruction, inotropes are avoided; β-blockers are used if HF is present (carefully), while IV fluids and α-agonists are used if shock is present. Functional MR is seen in ~20% of TCs, and results from either LV dilatation or LVOT obstruction/SAM.

I. Other stress-related transient cardiomyopathies
- *Neurogenic stress cardiomyopathy* is seen in up to 20–30% of patients with subarachnoid hemorrhage, and less often in ischemic stroke. As opposed to TC, it usually involves the basal and mid-ventricular segments and spares the apex (inverted TC pattern).
- *Septic or acute medical illness cardiomyopathy:* ~50% of septic patients develop a septic cardiomyopathy. It results from the myocardial depressant effect of cytokines (TNF-α) and is usually characterized by diffuse global hypokinesis rather than a TC pattern. A subgroup of patients develop a typical TC pattern, depending on the relative effect of catecholamine surge vs. cytokines. The RV is involved as well. Septic cardiomyopathy always normalizes within 7–10 days.

II. Specific infiltrative restrictive cardiomyopathies
A. Amyloidosis
There are three forms of cardiac amyloidosis:

1. Amyloid light-chain (AL) amyloidosis results from myocardial light chain deposition and may be primary or secondary to multiple myeloma. It is the usual and most common form of cardiac amyloidosis, and is seen at an age over 40–50.[27] It is associated with amyloid renal failure and nephrotic syndrome.
2. Genetic familial amyloidosis is related to the deposition of an abnormal transthyretin (autosomal dominant). It leads to cardiomyopathy and neuropathy (no renal involvement).
3. Senile amyloidosis occurs ~ exclusively in elderly men (>90% men, median age 75) and is more slowly progressive than AL amyloidosis (survival 5 years vs. 15 months after HF onset). It results from aberrant deposition of normal, wild-type transthyretin and usually only affects the myocardium. Carpal tunnel syndrome frequently coexists with all forms of cardiac amyloidosis.

Amyloid A (AA) amyloidosis (inflammatory amyloidosis) does not usually affect the myocardium.

Amyloidosis is diagnosed by performing a **peripheral biopsy** (periumbilical fat pad biopsy, sensitivity 80% for AL amyloidosis, 70% for genetic amyloidosis) and urine and serum immunofixation looking for a monoclonal peak (AL amyloidosis). Genetic testing may diagnose genetic amyloidosis. **A nuclear scan using technetium pyrophosphate**, which is taken up by the cardiac amyloid tissue, is particularly sensitive and specific for transthyretin amyloidosis. **Cardiac MRI**, showing **global subendocardial LGE**, is 90% sensitive and specific for any cardiac amyloidosis. **Endomyocardial biopsy** is done when the prior tests are inconclusive, or when a tissue diagnosis is still needed (~100% sensitivity for the diagnosis of cardiac amyloidosis). The tissue sample should be subjected to protein analysis to confirm the subtype of amyloid (light chain vs. transthyretin). Once the diagnosis of AL amyloidosis is made, a bone marrow biopsy is often performed to confirm AL amyloidosis and to look for myeloma.

Amyloidosis has a very poor prognosis. The LV compliance curve is severely shifted leftward, and thus PCWP is severely elevated despite a normal or reduced preload, which precludes the use of significant doses of diuretics. *Digoxin should be avoided as it has a high affinity for the amyloid material and thus a high toxicity even at therapeutic doses.* In light of the autonomic dysfunction and the severely limited cardiac output reserve, vasodilators like ACE-Is are poorly tolerated and lead to profound hypotension. AL amyloidosis is treated with chemotherapy and bone marrow transplant. When cardiac involvement is advanced with severe, refractory HF, the prognosis is guarded and the patient is unlikely to tolerate high-dose chemotherapy.

B. Sarcoidosis
See Section 1.I.F.

C. Hemochromatosis
Hemochromatosis is characterized by multi-organ iron deposition leading to infiltrative cardiomyopathy, diabetes, and cirrhosis. Ferritin and iron saturation are elevated.

D. Genetic metabolic storage disorder
Fabry disease, an X-linked deficiency of α-galactosidase, leads to deposition of sphingolipids in the myocardium (LV ± RV thickening) and the kidneys (advanced renal failure), and sometimes the skin and the nervous system. It manifests in men but also heterozygous women. Accessory pathways are common. **As opposed to the low QRS voltage of amyloidosis, high voltage (LVH) is seen in Fabry**. The severe manifestations are usually seen in the third or fourth decade of life, but sometimes later, especially in women. The diagnosis may be established by a tissue biopsy, but also by checking galactosidase activity on peripheral leukocytes. The disease is treatable with α-galactosidase infusions.

In a patient with ventricular thickening and restrictive filling, three diagnoses are possible: hypertrophic, hypertensive, or infiltrative cardimyopathy. MRI helps in the differential diagnosis and reveals *global subendocardial late gadolinium enhancement in amyloidosis* versus *patchy mid-wall enhancement in HCM, and patchy mid-wall or subepicardial enhancement in Fabry disease*. While concomitant renal failure frequently suggests hypertensive disease, Fabry or amyloidosis should be considered in the right setting.

In a *young* patient with biventricular thickening and restrictive filling, consider the possibility of Fabry disease, genetic familial amyloidosis, or hypertrophic cardiomyopathy with restrictive phenotype.

E. Loeffler endocarditis–hypereosinophilic syndrome is secondary to severe systemic eosinophilia (Churg-and-Strauss disease or systemic parasitic infection). It leads to severe eosinophilic endocardial infiltration with secondary restrictive cardiomyopathy, MR/TR, and cavitary thrombus formation. It is treated with steroids ± antiparasitic agents in case of systemic parasitic infection.

An overlapping disorder, *endomyocardial fibrosis*, is a form of Loeffler endocarditis that progresses to extensive endocardial fibrosis. It is seen in tropical Africa, America, and the Middle East.

The three cardiomyopathies with the worst prognosis are: HIV cardiomyopathy, infiltrative cardiomyopathy from hemochromatosis or amyloidosis, and doxorubicin cardiomyopathy. The survival is <50% at 2 years.[13]

2. ADVANCED HEART FAILURE: HEART TRANSPLANT AND VENTRICULAR ASSIST DEVICES (VADS)

I. Stages of HF
- Stage A: Patients at risk for HF, but without HF symptoms or structural heart disease (e.g., HTN, CAD without MI, diabetes)
- Stage B: Structural heart disease but no HF (e.g., previous MI, LVH, reduced EF, or severe valvular disease)
- Stage C: Structural heart disease with prior or current HF functional class II, III, or IV (unlike stage D, it is not refractory to medical therapy)
- Stage D: HF functional class IV or advanced class III *refractory to medical therapy*, recurrently hospitalized

Neurohormonal therapies (ACE-Is, β-blockers, spironolactone) should be sequentially tried at very low doses in stage D patients if SBP ≥80 mmHg and in the absence of severe signs of hypoperfusion. Medical therapy is, however, poorly tolerated at this stage (hypotension and worsening of renal failure occur with ACE-Is; hypotension and worsening of HF occur with β-blockers).

In addition, stage D patients may not be able to be weaned off inotropic therapy because of severe low output and low organ perfusion, and these patients may require chronic outpatient inotropic support.

II. Cardiac transplantation
A. Indications
The 5-year survival after cardiac transplantation is ~70–75%. Transplant is indicated in HF patients whose 2-year survival is <50% (ACC and transplant society):[28,29]

- Patients with class III or IV HF that is refractory to medical therapy (stage D), *peak O$_2$ consumption ≤10 ml/kg/min on a maximal cardiopulmonary stress testing* where anaerobic threshold is achieved, and objective evidence of impaired hemodynamics on right heart catheterization (high filling pressures, reduced CO). Anaerobic threshold may be quickly achieved in patients with severe HF (e.g., 1 min). A severely reduced LVEF <30% is usual but not necessary (e.g., restrictive cardiomyopathy). These patients have typically had multiple HF hospitalizations in the last year.
- Patients who are dependent on inotropes and/or IABP (higher priority for transplantation).
- Patients with peak O$_2$ consumption of 11–14 ml/kg/min or ≤50% of predicted O$_2$ consumption have a relative indication for transplant.* A young patient may have a large predicted O$_2$ consumption, such that a higher value may qualify him for transplant. Ideal body weight is used in this calculation.

B. Contraindications
- Severe precapillary pulmonary hypertension with PVR >5 Wood units. These patients have a high risk of postoperative RV failure. Patients with any PVR elevation should undergo a vasodilator challenge (e.g., nipride) to assess PVR reduction. If PVR does not decrease acutely, short-term (24–48 hours) therapy with inotropes, diuretics, and vasodilators (milrinone, nipride) may be performed with continuous hemodynamic monitoring. If PVR can be reduced to <2.5 Wood units, the patient remains a transplant candidate with perioperative vasoactive therapy.[29] In those with refractory pulmonary hypertension, the complete LV unloading with LVAD is often effective in reversing pulmonary hypertension and bridging the patient to transplant.
- Uncontrolled diabetes, irreversible renal dysfunction (GFR <40), cirrhosis, or treated cancer in the last 5 years.
- Active tobacco use in the last 6 months, current or ± recent (2 years) alcohol or drug use.
- Obesity (BMI >30) is a strong relative contraindication, as it is associated with twice the 5-year mortality and a higher risk of rejection and allograft vasculopathy.
- Age >70 is a relative contraindication.

---

*1 metabolic equivalent (MET) corresponds to 3.5 ml/kg/min. Inability to reach peak O$_2$ consumption of 14 ml/kg/min implies an inability to perform 4 METs from a cardiorespiratory standpoint, rather than from joint or pain limitation, as evidenced by the fact that the patient reaches the anaerobic threshold.

C. Notes

ABO compatibility is important but not Rh compatibility (Rh is not expressed on myocardial cells). Testing for preformed HLA-reactive antibodies, or panel reactive antibodies, is performed in the recipient, and is repeated after blood transfusions, as those can trigger HLA antibodies (anti-leukocytes).

A hyperacute rejection occurs within minutes to hours and results from ABO incompatibility or anti-HLA antibodies, and is usually fatal unless treated urgently with retransplantation or mechanical support. Acute cellular rejection is T-cell mediated and is the most common type of rejection, the one for which immune therapies are used. It is most common in the first 3 months, but late rejections can occur. It is caught early on surveillance biopsies.

D. Immune therapies

Immune therapies consist of a calcineurin inhibitor (cyclosporine, tacrolimus) and an antimetabolite (azathioprine, mycophenolate), an inhibitor of cell proliferation. Steroids are used early on but are tapered and sometimes discontinued later on. Sirolimus is frequently used instead of a calcineurin inhibitor. Sirolimus has the advantages of less allograft vasculopathy and less renal failure than calcineurin inhibitors. Sirolimus needs to be stopped 1 week before and 4–6 weeks after elective surgery and replaced by calcineurin inhibitors to allow wound healing.

Statin therapy started early after transplantation reduces mortality, rejection, and cardiac allograft vasculopathy.[30]

E. Complications

1. Acute rejection occurs most frequently in the first few months after transplant, but may occur later. It is the leading cause of death in the first month after transplant. Surveillance biopsies are performed weekly early on, then monthly up until 6 months, then every 3–6 months. *A clinical acute rejection is an emergency. It should be suspected in any transplant patient presenting with acute HF, especially if fever is present*. When suspected clinically, it should be treated emergently with IV steroids, even before a biopsy is performed.

2. RV failure is the second leading cause of death in the first month, particularly in patients with irreversible pulmonary hypertension.

3. Nosocomial infections occur in the first 30 days and are followed by opportunistic infections, such as pneumocystis, cytomegalovirus, toxoplasmosis, especially in the first 6 months. The latter are prevented by Bactrim and antiviral prophylaxis.

4. Malignancy, especially skin cancers and lymphomas.

5. Renal dysfunction, mainly from calcineurin inhibitors.

6. Cardiac allograft vasculopathy: this is a diffuse and progressive coronary arteriopathy characterized by excessive proliferation of the intimal layer. The mechanism is both immune and non-immune (metabolic syndrome, hyperlipidemia, older age, prolonged ischemic time), and it is the leading cause of death beyond the first year of cardiac transplantation, with an estimated incidence of 8% in the first year, 30% within 5 years, and 50% within 10 years. Since it is a progressive process, the definitive treatment is eventually retransplantation, which is required when the diffuse disease becomes severely obstructive. Being diffuse, the disease is missed or underestimated by coronary angiography and is better assessed by IVUS. Preliminary therapy consists of PCI for focal stenoses, statin, switching to sirolimus, and aggressive therapy of the metabolic syndrome. Many centers recommend yearly coronary angiography with IVUS as a screening modality for this vasculopathy. IVUS is more sensitive than angiography for detection of this diffuse process, which is characterized by an intimal thickness >0.5 mm.[31] Also, IVUS can assess the true severity of coronary obstruction.

III. Left ventricular assist devices (LVADs)

LVADs may be used as a **bridge to transplant**. They help stabilize patients hemodynamically so they can tolerate medical therapy (ACE-Is, β-blockers, spironolactone). They improve organ perfusion and kidney function, PA pressure and survival rate, and make patients better candidates for transplant. LVADs may also be used as a **destination therapy** in patients ineligible for heart transplant, or a **bridge to a possible myocardial recovery** (e.g., reperfused MI with cardiogenic shock, severe myocarditis, post-cardiac surgery shock, severe but possibly reversible non-ischemic cardiomyopathy). The destiny of the LVAD is sometimes only elucidated with time. Many patients with non-ischemic cardiomyopathy improve significantly with the combination of LVAD and medical therapy, their ventricles recover, and LVAD may be explanted after 1–2 years (~15–20%).[32]

In the REMATCH trial of refractory class IV HF, HeartMate LVAD drastically improved survival at 1 and 2 years in patients with any advanced cardiomyopathy who were not transplant candidates (survival at 1 year was 52% with LVAD vs. 25% without LVAD).[33]

A. Types of ventricular assist devices

LVAD supports the LV and consists of a pump, an inflow cannula inserted in the apex and an outflow cannula inserted in the ascending aorta. Those three components are intracorporeal, with the pump in the preperitoneal or pericardial space; in older devices, the pump was extracorporeal. The pump is connected to an external battery through a transcutaneous driveline, a potential source of infection.

A right ventricular assist device (RVAD) supports the RV, the inflow cannula being inserted in the RA or RV and the outflow cannula in the PA. BiVAD consists of LVAD and RVAD. RVAD is not as effective in supporting the right circulation as LVAD is for the left circulation. This is because the RVAD pump often leads to a severe increase in PA pressure, particularly over long-term use.

There are several pump designs:

1. The first-generation devices, such as HeartMate, have a pulsatile pump with two valves. Despite improving mortality, the HeartMate device had a high malfunction rate of 35% at 2 years in the REMATCH trial, which translated into a drop of 2-year survival to 24% (albeit much better than no device).

2. Continuous-flow axial pump, such as HeartMate II: since no reservoir is needed, these devices are much smaller and require less energy, with less risk of malfunction. In the HeartMate II trial, the HeartMate II device was associated with a substantially lower rate of reoperation to repair or replace the pump at 2 years (10% vs. 36%), and less infection and bleeding (less surgical dissection), which translated into a better 2-year survival in comparison with HeartMate (58% vs. 24%).[34]

3. Continuous-flow centrifugal pump.

The flow generated by the continuous-flow devices depends on the pump's "*delta pressure*," which is the uphill outflow pressure (aorta) minus the inflow pressure.[35] The lower this delta pressure, the higher the flow. A higher outflow pressure translates into a lower pump flow, hence the importance of keeping a low afterload (mean BP <90 mmHg) and a high preload.

Depending on the remaining intrinsic cardiac output, some pulsatility may be seen with non-pulsatile devices. The residual LV contraction generates an inflow pressure that is higher in systole than diastole, and thus flow through the pump is higher in systole than diastole. Hypotensive patients with severely reduced LV systolic pressure and increased LVEDP have the lowest pulsatility: the aortic minus LV pressure is low in diastole, leading to a high diastolic flow that approximates the high systolic flow. Overall, the extra flow provided by the pump is highest in patients with the most depressed intrinsic function, where aortic pressure is reduced and inflow is high in diastole. A centrifugal pump is more sensitive to delta pressure changes and may shut off its flow if delta pressure is high.[35]

B. Indications for LVAD and other considerations

The hemodynamic indications for LVAD are similar to those for transplant:

- Refractory NYHA class IIIB or IV, including patients with frequent readmissions for HF despite appropriate medical therapy, or low-output patients who cannot tolerate β-blocker/ACE-I therapy
- *and* EF ≤25%
- *and* Peak O_2 consumption ≤14 ml/kg/min or inotrope dependence for over 2 weeks or IABP dependence for over a week (HeartMate II trial criteria).[34,36]

The most definitive indication for LVAD is inotrope dependence. It is unclear whether the risk of LVAD therapy (stroke, bleeding, sepsis, AI) is warranted in patients who are not inotrope-dependent (ROADMAP study).[37]

Age and obesity are not significant contraindications to LVAD.

Fixed pulmonary hypertension, a contraindication to cardiac transplantion, is not a contraindication for LVAD, which frequently allows the reversal of pulmonary hypertension. On the other hand, it is important to address baseline RV failure prior to LVAD implantation. In fact, in patients with RV dysfunction, *a high PA pressure may be more favorable for LVAD implantation than a normal PA pressure, as a high PA pressure predicts better RV function*. RV failure is a major complication that occurs in up to 20% of patients post-LVAD and is predicted by the presence of elevated RA pressure (RA pressure >20 mmHg or RA pressure >0.65 × PCWP), reduced RV stroke work index,* or preoperative signs of RV dysfunction on echocardiography. LV unloading by LVAD is beneficial for the RV, and the RV eventually improves in most of these patients. Early on, however, total LV unloading can shift the septum to the left and further exaggerate RV dilatation and reduce the septal contribution to RV function. RV failure is treated conservatively with inotropes and pulmonary vasodilators, but may require RVAD if refractory.[36]

Patients with severe AI need to have AVR concomitant to LVAD placement, to avoid a closed loop circulation between the LV and the aorta. Bioprosthetic rather than mechanical AVR is used to reduce the risk of thrombosis of this unloaded valve; if the patient has a prior mechanical AVR, it may need to be replaced with a bioprosthetic AVR.

C. Some technical aspects

The following LVAD parameters are displayed:

1. *Pump speed*, in rpm, is the only adjustable LVAD variable.
2. *Power* is the energy generated by the LVAD. Power inversely correlates with the resistance that opposes the LVAD pump (delta pressure).
3. *Pulse index* corresponds to how much cardiac output is generated by the native LV. The lower the pulse index, the higher the amount of support provided by the pump.
4. *Flow* correlates with power and is estimated based on pump power and speed, and blood viscosity (hemoglobin).

Power and pulse index are measured by LVAD; flow is not directly measured but calculated.

Causes of increased power – For the same speed, an increase in power may correspond to an increase in flow. This may result from high metabolic demands or vasodilatation, in which case the pulse index is also high as the intrinsic LV flow also increases; or may simply be an excessive pump flow with a resultant HTN. The latter case dictates a reduction of the pump speed. An increase in power may also indicate rotor pump thrombosis; the flow reading is paradoxically and falsely increased, and the pulse index is low.

Causes of reduced power – Reduced power correlates with reduced flow and indicates low preload or high afterload. For example, it may indicate an empty LV with a suckdown of the LV walls. It may also indicate RV failure, tamponade, inflow or outflow obstruction (kink or thrombosis), or HTN (mean BP should be kept <90 mmHg).

Since pulsatility is significantly attenuated with continuous-flow devices, the pulse is often not palpable and blood pressure measurement may be difficult non-invasively. An arterial Doppler is used during non-invasive BP measurement; the continuous noise heard during BP cuff deflation corresponds to mean BP. The mean BP goal is 65–90 mmHg.

In a patient with VAD, ***hypotension*** may be:

- VAD-related: RV failure; VAD pump failure, malposition, or obstruction (thrombosis); LV suction or excessive pump speed
- Not VAD-related: sepsis, tamponade, hemorrhage

LV suction, per se, is secondary to hypovolemia, RV failure, or high pump speed and is treated with fluid administration and slowing the pump speed. On echo, the septum should be kept in the middle; a septum that is excessively pulled towards the LV mandates a reduction of the LVAD speed. A dilated LV may imply LVAD pump failure.

---

*RV stroke work index = stroke volume × (mean PA pressure – RA pressure)/BSA. Must normally be >300 mmHg.ml/m².

D. Complications

1. Device failure:
- Continuous-flow axial pumps: the failure of axial pumps can be catastrophic, as these pumps lack valves, which creates the equivalent of severe AI.
- Pulsatile pumps: failure of the pump is less catastrophic than with an axial pump, as the valves protect from severe regurgitation of flow. However, failure of one of the valves can create the equivalent of severe AI.

2. Sensitivity to low preload: axial pumps generate such a negative pressure that there is a risk of collapse of the ventricle leading to flow cessation, thrombus formation, and VF. This issue is further compounded by the fact that the flow of axial pumps does not cease with a low inflow pressure and keeps sucking. Conversely, centrifugal pumps stop pumping when the inflow pressure is very low and the inflow–outflow uphill gradient is high (better response to physiology). Thus, preload needs to be appropriately maintained.

3. RV failure (~20% at 2 years).

4. Infections (~20% at 2 years).

5. Thromboembolic complications: except for HeartMate, LVAD implants require warfarin therapy. HeartMate II requires INR 2–3.[34] In the Heart-Mate II post-approval study, ~12% of patients had a stroke at 2 years.

6. Hemorrhagic complications (54% at 2 years), including a high risk of postoperative bleeding because of liver congestion, poor nutrition, and warfarin therapy. Also, the continuous flow may lead to arteriovenous malformations and may degrade von Willebrand factor, resulting in GI bleed. If bleeding persists, urgent cardiac transplantation may be needed to allow withdrawal of LVAD and anticoagulation.

7. AI: blood flows through the LVAD, bypassing the aortic valve, which remains closed and may eventually fuse. Aortic fusion leads to AI, a serious complication that may develop in up to 30% of LVAD patients at 3 years and requires AVR.

8. Hemolysis with continuous pumps.

9. Arrhythmias such as VF. When stable LVAD patients develop VF, they feel tired but they do not develop circulatory arrest. The LV becomes fully dependent on the pump. The RV arrests but in stable patients with low PA pressure, blood flows passively through the arrested RV, similarly to a Fontan circulation. This does not apply to the early postoperative period, where the RV function is critical in surpassing the left septal pull and the high PA pressure.

3. PATHOPHYSIOLOGY OF HEART FAILURE AND HEMODYNAMIC ASPECTS

I. LV diastolic pressure in normal conditions and in HF (whether systolic or diastolic)

Normally, LV diastolic pressure slightly increases throughout diastole and has an initial dip in early diastole that "sucks" blood from the LA, particularly in young patients with a highly compliant LV ("suckers"). LV end-diastolic pressure (LVEDP) is the LV pressure that immediately follows the A wave; in normal individuals, this pressure approximates LV diastolic pressure before the A wave.

An elevated LVEDP (>16 mmHg) usually signifies LV dysfunction and is the most commonly used surrogate of LV dysfunction (systolic or diastolic dysfunction). In fact, **an elevated LVEDP with normal EF and normal LV volume equates with LV diastolic dysfunction and is a prerequisite for defining diastolic heart failure**. In patients with clinically compensated LV systolic or diastolic dysfunction, LV pressure only increases significantly at the end of diastole, particularly after atrial contraction, which may lead to an elevated LVEDP and an increased LV "A" wave despite a normal or mildly elevated pre-A LV diastolic pressure and mean LV diastolic pressure (Figure 5.1). This correlates with S_4 on physical exam and transmitral E/A reversal on echocardiography. A compliant LA will accommodate the volume load during systole and early diastole, keeping its pressure normal or minimally elevated until late diastole. Thus, mean LA pressure is normal and is discrepant with the elevated end-diastolic LV and LA pressure. The patient is not in pulmonary edema at rest but may very well increase LA pressure with any stress.

In decompensated or acute LV failure (systolic or diastolic failure), the early diastolic LV compliance is overwhelmed, leading to increased LV pressure throughout diastole. LA compliance is also overwhelmed, which increases LA pressure and allows it to "push" flow into the LV. A high early diastolic LA–LV gradient corresponds to a large E wave and a high E/A ratio on echocardiography. The large early filling leads to S_3 on physical exam, which is heard at the end of the LV diastolic dip, when the LV reaches its limit of distensibility. Thus, isolated S_4 represents elevated LVEDP but normal pre-A LV diastolic pressure, while S_3 represents LV decompensation with volume overload of the LV and LA and a "push" from LA to LV in early diastole.[38]

> Patients with compensated LV systolic or diastolic dysfunction have normal LA pressure/PCWP at rest but are prone to raising LA pressure and E/A ratio during exercise or tachycardia, *and* are less capable of increasing stroke volume, which explains exertional dyspnea and fatigue in these patients despite the normal resting LA pressure.

II. Definition of afterload

Ventricular afterload corresponds to the tension the myocardium is pumping against during systole, called *ventricular wall tension or stress*. **Afterload is not simply the aortic pressure.** Afterload depends on the intracavitary systolic pressure but also the intracavitary size, i.e., the intracavitary stretch (the more the myocardium is stretched, the higher the tension against the myocardial wall). At a given pressure, afterload or wall stress increases as the ventricle further dilates. Moreover, the intracavitary pressure is not the only pressure affecting afterload; a positive pressure surrounding the myocardium negates some of the intracavitary pressure and reduces the tension against the inner myocardial wall. Therefore, the transmural pressure, which equals the intraventricular pressure minus the pericardial pressure, is the afterload pressure.

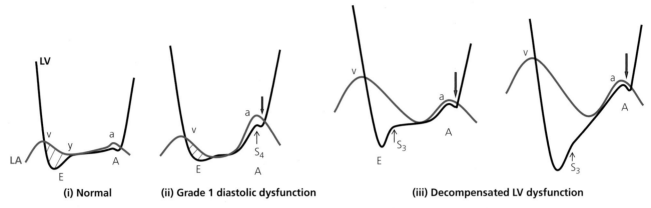

Figure 5.1 Simultaneous LA and LV pressure recordings in diastole.

i. Normal. Assess:

  1. *LV relaxation pattern,* as manifested by the sharpness of LV descent. The relaxation descent of the LV is evaluated by the variable tau, which corresponds to the full duration of relaxation. On tissue Doppler, LV relaxation is best characterized by the annular velocity E' (E' = myocardial recoil/relaxation).

  2. *LV stiffness and compliance,* as manifested by the slope of LV diastolic pressure (the sharper it is, the less compliant the LV is), and by the post-A LV pressure or LVEDP (*arrow*).

  3. *Early diastolic gradient between LA and LV.* This early gradient is determined by LV relaxation (sucking effect of the black curve) and by LA pressure (pushing effect of the blue curve), and corresponds to E wave on Doppler.

ii. Diastolic dysfunction is characterized by two features: poor LV relaxation and reduced LV compliance. *Poor LV relaxation* explains the absence of the LV dip in early diastole. This leads to poor early diastolic LV filling. *Reduced LV compliance* explains the elevated LVEDP: when the volume that has cumulated in the LA in early diastole suddenly rushes into the LV during A wave, LV pressure strikingly increases leading to elevated LVEDP. Note that LV diastolic pressure and LA pressure are normal outside A wave, particularly when LA is compliant enough to prevent an increase in LA pressure outside A wave. E/A is reversed and E' is reduced.

iii. In decompensated diastolic or systolic LV dysfunction, LA pressure is high with an early LA–LV diastolic gradient (= LA pressure is a "pusher" in early diastole). The LV relaxation slope is slow, hence the diminished early LV diastolic dip. LV is also poorly compliant, more so than in compensated dysfunction, and this manifests as a sharp increase in LV pressure after the dip, which quickly attenuates the LA–LV pressure gradient and LV filling. E is high but narrow because the flow is very brief, which explains the short E deceleration time. Despite the increase in LV pressure during A wave, there is no significant flow during A wave (small A with E/A >1.5–2). **Since E = LA pressure × LV relaxation; and E' = LV relaxation → E/E' = LA pressure.**

Afterload also depends on the ventricular wall thickness. The thicker the wall, the less tension is experienced by each sarcomere unit. This explains why the RV, being thinner than the LV, is more afterload-dependent than the normal LV.

In summary, the afterload is defined as ventricular wall stress and, according to Laplace's law, is equal to:

$$(\text{systolic LV radius} \times \text{systolic LV transmural pressure}) / 2 \times \text{myocardial thickness}$$

Beside reducing preload, diuresis reduces afterload by reducing systolic LV radius. Positive-pressure ventilation reduces afterload by reducing LV transmural pressure (pericardial pressure being positive in positive-pressure ventilation).

III. Cardiac output, relation to preload and afterload

The cardiac output depends on:

- *Inotropism.* Inotropism is the pure contractile function at a given length of the sarcomere, independent of loading conditions.
- *Chronotropism.* An acutely decompensated heart is unable to increase its contractility and stroke volume with longer filling times; thus, *tachycardia increases the cardiac output and should be respected in decompensated states.*
- *Preload.* Preload is the LV stretch in end-diastole (= LV end-diastolic volume). Increasing preload increases cardiac output up to a certain point, after which the cardiac output may decrease. In fact, a higher preload leads to LV dilatation, which increases systolic afterload and worsens functional MR, ultimately decreasing cardiac output (Frank–Starling curve, Figure 5.2).
- *Afterload.*

The failing heart is typically more afterload- than preload-dependent and is more afterload-dependent than a normal heart (Figure 5.3).[39,40] Small changes in afterload can produce large changes in stroke volume. Conversely, an increase in preload does not usually increase the cardiac output (flat cardiac output–preload curve), and may even decrease it because of the subsequent LV dilatation and rise in afterload.

A decrease in preload is usually well tolerated and improves pulmonary edema without affecting the cardiac output, explaining that diuresis is well tolerated (flat cardiac output–preload curve).[41] The only exceptions are diastolic HF and new-onset, acute systolic HF (e.g., massive MI), conditions in which LV end-diastolic volume is not increased, yet pulmonary edema develops at a normal preload because of a very poor ventricular compliance and a steep pressure–volume ventricular relationship. These patients are less tolerant of a decrease in their "normal" LV volume and should be carefully diuresed (Figure 5.4).

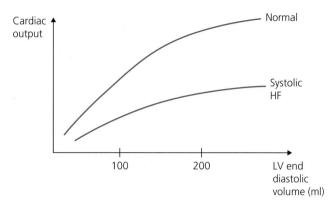

Figure 5.2 Cardiac output–preload relationship (Frank–Starling curve).
Note that preload is end-diastolic volume, not end-diastolic pressure.

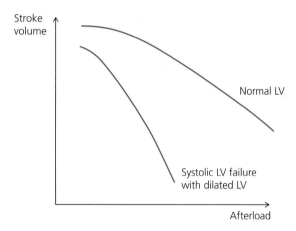

Figure 5.3 The failing LV is exquisitely sensitive to changes in afterload.
In systolic LV failure, note how the stroke volume varies sharply with afterload variation (much more than a normal LV). The normal RV is also exquisitely sensitive to afterload changes, like the failing LV.

IV. LV pressure–volume relationship in systolic versus diastolic failure: therapeutic implications

- *Systolic LV failure* is characterized by impaired LV contractility; as a result of the low volume ejected, the LV progressively dilates, which initially serves to maintain the stroke volume on the Frank–Starling curve, but eventually becomes harmful as LV dilatation increases afterload.
- *Diastolic LV failure* is characterized by two features: a slow LV relaxation (tau index) (Figure 5.1 [ii]) *and* a steep LV pressure–volume relationship in diastole (beta index) (Figure 5.1 [ii–iii]; Figure 5.4). LV is not dilated. In fact, a normal-size LV with elevated LVEDP indirectly suggests a steep pressure–volume relationship.

All patients with decompensated systolic LV failure are at a point on the pressure–volume curve where LV is stiff and thus have "diastolic failure" as well. In addition, all patients with systolic dysfunction, compensated or not, have impaired relaxation that is characteristic of diastolic dysfunction. Thus, *systolic LV failure has the two characteristics of diastolic failure, and every systolic heart failure is actually a combined systolic and diastolic heart failure*. Yet, less volume is necessary to overwhelm the LV compliance in diastolic dysfunction than in chronic systolic dysfunction, which is characterized by an LV that remains compliant up to a large volume load (Figure 5.4). Some patients with systolic failure only have a mild increase in LV volume yet a marked increase in LV diastolic pressure; this represents a form of systolic failure wherein the diastolic function is more impaired than usual and the LV pressure rises more steeply than usual, a form of predominant diastolic failure.

The goals of diuresis and preload and afterload therapy are to normalize PCWP and RA pressure. Even if severe or reactive, pulmonary hypertension usually reverses with reduction of PCWP but may lag several weeks behind PCWP normalization. **In the failing dilated LV, cardiac output is not reduced with preload reduction, because the cardiac output–LV volume curve is at a flat part (Figure 5.2).**[38–42] **In fact, PCWP of 15–18 mmHg corresponds to an unnecessary increase in LV end-diastolic volume (preload) and may be safely reduced to 12 mmHg in patients with chronic systolic LV failure, including acutely decompensated chronic systolic failure** (Figures 5.2, 5.5). Thus, diuresis does not reduce stroke volume in decompensated HF; in fact, **diuresis improves stroke volume as a result of the following:**[38] (1) diuresis reduces LV volume which, besides defining preload, is a major determinant of LV wall stress, i.e., LV afterload; (2) by reducing LV volume, diuresis reduces the severity of functional MR and, consequently, improves forward cardiac output; (3) in RV failure, diuresis reduces RV volume and thus reduces the compression of the LV by the RV. Therefore, patients with *decompensated systolic LV failure* should be treated with afterload and preload reduction and should tolerate PCWP <15 mmHg and a drastic reduction of their LV volume. Stroke volume is highest at a low PCWP. This may not apply to patients with poor LV compliance, such as patients with severe diastolic LV failure or new-onset, acute LV failure. In fact, patients with *severe restrictive cardiomyopathy* may require high PCWP to keep an adequate end-diastolic volume and cardiac output.

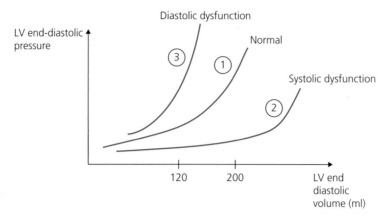

Figure 5.4 Compliance curve, i.e., pressure–volume relationship in diastole.
    LV is compliant in severe systolic dysfunction and is poorly compliant in severe diastolic dysfunction. In decompensated systolic dysfunction, however, the LV volume is high enough to be at the steep, non-compliant portion of the curve. In diastolic dysfunction, a normal 100–120 ml end-diastolic volume, which is necessary to maintain cardiac output on the Frank–Starling curve, leads to a high LV end-diastolic pressure and pulmonary edema. That is why such patients are less likely to tolerate diuresis; they are more preload-dependent than patients with systolic HF. An improvement in the relaxation pattern will move curve 3 to 1 and is called the *lusitropic effect; afterload reduction has a lusitropic effect.*

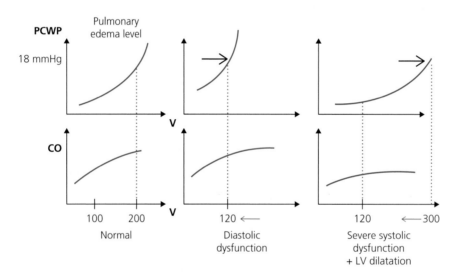

Figure 5.5 Important HF figure, showing a **diastolic superimposition of the Frank–Starling curve (= cardiac output–end-diastolic volume curve)** (*lower curve*) **and the pressure–volume curve (***upper curve***) in three situations.**
    In diastolic dysfunction, the pressure–volume curve is steep even at a normal diastolic volume. Diuresis to a volume of 100–120 ml corresponds to a PCWP of 15–18 mmHg, which may need to be accepted.
    In chronic systolic dysfunction, the pressure–volume curve is flat, i.e., LV is compliant at moderate volumes but becomes stiff at high volumes only. PCWP of 18 mmHg corresponds to a severely increased LV volume, and PCWP of 10–12 mmHg usually corresponds to the ventricular volume that provides maximal cardiac output. When the patient is in decompensated heart failure, whether from systolic or diastolic failure, the LV is at a steep and poorly compliant point of the pressure–volume curve (*arrows*).
    Modified from Gorlin R. Primary Cardiol 1980; 6: 84.

V. Decompensated LV failure: role of heart rate

Patients with compensated diastolic or systolic LV failure have impaired relaxation and E/A reversal on echo. They may decompensate with any volume load or mild exertion that increases preload and/or afterload (E/A changes from <0.8 to >1.5). Moreover, inappropriate tachycardia, the loss of atrial contraction with atrial fibrillation, or a very prolonged PR interval impedes atrial emptying and leads to volume overload of the LA and increased LA pressure.
    Thus, patients with compensated LV failure and reversed E/A decompensate with tachycardia or AF. However, once the patient is in decompensated failure (high E/A ratio), diastolic filling occurs only briefly in early diastole during the LA-to-LV "push" (E wave), with minimal filling in mid- and late-diastole. Except in cases of severe tachycardia >150 bpm, slowing the heart rate to prolong diastole or reestablishing atrial contraction does not help at this point, since LV fills minimally outside early diastole. In fact, tachycardia of up to 120 bpm may be helpful, as it serves to increase cardiac output and LV emptying by increasing the number of emptying cycles per minute (see Chapter 4,

Figure 4.2). The key here is to treat heart failure with diuresis and preload and afterload reduction; once LV failure is compensated and E/A reduced, slowing the heart rate and re-establishing atrial contraction (AF cardioversion) improves LA emptying and thus helps prevent decompensation.

VI. Mechanisms of exercise intolerance in HF

In normal individuals, LV end-diastolic volume and stroke volume increase and LVEDP decreases during exercise. LVEDP may slightly increase (≤2 mmHg) in elderly patients since the myocardial contractility fails to increase as much as in young individuals.

Also, during dynamic exercise, as during infectious states, both preload and inotropism increase, which allows cardiac output to increase and match the high metabolic demands. In systolic dysfunction with poor inotropic reserve, or in diastolic dysfunction, two untoward effects occur:

i. LV is unable to accommodate the increased preload, leading to an increase in filling pressures and a lack of appropriate increase in stroke volume.

ii. *Cardiac output may be normal at rest during a hemodynamic study but the cardiac output reserve is poor.* Patients with HF and reduced or even preserved EF are characterized by a blunting of the increase in stroke volume index in comparison to normal or hypertensive controls who do not have HF, which partly explains the early fatigue and exercise limitation of patients with HF.[43-45]

In a patient with HF and preserved EF, the LV cannot significantly increase its filling and its end-diastolic volume during exercise despite the increased venous return (small and stiff LV cavity with no preload reserve, inability to use the Frank–Starling mechanism).[44] This lack of preload reserve prevents the rise in stroke volume and induces a backup increase in LA pressure. Moreover, these patients have impaired capacity to increase LV contractility during exercise, despite a preserved baseline EF.[44] They also manifest a blunted exercise-induced vasodilatation; this elevated afterload during exercise further reduces stroke volume and subsequently increases PCWP during exercise.[43,44]

VII. Pressure–volume (PV) loops (advanced reading)

The PV loop expands on the pressure–volume relationship shown in Figure 5.4 to incorporate the systolic behavior. The PV loop is bounded inferiorly by the end-diastolic pressure–volume relationship, which is dictated by *chamber stiffness* and diastolic function; it is bounded on top by the end-systolic pressure–volume relationship (ESPVR) or elastance, which is dictated by *myocardial contractility* (Figure 5.6). *Stroke volume* corresponds to the width of the PV loop. The total PV area corresponds to the *stroke work* and closely correlates with the myocardial oxygen uptake as well as the overall pumping function of the ventricle.

VIII. Additional features of HF with preserved EF

HFpEF, often called diastolic HF, is differentiated from systolic HF by a normal EF, a non-dilated or only mildly dilated LV during decompensation (LV end-diastolic volume <75 ml/m² or <96 ml/m², respectively), and a different pressure–volume relationship. However, HFpEF is not simply diastolic HF; beside diastolic dysfunction, additional mechanisms are seen in a substantial proportion of patients:

a. Increased arterial stiffness and impaired capacity to vasodilate during exercise, with increased afterload and exaggerated hypertension during exercise.[43,44]

b. Pulmonary hypertension disproportionate to the rise of PCWP. One study documented a high prevalence of pulmonary hypertension in patients with HFpEF; 83% of patients in this study had pulmonary hypertension, the median PA systolic pressure being 48 mmHg.[46]

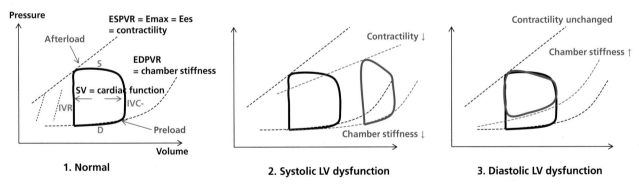

Figure 5.6 Pressure–volume loops.

1. Normal individuals, with pressure–volume relationship during diastole (D), systole (S), isovolumic contraction (IVC), and isovolumic relaxation (IVR). Four parameters determine the pressure–volume loop: (1) chamber stiffness line; (2) contractility line or end-systolic line; (3) preload, which is the end-diastolic volume, a point on the chamber stiffness line; (4) afterload, which is the end-systolic volume and pressure. For the same preload, a stiffer chamber will have a higher pressure. For the same contractility, afterload reduction moves the curve down along ESPVR, which increases stroke volume. Ejection fraction (= stroke volume/end-diastolic volume) is affected not only by contractility but by preload and afterload.

2. Systolic LV dysfunction: the contractility line (end-systolic line) is tilted down. In decompensated failure, the preload is severely increased so that the end-diastolic volume is on the steep portion of the chamber stiffness line, contractility is reduced, and afterload is increased. The loop is narrow (low stroke volume), with *contractility/afterload mismatch*. The end-systolic line being down, *changes in afterload more strikingly affect stroke volume than changes in preload.*

3. Diastolic LV dysfunction: the chamber stiffness line is up. As opposed to systolic dysfunction, a decrease in afterload results in less increase in stroke volume and more decrease in systolic pressure.

EDPVR, end-diastolic pressure–volume relationship; ESPVR, end-systolic pressure–volume relationship; Ees, end-systolic elastance; SV, stroke volume.

Interestingly, PA pressure was out of proportion to what would be expected from the rise in PCWP. For the same PCWP, patients with HFpEF had a much higher PA pressure than patients with hypertension and no heart failure. Thus, beside the postcapillary pulmonary hypertension, a precapillary pulmonary arterial hypertension frequently coexists or develops during the course of HFpEF, and may be an independent contributor to the symptomatology of HFpEF.

c. Mild impairment of LV contractility is common in HFpEF. In particular, the capacity to increase contractility and EF with exercise is significantly impaired.[47] EF, which equals stroke volume/end-diastolic volume, is determined not only by contractility but also by loading conditions. For the same contractility, a reduction in preload reduces the EF denominator and thus increases EF; a reduction in afterload increases stroke volume and thus increases EF. Thus, a normal EF may be seen in a patient with impaired contractility but a small LV with low afterload. EF is more a marker of remodeling than of contractility. Impaired systolic function is diagnosed by: (i) reduced LV strain on echo, which is highly prevalent in HFpEF (~50% in TOPCAT trial); (ii) impaired capacity to reduce end-systolic volume with exercise.

d. As opposed to the dilated LV of systolic HF and the normal-size LV of HFpEF, a subgroup of patients with HFpEF have a small, and sometimes hypercontractile LV. Despite being hypercontractile, the small LV size implies severe LV diastolic dysfunction with inability of the LV to distend and provide stroke volume; in fact, as compared to matched controls or hypertensive patients, HFpEF patients have a smaller LV diastolic volume,[48] and an impaired capacity to increase LV volume during exercise (limited preload reserve).[44,49] In addition, LVOT obstruction may result from the hyperdynamic, hypertrophic walls. A prototype is the hypertensive hypertrophic cardiomyopathy of the elderly.

> β-Blockers may be harmful in patients with small LV, i.e., patients whose preload reserve and stroke volume are limited and who depend on heart rate to increase their cardiac output.

e. While the LV is normal in size in the majority of patients, in a subgroup of patients with HFpEF, LV is mildly dilated and *hypervolemia* is the mechanism of HF. As may be seen on the pressure–volume relationship in Figures 5.4 and 5.5, even patients with normal LV function can have an increase in LVEDP and PCWP when the LV volume is excessive, e.g., over 250 ml, as in advanced kidney disease and high-output states (high-output HF).

f. Tachycardia, whether induced by pacing or exercise, is associated with a more potent relaxation in normal individuals, but further impairment of relaxation and LV filling in patients with diastolic dysfunction.[50] **Yet blunting of the heart rate may be harmful, as some patients cannot increase their ventricular filling with a longer diastole and rely on their heart rate to maintain cardiac output.** Also, *50% of HFpEF patients actually have chronotropic incompetence that may be a major contributor to their exercise intolerance.*[44,51,52] Patients with systolic or diastolic dysfunction have chronic β-receptor overstimulation with subsequent β-desensitization and blunted response to exercise, even if the baseline heart rate is increased.[52] β-blockers may improve this phenomenon but may also worsen symptoms if chronotropic incompetence is due to autonomic dysfunction, a common process in any HF.

g. *Vasodilators are more likely to reduce systolic BP and less likely to improve stroke volume in patients with diastolic HF than systolic HF, and thus they may not be tolerated in diastolic HF with normal or low-normal BP.*[53] The latter is the result of three mechanisms: (1) Vasodilators are also venodilators that reduce preload; diastolic HF is more preload-sensitive than systolic HF, and thus the stroke volume is less likely to increase with vasodilators in diastolic vs. systolic HF. (2) BP decreases while the stroke volume increases with vasodilation, and the extent of change in each is dictated by the afterload sensitivity. Afterload reduction results in less stroke volume increase and more BP drop in diastolic HF than systolic HF (Figure 5.3). However, this equation also depends on how elevated the baseline afterload is. Patients with hypertension or severely increased afterload benefit from vasodilators regardless of the type of HF. (3) In addition to ventricular stiffening, diastolic HF is characterized by arterial stiffening, making BP more sensitive to small afterload changes. A small increase in afterload is harmful as a result of the striking increase in BP, but excessive reduction in afterload may not be tolerated either. Patients without HTN and with severe restrictive cardiomyopathy, such as amyloidosis, very poorly tolerate vasodilators.

IX. High-output HF

High-output HF is characterized by elevated left ± right filling pressures, yet a cardiac index that is at the upper limit of normal or elevated (>4 l/min/m²), and a wide rather than a narrow pulse pressure. High-output HF is seen with morbid obesity, severe anemia, hyperthyroidism, cirrhosis, lung disease with hypercapnia, large AV fistula (including dialysis fistula, Paget bone disease), thiamine deficiency (beriberi, especially in an alcoholic), or volume overload in a patient with advanced kidney disease.

The high output is typically related to a high-volume state or to significant systemic vasodilatation or AV fistula. High-output HF has two pathophysiological characteristics:

1. The systemic vasodilatation or the fistula requires a high cardiac output to maintain the systemic pressure, which eventually leads to renal salt retention and a **high venous return/preload**. *As a result of this severely increased preload, the left- and right-sided filling pressures increase.* Even if LV compliance is normal, the LV diastolic pressure increases when LV diastolic volume exceeds 250–300 ml (Figures 5.4, 5.5). In many cases, these patients also have a degree of ventricular dysfunction that further makes them sensitive to the rising preload.

2. While increased in absolute value, the cardiac output may not be high enough to fill the vasodilated circulation, meaning it is a relatively low cardiac output. This is similar to the exertional response of any HF: **cardiac output increases in absolute value (e.g., 2× the baseline), but is far below the required increase (4–5 times the baseline), with inability to accommodate the high venous return**. Although high, this inappropriate cardiac output is associated with tissue ischemia and a low mixed venous O_2 saturation.

LV is usually dilated or at the upper limit of normal. LVEF may be normal or reduced as a result of the increased ventricular volume (EF denominator). In fact, a low LVEF is common in high-output HF.

References

Cardiomyopathies

1. Nerheim P, Birger-Botkin S, Piracha L, Olshansky B. Heart failure and sudden death in patients with tachycardia-induced cardiomyopathy and recurrent tachycardia. Circulation 2004; 10: 247–52.

2. Simantirakis EN, Koutalas EP, Vardas PE. Arrhythmia-induced cardiomyopathies: the riddle of the chicken and the egg still unanswered? Europace 2012; 14: 466–73.

3. Cha YM, Lee GK, Klarich KW, et al. Premature-induced ventricular contraction-induced cardiomyopathy: a treatable condition. Circ Arrhythm Electrophysiol 2012; 5: 229–36.

4. Medi C, Kalman JM, Haqqani H, et al. Tachycardia-mediated cardiomyopathy secondary to focal atrial tachycardia. J Am Coll Cardiol 2009; 53: 1791–7.

5. Redfield MM, Kay GN, Jenkins LS, et al. Tachycardia-related cardiomyopathy: a common cause of ventricular dysfunction in patients with atrial fibrillation referred for atrioventricular ablation. Mayo Clin Proc 2000; 75: 790–5.

6. Imazio M, Brucato A, Barbieri A, et al. Good prognosis for pericarditis with and without myocardial involvement: results from a multicenter, prospective cohort study. Circulation 2013; 128: 42–9.

7. McNamara DM, Holubkov R, Starling RC, et al. Controlled trial of intravenous immune globulin in recent-onset dilated cardiomyopathy. Circulation 2001; 103; 2254–9.

8. Magnani JW, Dec JW. Myocarditis: current trends in diagnosis and treatment. Circulation 2006; 113: 876–90.

9. Grogan M, Redfield MM, Bailey KR, et al. Long-term outcome of patients with biopsy-proved myocarditis: comparison with idiopathic dilated cardiomyopathy. J Am Coll Cardiol 1995; 26: 80–84. *Myocarditis and DCM have the same 5-year mortality (~50%).*

10. McCarthy RE, Boehmer JP, Hruban RH, et al. Long-term outcome of fulminant myocarditis as compared with acute (non-fulminant) myocarditis. N Engl J Med 2000; 342: 690–5.

11. Felker GM, Boehmer JP, Hruban RH, et al. Echocardiographic findings in fulminant and acute myocarditis. J Am Coll Cardiol 2000; 36: 227–32.

12. Barbaro G, Di Lorenzo G, Grisorio B, Barbarini G. Incidence of dilated cardiomyopathy and detection of HIV in myocardial cells of HIV-positive patients. N Engl J Med 1998; 339: 1093–9.

13. Felker CM, Thompson RE, Hare JM, et al. Underlying causes and long-term survival in patients with initially unexplained cardiomyopathy. N Engl J Med 2000: 342: 1077–84.

14. Currie PF, Jacob AJ, Foreman AR, et al. Heart muscle disease related to HIV infection: prognostic implications. BMJ 1994; 309; 1605–7.

15. Biolo A, Ribeiro AL, Clausell N. Chagas cardiomyopathy: where do we stand after a hundred years? Prog Cardiovasc Dis 2010; 52: 300–16.

16. Mcdlvit AM, Askari AT. A middle-aged man with progressive fatigue. Clev Clin J Med 2009; 76: 10: 564–74.

17. Oechslin EN, Attenhofer Jost CH, Rojas JR, Kaufmann PA, Jenni R. Long-term follow-up of 34 adults with isolated left ventricular noncompaction: a distinct cardiomyopathy with poor prognosis. J Am Coll Cardiol 2000; 36: 493–500.

18. Murphy RT, Thaman R, Blanes JG, et al. Natural history and familial characteristics of isolated left ventricular non-compaction. Eur Heart J 2005; 26: 187–92.

19. Nieman M, Stork S, Weidemann F. Left ventricular noncompaction cardiomyopathy: an overdiagnosed disease. Circulation 2012; 126: e240–3.

20. Kohli SK, Pantazis AA, Shah JS, et al. Diagnosis of left-ventricular non-compaction in patients with left-ventricular systolic dysfunction: time for a reappraisal of diagnostic criteria? Eur Heart J 2008; 29: 89–95.

21. Thavendiranathan P, Dahiya A, Phelan D, et al. Isolated left ventricular non-compaction controversies in diagnostic criteria, adverse outcomes and management. Heart 2013; 99: 681–9.

22. Gati S, Papadakis M, Papamichael ND, et al. Reversible de novo left ventricular trabeculations in pregnant women. Circulation 2014; 130: 475–83.

23. Zemrak F, Ahlman MA, Captur G, et al. The relationship of left ventricular trabeculation to ventricular function and structure over a 9.5-year follow-up. J Am Coll Cardiol 2014; 64 : 1971–80.

24. Bybee KA, Kara T, Prasad A, et al. Systematic review: transient left ventricular apical ballooning: a syndrome that mimics ST segment elevation myocardial infarction. Ann Intern Med 2004; 141: 858–65.

25. Gianni M, Dentali F, Grandi AM, et al. Apical ballooning syndrome or Takotsubo cardiomyopathy: a systematic review. Eur Heart J 2006; 27: 1523–9.

26. Elesber AA, Prasad A, Lennon RJ, et al. Four-year recurrence rate and prognosis of the apical ballooning syndrome. J Am Coll Cardiol 2007; 50: 448–52.

27. Falk RH. Diagnosis and management of the cardiac amyloidosis. Circulation 2005; 112: 2047–60.

Advanced HF

28. Yancy CW, Jessup M, Bozkurt B, et al. 2013 ACCF/AHA guideline for the management of heart failure. Circulation 2013; 128: e240–327.

29. Mehra MR, Kobashigawa J, Starling R, et al. Listing criteria for heart transplantation: International Society for Heart and Lung Transplantation guidelines for the care of cardiac transplant candidates: 2006. J Heart Lung Transplant 2006; 25:1024–42.

30. Kobashigawa JA, Katznelson S, Laks H, et al. Effect of pravastatin on outcomes after cardiac transplantation. N Engl J Med 1995; 333: 621–7.

31. Kobashigawa JA, Tobis JM, Starling RC, et al. Multicenter intravascular ultrasound validation study among heart transplant recipients: outcomes after five years. J Am Coll Cardiol 2005; 45: 1532–7.

32. Birks EJ, Tansley PD, Hardy J, et al. Left ventricular assist device and drug therapy for the reversal of heart failure. N Engl J Med 2006; 355: 1873–84.

33. Rose EA, Gelijns AC, Moskowitz AJ, et al. Long-term use of a left ventricular assist device for end-stage heart failure. N Engl J Med 2001; 345: 1435–43.

34. Slaughter MS, Rogers JG, Milano CA, et al. Advanced heart failure treated with continuous-flow left ventricular assist device. N Engl J Med 2009; 361: 2241–51.

35. Moazami N, Fukamachi K, Kobayachi M, et al. Axial and centrifugal continuous-flow rotary pumps: A translation from pump mechanics to clinical practice. J Heart Lung Transplant 2013; 32: 1–11.

36. Miller LW, Guglin M. Patient selection for ventricular assist devices. J Am Coll Cardiol 2013; 61: 1209–21.

37. Estep JD, Starling RC, Horstmanshof DA, et al. Risk assessment and comparative effectiveness of left ventricular assist device and medical management in ambulatory heart failure patients. J Am Coll Cardiol 2015; 66: 1747–61.

Pathophysiology of HF

38. Hanna EB. Pressure tracings and left ventricular failure. In: Hanna EB, Glancy DL. Practical Cardiovascular Hemodynamics. New York, NY: Demos Medical, 2012, pp. 7–74.
39. Little RC, Little WC. Cardiac preload, afterload, and heart failure. Arch Intern Med 1982; 142: 819–22.
40. Mason DT, Awan NA, Jaye JJ, et al. Treatment of acute and chronic congestive heart failure by vasodilators: Afterload reduction. Arch Intern Med 1980; 140: 1577–81.
41. Stevenson LW, Tillisch JH. Maintenance of cardiac output with normal filling pressures in patients with dilated heart failure. Circulation 1986; 74: 1303–8.
42. Rosario LB, Stevenson LW, Solomon SD, Lee RT, Reimold SC. The mechanism of decrease in dynamic mitral regurgitation during heart failure treatment: importance of reduction in the regurgitant orifice size. J Am Coll Cardiol 1998; 32: 1819–24.
43. Maeder MT, Thompson BR, Brunner-La Rocca HP, Kaye DM. Hemodynamic basis of exercise limitation in patients with heart failure and normal ejection fraction. J Am Coll Cardiol 2010; 56: 855–63. *Catheterization study showing an impaired increase of stroke volume index at peak exercise, with impaired reduction of SVR, and excessive rise of PCWP.*
44. Borlaug BA, Olson TP, Lam CSP, et al. Global cardiovascular reserve dysfunction in heart failure with preserved ejection fraction. J Am Coll Cardiol 2010; 56: 845–54. *Echo study showed that HFpEF, as compared to controls, had an impaired increase in cardiac output, LV end-diastolic volume (trend; only mild increase of end-diastolic volume compared to baseline), and chronotropy with exercise. Also, impaired vasodilatation and impaired contractility (impaired reduction of LV end-systolic volume with exercise).*
45. Paulus WJ. Culprit mechanism for exercise intolerance in heart failure with normal ejection fraction. J Am Coll Cardiol 2010; 56: 864–6.
46. Lam CS, Roger VL, Rodeheffer RJ, et al. Pulmonary hypertension in heart failure with preserved ejection fraction: a community-based study J Am Coll Cardiol 2009; 53: 1119–26.
47. Borlaug BA, Lam CSP, Roger VL, et al. Contractility and ventricular systolic stiffening in hypertensive heart disease. Insights into the pathogenesis of heart failure with preserved EF. J Am Coll Cardiol 2009; 54: 410–18.
48. Lam CS, Roger VL, Rodeheffer RJ, et al. Cardiac structure and ventricular-vascular function in persons with heart failure and preserved ejection fraction from Olmsted County, Minnesota. Circulation 2007; 115: 1982–90.
49. Kitzman DW, Higginbotham MB, Cobb FR, et al. Exercise intolerance in patients with heart failure and preserved left ventricular systolic function: failure of the Frank–Starling mechanism. J Am Coll Cardiol 1991; 17: 1065–72.
50. Selby DE, Palmer BM, LeWinter MM, Meyer M. Tachycardia-induced diastolic dysfunction and resting tone in myocardium from patients with a normal ejection fraction. J Am Coll Cardiol 2011; 58: 147–54.
51. Borlaug BA, Melenovsky V, Russell SD, et al. Impaired chronotropic and vasodilator reserves limit exercise capacity in patients with heart failure and a preserved ejection fraction. Circulation 2006; 114: 2138–47.
52. Phan TT, Shivu GN, Abozguia K, et al. Impaired heart rate recovery and chronotropic incompetence in patients with heart failure with preserved ejection fraction. Circ Heart Fail 2010; 3: 29–34.
53. Schwartzenberg S, Redfield MM, From AM, et al. Effects of vasodilation in heart failure with preserved or reduced ejection fraction. J Am Coll Cardiol 2012; 59: 442–51.

Part 3   VALVULAR DISORDERS

6   Valvular Disorders

Practical Cardiovascular Medicine, First Edition. Elias B. Hanna.

© 2017 John Wiley & Sons Ltd. Published 2017 by John Wiley & Sons Ltd.

1. MITRAL REGURGITATION

I. Mechanisms of mitral regurgitation

The mitral valve anatomy is shown in Figure 6.1. Normally, each papillary muscle provides chordae to both leaflets. The free edges of the leaflets coapt over several millimeters, at a depth of 5–10 mm from the mitral annular plane.

Mitral valve competence depends on: (a) appropriate ventricular contractility that pushes the papillary muscles, chordae, and valvular leaflets up (mitral closing force); (b) appropriate chordal length and tension that restrain the leaflets from prolapsing in the LA; (c) slim leaflet tissue that allows a tight seal in systole (as opposed to a bumpy, redundant tissue).[1]

There are four major mechanisms of mitral regurgitation (Carpentier's classification) (Figure 6.2):[2]

Type I: MR occurs despite normal leaflet motion and leaflet tip position. Type I MR may occur with leaflet tear(s) secondary to endocarditis or blunt trauma.

Type II: *Prolapse* of one or both leaflets, i.e., the billowing body of the leaflet is >2 mm above the annular plane (the free edge of the leaflet is at the annular plane or above it). If, in addition to the prolapse of the leaflet body, the free edge is overriding the other leaflet and turned towards the LA rather than the LV, the leaflet is called a *flail leaflet*; this is usually secondary to chordal rupture (a piece of chordae is usually seen flopping in the LA). Type II MR may result from mitral valve prolapse, chordal rupture (from mitral valve prolapse, endocarditis, trauma), or papillary muscle rupture (MI, trauma).

Type IIIa: The leaflets and chordae are thickened, retracted, and shortened, with chordal fusion (rheumatic or rheumatic-like process). The mitral motion is restricted in both systole and diastole, potentially leading to both MS and MR.

Type IIIb: Functional MR. A localized, inferior ventricular dysfunction pulls the papillary muscle(s) and chorda(e) posterolaterally, predominantly restricting the motion of the posterior leaflet (leaflet tethering). In severe global LV dysfunction, the ventricular geometry changes from an ellipse to a sphere, which pulls both leaflets posterolaterally and apically, restricting their closure. Three additional mechanisms contribute to MR: (a) annular dilatation, which reduces leaflet coaptation; (b) reduced LV systolic pressure, which reduces the mitral valve closing force and sometimes leads to MR even when tethering is mild; (c) papillary muscle dyssynchrony in some patients with LBBB or RV pacing: one papillary muscle contracts while the other is relaxed; therefore, one leaflet is pushed up while the other is still down, which creates a gap between the two leaflets.

II. Specifics of various causes of mitral regurgitation

A. Acute MR

Causes of acute MR:

a. Mitral valve endocarditis: the vegetations may interfere with proper leaflet coaptation or may destroy and perforate the leaflet(s) or chorda(e)

b. Papillary muscle rupture or acute functional MR occurring in the context of an acute MI

c. Chordae tendinae rupture. Causes: idiopathic, mitral valve prolapse, endocarditis, trauma

d. Acute functional MR secondary to an acute ventricular process (MI, myocarditis)

In acute MR, *EF increases* to allow an increase in total stroke volume, the forward stroke volume remaining, however, low. The patient is in shock with pulmonary edema, LA pressure is severely increased, yet the intrinsic LV function is normal and the LV diastolic pressure may be normal.

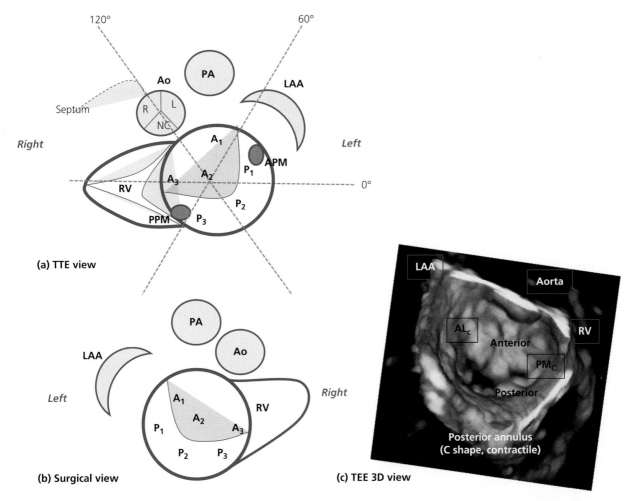

Figure 6.1 (a) Illustration of a horizontal cut across the mitral plane on transthoracic echocardiography, showing the relationship of the cusps with the papillary muscles, aortic valve, and left atrial appendage (LAA). Also, illustration of how various TEE rotations cut the mitral valve. Note that the anterolateral and posteromedial papillary muscles (APM and PPM) are located between the two leaflets rather than underneath the corresponding leaflet (they are underneath the commissures). A_1–A_3 are various anterior leaflet cusps, and P_1–P_3 are various posterior leaflet cusps (A_3 and P_3 are the ones attached to the septum). The mitral annulus surrounding the anterior leaflet and separating the anterior leaflet from the aortic valve is fibrous and relatively straight, and forms the mitroaortic curtain or fibrous trigone. The posterior mitral annulus has a C shape and is muscular. **(b)** Illustration of how the mitral valve looks surgically when approached from inside the LA through the anterior heart. A_3 and P_3 are on the right (flipped view in comparison with TTE). **(c)** 3D TEE view of the mitral valve (en face view). This view is similar to the surgical view. For orientation, identify the anterior leaflet (leaflet with the convex border) and the posterior annulus. The posterior annulus has a C shape, is muscular and contractile. It contracts in systole and contributes to the mitral valve competence. There are two commissures: anterolateral (AL_c) and posteromedial (PM_c).

Blunt chest trauma during the isovolumic contraction may also lead to acute MR (rupture of the papillary muscles, chordae, or leaflets).

B. Degenerative mitral valve disease or mitral valve prolapse (MVP)

MVP (Figure 6.3) is defined as:

i. One or two cusps prolapse >2 mm into the LA above the annulus level, in the long-axis view
ii. Thick cusps ≥2 mm (myxomatous, redundant valve)
iii. Cusp/chordae elongation

There are two forms of MVP:[1,3] (1) mitral fibroelastic deficiency, wherein the prolapsed leaflet(s) are thin (i + iii); (2) Barlow disease or classic MVP, wherein the prolapsed leaflets and chordae are thick (i + ii + iii). Fibroelastic deficiency is a local disease that usually affects a single cusp, with the remaining cusps being normal and non-prolapsed. These patients typically do not have a long history of murmur, and MR may appear and progress rapidly (months), with a frequent chordal rupture. Conversely, Barlow's disease is a chronic process (years) associated with a long history of click or murmur and with thickening of the whole valve. Fibroelastic deficiency is most common in older patients (>50 years old), while Barlow's disease is most common in patients <50 years of age, often women, may be associated with connective tissue disorders (e.g., Marfan), and may have a familial predisposition.

Fibroelastic deficiency is the most common cause of severe intrinsic MR requiring surgery.

A prolapse seen in the apical four-chamber view is less specific and should not be used to define MVP.

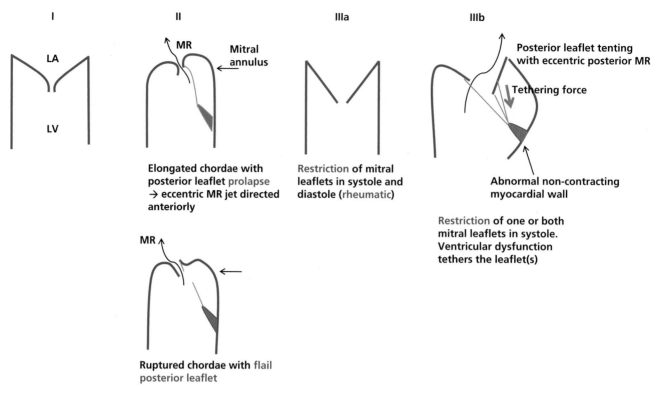

Figure 6.2 Carpentier's classification of the mechanisms of mitral regurgitation.

Type I: Normal mitral leaflet motion with the free edges positioned 5–10 mm below the mitral annular plane. Normally, the leaflets coapt over a minimum length of 2 mm. Type I MR may occur with a leaflet tear secondary to endocarditis or blunt trauma.

Type II: Prolapse of one or both leaflets. The billowing body of the prolapsed leaflet is over 2 mm above the annular plane. The free edge may be above the annular plane, less markedly than the leaflet body. When the free edge is significantly prolapsed and looking into the LA rather than the LV, the leaflet is called a *flail leaflet*.

Type IIIa: Rheumatic or rheumatic-like process. The leaflets and chordae are thickened, retracted, and shortened, with chordal fusion. The mitral motion is restricted in systole and diastole, potentially leading to both MS and MR.

Type IIIb: Ventricular dysfunction pulls the papillary muscle(s) and chorda(e) posterolaterally, restricting the motion of one or both leaflets, predominantly the posterior leaflet.

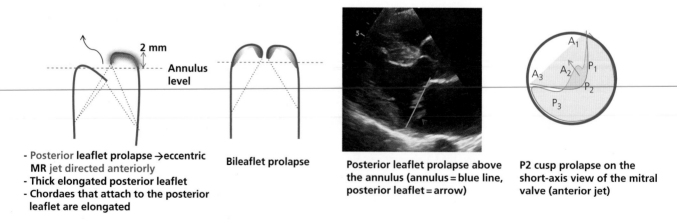

Figure 6.3 Mitral valve prolapse. The long-axis view defines prolapse, while the short-axis view defines which cups are involved (particularly when color Doppler is added).

Notes on MVP (degenerative MV disease)

- MVP is usually benign and occurs in 1–2% of the population with a familial trend. Female-to-male ratio = 2:1.
- MVP most commonly involves the posterior leaflet, especially the posterior cusp P$_2$. While two-thirds of MVPs are posterior MVPs, the anterior leaflet (often A$_2$) or both leaflets are involved in one-third of the cases. When confined to a single cusp, the prolapsed or the flail leaflet may be missed by TTE: TTE shows MR, often very eccentric, hugging the LA wall and underestimated in some views, without obvious structural abnormality. The jet is directed opposite to the prolapsed leaflet.
- MVP may be associated with tricuspid prolapse (in ~40%) and aortic valve prolapse (in ~10%).
- 15% of MVP cases are severe, meaning that they progress to severe MR at a mean follow-up duration of 15 years.
- Risk factors for severe MVP:
  - Man > 50 years old. MVP in an elderly patient is generally more serious than MVP in a young woman
  - Very thick valve (≥5 mm)
  - Significant MR at baseline with MR murmur
- Possible complications in the serious MVP subgroup: (1) severe MR; (2) endocarditis; (3) VT/sudden death (rare)
- MVP, regardless of its severity, can be associated with autonomic dysfunction (e.g., orthostatic intolerance) and atypical complaints (chest pain, fatigue, palpitations).

C. Functional ischemic MR and functional non-ischemic MR (Figures 6.4, 6.5)

Ischemic MR is not a valvular problem; it is a problem of segmental ventricular distortion and, to a lesser extent, increased ventricular sphericity. ***A posterior change in LV geometry tethers the posterior papillary muscle posterolaterally; subsequently, both leaflets are tethered, predominantly the posterior leaflet.*** In fact, *local geometric remodeling that specifically tethers the posterior papillary muscle* is a more important determinant of ischemic MR than global LV remodeling, global LV sphericity, LV dilatation, or EF.[3] Severe MR may be seen with a relatively preserved EF: the majority of patients with ischemic MR secondary to inferior MI have a normal or a mildly reduced EF and a normal LV volume. Studies have shown a higher incidence and greater severity of ischemic MR in patients with inferior as opposed to anterior MI, despite a lower EF and more LV dilatation in anterior MI.[4] This is related to the greater local geometric remodeling seen with inferior MI causing greater posterior papillary muscle displacement. For a given LV volume, local posterior LV remodeling is the determinant of MR severity.[5]

Overall, ~80% of cases of ischemic MR are associated with inferior or inferolateral MI (RCA or LCx), while 20% are associated with anterior MI (LAD),[4,5] although some series found that anterior MI is responsible for ~50% of ischemic MR.[6–8] In two studies of ischemic MR, approximately half the patients had inferior MI, half had anterior MI, and a quarter had infarcts in both territories, with a mean EF of 35–40%.[6,8]

In anterior MI, anterior ventricular dysfunction, which exerts longitudinal tension on the anterior papillary muscle and the leaflets, does not lead to enough tethering to provoke MR. Tethering relates to posterior and apical rather than anterior shift of the papillary muscles, directing papillary muscle tension away from the axial direction that closes the leaflets.[4,9,10] This explains why anterior MI cannot provoke ischemic MR unless global remodeling and posterolateral and apical tethering, usually of both papillary muscles, occurs.[7] Ischemic MR that occurs with anterior MI is, thus, associated with a much lower EF, a larger LV volume, and a larger and more symmetric annular dilatation.[7] Global remodeling may apically tether both leaflets equally (symmetric tethering with central jet); it may also tether the posterior leaflet more prominently, leading to a posterior jet (asymmetric tethering).[10] Conversely, inferior MI tethers the posterior papillary muscle, and consequently both the posterior and anterior leaflets through their attachments to the posterior papillary muscle. Being orthogonal to the posterior papillary muscle, the posterior leaflet is more significantly tethered than the anterior leaflet.

An eccentric, anteriorly directed jet cannot be seen with ischemic MR.

Note that annular dilatation, by itself, does not lead to functional MR. The ratio of leaflet area to annular surface area being normally >2:1, very severe annular dilatation would be required to cause inadequate mitral coaptation. Annular dilatation is, however, a contributing factor in ischemic MR. In addition, the annulus normally has a contractile function in systole. The loss of annular contraction reduces the coaptation of the tented leaflet and contributes to MR.

Contrary to an older belief, ischemic MR is not related to ischemic papillary muscle dysfunction. In fact, papillary muscle ischemia, per se, does not usually produce MR; it is the underlying wall dilatation that produces MR.

In summary: With either inferior or anterior MI, local posterior remodeling or global remodeling with posterior involvement is necessary to produce ischemic MR. The posterior remodeling tethers the posterior papillary muscle, which tethers both leaflets, predominantly the posterior leaflet, and leads to a posteriorly directed MR. Apical tethering of both papillary muscles and leaflets may also occur, especially with a globally remodeled anterior MI.

Functional MR may be secondary to ischemic or non-ischemic global LV dysfunction, with an MR jet that is central or posteriorly directed. Approximately 20% of patients with severe systolic HF have severe MR.

In the setting of acute inferior MI, acute ischemic MR related to leaflet restriction should be distinguished from papillary muscle rupture (the leaflet is restricted in the former vs. prolapsed in the latter). Any process leading to acute ventricular dysfunction may be associated with acute leaflet tethering and acute functional MR. Examples include acute inferior or anterior ischemia or infarction, but also takotsubo cardiomyopathy, myocarditis, and postpartum cardiomyopathy.

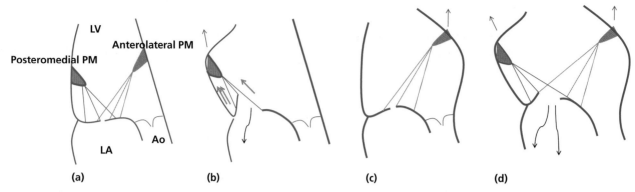

Figure 6.4 Illustration of ischemic MR on longitudinal views. **(a)** Normal valvular anatomy. Both papillary muscles (PM) provide chordae to both mitral leaflets. **(b)** Inferior akinesis with posterolateral displacement of the posterior papillary muscle (PM). This leads to major restriction of the posterior leaflet and minor restriction of the anterior leaflet. The tethering force being more orthogonal to the posterior leaflet, the latter is more restricted than the anterior leaflet. In fact, the anterior leaflet overrides the posterior leaflet. **(c)** Anterior akinesis, by itself, does not lead to major restriction of any leaflet as it pulls the leaflets axially rather than sideways. **(d)** Anterior MI with global remodeling and global LV dilatation pulls both the anterior and posterior papillary muscles apically and posterolaterally. The more the LV is dilated and spherical, the more laterally the leaflets are pulled, the more severe the MR. Both leaflets are tethered, and the jet may be central or predominantly posterior (if the posterior leaflet is more tethered than the anterior leaflet). Note that ischemic MR cannot be anteriorly directed (it is either central or posterior).

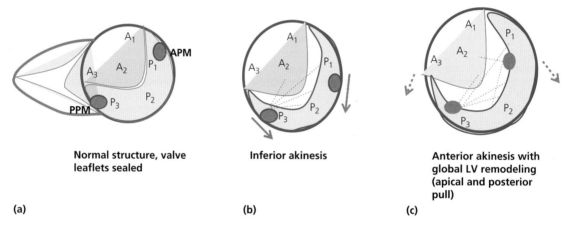

Figure 6.5 (a) Horizontal cut across the mitral valve. Normal ventricular, papillary muscle, and leaflet structures. **(b)** Inferior and inferolateral akinesis with posterior displacement of the posterior papillary muscle. As a result, the posterior leaflet is getting tethered with a posteriorly directed MR. The anterior leaflet is less affected. **(c)** Anterior akinesis with global spherical remodeling of the LV and posterolateral displacement of both the anterior papillary muscle (APM) and posterior papillary muscle (PPM). In addition, the apical remodeling leads to apical tethering of both papillary muscles. As a result, the posterior and anterior leaflets are getting tethered with a jet that is central (symmetric tethering of both leaflets) or posterior (predominant tethering of the posterior leaflet). Thus, posterior leaflet tethering may occur with anterior MI.

Functional MR is dynamic

Ischemic MR (or any functional MR) may vary with dynamic changes in LV volume and geometry. Symptomatic patients with an ischemic mild or moderate MR at rest may have *dynamic MR* that worsens with exercise, i.e., with increased venous return and LV volume.[6,8] The increase in venous return increases LV dimension, leaflet tethering, and annular dilatation, which worsens functional MR. The concept of dynamic MR is an important concept, as it may explain exertional or nocturnal symptoms and pulmonary edema in patients with mild ischemic MR at rest. In this case, MR, LA pressure, and PA pressure increase during exercise or during sleep with the increase in venous return. *In fact, as opposed to patients with mild ischemic MR and no pulmonary edema, patients with mild or moderate ischemic MR who present with pulmonary edema usually have dynamic MR that worsens with exercise or at night*; this apparently "mild" MR is actually a major contributor to their pulmonary edema. This is proven by stress echocardiography, wherein MR severity and PA pressure increase without any ECG or echocardiographic signs of ischemia (effective regurgitant orifice area increases by $\geq 13\,mm^2$).[8]

On the other hand, the minority of patients with inferior MI who have a significant improvement in global myocardial contractility and LV volume with exercise may have a reduction in the severity of the resting functional MR and in leaflet tethering,[8] and those are the patients who may have improvement of ischemic MR purely with revascularization (~10% of patients with ischemic MR).[8]

However, before presuming that dynamic MR is due to a combination of baseline tethering and added loading, always rule out another cause of dynamic MR: off-and-on ischemia secondary to preload change, ACS, or exercise. In the latter case, the wall motion abnormality that drives MR is fleeting rather than persistent, and revascularization will reverse MR. Stress echo will show a dynamic wall motion abnormality, beside the dynamic MR.

> Ischemic MR is typically characterized by chronic, unchanging LV dysfunction/infarction with MR that varies according to the loading conditions. Conversely, another form of ischemic MR is induced by off-and-on ischemia and is characterized by off-and-on LV wall motion abnormality without infarction.

> *Dynamic MR may explain the puzzle of patients who only have an old inferior infarct with an overall preserved EF, no residual ischemia, and mild MR at rest, yet present with pulmonary edema or significant dyspnea on exertion.[6]*

Avoid assessing ischemic MR intraoperatively. The unloading conditions of anesthesia convert the dynamic, severe ischemic MR into mild MR.

D. Severe HTN as an aggravating factor in functional MR; other forms of functional MR

Severe acute or chronic HTN aggravates functional MR. HTN makes it harder for the LV to pump forward, which creates the backward leak. This functional MR quickly improves with HTN control.

Severe functional MR may also be seen with restrictive or hypertensive cardiomyopathy, as a result of the severe LA dilatation, even if LV systolic function and size are relatively preserved.

Functional MR results not only from LV dilatation but also from LA dilatation. LA dilatation pulls the annulus up, which pulls the insertion of the leaflets upwards, resulting in leaflet tethering. It also dilates the annulus.

> HTN worsens *functional MR*, while reduction in preload and afterload improves functional MR. Changes in loading conditions (HTN, exercise) do not affect the severity of an *organic MR*, yet they do affect the regurgitant volume, the LA pressure, and the degree of pulmonary edema.

E. Rheumatic fever

Rheumatic fever leads to scarring and constriction of the leaflets and the subvalvular apparatus, restricting mitral valve closure (→ MR) and opening (→ MS). A predominant or isolated MR may be seen with rheumatic heart disease.

F. Other causes of MR

- Healed, old endocarditis with progressive scarring and retraction of the mitral leaflet(s) may lead to late MR.
- Systolic anterior motion of the anterior leaflet and chordae in HOCM.
- Severe posterior mitral annular calcifications (MAC). MAC may immobilize the basal portion of both mitral leaflets, preventing their normal excursion in diastole (→ MS) and coaptation in systole (→ MR). Also, the mitral annulus loses its expansile function (→ MS) and contractile function (→ MR).

> **Causes of transient severe MR**
>
> **1.** Acute ischemic MR that results from *acute, transient* LV dysfunction.
> **2.** Dynamic ischemic/functional MR that results from *chronic, persistent* LV dysfunction. This MR worsens with an increase in loading conditions (acute HF decompensation, exercise, prolonged supine position, HTN). The acute increase in preload and/or afterload worsens a mild ischemic/functional MR.

> **Important situation: severe MR with severe LV dysfunction**
>
> MR could be the cause of LV dysfunction (intrinsic MR) or, much more commonly, the result of it (functional or ischemic MR). These two conditions are treated differently: intrinsic MR requires valvular repair, whereas the first-line therapy of functional MR is treatment of the underlying LV dysfunction.
>
> Severe organic MR leads to symptoms long before the occurrence of LV dysfunction, and very long before severe LV dysfunction. *Thus, **when severe LV dysfunction is associated with severe MR, LV dysfunction is usually the primary issue and MR is usually functional, unless there is a long history of severe MR**.* The definite diagnosis relies on assessment of the mitral valve structure. If the valve leaflets are thick and prolapsed, MR is organic, whereas if the valve leaflets are thin and normal but restricted in their motion, MR is functional. TEE often helps in that regard, as it provides better leaflet visualization.
>
> Another hint: in acute MR, LV is hypercontractile, i.e., EF is increased rather than decreased. *Acute HF with low EF and severe MR usually implies functional rather than primary MR.*

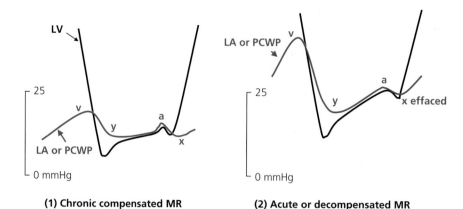

(1) Chronic compensated MR   **(2) Acute or decompensated MR**

Figure 6.6 Difference in V wave and LV diastolic pressure between (1) chronic compensated MR and (2) acute or decompensated MR. In decompensated MR, V wave gets larger, Y descent gets deeper, while X descent gets shallower. LA pressure may switch from (1) to (2) with simple maneuvers: handgrip (↑ afterload), small volume loading, exercise. LA pressure may switch from (2) to (1) with sedation, acute hypertension control, or nitroprusside infusion (↓ preload and afterload). Reproduced with permission from Hanna EB. Mitral regurgitation. In: Hanna EB, Glancy DL. Practical Cardiovascular Hemodynamics. New York, NY: Demos Medical, 2012, p. 112.

III. Assessment of MR severity

A. Severe MR on echo (see also Chapter 32)
Severe MR criteria:

a. Regurgitant color jet fills >40% of the area of the LA, at a proper color gain and a Nyquist limit of 50–60 cm/s. Eccentric MR is underestimated by the jet area.

b. Pulmonary vein systolic flow reversal.

c. High early mitral inflow velocity (E wave >1.2 m/s). Also, *LA must be enlarged* in chronic severe MR.

d. Large PISA radius ≥ 0.9 cm (at 40 cm/s Nyquist limit) and effective regurgitant orifice (ERO) area ≥ 40 mm^2. Note that *20 mm^2 better defines severe ischemic MR*, which tends to be dynamic and underestimated at rest.[6,8]

Acute severe MR may look mild on TTE. The increased LA pressure reduces the LV–LA pressure gradient and the MR velocity, which may reduce the color signal and turbulence; also, acute MR may be eccentric. Thus, if a patient with a questionable MR severity and a normal or hyperdynamic LV has severe pulmonary edema, think of severe MR and perform TEE or left ventriculography.

B. TEE
TEE is performed if the severity or the cause of MR is unclear by TTE. It is also valuable in assessing which cusp(s) is involved and whether repair is feasible.

C. Left ventriculography
Left ventriculography is indicated if the echo data are inconclusive or when there is discrepancy between the echo data and the clinical findings. When properly done, ventriculography is highly accurate in MR grading, as it semi-quantitatively addresses the regurgitant volume rather than velocity.

In severe MR, LA entirely fills with contrast, as intensely as LV (=3+ MR), or more intensely than LV, sometimes with pulmonary venous filling (=4+ MR).

D. Right heart catheterization
Right heart catheterization may be performed as an adjunct to left ventriculography when the severity of MR is unclear. The finding of an ample V wave that exceeds 45 mmHg or is twice the mean PCWP suggests severe MR. However, the V wave may not be that ample in severe but compensated MR (Figure 6.6). An ample V wave may also be seen with decompensated HF, even without MR.

In addition, the invasive measurement of PA pressure and PCWP *at rest and with stress* is valuable in addressing the surgical indication when MR is severe but symptoms are mild and non-specific. An elevated PCWP implies that MR is likely functionally limiting, even if the patient denies any symptom.

E. Stress testing and BNP
Beside an elevated PCWP and PA pressure, a stress test showing a limited exercise tolerance (*class IIa*) or an elevated BNP may indicate surgery in patients who deny symptoms.

IV. Natural history and pathophysiology of organic MR
Even among asymptomatic patients with normal LV function, severe MR leads to symptoms or LV dysfunction in 100% of patients at ~5 years. Asymptomatic severe MR is associated with the following yearly risks: 0.8% sudden death, 5–6% cardiac death, 10% combined cardiac death, HF, or AF, and ~20% death or requirement for valvular surgery (fast progression).[11]

Once symptomatic, the mean survival of severe MR is ~3 years without surgical correction.

In chronic MR, the LV pumps a double stroke volume in two directions, including an "easy" low-pressure LA. This explains how EF is increased if LV is normal and is helped early on by the low afterload. LV diastolic size increases to allow an increase in total stroke volume and the maintenance of a forward stroke volume, whereas LV end-systolic size decreases (EF ↑). Once LV intrinsic contractility starts to fail, EF decreases towards the normal range and LV end-systolic size starts to increase. *An EF of 50–60% is already abnormal and indicates an intrinsic myocardial dysfunction that may not be fully reversed with surgery.* LV afterload is reduced early on in MR, but increases with time as LV systolic size increases (wall stress being proportional to LV systolic size).

V. Treatment of organic (primary) MR

A. Surgical indications in primary MR

The patient must have severe MR *and* one of the following findings:[12]

a. Symptoms (functional limitation class II–IV) (*class I indication*).

b. EF of 30–60% or LV end-systolic diameter (LVESD) ≥ 40 mm (*class I indication*).

c. Asymptomatic patient with normal EF but moderate pulmonary hypertension (systolic PA pressure >50 mmHg at rest or >60 mmHg with exercise) or new-onset AF (*class IIa indication if high likelihood of durable repair*). Pulmonary hypertension implies a risk of HF and symptomatic progression in pauci-symptomatic patients; even lesser degrees of pulmonary hypertension are associated with impairment of long-term survival.[13] As compared to sinus rhythm, AF is associated with excess mortality under watchful management.[14] Also, as opposed to patients with AF >3 months, patients with AF <3 months have a very low recurrence of AF on long-term follow-up after mitral repair, as early LA remodeling is reversed.[15]

d. When EF is <30%, MR is usually secondary to LV dysfunction rather than primary. If primary, mitral surgery remains reasonable (*class IIb*), especially if MV repair is likely. Mitral surgery is still reasonable if MV repair is not likely but MV replacement with chordal preservation is feasible.

e. Severe primary MR (*class I*) or moderate primary MR (*class IIa for mitral repair*) undergoing cardiac surgery for another indication. In a patient undergoing AVR, AVR + mitral repair is preferred to double valve replacement (lower operative risk).

f. *MV repair is reasonable in asymptomatic severe MR with EF >60%, normal LV size, and normal PA pressure, as long as the likelihood of successful repair is >95% and the operative mortality <1% (class IIa, mainly posterior leaflet prolapse).* In fact, there is a significant risk of events associated with severe MR during the watchful waiting period, with a doubling of cardiac mortality and quadrupling of cardiac events.[11,16–20] Furthermore, when surgery is performed in symptomatic patients or those with early LV dysfunction, it frequently leaves residual postoperative LV dysfunction, which carries a poor long-term prognosis. In light of the reduced afterload early on, any EF reduction is a sign of advanced intrinsic LV dysfunction that may not improve postoperatively. Excess mortality persists after surgery in patients operated with EF ≤60% (especially <50%) or severe symptoms III/IV, whereas life expectancy is restored to normal in patients operated with no or minimal symptoms and EF >60%.[21,22] The 5-year mortality of patients who undergo surgery with EF of 50–60% is almost double the mortality of those with EF >60%. Data suggest an improvement in long-term survival and risk of HF with early intervention in these asymptomatic patients (vs. watchful waiting), as long as mitral repair is performed.[18,20] An increase in BNP ≥ 31 pg/ml is also predictive of increased long-term mortality under conservative management.[23] Early surgery may prevent the risk of adverse LV remodeling that occurs in the waiting period or postoperatively.

LV function may deteriorate after mitral surgery:

i. This is partly related to damaging the subvalvular annular–chordal–papillary muscle continuity during mitral valve replacement, which leads to a change in the LV geometry and the effectiveness of LV contraction. In fact, the LV changes from elliptical to spherical, which strongly limits longitudinal motion.

ii. LV deterioration is also related to the fact that, in MR, mild EF reduction is a sign of advanced LV contractile dysfunction that is unlikely to improve postoperatively, particularly since afterload may increase with closing the low resistance leak.

iii. Closing the low-resistance leak increases afterload in the immediate postoperative period. This *"afterload mismatch"* contributes to early EF deterioration. In fact, ~25% of patients with baseline LV dysfunction experience immediate EF deterioration after mitral valve repair, related to this afterload mismatch. This may even happen in a small number of patients (<10%) with normal EF. Yet, afterload mismatch is unlikely to affect long-term EF, as reducing MR also reduces LV volume and improves long-term EF (EF often returns to baseline before hospital discharge).

Mitral valve repair or chordal preservation during mitral replacement lessens LV deterioration. Chordal preservation consists of fixing the chordae and attached leaflet pieces to the annulus before implanting the new valve; this way, the chordae suspend the LV to the annulus and prevent sagging and ballooning of the LV.

B. MV repair is preferred to MV replacement in isolated posterior leaflet prolapse limited to less than half of the posterior leaflet, where MV repair should be attempted and MV replacement restricted to unsuccessful repair (*class I*). It is also indicated with anterior or bileaflet prolapse, when durable repair seems probable (*class I*).

a. MV repair preserves the subvalvular apparatus and the LV geometry. Even if MV replacement is performed, the MV apparatus should be preserved and fixed to the annulus rather than resected to preserve the ventricular geometry.

b. MV repair protects from the LV deterioration that commonly occurs after MV replacement, especially with EF ≤60% but even with EF >60%. MV repair is associated with over 50% improved long-term survival, whether performed for posterior or anterior MVP (vs. MV replacement). In addition, the postoperative mortality after MV repair may be very low (<1%) and approximates half the mortality of MV replacement when expeditiously done (meta-analysis that included Mayo Clinic data).[24]

c. MV repair does not necessitate chronic anticoagulation therapy.

d. MV repair is feasible in MVP, mainly posterior leaflet MVP, but also leaflet perforation secondary to endocarditis, when the annulus is not involved and tissue destruction is limited. MV repair is also recommended for anterior leaflet prolapse, albeit the success rate is lower. MV repair is least successful in rheumatic, calcified MR.

e. *Reoperation rate is ~5–10% at 10 years with posterior MVP, and 20–30% with anterior or bileaflet MVP.* Reoperation is performed for progressive, recurrent MR, often (70%) related to initial technical failure.

f. MV repair of a posterior prolapse typically involves resection of the redundant cusp and placement of an annuloplasty ring. Conversely, anterior prolapse consists of a larger area of cusp prolapse that is more difficult to correct. As opposed to resection of the abnormal cusp, repair of an anterior prolapse consists of chordal transfer: a normal segment of the posterior leaflet is identified, cut and attached with its chordae to the unsupported, prolapsed portion of the anterior leaflet (the cut posterior leaflet is then repaired in a sliding fashion). Chordal transfer may also be performed from the belly of the anterior leaflet to its edge; chordal replacement with PTFE chords may also be performed. An annuloplasty ring is placed at the end. Anterior leaflet repair is improved with these techniques, but there is a higher need for reoperation at 10 years (30% vs. 10% for posterior leaflet).

MV repair may, therefore, be more technically challenging than MV replacement and, in case of failure, requires longer pump time, which may not be tolerated in the sickest patients.

g. *Immediately postoperatively, ~10% of patients undergoing MV repair for MVP develop significant SAM of the anterior leaflet* with LVOT obstruction and significant MR. This MR may be misdiagnosed as failed repair. SAM is secondary to the anterior leaflet being "squeezed" down into the LV by the narrow annuloplasty ring and therefore touching the septum, particularly if the LV cavity is small and the anterior leaflet is long and redundant. Moreover, the increase in steepness of the mitroaortic angle moves the leaflet coaptation line anteriorly towards the LVOT. SAM immediately improves with fluid administration and cessation of inotropic drugs.

C. Medical therapy

Medical therapy does not have a role in primary severe MR, except for the use of ACE-Is and CCBs preoperatively or for an associated hypertension.

VI. Treatment of secondary MR (ischemic and non-ischemic functional MR)

While ischemic MR is initiated by ventricular disease, the ventricular function is frequently normal or mildly/moderately reduced. Therefore, ischemic MR frequently becomes the primary driver of functional limitation, pulmonary edema, and progressive LV remodeling, which begets worsening of MR.[6,8] Treating MR may stop this deleterious process. Three questions need to be addressed before deciding to surgically target functional MR.

A. What is the primary driver of HF (MR vs. underlying LV failure)?

MV repair is not likely to help patients with underlying severe LV enlargement (LV end-diastolic diameter >65 mm) or scarring and non-viability, in which case LV is the primary driver of symptoms and events. LV is irreversibly remodeled and will continue to dilate even after mitral correction.

B. Will revascularization alone reverse MR?

In most patients, coronary revascularization alone does not correct moderate or severe MR. In two registries of severe MR, only ~50% of patients improved their MR with CABG and <10% became mild MR or no MR.[25,26] Up to 70% of patients with moderate MR show an improvement with CABG. The evidence is less compelling for PCI.

Standalone revascularization is expected to improve dynamic MR that is associated with *off-and-on* ischemic dysfunction of a myocardial segment (e.g., ACS) without chronic infarction. This has to be distinguished from dynamic MR that results from fluctuations of loading conditions on top of a *fixed, chronic* myocardial dysfunction. The latter MR usually does not reverse with revascularization, except when it improves with exercise or low-dose dobutamine.

Off/on inferior akinesis with off/on MR → revacularize without MV repair
Steady inferior akinesis with off/on or steady MR → revascularize with MV repair

C. Can MR therapy reverse the underlying tethering process?

Mitral valve reduction annuloplasty consists of suturing a downsized ring to the endocardial surface of the mitral annulus in order to reduce the annular size. Thus, ***rather than addressing the underlying LV dysfunction and tethering, annuloplasty attempts to compensate by addressing the other end of the mitral apparatus***. This explains the inconsistent and sometimes suboptimal long-term results of annuloplasty. The best results are obtained when a rigid or semi-rigid full-circumference annuloplasty is performed with a ring measured to the anterior leaflet area and downsized two sizes (24–28 mm). Posterior bands were used with the thought that the posterior (muscular) annulus is the one that dilates; however, the fibrous anterior annulus dilates as well. In an older Cleveland Clinic series, CABG + mitral annuloplasty (mostly using the posterior flexible Cosgrove–Edwards band) did not show any improvement in functional status or survival compared with CABG only.[27] In addition, one study has suggested that annuloplasty may lead to functional mitral stenosis.[28]

More recently, in a series of patients with severe ischemic MR and mean EF ~30%, CABG + downsized complete annuloplasty showed a sustained improvement in MR, functional status, and reverse remodeling.[29] This benefit mainly applied to patients with LVEDD <65 mm, wherein reverse remodeling occurred and 5-year survival was high (80%); patients with enlarged LV were at an irreversible stage of remodeling and had a low 5-year survival rate (49%) despite annuloplasty. The benefit in moderate ischemic MR is less clear, with one trial showing a lack of benefit and an early hazard of adjunctive annuloplasty, MR improving in 70% of patients undergoing CABG only; another trial of moderate ischemic MR and non-severe LV dilatation (mean EF ~40%) has shown that CABG+complete rigid annuloplasty reduces LV remodeling (LV end-systolic volume) and strikingly improves functional class and peak O_2 consumption in comparison to CABG only, at the expense of higher postoperative complications (length of stay and transfusions) (RIME trial).[30] Other techniques that relieve tethering, such as chordal cutting or papillary muscle repositioning, have been used. The perioperative mortality of CABG+mitral annuloplasty is 3% (RIME) to 8%.[29,30]

In a recent trial of patients with severe ischemic MR and moderate EF reduction (40±10%), *mitral valve replacement with chordal preservation proved equivalent to annuloplasty repair in terms of clinical outcomes and reverse remodeling*, with a more durable MR correction.[31] Most of these patients underwent concomitant CABG (~75%).

All the above data address adjunctive mitral surgery in patients who, for the most part, are undergoing CABG, and mainly show a benefit in patients without a severely enlarged LV. The value of annuloplasty is even more questionable in patients who do not have an indication for CABG. In the latter patients, *severe symptoms without severe LV dysfunction/dilatation* and with a viable myocardium are compelling evidence that MR is the primary driver of symptoms and LV remodeling; surgical correction of MR may, therefore, be beneficial even if CABG is not feasible, as long as the surgical morbidity is low. Medical therapy and CRT, when indicated, are first-line therapy. In fact, CRT improves MR in over 60% of patients with severe functional MR, but may also worsen MR in ~10% of patients.[32,33] This is related to the degree of reverse remodeling (reduction of LV volume) achieved with CRT. An immediate improvement results from coordinated papillary muscle contraction and increased LV pressure, followed by further improvement over the ensuing 3 months.

D. Guidelines for the management of ischemic or non-ischemic functional MR

Guidelines recommend adjunctive mitral annuloplasty or replacement in patients undergoing CABG or AVR who have functional severe MR (*class IIa*) or moderate MR (*class IIb for repair*). In patients with mild or moderate ischemic MR, an exercise test addressing dynamic MR further selects patients who are most likely to benefit. ***Also, as opposed to the ERO cutoff of 40 mm² used to define severe primary MR, a cutoff of 20 mm² better defines severe ischemic MR. This is because ischemic MR is a dynamic MR, and therefore a resting ERO of 20 mm² generally corresponds to a much larger exertional ERO and hemodynamic impact.*** The 20 mm² cutoff has been prognostically validated in registries.[6,8,34]

Patients with severe functional MR who do not have an indication for CABG should receive HF therapy, aggressive hypertension control, and CRT (if indicated) as first-line therapy. Mitral annuloplasty or replacement may be performed if symptoms are class III–IV despite medical therapy and CRT, EF is >30%, and perioperative morbidity is expected to be low (*class IIb* in European and ACC guidelines). In patients with EF <30% and no indication for CABG, annuloplasty is even less compelling, as MR may not be the driver of symptoms or the negative remodeling process, and progressive LV dilatation and deterioration may continue despite mitral surgery. Yet annuloplasty may be considered, particularly if LV is not severely enlarged (*class IIb* recommendation in the ACC guidelines). Percutaneous repair with the Mitraclip appears to be a viable option for these high-risk patients with cardiomyopathy and no plans for CABG.

VII. Treatment of acute severe MR related to acute MI

In case of papillary muscle rupture, perform emergent valvular surgery+CABG. Place IABP preoperatively and consider IV vasodilators (nitroprusside) if blood pressure allows, as in all cases of acute severe MR. MV replacement is often performed, as it is more expeditious than repair, but repair may be performed in select cases.

In acute severe MR secondary to acute mitral leaflet tethering, treat the patient medically with vasodilators and place IABP for temporary support. It is expected that leaflet tethering will improve once the function of the reperfused territory improves. Surgery should be considered as a second-line therapy for those patients who do not improve with medical therapy.

VIII. Percutaneous mitral valve repair using the Mitraclip device

The Mitraclip consists of a clip that approximates the edges of both mitral valve leaflets. This creates a double mitral orifice (edge-to-edge repair) and stabilizes the anteroposterior annular dilatation. It is delivered percutaneously through a trans-septal puncture. One or sometimes two clips (~40%) may be needed. The EVEREST II trial randomized patients with both organic (73%) and functional (mostly ischemic) (27%) severe MR to Mitraclip vs. mitral surgery, mostly mitral repair.[35] At 1 year, a substantial proportion of Mitraclip patients had residual moderate (27%) or severe (~20%) MR, and 22% had to undergo mitral valve surgery at 1 year. However, three subgroups of patients seemed to achieve equivalent benefit and equivalent freedom from death and mitral reoperation with Mitraclip: functional MR, patients >70 years old, and patients with EF <60%. *Thus, Mitraclip may be more suited for functional MR or high-surgical-risk cases.*[36] In addition, two series addressed the use of Mitraclip in patients with severe ischemic or non-ischemic LV dysfunction (EF ~25%), severe LV enlargement, class III/IV HF, and severe functional MR who were refractory to CRT therapy. In these series, Mitraclip led to a significant improvement of MR, LV size, and functional class: ~80% of patients improved to a functional class of I–II at 1 year, and EF improved by >5% on follow-up.[37,38] The majority of patients were left with a moderate degree of MR, but less than 10% had residual severe MR.

Anatomically, when Mitraclip is used for functional MR, the coaptation depth must be <11 mm below the annulus and the leaflets must coapt over >2 mm. When used for degenerative MR, the following are exclusion criteria: severe flail (gap between leaflets ≥ 10 mm in height or ≥15 mm in width), bileaflet flail, or severe bileaflet prolapse.

2. MITRAL STENOSIS

I. Etiology and natural history

- Mitral stenosis (MS) is usually secondary to rheumatic fever and occurs a couple of decades after the initial infection, as the injured valve gets progressively traumatized by the turbulent blood flow. Rheumatic MS is more common in women (2:1), and occurs at a young age in third-world countries (20s–30s) vs. a later age in developed countries (role of recurrent infections?).
- The fibrotic process initially involves the mitral commissures and the leaflet edges, and manifests as commissural fusion. The process then progressively involves the whole valve and subvalvular apparatus with progressive calcifications. The leaflets and subvalvular apparatus (chordae) are thickened, fused, and progressively calcified.

The subvalvular apparatus shortens and pulls on the leaflets, potentially creating rheumatic MR beside MS.

- Symptoms progress more slowly than with other valvular disorders (it takes 5–10 years to progress from early functional class II to functional class III–IV). Asymptomatic or minimally symptomatic patients with moderate/severe MS often remain so for many years.
- Without surgical or percutaneous therapy for class II or III symptoms, the survival is ~50% at 10 years, which is low yet better than other valvular disorders left untreated. However, class IV patients have a mean survival of <1 year without invasive therapy.[39,40]
- Other rare causes of MS:
  - *Mitral annular calcification* (MAC) or *senile MS* – MAC occurs with age and HTN and initially develops at the posterior annulus without causing any inflow obstruction. MAC can progress from the posterior annulus and involve the base of both mitral leaflets and the papillary muscles; the valvular edges remain freely mobile.[41] This is opposite to rheumatic MS, which starts at the valvular edges and commissures. Severe MAC may lead to mild or moderate MS, but also MR (sometimes severe), as MAC impairs the overall leaflet mobility and coaptation. Severe MAC is particularly common in end-stage renal disease. Calcifications may also extend into the mitroaortic interannular fibrosa and tricuspid annulus (Lenegre disease). Since it does not consist of commissural fusion, valvuloplasty is not an effective therapy. Also, annular calcium precludes placement of an adequately sized prosthesis, unless calcium is debrided.
  - *Rheumatic-like inflammatory process* – rheumatoid arthritis, lupus, carcinoid syndrome.
  - *Congenital MS* usually consists of a single papillary muscle to which all chordae converge (parachute mitral valve). This chordal convergence restricts valvular opening. It usually presents early in life.

II. Diagnosis (Table 6.1)

A. Echocardiographic features (see also Chapter 32)

a. Early on, the commissures are fused and the free edges are immobilized, while the body of the anterior leaflet is free-moving. This gives the anterior mitral leaflet a hockeystick shape. The posterior leaflet appears stiff, immobile (Figure 6.7).

b. On the mitral valve M-mode, the E–F slope is flattened because there is no diastasis in mid-diastole. The posterior leaflet is pulled towards the anterior leaflet because of the commissural fusion.

c. The valve and subvalvular apparatus are thick ± calcified. The chordal thickening is particularly well visualized on the apical views (Figure 6.7).

Table 6.1 Severity of MS.

	Mitral valve area	Mean mitral gradient at a normal heart rate (60–80 bpm)
Moderate MS (formerly mild MS)	>1.5 cm²	<5 mmHg
Severe MS	1–1.5 cm²	5–10 mmHg
Very severe MS	≤1 cm²	>10 mmHg

The mitral valve area (4–6 cm²) is normally larger than the aortic valve area (3–4 cm²). As a result, severe AS is classified as valvular area ≤ 1 cm², while severe MS is classified as valvular area ≤ 1.5 cm². Percutaneous or surgical intervention is indicated in severe MS with symptoms or pulmonary hypertension (systolic PA pressure > 50 mmHg at rest or > 60 mmHg with exercise).

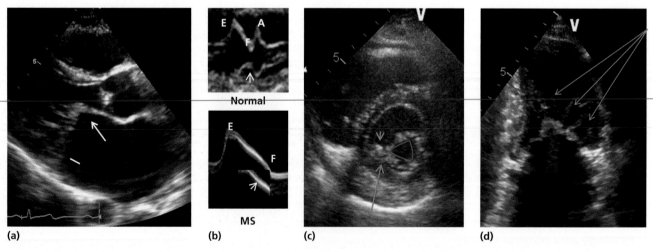

(a)   (b)   (c)   (d)

Figure 6.7 **(a)** Long-axis view in diastole. See the hockeystick shape of the anterior leaflet (*arrow*), the tip of which looks attached to the stiff posterior leaflet (*line*), with no diastolic opening. In fact, **both leaflets are tied together by the commissural fusion. (b)** M-mode across the mitral valve. The E–F slope is flattened and the posterior leaflet is dragged towards the anterior leaflet (*arrowhead*). **(c)** Commissural fusion on the mitral short-axis view (*arrow*). Commissural calcium is seen (*arrowhead*). Rather than oval, the mitral opening has a "fish mouth" shape. **(d)** Apical four-chamber view shows severe chordal thickening extending to the papillary muscles (*arrows*). The mitral leaflets are thickened, and the thickening and immobility extend beyond the edges into the body of the leaflets. The Wilkins score is 10 (leaflet thickness = 2, calcium = 2, leaflet mobility = 2, chordal thickening = 4).

d. Commissural fusion ± commissural calcium are seen on the mitral short-axis view and lead to a "fish mouth" shape of the mitral orifice (Figure 6.7).

e. Since it is easy to align the Doppler beam with the mitral inflow on the apical views, the echocardiographic determination of the transmitral gradient is highly accurate. However, the estimation of the mitral valve area (MVA) using one of the four echo methods (mitral inflow pressure half-time, continuity equation, PISA method, and planimetry) may be subject to measurement errors, and thus MVA is better assessed with invasive hemodynamics.

> ***MVA is a better determinant of MS severity than the mitral gradient.*** In fact, transmitral pressure gradient being proportional to the square of the transmitral flow per second, tachycardia or a high-output state (e.g., anemia, heavy vasodilator use, sepsis) may convert an *anatomically mild MS into a hemodynamically severe MS with a severely increased transmitral gradient. Hence, in any echo or invasive study of MS, it is always important to report the heart rate.* Heart rate reduction and diuresis may be appropriate first-line therapies in an anatomically mild MS, which underlines the importance of invasive assessment of cardiac output and MVA in selective cases. Overall, invasive hemodynamics are valuable for the assessment of MS whenever there is discrepancy between the echocardiographic MVA and transmitral gradient; and whenever it is not clear whether the patient's symptoms or pulmonary hypertension are purely secondary to MS, or rather secondary to mild MS + high-output state and tachycardia, mild MS + LV diastolic dysfunction, or intrinsic pulmonary arterial hypertension. ***The invasive calculation of MVA and cardiac output is invaluable in these cases, and is often performed in patients whose echocardiographic MVA is in the mild or moderate range.***
>
> Another case scenario: a patient with severe diastolic dysfunction and mild/moderate MS (MVA > 1.5 cm²) may have severe LVEDP elevation with a PCWP that is only slightly larger than LVEDP, implying a more dominant role of LV dysfunction in the patient's symptomatology. Stress testing may be performed: a disproportionate rise of PCWP and transmitral gradient in comparison to LVEDP implies significant MS.

B. Catheterization

Simultaneous LA–LV pressures should be obtained, and, ideally, LA pressure should be directly measured through a trans-septal puncture. PCWP is often used as a surrogate of LA pressure and PCWP–LV simultaneous recordings are often used to assess MS (Figure 6.8). Three pitfalls attend the use of PCWP and lead to overestimation of the transmitral gradient:

- PCWP tracing is delayed by 50–150 ms in comparison to LA pressure tracing.
- PCWP is more damped than LA pressure with less deep and steep Y descent.
- The obtained PCWP may not be a true PCWP and may rather be a damped PA pressure or a hybrid PA–PCWP. True PCWP has well-defined A and V waves with the following characteristics: (1) as opposed to the systolic PA pressure, the V wave of PCWP peaks after the T wave and its peak intersects the LV descent; (2) if a diastolic segment is well seen between pressure peaks, it is horizontal or upsloping in PCWP vs.

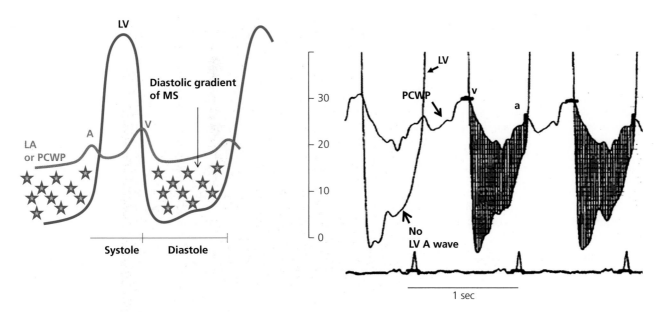

Figure 6.8 Two examples of mitral stenosis with a diastolic pressure gradient between PCWP and LV at a heart rate of 60 bpm (*dark filled areas*).

Due to phase delay, the tracing of PCWP has been shifted to the left so that the *peak of the V wave almost intersects the LV downslope.* There is no LA–LV diastasis, i.e., LA pressure remains higher than LV pressure throughout diastole, signifying severe MS. *LA A wave is pronounced but LV A wave is reduced because of ventricular underfilling.*

With more severe MS, the LA pressure tracing is higher and the intersection between V wave and LV occurs earlier; *this translates into an opening snap that is closer to S_2.*

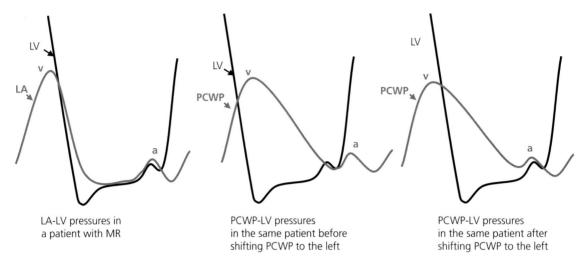

LA-LV pressures in
a patient with MR

PCWP-LV pressures
in the same patient before
shifting PCWP to the left

PCWP-LV pressures
in the same patient after
shifting PCWP to the left

Figure 6.9 False impression of MS resulting from the use of PCWP as a surrogate for LA pressure in a patient with severe MR. When LA–LV pressures are simultaneously recorded, an early diastolic gradient is seen between LA and LV and is quickly followed by diastasis. However, when PCWP–LV pressure recording is performed, the damped and prolonged Y descent creates the impression of a large pressure gradient and a lack of diastasis, even when PCWP is appropriately shifted to the left, thus creating the impression of MS. Also, in comparison to patients without concomitant MR, patients with combined MS and MR are more likely to have their transmitral gradient overestimated with the use of PCWP.

Note that LV A wave is still present and prominent, arguing against severe MS.

Reproduced with permission from Hanna EB. Mitral stenosis. In: Hanna EB, Glancy DL. Practical Cardiovascular Hemodynamics. New York, NY: Demos Medical, 2012, p. 101.

downsloping in damped PA pressure; (3) A wave is seen between V peaks on the PCWP tracing, whereas a dicrotic notch is seen on the PA tracing; (4) mean PCWP <mean PA pressure.

To correct for the phase delay, one may shift the PCWP leftward until the peak of the V wave is bisected by the LV downstroke (or slightly precedes it) (Figure 6.8). ***Two situations particularly exaggerate the PCWP pitfalls, mandating a trans-septal LA pressure measurement:***

- Large V wave, where the "spread-out," damped V downslope creates a false gradient (Figure 6.9).
- Pulmonary hypertension. Pulmonary hypertension makes it difficult to wedge the PA and obtain a true PCWP. Even when PCWP is obtained, it is usually a damped, flat tracing that falsely suggests a high PCWP–LV gradient.

A proper PCWP that is appropriately damped without a large V wave is usually a satisfactory substitute for LA pressure, with overestimation of the transmitral gradient by only 1.7 ± 0.6 mmHg according to some investigators.[42]

Typically in severe MS, LV and LA pressures do not equalize at the end of diastole (diastasis is not reached), even when the heart rate is controlled at 60–75 bpm. In fact, the lack of diastasis at a heart rate <75 bpm or a pause of 1 second implies severe MS. Also, a large LA A wave with a discrepantly absent LV A wave suggests MS (LV underfilling).

When MVA is 1–1.5 cm² but the heart rate is slow (≤60 bpm) and the cardiac output is low, diastasis may be reached at the end of diastole and the gradient may decline to 5 mmHg.

Conversely, tachycardia (or heart rate >80 bpm) may convert a mild MS gradient into a severe MS gradient with no diastasis.

In contrast to AS, the gradient of MS increases during tachycardia (short diastole) and decreases during long R–R cycles.

Note that patients with elevated LA pressure and ample V wave, such as patients with severe mitral regurgitation, have an early diastolic pressure gradient between LA and LV, but in contrast to severe MS, LA and LV pressures equalize at mid-diastole (diastasis) and there is no LA–LV end-diastolic gradient.

C. Echocardiographic Wilkins score
The Wilkins score is an assessment of the severity of the valvular and subvalvular distorsion and a rough estimate of suitability for percutaneous mitral valvuloplasty. It consists of the following four elements, each one being graded from 1 to 4:[43]

  i. valve thickness (only tips are thick vs. the whole valve is thickened)
 ii. valve mobility (only leaflet tips are immobile vs. tips and body vs. tips, body, and base are immobile)
iii. valve calcification (spots of calcium vs. the whole leaflet is calcified)
iv. chordal thickening and calcification (thickening only underneath the leaflets vs. thickening extends towards the papillary muscles).

A score ≤8 makes the valve appropriate for commissurotomy. An additional feature that determines suitability for commissurotomy is the presence of calcium at the commissures (Figure 6.7C). Commissural fusion is present in MS, but commissural calcium is only seen at a later stage and precludes successful commissurotomy, even if the Wilkins score is low. In general, Wilkins score is higher in patients older than 60–70 years of age.

D. TEE

In general, TEE does not offer additional information in regards to the severity and morphology of MS (Wilkins score). The apical TTE views "look" directly into the subvalvular apparatus and allow estimation of the subvalvular thickening better than TEE, which "looks" at the mitral valve through the enlarged LA.

However, TEE is indicated prior to percutaneous valvotomy, in order to assess (i) severity of MR, and (ii) presence of left atrial appendage thrombus.

E. Stress testing and other maneuvers for MS

Resting transmitral gradient may not reflect the true severity of MS. As expressed in Gorlin's equation, for the same mitral valve area, the transmitral gradient is directly proportional to the square of the per-second flow across the valve (MVA $\propto$ transmitral flow/$\sqrt{}$transmitral gradient). Thus, if the per-second diastolic flow doubles because the cardiac output increases and/or the diastolic filling time decreases (tachycardia), the pressure gradient across the valve quadruples.[44–46]

Stress testing is useful in symptomatic patients with *mild/moderate MS, after ruling out tachycardia or high-output state as an aggravating factor*, and helps sort out whether their symptoms are due to MS or LV failure. In MS, PCWP and transmitral gradient increase with exercise while LV diastolic pressure remains unchanged; in LV failure, both PCWP and LV diastolic pressure increase with exercise while the gradient remains unchanged. MS is clinically significant and would likely benefit from an intervention if the mean transmitral gradient increases to >15 mmHg; or if systolic PA pressure or PCWP increases to >60 mmHg or >25 mmHg, respectively, without a significant increase in LVEDP.

A second condition where stress testing is helpful is asymptomatic severe MS. An exertional increase of systolic PA pressure to >60 mmHg or a severe increase in transmitral gradient signifies that the patient is likely limited functionally and will likely benefit from an intervention to avoid the consequences of prolonged pulmonary hypertension.

Note that, similarly to exercise, the heavy use of vasodilators increases cardiac output and the mitral gradient. Also, passive leg raising increases venous return and the mitral gradient. In fact, passive leg raising is routinely performed during echo assessment of MS. Dobutamine may also be used.

III. Treatment

A. Medical therapy

- Diuretics and β-blockers often produce substantial symptomatic improvement. β-Blockers increase diastolic time, allowing more time for LA emptying. A heart rate of 60 bpm should be targeted. Medical therapy is not usually indicated as a standalone therapy, as even patients with class II symptoms have impaired long-term outcomes without mechanical relief of MS. Standalone medical therapy may, however, be used in select patients with class II symptoms:
  - Patients with class II symptoms who do not have appropriate morphological features for percutaneous mitral balloon valvotomy (PMBV). Class II symptoms are not severe enough to warrant surgery.
  - Patients who improve after PMBV but have residual symptoms.
  - Patients with mild/moderate MS that is symptomatic because of hemodynamic disturbances (tachycardia, high cardiac output).
  - Sedentary, elderly patients with mild symptoms on exertion.[47] This includes senile MS.
- Treatment of AF: β-blockers and/or digoxin are used for rate control. Rhythm control may be attempted after a new onset of AF, but repeated DC cardioversions should be avoided in light of the associated stroke risk and the fact that, over time, rhythm control is difficult to achieve in MS. The yearly risk of stroke with the AF–MS combination is 10–15% per year, implying a critical role of warfarin therapy.

Note the effect of β-blockers on the transmitral gradient (Figure 6.10). The reduction of PCWP and transmitral gradient with a longer diastole makes β-blocker therapy important in decompensated MS with pulmonary edema. A similar benefit of β-blockade is seen when pulmonary edema is related to HOCM. *No other case of decompensated left heart failure, whether systolic or diastolic, is acutely served by β-blockers.*

B. Indications for percutaneous or surgical therapy

A mechanical intervention is indicated for select patients with **severe** ($\leq$1.5 cm^2) **or very severe MS** ($\leq$1 cm^2):[12]

- Symptoms class II–IV for PMBV or III–IV for MV *surgery (class I indication)*.
- Asymptomatic patient with moderate pulmonary hypertension qualifies for PMBV (systolic PA pressure >50 mmHg at rest, >60 mmHg with exertion) *(class I indication in older guidelines)*. Pulmonary hypertension more readily indicates mechanical correction in MS than MR, as pulmonary hypertension of MS more quickly progresses to precapillary pulmonary hypertension and RV failure.
- Asymptomatic patient with very severe MS ($\leq$1 cm^2) qualifies for PMBV, as the patient likely has unnoticed functional decline and will develop progressive pulmonary hypertension *(class IIa)*.
- Asymptomatic patient with AF. PMBV may be performed, but the strength of this recommendation is weak *(IIb)*, as PMBV has not been universally successful in preventing or reverting rheumatic AF ($\neq$ MV replacement for MR).[47]

Also, as explained above, symptomatic patients with moderate MS (MVA 1.5–2 cm^2) and moderate gradient at rest need to be assessed with stress testing. A severe increase in transmitral gradient without a significant change in LVEDP implies that MS is hemodynamically significant and may benefit from PMBV *(class IIb)*. **On the other hand, patients with moderate anatomic MS who have a severe**

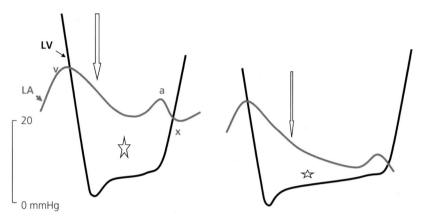

Figure 6.10 β-blockers slow the heart rate and allow more LA emptying, which ultimately reduces LA pressure, V and A waves.

The slope of the PCWP descent is unchanged (*arrows*); however, a longer diastole allows a longer duration of emptying and approximation of LA and LV pressures. Diastasis may be achieved if MS is not very severe. The height of LA pressure ↓ after several long R–R cycles as LA volume ↓.

Reproduced with permission from Hanna EB. Mitral stenosis. In: Hanna EB, Glancy DL. Practical Cardiovascular Hemodynamics. New York, NY: Demos Medical, 2012, p. 107.

gradient at rest need to be invasively assessed and treated for associated hemodynamic disturbances: tachycardia, high-output state (e.g., anemia, vasodilator therapy). In the absence of those hemodynamic disturbances, moderate MS may be the cause of the severe gradient and the severe pulmonary hypertension and may warrant PMBV (also, a valve area of 1.6 cm² may imply severe MS when indexed for body size).

For patients who are not PMBV candidates, mitral valve replacement is not usually considered unless symptoms are class III/IV, i.e., more severe than required for PMBV, as valve replacement has a higher operative mortality than PMBV. Patients with class II symptoms and a valve morphology that is not favorable for PMBV should undergo medical therapy with 6-month follow-ups rather than surgery. Yet, those patients with severe pulmonary hypertension and MVA <1 cm² are likely more symptomatic than they claim and likely qualify for valve replacement (*class IIa in older guidelines*).

On the other hand, patients who have class III/IV symptoms with a valve morphology that is not suitable for PMBV but who are at a high surgical risk may still undergo PMBV (*class IIa*).

C. Percutaneous commissurotomy (or percutaneous mitral balloon valvotomy [PMBV])
When feasible, PMBV is the therapy of choice for MS.

1. Mortality = 1–2%, stroke ~1%
2. Risk of severe MR ~2–5% (moderate MR ~15%)
3. A successful PMBV is defined as a post-PMBV valvular area ≥ 1.5 cm² with ≤ moderate (2+) MR
4. PMBV should be considered if:

    i. Wilkins score ≤ 8 with no commissural calcium. The extent of calcifications and the subvalvular involvement are the two most important features of Wilkins score.

    ii. No MR, or mild MR.

    iii. No thrombus in the left atrium or left atrial appendage (ruled out by TEE). If thrombus is present, give 1–3 months of anticoagulation then reassess and attempt PMBV if the thrombus resolves. Surgical commissurotomy is an alternative.

Valvotomy works by splitting the fused commissures. Unlike AS, early MS mainly consists of a ***commissural fusion that is not calcified***. Tearing this fusion opens the mitral orifice, and thus balloon valvotomy is effective in treating early MS. Once the fibrosis and the immobility extend to the body of the leaflets or the subvalvular apparatus, or once calcium develops, valvotomy becomes less effective and risks tearing the stiff unyielding valve or the subvalvular apparatus in the process of dilating the orifice. Also, the balloon may get stuck in the thick subvalvular apparatus and tear it upon inflation. This is how Wilkins score and commissural calcium predict outcomes with PMBV.

In its original description, a Wilkins score ≥ 12 particularly predicted poor results with PMBV, while over a third of patients with an intermediate Wilkins score of 9–11 had a good result with PMBV.[43] In one large analysis, ~60% of patients with Wilkins scores 9–11 achieved a successful result with PMBV, and even patients with Wilkins score ≥ 12 achieved significant improvement of MVA, although a full success was uncommon (30%).[48] In an analysis of elderly patients >70 years of age, MVA and symptoms improved in most patients, even those with Wilkins score >8; half of patients with Wilkins score >8 had improvement of MVA to >1.2 cm², and most patients, even those with scores >10, had some improvement of valve area and functional class with PMBV.[49] Also, while moderate 2+ MR predicts a 4× higher failure rate, it does not prohibit PMBV.[43,48] In the original Wilkins paper, no patient with moderate MR developed severe MR after PMBV.[43] In a large PMBV series, ~6.5% of patients had moderate baseline MR.[48] Balance Wilkins score with the degree of MR (Wilkins score of 10 without any MR may be as amenable to PMBV as Wilkins score of 8 with mild-to-moderate MR).

Thus, while a surgical approach is advisable in most patients with high scores, PMBV may still be beneficial in patients with an intermediate (9–11) or even high score, or patients with 2+ moderate MR when serious comorbidities are present or the surgical risk is high.[48–50] Hence, the ACC guidelines consider PMBV a reasonable therapy for patients with class III/IV symptoms and a valve morphology that is not favorable for PMBV if the surgical risk is high (*class IIb indication*).

After a successful PMBV, restenosis occurs at a rate of ~20% at 10 years, more so in patients with a suboptimal early result and in those with unfavorable Wilkins score, which is associated not only with short-term but also with long-term failure.[51,52] Overall, ~25% of patients require MV replacement within 5 years, whether for restenosis, progression of a suboptimal result, or progression of MR; this risk is higher in patients with an unfavorable early result or a high Wilkins score (up to 50%).[48,52] Redo PMBV may be performed with a high success rate (~75%) in the presence of favorable echocardiographic features.[51]

Beside a young age < 60–70 years, two clinical findings imply that the valve is pliable and is likely to be responsive to PMBV: loud S$_1$ *and* the presence of an opening snap.

D. Surgical mitral commissurotomy
1. Perioperative mortality = 1–2%
2. Indications: pliable mitral leaflets with no severe subvalvular involvement, but with a left atrial appendage thrombus that precludes percutaneous therapy, CAD that necessitates CABG, or unavailability of percutaneous therapy. In general, for the same patient, surgical commissurotomy has the same success rate as PMBV.

E. Mitral valve replacement; AF procedures
MV replacement is necessary in the case of extensive mitral valve calcification, high Wilkins score, or combined MS and MR. The operative mortality is ~4–6%, which increases to ~12% if significant pulmonary hypertension has developed. Since MV replacement has a higher risk than PMBV, patients who do not qualify for PMBV qualify for MV replacement later in the course of disease, i.e., for more severe symptoms (III–IV).

When surgery is performed for MS or MR associated with persistent AF or paroxysmal symptomatic AF, biatrial ablation lines that include the pulmonary veins, the venae cavae, and the valvular annuli (maze procedure) may be performed and are associated with a high success in maintaining sinus rhythm (up to 80%), even in patients with left atrial enlargement (*class II indication, class IIb in non-mitral surgery*).[53] Maze procedure may not significantly add to the complexity and risk of a mitral valve procedure as the LA is already open.[12] A less invasive uniatrial ablation or isolated pulmonary vein ablation (mini-maze) may be performed in paroxysmal AF or along non-mitral surgeries.[12] Excision of the left atrial appendage may also be performed, although the benefit on stroke reduction is unclear.

Patients with severe MS and chronically elevated PCWP > 25 mmHg may develop reactive changes in the pulmonary arteriolar bed, severe increases in the pulmonary vascular resistance (PVR), as high as 25 Wood units, and very severe pulmonary arterial hypertension disproportionate to the PCWP. This may be associated with severe RV failure. Even at this stage, however, patients usually respond to correction of MS; the elimination of the passive postcapillary component of pulmonary hypertension results in an immediate drop in PA pressure, followed by a slow and gradual decline in the reactive and hypertrophic component.[54–56] In fact, PA pressure and PVR decline towards normal over the course of several weeks to months. Therefore, invasive treatment is still warranted at the stage of severe pulmonary hypertension. In the majority of patients, an almost complete normalization of pulmonary hypertension is expected. Pulmonary vasodilators (endothelin antagonist, intravenous prostacyclin) may be temporarily used in the early postoperative period.

---

3. AORTIC INSUFFICIENCY

I. Etiology

A. Acute AI
a. *Endocarditis:* the vegetation may perforate the leaflet(s) or prevent valvular coaptation.
b. *Aortic dissection* leads to AI through three potential mechanisms: (i) dilatation of the sinotubular junction; (ii) dissection extends into the leaflet attachment at the sinotubular junction, resulting in leaflet prolapse and eccentric AI; (iii) dissection flap prolapses through the aortic orifice and prevents leaflet coaptation. AI may also be pre-existent, secondary to a bicuspid aortic valve.
c. *Closed chest trauma* may lacerate the aortic leaflet or its sinotubular insertion, causing it to prolapse. Being anterior, the aortic valve is the valve most commonly involved in chest trauma.

B. Chronic AI
a. *Dilatation of the ascending aorta with secondary AI:* this is the most common cause of severe AI. Dilatation of the ascending aorta may lead to dilatation of the junction between the aortic root and the sinuses of Valsalva, called the *sinotubular junction*, precluding the coaptation of the aortic leaflets (Figure 6.11). Rather than being secondary to AI or AS, aortic dilatation is a primary process that can cause AI or coexist with bicuspid aortic valve disease. While potentially causing AI, aortic dilatation is reciprocally worsened by the high stroke volume of AI; it is also worsened by the high post-stenotic jet of AS (post-stenotic dilatation).
Causes of ascending aortic disorders:

i. Degenerative aortic dilatation, related to age and HTN, is the most common cause of ascending aortic dilatation.
ii. Cystic medial necrosis, which occurs in younger patients: (1) Marfan or Marfan fruste, (2) bicuspid aortic valve, (3) spondyloarthropathies.

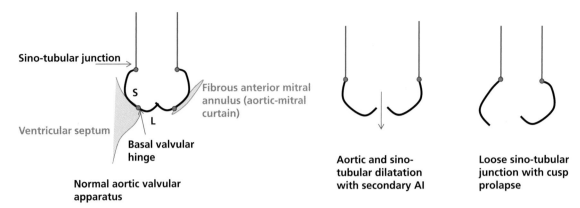

Figure 6.11 Aortic leaflets and their relation to the ascending aorta. A normal valve apparatus consists of aortic tissue that extends from the *sinotubular junction*, forms local aortic dilatations called *aortic root or sinuses of Valsalva (S)*, then touches the ventricle and suspends the aortic *leaflets (L)* (also called semilunar *cusps*). The sinuses of Valsalva are an extension of the aortic wall tissue. The sinotubular junction, rich in elastic tissue, provides the main support for the sinuses. The coronary arteries originate from the sinuses of Valsalva or just above them. Two-thirds of the circumference of the aortic valve is connected to the muscular ventricular septum, while the remaining one-third is in fibrous continuity with the anterior mitral leaflet (fibrous trigone, close to the non-coronary posterior cusp) (see Figure 6.1). At one point posteriorly, the aortic valve is in continuity with the interatrial septum. The *annulus* is a ring formed by the junction of the basal valvular hinges (leaflets' insertion on the ventricle).

b. *Aortic valve disorders*

   i. Bicuspid aortic valve is the most common valvular cause of severe AI. AI results from prolapse of a leaflet or incomplete closure of a thickened redundant valve.

   ii. Old, healed endocarditis. Subacute endocarditis may only be associated with mild or moderate AI early on, but progressive valvular deformity results from the healing process and leads to progressive AI (progressive widening of a perforation or progressive retraction of the scarred leaflet(s) with malcoaptation).

   iii. Idiopathic degeneration of the aortic valve with increased and disorganized collagen and elastic fibers. Anatomically, a mild degree of thickening/retraction, redundancy, or myxomatous degeneration may be seen. This was the most common cause of isolated AI in one study.[57]

   iv. Rheumatic fever with fibrosis and retraction of the leaflets. Fibrosis and fusion of the commissures also leads to AS. The aortic valve is immobile and does not open or close (combined AS/AI).

   v. Prolapse of an aortic valve leaflet in the context of bicuspid aortic valve, endocarditis, trauma, or myxomatous degeneration.

   vi. Degeneration of a bioprosthesis.

II. Pathophysiology and hemodynamics (Figure 6.12)

A. Acute AI

In acute AI, LV is non-compliant and LV volume is normal. Thus, the regurgitant volume leads to a severe increase in LVEDP and the aortic and LV diastolic pressures come close together (Figure 6.12). LV diastolic pressure exceeds LA pressure in mid- or late-diastole (Figure 6.12), leading to a reverse LV–LA gradient and forcing the mitral valve to close prematurely (functional MS), a finding typical of decompensated AI.[58,59] Since LV is not dilated, the stroke volume is reduced in acute AI. Therefore, in addition to the low DBP, SBP is usually low (e.g., BP 90/40 mmHg). **As opposed to chronic AI, pulse pressure is only mildly widened, but this already suggests acute AI in a patient with acute heart failure, wherein the arterial pulse pressure is typically narrow. Tachycardia is an important compensatory response** in acute AI as it increases the cardiac output and reduces the regurgitant time, and thus should be respected.

B. Chronic compensated AI

In chronic compensated AI, LV volume increases, the total stroke volume increases, leading to a high pulse pressure (e.g., 160/60 mmHg), and the forward stroke volume is maintained. The LV is large and compliant in a way that it accommodates the regurgitant volume without an increase in LVEDP. The aortic and LV pressures do not approximate at the end of diastole; on Doppler, this corresponds to a gradual rather than steep drop of the regurgitant flow velocity with a pressure half-time that is >250 ms, even if AI is severe. While a wide pulse pressure (>½ SBP or >60–80 mmHg) is a very sensitive finding in chronic severe AI, it is not a specific finding and may be seen in a poorly compliant aorta and in high-output states with low afterload (patent ductus arteriosus, hyperthyroidism, anemia, fever, and arteriovenous fistula).

   The peripheral femoral pressure may get excessively amplified and may exceed the central systolic pressure by 50 mmHg or more. This is an exaggeration of a normal effect and is due to the hyperdynamic state and the excess of reflected waves in the periphery. These reflected waves may explain a second systolic pressure peak in the peripheral arteries and aorta (pulsus bisferiens).

C. Chronic decompensated AI

In chronic decompensated AI, the LV function starts to decline, and EF decreases such that the forward stroke volume declines and the LV volume further increases. This leads to increased LVEDP despite good LV compliance. Similarly to acute AI, LV and aortic pressures approximate in end-diastole.[58,59] On Doppler, this corresponds to a steep drop of regurgitant flow velocity throughout diastole with a short pressure half-time <250 ms. Total stroke volume remains elevated, and thus the pulse pressure remains elevated. At an advanced stage, when EF is severely reduced, total stroke volume and pulse pressure may decline.

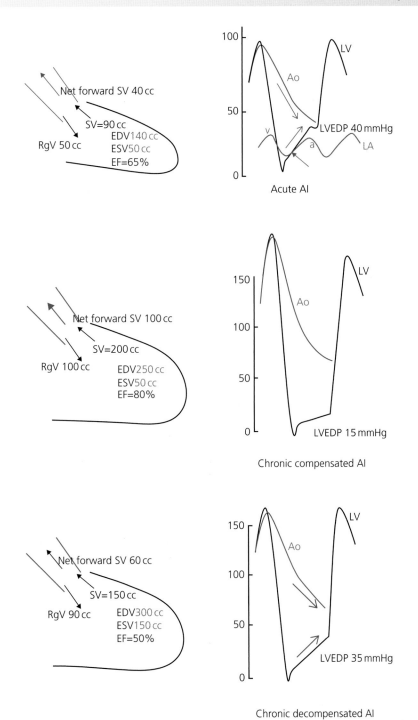

Figure 6.12

1. In acute AI, LV volume is normal and the regurgitant volume leads to a severe increase in LVEDP. The LV and aortic pressures approximate in end-diastole (*blue arrows*). LV diastolic pressure exceeds LA pressure in mid- or late-diastole (*black arrow*).

2. In chronic AI, LV volume increases and the total stroke volume increases, thus leading to a high pulse pressure, and the forward stroke volume is maintained. The LV is large and compliant in a way that it accommodates the regurgitant volume without an increase in LVEDP.

3. In chronic decompensated AI, the LV function starts to be impaired, EF is reduced in a way that the forward stroke volume is reduced, and the LV volume increases, leading to increased LVEDP. Total stroke volume remains elevated, and thus, the pulse pressure remains elevated.

Note the attenuation or loss of the dicrotic notch in all severe AI, especially acute. EDV, end-diastolic volume; EF, ejection fraction; ESV, end-systolic volume; RgV, regurgitant volume; SV, stroke volume.

Reproduced with permission from Hanna EB. Aortic regurgitation. In: Hanna EB, Glancy DL. Practical Cardiovascular Hemodynamics. New York, NY: Demos Medical, 2012, p. 115.

As opposed to other valvular disorders, chronic AI is well tolerated during exercise. In fact, tachycardia reduces diastole and the time available for regurgitation, and the vasodilatation associated with exercise reduces the regurgitant volume, which allows an increase in cardiac output during exercise. That is why severe AI, as opposed to MR, is well tolerated for years before symptoms develop. In addition, in AI, volume overload must surpass the compliance of the LV then the compliance of the LA to provoke pulmonary edema, whereas in MR only surpassing the compliance of the LA is necessary. Symptoms develop very gradually and the patient adapts to them over the years, sometimes not realizing the change in functional status.

Note that both preload and afterload are increased in severe AI. The LV dilatation increases wall stress, i.e., afterload, which is proportional to both the LV systolic pressure and the LV radius. Eccentric LV hypertrophy allows the LV to adapt to this load increase. Initially, the EF reduction results from the progressive increase of LV size and afterload rather than an intrinsic LV contractile dysfunction (**afterload mismatch**). *This process is fully reversible with AVR and is different from the early decline of EF in MR, which already implies a significant contractile dysfunction that may be irreversible, LV afterload not being increased with MR early on.* With time, however, even in AI, impaired contractility progressively becomes a major contributor to the decline in EF and may not be fully reversed with surgery, particularly when EF is <25% or the decline has persisted over 18 months preoperatively.

III. Diagnosis

A. TTE
TTE is useful to diagnose the severity and etiology of AI. The following features suggest severe AI:

- The width of the regurgitant jet *just below the aortic valve* level is >60% of the LVOT diameter (long-axis view), or >60% of the aortic area (short-axis view). The narrowest AI neck, measured *at the aortic valve* level and called vena contracta, is >6 mm (long-axis view). Bicuspid AI jet may be eccentric and may thus be underestimated.
- Holodiastolic flow reversal in the descending aorta (most important feature).
- On the spectral Doppler, pressure half-time of the regurgitant flow is <250 ms; this correlates with AI acuity and the status of the LV. Pressure half-time may be >250 ms if AI is severe but chronic and compensated. Conversely, pressure half-time may be <250 ms in patients with moderate AI but underlying severe LV dysfunction (from CAD, HTN).
- Also, *to diagnose chronic severe AI, LV must be dilated.*

B. TEE
TEE is not significantly superior to TTE for the assessment of the severity of AI. TEE is superior for the anatomical assessment of the aortic valve and aortic annulus (bicuspid morphology, endocarditis), and for the assessment of the ascending aorta.

C. Invasive assessment (aortic root angiography and hemodynamic measurements)
As in other valvular disorders, invasive assessment of AI is indicated when echo is inconclusive in regards to the severity of AI or when there is discrepancy between clinical findings and echo results.

On aortic root angiography, severe AI is characterized by LV filling that is as dense (3+) or more dense (4+) than aortic filling.

Hemodynamically, severe AI is characterized by four features (Figure 6.12): (1) wide aortic pulse pressure, particularly seen in chronic AI; (2) loss of the aortic dicrotic notch, particularly seen in acute AI; (3) LV end-diastolic pressure approximates aortic pressure; (4) LV end-diastolic pressure exceeds mean PCWP and even end-diastolic PCWP (the last two findings are seen with acute or chronic decompensated AI).

IV. Natural history and symptoms
Asymptomatic severe AI with normal LV function has a slow progression: <0.2% sudden cardiac death per year, 4.5% progression to symptoms and/or LV dysfunction per year.[12] Patients with LVESD >50 mm or LVEDD >70 mm have the highest risk of progression to symptoms and/or LV dysfunction (10–20% per year).

Conversely, symptomatic AI or AI with LV dysfunction has a mean survival rate of 2–3 years without surgical intervention: yearly mortality 5–10% if NYHA class II dyspnea, >10% if angina, >20% if class III–IV HF, wherein the mean survival is 1.5 years.[60]

AI symptoms appear late in the disease process, usually after LV has severely enlarged. Class II *dyspnea* appears earlier than *angina* and *severe HF*. Subendocardial coronary flow being driven by the gradient between aortic diastolic pressure and LVEDP, angina is often functional and related to the severe drop in aortic diastolic pressure and the increase in LVEDP. Moreover, O_2 demands of the large LV are severely increased. Angina may be nocturnal rather than exertional, aggravated by bradycardia, wherein the aortic diastolic pressure decreases to very low levels. Diastolic reversal of coronary flow may be seen in severe cases. *Palpitations* may appear early on and are related to the ejection of a large LV volume, especially after a PVC; they are not, per se, an indication for surgery.

V. Treatment

A. Medical therapy
Aortic valve surgery is the only effective therapy for severe AI that requires treatment. Vasodilators (ACE-I, CCBs) may be useful for systolic HTN and are used as a temporizing measure preoperatively. Vasodilators, as well as β-blockers, may be used in patients who are not undergoing surgery because of high risk (*class IIa*). By prolonging diastole, β-blockers may aggravate symptoms, but if tolerated, they may prevent the deleterious LV dilatation and remodeling, according to one retrospective analysis.

In severe asymptomatic AI with dilated LV and no indication for surgery, vasodilators may slow LV dilatation; however, a randomized trial has disproved this theory, and thus vasodilators have a questionable value in severe asymptomatic AI (not recommended).[61] Also, it is important to avoid a harmful drop in DBP with these agents; a slightly increased SBP may be accepted if SBP reduction would come at the price of excessive DBP reduction (per guidelines). Mild exercise is allowed in asymptomatic severe AI. Athletic activity may be allowed in some cases, after performing stress testing for safety purposes; the long-term effect of exercise on severe AI is, however, unknown.

B. Indications for surgery

Aortic valve surgery is indicated for severe AI with any of the following:

- Symptoms (NYHA functional class ≥ II)
- EF <50% (as compared to EF ≤ 60% for MR)
- LVESD >50 mm (as compared to ≥ 40 mm for MR) or >25 mm/m² of BSA
- Asymptomatic severe AI while undergoing CABG or other cardiac/aortic surgery. AVR is also reasonable for moderate AI while undergoing cardiac/aortic surgery (*class IIa indication*)

Similarly to LVESD, LVEDD correlates with AI volume overload but less strongly with LV systolic function. Surgery may be considered for LVEDD >65 mm, particularly when LV dilatation is rapidly progressive and the surgical risk is low (*class IIb indication*). In general, asymptomatic patients with less severely enlarged LV (LVESD 40–50 mm or LVEDD 55–65 mm) should be re-evaluated by echo in 3 months then every 6–12 months if the LV dimensions are stable. If unstable, echo should be repeated every 3 months.

AI is tolerated for a long period of time before symptoms develop. Even when symptoms develop, they are insidious in a way that the patient may not realize his functional limitation. *Before considering AI asymptomatic, exercise testing is often warranted.*

Patients with advanced symptoms or LV dysfunction. As opposed to MR, LV function does not usually deteriorate postoperatively and is likely to improve even with markedly reduced EF.[62] Early on in AI, the reduced EF is secondary to the high afterload rather than intrinsic dysfunction (afterload mismatch). AVR reduces regurgitant flow, which reduces LV wall stress/afterload and allows an improvement of EF, the earliest sign being a reduction of LV size. However, long-term postoperative survival is significantly reduced, ~ in half, in patients with NYHA class III–IV symptoms or EF <50% preoperatively, especially if LV dysfunction has been prolonged >18 months, severe (EF <25%), or not recovering early postoperatively (long-term mortality 5–10% per year).[60,63,64] Patients with EF <25% may have irreversible myocardial damage and persistent LV dysfunction postoperatively, yet most of these patients have a meaningful postoperative recovery, particularly if symptoms are class II/III, LV dysfunction is recent, and HF significantly improves with preoperative diuretics and vasodilators.[12,62] *No EF cutoff is prohibitive of AVR.* Postoperatively, the earliest sign of LV improvement is a decrease in LV diastolic size, which should occur within 2 weeks of surgery. In fact, 80% of LVEDD decline occurs within 2 weeks, and correlates with the eventual improvement of EF that ensues within 6–12 months.[12] A lack of early reduction of LV size implies intrinsic LV dysfunction.

C. AI and ascending aortic dilatation

Ascending aortic replacement is indicated for: (i) ascending aortic dilatation, ≥ 5.5 cm in most patients, including bicuspid valve patients, or ≥ 5 cm in patients with Marfan syndrome or bicuspid valve with family history of aortic dissection; or (ii) ascending aortic dilatation ≥ 0.5 cm/ year. The same 5.5 cm cutoff is used for aortic dilatation at the level of the sinuses of Valsalva or beyond the sinotubular junction. In the absence of significant AI, the ascending aorta is replaced with an aortic graft that is sutured to the aortic ring, and the valve is spared (valve-sparing aortic root replacement or reimplantation technique [David's surgery]); the coronaries are reimplanted, sometimes with an interposition graft.[65–67]

Patients with combined ascending aortic disease and severe AI may undergo a composite graft replacement of both the aortic root and the aortic valve (Bentall procedure, or Cabrol procedure if an interposition graft is used for coronary reimplantation); the composite graft typically has a mechanical valve. The valve may be spared and reimplanted rather than replaced if the cusp's tissue quality is good and the valve is not calcified, this being associated with an acceptable long-term result and a 5–15% risk of reoperation for AI at 10 years.[65–67] Even a bicuspid valve may be repaired if non-calcified and regurgitant rather than stenotic.

In patients with less than severe AI and/or less than severe aortic root dilatation, the following situations may be encountered:

- Severe ascending aortic dilatation with moderate AI: beside ascending aortic replacement, aortic valve replacement may be performed if the valve is severely abnormal. Aortic valve reimplantation may be performed if the cusp tissue quality is good, sometimes along with resuspension of a prolapsed cusp (*class IIa*).
- Moderate ascending aortic dilatation along with severe AI or AS that has a surgical indication: beside aortic valve replacement, replace the ascending aorta when it is ≥ 4.5 cm rather than 5.5 cm (*class I*). If unoperated, ~60% of patients with a bicuspid valve and an aorta of 4.5–4.9 cm go on to develop significant aortic events requiring aortic surgery over the next 15 years, mainly progressive aortic dilatation;[67] thus, in this range, concomitant aortic surgery is particularly applied to young patients and those at a low operative risk.

D. Aortic valve repair

Aortic valve reimplantation, a form of aortic valve repair, may be performed in patients with severe or moderate AI whose primary disorder is aortic root disease and whose cusp tissue quality is good. Resuspension of a prolapsed cusp may additionally be performed.

While aortic valve replacement remains the standard surgery for AI due to aortic valve disease, aortic valve repair may be performed for a minority of cases, such as prolapse of an elongated, non-calcified leaflet (cusp resuspension with resection or plication of the edge) or leaflet perforation from healed endocarditis (patch repair). The prolapsed valve is commonly bicuspid, wherein the conjoint cusp elongates and prolapses; this cusp is resuspended and the raphe of the conjoint cusp resected. Since annular dilatation is common in these patients, subcommissural annuloplasty is often performed.

4. AORTIC STENOSIS

I. Etiology

A. Age-related calcific degeneration

This is the most common cause of AS. It is related to endothelial valvular injury and has the same risk factors as atherosclerosis/CAD. Calcifications develop throughout the valve leaflets *rather than specifically over the commissures*. Non-stenotic aortic valve sclerosis (thickening) precedes AS, is present in ~20% of patients older than 65 years, is associated with an increased risk of cardiovascular death and CAD, and progresses to some degree of AS in ~10% of patients at 5 years.

B. Bicuspid aortic valve

a. Bicuspid aortic valve is the most common congenital heart disease (~1.3% of the population). It is present in >50% of patients with aortic coarctation and in ~10% of women with Turner syndrome. It has a familial trend (36% have at least one first-degree relative affected) and is more prevalent in men (3:1).[68] Screening of the patient's children is appropriate.

b. Two of the three cusps are fused, most commonly the right and left cusps (80%), followed by the right and non-coronary cusps (20%). A residual raphe is often seen at the fusion site (Figure 6.13). A pliable bicuspid valve does not usually impede aortic flow, per se. However, the presence of two rather than three leaflets leads to a smaller surface in contact with the high-pressure stroke volume and marked leaflet bending, making the bicuspid valve more susceptible to shear stress. Progressive stress leads to calcific degeneration and AS later in life. The more asymmetrical the cusps are, the higher the stress is, and the faster AS develops.

c. Yet bicuspid valves may be stenotic at birth, in childhood, or in early adulthood, before calcium develops, when a significant degree of commissural fusion is present or when the valve is, in fact, unicuspid. This early AS may be treated with valvuloplasty.

d. Later on, in early adult life (between the ages of 20 and 50 years), 20% of bicuspid valves develop AI.[69] The remaining patients develop progressive aortic calcification and stenosis over time, as the bicuspid valve is more prone to mechanical and shear stress than a tricuspid valve. Severe AS usually appears in patients >40 years old, and 75% of bicuspid patients eventually develop severe AS over their lifetime (not all become severe AS).[69,70] Bicuspid aortic valve is the most common cause of AS in patients <70 years old (~two-thirds of AS), more so if <60 years old. In patients older than 70 years, bicuspid AS is the cause of 40% of severe AS.[69]

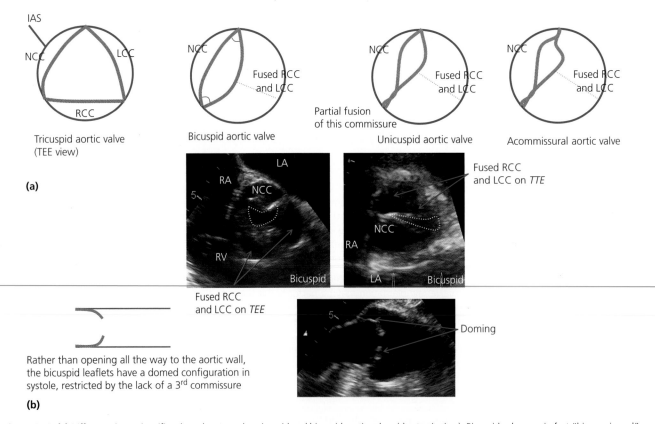

Tricuspid aortic valve (TEE view)

Bicuspid aortic valve

Unicuspid aortic valve

Acommissural aortic valve

(a)

Rather than opening all the way to the aortic wall, the bicuspid leaflets have a domed configuration in systole, restricted by the lack of a 3rd commissure

(b)

Figure 6.13 (a) Difference in aortic orifice shape between the tricuspid and bicuspid aortic valves (short-axis view). Bicuspid valves are in fact "bicommissural" valves, while unicuspid valves are "unicommissural" or "acommissural" valves. The commmissures of a bicuspid valve (*arc*) may be partially fused, leading to AS at an early age; otherwise, AS develops later in life. Note that aortic opening/closure becomes eccentric in bicuspid valves; this is seen on M-mode analysis of the aortic valve. On echo, instead of analyzing how many cusps are seen when the valve is closed, it is best to analyze how the aortic valve opens: an elliptical rather than a triangular opening is a hint to a bicuspid valve. RCC and LCC are often fused, NCC being the cusp looking towards the IAS. **(b)** Doming of the bicuspid aortic valve on a long-axis view.

IAS, interatrial septum; LCC, left coronary cusp; NCC, non-coronary cusp; RCC, right coronary cusp.

e. While AS is the most common result of a bicuspid valve, severe AI or the combination of AI/AS is also possible. AI, which often develops at a younger age than AS, may be related to a dilated aortic root, but also to: prolapse of the asymmetrically large cusp (can't support the extra weight of blood in diastole), myxoid degeneration with malcoaptation, endocarditis, or retraction of a fibrotic/calcified leaflet.

f. Patients with a bicuspid aortic valve have a high risk of *ascending aortic dilatation or dissection*. Aortic dilatation occurs in 50–60% of patients with bicuspid aortic valve by the age of 30, and occurs as frequently in young patients with a normally functioning aortic valve as in patients with aortic stenosis, regurgitation, or AVR.[71] This aortopathy is mainly secondary to cystic medial necrosis and is partly exaggerated by AS's post-stenotic dilatation or AI's volume and pressure load. As opposed to the ascending aortic dilatation that may be seen with age and HTN, this aortopathy frequently involves the aortic sinuses beside the tubular aorta. Patients with bicuspid valve should undergo, at least once, a screening with CT to assess the whole aorta. If dilatation is found to predominantly involve the sinuses, sinotubular junction, or early tubular aorta, TTE is usually appropriate for surveillance. A surveillance echo is recommended every year in patients with aortic size >4 cm at the sinuses or higher, and every 2 years in bicuspid patients with aortic size <4 cm. The lifetime risk of aortic dissection in bicuspid patients is ~3–6%, vs. 40% in Marfan patients. Dissection is often preceded by aortic dilatation, sometimes mild,[71] and in general, ~60% of all dissections occur at a diameter <5.5 cm.

C. Rheumatic fever (rare): in this case, AS almost always occurs with rheumatic involvement of the mitral valve and is often associated with severe AI.

II. Laboratory diagnosis and severity

The diagnosis of severe AS is often made by TTE (Table 6.2). An invasive hemodynamic study is only indicated when the physical exam suggests severe AS (absent A_2, pulsus parvus and tardus), yet the echocardiogram suggests a milder degree of AS or vice versa; or when the echocardiography data is inconclusive (for example, the gradient is elevated but the valve area is >1 cm²).

A. Echo and Doppler features of severe AS

Aortic valve velocity, which translates into transaortic pressure gradient ($4 \times \text{velocity}^2$), is the most important diagnostic feature of severe AS. However, Doppler may underestimate the pressure gradient if the cursor is not perfectly aligned with the transaortic flow. Therefore, the aortic velocity must be assessed in multiple views: the apical five- and three-chamber views, but also the suprasternal view and a special right parasternal view, wherein the transducer is aligned with the ascending aorta to the right of the sternum.

Aortic valve area (AVA) is calculated using the continuity equation and is subject to the additional pitfalls of measuring the LVOT diameter and velocity. ***Echocardiographic AVA measurement is even less accurate and reproducible than the transaortic gradient***.

The transaortic gradient is difficult to assess by TEE because only one view is aligned with the aortic flow, the transgastric long-axis view, a view that is not always obtainable.

> Doppler gradients rarely overestimate the severity of AS. *A high velocity/gradient is diagnostic of severe AS in a patient with a calcified, poorly mobile valve*, regardless of AVA calculation. Doppler may, however, underestimate AS.

> Note that, according to Hakki's equation for invasive AVA calculation ($\text{AVA} = \text{CO}/\sqrt{\text{mean gradient}}$), a patient with a normal cardiac output of 5.5 l/min and an AVA of 1 cm² will have a mean gradient of 30 mmHg. Therefore, a mean gradient of 30 mmHg may very well be consistent with severe AS in patients with normal output (resting conditions). This is particularly true in patients with a small body habitus, who have a relatively lower cardiac output. This gradient would strikingly increase with a slight increase in cardiac output, as the gradient is proportional to the square of the cardiac output. On Doppler, a gradient >40 mmHg is used as a more specific cutoff for defining severe AS, keeping in mind that a gradient of 30–40 mmHg may be consistent with a normal-output severe AS, and a gradient of 15–30 mmHg may be consistent with a low-output severe AS. Underestimation of gradient by Doppler is an additional possibility. Invasive confirmation of a small AVA is often needed in the latter two cases.

Other features suggestive of severe AS:

a. While aortic valve velocity ↑ (obstruction), LVOT velocity ↓ (reduced stroke volume). Typically, in severe AS:

- Peak LVOT velocity is <1 m/s.
- LVOT velocity/aortic valve velocity is ≤0.25. This is called the dimensionless index (DI) and is in fact a component of AVA calculation (AVA = LVOT area × DI). As opposed to AVA calculation, the dimensionless index is not subject to the bias of LVOT diameter measurement.

Table 6.2 Classification of AS severity.

	Mean transaortic gradient	Peak aortic velocity	Aortic valve area
Mild AS	<20 mmHg	2–2.9 m/s	>1.5 cm²
Moderate AS	20–40 mmHg	3–3.9 m/s	1–1.5 cm²
Severe AS	≥40 mmHg	≥4 m/s	≤1 cm² or indexed area ≤0.6 cm²/m²

Pitfalls – LVOT velocity may be higher than 1 m/s when AS is associated with moderate AI or high-output states (anemia, fever), but DI remains ≤ 0.25 if AS is severe. Moreover, up to 10% of patients with severe AS develop significant, sometimes severe, septal hypertrophy with septal bulge and LVOT obstruction. The LVOT velocity and DI may be increased, leading to the false calculation of a large AVA, but this obstruction is actually part of the AS anatomy and does not rule out severe AS; this high LVOT velocity and high DI should not be used in AVA calculation. Also, LVOT velocity may be falsely elevated if the pulsed cursor is placed too close to the aortic valve, in the aliasing zone.

Low-output states may lead to a low-gradient severe AS; the gradient is low, but LVOT velocity is <1 m/s and DI is low, providing a hint to severe AS. DI does not allow, however, the distinction between severe AS and pseudo-severe AS (see below), and, like any velocity assessment, it is angle-dependent.

b. *M-mode of the aortic valve shows flattening of the aortic box*. The aortic valve does not clearly open in the parasternal views.

However, a bicuspid aortic valve may appear to open moderately well on a parasternal view despite being severely stenotic. Since it only opens eccentrically between the non-coronary cusp and the fused cusp, the bicuspid valve is three-dimensionally more stenotic than it may appear on a two-dimensional view. This is similar to assessing eccentric coronary artery stenosis on angiography: the stenosis may appear mild in one view but severe in another.

c. *Small AVA by planimetry. Planimetry of the aortic valve area is performed on the TEE short-axis view, especially if the edges are well defined on TEE*. The cut may be slightly above or below the true valvular orifice, which overestimates AVA.

d. *A bicuspid valve is characterized by eccentric closure on M-mode and, when not severely stenotic, systolic doming on the long-axis view* (Figure 6.13).

e. The lack of LV hypertrophy is unusual but does not exclude AS. In fact, ~10% of AS patients do not develop concentric hypertrophy, and 4% do not even develop concentric remodeling, i.e., an increase in LV thickness (especially patients with small body habitus).[72] Those patients may have a higher mortality risk after AVR.

B. The three types of transaortic pressure gradients

The peak instantaneous gradient obtained by echocardiography is different from the peak-to-peak gradient obtained by catheterization and from the mean gradient (Figure 6.14). The mean and peak-to-peak gradients have almost equivalent values. The value of the mean gradient is ~65% that of the peak instantaneous gradient.

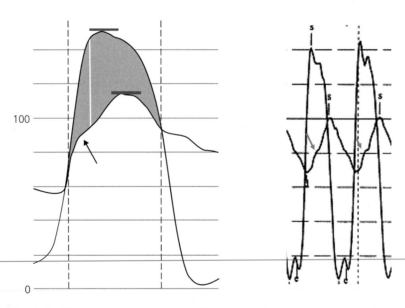

Figure 6.14 Peak-to-peak gradient is the difference between the two peaks (*horizontal bars*). Peak instantaneous gradient is the largest difference between the two curves (*white vertical line*). Mean gradient is the integration of all gradients (*gray area*). LV pressure peaks early and the aortic pressure peaks late, which is the opposite of what is found in HOCM.

Note the anacrotic notch beyond which the aortic upstroke is slowed (*arrows*). The aortic upstroke starts normally then is sharply impeded after the valve stops opening, creating this bend called the anacrotic notch. The aortic pressure has a *slow upstroke after the anacrotic notch and peaks late (pulsus tardus)*. Also, the pulse pressure is reduced because of reduced stroke volume (*pulsus parvus*). In elderly patients with reduced arterial compliance, the pulse pressure may be preserved and sharp without anacrotic notch.

The mean gradient usually approximates the peak-to-peak gradient and is about 65% the peak instantaneous gradient. *The mean gradient is usually slightly smaller than the peak-to-peak gradient; however, in severe AS with severely delayed aortic upstroke, the mean gradient area may be larger than the peak-to-peak gradient.*

Note that, in AS, **the aortic pressure upstroke is less steep than the LV pressure upstroke**; if the LV and aortic upstrokes are superimposed, suspect subaortic obstruction or error in zeroing creating a false gradient (e.g., the LV and aortic transducers were zeroed at two different levels).

Reproduced with permission from Hanna EB. Aortic stenosis. In: Hanna EB, Glancy DL. Practical Cardiovascular Hemodynamics. New York, NY: Demos Medical, 2012, p. 79.

C. Case of AF

Transaortic pressure gradient is reduced in case of inappropriate tachycardia or short R–R interval (AF), and is increased after a PVC or a long R–R interval. The opposite occurs in MS. Tachycardia may, however, be associated with an increase in transaortic gradient if inotropism and cardiac output are increased, as an increase in cardiac output strikingly increases the gradient. Try to control the rate before assessment of AS and average the mean gradient from 5–10 beats. For echocardiographic AVA calculation, use LVOT VTI and aortic valve VTI obtained after the same R–R cycle lengths. The invasive AVA calculation in AF is described in Chapter 36.

III. Low-gradient AS with aortic valve area (AVA) ≤1 cm² and low EF <50%

In the case of a moderate-range mean gradient (30–40 mmHg) and AVA ≤1 cm², the patient likely has a truly severe AS. In the case of a mean gradient <30 mmHg, AVA ≤1 cm², and EF <50% (especially <40%), the patient may have: (1) a truly severe AS with a low gradient resulting from the low cardiac output, or (2) a pseudo-severe AS with a valve that is mildly or moderately stenotic, the excursion of which is further limited by the reduced cardiac output, leading to underestimation of the true AVA. Gorlin's equation shows that the transvalvular pressure gradient directly correlates with the square of cardiac output (AVA ~ CO/√mean gradient); thus, a patient with AVA of 1 cm² and a cardiac output of 3.5 liters/minute will have a mean gradient of only 15 mmHg. On the other hand, a patient with a cardiac output of 3.5 liters/minute and a gradient of 15 mmHg may not have severe AS even if Gorlin's equation yields AVA ≤1 cm², as the valve opening is flow-dependent. A dobutamine study is indicated to increase the cardiac output and assess AS, and may be performed during *an echo or an invasive study*. Dobutamine is started as an infusion of 5 mcg/kg/min. The increase in cardiac output, AVA, and gradient are assessed then dobutamine up-titrated every 5–8 minutes if the diagnostic features are not met, the maximum dose being 20 mcg/kg/min. There are three possible responses: [73,74]

1. Stroke volume increases by ≥20%, gradient increases to >30 mmHg (especially if it increases to >40 mmHg or by >10 mmHg, or velocity increases to ≥4 m/s), AVA remains unchanged or increases but remains ≤1.2 cm² (or increases <0.2 cm²): truly severe AS with good contractile reserve. The reduced EF and output are due to afterload mismatch rather than intrinsic contractile abnormality and will reverse with surgery.
   LVOT and aortic valve velocities similarly ↑ → Ratio (DI) remains unchanged or ↓.
2. Stroke volume increases by ≥20%, gradient remains ≤30 mmHg, and AVA increases to >1.2 cm²: pseudo-severe AS.
   LVOT velocity ↑ more than aortic valve velocity → DI ↑.
3. Stroke volume does not significantly increase (<20%), gradient and AVA do not significantly change: poor contractile or flow reserve. This may represent an advanced stage of AS with poor LV systolic function, or a combination of AS and cardiomyopathy.

The last subgroup has the worst prognosis but may still benefit from AVR.[75] However, before considering that the patient has a poor and irreversible contractile reserve, make sure he is not hypovolemic. Hypovolemia, which is suggested by low cardiac filling pressures, may explain the lack of increase in cardiac output and may be solved by a small volume load. Also, make sure the patient does not have a severely increased afterload from hypertension and high SVR. In this case, a careful nitroprusside infusion with titration may allow an increase in cardiac output, prove a good flow reserve, and allow evaluation of the severity of AS. Nitroprusside may precipitously drop the systemic pressure in patients with truly severe AS who cannot increase their cardiac output to match the dilated circulation, and should be used with great caution.

IV. Low-gradient AS with aortic valve area (AVA) ≤1 cm² but normal EF (paradoxical low-flow/low-gradient severe AS)

A gradient is paradoxically low when it is <40 mmHg or peak velocity is <4 m/s despite AVA ≤1 cm² (ACC guidelines). However, even under normal flow, a severe AVA of 1 cm² may translate into a gradient of 30 mmHg; therefore, a gradient <30 mmHg, usually 15–30 mmHg, more definitely defines a paradoxical low gradient.[76–79]

A normal EF does not signify a normal cardiac output. Thus, even if EF is normal, patients with severe AS may have a reduced cardiac output that leads to a reduced gradient. This situation is seen in 10–20% of severe AS cases and usually reflects:

1. Severe preload reduction (e.g., hypovolemia)
2. Associated mitral valve disease that reduces the flow across the aortic valve
3. Most importantly, this situation is commonly seen in severe systemic HTN. Hypertensive patients may have severe AS with a paradoxically low flow and low gradient for the following reasons:[76–80]

   i. The global LV afterload is the sum of AS and HTN (this is called double load or valvuloarterial impedance). HTN leads to an increased total afterload which leads to a reduced stroke volume and cardiac output even if EF is normal. Subsequently, the transvalvular gradient but also the systemic pressure are reduced and "pseudo-normalization" of HTN may be seen in up to 30% of cases of high double load. Thus, both HTN and AS appear less severe in patients with a high total afterload and a low stroke volume. Calculate the stroke volume, using LVOT velocity and diameter, and the valvuloarterial impedance, which is equal to (systolic blood pressure + mean gradient)/stroke volume index. A low stroke volume <35 ml/m² and an elevated valvuloarterial impedance (>3.5–4.5 mmHg/ml/m²) suggest an increased total afterload and masked AS and HTN.
   ii. Patients with HTN may have significant concentric left ventricular hypertrophy with reduced LV cavity size, and thus reduced stroke volume even if EF is normal.
   iii. The gradient between the LV and the vena contracta (narrowest aortic area) is higher than the gradient between the LV and the aortic root. As a result of decreased vascular compliance, patients with HTN have increased pressure downstream of the valve, explaining the reduction in LV–aortic gradient when aortic pressure is measured downstream of the valve rather than at the valve. As opposed to pressure recovery, HTN does not reduce the overall afterload, in fact, it increases it; thus, the true gradient the LV generates is the LV–vena contracta gradient. Catheterization may further underestimate the gradient in this case, since it assesses the gradient between LV and the aortic root beyond the vena contracta.

Thus, in these cases, AS is likely a truly severe AS with a low gradient due to a low stroke volume (= low-flow, low-gradient AS), and it is likely that the patient will benefit from aortic valve replacement. ***Dobutamine testing is unlikely to be useful in these patients, as the preload and afterload are problematic, not contractility***.

Reassessing gradients after normalization of systemic pressure reduces the first and third caveats. This may be done acutely in the cath lab by the cautious administration of intravenous nitroprusside. While it may seem that a gradient of <30 mmHg is not high enough to allow benefit from valvular surgery, and that HTN control is the only treatment necessary, valve replacement is actually an important aspect of therapy. Valve replacement reduces the severe gradient that is seen after HTN is controlled and after cardiac output rises. Also, valve replacement improves cardiac output reserve, allowing cardiac output to increase under exertional conditions (as opposed to the static, limited output in severe AS). In fact, in comparison to a high transaortic gradient, a paradoxical low-flow, low-gradient severe AS is associated with a worse prognosis and a markedly lower survival with medical therapy compared to AVR.[72] Survival is markedly improved with AVR.[76–78,82,83] Two registry analyses have shown that one-third of patients with severe AS and normal EF have a low stroke volume secondary to a high total LV load, and 56% of these patients have a low mean gradient <30 mmHg.[72,75] In other studies, low-flow, low-gradient severe AS constituted ~10–20% of severe AS cases, particularly in elderly and female patients.[84]

When the diagnosis of severe AS with paradoxical low flow/low gradient is suggested by echocardiography, the following is performed:

1st step – Ensure appropriate echo measurements, particularly LVOT diameter measurement (which should generally be >2 cm). Also ensure acquisition of the highest aortic valve velocity, aligned with the flow.

2nd step – Ensure that the indexed AVA is reduced <0.6 cm²/m². AVA of 1 cm² may, in fact, correspond to moderate AS in a small patient.

3rd step – Measure the stroke volume index and valvuloarterial impedance. A low gradient associated with a normal stroke volume index >35 ml/m² and a normal valvuloarterial impedance suggests that AS is not severe (normal-flow, low-gradient AS → AVA miscalculation, pressure recovery, or non-severe indexed AVA).[83] A high LVOT velocity >1 m/s, with a properly placed LVOT cursor not too close to the aortic valve orifice, rules out low cardiac output and thus rules out low-gradient AS. Similarly, a dimensionless index >0.25 almost excludes low-gradient AS.

4th step – **Low-gradient AS with normal EF frequently requires invasive measurements to confirm accurate gradient and valve area calculation, especially after control of HTN.**

V. Pressure recovery phenomenon

In patients with AS, pressure (potential energy) is generated by the LV. A significant portion of this energy is lost across the narrow aortic valve orifice and becomes kinetic energy. Downstream from the valve, the flow becomes laminar again and there may be a reincrease in pressure and in potential energy, particularly in female patients with a narrow aorta (diameter at the sinotubular junction <2.6–3 cm) (Figure 6.15). This reincrease in pressure a few centimeters downstream of the valve, at the sinotubular level, is called pressure recovery. The true gradient is the gradient between LV pressure and the pressure downstream of the valve.[85–88] This gradient represents the true loss of energy the ventricle is subject to. In this case, the transaortic gradient obtained by echo is the pressure gradient between the LV and the vena contracta and overestimates the physiologic AS; in addition, AVA calculated by the echocardiographic continuity equation overestimates the severity of AS.[85–88] One study has shown that 45% of patients with moderate transaortic pressure gradient and severe AS per echocardiographic AVA, who do not have HTN or high valvuloarterial impedance, have, in fact, significant pressure recovery with milder degrees of AS.[85] The pressure recovery is less prominent at high gradients. This explains why catheter-calculated orifice area tends to be higher and gradient tends to be lower than Doppler-derived area/gradient in individuals with valve areas of 1–1.5 cm². When echocardiography suggests severe AS but significant pressure recovery is suspected in a patient with small tubular aorta <3 cm, recalculate AVA using an energy loss index (ELI) correction that takes into account the aortic diameter, or, better, perform cardiac catheterization. Ensure that this combination of moderate gradient with AVA in the severe range is not related to HTN or increased valvuloarterial impedance, in which case the AVA is truly small and the echo gradient between the LV and the aortic valve orifice is the true gradient (as opposed to pressure recovery, HTN does not reduce the overall afterload; in fact, it increases it and reduces stroke volume).

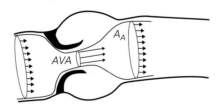

Figure 6.15 Pressure recovery phenomenon.
Pressure (potential or static energy) is generated by the LV (*left-sided arrows*). This pressure/energy is partially converted into kinetic energy across the narrow aortic valve area (AVA) (*middle arrows*). Downstream from the valve, the kinetic energy may be fully lost if the flow swirls around; however, if part of the flow is laminar, the kinetic energy may partially recover into pressure energy, so that the overall energy loss and the overall pressure drop are less severe. *While the true anatomic AVA may correlate better with the maximal pressure drop at the aortic orifice, the physiologic AVA better correlates with the net pressure drop after pressure recovery.* Pressure recovery is particularly seen when the aortic area (A$_A$) is small.
Reproduced with permission of Elsevier from Briand et al. (2005).[81]

Table 6.3 provides an overview of the causes of low-gradient AS. Table 6.4 lists the causes of a high gradient with an AVA that is, nonetheless, calculated >1 cm². **In practice, echocardiography much more often underestimates than overestimates AS gradient, and thus, *gradient >40 mmHg is usually severe AS even if AVA is calculated as >1 cm²*.**

VI. Symptoms

The following symptoms may be seen in AS:

1. Dyspnea and reduced functional capacity: related to the elevated LVEDP and the inability to raise cardiac output with exercise.

2. Syncope: related to the fixed cardiac output that cannot increase with exertion or to the occurrence of arrhythmias. Vasodilatation occurs during exertion, but cardiac output cannot increase because of the fixed, severe outflow obstruction. Thus, the systemic pressure drops (pressure = CO × SVR).

3. Angina occurs in two-thirds of the patients and is associated with CAD in 50% of these patients. In the other 50%, it results solely from increased O_2 demands (LVH) and reduced myocardial capillary perfusion (↑ LVEDP compresses the subendocardial microcirculation).

4. Bleeding tendency is seen (especially GI bleed from AV malformations). It is due to the disruption of von Willebrand molecules as they cross the stenotic valve. This improves with AVR.

VII. Natural history

Severe asymptomatic AS almost always becomes symptomatic within 5 years (fast progression, similar to MR); ~50% of patients become symptomatic within 2 years, particularly if the valve is heavily calcified or the transaortic velocity increases >0.3 m/s/yr.[89] Severe AS is, however, associated with low morbidity and mortality as long as the patient is asymptomatic. Sudden cardiac death rate is <0.5–1% per year in truly asymptomatic AS.[89]

Severe symptomatic AS, on the other hand, is associated with a survival of 2–3 years only. Classically, the survival is ~3 years in patients with syncope, angina, or early dyspnea, and 1–2 years in patients with HF. *Sudden death is a frequent cause of death* in symptomatic patients, thus justifying prompt surgery.

In moderate or severe AS, AVA ↓ by ~0.12 cm², aortic velocity ↑ by 0.3 m/s, and aortic mean gradient ↑ by 7 mmHg per year. AS progresses faster in patients with heavy calcifications or advanced renal failure. Some of the latter patients may progress from mild/moderate AS to severe AS within 3–4 years.

VIII. AS should be differentiated from subvalvular and supravalvular AS in children or young adults

While the majority of congenital aortic obstructions are due to bicuspid AS, 14% are due to fixed subvalvular AS, and a minority are due to supravalvular AS. The latter two conditions mainly present in children or young adults.

Table 6.3 Causes of low-gradient AS (AVA ≤ 1 cm² with a mean gradient < 40 mmHg).

In patients with low EF (particularly <40%)[a]
- Low EF with truly severe AS. Low gradient is explained by a low cardiac output
- Low EF with mild/moderate AS. Low cardiac output leads to poor valve excursion and a small calculated AVA (pseudo-severe AS)

In patients with normal EF[a]
- Truly severe AS with false measurement of the aortic gradient: if Doppler beam is not parallel to LV–aortic flow, the gradient obtained is an underestimation of the true gradient. In this case, true gradient is higher.
- Truly severe AS with **hypertension** at the time of the study, particularly if concentric LV hypertrophy is present. In this case, the low gradient is due to a low output despite a normal LVEF
- Truly severe AS with hypovolemia
- Truly severe AS with severe mitral regurgitation or stenosis (i.e., low forward cardiac output)
- A gradient of 30–40 mmHg is consistent with normal-flow severe AS (cardiac output of 5.5 l/min with AVA of 1 cm² translates into a mean gradient of 30–40 mmHg)
- On echo, a low gradient associated with a small AVA may be related to **moderate AS with indexed AVA > 0.6 cm²/m², moderate AS with false AVA measurement, or moderate AS with pressure recovery. Moderate AS is suggested in patients with normal flow (normal stroke volume), normal valvuloarterial impedance, or high dimensionless index:**
  ○ Erroneous measurement of LVOT diameter or LVOT velocity (leading to a falsely small AVA)[b]
  ○ Pressure recovery phenomenon in patients with a small aorta: true gradient is smaller and true AVA is larger than obtained by echocardiography. Catheterization is more accurate in this case.

---

[a] Unless otherwise specified, the listed causes of low-gradient AS apply to AS evaluated by both invasive and echocardiographic means.
[b] LVOT diameter should be measured at the aortic annulus, i.e., at the insertion of the aortic valve leaflets, in early systole (largest diameter). LVOT is often oval and is frequently underestimated on the echo long-axis view; LVOT area is more accurately assessed by CT.

Table 6.4 Causes of AVA > 1 cm² with a mean gradient > 40 mmHg.

- Severe AS in a patient with a large body size: AVA > 1 cm² but indexed AVA < 0.6 cm²/m²
- Severe AS with overestimation of AVA when secondary septal hypertrophy and high LVOT velocity are present[a]
- Severe AS with overestimation of AVA when LVOT diameter or LVOT velocity is overestimated (misplacement of the LVOT cursor)[a]
- Moderate AS with a high gradient in high-output states (anemia, sepsis, associated AI). In associated AI, the high gradient describes the combined effect of AS/AI and still indicates surgery
- Less likely: moderate AS with pressure recovery (less common at high gradients)

---

[a] Remember that AVA = LVOT area × LVOT velocity/aortic valve velocity.

A. Subvalvular AS

Fixed subvalvular aortic stenosis is present at birth and is most often caused by a discrete fibrous membrane that encircles the outflow tract beneath the aortic valve. The aortic valvular leaflets are commonly thickened and regurgitant as a result of the turbulent blood flow jet caused by the subvalvular stenosis. Less commonly, a thick fibromuscular ridge or a prolonged segment of LVOT thickening (tunnel obstruction) is seen. It is commonly associated with VSD. Surgical therapy is indicated in fixed subvalvular stenosis to prevent the progressive AI that is seen in >80% of untreated patients, regardless of symptoms (as long as mean gradient >30 mmHg).

B. Supravalvular AS

Supravalvular stenosis results from aortic narrowing at the superior margin of the aortic sinuses. Stenosis may be a focal hourglass type of narrowing (most common form), a discrete supravalvular membrane, or diffuse hypoplasia of the ascending aorta (the least common form). It results from medial thickening that may also be seen in the thoracic and abdominal branches of the aorta and may cause focal luminal narrowing in these arteries (e.g., subclavian, carotid artery). Like the aortic sinuses, the coronary arteries are subject to large systolic and pulse pressures, as the stroke volume overfills the small aortic chamber prior to the obstruction. Frequently, the coronary arteries are diffusely dilated and develop ostial stenoses. Aortic valve thickening and regurgitation may develop. This condition is frequently associated with peripheral pulmonary artery stenosis. Surgical therapy is indicated in supravalvular AS that is symptomatic, associated with LVH, or asymptomatic with mean gradient >50 mmHg. Supravalvular AS is often non-syndromic but may be associated with Williams syndrome (hypercalcemia, elfin facies, mild mental retardation) and may be genetically transmitted.

In both those conditions, Doppler shows high velocity across the transaortic plane with a structurally normal aortic valve. The actual site of narrowing/membrane may be seen. On color Doppler, the turbulence is seen below or above the aortic valve. TEE may be required in young patients with aortic obstruction to further define this anatomy. Invasively, pressure pullback with an end-hole catheter confirms the site of obstruction; in contrast to HOCM, the gradient is not dynamic and does not have a dagger shape. *On exam*, A_2 is loud rather than attenuated (≠ AS) and a systolic click is not heard (≠ bicuspid AS). In subvalvular AS, the murmur does not consistently radiate to the carotids. In supravalvular AS, the narrow jet goes preferentially towards the right side of the aorta as it abuts the aortic wall, and thus the pulses are stronger in the right vs. left arm, and the murmur only radiates to the right carotid with suprasternal thrill.

IX. Treatment

A. Antihypertensives

Antihypertensives, such as vasodilators or β-blockers, may be harmful in AS but should be carefully used if HTN coexists. Normally, when vasodilators are administered, the systemic pressure is maintained thanks to an increase in cardiac output (pressure = cardiac output × resistance). Severe AS may limit the increase in cardiac output, and thus severe hypotension may ensue. Conversely, HTN is common in AS (~1/3 of patients), worsens LV afterload, and leads to double loading of the LV with a low-flow/low-gradient state. Thus, careful antihypertensive therapy is beneficial as it reduces the total afterload and increases cardiac output.

B. Indications for aortic valve replacement (AVR)

a. Severe, symptomatic AS (syncope/pre-syncope, dyspnea, or angina). GI bleed, per se, is not an indication for AVR.

b. Severe asymptomatic AS with reduced LV function (EF <50%) that is not due to another cause.

c. Symptomatic, low-gradient severe AS with a low EF, as long as the patient has contractile reserve. EF reduction is mostly due to *afterload mismatch* and improves or normalizes in most of these patients after AVR. In the absence of contractile reserve, AVR has a high operative mortality (~32%), but superior long-term survival and EF and symptomatic improvement vs. no AVR; AVR may be considered in individual cases (*class IIb* in ESC guidelines).[90]

d. Symptomatic, low-flow, low-gradient severe AS with normal EF (ensure indexed AVA ≤ 0.6 cm²/m², stroke volume <35 ml/m², and ensure no echo measurement error).[91]

e. Severe AS that is initially considered asymptomatic, but an abnormal response is seen during exercise testing: low functional capacity for age and sex, or drop in SBP below baseline.

f. Severe (*class I*) or moderate (*class IIa*) asymptomatic AS undergoing CABG, aortic surgery for ascending aortic aneurysm, or other valvular surgery. In moderate AS, AVR is performed to prevent the need for redo cardiac surgery in ~5 years (long-term benefit).

g. Symptoms associated with a combination of moderate AS (AVA 1.0– 1.5 cm²) and moderate AI.[92]

The mortality risk of AVR is ~3%, and may be as low as 1–2% in low-risk young patients and as high as 10% in patients with low EF, especially low EF with low-gradient AS.[90] AVR may be performed safely in octogenarians, albeit at a higher perioperative mortality risk (~6–9%). Concomitant CAD, particularly multivessel CAD requiring CABG, increases the perioperative mortality, especially in octogenarians (up to 18%). Rather than CABG, it is the underlying CAD and comorbidities of those patients that explain the increased surgical risk. In fact, leaving CAD untreated increases the perioperative risk of ischemia and MI, and thus, CABG is rather salutary for these patients.

LV dysfunction is seen in many symptomatic, high-risk AS cases (e.g., PARTNER trial). Yet, as opposed to valvular regurgitation, LV dysfunction very rarely develops in AS before symptoms (unless due to other causes, e.g., CAD). LV dysfunction improves more readily in patients with AS than in those with AI or MR, as it is usually due to *afterload mismatch* rather than contractile/fibrotic dysfunction. LV mass decreases over the course of one to several years postoperatively.

C. Ross procedure

The Ross procedure consists of pulmonary artery + pulmonic valve autograft placement in the aortic position, while a homograft valve is placed in the pulmonary position. This procedure is mainly used in young patients. It has the advantage of not requiring anticoagulation. Moreover, the autograft grows when used in children.

However, this procedure should be avoided in cases of AI with dilated ascending aorta, as the dilated aorta will put tension on the grafted pulmonary artery, with a risk of neoaortic root dilatation and late AI.

Also, a long-term risk of pulmonic stenosis and/or regurgitation of the homograft and AI of the neoaorta is seen.

D. Surgery for severe asymptomatic AS with normal EF

As long as they remain asymptomatic, patients with asymptomatic AS and normal EF have a very low yearly risk of sudden cardiac death, and thus watchful waiting is recommended. *Once symptoms develop, even for a few months, the prognosis becomes guarded with a significant risk of sudden death and death from severe heart failure* (>20% per year).[89,93] Thus, patient education and echo and clinical follow-up (every 6–12 months) are recommended.

Moreover, it is reasonable to verify that these patients are truly asymptomatic by performing stress testing with monitoring of symptoms and blood pressure response. Since exercise limitation may be related to reduced fitness or concomitant CAD, stress testing is mainly useful in physically active young patients (<70 years old) and is considered abnormal if symptoms of angina, dyspnea, or dizziness develop, particularly at <7 METs, if SBP drops below baseline, or if functional capacity is below the standard for age and sex.[94] During testing, truly severe dyspnea should be distinguished from mild transient breathlessness. Dizziness is the most specific symptom and the one most likely to predict symptomatic progression over the next year.[94]

Other patients also have a fast progression, which may justify earlier surgery:[95]

- Very severe AS (mean gradient >60 mmHg, peak velocity >5 m/s) with an expected perioperative mortality of ≤ 1.5% (ACC, class IIa).
- Severe valve calcification with peak velocity progression ≥0.3 m/s/yr (ESC, class IIa). Valve calcification may be better quantified by CT imaging. An aortic valve calcium score >1000 Agatston units defines severe calcification.[12]
- Markedly elevated BNP (>130 pg/ml) or excessive LVH (ESC, class IIb).
- Mean gradient increases >20 mmHg with exercise (ESC, class IIb).
- Patients with associated CAD that requires CABG should undergo concomitant AVR.

A recent Japanese registry suggested that, in very low-surgical-risk patients with severe AS, watchful waiting was associated with a significant increase in 5-year mortality compared with initial AVR. This was driven by an increased rate of HF during the waiting period, including severe HF as first presentation, and a higher operative risk once AS was symptomatic.[96]

E. MR associated with severe AS

MR frequently coexists with severe AS and is often functional, secondary to LV and LA remodeling and the increased LV systolic pressure (>15% of AS patients have moderate or severe MR). MR often improves by ≥ 1 grade in 50–90% of patients after AVR, especially if functional and not severe. MR improves in two waves (immediate and late).[97]

Mitral annuloplasty repair is generally performed concomitantly to AVR if MR is severe, or moderate with pulmonary hypertension, LA enlargement/AF, or intrinsic mitral valve disease, and the surgical mortality is low.[97] If the surgical mortality is intermediate or high, only AVR is generally performed.

F. Percutaneous aortic valvuloplasty

Valvuloplasty, which consists of inflating a balloon across the aortic valve, is only a palliative therapy and is not effective over the long term. Valvuloplasty may be performed as a bridge to eventual AVR in patients with severe AS who are hemodynamically unstable with multiple organ failure. Once the patient is stabilized, surgical or transcutaneous AVR may be performed at a lower risk.

> In early rheumatic MS, valvuloplasty is effective as it opens the *fused* but *non-calcified* commissures. In calcific AS, the whole valve is calcified and the process is not limited to the commissures. Aortic valvuloplasty temporarily fractures the calcified framework of the valve, making it more flexible/pliable; also, it mildly tears the valve and opens the commissures. It is usually moderately effective and converts critical AS into severe AS, with a high risk of complications (>10%, including AI and stroke). Calcium quickly regrows and leads to recurrence of AS within 6–12 months.

Valvuloplasty may be used as a long-term therapy in children or young adults with *non-calcified bicuspid AS* wherein commissural fusion is the cause of stenosis, and where valvuloplasty produces small commissural tears. The results usually last 10–20 years, and most patients eventually require AVR later in adulthood. Moreover, there is an early and late risk of AI (~15% at 3–4 years). Valvuloplasty is indicated in children or young adults with a peak-to-peak or mean gradient >50 mmHg who are symptomatic, or asymptomatic with ST–T changes of LVH (*class I*), asymptomatic with a peak-to-peak gradient >60 mmHg (*class I*), or asymptomatic and planning pregnancy or athletic activity (*class IIa*).

G. Transcutaneous aortic valve replacement (TAVR)

TAVR may be performed through a transfemoral, transaxillary, or transcaval approach. It may also be performed surgically through a transapical or direct ascending aortic approach. The valve is a balloon-expandable valve (Edwards Sapien valve, Sapien 3 valve) or a self-expanding valve (Corevalve). In high-surgical-risk patients (STS score ≥ 8%), TAVR was associated with a postoperative mortality similar to that of surgical AVR (~6.5%). In inoperable, high-risk patients, TAVR drastically reduced 1-year mortality in comparison with conservative management (30% vs. 50% one-year mortality) (PARTNER trial).[98] The mean age in the PARTNER trial was 84 years (84±7), functional class was mainly III–IV, and prior CABG, stroke, or advanced COPD was common; ~20% of patients had associated moderate or severe MR. Therefore TAVR was mainly applied to advanced-stage, often octogenarian patients. Approximately 9% of patients had radiation heart disease and ~20% had extensively calcified aorta. The mean transaortic gradient was 43±15 mmHg; in fact, the PARTNER trial included a significant proportion of patients with low-flow/low-gradient AS (with low EF [15%] or normal EF/paradoxical low gradient [14%]). Those demonstrated the highest mortality and the most drastic survival improvement with TAVR in comparison with conventional management, whether EF was reduced or not.[99]

The Corevalve trial of self-expanding valve was even more impressive than the PARTNER trial. TAVR with Corevalve was associated with *better 1-year survival than surgical AVR,* in intermediate and high-surgical-risk patients (most patients had STS score between 4 and 10, mean age was 83).[100] Corevalve impinges on the AV nodal area, hence the frequent need for permanent pacing (~20%).

The PARTNER 2A trial used a lower-profile, newer balloon expandable valve (Sapien) in intermediate-surgical-risk patients with STS score 4–8%. It suggested a better 1-year survival with transfemoral TAVR vs. surgical AVR, potentially expanding the use of TAVR to these lower-risk patients.[101]

The transcutaneous valve consists of a thin stent frame that actually contains stentless bioprosthetic leaflets. Without the bulk of the sewing ring and the stented struts, the transcutaneous valve has a larger orifice area and less gradient than a surgical bioprosthesis (~0.4 cm² larger), with less patient/prosthesis mismatch.

TAVR is *not* typically used in patients with a *clearly bicuspid* valve, where the aortic opening is elliptical rather than circular, which prevents symmetrical apposition of the cylindrical prosthesis and allows paravalvular leaks. This is only a relative contraindication, particularly because in many critical AS cases, the tight residual orifice does not allow distinction between tricuspid and bicuspid valves.

The use of TAVR in severe AI is limited by: (1) coexistent aortic root disease and large annular size, which increases the risk of dehiscence and persistent AI; (2) frequent lack of significant valvular calcifications, which serve as a fluoroscopic landmark for valve positioning and as an anchor at the lower part of the stent frame; (3) difficulty in positioning in a patient with regurgitant jet.

TAVR is associated with a 5% rate of postoperative stroke. Moderate or severe paravalvular regurgitation is common (10%) and is associated with early and long-term increase in mortality, particularly with the balloon-expandable valves. Conversely, the Corevalve trial revealed that paravalvular AI improves at 1 year to less than mild in 75% of patients with moderate/severe AI, thanks to the sustained expansion of the self-expanding frame.

5. TRICUSPID REGURGITATION AND STENOSIS

I. Etiology of tricuspid regurgitation (TR)

A. TR is often secondary to RV pressure or volume overload

i. PA pressure >55 mmHg *or* PVR >3 Wood units implies that TR is secondary to pulmonary hypertension:[102]
- LV dysfunction or left valvular disorders with pulmonary hypertension
- Pulmonary arterial hypertension or lung disease with pulmonary hypertension

The high RV pressure as well as the secondary RV dilatation, annular dilatation, and leaflet tethering lead to TR. As opposed to functional MR, annular dilatation is the more important factor in functional TR (the right papillary muscles are highly placed and less severely tether the tricuspid leaflets). The tricuspid annulus is very dynamic and may considerably "shrink" with volume unloading.

ii. PA pressure <40–50 mmHg with normal PVR favors either primary TR or TR secondary to a pure RV volume overload (ASD, ARVD).

Secondary TR is always associated with an elevated RA pressure and a large V wave, as, by definition, decompensated RV failure is present. Conversely, in primary TR, the RA may be highly compliant and RA pressure may be normal.

B. Primary TR etiologies
- Rheumatic fever (beside secondary TR, one-third of rheumatic MS cases have intrinsic tricuspid involvement)
- Endocarditis
- Pacemaker wires causing TR
- Flail leaflet from blunt thoracic or abdominal trauma (abdominal trauma briskly increases IVC pressure, which may rupture the tricuspid valve)
- Carcinoid syndrome, tricuspid valve prolapse, Ebstein anomaly

In a Mayo clinic registry, pacemaker or ICD-related TR was the cause of severe TR in 26% of patients with pacemaker/ICD requiring tricuspid surgery.[103] Isolated RV failure was the mode of presentation in 50% of these cases, sometimes years after device implantation. Importantly, TTE and TEE diagnosed pacemaker-related injury as the cause of TR in only ~20% and 45% of the cases, respectively. Thus, the diagnosis is usually a diagnosis of exclusion. TR may result from valve perforation but more commonly results from impingement on the leaflets or apparatus by the lead, or lead adherence to the valve. When treatment is required for symptomatic RV failure, surgery is the only option (tricuspid repair or replacement).

II. Natural history of TR

A primary, severe TR is well tolerated for months or years before it leads to RV failure, as long as the pulmonary arterial pressure is normal (e.g., the case of valvectomy performed for tricuspid endocarditis). In fact, RV tolerates volume overload. However, TR secondary to pulmonary hypertension is not well tolerated and aggravates RV function and RV dilatation.

In TR secondary to left valvular disease, percutaneous or surgical correction of the left valvular problem reduces PA pressure and may eventually reduce TR. However, *TR often does not improve,* and rather leads to more annular dilatation, TR and RV failure, particularly in patients with underlying MS or ischemic MR and a dilated tricuspid annulus > 35–40 mm on TTE (or > 21 mm/m²). *Tricuspid annular dilatation is an ongoing progressive process that results in more annular dilatation,* such that an initially mild TR may progress over time and become the primary driver of RV failure. When the primary process is degenerative MR, < 20% are left with significant residual TR or late TR after correction of MR (vs. > 50% in MS or ischemic MR, several years after surgery).[104] Therefore, adjunctive tricuspid annuloplasty is reasonable in severe TR, or mild/moderate TR with severe annular dilatation, and is associated with improved functional capacity and reduced long-term risk of TR and HF (yet questionable survival benefit).[104] In general, tricuspid annuloplasty concomitant to mitral surgery does not significantly increase the surgical risk and pump time, whereas reoperation for severe progressive TR after mitral surgery is associated with a high mortality of 10–25%, further justifying early, concomitant surgery.[12]

III. Treatment of TR

A. Medical therapy of RV pressure or volume overload

This includes diuretics, treatment of LV failure, lung disease, or pulmonary arterial hypertension.

B. Surgical indications

a. Severe *and* symptomatic primary TR (fatigue, dyspnea, right HF with edema/ascites) (*class IIa*). Perform tricuspid repair with an annuloplasty ring (preferably) or tricuspid valve replacement with a bioprosthetic valve. A bioprosthesis is preferred to a mechanical prosthesis because of the high thrombotic risk on the right side, where the closing pressure is low. Also, a bioprosthetic valve lasts longer in a low-pressure system (i.e., tricuspid, or, even better, pulmonic position).

b. Severe primary TR with progressive RV dilatation or dysfunction, even if asymptomatic (*class IIb*).

c. In a patient undergoing mitral valve surgery, tricuspid valve surgery should be performed if secondary *severe TR* is present (*class I*). Tricuspid annuloplasty is preferred to replacement. Tricuspid annuloplasty should also be performed for *mild or moderate TR* associated with annular dilatation >40 mm or prior right HF,[12] as annular dilatation and TR may continue to progress after mitral surgery even if pulmonary pressure is eventually reduced (*class IIa*); this is particularly true if baseline PA pressure is not severely elevated and does not appear to be the driver of TR. When measured intraoperatively on an arrested heart, annular dilatation >70 mm, rather than 40 mm, indicates repair.

d. If the mitral valve is amenable to PMBV, PMBV may be performed and TR reassessed. If the mitral valve is treated surgically, TR is concomitantly repaired to avoid the risk of progressive TR and a second surgery.[12]

There are two types of tricuspid annuloplasty: (1) ring annuloplasty; (2) suture annuloplasty, which consists of a single suture tied circumferentially around the posterior and anterior aspects of the annulus (de Vega). A ring has more sustained long-term efficacy than a suture, lasting >5 years, but requires more surgical time (~30 minutes). De Vega annuloplasty usually requires <5 minutes and does not significantly add to the operative ischemic time.

IV. Tricuspid stenosis (TS)

Tricuspid stenosis is usually rheumatic and always associated with left valvular disorders. Other causes: carcinoid syndrome, cardiac tumors obstructing the tricuspid orifice. Carcinoid heart disease is related to the secretion of serotonin by a neuroendocrine tumor (usually a gastrointestinal tumor). This leads to thickening of the right-sided valves, particularly the tricuspid valve. Since serotonin is degraded by the lungs, the left valves are not involved unless right-to-left shunt or pulmonary metastasis is present. The tricuspid leaflets become thickened and completely immobile along their entire length, with lack of opening or closure, which explains the combined stenosis and regurgitation.

6. PULMONIC STENOSIS AND REGURGITATION

I. Pulmonic stenosis (PS)

PS is usually congenital. While the normal pulmonic valve is tricuspid, the stenotic pulmonic valve is often a domed valve with extensive commissural fusions, leading to an acommissural morphology with a small central orifice (no commissure, or one or two commissures). The domed appearance is recognized on angiography.[105] Rarely, the valve is tricuspid with diffuse myxomatous thickening and little or no commissural fusion (dysplastic valve, e.g., Noonan's syndrome). Other causes of PS: rheumatic, carcinoid (always in conjunction with other valvular diseases).

Pulmonic stenosis leads to RV hypertrophy but not RV dilatation and failure. In fact, RA pressure is characterized by a large A wave but a normal V wave. The congenital RV maintains its function for years even when the RV pressure is in the systemic range; thus, in RV failure, one should look for an associated "volume" lesion such as ASD, TR, or PR. Usually in PS, RV does not fail until later in life (fifth decade) or unless atrial arrhythmias develop. On chest X-ray, PS is characterized by a dilated main and left pulmonary arteries (post-stenotic dilatation). As opposed to Eisenmenger syndrome, the lung perfusion is normal (no oligemia).

PS is considered severe when the peak-to-peak gradient is >80 mmHg, and moderate when the peak-to-peak gradient is >40 mmHg. The gradient in PS, particularly mild or moderate PS, usually remains stable over the long-term follow-up. Severe PS is usually symptomatic and is treated with percutaneous balloon valvotomy with excellent long-term result (no recurrence over >20 years follow-up). Most patients with moderate PS eventually develop symptoms during a 25-year follow-up and require valvotomy.[106] In the ACC guidelines, percutaneous valvotomy is indicated for symptomatic PS with a peak-to-peak gradient >30 mmHg, or asymptomatic PS with a peak-to-peak gradient >40 mmHg. Moderate-to-severe pulmonary regurgitation may subsequently be seen in up to 20% of patients, but is not usually clinically significant; <10% eventually require surgery for PR, years later. Dysplastic PS does not respond to valvuloplasty, as the primary process is not commissural fusion.

Athletes with a PS gradient >40 mmHg can participate in low-intensity competitive sports or can be referred for intervention. Two to four weeks after valvuloplasty, asymptomatic athletes with no more than mild residual PS and normal ventricular function can participate in all competitive sports.[107]

Patients with PS have a hypertrophied RVOT. Following percutaneous valvuloplasty, the reduction in RV afterload reduces RV volume and may cause a dynamic obstruction across the hypertrophied RVOT and a residual gradient that is actually an intraventricular gradient. This gradient should not be confused with a persistent transpulmonic gradient, and the diagnosis is confirmed on a slow PA-to-RV pressure pullback. The RVOT obstruction may be severe ("suicide RV") and is initially treated with fluids, β-blockers, and calcium channel blockers. This gradient resolves gradually.

II. Pulmonic regurgitation (PR)

The most common cause of PR is pulmonary hypertension, which leads to a *secondary form of PR*. This is classically seen with MS. *Primary PR* may be seen decades after surgical therapy of tetralogy of Fallot, valvotomy for PS, or after Ross procedure. It may also be seen with endocarditis and carcinoid syndrome.

When associated with pulmonary hypertension, PR leads to Graham Steell's PR murmur, which is a diastolic murmur similar to AI, except that it is only heard at the left second intercostal space and increases with inspiration.

Isolated PR is seldom severe enough to require any specific therapy, particularly when secondary to pulmonary hypertension. Valve replacement may be required for severe PR related to endocarditis or surgical correction of tetralogy of Fallot if *symptomatic RV failure* ensues. Note that the RV usually tolerates PR for years, sometimes decades, before it fails. RV size tends to normalize and functional status improves when pulmonic valve replacement is performed for PR late after tetralogy of Fallot repair. However, RV function may not fully recover once marked enlargement and systolic dysfunction are evident.[108] Therefore, many experts recommend valve replacement in asymptomatic severe PR with RV dilatation/dysfunction.

7. MIXED VALVULAR DISEASE; RADIATION HEART DISEASE

I. Mixed single-valve disease

In mixed moderate or severe stenosis *and* moderate or severe regurgitation of the same valve, i.e., MS+MR or AS+AI, one lesion usually predominates over the other (stenosis or regurgitation) and the pathophysiology resembles the dominant lesion. However, the non-dominant lesion worsens the effect and the symptomatology of the dominant lesion, and these patients are more prone to elevate PCWP and develop pulmonary edema than patients with isolated stenosis or regurgitation. Since the flow across the valve is increased, the transvalvular gradient is increased in comparison to valvular stenosis without regurgitation. This leads to overestimation of the anatomic severity of the stenosis when assessed by gradient. **The gradient, however, correlates with the physiologic consequences of the mixed stenosis–regurgitation and properly correlates with the overall disease severity**. The valvular area is unchanged when calculated by Doppler echocardiography (continuity equation for AS or MS, or pressure half-time for MS). The valvular area may be underestimated, i.e., the stenosis may appear more severe, if Gorlin's equation is used with the net forward cardiac output rather than the total output across the valve.

In moderate mixed disease in a symptomatic patient, a hemodynamic study is useful in addressing the selective impact of valvular vs. myocardial disease. If mixed mitral disease is the cause of the patient's symptoms, PCWP and PA pressure will rise with exercise disproportionately to LVEDP. If mixed aortic valve disease is the cause of the patient's symptoms, LV and aortic end-diastolic pressures are approximated, the dicrotic notch is attenuated, the LV–aortic gradient is in the severe range even if the valve area is not, and an anacrotic notch may be seen.

II. Multiple valvular involvement (combined stenosis or regurgitation of two different valves)

Multiple valvular involvement may be caused by: rheumatic disease (MS with AI or AS, MR with AI), radiation, endocarditis, severe AS or AI with functional MR, myxomatous degeneration of both aortic and mitral valve, or AI due to aortic dilatation and MR due to MVP in patients with connective tissue disorders. Functional TR may occur secondarily to severe mitral disease.

Moderate or severe multiple valvular disease is poorly tolerated. One valvular lesion may mask the hemodynamic manifestation of the other. *The proximal lesion tends to mask the severity of the more distal lesion by reducing the flow across the distal lesion, whereas the distal lesion tends to exacerbate the hemodynamic effect of the proximal lesion because of increased backward volume and/or pressure.* In general, the clinical effect of the proximal lesion is more prominent than that of the distal lesion.

In **severe MR or MS associated with AS**, AS worsens the hemodynamic effects of MS or MR and may worsen the severity of MR (from moderate to severe). In combined AS and MR, the LV is exposed to both pressure and volume overload in systole. Aortic stenosis does not affect the assessment of severity of mitral valve disease, except that MVA may be falsely increased when calculated using the echocardiographic pressure half-time. On the other hand, the severity of AS may be underestimated by gradient assessment as a result of the low cardiac output, but may be overestimated by AVA assessment (low-flow/low-gradient pseudo-severe AS). If surgery is indicated for the mitral valve, consider anatomic assessment of the severity of AS during surgery (palpation of the aortic valve) to make a decision about concomitant aortic valve replacement. When MS is associated with mild AS and mitral balloon valvuloplasty is planned, reassess the aortic valve after treatment of MS.

In **severe MS with AI**, the hemodynamic effect of MS is exacerbated. In order to allow transmitral flow, LA pressure has to increase in parallel to the increase in LV diastolic pressure. On the other hand, the hemodynamic effect of AI is reduced. Overall, the patient has a higher LA pressure than a patient with isolated MS, but less LV dilatation and less elevated LVEDP than a patient with isolated AI. The severity assessment of MS or AI by catheterization and of AI by echo Doppler are not affected; MVA calculated by Doppler pressure half-time is falsely increased.

Combined *MR–AI* is the most poorly tolerated combination. The LV gets a double volume load in diastole and is more severely enlarged than with either lesion alone. MR is aggravated, and the regurgitant MR volume is more severely increased than with isolated MR. LV and LA filling pressures and volumes are more severely increased than with each lesion alone. The combination does not affect the echocardiographic or invasive assessment of either lesion. MR may be functional, secondary to LV dilatation; AVR alone often improves functional MR, but MV annuloplasty is usually warranted.

In combined ***severe AS–moderate-to-severe MR***, MR is often functional, related to the LV pressure overload, and often improves after aortic valve surgery. MR is worsened by AS, and AS severity may be underestimated by gradient assessment because of the low flow secondary to MR. If MR is severe, these patients often undergo mitral valve repair along with aortic valve replacement; if MR is moderate, mitral repair may be warranted when MR is organic rather than functional or when the surgical risk is low.

III. Radiation heart disease

Radiation heart disease leads to calcification of the cardiac valves and fibrous skeleton, with cardiac abnormalities becoming evident over 5–10 years, sometimes decades, after radiation. The pericardium is the cardiac structure that is most sensitive to radiation and is the most common site of clinical involvement (constrictive pericarditis). The aortic valve is the valve most commonly affected, the combination of AS and AI being the most common radiation-induced valvular disease. MR is also common (second in frequency), followed by TR. The early process consists of fibrosis of the aortic and mitral annuli with subsequent valvular retraction and regurgitation. This is followed by progressive thickening and calcification of the valves but also the cardiac skeleton and mitroaortic curtain.[109] As opposed to rheumatic disease, the mitral base is involved but the mitral leaflets' tips and commissures are spared. In addition, radiation leads to: (1) ostial or diffuse CAD, mainly involving the left main, ostial RCA, or LAD (anterior); (2) myocardial fibrosis with restrictive cardiomyopathy and sometimes LV systolic dysfunction (usually mild); and (3) heavily calcified porcelain aorta. All this complicates the valvular surgery and limits its efficacy. The severe calcifications limit the size of the aortic prosthesis that can be implanted. In addition, interstitial lung disease, recurrent pleural effusions, and impaired skin and sternal healing complicate the operation.[12]

> While senile mitral annular calcifications are usually posterior, anterior mitral annular calcifications on the long-axis view always suggest radiation heart disease. This corresponds to calcification of the mitroaortic intervalvular fibrosa.

8. PROSTHETIC VALVES

I. Bioprosthesis

A bioprosthesis can be a porcine trileaflet valve or a bovine pericardial trileaflet valve, with three components: ring, struts (both mounted over a stent frame), and leaflets arising from the struts. The leaflets, per se, do not contain any metal. Less commonly, stentless porcine or homograft valves are used: they have a thin ring and thin struts and are only available for the aortic position. The percutaneous aortic prosthesis consists of leaflets mounted inside a thin stent frame without bulky struts; the leaflets are stentless (Figures 6.16, 6.17).

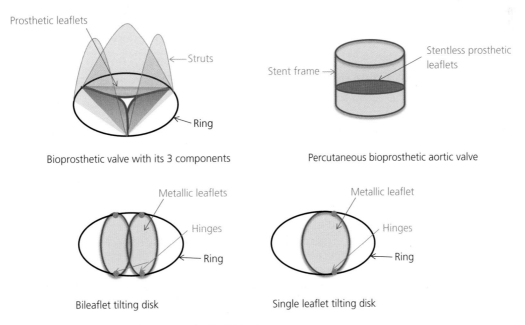

Bioprosthetic valve with its 3 components

Percutaneous bioprosthetic aortic valve

Bileaflet tilting disk

Single leaflet tilting disk

Mechanical prosthesis with its 3 components

Figure 6.16 Prosthetic valves. Surgical bioprostheses typically have a metallic stent frame that extends from the sewing ring to each strut. Stentless bioprostheses have very thin rings and struts without any metal.

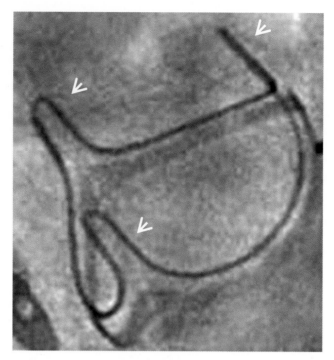

Figure 6.17 Bioprosthetic valve as seen on fluoroscopy. The ring and the three struts (*arrowheads*) are mounted over a metallic stent frame, which explains their visualization on fluoroscopy. The leaflets, per se, do not contain any metal and are not visualized.

One-third of bioprostheses degenerate in 10–15 years. Scarring/calcification and tears/perforations occur over time. Leaflet fibrosis and calcification may lead to stenosis but also regurgitation from leaflet retraction. Cuspal tears and perforations lead to regurgitation.

A bioprosthesis degenerates more quickly in younger patients (<60 years, high cardiac output) and in the mitral position (high valvular closing pressure). In patients older than 65 years, a bioprosthetic AVR has a risk of degeneration of <10% over 10 years.[110,111] Atherosclerotic risk factors accelerate degeneration, while statin therapy may slow it.

In aortic valve endocarditis, a homograft is preferred. In case of a small scarred annulus, a stentless bioprosthesis or a homograft is the best option (lowest profile). The main problem with homograft and stentless prostheses is the lack of long-term longevity data.

Advantages of a bioprosthesis over a mechanical prosthesis:[110]

- No need for anticoagulation.
- It is preferred in patients older than 70 years, in patients with bleeding diathesis, and possibly in women considering pregnancy (*class IIa* for the latter in ESC guidelines).

II. Mechanical valve: bileaflet tilting disk (St. Jude) or single-leaflet tilting disk (e.g., Medtronic-Hall)
A mechanical valve is preferred in the following cases:

- Age <60 years
- The patient requires anticoagulation for other conditions (e.g., AF)

Either a mechanical or a bioprosthetic valve is acceptable in patients 60–70 years of age (*class IIa*).[12] In particular, a bioprosthesis may be reasonable in the slowly degenerating aortic position. Should degeneration occur, valve-in-valve TAVR would be considered.

The stentless bioprosthesis, the TAVR bioprosthesis, and the bileaflet mechanical valve have the lowest profile (i.e., the largest orifice area and lowest gradient for the same ring size).

III. Determinants of valve degeneration and valve thrombosis; anticoagulation guidelines
A. Bioprosthetic valve degeneration depends on:
- *Cardiac output:* the higher stroke volume of the young active patient is associated with faster degeneration; also, the higher heart rate of the physically active patient means more frequent opening and closing of the valve, and thus more injury.[111]
- *Valvular closing pressure,* which is the difference between LV systolic pressure (e.g., 130 mmHg) and LA pressure (e.g., 10) for the mitral valve, or the difference between aortic diastolic pressure (e.g., 80) and LV diastolic pressure (e.g., 10) for the aortic valve. Thus, the closing pressure is highest for the mitral valve, which degenerates the fastest, followed by the aortic valve, then the right-sided valves (tricuspid then pulmonic valve). A bioprosthesis is often long-lasting in the right-sided position.

B. Prosthetic valve thrombosis depends on:
- *Valvular closing pressure.* The low closing pressure on the right side explains the high thrombotic risk of prosthetic valves in this position, *another reason why bioprosthesis may be favored.* Despite a higher closing pressure, the mitral valve has a higher thrombotic risk than the aortic valve, because of its proximity to the diseased, sluggish LA, prone to microthrombus formation.

Anticoagulation guidelines

Always try mitral valve repair instead of MVR: no need for long-term anticoagulation, better operative and long-term mortality, and better preservation of LV function.

Anticoagulation goals

- Aortic mechanical prosthesis, bileaflet tilting-disk type or current-generation single-leaflet type (e.g., Medtronic-Hall), without thromboembolic high-risk factors: warfarin with an INR goal of 2–3 + aspirin 81 mg. Thromboembolic risk is high with any of the following four factors: history of embolic events, AF, LV dysfunction, hypercoagulable state.
- Mitral mechanical prosthesis or aortic mechanical prosthesis outside the exception noted above: warfarin with an INR goal of 2.5–3.5 + aspirin 81 mg. The addition of aspirin reduces stroke and mortality and is given a class I recommendation.
- Bioprosthesis without thromboembolic high-risk factors: aspirin 81–325 mg/day. Give warfarin for 3 months postoperatively, until the sewing cuff endothelializes (*class II* recommendation). Anticoagulation for the first 3–6 months was associated with a mortality reduction in a large registry.[112]
- Bioprosthesis with thromboembolic high-risk factors: warfarin (INR 2–3) + aspirin.
- Stroke despite appropriate anticoagulation: increase the level of anticoagulation, i.e., increase the INR goal from 2.5–3.5 to 3.5–4.5; may also add aspirin if not used previously.
- Mitral valve repair: aspirin lifelong + warfarin for 3 months postoperatively.
- TAVR: lifelong aspirin + 3–6 months of clopidogrel. If TAVR patient has AF: warfarin ± one antiplatelet agent

Correction of excessive anticoagulation

- In case of a high INR (5–10) without bleeding, hold warfarin. If INR > 10, give oral vitamin K 1–2.5 mg. In case of bleeding, give fresh frozen plasma or prothrombin complex concentrate.
- While a high dose of vitamin K is used in bleeding patients without prosthetic valve, avoid this high dose in prosthetic valves, because it may overcorrect to a hypercoagulable state. A 1.0–2.5 mg dose of vitamin K is safe. Fresh frozen plasma is a safer option in case of bleeding.

Bridging for a planned procedure

- Hold warfarin 5 days before the procedure; start unfractionated heparin (UFH) infusion when INR falls below 2 (typically 36–48 hours after warfarin discontinuation) and continue heparin until 4–6 hours before the procedure, then restart it as soon as possible afterwards, (typically 24–48 hours) and restart warfarin on the day of the procedure. The use of LMWH instead of UFH is an acceptable alternative supported by data and ACC/ACCP guidelines (*class I*). LMWH is also an acceptable alternative to UFH in pregnancy (*class I*). For patients with bileaflet mechanical AVR without high-risk factors, bridging is not necessary; warfarin is stopped 2–4 days before and resumed 24 hours after the procedure.

IV. Particular cases: women who wish to become pregnant and dialysis patients

During pregnancy, the hypercoagulable state increases the risk of mechanical valve thromboembolic complications even with appropriate anticoagulation. The maternal mortality is 1–4% in patients with mechanical valves.[91] Moreover, warfarin has fetal risks between 6 and 12 weeks and has to be replaced with UFH or LMWH during this period. LMWH and UFH are not as effective as warfarin in pregnancy; most valvular thromboembolic events in pregnancy occur while the mother is receiving heparin. Yet even with warfarin anticoagulation throughout pregnancy, the risk of valve thrombosis is 4% (versus 9% if heparin is used between 6 and 12 weeks).[113] Therefore, knowing that the risk associated with valvular reoperation is low and only slightly higher than that of the first operation, bioprosthesis may be the best option in women who wish to become pregnant, despite the rapid bioprosthetic degeneration at this age (possibly accelerated by the high cardiac output of pregnancy).[91] Pre-pregnancy percutaneous valvuloplasty may be the best option for patients with non-calcified, severe AS, whether symptomatic or not. Pregnancy before valvular surgery is an option in patients with severe asymptomatic AI or MR and normal EF/LV dimensions, after confirming the asymptomatic status and the normal PA pressure by exercise testing.

Dialysis patients have a high mortality following valve replacement, whether with mechanical or biological prostheses. Although bioprosthesis degenerates faster in this population, it seems a reasonable choice given the high bleeding risk and the limited survival, except in the very young (<35 years).

V. Echocardiographic follow-up of prosthetic valves

Postoperative echo should be performed 6 weeks postoperatively, at the first outpatient visit, to obtain baseline function and gradient across the prosthesis. This baseline gradient provides a reference in case of any future deterioration. Follow-up echo is indicated at 6–12 months in patients with severe LV dysfunction to assess for improvement in LV size and function. Otherwise, echo is only indicated if there is a change in symptoms.

Routine echo is not indicated for a mechanical prosthesis, not even years after valve replacement. Conversely, yearly echo surveillance of bioprostheses is reasonable after 10 years, or 5 years in young patients, to detect severe deterioration early on before LV dysfunction or HF occurs (*class IIa*).

VI. Complications

(rate, ~2–3% per year)

A. Degeneration

Degeneration occurs with bioprosthetic valves and leads to valvular stenosis or regurgitation. Reoperation is necessary once symptoms develop (*class I*), or even in asymptomatic patients with severe regurgitant dysfunction (*class IIa*, ESC and ACC guidelines), or severe stenotic dysfunction (*class IIa*, ESC). Since dysfunction is progressive, sometimes suddenly so with further leaflet tearing/regurgitation, early reoperation at a stable stage reduces the risk of this second operation and thus may be justified. In fact, the risk associated with reoperation in a stable patient is only slightly higher than the risk of the first operation (ESC).[91] Treating bioprosthetic aortic valve failure by transcatheter valve-in-valve implantation has been shown to be feasible and is an alternative in high-risk patients.

B. Prosthetic valve thromboembolism and thrombosis

a. *Thromboembolic events:* without anticoagulation, the risk of thromboembolic events with a mechanical prosthesis is 8% per year, but up to 20% in the highest-risk patient, e.g., MVR with AF or history of embolic events. Anticoagulation reduces the risk to 1–2% per year, more so when aspirin is added. Many thromboembolic events are due to an intermittently subtherapeutic INR, but some of them occur despite a therapeutic INR.

b. *Valve thrombosis:* 0.2–0.5% per year. It is recommended that patients with a large valve thrombosis (>10 mm or 0.8 cm^2) or functional class III–IV undergo surgical removal of the thrombus or prosthesis replacement. Thrombolytic therapy is an alternative if surgery is deemed high-risk, e.g., if the patient has shock requiring multiple vasopressors (100 mg of r-tPA over 2 hours). Several series have shown that thrombolysis results in total dissolution of the thrombus in up to 71% of the cases, and partial dissolution in up to 17% of the cases, with a 7–16% incidence of clinical embolization. One-third of patients require repeated courses of thrombolysis, and 23% ultimately require surgery.[114,115] These series suggest that thrombolysis may be used as a first-line therapy in high-surgical-risk patients, while surgery may be reserved for thrombolysis failure.

On the other hand, in a patient with NYHA class I–II and a small clot burden <0.8 cm^2, thrombolysis is associated with a low embolization risk and is a first-line therapy. Alternatively, intravenous heparin infusion may be tried for a few days before proceeding with thrombolysis.

Thrombolysis is also first-line therapy for right-sided thrombosis, even if it is large or symptoms are advanced, as the success rate is high and systemic embolization is unusual.

C. Paraprosthetic leak

A paraprosthetic leak may cause severe regurgitation and hemolysis. It is frequently due to endocarditis (~50% in some series), which should always be carefully sought. It may also be due to loose sutures, or heavy annular calcium that prevents complete prosthetic apposition and suturing or leads to late suture dehiscence.[116] It is observed with both mechanical and bioprosthetic valves (more common with bioprosthetic valves in one study).[116]

Small, asymptomatic leaks are common early postoperatively (10–25%) and are seen on postoperative TEE. Those decrease or resolve in the ensuing days or months with the healing process. Rarely (~1.5%), paravalvular leaks may be severe and symptomatic, and may appear early postoperatively (loose suture) or months or years later if a suture suddenly dehisces from a calcified annulus, if early paravalvular channels enlarge and mature with the continuous flow, or if endocarditis develops.[116,117]

Valvular dehiscence is an extreme form of paravalvular leak that involves >20–40% of the sewing ring circumference and is often due to endocarditis. It manifests as a "rocking" movement of the prosthesis on echo and fluoroscopy.

Severe hemolysis may be seen with large paravalvular leaks but also with central leaks of degenerated bioprostheses or, rarely, with small, high-jet leaks even if the regurgitation is not severe.[118] Iron replacement may be an effective therapy.

Repair of the paraprosthetic leak with additional sutures or valvular re-replacement is indicated for a severe leak associated with HF or severe hemolysis requiring repeated transfusion (fortunately, the leak and the chronic hemolysis are often mild). Moderate-to-severe paravalvular leaks are associated with a late increase in mortality and progressive HF, particularly if the underlying LV is abnormal. A severe paravalvular leak without clear HF or symptoms does not, per se, have a clear indication for repair.[91]

D. Endocarditis
(~0.5% per year, the frequency being highest in the first 6–12 months)

a. Early endocarditis (<60 days to 1 year postoperatively, usually a complication of valve surgery): *Staphylococcus coagulase*-negative and -positive. Second in frequency are enterococcal and gram negative infections.

b. Late endocarditis (>1 year postoperatively): the microbiology resembles that of native valve endocarditis. *Streptococcus* species (*viridians*, *bovis*) are the most common, followed by staphylococci and enteroccoci. Coagulase-negative staphylococcus may still be seen, especially after central line placement.

E. Patient/prosthesis mismatch (PPM)

In this case, the prosthesis is small and obstructive. This occurs more commonly in patients with a small scarred mitral or aortic annulus, forcing the surgeon to place a small prosthesis. PPM is defined as an indexed prosthetic effective orifice area (EOA) ≤ 0.85 cm^2/m^2 in the aortic position and ≤ 1.2 cm^2/m^2 in the mitral position, and while it was classically described with aortic prostheses, it is actually seen with up to ~30–50% of both mitral and aortic prostheses.[110,119–121] This is more likely to occur with valvular replacement performed for aortic or mitral stenosis rather than regurgitation, as the annulus is usually scarred in these cases.

These patients have a relatively stenotic prosthesis with a pressure gradient across the prosthesis at rest and much more so with exercise. They often do well in the intermediate term but have a reduced functional capacity and an impaired long-term survival and prognosis, with frequent persistence of LV dysfunction, hypertrophy, or pulmonary hypertension. PPM has a particular impact on young active patients or patients with pre-existing LV dysfunction, especially when in the severe range (e.g., aortic EOA <0.75 cm^2/m^2, mitral EOA <0.9 cm^2/m^2); the effect of moderate PPM is significant but much less striking.[119,120]

PPM may be prevented by avoiding valves ≤ 21 mm in the aortic position, and ≤ 27 mm in the mitral position, if possible, taking into account the patient's body size. Charts correlating the in-vitro prosthetic diameter of each brand of prosthesis with the effective orifice area are available. For example, a 23 mm bioprosthesis in the aortic position has an EOA of 1.4 ± 0.3 cm^2; for a patient with a BSA of 2 m^2, the indexed EOA is 0.7 cm^2/m^2, consistent with PPM. A 25 mm bioprosthesis (EOA 1.7 cm^2), or a different prosthesis, such as a low-profile stentless prosthesis or a mechanical prosthesis (0.4 cm^2 larger EOA), should be selected for this patient.[110] Supra-annular implantation is another alternative. TAVR valves only have a thin stent frame without sewing ring and without stented struts, and thus have larger orifice areas and less PPM than surgical bioprostheses.

F. Mechanical valve obstruction

Mechanical valve obstruction occurs at a frequency of 0.5% per year. It leads to the loss of the prosthetic click on exam, and to HF and hemodynamic compromise clinically. Causes (all these processes may also be seen with a bioprosthetic valve, at a lower frequency):

a. Pannus formation = fibrosis that grows from the endocardium surrounding the sewing ring and extends onto the prosthesis. Compared to a thrombus, a pannus is smaller and sometimes missed by TEE (mean size 1 cm), symptoms develop more progressively (over a month or more), and anticoagulation is usually adequate.
b. Thrombosis (more common than pannus formation)
c. Early postoperative prosthetic obstruction may be due to severe annular calcification that impinges on leaflet motion.

G. Differential diagnosis of a high transvalvular prosthetic gradient

A high gradient, up to a certain degree, may be seen with a normally functioning prosthetic valve or may be due to four states:

a. prosthetic obstruction (thrombus, pannus, degenerative bioprosthesis)
b. PPM
c. pressure recovery in the case of a bileaflet valve
d. high flow state, subvalvular obstruction, or significant regurgitation across the valve

On the other hand, a falsely low gradient, within the normal range for a prosthesis, may be seen in patients with prosthetic obstruction but low-flow state. The following ideas help establish the diagnosis:[110,122]

1. A velocity of up to 3 m/s across the aortic prosthesis (mean gradient up to 20 mmHg) and 1.9 m/s across the mitral prosthesis (gradient up to 6 mmHg) is within the normal range unless the cardiac output is low, in which case a low dimensionless index will suggest valvular obstruction.
2. A high transvalvular velocity with a high LVOT velocity and a high dimensionless index (LVOT VTI/aortic or mitral VTI), >0.30 with aortic prosthesis and >0.45 with mitral prosthesis, usually implies a high flow state, an associated subvalvular obstruction, or prosthetic aortic regurgitation. The calculated EOA would be within normal range.
3. A valve with a small reference EOA on the manufacturer's chart and a small indexed EOA for the particular patient is diagnostic of *PPM, which is by far the most common cause of a high transprosthetic gradient*. In this case, *the small calculated EOA matches the manufacturer's EOA*.
4. Outside the above conditions, the patient may have a true obstruction or, in the case of a bileaflet valve, pressure recovery phenomenon. The smaller central orifice of the bileaflet valve gives rise to a high-velocity jet; this corresponds to a localized pressure drop that is largely recovered once the central flow joins flow originating from the two lateral orifices.

The analysis of leaflet motion and structure on TEE allows differentiation between a structurally normal prosthesis and a true obstruction that requires operative correction. TEE often demonstrates abnormal leaflet motion and may show a large thrombus. Conversely, a high transprosthetic gradient with a normal leaflet motion corresponds to a normally functioning valve with a high velocity (PPM, pressure recovery, high flow state). Also, cinefluoroscopy is a very helpful adjunctive technique that allows analysis of the mechanical prosthesis leaflet's excursion (to assess stenosis) and the prosthesis seating (to assess dehiscence and regurgitation).

9. AUSCULTATION AND SUMMARY IDEAS

I. Auscultation and other physical findings (see Table 6.5)

A. MR murmur
- Blowing, high-pitched holosystolic murmur at the apex. S_3 indicates severe MR.
- In posterior mitral leaflet prolapse, the regurgitant jet is directed anteriorly and radiates to the aorta. In anterior leaflet prolapse or posterior leaflet tethering (ischemic MR), the jet is directed posteriorly and radiates to the axilla, back, and sometimes skull. MR murmur does not radiate to the neck.
- Could be an end-systolic murmur in mitral valve prolapse. It becomes holosystolic with worsening of MR severity or chordal rupture. In fact, a **murmur that is only end-systolic argues against severe MR**.

Table 6.5 Auscultation features

		Systolic						Diastolic[a]		Continuous
	MR	**TR**	**AS**	**HOCM**	**VSD**	**PS**	**CoA**	**AI**	**MS**	**PDA**
Duration	Holo (may be early in ischemic MR, late in MVP)	Holo	Mid	Mid	Holo	Mid	Mid	Holo, or early	Mid, may extend to late	Continuous, peak at S_2
Location	Apex	LLSB	RUSB	LLSB	LLSB	LUSB	LUSB	LUSB	Apex	Left infraclavicular
Quality	Blowing	Blowing	Harsh	Harsh	Harsh	Harsh	Harsh	Blowing	Low pitch	Machinery
Radiation	Axilla + back vs. base	–	Carotids, ± apex	–	–	–	Back	–	–	–

[a] PR also leads to a diastolic murmur that is mainly heard if pulmonary hypertension is present.
LLSB, left lower sternal border; LUSB, left upper sternal border; RUSB, right upper sternal border.

- A mid-systolic click is heard after S_1 in mitral valve prolapse, sometimes simulating gallop or S_1 splitting.
- May become musical ("seagull cry" murmur) in case of a ruptured chorda that gets "shaken" by the regurgitant flow like a guitar chord.
- In acute MR or MR with severe LV dysfunction, the murmur may be soft or absent because of diminished LV–LA pressure gradient and flow. It also tends to be early-systolic only: left atrial pressure being so high, LV–LA pressure gradient diminishes quickly (large V wave).

B. MS murmur

- Low-pitched, diastolic rumble heard at the apex. It is best heard in mid-diastole. When it extends to late diastole, it suggests the persistence of gradient in late diastole and, thus, severe MS. It is best heard in a left lateral decubitus position that puts the apex against the chest wall, and *unveiled by exercise.*
- While the diastolic rumble may be difficult to hear, a *loud S_1* is the most characteristic finding in some patients (see explanation under paragraph L). S_1 is loud when the leaflets are pliable, and becomes muffled later on, as the leaflets fully immobilize. A mitral valve opening snap is also heard with pliable leaflets.
- Severe MS is characterized by: (i) short interval between S_2 and the opening snap; (ii) long MS murmur. The higher the LA pressure, the earlier the mitral valve opens during LV relaxation, which leads to a short S_2–opening snap interval.
- A diastolic mitral rumble may also result from the functional mitral obstruction caused by the regurgitant flow of AI (Austin–Flint murmur), or from the high flow recrossing the mitral valve in severe MR.

C. AS murmur

- Harsh, crescendo–decrescendo mid-systolic murmur best heard at the right upper sternal border (RUSB).
- Radiates to the carotids.
- Murmur of severe AS may radiate to the apex and be loudest at the apex. High-frequency vibrations may get transmitted through the LV cavity and lead to a predominant apical, "musical" murmur.
- *Signs of severe AS:*
  - Reduced, paradoxically split, or absent aortic component of S_2, i.e., reduced S_2 at the RUSB. *A normal aortic component of S_2 reliably excludes severe AS.*
  - Carotid upstroke characterized by pulsus parvus (weak) and tardus (slow and delayed). The carotid upstroke may, however, remain brisk in elderly patients with stiff arteries.
  - Murmur peaks late in systole and is prolonged.

D. AI murmur

- Blowing diastolic murmur best heard in a sitting/leaning-forward position that puts the aorta against the chest wall, particularly at end-expiration. Since the retrograde aortic flow goes to the left, the murmur is best heard at the left upper sternal border (LUSB) in intrinsic valve disease. As opposed to AI, the turbulent flow of AS is directed towards the aorta (right), hence the AS murmur is best heard at the RUSB. Only when AI is secondary to aortic root disease, which is on the right side of the chest, is the AI murmur best heard at the RUSB.
- ↓ S_1 with LV enlargement, ↓ S_2 (A_2).
- Duration of the murmur correlates with the severity of AI (severe = pandiastolic). However, in acute AI or in the case of a severely decompensated LV, the murmur may be soft and short.
- Pulse abnormalities in *chronic severe AI:*

  - A wide pulse pressure is seen with chronic severe AI, reflecting the large increase in stroke volume (e.g., 170/70). In acute AI, while the diastolic pressure is low, the LV is small and the stroke volume is low, which prevents the pulse pressure from being particularly wide (e.g., 90/40). *A wide pulse pressure is very sensitive for the diagnosis of chronic severe AI. In fact, a normal pulse pressure almost excludes chronic severe AI.* However, a wide pulse pressure is not a specific finding and may be seen in patients with stiff non-compliant arteries, wherein the systolic pressure quickly rises and falls, and in disease states with diastolic runoff (PDA, AV fistula). Rarely, the pulse pressure may not be wide in severe AI with severely reduced EF, an advanced stage where the total stroke volume is reduced.
  - The pulse may be double-peaked (bisferiens) as a result of the large pulse waves reflected from the peripheral arteries. This bisferiens pulse may also be seen in any high-output state and in HOCM.

E. TR murmur

- Holosystolic murmur heard at the left lower sternal border (fourth intercostal space). The murmur may extend and become prominent at the apex if the RV is severely enlarged, or may extend below the xiphoid in patients with COPD pushing the heart down.
- Loudness is related to the degree of pulmonary hypertension (murmur is mild and short in primary TR).
- The murmur increases in intensity with inspiration (Carvallo's sign).
- Associated with pulsatile hepatomegaly and large and prolonged V waves on JVP. These V waves may simulate the carotid pulsations and make it hard to distinguish carotid pulsations from JVP. *In fact, a JVP that mimics a carotid pulse is a hint to TR.*

F. HOCM murmur

- Harsh, mid-systolic, crescendo–decrescendo murmur, which may simulate AS but is heard at the left sternal border (as opposed to *AS: RUSB; MR: apex*).
- May radiate to the base but, in contrast to AS, *does not radiate to the carotids*.
- Carotid pulse is brisk (in contrast with severe AS, which weakens the carotid upstroke), and double-peaked (spike and dome).
- Usually associated with another type of murmur at the apex, an MR murmur related to SAM of the mitral valve.
- Varies with maneuvers (paragraph J).

G. Patent ductus arteriosus

- Continuous, crescendo–decrescendo murmur that peaks around S_2 and is loudest at the left infraclavicular region. The murmur becomes softer when severe pulmonary hypertension develops.
- ***A continuous murmur is different from a systolo-diastolic murmur***. In the latter, two peaks, one systolic and one diastolic, are heard. A systolo-diastolic murmur may be heard with combined AS/AI.
- A continuous murmur that peaks anywhere outside the LUSB suggests another fistula: coronary fistula to the RA/RV/PA, ruptured sinus of Valsalva aneurysm that communicates with the RA or RV.

H. Other pathological murmurs

- *VSD*: harsh holosystolic murmur at the left lower sternal border (in contrast to AS: harsh mid-systolic murmur).
- *Pulmonic stenosis*: mid-systolic murmur at the LUSB with early systolic click. In inspiration, the murmur increases while the click diminishes. In inspiration, the RV diastolic pressure increases and equalizes with the PA diastolic pressure, leading to premature soft opening of the pulmonic valve in diastole, which reduces the opening click. P_2 decreases in severe PS (like A_2 in severe AS).
- *Coarctation of the aorta*: mid-systolic murmur at the LUSB ($\neq$ AS), radiates to the back through the intercostal collateral flow.
- *Pulmonary regurgitation*: holodiastolic murmur is heard at the LUSB *mainly when pulmonary hypertension is present*, i.e., when there is a high gradient between PA and RV (Graham Steell). This diastolic murmur increases with inspiration.
- *Peripheral pulmonary artery stenosis* (e.g., associated with supravalvular AS): murmur is heard at the back.

I. Benign murmurs

- Benign murmurs are mid-systolic.
- In children or young adults, they are due to vibrations across the flexible pulmonic valve leaflets or the pulmonary trunk and are best heard at the LUSB. They may also be due to vibrations across the aortic leaflets and are heard at the mid-left precordium (Still's murmur). Those vibratory murmurs are musical and sound like a "guitar string."
- In older patients, a benign murmur is due to aortic valve sclerosis. Even if the leaflets open fully, fibrocalcific deposits create turbulence leading to a murmur. This murmur does not radiate to the carotids.
- A murmur is considered benign at any age, especially young age, when it is mid-systolic (not early systolic or holosystolic), grade 1 or 2/6 in loudness, without any associated clinical findings, without radiation to the carotids, and without worsening during Valsalva. Being a flow murmur, it may improve with the reduction of ventricular filling upon sitting, standing, or Valsalva. Echo is not needed in these cases. Conversely, a diastolic murmur is not benign and always requires echo assessment.

J. Effects of different maneuvers on murmurs

1. All right-sided murmurs increase with inspiration, except the systolic ejection click of pulmonic stenosis, which becomes softer with inspiration.

2. A reduction in LV volume further narrows the LVOT in HOCM, and further "squeezes up" the prolapsed mitral leaflet(s) in MVP. LV volume is reduced with a reduction in preload or afterload.

  Thus, the straining phase of Valsalva's maneuver, standing, or NTG:
  - ↓venous return and ↓ LV volume.
  - ↑ HOCM murmur, ↑ MVP murmur (+ the MVP click moves closer to S_1) and ↓ all other valvular murmurs (AS, severe MR).

3. Handgrip, squatting:
  - ↑ afterload.
  - ↓ HOCM murmur, ↓ MVP murmur (+ the MVP click moves further away from S_1), and ↑ regurgitant and VSD murmurs. If MVP has progressed to severe MR, the murmur would generally increase with handgrip.

4. ***A murmur that increases after a pause (as in the first beat after a PVC) is typical of HOCM and AS. The*** pulse decreases *after a pause in HOCM (Brockenbrough), whereas it increases after a pause in AS*. MR murmur does not increase after a pause.

K. Second heart sound (S_2) abnormalities and splits

- The aortic valve normally closes before the pulmonic valve. Thus, the aortic component A_2 (RUSB) usually occurs before the pulmonic component P_2 (LUSB) (***A_2 then P_2***). A_2 is normally the loudest and is the second heart sound heard all across the precordium. P_2 is mainly heard at the LUSB. Inspiration further increases RV volume and RV ejection time, and thus a *split S_2 can be normally heard during inspiration, especially in young patients,* and is best heard at the LUSB. Split abnormalities are generally best heard at the LUSB.
- A *persistently* split S_2 that is worse with inspiration suggests right-sided pathologies and is heard at the LUSB: RV failure, including pulmonary HTN associated with RV failure, PE, RBBB.
- A ***loud split S_2*** suggests pulmonary hypertension. In this case, the split is heard not only at the LUSB but also lower, at the left lower sternal border, and is loud. A loud split S_2 that is heard at the apex implies a systolic PA pressure >50 mmHg.
- A *paradoxically* split S_2, i.e., a split S_2 that is worse with expiration, suggests a pulmonic valve closure before the aortic valve closure: LBBB, RV pacemaker, advanced AS, or advanced HOCM.
- A fixed-split S_2 suggests ASD. Inspiration increases right-sided flow, which leads to a proportionate reduction in the left-to-right shunt and an unchanged overall right-sided flow. The right and left ventricular outputs remain unchanged with inspiration.
- A loud P_2 (on the left sternal border) suggests pulmonary hypertension.
- A loud A_2 (on the right sternal border) suggests systemic hypertension.
- ***A diffusely faint S_2 usually implies a faint A_2 and suggests AS.***

L. S₁, S₃, S₄

- S$_1$ may be soft in case of a depressed LV function or **loud in case of a short PR interval, MS, or tachycardia**:
  - When PR is short, ventricular contraction may occur before the end of atrial contraction, at a time when the mitral leaflets are wide open and would close more vigorously. In MS, the persistent LA–LV pressure gradient in late diastole keeps the mitral leaflets open until the ventricle contracts, which shuts them vigorously.
  - S$_1$ is variable in intensity in AF and in AV dissociation. If S$_1$ is variable in intensity and the patient has a regular tachycardia, the diagnosis is VT; if the patient is bradycardic, the diagnosis is AV block.
- S$_3$ occurs during the rapid diastolic filling phase, and implies that LA pressure is elevated and forcefully fills the LV ("pusher" effect). This corresponds to a decompensated LV systolic or diastolic failure. S$_3$ may, however, be normally heard in patients <40 years old and during pregnancy, wherein the LV is "supercompliant" and forcefully "sucks" blood from a normal-pressure LA.
- S$_4$ corresponds to an elevated LV end-diastolic pressure (LVEDP), i.e., elevated LV pressure after A wave. LV compliance is impaired, which leads to a striking rise of LV pressure after atrial contraction. S$_4$ is heard in any systolic or diastolic LV dysfunction (e.g., LVH with abnormal relaxation, active ischemia/acute MI, dilated cardiomyopathy). LVEDP generally approximates mean LA pressure, yet in compensated LV dysfunction, LVEDP may be elevated (= S$_4$) with a normal mean LA pressure. Thus, S$_4$ predicts an increase in LA pressure, but less reliably than S$_3$, and the increase in LA pressure with isolated S$_4$ is less than that seen with S$_3$. Approximately 35% of patients with S$_4$ have normal LA pressure and compensated HF.
- S$_4$ cannot be present in AF. S$_3$ and S$_4$ cannot be present in severe MS, as MS restricts diastolic LV filling

M. Precordial palpation of the apical impulse in the left lateral decubitus position: point of maximal impulse (PMI)

The PMI is normally located at or medial to the mid-clavicular line in the submammary space. PMI is normally smaller than the size of a quarter. The PMI is *enlarged and displaced laterally* and downward in LV dilatation (systolic HF, AI). A *double bulge* (early then late systolic bulge), or sometimes triple bulge, implies HOCM. A *forceful PMI* that is sustained throughout systole implies LV hypertrophy; the apex is not necessarily displaced laterally or enlarged. A *hyperkinetic PMI* implies a large stroke volume and is seen in severe AI and MR.

> Acute AI/MR, all severe valvular disorders, and low cardiac output states may be associated with a paradoxical reduction of murmur intensity.
>
> In any valvular disease, some common associated signs indicate complicated, severe disease: loud P$_2$ (= pulmonary hypertension), RV heave, LV enlargement (PMI is displaced laterally and is enlarged, i.e., larger than a coin), and S$_3$. S$_3$, however, is usually found with any severe MR and is not necessarily a sign of decompensated MR.

II. General ideas and workup

A. There is no role for medical therapy in symptomatic, severe valvular disorders or in valvular disorders associated with secondary LV dysfunction.
The only effective therapy at this point is surgery, the exceptions being MS with very mild symptoms in a debilitated patient and severe MR secondary to severe LV dysfunction.

B. Transthoracic echocardiography (TTE)
TTE diagnoses the severity and the cause of valvular disorders. In all valvular disorders, LA or LV enlargement or decreased EF is a sign of severity.

C. Transesophageal echocardiography (TEE)
- TEE is indicated in severe MR. It establishes the severity of MR, the anatomic cause of MR, the feasibility of mitral repair (cusps involved), and guides mitral repair.
- TEE is not superior to TTE in assessing the severity of AS or AI. In fact, it is difficult to get the aortic valve gradient by TEE. TEE is superior to TTE for the anatomic assessment of the aortic valve and for the diagnosis of endocarditis.
- TEE can identify a left atrial appendage thrombus in patients with MS or AF, the presence of which dictates the deferral of percutaneous valvuloplasty.

> **Intraoperative TEE** is indicated in all cases of valvular surgery, particularly mitral valve repair. It immediately detects a suboptimal result or postoperative technical problems, especially in the case of mitral repair or valvular endocarditis with abscess. In the immediate preoperative setting, it should not be relied upon for the assessment of valvular disease severity, particularly functional MR, as general anesthesia decreases the cardiac loading conditions and may make valvular regurgitation appear less severe. A mild ischemic MR on preoperative TEE may actually be moderate or severe, especially during exertion.

D. Exercise testing
Patients with severe valvular disease and equivocal symptoms should undergo exercise testing to assess for dyspnea and functional capacity impairment. A functional capacity 1–2 METs below average is concerning for symptomatic valvular disease.

> Predicted METs for men: $18 - (0.15 \times age)$; women: $14.7 - (0.13 \times age)$.[123,124]

Exercise testing is also used to assess the exertional PA pressure in mitral valve disorders and the dynamic worsening of ischemic MR. It is valuable for the assessment of blood pressure response to exercise in asymptomatic, severe AS. Stress testing may be risky in severe AS and needs to be carefully monitored by a cardiologist.

E. Preoperative coronary angiography, and preoperative angiographic and hemodynamic assessment of valvular disease

- Coronary angiography is used to identify CAD in cases of angina, man >40 years old or postmenopausal woman, or patients with >1 CAD risk factor. The presence of CAD dictates a combined CABG + valvular surgery. Beside being an appropriate therapy for CAD, CABG reduces the risk of postoperative infarction and LV failure. Coronary angiography may be forgone in emergent valvular surgery (acute regurgitation, endocarditis, aortic dissection).
- A hemodynamic study of AS or MS and a hemodynamic and angiographic study of MR or AI can help define the severity of the valvular disorder. This invasive valvular assessment is indicated if the echo data are inconclusive *or* if there is discrepancy between the echo and the clinical findings.

F. Endocarditis prophylaxis

- Not routinely indicated for native valvular disease of any severity.
- Only indicated in patients with high-risk cardiac conditions who are undergoing an invasive gingival, dental, or respiratory procedure:
  - Prosthetic valve or history of valvular repair using a prosthetic material.
  - History of infective endocarditis.
  - Unrepaired cyanotic congenital heart disease, partially repaired congenital heart disease with persistent defects adjacent to a prosthetic material, or in the first 6 months after full repair of any congenital heart disease.
  - Transplant valvulopathy.

G. Follow-up echo

- Q6–12 months for severe valvular disease without symptoms and without surgical indication (more spaced for MS: Q1 year for very severe MS, Q1–2 years for severe MS)
- Q1–2 years for moderate valvular disease without symptoms and without surgical indication (more spaced for MS: Q3–5 years for moderate MS)
- Q3–5 years for mild valvular disease

H. Surgical mortality

- CABG: ~1–5%
- Redo CABG: ~10%
- AVR: ~3–4%; 1–2% in low-risk patients, up to 8% in patients with low EF
- AVR + CABG: 6%
- AVR in octogenarians: ~6–9% (6.4% in PARTNER trial), increases to 18% if AVR + multivessel CABG
- MVR: ~6%; MV repair: ~1–3% (half the mortality of MVR)
- MVR in patients >70 years old: 14%
- MVR + CABG: 11% (mainly due to the higher baseline comorbidity of these patients; the risk is related to CAD rather than CABG itself and is potentially higher if CAD is left untreated)
- AVR + aortic aneurysm repair: 9%
- Multiple valve replacement: 9%
- Redo valve replacement: 5–15% (depending on age and comorbidities)

I. Volume and pressure overload with valvular disease

- MR leads to an increase in LV preload. LV afterload is initially reduced because of the low-pressure leak. However, at an advanced stage, LV afterload (= wall stress) increases because of LV dilatation.
- AS leads to an increase in LV pressure afterload.
- AI leads to an increase in preload but also a severe increase in afterload from the LV dilatation and the increased pulse pressure. This increase in preload, volume afterload, and pressure afterload explains the massive LV dilatation and the ensuing progressive rise in LV afterload. LV has eccentric hypertrophy. In comparison with AS, AI is associated with the highest afterload and the highest LV mass.
- In MS, HF results from mitral obstruction without any LV abnormality, unless intrinsic LV disease coexists.
- All severe valvular disorders lead to HF before LV systolic function is grossly affected.

QUESTIONS AND ANSWERS

Question 1. A 69-year-old woman presents with acute HF and severe HTN (SBP 180 mmHg). Echocardiography shows normal LVEF, AS with a mean gradient of 27 mmHg and AVA of 0.9 cm^2, and moderate MR. If this is severe AS, what can explain the paradoxically low gradient?

A. Hypertension at the time of the study, particularly if concentric LV hypertrophy is present. In this case, the stroke volume is reduced because of double afterload (HTN and AS), and the small LV cavity

B. MR, which reduces forward cardiac output

C. Truly severe AS with false measurement of aortic gradient (Doppler beam not parallel to aortic flow)

D. All of the above

Question 2. If the patient in Question 1 actually has moderate AS, what could explain the low AVA calculation?
A. Echocardiographic error in measurement (underestimation of LVOT diameter leads to a falsely low AVA)
B. Pressure recovery phenomenon in a patient with a small tubular aorta (true gradient is smaller and true AVA is larger)
C. The AVA is truly <1 cm^2 but the patient has a small body size and the indexed AVA is >0.6 cm^2/m^2, implying a truly moderate AS
D. All of the above

Question 3. In the above patient, how can one make a diagnosis of severe AS vs. moderate AS?
A. Try to obtain aortic gradient in multiple views, including right parasternal view, and try to be coaxial to the aortic flow. Ensure proper echo measurement of LVOT at the aortic annulus (early systole)
B. Measure aortic gradient after control of HTN
C. Measure stroke volume index and valvuloarterial impedance. A stroke volume index >35 ml/m^2 or a high LVOT velocity >1 m/s suggest that the stroke volume is preserved, ruling out low-output low-gradient AS and suggesting moderate AS.
D. Invasive measurements are frequently required to measure cardiac output, true gradient and AVA, especially after control of HTN
E. Dobutamine testing
F. A through D

Question 4. A patient has dyspnea on exertion and a mid-systolic murmur with absent A$_2$. Echo shows AS with calcified aortic valve, a mean gradient of 48 mmHg and AVA 1.1 cm^2. No AI is present. Is AS severe?
A. AS is severe. When the gradient is >40 mmHg on echo, AS is usually severe even if AVA >1 cm^2
B. AS is severe. AVA may be over-calculated in a patient with a septal hypertrophy and a high LVOT velocity
C. AS may be moderate, but this is unlikely. A pressure recovery phenomenon may falsely exaggerate the gradient and is suggested by a small aortic diameter <3 cm
D. All of the above

Question 5. A 76-year-old man with a prior history of CABG and low LVEF is admitted with severe HF. His echo shows severe LV dysfunction with EF ~25%, a severely calcified aortic valve with a mean gradient of 22 mmHg and AVA 0.8 cm^2. A dobutamine infusion is performed (started at 5 mcg/kg/min, and raised to 20 mcg/kg/min). His stroke volume increases from 50 ml to 65 ml, gradient increases to 35 mmHg, and AVA increases to 1 cm^2. Does he have severe AS?
A. AS is severe
B. AS is pseudo-severe (poor valve excursion related to the poor flow rather than severe AS)
C. Poor contractile reserve
D. Perform cardiac catheterization to establish the diagnosis

Question 6. In the patient of Question 5, what happens to the dimensionless index (DI) during dobutamine testing?
A. Remains the same or declines
B. Increases

Question 7. What is the best treatment of the patient in Question 5?
A. Surgical AVR
B. TAVR should be considered. TAVR is an option in low-gradient AS
C. Conservative management

Question 8. A 62-year-old man is admitted with acute HF. He is found to have severe LV dysfunction with global hypokinesis, inferior akinesis, and overall EF 25%. He has a posteriorly directed mitral regurgitation with a calculated effective regurgitant orifice (ERO) of 0.30 cm^2. His coronary angiogram shows severe three-vessel CAD with a subtotally occluded RCA. CAD appears amenable to PCI. Beside medical therapy, what is the best treatment option?
A. Medical therapy only
B. Repeat echo after diuresis. If MR improves, revascularize with PCI
C. CABG
D. CABG + MV repair using annuloplasty ring
E. CABG + MV repair using annuloplasty ring, or CABG + MV replacement

Question 9. A patient with a history of anterior MI presents with HF. He is found to have severe MR. Can a patient with anterior MI and no inferior MI have severe ischemic MR? If so, would it be anteriorly directed?
A. Yes, a centrally directed MR
B. Yes, an anteriorly directed MR
C. Yes, a posteriorly directed or centrally directed MR
D. No

Question 10. A patient presents with severe chest pain and dynamic, diffuse ST segment depression. BP is 170/93 mmHg. A holosystolic MR murmur is heard. Bedside echo shows inferior akinesis with severe MR. Troponin rises to 1.2 ng/ml. After aspirin, heparin, and nitrate therapy, chest pain resolves. The murmur is not heard anymore and a bedside echo performed a few hours later shows an improvement of the inferior akinesis. Coronary angiography is performed and shows a 90% thrombotic RCA stenosis and a 75% mid-LAD stenosis. Both lesions are amenable to PCI. What is the next step?
A. PCI of RCA and LAD
B. CABG with MR repair or replacement

Question 11. A 64-year-old asymptomatic woman is found to have an apical murmur radiating to the base. An echo shows posterior leaflet prolapse with severe, eccentric MR. The LV size is normal (LV end-systolic diameter is 37 mm) and LVEF is 65%. The LA is enlarged, with an anteroposterior diameter of 4.8 cm. Her PA pressure is 40 mmHg at rest. The patient is in sinus rhythm. She can perform her daily chores without limitation. What parameters help determine if MV surgery is appropriate now, as opposed to surveillance?

A. Exercise testing with determination of functional capacity (worrisome if <6 METs)

B. In the echo lab, measure PA pressure after isometric exercise or leg raising

C. TEE to assess the extent of posterior leaflet abnormality.

D. Right heart catheterization, with measurement of PA pressure and PCWP at rest and with leg raising and exercise

E. BNP >100 pg/ml

F. All of the above

Question 12. A 44-year-old woman presents with dyspnea on exertion. Echo shows a restricted posterior leaflet with a hockeystick anterior leaflet and immobile leaflet tips. The trasmitral gradient is 10 mmHg at rest, 15 mmHg with leg raising, and the MVA is 1.6 cm² by echo, at a heart rate of 100 bpm. The valve is pliable and the subvalvular apparatus is not heavily calcified (Wilkins score of 8). The patient has been having heavy menstruations and hemoglobin is 7.5 g/dl. What is the next step?

A. Transfusion and PMBV

B. Transfusion and right and left heart catheterization

C. TEE

Question 13. Heart catheterization is performed in the patient in Question 12. A good PCWP waveform is obtained. There is a lack of diastasis between PCWP and LV at end-diastole, the mean transmitral gradient is 12 mmHg at a heart rate of 100 bpm, cardiac output is 7.5 l/min, and the mitral valve area is 2 cm² by Gorlin's equation. PCWP is 24 mmHg and systolic PA pressure is 50 mmHg. What is the next step?

A. Transfusion, metoprolol, and diuresis, then reassess symptoms

B. Transfusion, metoprolol, diuresis and PMBV

Question 14. A patient has severe valvular disease and LVEF of 40%. He undergoes valvular replacement. In which valvular disease does EF more readily improve after surgical correction?

A. AS > AI > MR

B. AI > AS > MR

C. AS > MR > AI

Question 15. A 55-year-old man presents with HF. He has a history of mechanical bileaflet AVR performed 5 years previously. An echo is performed and shows a transaortic gradient of 30 mmHg and a peak velocity of 3.5 m/s, without a significant AI. Hemoglobin is 13 g/dl. What is the most likely cause of the gradient across the valve?

A. Normal gradient across a normally functioning valve

B. Patient/prosthesis mismatch

C. High flow state

D. Pressure recovery

E. Valvular obstruction, further suggested if metallic S₂ is muffled

Question 16. If the patient in Question 15 is presenting with atypical chest pain or a non-cardiac complaint rather than HF, what would the diagnosis be?

A. Normal gradient across a normally functioning valve

B. Patient/prosthesis mismatch

C. High flow state

D. Pressure recovery

E. Valvular obstruction, further suggested if metallic S₂ is muffled

Question 17. If the patient in Question 15 is presenting with HF, but a review of a postoperative echo shows a similarly increased velocity and gradient across the prosthetic valve, what would the diagnosis be?

A. Normal gradient across a normally functioning valve

B. Patient/prosthesis mismatch

C. High flow state

D. Pressure recovery

E. Valvular obstruction, further suggested if metallic S₂ is muffled

Question 18. What is the next step for the patient in Question 15?

A. TEE

B. Cinefluoroscopy

C. A and B

D. No further workup, as the cause is benign

Question 19. A 60-year-old patient presents with shock and pulmonary edema. He is intubated and requires vasopressor support. He has a history of mechanical MVR 5 years previously. An echo shows a large gradient across the prosthetic valve (35 mmHg). On fluoroscopy, one mechanical leaflet is totally immobile, while the other one has restricted motion. INR is 1. What is the next step in management?

A. Thrombolytic therapy

B. Valvular surgery

C. Anticoagulation with heparin

Question 20. Which of the following patients with severe MR does not have an indication for mitral valve surgery?
A. LV end-systolic diameter 40 mm
B. LVEF 60%
C. Recently diagnosed HF with LVEF 20% and severe MR
D. LVEF 45%

Question 21. Answer each option as true or false:
A. S_3 and S_4 are present in MS
B. Persistently split S_2 suggests RV failure
C. Loud P_2 (= loud S_2 split) suggests pulmonary hypertension
D. Absent A_2 with midsystolic murmur suggests severe AS
E. A loud S_1 characterizes MS or a short PR interval
F. A short S_2-opening snap interval implies severe MS
G. A wide pulse pressure with a diastolic murmur implies severe AI
H. A high JVP that peaks simultaneously with the pulse suggests TR
I. HOCM murmur changes in an opposite direction to preload and afterload

Question 22. A 55-year-old man with a history of radiation for lymphoma 20 years ago presents with hypoxia and peripheral edema. On exam, he has lung crackles, an elevated JVP with a high V wave peaking along with the pulse, and a pulsatile liver. He has a holosystolic murmur at the LLSB that increases with inspiration. A holosystolic murmur is also heard at the apex and radiates to the axilla. At the RUSB and LUSB, a mid-systolic murmur is heard. An early, decrescendo diastolic murmur is heard at the LUSB. S_2 is normal. Carotid upstroke is weak. RV heave is present. PMI is not enlarged. BP is 105/75 mmHg. What abnormalities does this patient have? (multiple choices)
A. Severe TR, severe MR, severe AS
B. Severe TR, moderate MR, severe AS
C. Severe TR, severe MR, moderate AS and moderate AI
D. On echo, AS gradient will seem less severe because of MR and TR. Conversely, MR severity is exaggerated by AS and AI. AI does not affect the severity assessment of MR
E. Restrictive cardiomyopathy is likely present

Question 23. Once symptoms arise in severe AS, AI, or MR, what is the mean survival without surgical correction?
A. 1 year
B. 2–3 years
C. 5 years

Question 24. A patient with a mechanical aortic prosthesis presents with hypotension. Echo is performed and shows increased velocity across the aortic valve (Figure 6.18). Is it cardiogenic shock? What is the cause of the elevated aortic valve velocity?

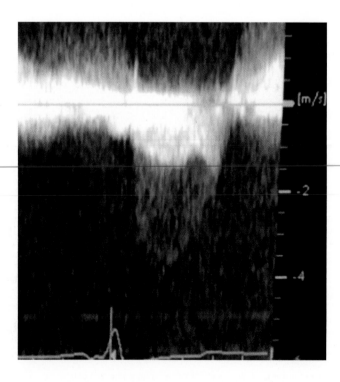

Figure 6.18

Question 25. A 44-year-old obese, hypertensive woman presents with dyspnea on exertion. On exam, she has a diastolic rumble and a loud S_1. Echo shows LA dilatation with typical MS. The mean gradient at rest is 6 mmHg (heart rate 85 bpm) and the MVA is calculated as 1.7 cm^2 by PHT method. Systolic PA pressure is ~35 mmHg at rest. The valve is pliable, not heavily calcified, with a Wilkins score of 7. With exercise testing, the gradient increases to 12 mmHg and systolic PA pressure increases to 45–50 mmHg. What is the next step?

A. MV replacement

B. Percutaneous mitral balloon valvuloplasty

C. Diuretic therapy

D. β-Blocker therapy and clinical follow-up in 6–12 months

Question 26. A 47-year-old man has a history of bicuspid aortic valve with AI. He is active and asymptomatic with excellent functional capacity. A surveillance echo shows severe AI, LVEF 50%, LVESD 52 mm, and LVEDD 68 mm. Note that LV dimensions have increased by ~4 mm over the last 6 months. The aortic root size is 46 mm. What is the next step?

A. AVR + ascending aortic replacement

B. AVR

C. Continue surveillance

D. Exercise testing

Question 27. A 70-year-old woman presents with severe dyspnea. She is found to have AF at a rate of 110 bpm, BP 110/70, and pulmonary edema. Echo shows normal LV systolic function, mitral thickening, biatrial enlargement, and mild RV dilatation. After rate control,

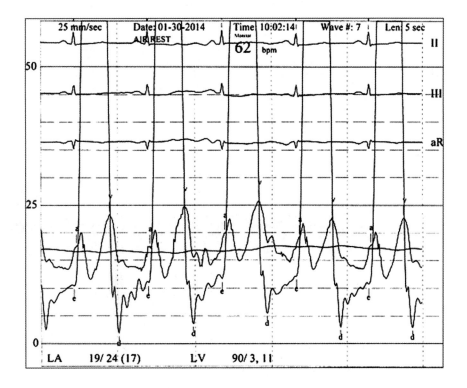

Figure 6.19

diuresis, and cardioversion, a hemodynamic study is performed (Figure 6.19). What is the diagnosis?

A. Severe MR

B. Severe MS

C. LV diastolic dysfunction and restrictive cardiomyopathy

Question 28. A 70-year-old woman presents with progressive dyspnea. She is severely hypertensive (BP 180/95 mmHg). Echo shows normal LVEF, biatrial enlargement, and mild MR. A hemodynamic study is performed (Figure 6.20). What is the diagnosis and what is the next step?

A. Severe MR (underestimated by echo)

B. Severe MS

C. Severe LV diastolic dysfunction and restrictive process from severe HTN

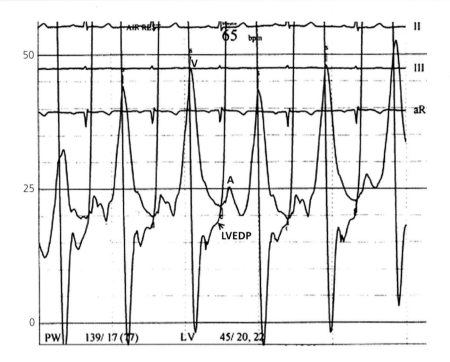

Figure 6.20

Question 29. A 67-year-old man has end-stage renal disease. He presents with pulmonary edema, SBP 85 mmHg, and two episodes of syncope over the last 3 weeks. On exam, 3/6 midsystolic murmur is heard throughout the precordial area, with absent A_2, and delayed and narrow carotid pulse. ECG shows anterloateral Q waves. Echo performed 2.5 years previously showed mild AS with AVA >2 cm².
A. Ischemic HF. AS is unlikely, as AVA declines by 0.12 cm²/year and it takes >5 years to progress from mild AS to severe AS
B. Combination of ischemic HF and severe AS. AS may progress faster in end-stage renal disease

Question 30. In the prior patient (Question 29), echo shows severe AS and EF 25%, and coronary angiography shows a totally occluded LAD without significant anterior wall viability on thallium testing. Attempts to perform hemodialysis and ultrafiltration are impeded by the occurrence of severe hypotension during hemodialysis. His surgical STS score for AVR is 14%. What is the best management option?
A. Perform CABG + AVR urgently
B. Perform hemodialysis with the support of norepinephrine. Perform CABG + AVR once pulmonary edema has resolved
C. Perform hemodialysis with the support of norepinephrine. Perform TAVR once pulmonary edema has resolved

Question 31. Which of the following statements is *incorrect*?
A. MR is associated with reduced afterload early on, then LV dilatation and increased afterload later on
B. AI is associated with a rise in preload and afterload
C. AI is associated with more rise in afterload than AS
D. In MR, the earliest EF reduction reflects intrinsic LV dysfunction and may be irreversible
E. In AI and AS, the earliest EF reduction reflects afterload mismatch rather than intrinsic LV dysfunction and is reversible with AVR
F. In acute AI, pulse pressure is severely widened and peripheral systolic pressure is much higher than central aortic pressure

Question 32. The valve shown in Figure 6.21 is seen on fluoroscopy. What type of valve is it?
A. Surgical bioprosthesis
B. Transcutaneous bioprosthesis
C. Mechanical prosthesis (St. Jude)
D. Mechanical prosthesis (single-leaflet tilting disk)

Question 33. A 67-year-old man has dyspnea on exertion. On exam, a mid-systolic murmur is heard, A_2 is absent, and pulsus parvus and tardus is present. His echo shows a mean aortic gradient of <40 mmHg and an aortic valve area of >1 cm². What is the diagnosis and what is the next step?
A. AS is moderate. No need for further workup
B. AS is probably severe. Cardiac catheterization and invasive AVA calculation are indicated

Question 34. A 67-year-old man has dyspnea on exertion. He has a loud holosystolic apical murmur with S_3. Echo shows a small eccentric MR jet. What is the diagnosis and what is the next step?
A. MR is mild or moderate. No further workup is needed
B. MR is likely severe. Perform TEE

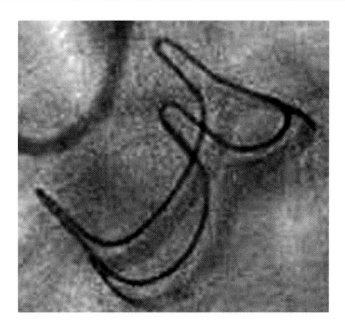

Figure 6.21

Question 35. A 60-year-old man is asymptomatic. He has a mild end-systolic murmur at the apex without S_3. Echo is performed and shows mitral valve prolapse with severe MR by jet area and ERO. LA size is normal. What is the diagnosis?
A. Severe MR from mitral valve prolapse
B. Mild-to-moderate end-systolic MR from mitral valve prolapse

Question 36. A 60-year-old man has dyspnea on exertion, with holodiastolic murmur at the base, enlarged PMI, and wide pulse pressure. Echo shows a bicuspid aortic valve with mild-to-moderate AI jet. AI pressure half-time is 320 ms. LV is enlarged. What is the diagnosis?
A. Severe AI. Further testing is needed (TEE, invasive aortogram)
B. Mild-to-moderate AI

Question 37. A 68-year-old hypertensive woman has dyspnea on exertion and a long diastolic murmur at the apex extending into end-diastole. Echo shows a rheumatic mitral valve with transmitral pressure gradient of 12 mmHg at rest and systolic PA pressure of 55 mmHg (heart rate of 70 bpm). The mitral valve area is calculated at 1.7 cm^2.
A. MS is severe
B. MS is mild/moderate anatomically, and the gradient is exaggerated because of a high cardiac output

Question 38. A 72-year-old man with a bioprosthetic mitral valve is presenting with dyspnea on exertion and a holosystolic apical murmur. Echo shows thickened prosthetic leaflets, mild mitral regurgitation, and a peak E velocity of 2.4 m/s. What is the diagnosis?
A. Prosthetic valve obstruction
B. Prosthetic valve regurgitation
C. Normally functioning mitral prosthesis

Question 39. A 67-year-old woman has mild dyspnea on exertion. On exam, he has a mid-systolic murmur with a well-heard A_2 and a preserved carotid upstroke. His echo shows a mean aortic gradient of 38 mmHg and an aortic valve area of 0.9 cm^2. What is the diagnosis, and what is the next step?
A. AS is severe. No need for further work-up
B. AS is likely moderate. Cardiac catheterization is indicated

Answer 1. D.

Answer 2. D.

Answer 3. F. The indexed AVA in this patient is calculated at 0.45 cm^2/m^2. The stroke volume index is calculated at 25 ml/m^2, suggestive of low flow. After control of HTN, the flow increased and the aortic gradient increased to 39 mmHg, confirming the effect of low flow on her gradient. Thus, she has a paradoxical low-flow, low-gradient severe AS related to severe HTN. In patients with normal EF and paradoxical low-gradient AS, the reduction in flow is secondary to the high afterload and the small underfilled ventricular cavity rather than impaired contractility. In this setting, dobutamine testing is not a suitable way of increasing cardiac output.

Answer 4. D. Echo rarely overestimates aortic valve gradient. It rather frequently underestimates the gradient. If the aortic valve is calcified and poorly mobile on echo imaging, a high gradient implies severe AS, even if AVA is calculated as >1 cm^2. An exaggeration of LVOT velocity or diameter may exaggerate the calculated AVA: AVA = LVOT area × LVOT velocity/aortic valve velocity.

Answer 5. A. The patient has low-gradient AS related to poor EF. The low gradient here is likely related to poor flow rather than errors in echo measurements. Dobutamine testing is appropriate. The stroke volume rose >20%, implying proper contractile (or flow) reserve. The gradient rose >10 mmHg to >30 mmHg, and the AVA remained <1.2 cm^2, implying a truly severe AS. In a pseudo-severe AS, the increase in flow leads to more valvular opening: gradient does not significantly increase, while the valve area dramatically increases, usually to >1.2 cm^2.

Answer 6. A. In truly severe AS, LVOT velocity increases with dobutamine, but aortic velocity increases similarly or further. DI, which is LVOT velocity/aortic velocity, remains unchanged or declines. In pseudo-severe AS, the aortic velocity increases less than LVOT (→ DI increases).

Answer 7. B. In light of the low-gradient/low-EF AS and the prior cardiac surgery, the surgical mortality is elevated, at least 8%. Formal STS score calculation should be performed and the patient referred for TAVR. In the PARTNER trial, patients with a low-gradient AS derived the largest mortality benefit from TAVR, as compared to conservative management.

Answer 8. E. The patient has ischemic MR due to an akinetic inferior wall. The presentation is HF, rather than acute ischemia; the inferior wall akinesis is a steady, persistent abnormality rather than an off/on ischemia and does not have a high likelihood of fully reversing with revascularization. As a result, MR only has a 50% chance of improving with revascularization. CABG along with mitral surgery is indicated in a patient with multivessel CAD and severe MR. The inferior wall akinesis is steady but ischemic MR is dynamic and may improve with diuresis and improvement of preload and afterload. However, MR easily reverses back to severe with a reversal of loading conditions, such as exercise or supine position (night), further attesting to the need for mitral surgery.

Answer 9. C. Anterior wall akinesis, per se, does not produce enough leaflet tethering and MR. Anterior MI may, however, lead to global remodeling with posterolateral and apical tethering of the papillary muscles and leaflets. This leads to ischemic MR, which may be centrally or posteriorly directed.

Answer 10. A. As opposed to Question 8, where the patient had a chronic persistent dysfunction of the inferior wall with HF presentation, this patient is having acute, fleeting ischemic dysfunction of the inferior wall with MR. The dynamic MR is dictated by ischemia, not just loading conditions. It is expected that this MR will reverse with revascularization of the acute RCA lesion. MV surgery is not immediately required here.

Answer 11. F. All these tests are reasonable in the asymptomatic patient with severe MR. On stress testing, if the patient develops severe dyspnea that persists into late recovery, or if her functional capacity is below expected (14.7 − [0.13 × age]), she is unlikely to be NYHA class I and MV surgery is reasonable. If the prolapse is limited to P$_2$ cusp, MV repair is likely to be successful and durable, and is reasonable even in an asymptomatic patient (class IIa). Elevated BNP, pulmonary hypertension, or elevated PCWP suggests that MR is starting to have hemodynamic repercussions and implies a high risk of HF and symptomatic deterioration, as well as an impairment of long-term outcomes; MV surgery is reasonable.

Answer 12. B. MVA is a better determinant of MS severity than the mitral gradient. In fact, transmitral pressure gradient being proportional to the square of the diastolic mitral flow, tachycardia or a high-output state may convert an *anatomically mild MS into a hemodynamically severe MS with a severely increased transmitral gradient*. Invasive hemodynamics are valuable for the assessment of MS whenever there is discrepancy between the echocardiographic MVA and transmitral gradient; and whenever it is not clear whether the patient's symptoms or pulmonary hypertension are purely secondary to MS, or rather secondary to mild MS + high-output state and tachycardia.

Answer 13. A. The cardiac output is markedly increased because of anemia and the heart rate is increased, both of which converted an *anatomically mild MS* (valve area 2 cm^2) into a *hemodynamically severe MS*, with a high gradient and lack of diastasis. Anemia should be corrected, the heart rate should be reduced to 55–60 bpm with β-blockade, and a small dose of diuretic may be administered. PA pressure and transmitral gradient should be assessed afterward. Once exacerbating factors are treated, valvuloplasty is considered for mild MS (MVA >1.5 cm^2) only if the patient remains symptomatic with exertional increase in PA pressure and transmitral gradient (>15 mmHg) (class IIb).

Answer 14. A. In AS and AI patients with LV dysfunction, the low EF is usually related to the high afterload rather than an intrinsic LV dysfunction (afterload mismatch). Thus, valvular surgery improves afterload and EF. This is not the case in MR: (1) afterload is usually reduced in MR, and thus the low EF is often due to intrinsic myocardial dysfunction; (2) MV surgery may disrupt the subvalvular apparatus and LV geometry, further reducing EF.

Answer 15. E. The five listed causes are the main causes of a high gradient across a prosthetic valve. The severity (>3 m/s) makes normal gradient less likely (not option A). The fact that he is presenting with HF implies a need to rule out valvular obstruction.

Answer 16. B or D. C is unlikely in the absence of anemia or sepsis.

Answer 17. B or D.

Answer 18. C. The next step consists of assessing the leaflet structure and excursion. This is done by using both TEE and fluoroscopy. If the structure and excursion are normal, PPM or pressure recovery is the cause of the valvular gradient.

Answer 19. A. The mitral obstruction is the cause of shock in this patient. The differential diagnosis includes thrombus or pannus formation. The acuity of onset and the normal INR are suggestive of thrombus. TEE may be performed to show the large thrombus but is not mandatory at this point. Patients with large prosthetic thrombosis or functional class III–IV should undergo surgical replacement or thrombolytic therapy if surgery is deemed high-risk. Surgery is high-risk in a patient with shock requiring multiple vasopressors. Serial echocardiograms need to be performed to document a reduction of gradient. Fluoroscopy may document improvement of disk mobility.

Answer 20. C. MR that occurs with a very low EF is likely a functional MR (unless a longstanding history of severe symptomatic MR precedes HF and low EF). Surgery is not first-line therapy for functional MR, particularly functional MR from a non-ischemic cardiomyopathy. Surgery is indicated in patients with MR and secondary LV dysfunction, manifested as EF ≤ 60%.

Answer 21. A is false (S_3 and S_4 cannot be present in MS). All the remaining statements are true.

Answer 22. C, D, and E. The patient has clinical signs of severe TR. He has MR that is likely severe, as he has pulmonary edema. AS is not severe by the fact that S_2 is not attenuated. The weak carotid pulse is due to the low-output state from the combined valvular disease rather than severe AS. AI is unlikely to be severe as the pulse pressure is narrow; however, a concomitant MR, TR, and cardiomyopathy may attenuate the total stroke volume and the pulse pressure of severe AI. PMI is not enlarged, strongly arguing against severe AI, especially AI combined with MR, where LV would be severely dilated. In combined mitral and aortic valvular disease, the aortic disease exaggerates the severity of the mitral disease and the rise in LA pressure. Conversely, the mitral disease reduces AS gradient and leads to underestimation of true AS severity. Despite MR and moderate AS/AI, LV is not enlarged by PMI. This suggests a concomitant restrictive cardiomyopathy from radiation.

Answer 23. B.

Answer 24. First, ensure the tracing obtained is truly an aortic tracing rather than MR. It is a true aortic tracing by the fact that is starts some time after the peak of the electrocardiographic R wave (this is opposite to MR, which starts exactly at the peak of R, i.e., at the isovolumic contraction). Second, address why the velocity is increased. The contour of the transaortic envelope is round and symmetrical, consistent with AS. However, within this envelope, there is another envelope that is late-peaking and consistent with an increased LVOT velocity ("whiter" envelope). Thus, the aortic velocity is ~4 m/s, but the LVOT velocity is ~2 m/s, implying a dimensionless index of ~0.5 (>0.3), which is not consistent with severe valvular or prosthetic obstruction. In addition, by using the true Bernoulli equation, the peak gradient across the prosthesis is not in the severe range: gradient $= 4\ (V_{aortic\ valve}^2 - V_{LVOT}^2)$ rather than $4\ V_{aortic\ valve}^2$. The velocity across the prosthesis is likely mildly increased at baseline (e.g., some degree of patient/prosthesis mismatch), and is now worsened by the increased LV velocity (hypercontractile state from sepsis, hypovolemia, or fever).

Answer 25. D. This patient has mild MS by MVA (>1.5 cm²). For this MVA, intervention is only considered if the mean gradient increases to >15 mmHg with stress or PA pressure increases to >60 mmHg with stress, after ruling out tachycardia or a high-output state as a cause of the high gradient. In this patient, obesity or diastolic LV dysfunction may be the cause of dyspnea. It is reasonable to perform heart catheterization and verify that MVA is truly in the mild/moderate range. Heart catheterization will also allow a diagnosis of LV diastolic dysfunction (LVEDP rises with stress more than the transmitral gradient does).

Answer 26. A. EF is still above the surgical cutoff (EF <50% being an indication for AVR). However, LVESD >50 mm and LVEDD >65 mm are class II indications for surgery. This is even more worrisome when progressive LV dilatation is noted.

Answer 27. B. This tracing represents simultaneous PCWP–LV pressure recording. Despite a rate of 60–75 bpm (in this case 62 bpm), there is a lack of PCWP and LV diastasis at end-diastole, which suggests severe MS. Also, PCWP A wave is prominent while LV A wave is attenuated, which further suggests MS. V wave is prominent; this does not necessarily imply MR and is common in MS.

Answer 28. A. This tracing represents simultaneous PCWP–LV pressure recording. Note the very large V wave (~47 mmHg), which mainly suggests severe MR, but may also be seen with severe LV failure. One may get the false impression of a gradient between PCWP and LV in diastole. Yet note that, when using PCWP as a surrogate of LA pressure, a large V wave exaggerates the transmitral gradient and may falsely suggest MS. In fact, the large V wave of PCWP has a slower downslope than the V wave of LA pressure, which exaggerates the space between PCWP and LV. Severe MR may have been missed on TTE for various reasons: (1) dynamic functional MR from hypertensive cardiomyopathy and severe LA enlargement (MR may have been milder at the time of the echo and got worsened by HTN); (2) extremely eccentric MR, such as MR related to MVP, underestimated on many TTE views.

Answer 29. B. The exam suggests severe AS, and ECG suggests anterior infarct. It is true that AVA only declines by 0.12 cm²/year and mean gradient only increases by 7 mmHg per year, but those are only average numbers. Progression is faster in renal patients and in those with heavy valvular calcifications.

Answer 30. C. While decongestion improves cardiac output, quick fluid removal during dialysis (2–3 liters in 3 hours) exceeds plasma refill time and creates transient reduction of intravascular volume. In patients with *limited cardiac output reserve*, the LV cannot increase its stroke volume and EF to fill the empty circulation. BP will precipitously drop during dialysis. Norepinephrine may be used to constrict the empty circulation and maintain BP during dialysis; in hypotensive patients, norepinephrine does not increase afterload untowardly as it only raises the SBP to 90–100 mmHg. In order to reduce perioperative complications, it is important to properly decongest the patient before a cardiac intervention. Considering his STS surgical risk score of ≥8%, TAVR is an acceptable alternative to surgical AVR. While non-viability does not preclude a benefit from CABG revascularization (STICH trial), non-viability associated with Q waves further reduces the likelihood of benefit.

Answer 31. F. Pulse pressure is severely widened when the stroke volume is markedly increased, as in chronic AI, where the LV is dilated, not acute AI. In AI, the early EF reduction reflects a reduction of stroke volume from the high afterload (stroke volume is the EF numerator).

Answer 32. A. The leaflets are not visualized (bioprosthetic leaflets). The metallic ring and struts of a bioprosthesis are seen on this image.

Answer 33. B. The echo findings should always be analyzed in the context of the physical exam. Since the exam suggests severe AS, echo may have underestimated the gradient because of poor alignment of the Doppler beam with the transaortic flow.

Answer 34. B. The exam suggests severe MR. On color Doppler, an eccentric MR (mitral valve prolapse) jet occupies a smaller area of the LA than a central jet of similar severity; MR may be underestimated. E velocity should remain elevated at >1.2 m/s and remains a hint to severe MR.

Answer 35. B. The color assessment of MR, whether by color jet area or color PISA calculation, assumes that MR occurs throughout systole. Inherently, an end-systolic MR that looks severe by color and PISA may only be mild or moderate when one accounts for the fact that it only occurs at the end of systole. The auscultation (end-systolic rather than holosystolic murmur, no S_3), and the normal LA size suggest that MR is overestimated by color. Also, color M-mode across the mitral valve shows that MR is limited to a portion of systole. LA size cannot be normal in chronic severe MR.

Answer 36. A. In a patient with a bicuspid aortic valve, AI may be eccentric and may appear mild by color Doppler. Pressure half-time is typically <250 ms in severe AI, but may be >250 ms in chronic compensated AI. The physical exam and the enlarged LV suggest severe AI. Holodiastolic flow reversal of the descending aorta on the suprasternal view would confirm severe AI.

Answer 37. A. MS is severe, as suggested by physical exam and by the high transmitral gradient and PA pressure despite a heart rate of <80 bpm. MVA measurement by echo is less reliable than transmitral gradient. The high MVA is likely a miscalculation by the pressure half-time method; for the same MVA, impaired LV compliance leads to quicker rise of LV pressure and a quicker approximation of LA and LV pressures, and thus a shorter pressure half-time (MVA is calculated as 220/pressure half-time).

Answer 38. B. The high velocity across the mitral prosthesis (>1.9 m/s, especially if >2.2 m/s) is abnormal and suggests prosthetic obstruction but also, as implied by exam, regurgitation across the prosthesis. Regurgitation is underestimated because prosthetic struts lead to acoustic shadowing into the LA.

Answer 39. B. While echo suggests severe AS, the auscultation suggests mild-to-moderate AS, In light of the physical exam, this is likely moderate AS with pressure recovery exaggerating the gradient and falsely reducing the calculated AVA.

References

MR

1. O'Gara P, Sugeng L, Lang R, et al. The role of imaging in chronic degenerative mitral regurgitation. J Am Coll Cardiol 2008; 1: 221–37.
2. Carpentier A, Adams DH, Filsoufi F. Carpentier's Reconstructive Valve Surgery. Maryland Heights, MO: Saunders, 2010.
3. Anyanwu AC, Adams DH. Etiologic classification of degenerative mitral valve disease: Barlow's disease and fibroelastic deficiency. Semin Thorac Cardiovasc Surg 2007; 19: 90–6.
4. Kumanohoso T, Otsuji Y, Yoshifuku S, et al. Mechanism of higher incidence of ischemic mitral regurgitation in patients with inferior myocardial infarction: quantitative analysis of left ventricular and mitral valve geometry in 103 patients with prior myocardial infarction. J Thorac Cardiovasc Surg 2003; 125: 135–43.
5. Yiu SF, Enriquez-Sarano M, Tribouilloy C, et al. Determinants of the degree of functional mitral regurgitation in patients with systolic left ventricular dysfunction: a quantitative clinical study. Circulation 2000; 102: 1400–6.
6. Piérard LA, Lancellotti P. The role of ischemic mitral regurgitation in the pathogenesis of acute pulmonary edema. N Engl J Med 2004; 351: 1627–34.
7. Watanabe N, Ogasawara Y, Yamaura Y, et al. Mitral annulus flattens in ischemic mitral regurgitation: geometric differences between inferior and anterior myocardial infarction: a real-time 3-dimensional echocardiographic study. Circulation 2005; 112: I458–62.
8. Lancellotti P, Troisfontaines P, Toussaint AC, Pierard LA. Prognostic importance of exercise-induced changes in mitral regurgitation in patients with chronic ischemic left ventricular dysfunction. Circulation 2003; 108: 1713–17.
9. Otsuji Y, Handshumacher MD, Liel-Cohen N, et al. Mechanism of ischemic mitral regurgitation with segmental left ventricular dysfunction: three-dimensional echocardiographic studies in models of acute and chronic progressive regurgitation. J Am Coll Cardiol 2001; 37: 641–8.
10. Agricola E, Oppizzi M, Pisani M, et al. Ischemic mitral regurgitation: mechanisms and echocardiographic classification. Eur J Echocardiogr 2008; 9: 207–21.

Survival in asymptomatic severe MR

11. Enriquez-Sarano M, Avierinos JF, Messika-Zeitoun D, et al. Quantitative determinants of the outcome of asymptomatic mitral regurgitation. N Engl J Med 2005; 352: 875–83.

Guidelines

12. Nishimura RA, Otto CM, Bonow RO, et al. 2014 ACC/AHA guideline for the management of patients with valvular heart disease. A report of the American College of Cardiology/American Heart Association Task Force on Practice Guidelines. J Am Coll Cardiol 2014; 63: 2438–88.

AF and pulmonary hypertension as indication for MV surgery

13. Ghoreishi M, Evans CF, DeFilippi CR, et al. Pulmonary hypertension adversely affects short- and long-term survival after mitral valve operation for mitral regurgitation: implications for timing of surgery. J Thorac Cardiovasc Surg 2011; 142: 1439–52.
14. Grigioni F, Avierinos JF, Ling LH, et al. Atrial fibrillation complicating the course of degenerative mitral regurgitation: determinants and long-term outcome. J Am Coll Cardiol 2002; 40: 84–92.

AF <3 months restored to sinus rhythm with surgery

15. Chua YL, Schaff HV, Orszulak TA, Morris JJ. Outcome of mitral valve repair in patients with preoperative atrial fibrillation. Should the maze procedure be combined with mitral valvuloplasty? J Thorac Cardiovasc Surg 1994; 107: 408–15. *High risk of events in patients with severe MR even if asymptomatic, and restoration of expected survival with surgery.*
16. Enriquez-Sarano M, Sundt TM. Early surgery is recommended for mitral regurgitation. Circulation 2010; 121: 804–12.
17. Avierinos JF, Gersh BJ, Melton LJ III, Bailey KR, Shub C, Nishimura RA, Tajik AJ, Enriquez-Sarano M. Natural history of asymptomatic mitral valve prolapse in the community. Circulation 2002; 106: 1355–61.
18. Kang DH, Kim JH, Rim JH, et al. Comparison of early surgery versus conventional treatment in asymptomatic severe mitral regurgitation. Circulation 2009; 119: 797–804. *Also very low postoperative mortality for repair.*
19. Ling L, Enriquez-Sarano M, Seward J, et al. Early surgery in patients with mitral regurgitation due to partial flail leaflet: a long-term outcome study. Circulation 1997; 96: 1819–25.

20. Suri RM, Vanoverschelde JL, Grigioni F et al. Association between early surgical intervention vs watchful waiting and outcomes for mitral regurgitation due to flail mitral valve leaflets. JAMA 2013; 310: 609–16. *Most patients underwent MV repair (93%). Postoperative mortality was very low (1%), and surgery was associated with improved survival in asymptomatic severe MR without classic surgical indication (vs. watchful waiting).*

Role of symptoms and EF in determining long-term outcomes

21. Enriquez-Sarano M, Tajik A, Schaff H, et al. Echocardiographic prediction of survival after surgical correction of organic mitral regurgitation. Circulation. 1994; 90: 830–7.
22. Tribouilloy C, Enriquez-Sarano M, Schaff H, et al. Impact of preoperative symptoms on survival after surgical correction of organic mitral regurgitation: rationale for optimizing surgical indications. Circulation 1999; 99: 400–5.
23. Detaint D, Messika-Zetoun D, Avierinos JF, et al. B-type natriuretic peptide in organic mitral regurgitation: determinants and impact on outcome. Circulation 2005; 111: 2391–7.

MV repair improves early and late mortality

24. Shuhaiber J, Anderson RJ. Meta-analysis of clinical outcomes following surgical mitral valve repair or replacement. Eur J Cardiothorac Surg 2007; 31: 267–75.

MV surgery for functional MR

25. Aklog L, Filsoufi F, Flores KQ, et al. Does coronary artery bypass grafting alone correct moderate ischemic mitral regurgitation? Circulation 2001; 104: I68–75.
26. Campwala SZ, Bansal RC, Wang N, et al. Factors affecting regression of mitral regurgitation following isolated coronary artery bypass surgery. Eur J Cardiothorac Surg 2005; 28: 783–7.
27. Mihaljevic T, Lam BK, Razzouk A, et al. Impact of mitral valve annuloplasty combined with revascularization in patients with functional ischemic MR. J Am Coll Cardiol 2007; 49: 2191–201.
28. Magne J, Senechal M, Mathieu P, et al. Restrictive annuloplasty for ischemic mitral regurgitation may induce functional mitral stenosis. J Am Coll Cardiol 2008; 51: 1692–701.
29. Braun J, van de Veire NR, Klautz RJ, et al. Restrictive mitral annuloplasty cures ischemic mitral regurgitation and heart failure. Ann Thorac Surg 2008; 85: 430–6.
30. Chan KMJ, Punjabi PP, Flather M, et al. Coronary artery bypass surgery with or without mitral valve annuloplasty in moderate functional ischemic mitral regurgitation: final results of the Randomized Ischemic Mitral Evaluation (RIME) trial. Circulation 2012: 126: 2502–10.
31. Acker MA, Parides MK, Perrault LP, et al. Mitral-valve repair versus replacement for severe ischemic mitral regurgitation. N Engl J Med. 2014; 370: 23–32.

Improvement of MR with CRT

32. Breithardt OA, Sinha AM, Schwammenthal E, et al. Acute effects of cardiac resynchronization therapy on functional mitral regurgitation in advanced systolic heart failure. J Am Coll Cardiol 2003; 41: 765–70.
33. Di Biase L, Auricchio A, Mohanty P, et al. Impact of cardiac resynchronization therapy on the severity of mitral regurgitation. Europace 2011; 13: 829–36.
34. Grigioni F, Enriquez-Sarano M, Zehr KJ, Bailey KR, Tajik AJ. Ischemic mitral regurgitation: long-term outcome and prognostic implications with quantitative Doppler assessment. Circulation 2001; 103: 1759–64.

Mitraclip

35. Feldman T, Foster E, Glower DD, et al.; EVEREST II Investigators. Percutaneous repair or surgery for mitral regurgitation. N Engl J Med 2011; 364: 1395–406.
36. Whitlow PL, Feldman T, Pedersen WR, et al. Acute and 12-month results with catheter-based mitral valve leaflet repair: the EVEREST II (Endovascular Valve Edge-to-Edge Repair) High Risk Study. J Am Coll Cardiol 2012; 59: 130–9. *EVEREST II high-risk registry showed that high surgical risk patients, most of whom had functional MR (~60%), derived significant improvement of HF, mortality, and LV remodeling with Mitraclip in comparison to conservative management, at a relatively low periprocedural mortality (~7%). European registries with mostly high-risk functional MR (~70%), mostly ischemic MR (>85%), like TRAMI, only had 2.5% periprocedural mortality.*
37. Franzen O, van der Heyden J, Baldus S, et al. MitraClip therapy in patients with endstage systolic heart failure. Eur J Heart Fail. 2011; 13: 569–76.
38. Auricchio A, Scillinger W, Meyer S, et al. Correction of mitral regurgitation in nonresponders to cardiac resynchronization therapy by mitraclip improves symptoms and promotes reverse remodeling. J Am Coll Cardiol 2011: 58: 2183–9.

MS

39. Olesen KH. The natural history of 271 patients with mitral stenosis under medical treatment. Br Heart J 1962; 24: 349–57.
40. Horstkotte D, Niehues R, Strauer BE. Pathomorphological aspects, aetiology, and natural history of acquired mitral valve stenosis. Eur Heart J 1991; 12 (suppl): 55–60.
41. Bittrick J, D'Cruz IA, Wall BM, et al. Differences and similarities between patients with and without end-stage renal disease, with regard to location of intracardiac calcification. Echocardiography 2002 Jan; 19: 1–6.
42. Lange RA, Moore DM, Cigarroa RG, Hillis LD. Use of pulmonary capillary wedge pressure to assess severity of mitral stenosis: is true left atrial pressure needed in this condition? J Am Coll Cardiol 1989; 13: 825.
43. Wilkins GT, Weyman AE, Abascal VM, Block PC, Palacios IF. Percutaneous balloon dilatation of the mitral valve: an analysis of echocardiographic variables related to outcome and the mechanism of dilation. Br Heart J 1988; 60: 299–308.
44. Schwammenthal E, Vered Z, Agranat O, et al. Impact of atrioventricular compliance on pulmonary artery pressure in mitral stenosis: an exercise echocardiographic study Circulation 2000; 102: 2378–84.
45. Picano E, Pibarot P, Lancelotti P, et al. The emerging role of exercise testing and stress echocardiography in valvular heart disease. J Am Coll Cardiol 2009; 54: 2251–60.
46. Leavitt JI, Coats MH, Falk RH, et al. Effects of exercise on transmitral gradient and pulmonary artery pressure in patients with mitral stenosis or a prosthetic mitral valve: a Doppler echocardiographic study. J Am Coll Cardiol 1991; 17: 1520–6.
47. Carabello BA. Modern management of mitral stenosis. Circulation 2005; 112: 432–7.

Wilkins score and PMBV results

48. Palacios IF, Sanchez PL, Harrell LC, et al. Which patients benefit from percutaneous mitral balloon valvuloplasty? Prevalvuloplasty and postvalvuloplasty variables that predict long-term outcomes. Circulation 2002; 105; 1465–71.

49. Sutaria N, Elder AT, Shaw TRD. Long term outcome of percutaneous mitral balloon valvotomy in patients aged 70 and over. Heart 2000; 83: 433–8.

50. Reid CL, Otto CM, Davis KB, et al. Influence of mitral valve morphology on mitral balloon commissurotomy: immediate and six-month results from the NHLBI Balloon Valvuloplasty Registry. Am Heart J 1992; 124: 657–65.

51. Pathan AZ, Mahdi NA, Leon MN, et al. Is redo percutaneous mitral balloon valvuloplasty (PMV) indicated in patients with post-PMV mitral restenosis? J Am Coll Cardiol 1999; 34: 49–54.

52. Cohen DJ, Kuntz RE, Gordon SPF. Predictors of long-term outcome after percutaneous mitral valvuloplasty. N Engl J Med 1992; 327: 1329–35.

53. Abreu Filho CAC, Lisboa LA, Dallan LA, et al. Effectiveness of the maze procedure using cooled-tip radiofrequency ablation in patients with permanent atrial fibrillation and rheumatic mitral valve disease. Circulation 2005; 112: I20–5.

54. Levine MJ, Weinstein JS, Diver DJ, et al. Progressive improvement in pulmonary vascular resistance following percutaneous mitral valvuloplasty. Circulation 1989; 79: 1061–7.

55. Dev V, Shrivastava S. Time course of changes in pulmonary vascular resistance and the mechanism of regression of pulmonary arterial hypertension after balloon mitral valvuloplasty. Am J Cardiol 1991; 67: 439–42.

56. Vincens JJ, Temizer D, Post JR, Edmunds LH, Herrmann HC. Long-term outcome of cardiac surgery in patients with mitral stenosis and severe pulmonary hypertension. Circulation 1995; 92: II137–42.

AI

57. Lakier JB, Copans H, Rosman HS, et al. Idiopathic degenration of the aortic valve: a common cause of isolated aortic regurgitation. J Am Coll Cardiol 1985; 5: 347–57.

58. Hanna EB. Aortic insufficiency. In: Hanna EB, Glancy DL. Practical Cardiovascular Hemodynamics. New York, NY: Demos Medical, 2012.

59. Carabello BA. Progress in mitral and aortic regurgitation. Curr Probl Cardiol 2003; 28: 553–82.

60. Dujardin KS, Enriquez-Sarano M, Schaff HV, Bailey KR, Seward JB, Tajik AJ. Mortality and morbidity of aortic regurgitation in clinical practice: a long-term follow-up study. Circulation 1999; 99: 1851–7.

61. Evangelista A, Tornos P, Sambola A, Permanyer-Miralda G, Soler-Soler J. Long-term vasodilator therapy in patients with severe aortic regurgitation. N Engl J Med 2005; 353: 1342–9.

62. Chaliki HP, Mohty D, Avierinos J, et al. Outcomes after aortic valve replacement in patients with severe aortic regurgitation and markedly reduced left ventricular function. J Am Coll Cardiol 2002; 106: 2687–93.

63. Klodas E, Enriquez-Sarano M, Tajik AJ, et al. Optimizing timing of surgical correction in patients with severe aortic regurgitation: role of symptoms. J Am Coll Cardiol 1997; 30: 746–52.

64. Bonow DO, Rosing DR, Maron BJ, et al. Reversal of left ventricular dysfunction after aortic valve replacement for chronic aortic regurgitation: influence of the duration of preoperative left ventricular dysfunction. Circulation 1984; 70: 570–9.

65. Kallenbach K, Karck M, Pak D, et al. Decade of aortic valve sparing reimplantation. Are we pushing the limits too far? Circulation 2005; 112: I253–9. *Reoperation with sparing, good long-term result.*

66. Shimizu H, Yozu R. Valve-sparing aortic root replacement. Ann Thorac Cardiovasc Surg 2011; 17: 330–6.

67. Borger MA, Preston M, Ivanov J et al. Should the ascending aorta be replaced more frequently in patients with bicuspid aortic valve disease? J Thorac Cardiovasc Surg 2004; 128: 677–83.

AS

68. Huntington K, Hunter AG, Chan KL. A prospective study to assess the frequency of familial clustering of congenital bicuspid aortic valve. J Am Coll Cardiol. 1997; 30: 1809–12.

69. Lewin MB, Otto, CM. The bicuspid aortic valve. Adverse outcomes from infancy to old age. Circulation 2005; 11: 832–4.

70. Fenoglio JJ, McAllister HA, DeCastro CM, et al. Congenital bicuspid aortic valve after age 20. Am J Cardiol 1977; 39: 164–9. *27% of patients >70 had a normally functioning bicuspid aortic valve.*

71. Ward C. Clinical significance of the bicuspid aortic valve. Heart 2000; 83: 81–5.

72. Seiler C, Jenni R. Severe aortic stenosis without left ventricular hypertrophy: prevalence, predictors, and short-term follow up after aortic valve replacement. Heart 1996; 76: 250–5.

73. Nishimura RA, Grantham JA, Connolly HM, et al. Low-output, low-gradient aortic stenosis in patients with depressed left ventricular systolic function: the clinical utility of the dobutamine challenge in the catheterization laboratory. Circulation 2002; 106: 809–13.

74. Picano E, Pibarot P, Lancellotti P, et al. The emerging role of exercise testing and stress echocardiography in valvular heart disease. J Am Coll Cardiol 2009; 54: 2251–60.

75. Monin JL, Quere JP, Monchi M, et al. Low-gradient aortic stenosis: operative risk stratification and predictors for long-term outcome: a multicenter study using dobutamine stress hemodynamics Circulation 2003; 108: 319–24.

76. Hachicha Z, Dumesnil JG, Bogaty P, Pibarot P. Paradoxical low-flow, low-gradient severe aortic stenosis despite preserved ejection fraction is associated with higher afterload and reduced survival. Circulation 2007; 115: 2856–64.

77. Barasch E, Fan D, Chukwu EO, et al. Severe isolated aortic stenosis with normal left ventricular systolic function and low transvalvular gradients: pathophysiologic and prognostic insights. J Heart Valve Dis 2008; 17: 81–8.

78. Dumesnil JG, Pibarot P, Carabello B. Paradoxical low flow and/or low gradient severe aortic stenosis despite preserved left ventricular ejection fraction: implications for diagnosis and treatment. Eur Heart J 2010; 31: 281–9.

79. Cramariuc D, Cioffi G, Rieck AE, et al. Low flow aortic stenosis in asymptomatic patients. Valvular-arterial impedance and systolic function from the SEAS substudy. JACC Cardiovasc Imaging 2009; 2: 390–9.

80. Hachicha Z, Dumesnil JG, Pibarot P. Usefulness of the valvulo-arterial impedance to predict adverse outcome in asymptomatic aortic stenosis. J Am Coll Cardiol 2009; 54: 1003–11.

81. Briand M, Dumesnil JG, Kadem L, et al. Reduced systemic arterial compliance impacts significantly on left ventricular afterload and function in aortic stenosis: implications for diagnosis and treatment. J Am Coll Cardiol 2005; 46: 291–8.

82. Ozkan A, Hachamovitch R, Kapadia SR, Tuzcu EM, Marwick TH. Impact of aortic valve replacement on outcome of symptomatic patients with severe aortic stenosis with low gradient and preserved left ventricular ejection fraction. Circulation 2013; 128: 622–31.

83. Eleid M, Sorajja P, Michelena HI, et al. Flow-gradient patterns in severe aortic stenosis with preserved ejection fraction: clinical characteristics and predictors of survival. Circulation 2013; 128: 1781–9. *In this Mayo Clinic paper, normal-flow low gradient AVA <1 cm² did not benefit from AVR. This is moderate rather than severe AS, with measurement errors, pressure recovery, or non-severe indexed AVA, and it included patients with a small body habitus and LVOT. In other papers, these patients benefited from AVR because they only included small indexed AVA.*

84. Pibarot P, Dumesnil JG. Paradoxical low-flow, low-gradient aortic stenosis: new evidence, more questions. Circulation 2013; 128: 1729–32.

85. Rahimtoola SH. Determining that aortic valve stenosis is severe: back-to-the-future: physical examination and aortic valve area index/energy loss index≤0.6 cm²/m². JACC Cardiovasc Imaging 2010; 3: 563–6. *Also, this original paper by Braunwald defines AS by the gradient after pressure recovery: Braunwald E, Goldblatt A, Aygen MM, et al. Congenital aortic stenosis. I. Clinical and hemodynamic findings in 100 patients. II. Surgical treatment and the results of operation. Circulation. 1963; 27: 426–46.*

86. Bahlmann E, Cramariuc D, Gerdts E, et al. Impact of pressure recovery on echocardiographic assessment of asymptomatic aortic stenosis: a SEAS substudy. JACC Cardiovasc Imaging 2010; 3: 555–62.

87. Levine RA, Jimoh A, Cape EG. Pressure recovery distal to a stenosis: potential cause of gradient "overestimation" by Doppler echocardiography J Am Coll Cardiol 1989; 13: 706–15.

88. Baumgartner H, Stefanelli T, Niederberger J, Schima H, Maurer G. "Overestimation" of catheter gradients by Doppler ultrasound in patients with aortic stenosis: a predictable manifestation of pressure recovery J Am Coll Cardiol 1999; 33: 1655–61.

89. Rosenhek R, Binder T, Porenta G, et al. Predictors of outcome in severe, asymptomatic aortic stenosis. N Engl J Med 2000; 343: 611–17.

90. Monin JL, Quere JP, Monchi M, et al. Low-gradient aortic stenosis: operative risk stratification and predictors for long-term outcome: a multicenter study using dobutamine stress hemodynamics. Circulation 2003; 108: 319–24.

91. Vahanian A, Alfieri O, Andreotti F, et al. Guidelines on the management of valvular heart disease (version 2012). Joint Task Force on the Management of Valvular Heart Disease of the European Society of Cardiology (ESC); European Association for Cardio-Thoracic Surgery (EACTS). Eur Heart J 2012; 33: 2451–96.

92. Otto CM, Pearlman AS. Doppler echocardiography in adults with symptomatic aortic stenosis. Arch Intern Med 1988; 148: 2553–60.

93. Lund O, Nielsen TT, Emmertsen K, et al. Mortality and worsening of prognostic profile during waiting time for valve replacement in aortic stenosis. Thorac Cardiovasc Surg 1996; 44: 289–95.

94. Das P, Rimington H, Chambers J. Exercise testing to stratify risk in aortic stenosis, Eur Heart J 26 2005 1309–13.

95. Dal-Bianco JP, Khandharia BK, Mookadam F, et al. Management of asymptomatic severe aortic stenosis. J Am Coll Cardiology 2008; 52: 1279–92.

96. Taniguchi T, Morimoto T, Shiomi H, et al. Initial surgical versus conservative strategies in patients with asymptomatic severe aortic stenosis. J Am Coll Cardiol 2015; 66: 2827–38.

97. Unger P, Dedobbeleer C, Van Camp G, et al. Mitral regurgitation in patients with aortic stenosis undergoing valve replacement. Heart 2010; 96: 9–14.

98. Leon MB, Smith CR, Mack M, et al. Transcatheter aortic-valve implantation for aortic stenosis in patients who cannot undergo surgery. N Engl J Med 2010; 363: 1597–607.

99. Herrmann HC, Pibarot P, Hueter I, et al. Predictors of mortality and outcomes of therapy in low flow severe aortic stenosis: A PARTNER trial analysis. Circulation 2013; 127: 2316–26.

100. Adams DH, Popma JJ, Reardon MJ, et al. Transcatheter aortic-valve replacement with a self-expanding prosthesis. N Engl J Med 2014; 370: 1790–8.

101. Leon MB, Smith CR, Mack MJ, et al. Transcatheter or surgical aortic –valve replacement in intermediate-risk patients. N Engl J Med 2016; 374: 1609–20.

TR

102. Ling LF, Marwik TH. Echocardiographic assessment of right ventricular function. JACC Cardiovasc Imaging 2012; 5: 747–53.

103. Lin G, Nishimura RA, Connolly HM, et al. Severe symptomatic tricuspid valve regurgitation due to permanent pacemaker or implantable cardioverter-defibrillator leads. J Am Coll Cardiol 2005; 45; 1672–5.

104. Shiran A, Sagie A. Tricuspid regurgitation in mitral valve disease. J Am Coll Cardiol 2009; 53: 401–8.

PS

105. Kan JS, White RI, Mitchell SE, et al. Percutaneous transluminal valvuloplasty for pulmonary valve stenosis. Circulation 1984; 69: 554–60.

106. Hayes C, Gersony W, Driscoll D, et al. Second natural history study of congenital heart defects: results of treatment of patients with pulmonary valvar stenosis. Circulation 1993; 87 (suppl): I-28–37.

107. Graham T, Driscoll D, Gersony W, et al. Task Force 2: congenital heart disease. J Am Coll Cardiol 2005; 45: 1326–33.

PR

108. Bruce CJ, Connolly HM. Right-sided valve disease deserves a little more respect. Circulation 2009; 119: 2726–34.

Radiation heart disease

109. Jaworski C, Mariani JA, Wheeler J, Kaye DM. Cardiac complications of thoracic radiation. J Am Coll Cardiol 2013; 61: 2319–28.

Prosthetic valves

110. Pibarot P, Dumesnil JG. Prosthetic heart valves. Selection of optimal prosthesis and long-term management. Circulation 2009; 119: 1034–48.

111. Banbury MK, Cosgrove DM, White JA, et al. Age and valve size effect on the long-term durability of the Carpentier–Edwards aortic pericardial prosthesis. Ann Thorac Surg 2001; 72: 753–7.

112. Merie C, Kober L, Skov OP, et al. Association of warfarin therapy duration after bioprosthetic aortic valve replacement with risk of mortality, thromboembolic complications, and bleeding. JAMA 2012; 308: 2118–25.

113. Chan WS, Anand S, Ginsberg JS. Anticoagulation of pregnant women with mechanical heart valves: a systematic review of the literature. Arch Intern Med 2000; 160: 191–6.

Thrombosis

114. Shapira Y, Herz I, Vaturi M, et al. Thrombolysis is an effective and safe therapy in stuck bileaflet mitral valves in the absence of high-risk thrombi. J Am Coll Cardiol 2000; 35: 1874–80.

115. Roudaut R, Lafitte S, Roudaut MF, et al. Fibrinolysis of mechanical prosthetic valve thrombosis: a single-center study of 127 cases. J Am Coll Cardiol 2003; 41: 653–8.

116. Maraj R, Jacobs LE, Ioli A, Kotler MN. Evaluation of hemolysis in patients with prosthetic heart valves. Clin Cardiol 1998; 21: 387–92.

117. O'Rourke DJ, Palac RT, Malenka DJ, et al. Outcome of mild periprosthetic regurgitation detected by intraoperative transesophageal echocardiography. J Am Coll Cardiol 2001; 38: 163–6.

118. Garcia, MJ, Vandervoort, P, Stewart, WJ, et al. Mechanisms of hemolysis with mitral prosthetic regurgitation: study using transesophageal echocardiography and fluid dynamic simulation. J Am Coll Cardiol 1996; 27: 399–406. *Hemolysis may occur with any degree of paravalvular leak, although patients in the study had severe leaks; equal bioprosthetic and mechanical valve.*

119. Magne J, Mathieu P, Dumesnil JG, et al. Impact of patient–prosthesis mismatch on survival after mitral valve replacement. Circulation 2007; 115: 1417–25.

120. Rao V, Jamieson WR, Ivanov J, Armstrong S, David TE. Prosthesis–patient mismatch affects survival after aortic valve replacement. Circulation 2000; 102: III5–9.

121. Lam BK, Chan V, Hendry P, et al. The impact of patient–prosthesis mismatch on late outcomes after mitral valve replacement. J Thorac Cardiovasc Surg 2007; 133: 1464–73.

122. Zoghbi WA, Chambers JB, Dumesnil JG, et al. Recommendations for evaluation of prosthetic valves with echocardiography and Doppler ultrasound. J Am Soc Echocardiogr 2009; 22: 975–1014.

123. Gulati M, Pandey DK, Arnsdorf MF, et al. Exercise capacity and the risk of death in women: the St James Women Take Heart Project. Circulation 2003; 108: 1554–9.

124. Morris CK, Myers J, Froelicher VF, et al. Nomogram based on metabolic equivalents and age for assessing aerobic exercise capacity in men. J Am Coll Cardiol 1993; 22: 175–82.

Part 4   HYPERTROPHIC CARDIOMYOPATHY

7   Hypertrophic Cardiomyopathy

I. Definition and features of HCM

A. Definition

Hypertrophic cardiomyopathy (HCM) is characterized by LV hypertrophy without an identifiable cause (no valvular disease, no hypertension, or the degree of hypertrophy is disproportionate to the severity of hypertension). The prevalence in the general population is 1 in 500. HCM is genetic. It is familial, autosomal dominant, in 50% of the cases; the remaining 50% are due to new mutations.

B. Asymmetry

The septal thickness is usually greater than 13–15 mm. The hypertrophy is usually asymmetric and involves the septum and the anterolateral wall with a septal-to-posterior wall thickness ratio of >1.3:1, and more specifically >1.5:1, but it may be symmetric and diffuse, involving the posterior wall in 10–20% of the cases (= concentric hypertrophy).[1–3] One report suggests that the posterior wall is involved in cases of diffuse hypertrophy,[3] while another report suggests that posterobasal wall involvement is very unusual even when hypertrophy is diffuse.[4] Either way, the posterior wall is the site *least* frequently thickened in HCM. Hypertrophy most often involves two or more myocardial segments in an asymmetric and sometimes "bumpy" fashion, but may involve only one segment.

Severe LVOT obstruction leads to severe afterload elevation that may result in a global LV hypertrophy with time; hence, septal reduction not only reduces septal thickness but also the LV thickness at distant segments.

C. LVOT obstruction

When obstructive, HCM is called *hypertrophic obstructive cardiomyopathy* (HOCM) and is usually characterized by septal hypertrophy that narrows the left ventricular outflow tract (LVOT). The increased velocity across the LVOT draws the anterior mitral leaflet and its chordae during systole, which further narrows the LVOT and creates LVOT obstruction. This process is called systolic anterior motion (SAM) of the anterior leaflet (both the leaflet edge and chordae). A significant obstruction is characterized by a resting gradient >30 mmHg or a gradient >50 mmHg with provocative maneuvers (peak instantaneous gradient).[1,2] Only 30% of patients with hypertrophic cardiomyopathy have a resting gradient, while 45% have a gradient with provocative maneuvers; the remaining patients have non-obstructive hypertrophic cardiomyopathy.

Practical Cardiovascular Medicine, First Edition. Elias B. Hanna.
© 2017 John Wiley & Sons Ltd. Published 2017 by John Wiley & Sons Ltd.

The gradient is within the LV, i.e., pressure is elevated throughout the LV body and a portion of the LVOT then drops at one point in the LVOT rather than across the aortic valve. On echo-Doppler, the velocity is increased across the point of LVOT obstruction and is decreased proximal to this point (LV inflow and mid-LV cavity) and distal to this point (aortic valve) (Figure 7.1). Mild or moderate MR is usually seen and is associated with SAM of the mitral valve. In up to 10% of HOCM cases, the hypertrophy and the obstruction may be mid-ventricular, as is the case with mid-ventricular HOCM, apical HOCM, or HOCM with anterolateral papillary muscle inserting directly onto the mitral leaflet. The marked septal hypertrophy may also contribute to RV outflow tract obstruction, particularly in children with HOCM.

LVOT obstruction is associated with more symptoms and a higher HF-related mortality, but only a weak correlation with sudden death.

D. Causes of MR in HOCM; mitral valve abnormalities in HOCM

MR is mainly related to SAM; it is ***directed posteriorly*** and peaks in mid and late systole (Figures 7.1–7.3).[5–7] The severity of MR correlates with the severity of the LVOT gradient.[5] MR may be severe (in ~10%) if the posterior leaflet is not elongated enough to meet with the "sucked" anterior leaflet. Severe MR with a relatively short posterior leaflet is expected to improve after myectomy, while severe MR despite an elongated posterior leaflet, or central or anteriorly directed MR, is concerning for a structural mitral abnormality.[8]

- ***Mitral valve abnormalities that aggravate SAM and LVOT obstruction***. Structural valvular abnormalities are common (~20%) and may consist of:
  - **i.** *Anterior leaflet elongation >30 mm*, which provides extra slack and facilitates SAM and LVOT obstruction
  - **ii.** *Central/anterior papillary muscle malposition* (as opposed to anterolateral position)
  - **iii.** *Chordal insertion at the base rather than the tip of the anterior leaflet*

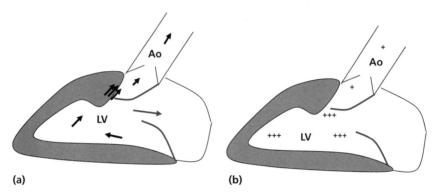

(a)   **(b)**

Figure 7.1 (a) Asymmetric septal hypertrophy with increased velocity across the LVOT (*3 arrows*). This increased systolic velocity creates a Venturi effect that pulls the anterior mitral leaflet (SAM) and creates LVOT obstruction as well as a posteriorly directed MR (*blue arrow*). Note the anatomic contiguity of the mitral and aortic valves. Pulsed-wave Doppler should be used to sequentially interrogate the LV from apex up to the LVOT in order to confirm the anatomical level of obstruction. Note the normal velocity across the LV body, LVOT proximal to the obstruction and distal to it, and aorta (*single arrows*). **(b)** Pressure is increased throughout LV inflow, LV body, LVOT (+++), and drops beyond the LVOT obstruction (+). Even pressure at the mitral valve level (inflow tract pressure) is elevated.

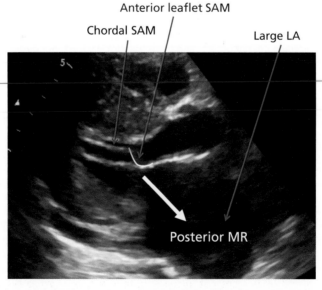

Figure 7.2 Parasternal long-axis view of a patient with HOCM, showing SAM of the anterior leaflet tip. Not just the leaflet gets drawn to the septum, but also the chordae (chordal SAM).

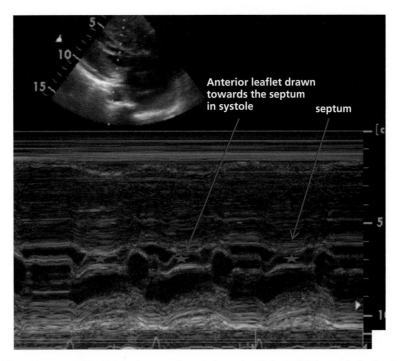

Figure 7.3 M-mode of SAM. The *star* corresponds to the gap between the anterior and posterior leaflets in systole, leading to severe MR in this patient.

(ii) and (iii) lead to tenting of the anterior leaflet anteriorly, into the LVOT stream. All these abnormalities facilitate SAM and LVOT obstruction, even in patients with milder degrees of septal hypertrophy ≤ 18 mm. Papillary muscle insertion directly on the anterior leaflet, without chordae, may cause LVOT obstruction (as it directly abuts the septum with each beat) and anterior tethering/MR.

- ***Mitral valve abnormalities that can cause a primary form of MR***. Some primary valvular abnormalities can cause MR independent of SAM, and these are seen in 10–20% of HOCM:[5] (i) extreme elongation and prolapse of the posterior mitral leaflet (~9% of operated HOCM);[8] (ii) chordal rupture; (iii) papillary muscle insertion directly onto the anterior leaflet. This primary MR is characterized by a *central or anteriorly directed jet that is usually holosystolic* and is not expected to resolve with septal reduction.[5,6]

E. Less common forms of HCM
- *Mid-cavitary HCM* consists of thickening of the mid-portion of the LV, with associated apical thinning and aneurysm formation, simulating apical MI; the hypertrophy was probably more diffuse, but the apex infarcted as a result of the severe pressure rise and diffusely increased O_2 demands that accompanied cavity obliteration. This form of HCM has a particularly unfavorable prognosis with a high risk of sudden death and LV thrombus. Mid-cavitary HCM may also be due to anomalous basal position of the anterior papillary muscle that inserts directly onto the anterior leaflet.
- *Apical HCM* is a common form of HCM in the Asian population, has a benign prognosis with <1% yearly mortality, and is not associated with an intracavitary gradient. It may evolve into an apical aneurysm.

II. Natural history and mortality
The HCM phenotype usually develops at the end of the second decade, and screening in adolescence may therefore miss it. Hypertrophy does not usually worsen in the adult. However, progressive global LV hypertrophy may develop as a result of the LVOT obstruction and increased LV workload, which leads to a vicious circle of more LVOT obstruction and LV hypertrophy. Approximately 5% of patients eventually succumb to this chronically elevated afterload and develop a late phase of LV cavity dilatation with reduced systolic function (*burned-out phase* of HCM).

HCM onset may occur late, in the elderly. Moreover, it is not uncommon for an early HCM to present and be diagnosed late. In fact, in alcohol ablation studies, the median age was 64. In a cohort study, ~25% of HCM patients were elderly (≥75 years old).[9] Elderly presentations are usually associated with milder LVH yet more obstruction.

A population study has shown that the mortality of unselected HCM patients is ~1% per year, which is not different from the mortality of the general population.[9] On the other hand, the annual mortality is 3–6% in high-risk patients with multiple predictors of sudden death or in patients with LVOT obstruction, which is predictive of HF-related death.[10]

The gradient is strongly associated with symptom progression, progressive HF, and cardiac death secondary to HF and stroke (AF).[11–13] In fact, in observational studies, patients with obstructive HCM had a higher mortality than patients with non-obstructive HCM or operated obstructive HCM.[11,12] *This is particularly true for patients with severe resting gradient (>100 mmHg, even if asymptomatic), symptoms (NYHA II or III–IV), or functional limitation*.[13,14] A gradient <100 mmHg without symptoms and with a normal functional capacity (>85% of predicted METs) does not impair long-term survival.[13] While LVOT obstruction is associated with HF-related death, the specific relation of obstruction to sudden cardiac death (SCD) is significant but weak. The positive predictive value for sudden death is low.

A large cohort analysis has shown that there are three modes of death in HCM: SCD (~50%, age 45±20), progressive HF (~36%, age 56±19), and AF-related stroke. SCD, while a relatively more common cause of death in young patients <50 years old, actually has a similar yearly incidence in the older population; neither sudden nor heart-failure-related death showed a statistically significant, disproportionate age distribution.[15]

III. Symptoms and ECG

Most patients with HCM or HOCM are asymptomatic. *Dyspnea* and HF may result from LVOT obstruction and/or LV diastolic dysfunction. *Angina* may result from increased demands and from the elevated LVEDP, which impairs coronary microcirculatory flow; myocardial bridging is also common and may contribute to ischemia. Severe functional limitation (class III or IV) is uncommon but may eventually develop in up to 45% of patients with LVOT obstruction, over the course of 10-year follow-up.[11] Conversely, up to 23% of patients may have a paradoxical reduction of gradient with exercise, which partly explains how some patients are asymptomatic.[16]

Two types of *syncope* must be distinguished: (i) exertional and (ii) post-exertional. Exertional syncope is more ominous and is secondary to arrhythmia (e.g., VT or AF) or dynamic LVOT obstruction that worsens with exertion. Conversely, in the post-exertional phase, the reduced peripheral venous pumping reduces venous return to the hypercontractile LV. This increases LVOT obstruction and may lead to syncope, but may also activate the myocardial C receptors of the small hypercontractile cavity, leading to a vasovagal syncope. *HOCM is sensitive to the post-exertional preload reduction and is prone to vasovagal syncope in light of the small, hypercontractile LV cavity.*

Unfortunately, ~70% of patients who die suddenly have no or only mild symptoms prior to SCD, and thus SCD is often the first manifestation in patients who die suddenly. SCD often occurs at rest or with mild activities, but 15% of SCDs occur during moderate or heavy activity (relatively more so in athletes).[15]

ECG shows LVH voltage with a strain pattern, and/or deep T-wave inversion in leads V_2–V_6 even without LVH voltage. Prominent septal depolarization may lead to large Q waves in the lateral and inferior leads (pseudoinfarct pattern). Approximately 10% of HCM patients have a normal ECG, which is a limitation of pre-athletic ECG screening.

IV. Exam (see Table 7.1)

Table 7.1 Exam findings in HOCM versus AS.

	HOCM[a]	AS
Quality	Harsh, crescendo–decrescendo mid-systolic murmur	Harsh, crescendo-decrescendo mid-systolic murmur
Location	LLSB	RUSB
Radiation	Apex/axilla, not carotids	Carotids
Carotid pulse	Brisk, double-peaked (bisferiens)	Slow, small amplitude
Dynamic with maneuvers (Valsalva, handgrip, standing)	++++	+ (changes are not usually audible)
Apical impulse	**Enlarged, triple ripple** (systolic ejection, systolic obstruction, and S_4)	Enlarged, single impulse

[a] MR murmur (SAM) may also be heard with HOCM: blowing, holosystolic murmur at the apex (while HOCM murmur is best heard at the LLSB). This MR murmur is also worse with Valsalva. The two murmurs are heard at two different locations and are both dynamic.

V. Invasive hemodynamic findings

In the presence of a gradient between the LV and aorta and if HOCM is suspected, use an end-hole catheter, rather than a multihole catheter, and slowly pull back across the LVOT to localize the site of pressure drop. In addition to the subaortic pressure gradient, the aortic and LV pressure tracings are characterized by the following (Figure 7.4):

1. Systolic aortic pressure has an early "spike" and a late "dome" ("spike and dome" appearance). In fact, LVOT obstruction is dynamic and is less severe in early systole when LV volume is largest, allowing a "peak" in aortic pressure. Obstruction is worst in mid- and late systole when LV volume is reduced, explaining the late "dome."

2. Since LV obstruction is worst in late systole, LV pressure proximal to the obstruction peaks late and has a *late-peaking* "dagger" shape (similar to the spectral Doppler "dagger" shape velocity across the LV).

3. After a premature beat, LV volume increases, but LV contractility increases even more and overwhelms the benefit derived from LV volume, producing an increase in LVOT obstruction. LV pressure increases but the stroke volume decreases, and thus the aortic pulse pressure decreases (*Brockenbrough phenomenon*); the aortic systolic pressure decreases as well. This contrasts with AS, wherein the fixed obstruction does not prevent the increase in stroke volume and aortic pulse pressure after a premature beat; the gradient increases with the increase in flow, as per Gorlin's equation, but the aortic pressure increases as well (Figure 7.5). In both HOCM and AS, the gradient and the murmur increase after a premature beat, but more so in HOCM, and the pulse only decreases in HOCM.

4. Pressure gradient is dynamic with provocative maneuvers. Being dynamic, the gradient may be labile and varies with changes of loading conditions.

VI. Echocardiographic findings

Beside the often asymmetric LV hypertrophy, the obstructive form of HCM is characterized by SAM. SAM is seen on the parasternal long-axis view and on the M-mode of the mitral valve (Figures 7.2, 7.3). The greater the degree and duration of mitral–septal contact (e.g., > 30% of systole), the more severe the obstruction. In addition, M-mode of the aortic valve shows mid-systolic closure due to the mid-systolic obstruction. LA enlargement is universal in HCM (*a normal LA size makes HCM unlikely*).

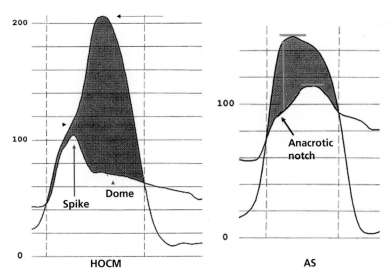

Figure 7.4 HOCM hemodynamics.

Note the early aortic pressure peaking (*blue vertical arrow*), the late LV pressure peaking (*horizontal arrow*), and the late gradient (*gray area*). The aortic pressure peaks in the first 80 ms of systole; then, LVOT obstruction worsens, the LV pressure tracing "bends" then peaks in mid- to late systole while the aortic systolic pressure adopts a "dome" appearance (LV pressure bend, *black arrowhead*). This contrasts with AS, where the aortic pressure bends and peaks late while the LV pressure peaks early.

As opposed to AS, the mean gradient in HOCM does not characterize the obstruction well, as it integrates the unobstructed early part of systole and under-represents the LVOT obstruction. As opposed to AS, **the peak-to-peak gradient approximates the peak instantaneous gradient in HOCM, and both those gradients are used to classify the severity of HOCM (≠ AS, where mean gradient is used).**

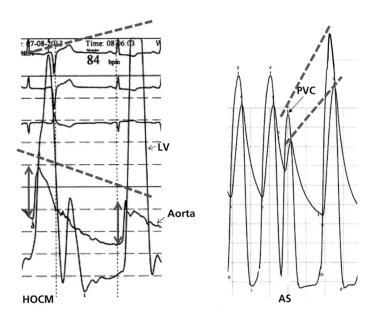

Figure 7.5 Brockenbrough phenomenon after a premature beat in HOCM. Note the increase in pressure gradient (*interrupted lines*) but the reduction in aortic pulse pressure (*double arrows*) after a pause in HOCM, vs. the increase in pressure gradient with an increase in aortic pulse pressure in AS. Note the "spike and dome" appearance of the aortic pressure in HOCM, which becomes more pronounced with worsening obstruction (after the pause).

Pulsed-wave Doppler interrogation reveals that the velocity is increased across one point in the LVOT, but is normal (~1 m/s) or low in the LV body and distally across the aortic valve. However, the velocity may also increase in the LV body when hypertrophy is generalized with cavity obliteration, even if the obstruction is mainly at the LVOT level. The LVOT gradient is late peaking, with a "dagger" shape on spectral Doppler. It is dynamic and may be unveiled or worsened by Valsalva maneuver, which should be performed in all cases of HCM (Figure 7.6). Aliasing typically occurs across the point of LVOT obstruction rather than the aortic valve. After localizing the site of obstruction with pulsed-wave Doppler, continuous-wave Doppler is required to capture the actual velocity.

Cardiac MRI may be used to further delineate the LV geometry and thickness and mitral geometry when echo is inconclusive (class I recommendation).

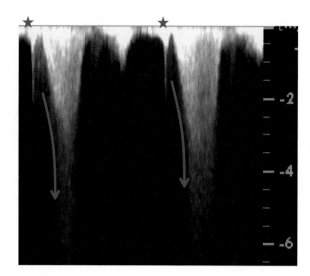

Figure 7.6 LVOT velocity in HOCM: late-peaking dagger-shape LVOT velocity (*arrows*). This is opposed to the parabolic, symmetrical AS Doppler. Occasionally, an older patient may have both AS and HOCM. The continuous-wave Doppler will show two superimposed but distinct ejection envelopes (e.g., AS envelope within the HOCM envelope).

Note the notch in early systole, before the LVOT envelope (*stars*). This notch corresponds to MR and is characteristic of LVOT interrogation in HOCM. In fact, in HOCM, MR is frequently captured on LVOT interrogation, as the mitral flow is in close proximity to the LVOT. Also, LVOT may be captured on MR interrogation.

VII. Provocative maneuvers

Patients without any gradient at rest may develop a significant gradient with maneuvers. The gradient increases with decreased preload (Valsalva maneuver, hypovolemia, nitroglycerin), decreased afterload (vasodilators), or increased inotropism (exercise, inotropic drugs such as dobutamine). Each of these changes results in closer approximation of the ventricular septum and anterior mitral leaflet during systole. For instance, a reduction in preload or afterload reduces LV volume and the high LV end-systolic pressure that holds the LVOT walls apart. Also, when the heart rate rises or when the atrial systole is lost, as in atrial fibrillation, the gradient increases as a result of the reduced diastolic filling time (preload).

While dobutamine increases the intraventricular gradient in patients with HOCM, dobutamine also induces a significant gradient in up to 20% of patients undergoing dobutamine echocardiography without suspected HOCM or even without LV hypertrophy.[17,18] *Dobutamine-induced gradient does not necessarily imply exertional gradient and should not be used to diagnose HOCM.* In fact, exercise increases myocardial contractility but also preload, which reduces cavity obliteration and the potential for intracavitary obstruction; dobutamine increases myocardial contractility but does not increase preload, and thus more readily creates intracavitary obstruction even in the absence of HOCM. Physiological maneuvers rather than pharmacological interventions should be used to assess provocable gradient (exercise, Valsalva).

VIII. Genetic testing for diagnosis; screening of first-degree relatives

Genetic testing identifies definite pathogenic mutations in only 60–70% of HCM cases. While the genes affected in HCM are known, the actual nucleotides affected vary widely; some sequences represent definite pathogenic mutations of the gene, while others may represent normal variants. Therefore, a positive test definitely establishes the HCM genotype, but a negative test is unhelpful.

Genetic testing of an index patient is indicated for family screening purposes. If the patient tests positive for a definite mutation, first-degree family members should be screened for that same mutation. The absence of this mutation excludes the risk of HCM occurrence in these relatives and is reassuring. A positive genotype with a negative phenotype in a family member indicates a considerable risk of developing HCM; routine ECG and echo follow-up is performed throughout life. The risk of SCD is unclear, and decisions about athletic activities are individualized.

Short of genetic testing, first-degree relatives of HCM patients should undergo yearly ECG and echocardiograms starting in early adolescence and until the age of 21.[19] Approximately 25% of those patients will develop HCM. Afterwards, they need to be screened every 5 years for the late development of HCM (more frequent interval in case of athletic activity or family history of SCD).

IX. Differential diagnosis of LVOT obstruction

The differential diagnosis of dynamic LVOT obstruction includes the following:

1. Patients with hypertension and generalized *or* asymmetric LV hypertrophy may develop intracavitary LV obstruction, particularly in case of hypovolemia. LVOT obstruction and a true LVOT gradient, sometimes exceeding 100 mmHg, may be seen, with occasional SAM of the mitral valve. This is called "**hypertensive hypertrophic cardiomyopathy**" or "**hypertensive obstructive cardiomyopathy**," and unlike HOCM, is not associated with myofibrillar disarray.[20,21]
- *Similarities with HOCM.* The invasive hemodynamics are similar to those of a typical HOCM (late-peaking pressure gradient, Brockenbrough phenomenon). While hypertensive obstructive cardiomyopathy is typically symmetric,[21] ~5% of all hypertensive patients have asymmetric septal hypertrophy and up to 34% of cases of severe hypertensive LV hypertrophy are asymmetric and predominantly septal (septal-to-posterior wall thickness >1.5), particularly in elderly patients with sigmoid septum, which further mimics HCM.[22–24]

- *Differences from HOCM.* As opposed to HCM, the septal thickness in hypertensive cardiomyopathy does not usually exceed 20 mm,[21] the hypertrophy does not have a bumpy heterogeneous morphology, SAM is less common,[21] and there is usually a diffuse increase in velocity throughout the LV, including the mid-cavity, directing the attention toward globally abnormal ejection hemodynamics. Occasionally, however, the septal thickness may be >20 mm (mean 21 mm in Topol et al.).[20,22,25] Ancillary signs of severe HTN are typically present and help distinguish this entity from HOCM (aortic sclerosis, aortic dilatation, mitral annular calcification, nephropathy). This obstructive cardiomyopathy is more prevalent in the elderly female, particularly black female, in whom the LV cavity is small (Table 7.2).[20,21]

In a patient with systemic HTN, a diagnostic dilemma frequently arises in determining whether the markedly increased LV wall thickness is solely a reflection of HTN or, alternatively, whether it is a manifestation of a coexistent, genetically determined HCM.[22] In addition, it is possible that some of these patients have a genetic HCM substrate that evolves into a HCM phenotype when exposed to longstanding HTN.[21] Genetic testing, if positive, or a family history of HCM helps point towards genetic HCM. On the other hand, ancillary manifestations of HTN, such as aortic dilatation or nephropathy, support the diagnosis of chronic severe HTN. One study, however, has shown that hypertrophic cardiomyopathy with LVOT gradient in severely hypertensive patients is indistinguishable from hypertrophic cardiomyopathy in normotensive patients, with similar SAM rates, pressure gradient (frequently exceeding 100 mmHg), and septal thickness, implying that "hypertensive obstructive cardiomyopathy" may, in fact, be a genetic HOCM with coexistent HTN rather than a hypertensive cardiomyopathy.[25]

For practical purposes, LVH >15–20 mm with significant SAM and LVOT obstruction, in the absence of severe hypovolemia or sepsis, is pathophysiologically a HOCM, even in a hypertensive patient and even if hypertrophy is symmetric, and is managed as HOCM.[25] In fact, a firm diagnosis of genetically determined HOCM is not always present in patients treated for the disease, even in HOCM studies and even when invasive therapies are used. This is related to the phenotypical overlap of HOCM and severe hypertensive cardiomyopathy and the limitations of genetic testing. Over 50% of patients in HOCM studies are hypertensive.

2. Severe asymmetric septal hypertrophy with subaortic obstruction is also seen in ~10% of patients with severe AS and is unmasked after aortic valve replacement (septal thickness up to 22 mm).[26] Doppler flow acceleration develops postoperatively and is attributed to LVOT obstruction and SAM in some series, while other series attribute it to the hyperdynamic small LV cavity that totally obliterates in systole. This obstruction is associated with postoperative hypotension, increased morbidity and mortality, and long-term persistence of a gradient in some patients. It is mainly treated medically (β-blockers, avoidance of inotropes, fluid resuscitation); a limited pre-emptive myectomy has been selectively used in patients with septal bulge, with good results.[27]

3. LVOT obstruction is frequently seen in patients receiving dobutamine regardless of the presence of LV hypertrophy and does not signify HOCM per se, as the obstruction may not be reproduced during exercise in most of these patients. It may also be seen in hospitalized patients with severe hypovolemia or sepsis and an empty, hypercontractile LV cavity, even if LVH is mild.

4. A pattern of LVOT obstruction and mitral SAM may also be seen in patients with apical dyskinesis and hypercontractile LV base, as in large anteroapical infarction or takotsubo cardiomyopathy.

Another form of subvalvular obstruction is subvalvular aortic stenosis that results from a discrete fibrous membrane or fibromuscular thickening within the outflow tract, just below the aortic valve (see Chapter 6). It leads to a fixed obstruction, the characteristics of dynamic LVOT obstruction being absent: no dagger-shaped LV pressure, no spike-and-dome aortic pressure, and no Brockenbrough phenomenon. *As opposed to HOCM, the gradient does not worsen with maneuvers such as Valsalva.*

Table 7.2 Differentiate LVOT obstruction of HOCM from hypertensive obstructive cardiomyopathy.

	HOCM	Hypertensive obstructive cardiomyopathy
Invasive hemodynamics: late-peaking gradient, Brockenbrough, gradient dynamic with maneuvers	+	+
Gradient >100 mmHg	Possible	Less common
SAM	+	Less common
		The increase in velocity is more global, involving LVOT but also mid-LV
Septal thickness >20 mm	Frequent	Rare
Asymmetric septal hypertrophy >1.5:1	Common (but 10–20% concentric)	Less common (but present in up to 1/3 of severe hypertensive hypertrophy)
Genetics and family history of HCM or SCD	Frequently +	–
Severe and chronic HTN, with other evidence of hypertensive disease (e.g., nephropathy, aortic dilatation)	± HTN, sometimes severe, may coexist	+
Hypovolemia	±	Common trigger of LVOT obstruction

X. Differential diagnosis of severe LV hypertrophy

Severe LV hypertrophy (septal thickness >15 mm, sometimes >20 mm) may be seen in **hypertension or AS** and may be asymmetric and/or obstructive.

In older patients, elongation of the aorta changes the angle of the aortic–septal junction and leads to a **sigmoid septum**. A sigmoid septum exaggerates the degree of asymmetric septal hypertrophy and may lead to LVOT obstruction (Figure 7.7).

A severe increase in septal thickness may also be seen with infiltrative disorders such as **amyloidosis**; in this case, thickening of the valve leaflets and the interatrial septum is often seen, along with a pericardial effusion. The increase in LV thickness is related to infiltration rather than true hypertrophy and is usually diffuse but may be asymmetric and obstructive. The familial form of amyloidosis may be seen at a young age and is, therefore, more likely to simulate HCM than the AL amyloidosis occurring in the elderly. An ECG showing a disproportionately low voltage differentiates amyloidosis from HCM but is insensitive. Cardiac MRI and endomyocardial biopsy may distinguish hypertrophic from amyloid cardiomyopathy.

While the septal thickness is usually >15 mm in HCM, it can be 12–15 mm in up to 15% of the patients, overlapping with the degree of wall thickening commonly found in hypertensive cardiomyopathy and occasionally found in normal athletes (Table 7.3). Hypertrophy can also be concentric in 10–20% of patients. *In these cases, a mild hypertrophy that is otherwise unexplained in a young patient suggests HCM.*

XI. Treatment of symptoms

A. Chronic medical therapy

(applies to HOCM *and* to the hypertensive obstructive cardiomyopathy)

Medical therapy consists of agents that reduce inotropism and chronotropism: **β-blockers** or **non-DHP CCBs**. By reducing inotropism and the LV ejection speed, they reduce the mitral valve drag. By reducing the heart rate, they increase preload and diastolic filling time, and reduce functional ischemia. A third agent, **disopyramide**, may be used (class Ia antiarrhythmic drug with potent negative inotropic effect and mild vasoconstrictive effect).[7] These drugs do not affect SCD.

β-Blocker therapy titrated to a heart rate of 60 bpm is the first-line therapy. It mainly blunts the provocable gradient with little effect on the resting gradient, unless the patient has baseline tachycardia. Thus, it is mostly effective in patients who have a provocable gradient

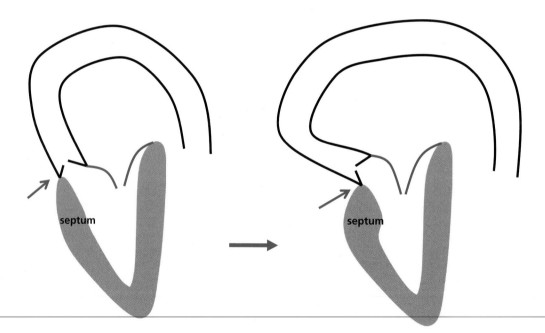

Figure 7.7 In the elderly, elongation of the aorta sharpens the angle between the aorta and the septum (*arrow*) and leads to a sigmoid "stocky" septum. A mild septal hypertrophy is transformed into a more severe, discrete septal thickening (DUST: discrete upper septal thickening).

Table 7.3 Athlete's heart vs. HOCM.

	Athlete's heart	HOCM
Septum thickness	<13 mm, gray zone: 13–15 mm	>15 mm, but can be less (gray zone)
LV diastolic diameter	Normal (>45 mm)	<45 mm (small cavity)
LA enlargement	None	Present
LV filling (diastology)	Normal	Abnormal diastology
Family history	None	(+) for HCM, SCD
LVH response to deconditioning (weeks)	↓ LVH	No ↓ LVH
SAM	No SAM	(+) SAM

with no or mild gradient at rest,[28,29] or patients with baseline tachycardia. Verapamil has more vasodilating and hypotensive effects than β-blockers and may paradoxically worsen the gradient through a reduction of afterload (rare). In fact, verapamil is associated with an early mortality risk when used in patients with severe HF or severe LVOT gradient and should be reserved for patients with mild gradients.

β-Blocker therapy is associated with a 50–60% initial success. This success is higher in patients whose main gradient is a provocable gradient, and is lower in patients with severe resting gradient or class III–IV symptoms at baseline.[28,29] In non-responders who have a mild resting gradient, a switch to verapamil may control symptoms. In non-responders who have a high resting gradient, β-blockade may be combined with disopyramide.

Disopyramide has a minimal bradycardic effect and is the most effective agent in reducing the resting gradient. In one study, the addition of disopyramide reduced the resting gradient by ~50% and controlled symptoms in two-thirds of patients, without any proarrhythmia or safety concern.[30] The combination of a β-blocker and a CCB is best avoided.

While heart rate reduction is useful, severe bradycardia (<50 bpm) or long pauses are harmful as they lead to increased myocardial contractility and thus increased gradient (similar to Brockenbrough phenomenon).

Hypovolemia should be avoided in these patients at all times. ***Diuretics and vasodilators worsen LVOT obstruction by reducing preload and afterload, respectively, and thus should be avoided.*** In fact, a symptomatic patient who is receiving a diuretic and/or a vasodilator experiences a significant symptomatic improvement upon cessation of these agents.

Patients with hypertensive obstructive cardiomyopathy or HTN coexistent with HOCM, whose HTN is not controlled with a β-blocker or a non-DHP, may require the careful use of a small diuretic dose. Similarly, a small diuretic dose may be carefully used in HOCM patients with persistent congestive symptoms (class IIb).

B. AF

Paroxysmal or chronic AF eventually develops in 20% of patients with HCM. AF is associated with a striking increase in the risk of HF, HF-related death, and stroke (>2%/year), especially in patients <50 years old or patients with LVOT obstruction.[31] Chronic AF is associated with a worse prognosis than paroxysmal AF in HCM, and thus rhythm control is preferred as a first-line therapy (AF guidelines).[31] Amiodarone is the most effective antiarrhythmic drug, but disopyramide may be used first. Digoxin is preferably avoided in light of its positive inotropic effect.

HCM-related AF is associated with a high risk of thromboembolic events regardless of CHADS2 score, and thus warrants chronic anticoagulation.

C. Acute therapy of acute HF or shock

Patients with HOCM or hypertensive obstructive cardiomyopathy who develop pulmonary edema are acutely treated with *β-blockers*. Diuretics may worsen LVOT obstruction and thus, paradoxically, worsen pulmonary edema.

Mitral stenosis and HOCM are the only two conditions wherein acute pulmonary edema is treated with β-blockers.

Patients with HOCM who develop hypotension are treated with *intravenous hydration*. If pulmonary edema is also present, *α-agonists* may be used, as they increase afterload and thus reduce LVOT obstruction. Positive inotropes should be avoided.

D. AV sequential ventricular pacing

Ventricular apical pacing leads to a delayed and less effective contraction of the basal septum, which reduces the LVOT narrowing. AV delay must be programmed short enough to ensure ventricular pacing without A truncation (~100 ms). Studies have shown a moderate efficacy of DDD pacing on the reduction of gradient (40–50% gradient reduction, with substantial variability). However, despite a real reduction of gradient in most patients, the effect of pacing on symptoms is more controversial: 40–60% of patients show symptomatic improvement with DDD pacing, yet the same number of patients show symptomatic improvement with atrial pacing (placebo), and the objective functional capacity only shows limited improvement.[7,32,33] This implies that most of the symptomatic benefit from pacing is a placebo effect. Pacing appears more efficacious in patients over 65 years of age, where objective improvement is seen.[32] DDD pacing with ventricular capture is recommended in patients who otherwise have an indication for pacing or patients who are not candidates for septal reduction.

Severe bradycardia (<50 bpm) is less likely to be tolerated in HOCM than in normal individuals, as it leads to increased contractility and increased gradient. In symptomatic patients whose rate is <50 bpm or even 50–60 bpm, and who cannot tolerate β-blockade because of rate, pacing followed by aggressive β-blockade may be used, especially if an ICD, which has pacing capacity, is required for sudden death prevention. However, septal ablation may be a better alternative for the latter patients.

E. Invasive septal reduction

Septal reduction is indicated in patients with class III/IV dyspnea or angina refractory to medical therapy, septal thickness ≥ 16 mm, and a peak instantaneous gradient of >50 mmHg at rest or with physiological maneuvers (not dobutamine). Also, recurrent syncope or near-syncope, whether exertional or post-exertional in nature but not clearly vasovagal, is an indication for septal reduction.

Septal reduction strikingly improves symptoms and the long-term risk of HF-related death. Myectomy may also reduce the risk of SCD.

There are two modalities of septal reduction:
1. **Surgical myectomy.** Myectomy consists of resecting the septal bulge through the aortic valve and has a low operative mortality (<1%). It is associated with a total abolition of gradient and symptom resolution in >90% of patients, with normalization of long-term survival.[12]

In addition, it appears to be associated with a reduction of the risk of ventricular arrhythmia (reduction of yearly ICD discharges). MR, even when severe, totally resolves with septal ablation. Yet, the minority of patients with severe independent MR (e.g., MR related to posterior leaflet prolapse), or LVOT obstruction related to mitral abnormalities may require concomitant mitral plication or papillary muscle/chordal release.[6,34] The latter is particularly suggested when LVOT obstruction is associated with a relatively thin septum ≤ 18 mm.[34]

Cutting the left septum is associated with a high risk of LBBB (~40%) and a low risk of complete AV block (~2%).

2. Alcohol septal ablation. Alcohol septal ablation is a percutaneous coronary procedure that consists of wiring the first or large septal branch that supplies the basal septum and injecting it with alcohol through a balloon catheter. This leads to infarction of the basal septum. The operative mortality is ~1%, and the symptomatic improvement is similar to that of myectomy. A retrospective analysis has shown that alcohol ablation is associated with a 4-year survival free of death or severe symptoms similar to myectomy (~80%) but may be less effective on symptoms and survival in patients <65 years of age.[35,36] An acute response with a striking gradient reduction (due to stunning of the myocardium) is followed by a gradient rise to about 50% of the pre-procedural level the next day(s), then a progressive septal remodeling and a great reduction of the gradient over 3 months. MR also improves with septal ablation.[36]

Limitations – Alcohol ablation abolishes the gradient (83%) less commonly than myectomy and is associated with an early risk of VT/VF (as with any MI). Its value is more limited in patients with one, and particularly two, of the following: severe septal hypertrophy (>25 mm), LVOT gradient >100 mmHg, age <65 years.[35,37] It is also limited in patients with mitral valve abnormalities that are contributing to LVOT obstruction, *hence the **importance of careful preoperative assessment of anterior leaflet length, papillary malposition, and chordal insertion, using TEE and MRI if needed.*** The success is dependent on identifying a major septal branch supplying the focal hypertrophy, as proven by contrast echocardiography (echocardiographic contrast injected in the septal artery while echo is performed). Since it induces a myocardial scar, there is a concern about a long-term arrhythmogenic potential, not seen with myectomy.[38] This was shown in one analysis of alcohol septal ablation, but not in others.[35,38]

Conduction abnormalities – Since the first septal branch supplies the right bundle, alcohol ablation is associated with a high risk of RBBB (~50% RBBB, vs. LBBB with myectomy). It is also associated with a risk of high-grade AV block requiring pacing (~12%, higher than the risk of AV block with myectomy).

In light of the complications and the less established success and long-term safety of alcohol septal ablation, myectomy is the preferred septal reduction strategy in patients without comorbidities, especially young patients.

Note that, following septal reduction, there is a reduction of LV thickness in remote (non-ablated) areas, and a decrease in the overall LV mass. In fact, severe LVOT obstruction, whether due to symmetric or asymmetric LV hypertrophy, increases LV workload and thus potentiates a vicious circle of progressive LV hypertrophy. Therefore, in HOCM, a component of LVH is secondary to the LVOT obstruction itself. Thus:[39–41]

1. Septal reduction therapies are likely useful in patients with symmetric global hypertrophy who exhibit LVOT obstruction.[39]
2. While septal reduction studies have only aimed to treat genetically determined HOCM, it is likely that many patients with hypertensive obstructive cardiomyopathy were inadvertently included in these studies, particularly given that distinguishing these two disease entities is not always possible. In fact, in a large registry that proved the efficacy of alcohol septal ablation, the mean age was 64 (mostly women), 54% of patients had hypertension, and 37% of patients had concentric hypertrophy (mean LV thickness 20 mm), implying that some of these patients who were labeled HOCM and who benefited from septal ablation may in fact have had hypertensive obstructive cardiomyopathy.[35] *Thus, in the right patient with severe hypertrophy and LVOT obstruction, septal ablation may be considered for a HOCM pathophysiology even if the diagnosis of genetic HOCM is uncertain.* Two small studies have shown positive results of alcohol septal ablation in the treatment of obstructive hypertensive hypertrophy that is concentric and severe and in the treatment of obstructive hypertrophy with sigmoid septum, which is not usually a genetic form of HOCM.[39,40]

F. Activity restriction

HCM patients, even those deemed at low risk for SCD, should not participate in any high-intensity sport. Patients at low risk of SCD or those at high risk who have already received an ICD may participate in low-intensity recreational sports, such as brisk walking, biking, modest hiking, modest swimming, or modest treadmill ± modest jogging.

XII. Treatment: sudden cardiac death risk assessment and ICD therapy

In a retrospective analysis of a large cohort of patients with HCM who received an ICD, ICD therapy for VT/VF occurred at a rate of ~11% per year in patients with a prior SCD, and ~3.5% per year in patients with any one of the following: HCM-related death in first-degree relative(s) younger than 50 years, prior unexplained syncope (inconsistent with vasovagal syncope), massive LVH ≥ 30 mm, or one or more runs of NSVT on Holter.[42] A study of unselected HCM patients suggests that the combination of two or more risk factors, including an abnormal BP response to exercise, more specifically predicts an increase in SCD.[43]

The ACC guidelines recommend ICD placement in HCM patients who have any one of the following:[18]

1. Prior history of SCD or sustained VT (class I)
2. Family history of SCD in one or more first-degree relatives (IIa)
3. LV wall thickness ≥ 30 mm (IIa)
4. Unexplained, recent syncope (IIa). Being preload-dependent, HCM patients are prone to neurally mediated syncope, such as syncope occurring after a rapid change in posture, emotion, micturition, prolonged standing, or sometimes *after* exertion. Syncope occurring in these contexts is not associated with an increased risk of SCD.[44] Unexplained syncope is a syncope that occurs at rest, during sitting, lying,

light activity, or during peak exercise. Unexplained syncope that is recent (<6 months) is associated with a fivefold increase in SCD; unexplained, remote syncope may also be associated with some increase in SCD (unless remote >5 years, or remote >6 months in a patient >40 years old).[44]

5. NSVT or lack of BP increase by 20 mmHg during exercise, along with one of the following minor factors: LVOT obstruction or late gadolinium hyperenhancement on MRI (IIa).Without these minor risk factors, the recommendation is weaker (IIb).

QUESTIONS AND ANSWERS

Question 1. A 68-year-old man with a history of severe HTN and CKD presents with progressive dyspnea on exertion (class III). He takes metoprolol, HCTZ, and lisinopril. On exam, BP is 110/65 mmHg, heart rate is 70 bpm, and a mid-sytolic murmur is heard at the LLSB. The murmur increases with Valsalva and improves with handgrip. Echo shows asymmetric septal hypertrophy with septal thickness of 19 mm, posterior wall thickness of 13 mm, and SAM of the mitral valve with LVOT gradient of 75 mmHg at rest and 120 mmHg with Valsalva. ECG shows LBBB. What is the appropriate next step?
A. Myectomy
B. Alcohol septal ablation
C. The patient has hypertensive cardiomyopathy. Discontinue HCTZ and lisinopril, titrate metoprolol, then add disopyramide
D. The patient has genetic hypertrophic cardiomyopathy. Discontinue HCTZ and lisinopril, titrate metoprolol, then add disopyramide
E. Add disopyramide

Question 2. Drug changes were performed in the patient of Question 1. Two months later, his symptoms have improved but he still gets dyspneic on activities of daily living. On Doppler, LVOT gradient is 40 mmHg at rest and increases to 75 mmHg with Valsalva. What is the next step?
A. Titrate disopyramide
B. Myectomy
C. Alcohol septal ablation
D. AV sequential pacing with short AV delay

Question 3. A 75-year-old man who has a history of severe HTN presents with exertional dyspnea (class III) and chest pain. He receives chronic metoprolol. On exam, he has two murmurs: (1) a holosystolic murmur heard at the LLSB, apex, axilla, worse with Valsalva, (2) a mid-systolic murmur heard at the base with radiation to the carotids. S_2 is normal and carotid upstrokes are normal. Echo shows asymmetric septal hypertrophy, with a septal thickness of 17 mm and a posterior thickness of 11 mm. SAM is present with a posteriorly directed, severe MR. A high LVOT gradient is present: 100 mmHg at rest and 160 mmHg with Valsalva. The aortic valve is calcified. The color Doppler shows aliasing at both the LVOT level and the aortic valve level. The continuous-wave (CW) spectral envelope shows two superimposed but distinct envelopes: one is dagger-shaped with a peak velocity of 5 m/s, and the other is parabolic with a peak velocity of 2.5 m/s. What is the patient's diagnosis?
A. Severe AS
B. Severe AS and HOCM
C. HOCM with mild–moderate AS
D. Hypertensive cardiomyopathy with mild–moderate AS

Question 4. What is the next step for the patient of Question 3?
A. TEE
B. Right and left heart catheterization with maneuvers + coronary angiography
C. Myectomy

Question 5. What is the best treatment for the patient of Question 3?
A. Myectomy
B. Myectomy + MVR
C. Myectomy + AVR
D. Alcohol septal ablation
E. C or D

Question 6. Patient X has a mid-systolic murmur that drastically increases after a pause (on the beat that follows a pause). His radial pulse, however, decreases after this pause. Patient Y has a mid-systolic murmur that increases after a pause (less than patient X); his radial pulse also increases in intensity after the pause.
A. Patient X has HOCM, patient Y has AS
B. Patient X has AS, patient Y has HOCM

Question 7. A 72-year-old man presents with dyspnea, NYHA class III. He has asymmetric septal hypertrophy (~19 mm) with SAM of the anterior leaflet. The LVOT gradient is 25 mmHg at rest and rises to 130 mmHg with Valsalva. He has severe MR at rest, directed anteriorly. Beside the anterior leaflet elongation, the posterior leaflet is excessively elongated and overrides the anterior leaflet. He does not have CAD. What is the best strategy?
A. Alcohol septal ablation
B. Septal myectomy
C. Septal myectomy + MV repair
D. No septal ablation as the gradient at rest is <50 mmHg

Question 8. Which statement concerning myectomy vs. alcohol septal ablation is *incorrect*?

A. The reduction of gradient after alcohol septal ablation is less immediate than after myectomy. Some of the gradient declines immediately, but the gradient reduction may take 12 months to catch with myectomy.

B. RBBB is common after alcohol septal ablation (60%). Thus, alcohol ablation is not favored in patients with underlying LBBB

C. LBBB is common after myectomy (~40%)

D. Transient complete AV block is common after alcohol ablation (~50%), and typically develops within 72 hours. This justifies placing a temporary pacing wire before alcohol ablation in all patients, and leaving it for 72 hours

E. The risk of lethal ventricular arrhythmias is similar with alcohol septal ablation vs. myectomy

Answer 1. D. The differential diagnosis includes genetic HOCM (elderly presentation), hypertensive cardiomyopathy, or discrete upper septal thickening in the hypertensive elderly. An ancillary sign of HTN is present (CKD), yet this does not rule out HOCM. HOCM is the likely diagnosis in light of SAM and the severe gradient >100 mmHg. HOCM may be difficult to distinguish from hypertensive obstructive cardiomyopathy; in fact, in a genetic HOCM patient, the phenotype of HOCM is more readily expressed if severe HTN is present. For practical purposes, severe LVH with LVOT obstruction and SAM is pathophysiologically considered HOCM and treated as such. Before considering ablative therapies, the medical regimen needs to be optimized. HCTZ (preload reduction) and lisinopril (afterload reduction) aggravate the gradient and symptoms in HOCM. The discontinuation of those drugs may drastically improve symptoms.

Answer 2. B. The patient has refractory symptoms and a gradient >50 mmHg despite proper medical therapy. Myectomy is the first-line ablative therapy, unless the surgical risk is high. Moreover, in a patient with LBBB, alcohol septal ablation will lead to RBBB in 50–60% of the cases and thus complete AV block.

Answer 3. C. The exam suggests HOCM and AS. The holosystolic dynamic murmur at the LLSB and apex is the combination of HOCM and its MR murmur. The murmur that radiates to the carotids is not characteristic of HOCM, and rather implies AS. The normal S_2 and the normal carotid upstroke imply that AS is not severe. The echo confirms this diagnosis. The two envelopes within the LVOT CW Doppler correspond to the LVOT envelope (dagger-shaped) and AS envelope (parabolic). The LVOT velocity is very high, implying severe HOCM obstruction rather than AS obstruction. The severity of the SAM and the gradient suggests HOCM rather than hypertensive cardiomyopathy.

Answer 4. B. An end-hole catheter is positioned in the LV and pulled back slowly across the LVOT and aortic valve, allowing the measurement of the LVOT gradient (between LV and LVOT) and the AS gradient (between LVOT and aorta). This study is performed and confirms the severity of the LVOT gradient (peak-to-peak 100 mmHg), and the rather mild AS gradient (peak-to-peak 18 mmHg, AVA 1.5 cm² using Gorlin's equation). Since most of the gradient is determined to be across the LVOT, simultaneous LV–aortic recording is subsequently performed using a double-lumen pigtail catheter, and maneuvers are performed. Coronary angiography is necessary to see if a large proximal septal branch is available for alcohol septal ablation. Conversely, extensive CAD would favor CABG+ myectomy. TEE may be performed to calculate the AVA by planimetry and determine the severity of AS, but has a lower yield than catheterization.

Answer 5. E. The MR is severe but posteriorly directed, suggesting it is purely related to SAM. Unless posterior leaflet prolapse is present (anterior or central jet), MR usually resolves with septal ablation. The patient has moderate AS by catheterization, and thus, *if* he is undergoing cardiac surgery, AVR would be reasonable (class IIa). Note that the AS gradient will increase once the LVOT obstruction is relieved (aortic flow will increase → gradient increases). Yet this non-severe AS should not necessarily drive the choice between myectomy or alcohol septal ablation. Alcohol septal ablation is an acceptable option, especially in a patient >65 years old with a septal thickness <30 mm and no LBBB.

Answer 6. A. This case illustrates how the Brockenbrough phenomenon may be assessed by physical exam.

Answer 7. C. The patient has LVOT gradient >50 mmHg (rest or stress) and septal thickness >15 mm; thus, he qualifies for septal ablation. As opposed to the patient in Question 3, this patient has abnormalities of the posterior mitral leaflet and an anteriorly directed MR, implying a form of primary MR (this MR is not simply secondary to SAM). Septal reduction, per se, will not abolish MR

Answer 8. E.

References

1. Maron BJ, McKenna WJ, Danielson GK, et al. ACC/ESC expert consensus document on hypertrophic cardiomyopathy. J Am Coll Cardiol 2003; 42: 1687–713.
2. Wigle ED, Rakowski H, Kimball BP, et al. Hypertrophic cardiomyopathy: clinical spectrum and treatment. Circulation 1995; 92: 1680–92.
3. Shapiro LM, McKenna WJ. Distribution of left ventricular hypertrophy in hypertrophic cardiomyopathy: a two-dimentional echocardiography study. J Am Coll Cardiol 1983; 2: 437–44.
4. Louie EK, Maron BJ. Hypertrophic cardiomyopathy with extreme increase in left ventricular wall thickness: functional and morphologic features and clinical significance. J Am Coll Cardiol 1986; 8: 57–65.
5. Yu EHC, Omran AS, Wigle ED, et al. Mitral regurgitation in hypertrophic obstructive cardiomyopathy: relationship to obstruction and relief with myectomy. J Am Coll Cardiol 2000; 36: 2219–25.
6. Grigg LE, Wigle ED, Williams WG, Daniel LB, Rakowski H. Transesophageal Doppler echocardiography in obstructive hypertrophic cardiomyopathy: clarification of pathophysiology and importance in intraoperative decision making. J Am Coll Cardiol 1992; 20: 42–52.
7. Fifer MA, Vlahakes GJ. Management of symptoms in hypertrophic cardiomyopathy. Circulation 2008; 117: 429–39.
8. Schwammenthal E, Nakatani S, He S, et al. Mechanism of mitral regurgitation in hypertrophic cardiomyopathy: mismatch of posterior to anterior leaflet length and mobility. Circulation 1998; 98: 856–65.
9. Maron BJ, Casey SA, Pollac LC, et al. Clinical course of hypertrophic cardiomyopathy in a regional United States cohort. JAMA 1999; 281: 650–5.
10. Maron BJ. Hypertrophic cardiomyopathy: a systematic review. JAMA 2002; 287: 1308–20.
11. Maron MS, Olivotto I, Betocchi S, et al. Effect of left ventricular outflow tract obstruction on clinical outcome in hypertrophic cardiomyopathy. N Engl J Med 2003; 348: 295–303.

12. Ommen SR, Maron BJ, Olivetto I, et al. Long-term effects of surgical septal myectomy on survival in patients with obstructive hypertrophic cardiomyopathy. J Am Coll Cardiol 2005; 46: 470–6.

13. Sorajja P, Nishimura RA, Gersh BJ, et al. Outcome of mildly symptomatic or asymptomatic obstructive hypertrophic cardiomyopathy. A long-term follow-up study. J Am Coll Cardiol 2009; 54: 234–41. *In this study study of class I (60%) or class II patients, a severe resting gradient (peak velocity >4 m/s) was associated with a striking increase in mortality and HF. A less severe gradient was neutral on mortality.*

14. Desai MY, Bhonsale A, Patel P, et al. Exercise echocardiography in asymptomatic HCM. Exercise capacity, and not LV outflow tract gradient predicts long-term outcomes. JACC Cardiovasc Imaging 2014; 7: 26–36. *In this study of patients who are asymptomatic or minimally symptomatic, resting or stress LVOT gradient up to 100 mmHg did not appear to predict outcomes; rather, a limited exercise capacity on treadmill testing (<85% of predicted METs) predicted adverse outcomes in those presumably asymptomatic patients.*

15. Maron BJ, Olivotto I, Spirito P, et al. Epidemiology of hypertrophic cardiomyopathy-related death : revisited in a large non-referral-based patient population. Circulation 2000; 102: 858–64.

16. Lafitte S, Reant P, Touche C, et al. Paradoxical response to exercise in asymptomatic hypertrophic cardiomyopathy. J Am Coll Cardiol 2013; 62: 842–50.

17. Pellikka P, Oh J, Bailey K, et al. Dynamic intraventricular obstruction during dobutamine stress echocardiography. A new observation. Circulation 1992; 86: 1429–32.

18. Luria D, Klutstein MW, Rosenmann D, et al. Prevalence and significance of left ventricular outflow gradient during dobutamine echocardiography. Eur Heart J 1999; 20: 386–92.

19. Gersh BJ, Maron BJ, Bonow RO, et al. 2011 ACCF/AHA Guideline for the diagnosis and treatment of hypertrophic cardiomyopathy. J Am Coll Cardiol 2011; 58: e212–60.

20. Topol EJ, Traill TA, Foruin NJ. Hypertensive hypertrophic cardiomyopathy of the elderly. N Engl J Med 1985; 312: 277–82.

21. Pearson AC, Gudipati CV, Labovitz A. Systolic and diastolic flow abnormalities in elderly patients with hypertensive hypertrophic cardiomyopathy. J Am Coll Cardiol 1988; 12: 989–95. *Describes 28 consecutive patients with HTN, old >65 (mean 75) and significant LVH with small cavity. Most of them had dagger-shaped elevated velocity, mean septum 16 mm. SAM rare, ~like Ref. 20*

22. Lewis J, Maron B. Diversity of patterns of hypertrophy in patients with systemic hypertension and marked left ventricular wall thickening. Am J Cardiol 1990; 65: 874–81. *Thirty-four percent of asymmetry in severe LVH in hypertensive patients, mean peak SBP 200, DBP 110.*

23. Wicker P, Roudaut R, Haissaguere M, et al. Prevalence and significance of asymmetric septal hypertrophy in hypertension: An echocardiographic and clinical study. Eur Heart J 1983; 4 (suppl G): 1–5.

24. Kansal S, Roitman D, Sheffield LT. Interventricular septal thickness and left ventricular hypertrophy: an echocardiographic study. Circulation 1979; 60: 1058–65.

25. Karam R, Lever HM, Healy BP. Hypertensive hypertrophic cardiomyopathy or hypertrophic cardiomyopathy with hypertension? J Am Coll Cardiol 1989; 13: 580–4. ***A study of 78 patients with HOCM morphology (>15 mm with SAM and gradient at rest or exertion) and HTN vs. patients with HOCM morphology and no HTN: both have the same echo features, implying that HTN is not the main cause of the hypertrophy in those patients.***

26. Aurigemma G, Battista S, Orsinelli D, et al. Abnormal left ventricular intracavitary flow acceleration in patients undergoing aortic valve replacement for aortic stenosis. Circulation 1992; 86: 926–36.

27. Kayalar N, Schaff HV, Daly RC, et al. Concomitant septal myectomy at the time of aortic valve replacement for severe aortic stenosis. Ann Thorac Surg 2010; 89: 459–64.

28. Stenson R, Flamm M, Harrison D, Hancock E. Hypertrophic subaortic stenosis. Clinical and hemodynamic effects of long-term propranolol therapy. Am J Cardiol 1973; 31: 763–73.

29. Adelman A, Shah P, Gramiak R, Wigle E. Long-term propranolol therapy in muscular subaortic stenosis. Br Heart J 1979; 32: 804–11.

30. Sherrid MV, Barac I, McKenna WJ, et al. Multicenter study of the efficacy and safety of disopyramide in obstructive hypertrophic cardiomyopathy. J Am Coll Cardiol 2005; 45: 1251–8.

31. Olivotto I, Cecchi F, Casey SA, et al. Impact of atrial fibrillation on the clinical course of hypertrophic cardiomyopathy. Circulation 2001; 104: 2517–24.

32. Maron BJ, Nishimura RA, McKenna WJ, et al. Assessment of permanent dual-chamber pacing as a treatment for drug-refractory symptomatic patients with obstructive hypertrophic cardiomyopathy: a randomized, double-blind, crossover study (M-PATHY). Circulation 1999; 99: 2927–33.

33. Nishimura RA, Trusty JM, Hayes DL, et al. Dual-chamber pacing for hypertrophic cardiomyopathy: a randomized, double-blind, crossover trial. J Am Coll Cardiol 1997; 29: 435–41.

34. Patel P, Dhillon A, Popovic ZB, et al. Left ventricular outflow tract obstruction in hypertrophic cardiomyopathy patients without severe septal hypertrophy: implications of mitral valve and papillary muscle abnormalities assessed using cardiac magnetic resonance and echocardiography. Circ Cardiovasc Imaging 2015; 8: e003132.

35. Sorajja P, Valeti U, Nishimura RA, et al. Outcome of alcohol septal ablation for obstructive hypertrophic cardiomyopathy. Circulation 2008; 118: 131–9.

36. Kwon DH, Kapadia SR, Tuzcu EM, et al. Long-term outcomes in high-risk symptomatic patients with hypertrophic cardiomyopathy undergoing alcohol septal ablation. JACC Cardiovasc Interv 2008; 4: 432–8.

37. Sorraja P, Binder J, Nishimura RA. Predictors of an optimal clinical outcome with alcohol septal ablation for obstructive hypertrophic cardiomyopathy. Cath Cardiovasc Interv 2013; 81: 58–67.

38. ten Cate FJ, Soliman OI, Michels M, et al. Long-term outcome of alcohol septal ablation in patients with obstructive hypertrophic cardiomyopathy: a word of caution. Circ Heart Fail 2010; 3: 362–9. *Alcohol ablation of patients without ICD is associated with a significant increase in the long-term risk of sudden death (~14% at 5 years).*

39. Kovacic JC, Khanna D, Kaplish D, et al. Safety and efficacy of alcohol septal ablation in patients with symptomatic concentric left ventricular hypertrophy and outflow tract obstruction. J Invasive Cardiol 2010; 22: 586–91.

40. Veselka J, Tomasov P, Zemanek D. Mid-term outcomes of alcohol septal ablation for obstructive hypertrophic cardiomyopathy in patients with sigmoid versus neutral ventricular septum. J Inv Cardiol 2012; 24: 636–40.

41. Naidu SS. Rethinking the selection criteria for alcohol septal ablation: is it time to push the envelope? J Inv Cardiol 2010; 22: 592–3.

42. Maron BJ, Spirito P, Shen WK, et al. Implantable cardioverter defibrillators and prevention of sudden cardiac death in hypertrophic cardiomyopathy. JAMA 2007; 298: 405–12.

43. Elliott PM, Poloniecki J, Dickie S, et al. Sudden death in hypertrophic cardiomyopathy: identification of high risk patients. J Am Coll Cardiol 2000; 36: 2212–18.

44. Spirito P, Autore C, Rapezzi C, et al. Syncope and risk of sudden death in hypertrophic cardiomyopathy. Circulation 2009; 119: 1703–10.

Part 5   ARRHYTHMIAS AND ELECTROPHYSIOLOGY

8   Approach to Narrow and Wide QRS Complex Tachyarrhythmias

I. The unstable patient (shock, acute pulmonary edema)

In a hemodynamically unstable patient with supraventricular tachyarrhythmia (shock or severe HF), **always ask yourself: did the tachyarrhythmia cause the shock or did the shock cause an increase in heart rate with a secondary SVT or AF?** Typically, **to attribute a shock to SVT or AF, the heart rate must be >150 bpm.** In addition, clinical features suggestive of another primary process should be sought (sepsis, acute bleed/severe anemia, tamponade, massive PE); in these cases, tachycardia is not the isolated cause of the instability, it is rather the consequence.

For example, in a patient with BP 75/50 mmHg and AF rate of 125 bpm, AF is likely secondary to the shock rather the cause of the shock.

If a tachyarrhythmia faster than 150 bpm is assumed to be the cause of instability, emergent DC cardioversion should be performed.

II. Initial approach to any tachycardia

When analyzing a tachycardia, start by looking at three features:

1. Narrow QRS vs. wide QRS (≥120 ms) (choose the lead where QRS is widest)
2. Regular vs. irregular ventricular rate
3. Look for P waves and their relationship with QRS complexes. P waves are usually seen as notches or deflections that fall over the ST–T segments and have a *consistent morphology* and *timing*, i.e., those deflections are regularly placed and can be marched out. Try to confirm that these deflections are P waves, rather than artifacts or parts of T wave, by analyzing multiple leads. Once P waves are found, their relationship with QRS complexes is analyzed.

P waves are often best seen in lead II, which is generally parallel to the spread of atrial depolarization; and in the lead where T and QRS are smallest (opening up room to see the scattered P waves).

In wide QRS tachycardia, analyze: (i) AV dissociation, and (ii) the number of P waves compared to the number of QRS complexes. In narrow QRS tachycardia, assess the length of the RP interval.

Practical Cardiovascular Medicine, First Edition. Elias B. Hanna.
© 2017 John Wiley & Sons Ltd. Published 2017 by John Wiley & Sons Ltd.

III. Approach to narrow QRS complex tachycardias (see Figures 8.1, 8.2)

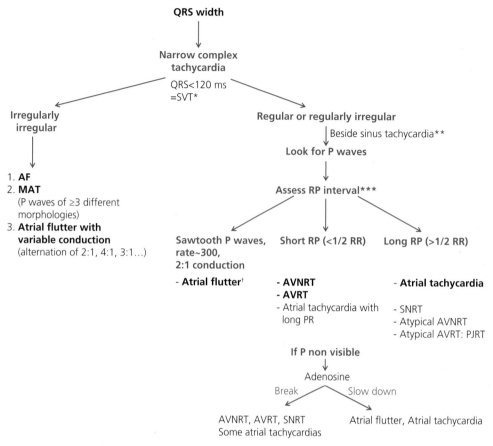

Figure 8.1 Approach to narrow QRS complex tachycardias.

*A narrow QRS tachycardia may occasionally be VT. If QRS is relatively narrow (~110–120 ms) but different in morphology from the baseline QRS, consider it VT or SVT with aberrancy.

**As opposed to other tachycardias, sinus tachycardia has a gradual onset and termination and does not have a fixed rate. *Tachyarrhythmias typically have a sudden onset and offset and a very fixed rate, although they may have a quick warm-up at the beginning*. For example, a tachycardia with a fixed rate of 122 bpm on a telemetry monitor suggests arrhythmia. The P wave of atrial tachycardia or SNRT may have a sinus P-wave morphology; the abrupt onset and the steady rate help differentiate these arrhythmias from sinus tachycardia.

***RP interval points to the interval between onset of QRS and onset of the following P wave. The P wave may be a retrograde P wave in AVNRT or AVRT. If this interval is <1/2 of the R–R interval, the tachycardia is a short RP tachycardia. A very short RP interval, i.e. < 90 ms, is diagnostic of AVNRT.

†**Atrial flutter** may mimic short RP tachycardia if only the flutter wave following the QRS is seen, or may mimic long RP tachycardia/atrial tachycardia if only the flutter wave preceding the QRS is seen. *Atrial tachycardia with negative P waves preceding the QRS complexes in the inferior leads may, in fact, be atrial flutter.* Look carefully for flutter waves to make the diagnosis.

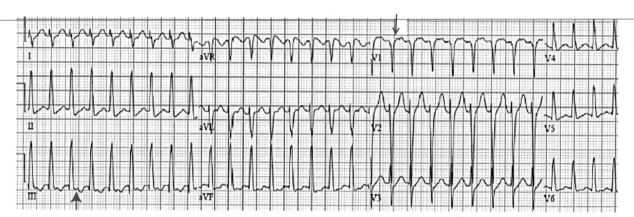

Figure 8.2 Narrow complex tachycardia, regular, rate ~200 bpm. Differential diagnosis: AVNRT, AVRT, atrial tachycardia with 1:1 conduction, or atrial flutter with 2:1 conduction.

1. Look for P waves: Ps are seen in leads III, aVF, and V$_1$ (*arrows*).

2. The RP interval is <1/2 R-R interval, so it is a short RP tachycardia. It is, thus, either AVNRT or AVRT. If RP interval is very short (<90 ms), and if P falls within or immediately past the QRS, looking like pseudo-S in the inferior leads or pseudo-r′ in V$_1$, the tachycardia is AVNRT rather than AVRT. On this ECG, RP is >90 ms, and therefore either AVNRT or AVRT is possible

IV. Approach to wide QRS complex tachycardias

The differential diagnosis of a wide QRS complex tachycardia includes:

1. VT.

2. SVT (including AF) with aberrancy. Aberrancy signifies the occurrence of a functional RBBB, LBBB, or RBBB+LAFB during a supraventricular tachycardia, leading to a wide complex morphology simulating VT. Aberrancy occurs when the refractory period of one of the bundles or fascicles is surpassed during the tachycardia (Figure 8.3). In addition, SVT with bundle branch block can be due to a pre-existing bundle branch block, in which case the QRS morphology during the tachycardia is similar to the QRS morphology during the sinus rhythm, sometimes slightly wider.

3. SVT (especially AF) with pre-excitation (Figure 8.4). This means that the SVT is conducted antegradely over an accessory pathway that connects one atrium to one ventricle, short-circuiting the AV node.

4. Other diagnoses: hyperkalemia; drug toxicity (class I antiarrhythmic agents, tricyclics); ventricular pacemaker tracking an atrial arrhythmia (lack of mode switch), or pacemaker- mediated tachycardia.

A wide complex tachycardia that is very grossly irregular is AF: AF with aberrancy, AF with pre-excitation, or AF with class I antiarrhythmic drug therapy. Polymorphic VT is a distant second possibility. On the other hand, a slightly irregular rhythm, with only slight variations of the R–R interval, may be seen with VT or any SVT at its onset (the first 20 beats).

A wide complex tachycardia is not necessarily "wide" (≥120 ms), as VT or aberrancy originating high in the septum near the His bundle or the bundle branches may be 110–120 ms wide, even narrower than a wide baseline QRS. The QRS morphology during tachycardia is, however, different from the baseline QRS morphology. *In particular, in patients with a wide baseline QRS, a tachycardia with a narrower QRS is VT.*

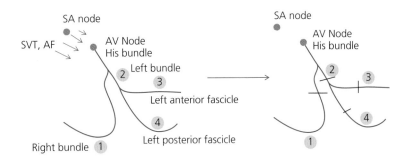

When rapid atrial activity reaches the bundles, one of these bundles or fascicles gets "tired" and blocks, leading to a functional bundle branch block = SVT with aberrancy

Figure 8.3 Explanation of how a wide QRS complex (aberrancy) may occur with SVT. RBBB, LBBB, or RBBB+LAFB may be seen. RBBB+LPFB is rare.

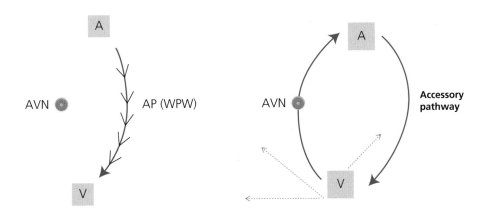

Atrial arrhythmia with pre-excitation

Antidromic AVRT

Figure 8.4 There are two types of SVT with pre-excitation, i.e., SVT with antegrade conduction over an accessory pathway (WPW syndrome):
- AF or any atrial arrhythmia with pre-excitation. The atrial waves are preferentially conducted through the fast accessory pathway, leading to a very fast ventricular rate.
- Antidromic AVRT. The electrical stimulus spreads down through the accessory pathway then up through the AV node. The ventricles get depolarized through the pre-excited ventricle (*dashed arrows*), not through the His bundle, and thus have a wide QRS morphology.

Approximately 80% of wide complex tachycardias are VTs (95% in case of CAD or HF). Thus, if one is unsure of the diagnosis, it is safer to consider the arrhythmia VT than SVT and treat it as such. However, it is best to look for features characteristic of VT and establish a definitive diagnosis.

V. Features characteristic of VT, as opposed to SVT with aberrancy

A. Four features are most helpful in differentiating VT from SVT. The presence of any one VT feature is immediately diagnostic of VT

a. *The presence of AV dissociation*. AV dissociation is characterized by P waves that do not have any consistent relationship with the QRS complexes. In tachycardia, AV dissociation is ~100% specific for VT. AV association, on the other hand, does not necessarily imply SVT and may be seen with VT. In fact, retrograde ventriculoatrial (VA) conduction is seen in ~25% of VTs, especially VTs slower than 170 bpm, leading to retrograde P waves that are regularly associated with the QRS complexes. This manifests as 1:1 AV association (1:1 retrograde conduction) that is indistinguishable from SVT. At times, other ratios of VA conduction may be seen (e.g., two QRS complexes with one P wave, three QRS complexes with two P waves), in which the number of QRS complexes is greater than the number of P waves, implying VT.

Thus, VT is diagnosed if either: (i) AV dissociation is present, or (ii) QRS complexes outnumber P waves (with AV association or AV dissociation). *P waves are often best seen in lead II, which is generally parallel to the spread of atrial depolarization, or leads with the smallest QRS and T wave.*

b. *QRS morphology*. A QRS morphology that is not consistent with a typical RBBB, LBBB, or RBBB + LAFB is characteristic of VT. In particular, a *QS or Qr pattern in V_4–V_6, i.e., deep Q wave in V_4–V_6, is particularly suggestive of VT.* In addition, in bundle branch blocks, the initial portion of the QRS complex corresponds to the quick localized depolarization at or near the septum and thus is narrow (LBBB → rS in V_1 with a narrow r; RBBB → rSR' in V_1 with a narrow r). On the other hand, in VT, the electrical activity often starts away from the septum, and thus the initial QRS deflection is not narrow (Figures 8.5, 8.6, 8.7).

Note that VT that starts in the septum has a narrower QRS than free wall VT and may simulate LBBB or RBBB morphology (e.g., idiopathic left ventricular VT). Also, bundle branch reentrant VT (macroreentry down the right bundle and up the left bundle), rarely seen in dilated non-ischemic cardiomyopathy, may have a typical LBBB morphology.

c. *The onset of the tachycardia on ECG or telemetry monitor*. A tachycardia that starts with a PVC and has a morphology similar to this PVC is VT. A tachycardia that starts with a wide aberrant PAC and has a morphology similar to this aberrant PAC is SVT. Also, a tachycardia that is similar in morphology to a previous PVC is VT. A tachycardia that starts with a PVC but does not have the morphology of that PVC is likely VT, but may be SVT initiated by the PVC.

How to distinguish a PVC from an aberrant PAC? A wide QRS complex which coincidentally falls on the top of a regularly occurring sinus P wave is a PVC (the regularly occurring sinus P wave shows up as a "blip" within the PVC). PVC may also fall after the regular sinus P wave

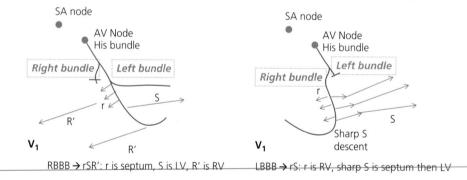

RBBB → rSR': r is septum, S is LV, R' is RV

LBBB → rS: r is RV, sharp S is septum then LV

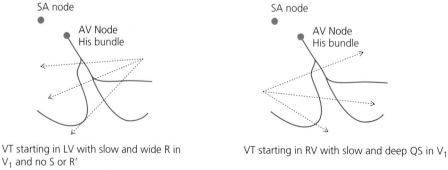

VT starting in LV with slow and wide R in V_1 and no S or R'

VT starting in RV with slow and deep QS in V_1

Figure 8.5 Difference in QRS morphology between bundle branch block and VT. The QRS description is in reference to lead V_1.

at a shorter PR distance. A PVC does not disrupt the underlying sinus/atrial rhythm, and P waves keep occurring regularly through it. On the other hand, an aberrantly conducted PAC starts after a premature and different-looking P wave that may fall within the preceding T wave and deform it. A deformation of the T wave preceding the premature complex suggests PAC.

d. *If the patient has a pre-existing RBBB or LBBB, or any intraventricular conduction delay, and the tachycardia has the* **exact morphology of the baseline QRS**, *the tachycardia is SVT.*

Figures 8.5 to 8.12 illustrate these concepts.

B. Other features (again, the presence of any one feature is suggestive of VT)

a. *Brugada criteria*. The Brugada criteria include four features, two of which have already been discussed: (1) AV dissociation, (2) QRS morphology inconsistent with a typical RBBB or LBBB, (3) onset of R-to-nadir of S >100 ms in any precordial lead, (4) monophasic QRS concordance in all precordial leads. The presence of *any one of these* is diagnostic of VT with a high sensitivity and specificity (~98%). The *lack of all four* is diagnostic of SVT with a high sensitivity and specificity (~98%).

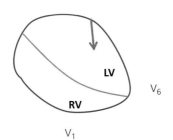

VT originating posteriorly. All QRSs in V$_1$–V$_6$ have a monophasic R morphology (positive concordance)

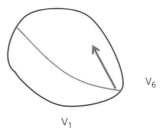

VT originating anteriorly close to the apex or at the distal septum. All QRSs in V$_1$–V$_6$ have a monophasic QS morphology (negative concordance)

Figure 8.6 QRS morphology when VT originates in the posterior wall or the apical wall.

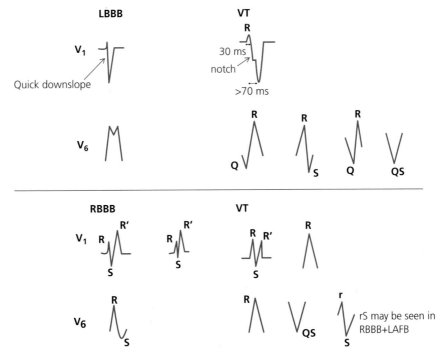

Figure 8.7 Differences in morphology between SVT with aberrancy and VT. SVT with aberrancy has a typical LBBB or RBBB morphology. Conversely, VT is suggested by:
- LBBB with a wide initial R wave >30 ms, R-to-nadir of S >70 ms, or notched S descent in V$_1$; or Q wave in V$_6$.
- RBBB with a wide R pattern in V$_1$ instead of RSR', R >R' in V$_1$, or monophasic R or QS in V$_6$. RBBB with a left axis or with a rS pattern in V$_6$ does not necessarily imply VT (could be RBBB + LAFB).

While rS pattern in V$_6$ is not typical of LBBB or RBBB, it may be seen with atypical LBBB (enlarged LV) or RBBB + LAFB. **Deep Q in V$_6$ (QS or Qr) implies VT.** Left QRS axis may be seen with LBBB or RBBB + LAFB. Right QRS axis, on the other hand, is not typically seen with either LBBB or RBBB and usually implies VT.

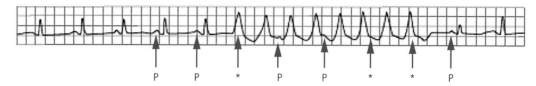

Figure 8.8 Run of wide complex tachycardia on a telemetry strip: is it VT or SVT?
1. See how it starts: the first wide complex is not preceded by any premature P wave and there is no deformation of the preceding T wave. This initial complex is a PVC, and the tachycardia has a morphology similar to this initial complex: this suggests that the tachycardia is VT.
2. Look for P waves. Some notches are visible inside the wide complex run. Try to march them out with the preceding and following sinus P waves → they do march out at the same rate as the sinus P rate, independently of the wide complex rhythm and scattered inside it. Some P waves are hidden within QRSs and cannot be seen (marked with an *asterisk* [*]). The two visible P waves that are dissociated from the QRS complexes imply AV dissociation, characteristic of VT.
3. The initial upslope of the wide QRS complex is slower and less steep than the upslope of the baseline QRS. This is suggestive of VT.

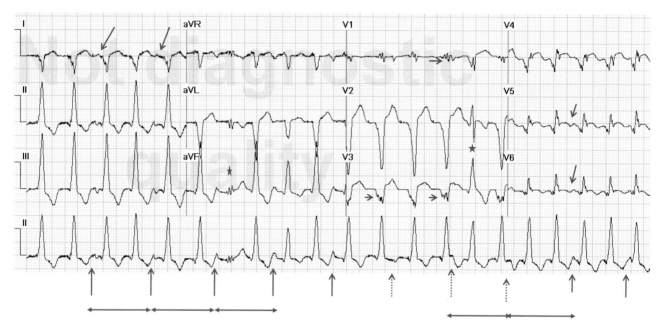

Figure 8.9 Wide complex tachycardia: VT or SVT?
1. Look for P waves, i.e., look for scattered "blips" that: (a) have a consistent morphology and timing, and (b) can be marched out. Blips are seen in lead II (*vertical arrows*). These blips can be marched out (*calipers*) and have a consistent morphology; they are not part of the T wave, as they do not consistently fall on every T wave. They are also seen in other leads (I, V_5, V_6, *arrows*), further adding to the evidence that these are P waves, not artifacts or parts of T wave. They do not have a consistent relationship with the QRS complexes, and some of them fall inside the QRS complexes and are not seen (*dashed arrows*). Thus, P waves are dissociated from QRS complexes and are less numerous than QRS complexes. This is diagnostic of VT. **The variable T-wave morphology is usually a hint to the presence of P waves that are dissociated from QRS/T and falling variably over some T waves.**
2. Analyse QRS morphology. QRS has a LBBB-like morphology in lead V_2. However, there is a QR pattern in V_5–V_6, QS pattern in lead I, and right-axis deviation (QRS negative in lead I), not consistent with LBBB. Besides, QRS has excessive notching, best seen in leads V_1 and V_3 (*horizontal arrows*). Thus, this is VT.
3. Additional findings:
- Wide QRS complexes of different morphology are scattered within the tachycardia (*stars*). Those may represent fusion complexes or PVCs. Being wide, they have no diagnostic value.
- ST-segment elevation, concordant with QRS, is seen in the anterolateral leads. This is concerning for STEMI.

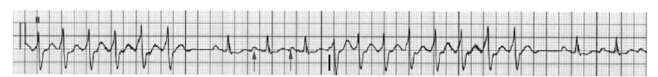

Figure 8.10 Two short tachycardia runs. The tachycardia starts after a regularly occurring sinus P wave (*bar*) at a shorter PR interval (the *bar* marches out with the *arrows*). This is typical of a PVC, which occurs without disrupting the timing of the underlying sinus P waves. PAC would have started with a premature P wave. Thus, the tachycardia starts with a PVC and has the same morphology as the PVC. This is VT.

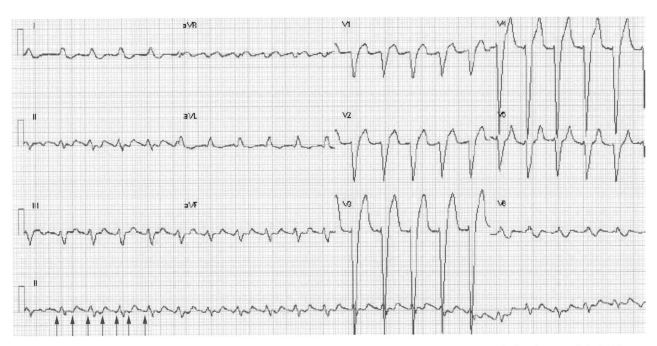

Figure 8.11 Wide complex, regular tachycardia, at a rate of ~135 bpm. QRS looks narrow in some leads; this is due to the fact that part of the QRS is isoelectric in those leads. That is why QRS should be measured in the lead where it is widest. QRS is wide (~140 ms) in lead V_3 in particular.

1. QRS looks like a typical LBBB in leads I, aVL, and V_1. This suggests SVT with LBBB aberrancy.

2. P waves are seen. A negative P wave is overlying the ST–T segment and another P wave is just preceding QRS (*arrows*); these deflections are recognized as P waves, as opposed to being fragments of T wave, by the fact that they have a *consistent morphology* and can be *marched out*. Thus, this tachycardia is an atrial tachyarrhythmia with 2:1 AV conduction, the atrial rate being 270. The atrial rate (>240) as well as the sawtooth shape seen in leads II and aVR and the lack of isoelectric baseline make the diagnosis atrial flutter.

Final diagnosis: Atrial flutter with 2:1 AV conduction and wide QRS due to LBBB aberrancy.

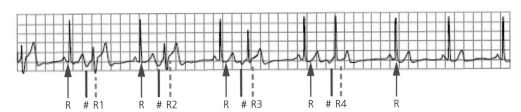

Figure 8.12 The baseline rhythm is sinus, consisting of QRS complexes (R) preceded by sinus P waves. Outside these complexes, there are premature complexes occurring in a bigeminal pattern (R1, R2, R3, R4). These could be PVCs or PACs with aberrancy. Look for P waves preceding these complexes: there is a P wave before each complex, marked #. It is an inverted, non-sinus P wave and occurs prematurely. This means that R1–R4 are PACs with aberrancy rather than PVCs. These PACs have aberrant conduction because they occur very prematurely, while the right bundle is still in its refractory period, which leads to RBBB morphology. Note that the aberrancy (QRS widening) is less pronounced when PAC is less premature. This is a form of ***Ashman's phenomenon***. R–R1 interval <R–R3 interval <R–R4 interval; hence, R4 is not aberrant.

Monophasic QRS concordance in the precordial leads signifies that all QRS complexes in V_1 through V_6 are monophasic and pointing in the same direction, either upward or downward. In other words, these QRS complexes are either monophasic R or monophasic QS complexes. Concordance is not present if any of the six leads has a biphasic QRS (e.g., qR or RS complex).

b. ***Northwest axis or right axis***. The typical forms of aberrancy, LBBB, RBBB, or RBBB+LAFB, are not associated with a right axis (RBBB may be associated with a right axis when RVH coexists, as seen on the baseline ECG). On the other hand, VT most frequently originates from the ventricle with the largest mass, i.e., LV, and therefore frequently has a right axis.

c. *In patients with a wide baseline QRS (LBBB or RBBB or non-specific intraventricular conduction delay),* **a tachycardia that is wide but narrower than the baseline QRS is VT.** Aberrancy can only widen QRS, not narrow it, whereas VT may paradoxically be narrower than the baseline rhythm. Also, a tachycardia with a bundle branch block morphology contralateral to a baseline bundle branch block is usually VT (e.g., in a patient with RBBB at baseline, a tachycardia with LBBB morphology is VT).

d. **QRS >160 ms suggests VT if the baseline QRS is narrow** and in the absence of class I antiarrhythmic drug therapy.

e. ***Presence of capture or fusion complexes***. When an impulse originating from the sinus node conducts down the AV node and captures the ventricles, instead of allowing the VT focus to capture the ventricles, the complex that results is a *capture complex squeezed within the VT*. If this impulse partially captures the ventricles, while the VT focus partially captures the rest of the ventricles, the resulting complex is a *fusion complex*. A capture complex has the same morphology as the baseline sinus beat, while a fusion complex has a morphology intermediate between the sinus beat and VT. A fusion complex may start like the sinus-originating beat and terminate like the VT beat, or vice versa. *Only when the beat squeezed in the tachycardia is narrow can one be certain that it is a capture or a fusion complex.* A QRS complex that is wide but of different morphology than the tachycardia (narrower or not) may be a fusion complex in a patient with VT or a PVC in a patient with SVT or VT.

f. *In VT, the QRS complex is wide in its initial portion and has a slow initial upslope or downslope*. Conversely, in SVT with aberration, QRS has a narrow initial deflection that corresponds to the septal depolarization, followed by widening of the terminal QRS portion. In addition, in VT, the impulse frequently spreads over a diseased, fibrotic myocardium and meets "bumps" on the road, creating *atypical notching of the QRS complex* (notching of S descent or R wave, different from bundle branch block).

g. *In aVR, VT is suggested by: (i) dominant, large or wide initial R wave (R or RS complex), or (ii) QR pattern with a slowly downsloping Q wave >40ms.* Normally, aVR consists of a sharp and deep negative deflection, sometimes preceded or followed by a small r wave (QS, rS, or Qr pattern).

VI. Features characteristic of SVT with pre-excitation

Once a diagnosis of VT is made using the above criteria of VT vs. aberrant SVT, step back and consider the diagnosis of pre-excited SVT before closing. Since the ventricular stimulation does not spread down from the His bundle, the QRS morphology of a pre-excited SVT resembles the QRS morphology of VT, i.e., not a typical LBBB or RBBB morphology. The initial portion of QRS is slurred, but this is seen with VT as well (slow upslope) and does not help differentiate VT from pre-excited SVT. *Seeing the slurred delta wave on the baseline ECG is diagnostic of pre-excitation; seeing it during tachycardia implies VT or pre-excited SVT.*

The most typical SVT with pre-excitation is AF with pre-excitation. In this case, the wide tachycardia is irregular, implying AF rather than VT, with a differential diagnosis that includes AF with aberrancy. AF with pre-excitation is diagnosed when AF has VT morphological features; or when AF is wide and polymorphic (QRS varies in height and width), bizarre looking, or very fast (>200 bpm) (Figure 8.13).

- When AF has the morphological features of VT or is too fast (>200 bpm), consider pre-excited AF (WPW syndrome).
- Also, as opposed to AF with aberrancy, where the QRS becomes more aberrant and wider after a shorter R–R interval (Ashman's phenomenon), pre-excitation may become more evident and the QRS may become wider after a longer R–R interval that allows recovery of the accessory pathway's refractory period.

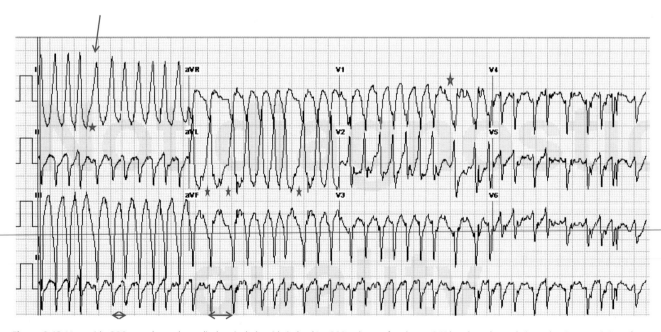

Figure 8.13 Very wide QRS complex tachycardia (particularly wide in lead I, ~200 ms), very fast (rate ~240 bpm), and grossly irregular. Because it is so fast, it may initially seem regular; but on careful assessment one sees that R–R intervals are grossly irregular, with some R–R intervals being half the size of other R–R intervals, without any particular pattern (irregularly irregular) (*double arrows*).

Differential diagnosis:

1. VT: VT is usually regular or slightly irregular, not grossly irregular. However, it may be grossly irregular in case of **polymorphic VT**, which is a very fast VT that quickly degenerates into VF. This could be the case here.

2. Being irregular, this tachycardia is likely **AF with wide QRS** complexes. AF is wide in the case of **(a)** aberrancy, or **(b)** accessory pathway (WPW). Aberrancy is unlikely because QRS morphology does not fit with a typical RBBB or LBBB. In fact, QRSs are too wide and polymorphic, with some complexes being ~200 ms wide (*arrow*). Thus, this is AF with VT features, implying AF with conduction over an accessory pathway. Note that QRS gets wider when the R–R interval increases (*stars*), which is consistent with pre-excitation rather than aberrancy.

A regular SVT with pre-excitation is less common than AF with pre-excitation (e.g., antidromic AVRT, atrial tachycardia with pre-excitation). Since the QRS morphology simulates VT, other features help differentiate VT from SVT with pre-excitation:

- AV dissociation *or* QRS complexes outnumbering P waves ($\rightarrow$ VT).
- A predominantly negative QRS complex in leads V_4–V_6 implies ventricular activity originating close to the apex, and thus VT rather than pre-excitation, as the accessory pathway cannot be apical. For the same reason, negative monophasic concordance in all precordial leads can only be VT, not pre-excitation. Positive monophasic concordance may be seen in pre-excitation from a left posterior or lateral accessory pathway.

Acutely, AF or any other SVT with pre-excitation is treated as VT. The administration of AV nodal blocking agents that are typically used for AF, particularly calcium channel blockers or digoxin, may shorten the accessory pathway's refractory period and allow more atrial activity to conduct over the accessory pathway, thus leading to a faster rate. Give procainamide if the patient is stable, then perform DC cardioversion if the arrhythmia does not respond or if the patient is unstable.

Table 8.1 summarizes the approach to wide QRS complex tachycardias.

VII. Role of adenosine in establishing a diagnosis

Adenosine may help differentiate various types of SVT. AVNRT, AVRT, SNRT, and a subgroup of atrial tachycardias often totally break with adenosine, but they may remain unchanged or may slightly and transiently slow down if the slow pathway (AVNRT) or the AV node (AVRT) is slowed rather than blocked. Atrial flutter and most subgroups of atrial tachycardia usually do not break but develop AV block with adenosine, which slows the QRS rate and allows one to see and assess the hidden P waves and make the diagnosis (Figure 8.14). AV block during tachycardia (e.g., 2:1 conduction) excludes AVRT and makes AVNRT less likely. The AVRT loop is dependent on both the atrial and ventricular myocardium; thus, a drop of atrial or ventricular activity leads to cessation of the arrhythmia.

VT is not affected by adenosine (except idiopathic VT). While potentially helpful in distinguishing SVT from VT, adenosine IV or verapamil or diltiazem IV should be avoided in wide complex tachycardias of uncertain diagnosis, because these should be presumed VT and treated as such. Diltiazem, verapamil, or adenosine are vasodilators that can lead to hemodynamic collapse in case of VT, in which the patient's systemic pressure is merely maintained by vasoconstriction. They can also lead to rate acceleration and VF in case of WPW (i.e.,

Table 8.1 Summary of the approach to wide QRS complex tachycardia.

---

(1) VT vs. **(2)** SVT (including AF) with aberrancy vs. **(3)** SVT (especially AF) with pre-excitation

1. VT is the most likely diagnosis (>80%), especially if history of heart disease. **Features that further support VT**:
- P waves are seen scattered within QRS complexes or ST–T segments and are unrelated to QRS complexes (**AV dissociation**); and/or number of P waves <number of QRS complexes
- Morphology of QRS is not consistent with a typical LBBB or a typical RBBB
- Tachycardia onset with a PVC rather than a PAC (no premature P wave)
- Exam: variable pulse despite a regular rhythm, off-and-on cannon A waves on JVP exam

2. SVT with aberrancy: this diagnosis is most confidently made if a baseline bundle branch block is present and the tachycardia has the same morphology as this baseline block. Otherwise, the lack of any VT feature supports the diagnosis of SVT

    Also, if the wide complex tachycardia is very grossly irregular, AF with aberrancy or pre-excitation is the likely diagnosis, rather than VT (VT may be slightly irregular, but not grossly irregular).

3. AF with pre-excitation: tachycardia is irregular, polymorphic, bizarre looking. The QRS morphology is wide but not consistent with aberrancy (not a typical RBBB or LBBB)

A wide complex tachycardia that is very grossly irregular is AF: AF with aberrancy or AF with pre-excitation. Polymorphic VT is a less likely possibility

---

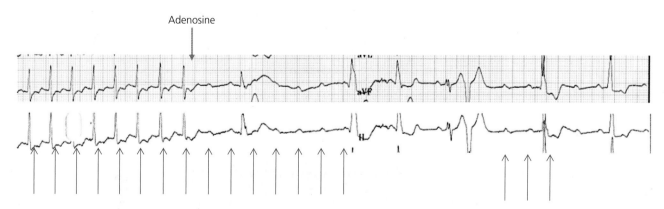

Figure 8.14 Short RP narrow complex tachycardia, initially suggestive of AVNRT or AVRT (*arrows* indicate P waves). After adenosine, the P waves keep marching out at the same rate unaffected by adenosine, while AV conduction is blocked and ventricular escape beats are seen. Thus, this is atrial tachycardia. Adenosine was helpful in establishing the diagnosis. Soon afterwards, the 1:1 AV conduction will resume.

SVT with pre-excitation). Adenosine can trigger AF in 12% of the treated patients, which destabilizes those with antegrade accessory pathway conduction.

VIII. Differential diagnosis of a wide complex tachycardia on a one-lead telemetry or Holter monitor strip

These features, selected from the preceding sections, suggest VT:

- AV dissociation.
- QRS >160 ms if the baseline QRS is narrow.
- Tachycardia similar in morphology to a prior PVC.
- Tachycardia starts with a PVC rather than a premature P wave and has the same morphology as the PVC.
- The initial portion of the wide QRS is wide, slurred or slow, sometimes with a notched descent. Conversely, the presence of a narrow initial deflection q or r (qR or rS, with narrow q or r <1 mm), or a fast downstroke of a QS pattern or a fast upstroke of an R pattern makes SVT more likely. In case of SVT with aberration, the QRS starts normal, then becomes slow, wide, and aberrant in its terminal portion.

IX. Various notes

A. Retrograde P wave

AVNRT and orthodromic AVRT have retrograde P waves, that is, negative P waves in the inferior leads II, III, and aVF. P waves may fall within the QRS or just after the QRS; P waves may not be visible if they fall within the QRS, as is common with AVNRT. VT may also lead to retrograde P waves; in fact, VA conduction, often 1:1 conduction, occurs in 25% of VTs.

P waves of atrial tachycardia may look retrograde in the case of a low atrial focus; otherwise, they are antegrade, upright in leads II, III, and aVF.

B. Ashman's phenomenon

Aberrancy of one or multiple consecutive beats can occur after a long–short QRS sequence in AF, or after a very premature PAC (Figure 8.12).

The QRS occurring at a short R–R interval may be wide and typically has an RBBB morphology, or RBBB+LAFB morphology. This is related to the fact that one of the bundles, often the right bundle, is still in a refractory period when the supraventricular stimulus comes early. The right bundle normally has a longer refractory period than the left bundle. A long R–R interval further prolongs the bundles' refractory period and makes a QRS that falls shortly after it aberrant (*long–short sequence*). The aberrancy may have an LBBB morphology, especially if the left bundle has underlying disease (such as incomplete LBBB). The aberrancy may be perpetuated for multiple beats, even if the R–R interval lengthens over the subsequent beats, as a result of the delayed trans-septal activation of the blocked bundle (see Chapter 13, Figure 13.25).

C. How the tachycardia starts

Looking at how the tachycardia starts helps distinguish VT from SVT in wide complex tachycardia, as discussed previously. A tachycardia that starts with a PVC and has the same QRS morphology as the PVC is VT; a tachycardia that starts with a PAC is usually SVT.

Once a diagnosis of SVT is made, whether narrow or wide SVT, focus on the P wave that initiates the tachycardia. If the premature P wave that starts the tachycardia has an identical morphology to the subsequent P waves of the tachycardia, and/or marches out with those subsequent P waves, the tachycardia is an atrial tachycardia (mainly the automatic form). However, if the P wave does not resemble subsequent P waves and does not march out with them, the tachycardia could be any SVT, including AVNRT, AVRT, or reentrant atrial tachycardia.

D. How the tachycardia ends

Examining how the tachycardia ends is helpful, although less so than examining how it starts:

- If it ends with a QRS complex – the tachycardia can be VT or any SVT.
- If it ends with a P wave – the tachycardia can be VT (with retrograde VA conduction), or any SVT except automatic atrial tachycardia. Automatic atrial tachycardia ends when the abnormal P wave vanishes rather than gets blocked. Reentrant atrial tachycardia or AVNRT ends when the slow pathway intrinsically slows down (vagal tone) or a PAC enters the reentry loop and blocks it (this PAC may or may not conduct to the ventricle).
- If it ends with a premature P wave, i.e., a P wave that does not march out with the P waves of the tachycardia and has a different morphology – the tachycardia is not VT. It can be any SVT except automatic atrial tachycardia.
- A tachycardia with 1:1 AV association that ends with a regularly occurring QRS, rather than P, is unlikely to be VT with 1:1 VA conduction.

E. Role of physical exam in the differential diagnosis of wide complex tachycardia

Two exam features are characteristic of AV dissociation and imply VT:

1. Cannon A waves on JVP exam. Forceful A waves are sometimes felt by the patient ("neck pounding") and imply that the atria and ventricles contract simultaneously. Regular, every-beat cannon A waves imply AVNRT, whereas *irregular cannon A waves imply AV dissociation (in this case, VT)*.

2. *Variable pulse and variable first heart sound despite a regular rhythm implies AV dissociation*. The variable pulse and variable first heart sound make VT mimic AF on exam; however, the monitored rhythm shows a regular rhythm, and this "irregular-sounding regular rhythm" is actually VT.

X. General management of SVT

A. Management of AF or atrial flutter (Table 8.2)

Table 8.2 Management of an acutely presenting, hemodynamically stable AF or atrial flutter.

1. Rate control
- If no acute systolic HF

  β-blocker (metoprolol 5 mg IV × 3 Q10min, then oral metoprolol)
  Diltiazem (0.25–0.35 mg/kg IV, then drip 5–15 mg/h, then oral diltiazem)

- If acute systolic HF

  Diuresis, ± digoxin and amiodarone

2. Start **acute anticoagulation** (UFH, LMWH)
3. 60% of acute AF cases spontaneously convert at 24 hours
   If AF persists at 24 hours, consider **TEE + DC cardioversion** (rhythm control for symptomatic AF)
+ Warfarin or novel oral anticoagulant for 1 month after DC cardioversion, then decide about longer-term anticoagulation based on CHA$_2$DS$_2$–VAS score
+ Typical atrial flutter may be ablated with >90% cure rate, obviating the need for long-term anticoagulation

Table 8.3 Management of focal atrial tachycardia.

1. Rate control (same protocol as AF and atrial flutter)
2. Rhythm control
   a. Adenosine, β-blockers, diltiazem: all may slow down atrial tachycardia or convert it to sinus rhythm. Antiarrhythmic drugs are used as second-line agents
   b. Digoxin is not usually used, because it can cause atrial tachycardia
   c. DC cardioversion may not be successful, as many atrial tachycardias are caused by enhanced automaticity rather than reentry. DC cardioversion is only attempted if the patient is unstable
3. Anticoagulation is not usually necessary for atrial tachycardia per se, but may be necessary in an older patient whose atrial tachycardia frequently coexists with AF

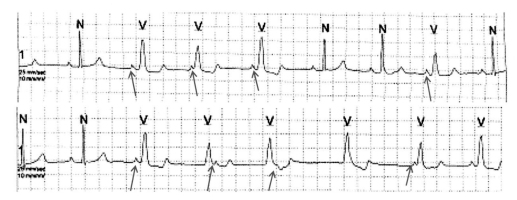

Figure 8.15 Two types of QRS complexes are seen: (1) narrow complexes preceded by sinus P waves; (2) wide complexes that seem to be preceded by sinus P waves (*arrows*) but are, in reality, coming too close to the P waves and dissociated from them, with a variable PR interval (ventricular complexes).

   The wide complex rate is close to the sinus rate, which makes those wide complexes fall around the sinus P waves. Whenever the sinus rate accelerates, P waves get conducted; when the sinus rate slows down, the wide rhythm expresses itself. The wide complex rhythm is an *accelerated idioventricular rhythm*, an automatic ventricular rhythm that competes with the sinus rhythm (rate ~65 bpm). The dissociation between P and QRS during those beats is *isorhythmic AV dissociation*.

B. AVNRT, AVRT
Convert with: vagal maneuvers, adenosine 6–12 mg IV (first-line therapy if no asthma), metoprolol 5 mg IV, diltiazem 20 mg IV.

C. Focal atrial tachycardia (Table 8.3)

Always remember to seek an underlying cause of the tachycardia and treat it. This alone may control the rate ± the rhythm:
- HF decompensation, hypovolemia, acute bleed, sepsis, PE, hypoxia, hyperthyroidism

XI. Non-tachycardic wide complex rhythms (see Figures 8.15, 8.16, 8.17)

QUESTIONS AND ANSWERS: Practice ECGs of wide complex tachycardias
Review every ECG and attempt to make a diagnosis of SVT vs. VT (Figures 8.18–8.25).

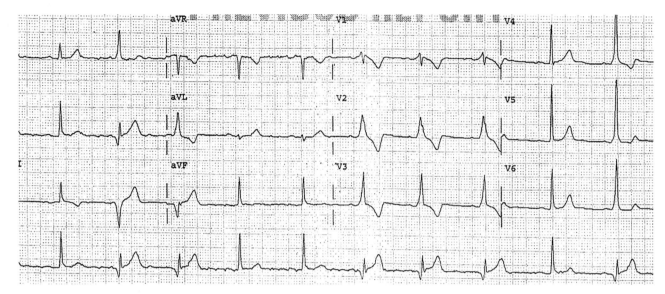

Figure 8.16 Again, two types of QRS complexes are seen: (1) narrow complexes preceded by a sinus P wave; (2) wide complexes preceded by the same sinus P wave (best seen in V$_2$–V$_6$). These wide complexes are not premature, hence they are not PVCs.

They may represent an idioventricular rhythm similar to Figure 8.15; however, the P and QRS relationship remains constant throughout those beats. *This intermittent widening of the QRS may represent intermittent bundle branch block or intermittent pre-excitation.* The lack of a change in rate argues against bundle branch block. The morphology of the wide QRS favors pre-excitation. A positive delta wave with a short PR interval is seen on the wide complexes in leads V$_5$–V$_6$ and I, while a negative delta wave (pseudo-Q wave) is seen in the inferior leads. This intermittent conduction across the accessory pathway implies a long refractory period and an inability to consistently conduct even at a normal rate (good prognosis).

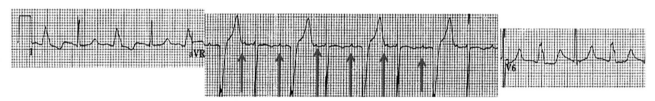

Figure 8.17 Alternation between wide and narrow QRS complexes. Both QRS complexes are occurring regularly after the regular sinus P waves (*arrows*), with a constant P–QRS relationship. The P–P interval and PR intervals are constant. The morphology suggests intermittent LBBB. Diagnosis: sinus rhythm with alternating LBBB.

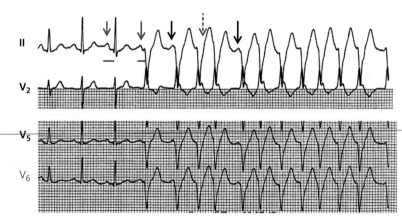

Figure 8.18 A run of wide complex tachycardia. It is irregular, but this does not necessarily imply AF. In a short run of VT or at the onset of VT, VT may be irregular.

1. See how it starts: tachycardia starts after a regularly occurring sinus P wave (*blue arrows*), at a shorter PR interval (*bars*). This implies that it starts with a PVC, a beat that does not interrupt the regularly occurring sinus P wave. The tachycardia has the same morphology as this PVC; thus, the tachycardia is VT.

2. Look for P waves: two P waves are seen within the tachycardia, in leads II, V$_5$, V$_6$ (*black arrows*). The first P wave has a similar morphology to the sinus P wave and comes at an interval that is equal to the sinus P–P interval. The second P wave falls at twice the sinus P–P interval. Another sinus P wave is expected to fall in between and is hidden in the QRS complex (*dashed arrow*). Those P waves fall around the QRS and ST–T segments at their own rate and are dissociated from QRS, implying VT.

3. Look at the QRS morphology. The QRS has a **QS morphology in V$_5$–V$_6$**, which is not seen with LBBB or RBBB, and is ***pathognomonic of VT***.
Final diagnosis: VT.

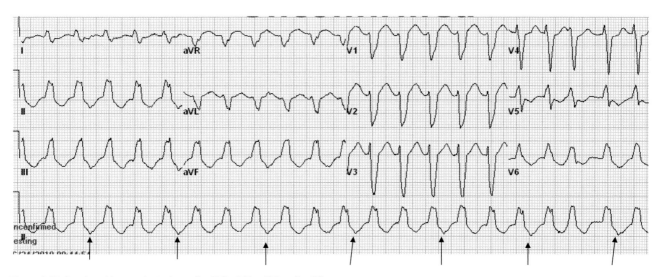

Figure 8.19 Regular wide complex tachycardia, QRS width ~180 ms (lead II).

1. QRS morphology is consistent with a typical LBBB in leads V$_1$–V$_6$.

2. Look for P waves in all leads. One can identify inverted blips that have a consistent *morphology* and *timing* and that can be marched out in lead II (*arrows*), and in leads III and aVF. They occur after every third QRS, and have a consistent relationship with QRS. Thus, there is AV association, with three QRS complexes for every P wave. Since the number of QRS complexes >number of P waves, this is VT. The P waves are retrograde P waves, secondary to a 3:1 ventriculoatrial conduction.

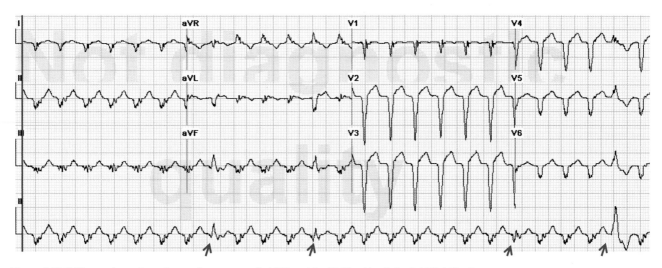

Figure 8.20 Wide complex tachycardia, regular, at a rate of ~155 bpm. The QRS is widest in lead aVF (~140 ms).

1. P waves are not seen. One cannot comment on AV dissociation.

2. QRS morphology. There is monophasic negative QRS concordance in V$_1$–V$_6$, with a QS pattern, pathognomonic for a VT that originates apically (likely from an apical MI scar). The axis is northwest (QRS negative in leads I and aVF), which is also suggestive of VT. QRS has a lot of notching, particularly seen in the inferior leads and in lead V$_1$, also characteristic of VT. A large dominant R wave is seen in lead aVR, also characteristic of VT.

Wide complexes of a different morphology are scattered in the tachycardia (*arrows*). The first three are likely fusion complexes, whereas the fourth is very wide and is likely a PVC from another focus.

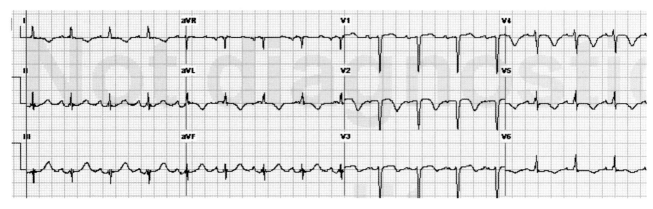

Figure 8.21 This is the baseline ECG of the patient in Figure 8.20. It shows an anterior MI pattern; however, the QS pattern does not extend all the way to V$_6$ and the axis is normal. Note the morphology of QRS in lead II, and see how the three different-looking complexes in Figure 8.20 are fusion between this narrow QRS and the VT's QRS.

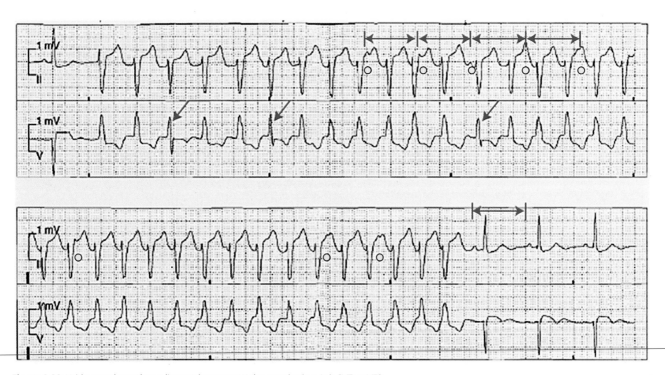

Figure 8.22 Wide complex tachycardia on telemetry or Holter monitoring. Is it SVT or VT?

1. See how it starts. The first complex is not preceded by a P wave or a deformation of the T wave, and thus is a PVC. The tachycardia starts with a PVC and has a morphology similar to the PVC → VT.

2. Look for AV dissociation: scattered notches are visible on the T waves (*blue dots*), and can be marched out (*blue calipers*). They are at equal distance from each other, and this distance is the same as the distance between two sinus P waves (marked by the last caliper). They are dissociated from QRS complexes. These are sinus P waves that keep marching through the tachycardia without any relation to it → VT. ***Deformation of a T wave is usually a hint to a hidden P wave***.

3. There are three narrower complexes scattered within the tachycardia (*arrows*). They start similarly to the tachycardia's QRS and end similarly to the sinus beat's QRS, suggesting fusion complexes in a patient with VT.

4. The tachycardia is irregular. This does not necessarily imply AF, as any SVT or VT may be irregular at its onset (the first 20 beats). Conclusion: VT.

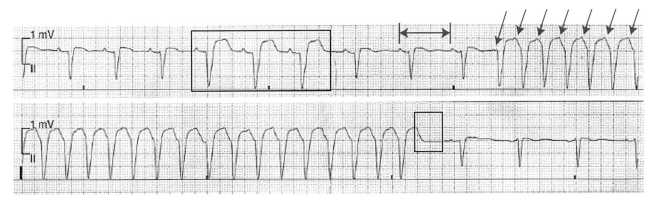

Figure 8.23 Run of wide complex tachycardia. Is it VT or SVT?

1. Look at how it starts. The first QRS of the tachycardia is preceded by a P wave (*first arrow*) that is premature in comparison to the sinus P waves (*caliper*); thus the first QRS is a PAC with aberrancy. A tachycardia that starts with a PAC and has a morphology identical to the PAC is SVT.

2. Throughout the tachycardia, one sees P waves (*arrows*) having a consistent 1:1 association with QRS. AV association does not prove the tachycardia is SVT, as it may also occur in up to 25% of VT.

3. What are the complexes in the area marked by the rectangle? Three wide complexes are preceded by sinus P waves with the same PR interval as the sinus rhythm. These are sinus beats conducted with aberrancy (LBBB aberrancy, QRS being negative in II). The patient probably has intermittent, rate-related LBBB. In fact, the sinus rhythm is a bit faster at the time of these three complexes. This proves that the left bundle is prone to rate-related block. The wide complex tachycardia is SVT having the same LBBB aberrancy.

4. Look at how the tachycardia ends (*box*). There is no P wave at the end; the tachycardia ends with a QRS complex. A presumed VT with 1:1 VA conduction usually ends with the retrograde P wave; thus, in this case, the lack of P wave at the end argues against VT.

So this is SVT. The next question is: what type of SVT? Is it AVNRT, AVRT, or atrial tachycardia?

1. Look at the RP interval. RP interval being over half the RR interval, this is a long RP tachycardia. The diagnosis includes atrial tachycardia vs. atypical AVNRT vs. SNRT.

2. The fact that the first P wave (PAC) marches out with the subsequent P waves means that each one of these P waves originates, like the PAC, from the same atrial focus and conducts antegradely. This favors automatic atrial tachycardia. The fact that the tachycardia ends with a QRS is also consistent with this diagnosis.

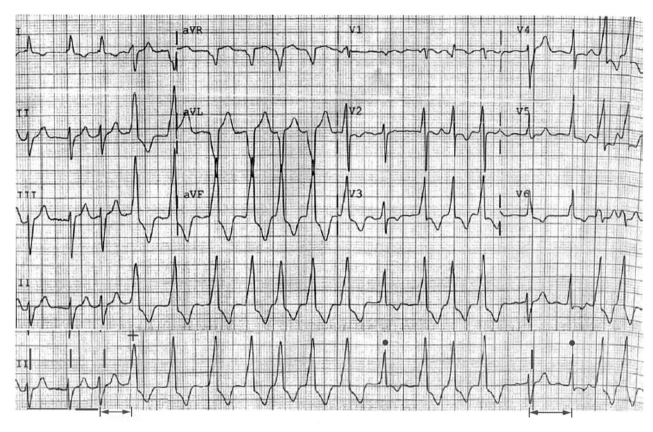

Figure 8.24 The baseline rhythm is AF and the baseline QRS is marked by *lines*. Runs of wide complexes are seen. **In a patient with baseline AF, are the wide complex runs VT or aberrant runs of AF?**

1. Use the rhythm strip with a different set of criteria, focused on Ashman's phenomenon:
   a. Does the wide run follow the Ashman rule, meaning it occurs after a long–short sequence? The first run (*cross*) starts after an interval that is not too short (*first caliper*), as there is, on the same ECG, a "longer–shorter" sequence without aberrancy (the sequence of the first two complexes, *underlined*). This argues against aberrancy. The second run (*second caliper*) starts after a long R–R interval. This again argues against aberrancy.
   b. Two complexes of intermediate morphology are seen (*dots*). These complexes are fusion complexes, further supporting VT (the complex starts similarly to the ventricular complex, and ends as a summation between the ventricular complex and the baseline QRS).
   c. If the coupling interval of the wide complexes was constant (timing of onset in relation to the normally conducted complex), it would have further supported VT (this is not the case here).
2. Use the 12-lead ECG to analyze the morphology of the wide complexes (i.e., the complexes that are not marked by a *line* or a *dot* on the rhythm strip) (e.g., Brugada criteria):
   - The wide QRS complex morphology does not fit with a typical LBBB or RBBB; it is close to LBBB in V_4–V_5, but the R wave of the RS complex in lead V_2 is wide (>30 ms), and QRS is negative in leads I and aVL, arguing against LBBB; the right-axis deviation of the wide complexes also argues against typical LBBB. This is VT.
   - The onset/initial part of QRS is more slurred than its later part (leads II, aVF, and V_3–V_5), which implies VT.
   - The notch on the descending limb of QS in leads aVR and aVL is consistent with VT.

Final diagnosis: AF with two runs of VT.

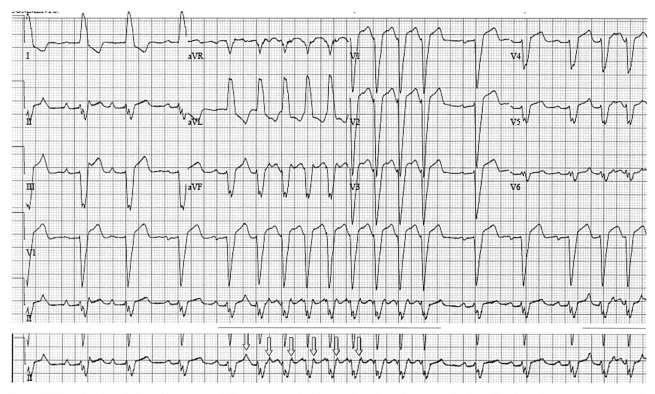

Figure 8.25 Baseline sinus rhythm with LBBB morphology. Two runs of wide complex tachycardia are seen (*horizontal lines*). Are these runs VT or SVT with aberrancy?

• Look at how the run starts. It starts with a P wave that occurs prematurely and deforms the preceding T wave, giving it a peaked appearance (*first arrow*), thus a PAC. The QRS of the tachycardia has the same morphology as this aberrant PAC. Thus, this is SVT.

• The morphology is similar to the baseline QRS morphology. A tachycardia that keeps the same bundle branch block morphology as the baseline is SVT.

• Look for P waves and for AV dissociation: there are notches after each QRS, likely P waves, associated with QRS in a 1:1 fashion (*arrows*). These notches are evident when the tachycardia's QRS morphology is compared to the baseline QRS. This 1:1 AV association implies SVT or VT with retrograde VA conduction (not here). The fact that the tachycardia ends with a QRS and no P wave argues against VT with 1:1 VA conduction.

This is SVT. What type of SVT is it? It is a short RP tachycardia, which could fit with AVNRT, AVRT, or atrial tachycardia. The P wave of the initial complex (PAC, *first arrow*) keeps marching out with the subsequent P waves, arguing that each one of these P waves is, like the first P wave, coming from the same atrial focus and conducting antegradely to the ventricles. Thus, the tachycardia is likely an automatic atrial tachycardia. Also, the upright P morphology in lead II indicates that the P wave is not a retrograde P wave, and thus the tachycardia is unlikely to be AVNRT or AVRT, which favors atrial tachycardia. The tachycardia ends with a QRS, as no P notch is seen at the last QRS complex. It is consistent with automatic atrial tachycardia, wherein the P vanishes as the automatic focus becomes quiescent.

Final diagnosis: sinus rhythm with LBBB, runs of a wide complex atrial tachycardia.

Further reading

Brugada P, Brugada J, Mont L, et al. A new approach to the differential diagnosis of a regular tachycardia with a wide complex. Circulation 1991; 83: 1649–59.

Strickberger SA, Man KC, Daoud EG, et al. Adenosine-induced atrial arrhythmia: a prospective analysis. Ann Intern Med 1997;127: 417–22. *Adenosine causes transient AF in 12% of patients after SVT therapy: transient AF lasts 5–20 minutes, but requires DCCV in 1/3 of those cases.*

ECC Committee, Subcommittees and Task Forces of the American Heart Association. 2005 American Heart Association guidelines for cardiopulmonary resuscitation and emergency cardiovascular care. Circulation 2005; 112 (suppl 24): IV1–203.

Vereckei A, Duray G, Szenazi G, et al. Application of a new algorithm in the differential diagnosis of wide QRS complex tachycardia. Eur Heart J 2007; 28: 589–600.

9 Ventricular Arrhythmias: Types and Management, Sudden Cardiac Death

I. Premature ventricular complexes

In the absence of heart disease, premature ventricular complexes (PVCs) are generally benign and do not clearly portend an increased risk of sudden or cardiac death, regardless of their frequency (>1 per minute) or pattern (e.g., couplets). Frequent PVCs are relatively common in an apparently healthy population (prevalence 1–4% at mean age of ~50). Benign PVCs generally occur at rest and improve with exercise; yet some idiopathic PVCs are triggered by exercise. Recent data suggest that a high PVC burden, exceeding 0.5 % of all QRS complexes, is associated with twice the risk of HF at 15-year follow-up, although no causal relationship is established. Very frequent PVCs (>5–10% burden) warrant echo±stress test to assess for heart disease. Even in the absence of underlying heart disease, very frequent PVCs may lead to a form of tachycardia-mediated cardiomyopathy. Among patients referred for PVC ablation, ~40% of those with PVC burden > 10% have reduced EF; EF fully normalizes with PVC ablation.[1,2]

In patients with heart disease, frequent or complex PVCs or non-sustained VT portend an increase in mortality independently of other baseline variables, according to most post-MI studies. However, targeted therapy of PVCs or non-sustained VT is not indicated. In fact, the use of class I antiarrhythmic drugs (AADs) to suppress PVCs worsens outcomes (as a result of the proarrhythmic side effects of AADs) and should be avoided in patients with underlying heart disease (CAST trial: in patients with a history of MI and normal or low EF, PVC suppression with class I AADs increases mortality).[3]

β-Blockers are the safest treatment for symptomatic PVCs and PVCs occurring in the context of structural heart disease. PVCs that originate from the same focus have a monomorphic appearance and may be treated with catheter ablation if the patient has refractory symptoms.

In the particular case of frequent PVCs (>5–10% burden on 24-hour Holter) with LV systolic dysfunction, there are three possible diagnoses: (1) ischemia causing both PVCs and LV dysfunction; (2) LV dysfunction causing PVCs; (3) frequent PVCs causing a form of tachycardia-mediated cardiomyopathy. Once ischemia is ruled out, it is reasonable to suppress PVCs using amiodarone or catheter ablation and see if EF improves. In fact, EF substantially improves in over 80% of these patients.[4,5]

How to differentiate PVC from PAC with aberrancy

PVC is a wide premature complex with ST–T changes opposite in direction to QRS. A PVC does not affect the sinus P waves, which keep marching through the PVC at approximately the same rate. Therefore a sinus P wave falls within the PVC and distorts it, or precedes the PVC at a PR interval shorter than baseline; *a wide premature complex preceded by a sinus P wave at a shorter PR interval is a PVC*. This also means that the PVC does not reset the sinus node. Hence the R–R interval between the complex before and the one after the PVC is equal to twice the regular R–R interval, and it looks like there is a pause after the PVC. PVC may, however, be *interpolated* between two normal QRS complexes, not affecting at all the sinus-conducted QRS complexes.

Practical Cardiovascular Medicine, First Edition. Elias B. Hanna.

© 2017 John Wiley & Sons Ltd. Published 2017 by John Wiley & Sons Ltd.

PAC with aberrancy (functional bundle branch block) mimics a PVC.* PAC, however, starts with a premature P wave of a different shape than the sinus P wave (may fall in the T wave and manifest as a change in the preceding T-wave morphology: deformity, peaking). PAC often conducts retrogradely to the sinus node and resets it, making it fire after the PAC at a rate close to baseline. Thus, the interval after a PAC is not a fully compensatory pause and is only slightly longer than the baseline R–R interval. The R–R interval between the complex before and the one after the PAC is less than twice the normal R–R interval. PAC with aberrancy is often of RBBB morphology. Interpolated PACs are possible but unusual, and may occur when the sinus node is not reset by the PAC.

While frequent PVCs are considered benign in patients with no identifiable heart disease, frequent PACs are associated with an increased risk of AF, stroke, and death in patients 55–75 years of age (prolonged rhythm monitoring may be warranted to detect periods of AF).

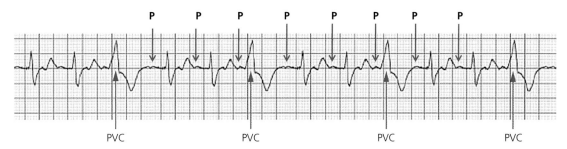

Figure 9.1 Wide premature complexes with a different morphology than the baseline QRS, and with prominent ST–T changes opposite to QRS, occurring in a trigeminal pattern. These are typically PVCs, but could be PACs with bundle branch block (aberrancy). They fall after normally occurring, non-premature P waves with a **_shorter PR interval than the sinus beats, which is typical of PVCs_**. Sinus P waves keep marching out through the PVCs.

- Frequent PVCs = PVCs > 30 per hour or > 1 per minute.
- Very frequent PVCs with a risk of tachycardia-mediated cardiomyopathy: total PVC burden > 5–10% of the total QRS complexes, or > 20,000 PVCs per day.
- Complex PVCs = polymorphic PVCs, or couplets or triplets of PVCs.
- Bigeminy means the alternation of one sinus beat with one PVC; trigeminy means the occurrence of one PVC after every two sinus beats (Figure 9.1). This is different from couplet (two PVCs in a row), or triplet (three PVCs in a row).
- Ventricular parasystole corresponds to an automatic ventricular focus that fires at a regular rate (~30–60 per minute), independently of the basic sinus or supraventricular rhythm and uninhibited by this rhythm (the parasystolic focus is protected by an entrance block). This focus impulse propagates to the ventricles whenever they are not in their refractory period. Parasystole manifests as PVCs that have no fixed relationship with the baseline QRS (non-fixed coupling), with interectopic intervals that are a multiple of the shortest interectopic interval. Fusion complexes are particularly common. Parasystole may be seen in the presence or absence of heart disease and does not affect prognosis. Even frequent parasystolic PVCs are benign, per se.

  In contrast to ventricular parasystole, typical PVCs are due to a reentrant circuit that is initiated by the supraventricular rhythm, and thus show fixed-interval coupling.
- **Site of origin of the PVC (PVC looks away, i.e., looks negative, from where it originates):**

(i) right vs. left:	right ventricular origin → LBBB morphology
	left ventricular origin → RBBB morphology
(ii) anterior vs. inferior:	anterior origin → QRS (+) in the inferior leads (vertical axis)
	inferior origin → QRS (–) in the inferior leads (left axis)
(iii) basal vs. apical:	basal origin → QRS complex is upright in all precordial leads, and (–) in I-aVL (if lateral origin)
	apical origin → QRS complex is negative in all precordial leads

II. Ventricular tachycardia (VT) (Figure 9.2)

A. Types
- Sustained VT = VT lasting > 30 seconds or VT associated with hemodynamic compromise (such as syncope/presyncope)
- Non-sustained VT: at least three consecutive ventricular beats, with a total VT duration < 30 seconds and no hemodynamic compromise

Also, by definition, the ventricular rate must be > 100 bpm. A ventricular rhythm slower than 100 bpm is accelerated idioventricular rhythm (AIVR); a ventricular rhythm slower than 40 bpm is a ventricular escape rhythm.

---

* PVC and PAC with aberrancy are wide, but may be narrow if the PVC or the aberrancy originates high in the septum close to the His bundle. They will, however, look different than the baseline QRS. In case of a wide baseline QRS, a PAC with aberrancy is wider than the baseline, with the same bundle branch block morphology as the baseline; a QRS narrower than baseline is diagnostic of PVC.

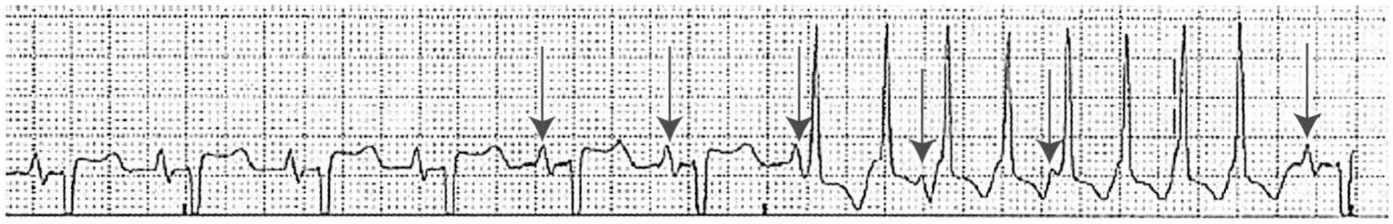

Figure 9.2 Tachycardia that seems narrow but has a different morphology than the native QRS and is associated with secondary ST/T abnormalities → VT or SVT with aberrancy. To differentiate, see how the tachycardia starts. It does not start after a premature P wave, but rather starts after a regularly occurring sinus P wave (*third arrow*) with a shorter PR interval than regularly: this means it starts with a PVC. It has the same morphology as this PVC → the tachycardia is VT. Also, one can regularly march out sinus P waves scattered within the tachycardia and dissociated from the QRS complexes, which is diagnostic of VT. These P waves are marked by *arrows*. One P wave falls within a QRS (marked by an *interrupted line*).

B. Causes of sustained VT

Sustained VT is typically secondary to an underlying heart disease:

- Acute or chronic ischemia. **Acute ischemia typically leads to polymorphic VT, whereas a prior ischemic scar/old infarct leads to monomorphic VT.** Occasionally, a scar may lead to polymorphic VT.
- Any cardiomyopathy, especially with EF < 35%. More specifically, the following *four cardiomyopathies are particularly prone to VT:* severe acute myocarditis, sarcoidosis, ARVD, and Chagas disease.
- Some forms of "benign" monomorphic VTs occur without heart disease in young patients with normal hearts (i.e., idiopathic left ventricular VT, right ventricular outflow tract VT). These VTs are benign as they do not lead to sudden death. They account for ~10% of all VT referral cases.
- Some "malignant" forms of VT/VF occur without obvious heart disease: Brugada syndrome, ARVD, idiopathic polymorphic VT (see Section VI, *Specific VTs*).
- Antiarrhythmic drugs and electrolyte abnormalities can trigger polymorphic VT. They can also trigger monomorphic VT but are not usually the sole cause of monomorphic VT (there is usually some underlying cardiac structural or electrical disease).

C. Causes and prognosis of non-sustained VT

Similarly to sustained VT, non-sustained VT typically occurs in patients with underlying heart disease; however, it occurs occasionally in healthy individuals, more so than sustained VT (prevalence of NSVT in the healthy population, ~1%). Approximately 1% of asymptomatic individuals without apparent heart disease develop NSVT during exercise testing; in the absence of ST changes on the sinus beats, NSVT does not affect long-term prognosis and is typically a form of monomorphic idiopathic VT.[6]

NSVT is likely an independent predictor of mortality in patients with cardiomyopathy. In the SCD-HeFT trial of ischemic and non-ischemic cardiomyopathies with EF < 35%, and in the MERLIN-TIMI trial of ACS with predominantly preserved EF, NSVT was independently associated with increased mortality.[7,8]

D. Acute management of sustained VT

- Acute DC cardioversion (DC cardioversion is a shock synchronized to R wave).
- Prior to DC cardioversion, if the patient is hemodynamically stable, one may attempt an IV bolus of amiodarone (150 mg over 10 minutes), lidocaine (1 mg/kg), or procainamide (20 mg/min for a total of 17 mg/kg, i.e., ~500–1000 mg). One drug is attempted one time only if the patient is stable. If the drug fails, DC cardioversion is performed.
- Then, after VT cardioversion (whether with DC cardioversion or drugs), and after a loading dose of one of these drugs, an IV drip of the drug is typically administered for 24 hours. Also, a β-blocker is started if BP can tolerate and in the absence of HF (e.g., metoprolol 5 mg IV repeated up to three times Q10 min, followed by oral metoprolol).
- Always look for an underlying heart disease. Coronary angiography and urgent coronary revascularization are performed if ACS is suspected. Also look for electrolyte abnormalities.
- In case of VF or pulseless VT, perform defibrillation. As opposed to DC cardioversion, defibrillation is a shock that is not synchronized to R wave.

> Electrical storm is defined as ≥ 3 episodes of sustained VT within 24 hours. The management includes ruling out and treating potential causes (including urgent coronary angiogram ± PCI), amiodarone, and β-blockers. The latter combination is usually the most effective antiarrhythmic therapy; however, if ineffective, amiodarone may be switched to lidocaine or procainamide. Sedation with propofol can assist in controlling the electrical storm.

E. Chronic management of sustained VT

- Place an ICD after any sustained VT, *except* in the following three cases:
  - Polymorphic VT/VF occurring within the first 48 hours of a STEMI.
  - Polymorphic VT occurring during active acute ischemia that eventually gets treated with revascularization. In that respect, any VT occurring in conjunction with low-level troponin elevation, or monomorphic VT, should not be considered as being due solely to the transient ischemic episodes, and revascularization of a lesion producing ischemia is not enough to prevent VT/VF. Rather than a purely reversible ischemia, an underlying irreversible scar is probably present. VT, by itself, often leads to low-level troponin elevation. As stated in the ACC guidelines, "Sustained monomorphic VT with prior MI is unlikely to be affected by revascularization."[9]
  - Idiopathic monomorphic VT: No underlying heart disease and no ECG suspicion of malignant electrical causes of VT.

- Treat any ongoing or recurrent ischemia potentially contributing to VT (revascularization).
- Chronic β-blocker therapy.
- Chronic antiarrhythmic therapy (mainly amiodarone or sotalol) is indicated in patients who already have an ICD but continue to have frequent, recurrent VT. Antiarrhythmic drugs are used to prevent symptoms and frequent shocks; they do not clearly reduce mortality. Amiodarone reduced mortality in patients with ischemic or non-ischemic HF in the older GESICA trial;[10] however, this was not shown in the more recent SCD-HeFT trial.[11] As opposed to class I agents, amiodarone is at least proven to be safe in the HF population.

> Note that a *monomorphic* VT occurring in the context of electrolyte abnormalities or antiarrhythmic drugs should be evaluated and treated similarly to VT occurring without electrolyte abnormalities or antiarrhythmic drugs. In general, monomorphic VT is not due solely to these factors. These factors, per se, can cause polymorphic rather than monomorphic VT. Keep a low threshold for placing an ICD for monomorphic VT, even in the context of seemingly reversible causes.[9]

F. NSVT management

No acute therapy is indicated. Underlying heart disease is sought (echo, stress testing).

Long-term treatment: NSVT does not dictate ICD by itself. ICD is dictated by the underlying cardiomyopathy (EF ≤ 35%).

G. Accelerated idioventricular rhythm (AIVR)

AIVR is defined as a slow VT that has a rate of 60–120 bpm. It usually competes with the underlying sinus rhythm with alternation of ventricular and sinus-originated complexes (Figure 9.3). AIVR may be seen in: (1) acute ischemia (including STEMI, whether reperfused or not), (2) up to 8% of HF cases and cardiomyopathies (including hypertensive or valvular cardiomyopathy), (3) digoxin or antiarrhythmic drug toxicity, and (4) electrolyte abnormalities (hyperkalemia). It may also be seen in patients with sinus node disease, where AIVR is a form of accelerated ventricular escape.

Treatment: there is no convincing evidence linking AIVR to VT/VF, and thus no specific treatment for AIVR is necessary. AIVR suppression is not indicated, particularly when AIVR is thought to be an escape rhythm. Only in symptomatic patients with sinus node disease and coexisting pauses or chronotropic incompetence is pacemaker therapy indicated.

See additional examples of wide complex rhythms in Chapter 8.

H. Workup of VT occurring without obvious heart disease on echo and coronary angiography

Rule out the following diseases by ECG, family history, and sometimes cardiac MRI:

- Brugada syndrome (diagnosed by ECG; dictates ICD placement).
- ARVD: ARVD is characterized by RV fatty infiltration and is diagnosed by ECG, echo, and cardiac MRI.
- Long QT syndrome.
- Sarcoidosis: severe AV blocks and ventricular arrrhythmias are common in cardiac sarcoidosis. Sarcoidosis is diagnosed by extracardiac involvement ± endomyocardial biopsy and cardiac MRI. ICD is indicated for secondary prevention, or primary prevention in patients with extensive myocardial involvement.
- WPW: leads to a pre-excited SVT that mimics VT. WPW is treated with ablation.
- Catecholaminergic polymorphic VT: characterized by polymorphic or bidirectional VT occurring during exercise testing. It dictates ICD.

If none of the above diagnoses is evident, and if VT is monomorphic, the patient is diagnosed with idiopathic VT and is treated with β-blockers or CCBs (idiopathic VT is the only VT in which CCBs are effective). Alternatively, the ventricular focus may be ablated.

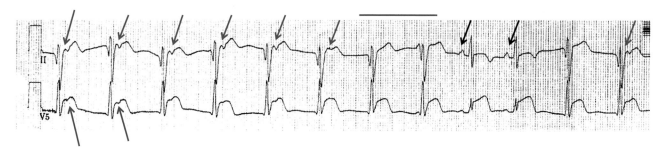

Figure 9.3 Wide complex rhythm at a rate of 70 bpm. P waves are initially seen after every QRS (*blue arrows*). This could be consistent with a ventricular rhythm with 1:1 VA conduction. However, further down the strip, those P waves start coming sooner and fall onto the QRS complexes (*two complexes under the bar*), then appear before the QRS complexes and get conducted (*black arrows*). Thus, these P waves are actually sinus P waves dissociated from the ventricular rhythm. This dissociation is an isorhythmic AV dissociation, wherein the ventricular and sinus rhythms have close rates: when the sinus rhythm speeds up, it takes over and P waves get conducted. When it slightly slows down, the ventricular rhythm takes over. This is AIVR in a patient with anterolateral STEMI. While classically seen after reperfusion, it may very well be seen in non-reperfused infarcts such as this one. ST elevation is seen on both the ventricular and sinus-originating complexes. ST elevation that is concordant to QRS is indicative of STEMI, even in ventricular complexes.

III. Polymorphic ventricular tachycardia

A. Morphology and types

Polymorphic VT is a VT that has two or more QRS morphologies:

1. The most common polymorphic VT is a **polymorphic VT without baseline QT prolongation.** In other words, the sinus rhythm's QTc interval is normal or only mildly prolonged. It is related to:

- Acute ongoing ischemia, from an acute coronary event or from severe shock of any origin
- Decompensated HF, with secondary ischemia and cellular stretch
- Metabolic abnormalities or drug toxicity (class I agents, tricyclics)

Acutely, polymorphic VT is treated similarly to monomorphic VT. The underlying metabolic abnormalities are treated and urgent ischemic evaluation and revascularization are performed. As opposed to TdP, amiodarone may be administered.

2. Torsades de pointes is a polymorphic VT with changing QRS polarity occurring in the context of a prolonged baseline QTc interval (often > 500 ms) or abnormal U wave. **VT with twisting QRS polarity similar to Figure 9.4, but normal baseline QTc interval, is a non-TdP polymorphic VT and is usually an ischemic rhythm.** TdP typically occurs in short runs < 20 seconds interceded with baseline rhythm, but may become persistent or degenerate into VF (Figures 9.4, 9.5, 9.6).

There are two types of TdP:

- *TdP secondary to congenital QT prolongation*, where TdP is often dependent on increased catecholaminergic tone. The long QT is secondary to a genetic channelopathy affecting potassium channels (LQT1 and 2), or, less often, sodium channels (LQT3), and leading to prolongation of repolarization with early afterdepolarizations. It is often inherited in an autosomal dominant fashion.
- *TdP secondary to acquired QT prolongation*, where TdP is related to a combination of:
  ○ Bradycardia, which further prolongs and disperses repolarization (pause-dependent TdP).
  ○ Long–short R–R sequences: a pause is followed by an early PVC that falls in the ventricular repolarization period and triggers TdP.
  ○ One of four factors causing prolonged QT:

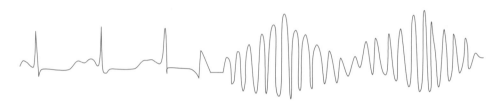

Figure 9.4 Torsades de pointes initiation.

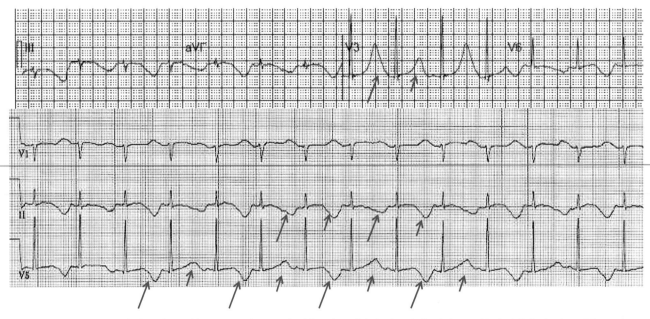

Figure 9.5 QT interval is markedly prolonged (QTc = 730 ms). T wave is wide and ample in lead V₃, is deeply inverted in the inferior leads, and demonstrates beat-to-beat alternation in morphology and amplitude, the so-called macroscopic T wave alternans. In addition, alternation in T-wave polarity is seen in lead V₅. T wave alternans may be seen with any cause of prolonged QT and implies severe heterogeneity of ventricular repolarization and an *imminent risk of TdP*; it is more characteristically seen in the congenital long QT syndromes. While this patient has hypokalemia, the wide and ample T-wave morphology without ST depression is not consistent with hypokalemia. The shape is consistent with long QT syndrome or ischemia. *Arrows* of two different lengths point to the two different T-wave morphologies.

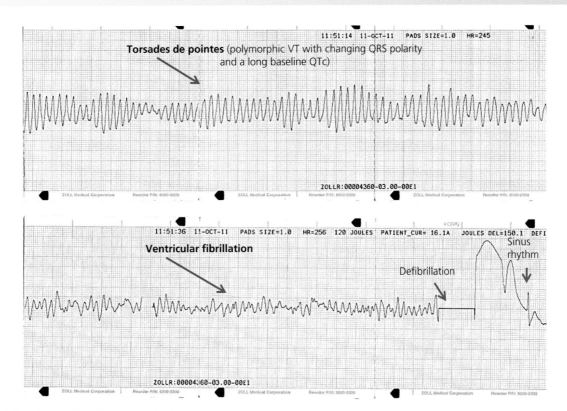

Figure 9.6 Torsades de pointes that degenerates into

    i. Electrolyte disorders (↓ K, ↓ Ca, ↓ Mg)
    ii. Drugs (AAD class I and III, neuroleptics, macrolides, cocaine)
    iii. Ischemia
    iv. Other: any cardiomyopathy, hypothyroidism, diabetic autonomic neuropathy, or cerebrovascular event (with tall or inverted T waves).
Acquired TdP is three times more common in women than men.

3. Even without QT prolongation, bradycardia and long pauses may lead to early afterdepolarizations and spontaneous action potentials that initiate reentry in a patient with underlying myocardial disease (acute ischemia, myocardial scar). Bradycardia not only prolongs but disperses repolarization across the myocardium, allowing the sustainment of reentry. Thus, bradycardia may trigger polymorphic VT or monomorphic VT even without QT prolongation.[12] In fact, in a patient with acute MI, frank bradycardia < 50 bpm can trigger VT/VF.

As opposed to a steady-state bradycardia, acute bradycardia that occurs after a period of tachycardia is associated with a more striking prolongation of repolarization that facilitates the induction of polymorphic VT.[13] For instance, this is seen when AV nodal ablation is performed in patients with AF. As a result, the latter patients are paced at a rate of 80–90 bpm for ~1 week to prevent VT.

B. Treatment

Acutely, three lines of therapies are applied:

- Defibrillation if TdP is sustained.
- IV magnesium 2 g bolus (effective in > 75% of patients, regardless of Mg levels).
- ***Acute pacing (between the episodes of TdP, rather than during TdP).*** IV isoproterenol (= β₁-agonist) may alternatively be used if pacing is not immediately available. ***Increasing the heart rate prevents the recurrence of the pause-dependent, non-sustained runs of TdP.*** Bradycardia further prolongs QT and further disperses repolarization delays across the myocardium. Bradycardia is a major trigger of TdP, particularly in patients with acquired long QT. Pacing to a rate of 80–100 bpm prevents TdP recurrence. This is different from "overdrive pacing," wherein an *ongoing* monomorphic tachyarrhythmia is paced at a rate faster than its rate with the hope of breaking into its reentry cycle (e.g., monomorphic VT, atrial flutter).

    Pacing does not apply to the patient in Figure 9.5 because he is tachycardic. Congenital long QT, as opposed to acquired long QT, is often triggered by a catecholamine surge and may be associated with tachycardia.

    In addition, offending agents are withheld and K is corrected to 4.5–5.0 mEq/l.

Long-term treatment:

- Congenital long QT with a history of TdP or syncope: ICD + β-blockers.
- Asymptomatic congenital long QT: β-blockers. In case of borderline QT prolongation but suspicious history, a stress test may be performed. Further prolongation of QT with exercise or T wave alternans (beat-to-beat alternation of T-wave morphology) establishes the diagnosis.
- Acquired bradycardia (pause)-dependent TdP or bradycardia-dependent polymorphic VT, persistent after potassium correction and after discontinuation of the offending drugs: permanent PM placement.

IV. Congenital long QT syndrome (LQT)

A. Types

The most common LQT syndromes are LQT1 (~35%), LQT2 (25%), and LQT3 (~5–10%). LQT1 and 2 are related to loss of function of K channels (I_{Ks} and I_{Kr} respectively), leading to prolongation of repolarization with a broad and long T wave in LQT1, and a broad and notched T wave in LQT2 (Figure 9.7).[14] LQT3 is related to a gain of function of Na channels, leading to increased depolarization and thus prolongation of the plateau phase of repolarization, i.e., prolongation of the ST segment with a normal-width T wave. The prolongation of repolarization (QT) elicits two untoward processes: (i) afterdepolarizations, and (ii) increased transmural dispersion of repolarization, which allows afterdepolarizations to propagate and sustain reentry and arrhythmias.

In LQT1 and 2, TdP is triggered by catecholaminergic activity, which increases the amplitude of early afterdepolarizations. In particular, swimming or physical or emotional stress may trigger TdP in LQT1. Sudden noise or emotion as well as pregnancy and postpartum may trigger TdP in LQT2 (not exercise), whereas sleep may trigger TdP in LQT3.

LQT is mainly autosomal dominant with variable penetrance (Romano–Ward syndrome).

B. Problems with the definition of long QT and with the diagnosis

A prolonged QT is defined as a QTc > 460 ms in women and > 450 ms in men. In the absence of reversible metabolic, drug, or ischemic causes, LQT syndrome is suspected, particularly if QTc > 480 ms. Up to 10% of normal individuals have QTc that is mildly prolonged (up to 480 ms), and 10–15% of patients with long QT syndrome have normal baseline QTc (mainly 400–460 ms).[15] Furthermore, 24-hour ambulatory monitoring of QTc has shown that the QTc of healthy individuals varies throughout the day by an average of 76 ms and may reach 480–490 ms at night or in the early morning.[16]

In patients with QTc prolongation, rule out the transient causes (e.g., drugs) and perform an echo to rule out underlying cardiomyopathy (any cardiomyopathy may prolong QT). If QTc > 480–500 ms without any reversible cause, the diagnosis of LQT is virtually established. In patients with borderline QTc prolongation of 450–480 ms, further testing may need to be performed, particularly in case of syncope or family history of sudden death: a further prolongation of QTc with exercise testing (measurement performed a few minutes into recovery, as the heart rate slows down), epinephrine infusion, Valsalva, standing, or post-PVC implies LQT1. In normal individuals, QTc is reduced with exercise or epinephrine infusion.[17] In addition, the presence of macroscopic T wave alternans supports the diagnosis of LQT. Other supportive features: syncope with borderline QTc prolongation, family history of LQT or sudden death, familial screening with ECG (marked prolongation of QTc in a family member may confirm the diagnosis in the index patient).

QT interval is best measured in the lead that shows a distinct T-wave termination with the best separation of T and U waves.[18] The QT interval may be artificially shortened in some leads, because an isoelectric segment may be recorded at the beginning of the QRS complex or at the end of the T wave in those leads. On the other hand, QT is often longest in leads V_2–V_3, but those leads show the least separation between the T wave and the normal U wave and may therefore overestimate the length of the QT interval. Leads I, aVR, and aVL do not have the normal diastolic U wave but do not always show a distinct T wave. Thus, QT interval is often best measured in leads II and V_5 or V_6.

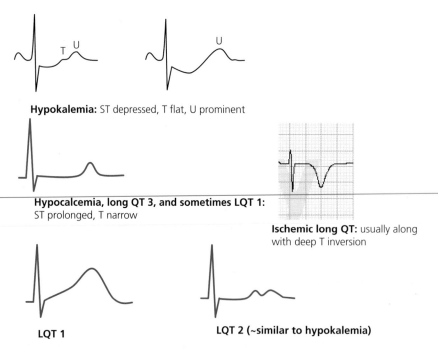

Hypokalemia: ST depressed, T flat, U prominent

Hypocalcemia, long QT 3, and sometimes LQT 1: ST prolonged, T narrow

Ischemic long QT: usually along with deep T inversion

LQT 1

LQT 2 (~similar to hypokalemia)

Figure 9.7 Typical ST–T morphologies in hypokalemia, hypocalcemia, and congenital long QT syndromes (LQT). In hypokalemia, ST segment is depressed and U wave is large while T wave is flattened. In hypocalcemia and LQT3, QT interval is prolonged as a result of ST-segment prolongation and, as opposed to other congenital LQT or QT prolongation secondary to drugs, there is no significant widening of the T wave. In LQT1, T wave is wide and ample without ST-segment depression, similar to Figure 9.5. In LQT2, T wave is wide and notched (double hump). LQT1 may have a morphology similar to LQT3 and is actually the most common LQT with this morphology. *In all long QT cases, particularly congenital LQT, the T wave may become notched after a pause, the notch representing the early afterdepolarization (EAD) wave that triggers TdP.*

Table 9.1 Risk of sudden death and cardiac events in patients with long QT syndrome before the age of 40.

	LQT1	LQT2 or LQT3
Risk of sudden death before the age of 40	10% Same risk in men and women[a]	20% Highest risk if woman LQT2 or man LQT3 (~25%)
Risk of sudden death or syncope before the age of 40 Highest risk when QTc>500ms, regardless of LQT type (70 % risk)	30%	~50%

Data from Priori et al. (2003).[19]
[a] Same risk in men and women in reference 19, higher risk in female in reference 20, where only adult patients were considered. QTc shortens with adult age in men (testosterone effect), and adult men are thus at lower risk of sudden death than women. Overall, the yearly risk of sudden death averages<0.5–1% per year.

A normal U wave (<25% of T wave) or an abnormal U wave that is not merging with the T wave should not be used in QT calculation. **In practice, a wave that exceeds 25% of the T wave and that merges with the T wave or gives a "bifid" T-wave appearance should be taken into account; this is a part of the T wave or a repolarization U wave (T2 wave) rather than a true diastolic U wave.** QT interval shortens with increasing heart rate; the corrected QT, which corresponds to the patient's predicted QT interval had the heart rate been 60 bpm, is often calculated using the Hodges formula: $QTc = QT + 1.75 \times (rate - 60)$.

C. Epidemiology and risk of sudden death

The long QT syndrome phenotype is more common in women than men (~1.5:1).

Sudden death and syncope mainly occur in childhood or early adulthood before the age of 40 (Table 9.1). QTc>500 ms, female sex with LQT2, or male sex with LQT3 confer the highest lifetime risk.[19] Female sex confers a higher risk of sudden death in adulthood, including LQT1, whereas male sex is a risk factor for sudden death in childhood.[20] Overall, ~ 50% of LQT syndrome patients experience cardiac events/TdP during their lifetime.

Patients with long QT syndrome genotype but normal phenotype (normal QTc) have a real risk of sudden death, albeit smaller than patients with prolonged QTc, and should be treated with β-blockers.

While the risk of sudden death attributed to long QT syndrome is highest in the first 40 years of life, this syndrome remains associated with a 2.65-fold increased risk of sudden death in patients 41–60 years of age, particularly in patients with LQT2 or 3, according to an LQT registry. The risk beyond the age of 60 is attenuated, partly because the risk of death from other illnesses increases at this stage.[21]

D. Genetic testing

Genetic testing is negative in 20–25% of patients with LQT1–3, because of unidentified mutations of identified genes. Thus, testing is not useful to rule out the diagnosis, but may rule it in when positive in a patient with borderline clinical criteria. Testing is useful for two more reasons: (i) identify the type of LQT, which has prognostic implications; (ii) once a mutation is identified in a proband, family members are checked for that same mutation with a very high rule-out yield.

E. Therapy

The mainstay of therapy of congenital LQT1 is β-blockade, the efficacy of which is assessed by blunting of the exertional heart rate. β-Blockers should be prescribed to all patients, including silent carriers. β-Blockade reduces the risk of sudden death by 64%, but is less effective in LQT2 (reduces the risk by ~1/3) and ineffective in men with LQT3.[22,23] In patients with prior syncope, β-blockers reduce the 5-year risk of recurrent syncope to 30%, and the 5-year risk of sudden death from long QTc to 3%.[23] In addition to β-blockade, long-term therapy of symptomatic or asymptomatic congenital LQT includes the maintenance of a normal electrolyte balance, avoidance of drugs that prolong the QT interval, and restriction from participation in athletic activities. LQT type is identified by genetic testing or by the effect of exercise or epinephrine on the QTc (in LQT1, QTc prolongs with exercise or epinephrine, while in LQT2 or 3, QTc shortens).

ICD is indicated in patients with LQT syndrome and prior cardiac arrest (class I indication). In patients with syncope, β-blockade therapy may be enough, with the use of ICD if syncope recurs. Note that TdP is self-terminating, so ICD may not be very helpful in patients with syncope; in fact, the ICD shock triggers anxiety and further catecholamine surge, which may provoke more TdP and VF. The use of ICD in patients with a prior syncope has a class IIa recommendation.[24] Those recommendations apply for young patients but also patients older than 40 years of age. ICD implantation may be considered in asymptomatic patients with the highest risk of sudden death, such as those with QTc>500 ms, or LQTS 2 or 3, the latter two being less responsive to β-blockade and having a high residual risk of cardiac events despite β-blockade (class IIb recommendation).

V. Indications for ICD implantation

A. Secondary prevention

ICD is indicated for sustained VT secondary to any structural heart disease, regardless of EF (AVID, CIDS trials),[25,26] *except*:

• Polymorphic VT or VF occurring the first 48 hours after a large MI or STEMI.
• Polymorphic VT secondary to active ischemia that can be treated with revascularization. The revascularization is urgent in this context.

In addition, ICD is not indicated for patients with sustained monomorphic VT, no structural heart disease, and no specific channelopathy/electrical disease (idiopathic monomorphic VT).

VT occurring in a patient with CAD but without acute MI or with only low-level troponin elevation qualifies for ICD regardless of EF and of the potential for complete revascularization (for the most part).[27] Outside acute MI, polymorphic VT with low EF and monomorphic VT usually signal an underlying scar and are unlikely to be affected by revascularization.[28]

B. Primary prevention means ICD implantation in a patient without a history of sustained VT or sudden death

It is indicated in ischemic or non-ischemic cardiomyopathy if EF is ≤ 35% and the patient is symptomatic, NYHA functional class II or III, despite optimal medical therapy (ACC class I recommendation). The following waiting periods are required before implanting the ICD:

- \> 40 days after acute MI.
- \> 3 months after revascularization for acute or chronic ischemia that did not lead to acute MI.
- \> 3 months of guideline-directed medical therapy for non-ischemic cardiomyopathy. This ensures the cardiomyopathy is not reversible before proceeding with ICD implantation (appropriateness criteria 2013).[27]

Note that, in ischemic cardiomyopathy with EF ≤ 30%, ICD is indicated even if the functional class is I, i.e., if the patient is asymptomatic (class I recommendation). Also, in ischemic cardiomyopathy, ICD is indicated if EF is 36–40%, NSVT is present, and VT is inducible on EP study (class I recommendation).

Those recommendations are based on the MADIT II and SCD-HeFT trials*.[11,29] The absolute yearly reduction in mortality was 3.5% in MADIT II, and 2% in SCD-HeFT. In these two trials, the survival curves of ICD therapy and placebo progressively diverged with time; however, in both trials, the curves did not begin to diverge until 9–12 months, indicating that **the benefit from ICD as a primary prevention therapy is a long-term benefit that is seen in patients healthy enough to survive several years**. The yearly number needed to treat (NNT) to prevent one death is 25 in the MADIT II trial.**

While the risk of sudden death is highest in the first 40 days after MI, ICD implantation is not beneficial during this time frame. One hypothesis is that, during this early period, patients at highest risk of VT/VF are patients with large infarctions and severe heart failure who may eventually succumb to pump failure even if resuscitated from VF (DINAMIT, IRIS trials).[31,32] Thus, ICD simply converts arrhythmic death into pump failure death or pulseless electrical activity (PEA) in many of those patients and does not prevent the eventual mortality. Also, the untoward effects of the periprocedural stress of ICD implantation may hinder the benefit. Building on this data, an analysis of the MADIT II trial has suggested that the benefit of ICD is mainly seen in patients whose MI is older than 1.5 years; while sudden death is highest in the early MI period, pump failure death, HF events, and recurrent acute coronary events are also highest during this period, reducing the effect of ICD on the overall mortality.[33] ICD is mainly effective in patients who have been stable for a prolonged duration after their MI, wherein the risk of isolated arrhythmic death from the arrhythmogenic scar becomes a relatively bigger concern.

The sickest patients with the highest risk of sudden death (e.g., class IV HF, recent MI, recurrent HF hospitalizations) also have a high risk of death related to pump failure and comorbidities. Preventing sudden death may not prevent the ultimate death, but rather converts it from sudden death to pump failure death or death related to comorbidities (e.g., MI, stroke, CKD). In fact, recent data suggest that old patients (> 65 years old) with ≥ 3 HF hospitalizations have a high mortality despite ICD placement, showing once more that ICD is mostly useful in stable patients, even though stable patients have a lower absolute sudden death risk.[34] The highest-risk patients in the MADIT II trial, such as those with advanced renal failure, did not benefit from ICD.[30]

The 3-month wait time after revascularization is derived from MADIT II, which excluded patients who received revascularization in the prior 3 months. The CABG-PATCH trial further supports this concept: patients with EF < 35% who received an epicardial ICD at the time of CABG surgery did not derive any mortality benefit, as revascularization by itself improved LV function and the risk of sudden death.[35] Hence, in stable CAD, the need for ICD should be reassessed several months after revascularization. Yet, similarly to the first 40 days after MI, the first 3 months after revascularization carry the highest risk of sudden death. Beyond 3 months, the risk of sudden death declines in revascularized patients.

ICD is not indicated for patients with a functional class of IV unless they also qualify for BiV pacemaker or unless they are transplant candidates. The COMPANION trial has shown that BiV–ICD, in comparison to BiV only or no device therapy, reduces mortality in HF patients with functional class III or ambulatory class IV.

C. Syncope of undetermined origin with inducible, hemodynamically significant, sustained VT or VF on EP study (performed as part of syncope evaluation) (class I recommendation).

D. Dilated cardiomyopathy with syncope of unknown origin (class IIa).

E. Hypertrophic cardiomyopathy

ICD is indicated if risk factors for sudden death are present (unexplained syncope, family history of sudden death, septum > 30 mm).

Note: Wearable, external cardioverter defibrillator (Lifevest)

A Lifevest may be temporarily used in patients who are at high risk of sudden death yet do not have an ICD indication. This includes patients with a newly diagnosed non-ischemic cardiomyopathy, in whom EF frequently improves, and patients in the first 40 days after MI. In the WEAR-IT registry, the latter groups received a Lifevest for up to 3 months; 1.1% of the patients, mainly ischemic cardiomyopathy patients,

---

* MADIT II: ischemic cardiomyopathy > 40 days post-MI, LVEF ≤ 30%, NYHA class I–III, 75% of patients had their MI > 1.5 years prior to randomization (median of ~5 years). SCD-HeFT trial: ischemic or non-ischemic cardiomyopathy, LVEF ≤ 35%, NYHA class II or III, placebo vs. amiodarone vs. ICD.

** MADIT II identified high-risk criteria that, combined with reduced EF, increase the likelihood of benefit from an ICD in primary prevention: AF, QRS > 120 ms, functional class II–III, mild renal failure, age > 70 years old. On the other hand, very high-risk patients with advanced renal failure, ≥ 3 high-risk features, or functional class IV seem less likely to benefit (U curve); ICD reduces their sudden death but does not reduce their ultimate death (pump failure, comorbidities).[30]

had a sustained VT/VF that was prolonged, unstable, and treated by Lifevest, with all of those VT/VF patients eventually surviving to the end of follow-up (they did not die of PEA or pump failure).[36] Another registry analysis has shown that Lifevest is associated with a dramatic mortality reduction in the first 3 months after PCI and after CABG in the setting of low EF, the first 3 months representing the highest risk period of sudden death (Cleveland Clinic registry).[37] Eventually, beyond the first 3 months, the risk of sudden death declines and EF improves to >35% in 40% of patients.[36] Only 40% of patients require ICD implantation at the end of 3 months.[36,37] While these data support the use of Lifevest in ischemic cardiomyopathy, there are no randomized data addressing it.

VI. Specific VTs that should be considered in the absence of obvious heart disease

A. Brugada syndrome

A *Brugada pattern* is defined by two ECG characteristics:

- ST elevation in V_1–V_3, typically coved and gradually descending. Less specifically, ST elevation may have a saddleback shape (Figure 9.8).
- True RBBB or pseudo-RBBB. In pseudo-RBBB, rSR' is seen in V_1–V_3 but the QRS is normal in the lateral leads. PR interval is frequently prolonged.

There are three types of Brugada patterns:

- Type 1: coved ST elevation ≥2 mm at the J point in ≥2 of the leads V_1–V_3, with T-wave inversion
- Type 2: saddleback ST elevation >1 mm with upright or biphasic T wave
- Type 3: coved ST <2 mm or saddleback ST <1 mm

Brugada patterns can be transient. Being due to a loss of function of Na channels, they can be unveiled by Na channel blockers, such as flecainide or procainamide (class I AAD) and can be simulated by fever, cocaine, propofol, or tricyclic drug use. Moving V_1–V_2 up to the second intercostal space may improve the detection of these abnormalities.

The spontaneous type 1 Brugada pattern is the one most specifically associated with sudden death and most specifically called *Brugada syndrome*. The other two patterns are suspicious patterns but may be seen in healthy individuals; they require provocative testing with class I drugs for confirmation. Provocation of type 1 pattern establishes the diagnosis; however, the prognosis of provoked type 1 Brugada is much better than the spontaneous type 1 Brugada. The prevalence of any Brugada pattern on the ECG of asymptomatic individuals is 0.01–0.1%, the higher prevalence being described in a Japanese population.[38] The syncope/sudden death rate for the spontaneous type 1 pattern is ~0.5% per year.[39,40] Types 2 and 3 are not clearly associated with an increased event rate.

Brugada syndrome is due to a sodium channel mutation with loss of function, predominantly at the level of the epicardial RV, creating the ECG abnormalities in V_1–V_3.* It is autosomal dominant but mainly expressed in men; 90% of affected patients are men.

Brugada syndrome leads to polymorphic VT or VF, not monomorphic VT. The arrhythmia occurs at rest or during sleep, or after triggers, such as fever. In fact, fever is a major trigger of sudden death in these patients, as fever further inactivates the Na channels. In one report, 51% of patients with a Brugada-type pattern on ECG during an acute illness, especially fever, developed cardiac arrest or syncope.[41] Unlike LQT, where the arrhythmia is often self-terminating, Brugada syndrome often manifests as sudden death, although self-termination of the arrhythmia is possible. ICD is indicated if there is a history of sudden death, or a history of syncope along with a spontaneous ± inducible type 1 pattern; quinidine reduces the risk of VT as it blocks the hyperactive I_{Kto} channel.

In asymptomatic type 1 pattern, an EP study may be performed; an inducible VF implies a higher risk of sudden death (controversial). Asymptomatic type 2 or 3 patterns do not require any specific workup and are normal variants rather than specific predictors of life-threatening ventricular arrhythmias.[42]

B. Arrhythmogenic right ventricular dysplasia or cardiomyopathy (ARVD/ARVC)

ARVD is a genetic cardiomyopathy characterized by progressive replacement of the RV by fibro-fatty tissue, leading to RV dilatation, localized RV aneurysms, then LV involvement. RV apex and anterior wall are most commonly involved.

ARVD presents between 10 and 50 years of age, more commonly in men, and is familial in 30% of the cases (usually autosomal dominant with 30% penetrance). ARVD manifests as ventricular arrhythmias early on, then progressive right and left HF.

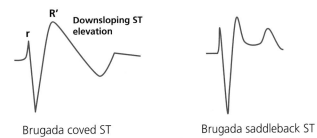

Brugada coved ST   Brugada saddleback ST

Figure 9.8 Brugada syndrome.

---

* This mutation reduces the sodium inflow current in phase 0 of the action potential, thereby reducing the action potential duration, which is opposite to LQT3 (SCN5A gene, Na ion channel). This effect is heterogeneous across the cardiac layers, which leads to dispersion of repolarization between the subepicardium and the myocardial M cells and subsequent reentrant circuits → VT–VF.

ECG features of the localized RV delay[43]

- T-wave inversion is frequently seen in leads V_1 through V_3, and in the absence of complete RBBB is highly suggestive of ARVD in both adult men and women. Normal women may have T-wave inversion in V_1 and V_2 that only rarely (4%) extends to V_3.
- ECG typically shows a prolongation of QRS $\geq$ 110 ms that is localized to leads V_1 through V_3, and more importantly, a delayed S upstroke (nadir of S to end of QRS $\geq$ 55 ms in 95% of patients). QRS is normal in lead V_6.
- A small positive deflection, called an *epsilon wave*, may be seen immediately after QRS.
- RBBB, whether complete or incomplete, is uncommon but may be seen in advanced stages.

VT that is due to ARVD originates from the RV and thus has an LBBB morphology. ECG abnormalities become more prevalent with time. Late potentials on signal-averaged ECG are also sensitive for ARVD diagnosis.

Echo features of ARVD[44]

- RVOT enlargement on the long- or short-axis views ($\geq$ 29 mm or 32 mm, respectively)
- Hyperreflective moderator band
- Hypertrabeculated RV
- Regional RV akinesis or aneurysms

Diagnosis of ARVD[44]

The diagnosis of ARVD requires $\geq$ 2 of the following:

a. Echo or MRI structural features
b. ECG features (epsilon, T inversion, or prolonged QRS with slow S upslope)
c. VT (sustained or non-sustained) of LBBB morphology or frequent PVCs (>500/24 hours)
d. Family history of ARVD or sudden death

Treatment of ARVD

Sudden death is common in ARVD; in fact, 25% of patients die suddenly. ICD is indicated in patients with one or more risk factors for sudden death: RV dysfunction, LV dysfunction, HF, syncope, sustained or even non-sustained VT. β-Blockers, sotalol, or amiodarone may be added to prevent VT. Since the ARVD process starts at the epicardial level, VT ablation is only effective if ablation is performed at both the endocardial and epicardial levels. When arrhythmic death is prevented, patients live long enough to develop severe right then left heart failure.

C. WPW

AF or atrial flutter that is conducted antegradely over an accessory pathway leads to a pre-excited, fast atrial arrhythmia that mimics polymorphic VT and may lead to sudden death.

D. Cardiac sarcoidosis

Cardiac sarcoidosis affects the electrical system early on and leads to tachy- or bradyarrhythmias, as well as bundle branch blocks. Inferobasal scarring is common.

E. Idiopathic catecholaminergic polymorphic VT

This is a form of polymorphic VT that occurs in the absence of ischemia, acute metabolic insults, or long QT. VT and sudden death occur during exercise or acute emotion, and most often manifest before the age of 20 and almost always before the age of 40. It is genetic and usually familial, related to excessive calcium release from the sarcoplasmic reticulum with subsequent delayed afterdepolarization. VT may look bidirectional as in digoxin toxicity (QRS alternation between left and right axis). It is treated with β-blockers and ICD. Flecainide is also a very effective therapy.

F. Idiopathic VTs: outflow tract VT (RVOT or LVOT VT, also called repetitive monomorphic VT) and idiopathic left ventricular fascicular VT

These VTs occur without any underlying heart disease. RVOT VT arises from the RVOT, LVOT VT arises from the LVOT or aortic sinus cusp, and LV fascicular VT arises from the left posterior fascicle (posterior septum, near the apex). The mechanism, ECG, and therapy of LVOT VT are closely related to RVOT VT.

Idiopathic VTs frequently present as palpitations and dizziness, usually in young patients (<50 years old); syncope is rare and sudden death is very rare. RVOT VT and LVOT VT most commonly (60–90%) manifest as repetitive, non-sustained salvos of VT or frequent monomorphic PVCs. RVOT VT and LVOT VT may occur with exertion, stress, or rest. LV fascicular VT typically occurs at rest but may be triggered with stress, and is more frequently sustained, occasionally leading to a tachycardia-mediated cardiomyopathy.

These VTs have specific ECG features (during VT, not during sinus rhythm):

- RVOT VT: LBBB with right axis. ARVD-associated VT may mimic RVOT VT.
- LVOT VT: RBBB, or LBBB with right axis and R transition in V_2, earlier than RVOT VT.
- Fascicular VT (Belhassen): RBBB with LAFB morphology. Since it originates near the normal conduction system, QRS is relatively narrow (~140 ms). Therefore, this VT is *difficult to differentiate from SVT*.

The ECG is typically normal between the VT episodes ($\neq$ ARVD).

Underlying heart disease, CAD, and the other specific VTs cited in this section must be ruled out. Therapy includes drugs (β-blockers or verapamil for RVOT VT and LVOT VT; verapamil for LV fascicular VT), or catheter ablation of the VT focus. Ablation may be used as first-line therapy in patients with severe symptoms or may be considered after drug failure. ICD is not indicated, as these VTs do not lead to sudden death. RVOT VT and LVOT VT represent cAMP-mediated triggered activity, and therefore may acutely resolve with adenosine; LV fascicular VT represents reentry across abnormally oriented posterior fascicular Purkinje fibers and only rarely responds to adenosine or β-blockers. ARVD does not respond to adenosine, and thus the response to adenosine helps differentiate RVOT VT from ARVD.

ARVD, sarcoidosis, Chagas disease, and giant-cell myocarditis are cardiomyopathies with predilection for arrhythmias and conduction blocks, even before overt myocardial disease.

VII. Causes of sudden cardiac death (SCD)
The mechanism of SCD is usually VT/VF.

A. Patients older than 35 years
- Ischemic heart disease is the most common cause of SCD
- Dilated and hypertrophic cardiomyopathies
- Severe valvular heart disease
- Electrical causes listed under *Patients younger than 35 years*

B. Patients younger than 35 years
1. Structural cardiac disease[45]
- Hypertrophic cardiomyopathy is the most common structural cause (10–30% of SCD at this age)
- ARVD: SCD mostly occurs during exertion
- Coronary artery anomalies
- Aortic stenosis secondary to a bicuspid aortic valve
- Myocarditis
- Dilated cardiomyopathy, including drug-related cardiomyopathy (cocaine)
- CAD

2. Electrical diseases explain up to 40% of SCDs at this age (also called sudden arrhythmic death syndrome or SADS)
- Long QT syndrome: SCD mostly occurs with exertion (especially swimming), emotion, or noise stimulation
- Brugada syndrome: SCD commonly occurs at rest, or during sleep, fever, or drug use
- Idiopathic catecholaminergic polymorphic VT: SCD occurs during exertion
- WPW
- Cardiac sarcoidosis
- Cocaine use
- Commotio cordis in athletes (blunt trauma to the chest during myocardial repolarization/T wave may lead to VF)

Pre-participation cardiac screening of athletes is a matter of controversy. The implementation of a systematic ECG screening strategy has led to a striking 90% reduction of SCD in Italy.[46] A screening ECG is fairly sensitive and specific for the detection of underlying cardiac disease. Normal ECG patterns seen in the athlete's heart need to be distinguished from pathological patterns:[47,48]

- *Normal athlete's heart patterns:* LVH by voltage criteria only, early repolarization pattern, incomplete RBBB, first-degree AV block.
- *Abnormal patterns:*
  - LVH with secondary ST–T abnormalities or LA enlargement rather than just LVH voltage criteria
  - RVH
  - ST-segment depression
  - Deep T-wave inversion beyond V_1 in white athletes and beyond V_4 in black athletes (worrisome for HCM or ARVD)
  - Pathological Q wave
  - QRS ≥ 120 ms, or complete RBBB or LBBB (which may suggest cardiomyopathy or progressive, premature conduction disorder)
  - Frequent PVCs (≥2 per 10s tracing)
  - Brugada pattern; long QTc (especially ≥ 470 ms in men, 480 ms in women)
- *Borderline patterns* (when isolated, they do not warrant further workup): right- or left-axis deviation; right or left atrial enlargement. Right-axis deviation in a young athlete is defined as axis > +115° rather than +90°.

The abnormal patterns are seen in 7–10% of athletes, more so black athletes, and warrant echo testing to rule out HCM, ARVD, or other structural abnormalities. The majority of patients with abnormal patterns are not found to have any structural abnormality on echo, but deserve close follow-up. Only 1–2% get disqualified from sport after echo assessment. Patients with bundle branch blocks may have HCM, ARVD, ASD, but may also have Lenegre AV conduction disease, in which AV block can develop with exertion (stress testing). A proportion of white athletes with deeply inverted T waves (≥2 mm) in the anterolateral precordial leads are at risk of having or developing cardiomyopathies or electrical problems, and thus are at risk of SCD. These T inversions are seen in ~3% of white athletes, of whom 6–25% end up having structural heart disease, sometimes not apparent on the initial echo.[49] In white athletes, these T-wave inversions are not always reflective of the "benign athlete's heart," and thus further workup (echo) and close follow-up is necessary. They are, however, commonly seen in leads V_1–V_4 in black athletes (~25%) and are benign in this group of patients, not warranting further investigation.[47]

Also, the ECG may identify a typical Brugada pattern, long QT, ARVD, or WPW patterns.

NSVT may be recorded in athletes without any heart disease and is considered a benign reflection of the "athlete's heart syndrome" when suppressed by exercise, after excluding cardiomyopathies and channelopathies.[50] An early repolarization pattern is very common in athletes; however, a downsloping ST-segment elevation or a J point that is notched and wide (≥1 mm) or elevated (≥2 mm) in the inferior leads identifies individuals at increased risk of sudden death (the absolute risk remains very low).[51]

ECG is highly sensitive and is reasonably reliable to exclude lethal cardiac disorders in young athletes. However, ~10% of HCMs have a totally normal ECG, and thus may be missed by ECG screening. The family history and symptoms help fill this 10% gap. The routine large-scale use of echocardiographic screening is not justified.

On echocardiography, some features differentiate "athlete's heart" hypertrophy from hypertrophic cardiomyopathy (see Chapter 7, Table 7.3).

Also, syncope or angina, family history of SCD, and murmur on exam are "red flags" that warrant the performance of an echocardiography. *If a teen or a young adult is found to have severe AS from a non-calcified bicuspid valve, or significant PS, valvuloplasty would be indicated even if the patient is asymptomatic. Afterwards, the patient may resume athletic activity in the absence of residual myocardial disease, significant valvular stenosis, or aortic dilatation (class IIa in the ACC valvular guidelines). Moderate AS or untreated severe AS is a contraindication to competitive sport.*

QUESTIONS AND ANSWERS

Question 1. (Questions 1 to 4 refer to the same case.) A 41-year-old with a history of hypertension presents with palpitations. His palpitations are sustained for one to several minutes and associated with near-syncope. During one of those episodes, the pulse checked by his wife was 150 bpm. ECG performed in the office shows sinus rhythm, borderline QRS width (~100 ms) with incomplete RBBB pattern, and biphasic T wave (mild terminal T inversion) in leads V_1–V_3. Echo shows a normal LV and borderline RV size, with no segmental akinesis. What is the next step?
A. Reassurance
B. 2-week event monitor
C. Cardiac MRI

Question 2. Event monitor reveals multiple runs of NSVT (3–12 beats, polymorphic) during the first 2 days of monitoring. What is the next step?
A. Admit the patient and perform coronary angiography
B. Cardiac MRI
C. Signal-averaged ECG

Question 3. Coronary angiography shows normal coronary arteries. A cardiac MRI is ordered next, and shows apical akinesis of the RV with late gadolinium enhancement of this portion of the RV. The RV is mildly enlarged by volume assessment, with RVEF 40–45% (mildly reduced, normal RVEF being > 45%). What is the diagnosis?
A. ARVD
B. Brugada syndrome
C. Idiopathic RVOT VT
D. Myocarditis

Question 4. What is the next step?
A. High dose of metoprolol, or sotalol. If this fails, switch to amiodarone and consider VT ablation
B. ICD
C. Genetic testing for the purpose of diagnosing the disease in his children
D. All of the above

Question 5. A 55-year-old woman presents with syncope. She had diarrhea for a week and her potassium is 3 mEq/l and calcium and magnesium are low. She has the ECG shown in Figure 9.5. What is the most likely underlying diagnosis?
A. Electrolyte abnormalities
B. Acute ischemia
C. Drug effect
D. Congenital long QT syndrome 1
E. Congenital long QT syndrome 2

Question 6. Which statement is *incorrect*?
A. VT with twisting QRS polarity is called TdP even if baseline QTc is normal
B. Bradycardia may elicit polymorphic VT even in the absence of a prolonged QTc (bradycardia-induced VT)
C. LQT1 and 2 are due to a loss of function (of K channel), while LQT3 is due to a gain of function (of Na channel)
D. Brugada syndrome is due to a loss of function of Na channel, while LQT3 is due to a gain of function of this same channel
E. If QTc > 480–500 ms without any reversible cause, the diagnosis of long QT syndrome is likely
F. In patients with borderline QTc 450–480 ms, further testing may need to be performed (e.g., effect of exercise or epinephrine on QTc)
G. In patients with QTc 430–450 ms who have syncope or a family history of sudden death, further testing may need to be performed

Question 7. A 30-year-old man who grew up in Mexico presents with syncope during basketball exercise. ECG and echo are normal. Stress testing reveals a monomorphic VT which appears to be originating from the LV inferolateral wall (QRS upright in V_1, negative in the inferior leads and lateral leads I-aVL). Coronary arteries are normal on angiography. What is the next step?
A. Ablation for idiopathic LV VT
B. Cardiac MRI

Question 8. Cardiac MRI is performed in the patient of Question 7. It shows a large inferolateral scar. In addition, the patient develops a complete RBBB on his ECG a few months later. What is the diagnosis?

A. Sarcoidosis
B. Chagas disease
C. ARVD
D. Giant-cell myocarditis
E. Some genetic cardiomyopathies (mutation of desmosomal genes)
F. A or B

Question 9. A patient experiences anterior MI and undergoes LAD PCI. His post-MI LVEF is 25%. Which of the following is true?

A. His highest risk of sudden death is in the first 40 days after MI. ICD is indicated in the first 40 days
B. His highest risk of sudden death is in the first 40 days after MI. But ICD implantation is not beneficial in the first 40 days. ICD is indicated at ≥40 days. Lifevest may be used in the first 40 days
C. His highest risk of sudden death is in the first year (risk equally spread throughout the year). ICD is indicated at ≥40 days

Question 10. A patient has LVEF 30% and is found to have severe LAD and RCA disease for which he undergoes PCI. Is the following statement true or false? The first 3 months after PCI constitute the highest-risk period of sudden death, yet ICD is only indicated beyond those 3 months (if EF remains ≤ 35%).

Question 11. A 40-year-old man has had daily palpitations described as "skipped beats" for 4 months, mostly at rest but also during emotional stress. He never had sustained palpitations or syncope. He is active and cycles 30 minutes every day without cardiac symptoms. ECGs capture frequent PVCs, of the same morphology (Figure 9.9). His baseline sinus rate is ~65 bpm. Echo is normal. What is the first-line therapy?

A. Metoprolol
B. Flecainide
C. Verapamil
D. Catheter ablation

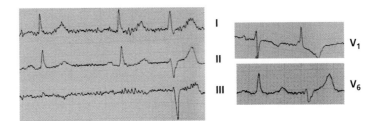

Figure 9.9

Answer 1. B. In patients with unsuspected cardiac disease, palpitations frequently correspond to non-arrhythmic awareness of one's heart beat (anxiety, stress) or to benign premature complexes. However, this patient has two worrisome elements in his history: (i) palpitations are sustained and associated with true near-syncope (in the absence of a myriad of functional complaints), and (ii) a fast pulse is documented. The ECG has borderline findings that, in an asymptomatic patient, may be considered normal (QRS being < 110 ms). However, in a patient with palpitations, the borderline RBBB pattern and the mild T inversion are suggestive of underlying structural heart disease (e.g., any cardiomyopathy), early ARVD, or even a hidden Brugada pattern. ST elevation must be present to make a Brugada diagnosis and may be unveiled with provocative testing or with moving the V₁–V₂ electrodes one interspace higher. One should attempt to document the cardiac rhythm during the index palpitations.

Answer 2. A. Based on the history of more sustained palpitations, the patient likely had, at times, more sustained episodes of VT. This warrants hospitalization. Polymorphic VT, even if non-sustained, is suspicious for myocardial ischemia.

Answer 3. A. The patient fulfills many criteria of ARVD, although none of them is a major criterion: (i) RV akinesis and scar on MRI; (ii) borderline but suggestive ECG; (iii) NSVT. RV involvement on MRI or echo would be a major criterion for ARVD if the RV were more than mildly dilated or EF were more severely reduced (<40%). Genetic testing and signal-averaged ECG, looking for late fragmented QRS potentials (microscopic epsilon waves), may further support the diagnosis. Myocarditis is possible but is a less likely diagnosis considering the constellation of findings.

Answer 4. D.

Answer 5. D. Electrolyte disturbances, acute ischemia, drug side effect and congenital long QT syndrome are the four major causes of a prolonged QT interval. While the electrolyte abnormalities accentuate the QT prolongation, the patient has another underlying cause of prolonged QT that explains the broad T-wave morphology, such as congenital long QT syndrome or acute ischemia. In long QT syndrome 1, T wave is wide and ample without ST-segment depression, similar to our patient. T wave alternans is most characteristic of congenital long QT syndrome.

Answer 6. A. VT with twisting QRS polarity, but normal baseline QTc, is a non-TdP polymorphic VT.

Answer 7. B. The normal ECG and echo suggest that VT may be idiopathic, but the occurrence of syncope and the inferolateral origin make idiopathic VT less likely.

Answer 8. F. All the five listed answers are specific causes of cardiomyopathy with focal scarring and a predilection for arrhythmia and conduction abnormality. In this case, ARVD is unlikely (no RV issue on imaging). The lack of HF and the slow course do not suggest giant-cell myocarditis. Sarcoidosis or Chagas is the most likely disease. Next, serologic testing for Chagas disease and a search for non-cardiac sarcoid involvement should be carried out.

Answer 9. B.

Answer 10. True.

Answer 11. C. The PVC has the morphology of RBBB + LAFB and is relatively narrow (~140 ms). It may get confused with an aberrant PAC. This PVC morphology and width is characteristic of idiopathic LV fascicular PVC originating from the left posterior fascicle. It is characteristically responsive to verapamil, as described by Belhassen. Catheter ablation is a second-line therapy (high success rate). As opposed to idiopathic RVOT PVC, this PVC is not usually responsive to metoprolol. The normal echo and the lack of other cardiac symptoms are necessary for the diagnosis of idiopathic fascicular PVC/VT; the same morphology may be seen with a scar PVC originating from an inferoseptal scar.

References

1. Bogun F, Crawford T, Reich S, et al. Radiofrequency ablation of frequent, idiopathic premature ventricular complexes: comparison with a control group without intervention. Heart Rhythm 2007; 4: 863–7.
2. Baman TS, Lange DC, Ilg KJ, et al. Relationship between burden of premature ventricular complexes and left ventricular function. Heart Rhythm 2010; 7: 865–9.
3. Echt DS, Liebson PR, Mitchell LB, et al. Mortality and morbidity in patients receiving encainide, flecain- ide, or placebo: the Cardiac Arrhythmia Suppression Trial. N Engl J Med 1991; 324: 781–8. *CAST trial = increased risk of sudden death with class I antiarrhythmics.*
4. Yarlagadda RK, Iwai S, Stein KM, et al. Reversal of cardiomyopathy in patients with repetitive monomorphic ventricular ectopy originating from the right ventricular outflow tract. Circulation 2005; 112: 1092–7.
5. Lu F, Benditt DG, Yu J, Graf B. Effects of catheter ablation of "asymptomatic" frequent premature complexes in patients with reduced (<48%) left ventricular ejection fraction. Am J Cardiol 2012; 110: 852–6.
6. Froelicher VF, Thomas MM, Pillow C, Lancaster MC. Epidemiologic study of asymptomatic men screened by maximal treadmill testing for latent coronary artery disease. Am J Cardiol 1974; 34: 770–6.
7. Moore HJ, Fletcher RD, Platt MD, et al. SCD-HeFT: non-sustained ventricular tachycardia on baseline holter monitor. Association with overall mortality. J Am Coll Cardiol 2011; 57: E41.
8. Scirica BM, Braunwald E, Belardinelli L, et al. Relationship between nonsustained ventricular tachycardia after non-ST-elevation acute coronary syndrome and sudden cardiac death: observations from MERLIN-TIMI 36 randomized controlled trial. Circulation 2010; 122: 455–62.
9. Epstein AE, DiMarco JP, Ellenbogen KA, et al. ACC/AHA/HRS 2008 guidelines for device-based therapy of cardiac rhythm abnormalities: a report of the American College of Cardiology/American Heart Association Task Force on Practice Guidelines. J Am Coll Cardiol 2008; 51: e1–62.
10. Doval HC, Nul DR, Grancelli HO, et al. Randomised trial of low-dose amiodarone in severe congestive heart failure. Grupo de Estudio de la Sobrevida en la Insuficiencia Cardiaca en Argentina (GESICA). Lancet 1994; 344: 493–8.
11. Kadish A, Dyer A, Daubert JP, et al. Prophylactic defibrillator implantation in patients with non-ischemic dilated cardiomyopathy. N Engl J Med 2004; 350: 2151–8. *SCD-HeFT trial.*
12. Scherlag BJ, Kabell G, Harrison L, Lazzara R. Mecahnisms of bradycardia-induced ventricular arrhythmias in myocardial ischemia and infarction. Circulation 1982; 65: 1429–34.
13. Satoh T, Zipes D. Rapid rates during bradycardia prolong ventricular refractoriness and facilitate ventricular tachycardia induction with cesium in dogs. Circulation 1996; 94: 217–27.
14. Roden DM. Long-QT syndrome. N Engl J Med 2008; 358: 159–68.
15. Vincent GM, Timothy KW, Leppert M, Keating M. The spectrum of symptoms and QT intervals in carriers of the gene for the long-QT syndrome. N Engl J Med 1992; 327: 846–52.
16. Molnar J, Zhang F, Weiss J, Ehlert FA, Rosenthal JE. Diurnal pattern of QTc interval: how long is prolonged? J Am Coll Cardiol 1996; 27: 76–83.
17. Shimizu W, Noda T, Takaki H, et al. Epinephrine unmasks latent mutation carriers with LQT1 form of congenital long-QT syndrome. J Am Coll Cardiol 2003; 41: 633–42.
18. Goldenberg I, Moss AJ, Zareba W. QT interval: how to measure it and what is normal? J Cardiovasc Electrophysiol 2006; 17: 333–6.
19. Priori SG, Schwartz PJ, Napolitano C, et al. Risk stratification in the long-QT syndrome. N Engl J Med 2003; 48: 1866–74.
20. Sauer AJ, Moss AJ, McNitt S. Long QT syndrome in adults. J Am Coll Cardiol 2007; 49: 329–37.
21. Goldenberg I, Moss AJ, Bradley J, et al. Long-QT syndrome after age 40. Circulation 2008; 117; 2192–201.
22. Priori SG, Napolitano C, Schwartz PJ, et al. Association of long QT syndrome loci and cardiac events among patients treated with beta-blockers. JAMA 2004; 292: 1341–4.
23. Moss AJ, Zareba W, Hall J, et al. Effectiveness and limitations of β-blocker therapy in congenital long-QT syndrome. Circulation 2000; 101: 616–23.
24. Zipes DP, Camm AJ, Borggrefe M, et al. ACC/AHA/ESC 2006 guidelines for management of patients with ventricular arrhythmias and the prevention of sudden cardiac death. J Am Coll Cardiol 2006; 48: 1064–108.
25. Connolly SJ, Gent M, Roberts RS, et al. Canadian implantable defibrillator study (CIDS): a randomized trial of the implantable cardioverter defibrillator against amiodarone, Circulation 2000; 101: 1297–302.
26. Antiarrhythmics versus Implantable Defibrillators (AVID) Investigators. A comparison of antiarrhythmic-drug therapy with implantable defibrillators in patients resuscitated from near-fatal ventricular arrhythmias, N Engl J Med 1997; 337: 1576–83.
27. Russo AM, Stainback RF, Bailey SR, et al. ACCF/HRS/AHA/ASE/HFSA/SCAI/SCCT/SCMR 2013 appropriate use criteria for implantable cardioverter-defibrillators and cardiac resynchronization therapy. J Am Coll Cardiol 2013; 61: 1318–68.
28. Brugada J, Aguinaga L, Mont L, et al. Coronary artery revascularization in patients with sustained ventricular arrhythmias in the chronic phase of a myocardial infarction: effects on the electrophysiologic substrate and outcome. J Am Coll Cardiol 2001; 37: 529–33.

29. Moss AJ, Zarebra W, Hall WJ, et al. Prophylactic implantation of a defibrillator in patients with myocardial infarction and reduced ejection fraction. N Engl J Med 2002; 346: 877–83. *MADIT 2.*

30. Goldenberg I, Vyas AK, Hall WJ, et al. Risk stratification for primary implantation of a cardioverter defibrillator in patients with ischemic left ventricular dysfunction. J Am Coll Cardiol 2008; 51: 288–96.

31. Hohnloser SH, Kuck KH, Dorian P, et al. Prophylactic use of an implantable cardioverter-defibrillator after acute myocardial infarction. N Engl J Med 2004; 351: 2481–8.

32. Steinbeck G, Andresen D, Seidl K, et al. Defibrillator implantation early after myocardial infarction. N Engl J Med 2009; 361: 1427–36.

33. Wilber DJ, Zareba W, Hall WJ, et al. Time dependence of mortality risk and defibrillator benefit after myocardial infarction. Circulation 2004; 109: 1082–4.

34. Chen C, Stevenson LW, Stewart GC, et al. Impact of baseline heart failure burden on post-implantable cardioverter-defibrillator mortality among Medicare beneficiaries. J Am Coll Cardiol 2013; 61: 2142–50.

35. Bigger JT. Prophylactic use of implanted cardiac defibrillators in patients at high risk for ventricular arrhythmias after coronary-artery bypass graft surgery. Coronary Artery Bypass Graft (CABG) Patch Trial Investigators. N Engl J Med 1997; 337: 1569–75.

36. Kutyifa V, Moss AJ, Klein H, et al. Use of the wearable cardioverter defibrillator in high-risk cardiac patients: data from the prospective registry of patients using the wearable cardioverter defibrillator (WEAR-IT registry). Circulation 2015; 132: 1613–19.

37. Zishiri ET, Williams S, Cronin EM, et al. Early risk of mortality after coronary artery revascularization in patients with left ventricular dysfunction and potential role of the wearable cardioverter defibrillator. Circ Arrhythm Electrophysiol 2013; 6: 117–28.

38. Matsuo K, Akahoshi M, Nakashima E, et al. The prevalence, incidence, and prognostic value of Brugada-type electrocardiogram. J Am Coll Cardiol 2001; 38: 765–70.

39. Eckardt L, Probst V, Smits JP, et al. Long-term prognosis of individuals with right precordial ST-segment-elevation Brugada syndrome. Circulation 2005; 111: 257–63.

40. Probst V, Veltmann C, Eckardt L, et al. Long-term prognosis of patients diagnosed with Brugada syndrome: Results from the FINGER Brugada Syndrome Registry. Circulation 2010; 121: 635–43.

41. Junttila MJ, Gonzales M, Lizotte E, et al. Induced Brugada-type electrocardiogram, a sign for imminent malignant arrhythmias. Circulation 2008; 117: 1890–3.

42. Junttila MJ, Raatikainen MJ, Karjalainen J, et al. Prevalence and prognosis of subjects with Brugada-type ECG pattern in a young and middle-aged Finnish population. Eur Heart J 2004; 25: 874–8.

43. Nasir K, Bomma C, Tandri H, et al. Electrocardiographic features of arrhythmogenic right ventricular dysplasia/cardiomyopathy according to disease severity: a need to broaden diagnostic criteria. Circulation. 2004; 110: 1527–34.

44. Marcus FI, McKenna WJ, Sherrill D, et al. Diagnosis of arrhythmogenic right ventricular cardiomyopathy/dysplasia: proposed modification of the task force criteria. Circulation 2010; 121: 1533–41.

45. Maron BJ. Sudden death in young athletes. N Engl J Med 2003; 349: 1064–75.

46. Corrado D, Basso C, Pavei A, et al. Trends in sudden cardiovascular death in young competitive athletes after implementation of a preparticipation screening program. JAMA 2006; 296: 1593–601.

47. Sheikh N, Papadakis M, Ghani S, et al. Comparison of electrocardiographic criteria for detection of cardiac abnormalities in elite black and white athletes. Circulation. 2014; 129: 1637–49.

48. Corrado D, Pelliccia A, Heidbuchel H, et al. Recommendations for the interpretation of the 12-lead electrocardiogram in the athlete. Eur Heart J 2010: 31: 243–59.

49. Pelliccia A, Di Paolo FA, Quattrinni FM, et al. Outcomes in athletes with marked ECG repolarization abnormalities. N Engl J Med 2008; 358: 152–61.

50. Biffi A, Pellicia A, Verdile L, et al. Long-term clinical significance of frequent and complex ventricular tachyarrhythmias in trained athletes. J Am Coll Cardiol 2002; 40: 446–52.

51. Tikkanen JT, Anttonen O, Junttila MJ, et al.Long Long-term outcome associated with early repolarization on electrocardiography. N Engl J Med 2008; 358: 2016–23.

Further reading

Frequent PVCs and NSVT in asymptomatic patients with unsuspected heart disease are benign

Kennedy HL, Whitlock JA, Sprague MK, et al. Long-term follow-up of asymptomatic healthy subjects with frequent and complex ventricular ectopy. N Engl J Med 1985; 312: 193–197.

Engstrom G, Hedblad B, Janzon L. Ventricular arrhythmias during 24-h ambulatory ECG recording: incidence, risk factors and prognosis in men with and without a history of cardiovascular disease. J Intern Med 1999; 246: 363–72. *Age 68, frequent PVCs in up to 30%, NSVT in 7%.*

Frequent PVCs may have a prognostic value

Bikkina M, Larson MG, Levy D. Prognostic implications of asymptomatic ventricular arrhythmias: the Framingham Heart Study. Ann Intern Med 1992; 117: 990–6. *Age 50s, frequent PVCs in 7%, association with mortality in men not women; but patients with underlying heart disease may not have been rigorously eliminated.*

Dukes JW, Dewland TA, Vittinghoff E, et al. Ventricular ectopy as a predictor of heart failure and death. J Am Coll Cardiol 2015; 66: 101–9. *In patients older than 65 with normal EF at baseline and with PVC burden > 0.5%, the risk of HF (frequently low EF) is 30% at 15 years; in those with PVC burden > 6% or > 10%, the risk of HF is ~35%. In those without or with minimal PVCs, the risk is ~20%.*

Prevalence of tachycardia-mediated cardimyopathy in patients with a high PVC burden

Baman TS, Lange DC, Ilg KJ, et al. Relationship between burden of premature ventricular complexes and left ventricular function. Heart Rhythm 2010; 7: 865–9. *Prevalence of reduced EF is ~33%, more so if PVC burden > 10%.*

The prognostic value of PACs

Beneci Z, Intzilakis T, Nielsen OW, et al. Excessive supraventricular ectopic activity and increased risk of atrial fibrillation and stroke. Circulation 2010; 121: 1904–11. *In patients 55–75 years old, frequent PACs (>30/hour) are associated with a threefold increase in stroke risk.*

10 Atrial Fibrillation

Atrial fibrillation (AF) is the most common sustained arrhythmia that requires treatment, with an estimated prevalence in the United States of 2.3 million in 2001.[1] Its prevalence increases with age, hypertension, and heart failure: 3–4% of patients aged 65–75 have AF and 10% of patients aged 80 years or older have AF; 4% of patients with heart failure (HF) functional class I and 50% of patients with functional class IV have AF.[2] On the other hand, HF is present in 34% of AF patients.[3] AF is typically initiated by one or more premature atrial complexes, often originating around the pulmonary veins, or by atrial tachycardia or atrial flutter.

I. Predisposing factors (see Table 10.1)

Hypertension is the most common factor associated with AF on a population basis; coronary artery disease (CAD) and HF are the most common associated features in hospital series.[4] Between 30% and 45% of paroxysmal AF cases, and 20–25% of persistent AF cases, are "lone AF," i.e., AF that occurs in patients younger than 65 years without underlying heart or lung disease and without hypertension.[5] Even in the case of lone AF, there are structural atrial abnormalities and some degree of atrial dilatation and dysfunction, as well as an increased prevalence of high-normal blood pressure (i.e., systolic pressure 130–140 mmHg), that are contributive to AF.[6,7] As they age, however, patients with lone AF may develop hypertension or heart disease that contributes to the progression of AF.

The most frequent histopathological feature of AF is atrial fibrosis, which may precede the onset of AF. Atrial dilatation is present in over 50% of patients with AF, with a mean left atrial diameter of ~40±8 mm in the Canadian Registry of non-valvular AF; atrial dilatation is less prevalent in patients with non-recurrent AF and lone AF.[7] Atrial dilatation may be not only a cause but also a consequence of AF, as evidenced by the fact that the left atrial size further increases with time, over months to years, in patients with persistent AF.[8,9] On the other hand, left atrial size decreases after AF cardioversion.[10,11]. Atrial electrical remodeling, i.e., *progressive shortening of the effective refractory period*, further explains how prolonged AF makes restoring and maintaining sinus rhythm less likely ("AF begets AF").[2]

AF requires a trigger that initiates the arrhythmia *and* a substrate that sustains it. The most common triggers are premature atrial beats originating from the pulmonary veins. Atrial stretch and atrial fibrosis shorten the atrial effective refractory period and disrupt the electrical interconnections between the muscle bundles, causing local conduction heterogeneity. This allows ectopic activity originating from the

Practical Cardiovascular Medicine, First Edition. Elias B. Hanna.
© 2017 John Wiley & Sons Ltd. Published 2017 by John Wiley & Sons Ltd.

Table 10.1 Factors predisposing to atrial fibrillation.

- Systemic arterial hypertension
- Coronary artery disease
- Heart failure
- Any acute or chronic structural heart disease
- Obesity and sleep apnea[a]
- Atrial inflammation: pericarditis, myocarditis
- Metabolic disorders: alcohol, hyperthyroidism, hypokalemia
- Pulmonary diseases: COPD, pulmonary embolism
- Postoperative state (cardiac, pulmonary, or esophageal surgeries)

---

[a] Sleep apnea is seen in 18% of patients with AF. CPAP therapy reduces the progression of AF.

pulmonary veins or elsewhere to get conducted and initiate multiple microreentry cycles (atrial wavelets). Those microreentrant cycles collide like "tornadoes" and generate new tornadoes that propagate throughout the atria.

The autonomic system may contribute to the initiation of AF, i.e., an increase in the sympathetic or parasympathetic drive may trigger ectopy in the pulmonary veins and AF.

II. Types of AF
There are three types of AF: paroxysmal, persistent, and permanent:[2,12]

- *Paroxysmal AF* is defined as AF that terminates spontaneously in less than 7 days (often 24–48 hours). AF that is terminated with cardioversion at ≤7 days of onset is also considered paroxysmal AF in the most recent classification.
- *Persistent AF* is AF that persists over 7 days or requires cardioversion at >7 days (or unknown duration). *Long-standing persistent AF* is continuous AF that persists greater than 12 months, yet the adoption of a rhythm-control strategy is still planned.
- *AF is considered permanent* or chronic in cases of failure of cardioversion attempts, early recurrences after cardioversion, or decision not to cardiovert. A decision may be made not to cardiovert a patient who is asymptomatic after rate control and has a high likelihood of recurrence (e.g., longstanding AF of over a year or severe left atrial enlargement >5 cm).

Paroxysmal and persistent AF may be recurrent. Over time, patients may alternate between paroxysmal and persistent AF. For example, in a particular patient, most of the AF episodes may be self-terminating, while some of them may require cardioversion. While a paroxysmal AF may recur as paroxysmal AF for years, AF is generally progressive over time, with a rate of progression to persistent or permanent AF of ~15% within the first year.

A newly diagnosed AF or "*first-detected AF*" could fall into either one of these categories. While the first-detected AF is often a symptomatic paroxysmal or recently persistent AF, 21% of patients in whom AF is newly diagnosed are asymptomatic, and AF is diagnosed by routine pulse exam during an office visit.[13] In the latter patients, AF is likely several weeks, months, or years old. Thus, a *newly diagnosed AF does not imply a new AF.*

The term "*valvular AF*" is used to describe AF associated with mitral stenosis, prosthetic heart valve (mechanical or bioprosthetic valve), or mitral valve repair, and portends a higher stroke risk than non-valvular AF.

III. General therapy of AF
There are three main consequences of AF: (i) thrombus formation in the left atrial appendage (LAA) followed by thrombus embolization, (ii) fast and irregular heart rate leading to compromised ventricular filling, and (iii) loss of the atrial kick that contributes to up to 40% of the cardiac output in stable HF patients. Also, a rapid ventricular response of 120 beats per minute or more that persists for over 2 weeks can cause tachycardia-mediated cardiomyopathy and HF.[14]

A. Anticoagulation
Administer an anticoagulant regardless of whether *AF is paroxysmal or permanent. AF often recurs, and asymptomatic recurrences are 12 times more common than symptomatic recurrences*.[15] In the AFFIRM study, the risk of ischemic stroke was strongly related to absent or suboptimal anticoagulation even in the rhythm-control strategy.[16] Drug therapy makes AF recurrences shorter and slower, hence less symptomatic; the stroke risk, however, is unchanged.

B. Rate control
Three classes of drugs may be used: β-blockers, non-dihydropyridine-type calcium channel blockers (CCBs), i.e., diltiazem or verapamil, and digoxin. A β-blocker or a CCB is used as a first-line agent.

β-blockers are the most effective rate-controlling agents chronically, are effective as monotherapy in up to 70% of patients with AF,[17] and are first-line therapy in compensated systolic HF. They also have an antiarrhythmic effect and may convert adrenergically mediated AF into sinus rhythm.

Digoxin is less effective as monotherapy and is poorly effective for rate control during exertion. Digoxin is only used as monotherapy in decompensated systolic HF, when the acute initiation of β-blockers is not possible. Digoxin is effective in combination therapy: the combinations digoxin–β-blocker and digoxin–CCB are at least as effective and safe as the combination β-blocker–CCB.[18]

If the rate is inadequately controlled with the maximum tolerated dose of a β-blocker, digoxin or diltiazem is added as a second-line agent; diltiazem is not an appropriate option in systolic HF. The combination of β-blocker and verapamil has a strong negative inotropic effect and should be avoided in all patients. Triple combination is required in ~15–20% of the cases, but increases the risk of excessive pauses. Pharmacological therapy can achieve rate control in >80% of patients.[17] The remaining patients cannot be rate-controlled with drugs and require rhythm control, provided that long-term success can be expected, or failing that, atrioventricular nodal ablation with ventricular pacing. Patients with AF, including AF with fast ventricular rates, may also have periods of sinus bradycardia or AF-related pauses that limit the use of rate-controlling agents: these patients may require rhythm control or pacemaker placement.

In symptomatic patients, the goal of therapy is to reduce the heart rate to <80 bpm at rest, <110 bpm with moderate activity or 6-minute walk, and to reduce the average heart rate to <100 bpm on 24-hour Holter monitoring. This goal has been adopted in the AFFIRM and RACE trials which established the efficacy of a rate-control strategy. However, in the RACE II trial, the strict rate-control goal did not offer any benefit over a more lenient control (a resting heart rate <110 bpm at rest) in patients with permanent AF, normal LV function, and mild or no AF-related symptoms.[19] There was no significant difference in hard outcomes (death, hospitalization for HF, stroke) or in symptom control at 3-year follow-up. The lenient strategy may reduce drug side effects and the occurrence of symptomatic AF pauses. Note, however, that most patients in the lenient group had a heart rate <100 bpm (85 ± 14 bpm), which implies that 100 bpm may be a better lenient goal than 110 bpm. In addition, these patients had normal LV function and mild or no symptoms.

In a patient with HF, or in a patient who is severely symptomatic despite lenient control (intolerable palpitations, unexplained dyspnea, or fatigue interfering with the quality of life), *a strict rate control should be adopted; if symptoms persist despite strict rate control, rhythm control should be considered*. Moreover, when lenient control is adopted, serial echocardiograms (Q6–12 months) need to be performed to ensure a stable LV function and the lack of progression to a tachycardia-mediated cardiomyopathy.

> **When AF becomes slow and regular, complete AV block with a junctional escape rhythm is diagnosed.** Also, AF pauses >3–5 seconds during wakefulness imply high-grade AV block. This may be related to excessive dosing of the rate-controlling drugs or to AV nodal disease. If this AV block persists after drug discontinuation, a permanent pacemaker is indicated.

C. Rhythm control

Rhythm control is generally the least important goal. Long-term rhythm control, as compared with rate control, has not been shown to improve mortality, stroke rate, or HF hospitalizations in patients at high risk of stroke or AF recurrences (AFFIRM and RACE trials),[20,21] and in stable HF patients with EF <35% (AF-CHF trial).[22] In fact, rhythm control was associated with a higher rate of hospitalization for recurrent AF and drug-related bradyarrhythmias and tachyarrhythmias. In addition, in the AFFIRM trial, rhythm control was associated with increased non-cardiac mortality, particularly when amiodarone was used (pulmonary and cancer mortality).[23,24] Amiodarone was the most commonly used drug in the AFFIRM trial, while sotalol was the most commonly used drug in the RACE trial. These studies enrolled persistent AF (RACE), and paroxysmal or persistent AF (AFFIRM, AF CHF).

This failure of rhythm control is partly related to the marginal efficacy of antiarrhythmic drugs and to their toxicity: only 62% of patients in the rhythm-control arm of the AFFIRM trial, compared to 34% in the rate-control arm, were in sinus rhythm at 3.5 years of follow-up (only 39% of patients in the rhythm-control arm of RACE were in sinus rhythm).[21] Secondary analyses of these trials showed that the presence of sinus rhythm on follow-up was associated with improved quality of life (RACE)[25] and survival (AFFIRM),[23] regardless of the treatment strategy or the use of antiarrhythmic drugs. Conversely, antiarrhythmic drugs, per se, were associated with reduced survival.[23]

> Rhythm control is still a valid strategy in patients who are **symptomatic despite rate control** *and* **who have a good likelihood of maintaining sinus rhythm** (Table 10.2 criteria without Table 10.3 criteria). Rate-control drugs should be continued during a rhythm-control strategy to ensure adequate rate control during AF recurrences.

> **AV nodal ablation with ventricular pacing is the ultimate and definite therapy for AF that cannot be rate- or rhythm-controlled.**

In patients with BMI >27 kg/m², *weight loss >10%, by itself, dramatically reduces the recurrence of AF*. Weight loss, by itself, is almost as effective as antiarrhythmic drugs in preventing AF recurrence, and it allows interruption of antiarrhythmic drug therapy in many patients (~50% freedom from AF and antiarrhythmic drug therapy over several years of follow-up, vs. <20% if no

Table 10.2 Cases in which a rhythm-control strategy should be considered (first four are most important).

- Intolerable symptoms despite rate control (fatigue, palpitations, or HF that correlates with AF episodes)
- Difficulty in achieving adequate rate control; or alternation of fast AF with sinus bradycardia, precluding the optimal use of rate-controlling drugs
- Newly diagnosed, symptomatic AF, even if symptoms get controlled with rate reduction[a]. This particularly applies to a young patient (ESC class IIa)[28]
- Decompensated HF (rhythm control after stabilization and diuresis); or advanced, class III–IV HF (not well represented in the AF-CHF trial)

- Other potential HF indications: diastolic HF; RV failure, where AV synchrony is critical[29]
- Age <65 years[b]
- AF secondary to a treated precipitant (ischemia, hyperthyroidism)[28]

---

[a] 21% of patients in whom AF is newly diagnosed are asymptomatic; these patients are unlikely to benefit from a rhythm-control strategy.[13]
[b] Most patients in the AFFIRM and RACE trials were older than 65. A recent meta-analysis suggests that rhythm control may improve mortality in patients younger than 65.[30]

Table 10.3 Risk factors associated with failure of direct-current cardioversion, recurrence of AF after cardioversion, or progression of paroxysmal AF to persistent AF (first five are most important). **The best candidate for rhythm control is the patient having Table 10.2 criteria with none of Table 10.3 criteria**.

- Severe left atrial enlargement, i.e., anteroposterior diameter >4.5–5 cm
- AF duration of more than 1 year
- Decompensated HF or decompensated medical condition that has not been treated, e.g., hyperthyroidism
- Previous recurrences of AF, especially ≥2 recurrences requiring cardioversion
- Morbid obesity

- Underlying HF or structural heart disease
- COPD
- Age >70–75 years

The Euro Heart Survey allowed the development of a risk score, somewhat similar to $CHADS_2$ score, that predicts the progression from paroxysmal to persistent or permanent AF: HAT_2CH_2 (**H**ypertension, **A**ge >75, **T**IA or stroke 2 points, **C**OPD, **H**F 2 points). HATCH score of 0 or 1 → <10% risk of progression; 2–5 → 25–30% risk of progression; 6 or 7 → 50% risk of progression at 1 year.[31] **Potentially harmful drugs and interventions, including cardioversion, may be avoided in patients with a high HAT_2CH_2 score.**

Table 10.4 Dosage of the drugs used for acute rate control.

1. Metoprolol 5 mg IV, to be repeated Q5 min up to 15 mg total. Then start oral metoprolol 25–50 mg Q6h if the IV doses have proven effective and tolerated. The IV metoprolol effect lasts a few hours. Alternatively, esmolol IV drip may be given (short-acting; effect lasts 10–20 min after the drip is off). Esmolol is the preferred agent if it is uncertain whether β-blockers will be hemodynamically tolerated
2. Diltiazem IV 0.25 mg/kg (~20 mg) bolus. May rebolus with 0.35 mg/kg (~25 mg) in 15 min if no response to 20 mg, then start 5–15 mg/h IV drip in responders.[a] The IV diltiazem effect lasts a few hours. In comparison with β-blockers, diltiazem has:
   - more hypotensive effects in general (vasodilatation)
   - similar hypotensive effects in pre-shock, wherein BP depends on both the adrenergic and vascular tone
   - less negative inotropic effects (than verapamil as well), but still not advised in systolic HF
3. Digoxin needs to be given as a load (0.5 mg, then 0.25 mg Q6–8 h × 2 = 1 mg load, oral or IV). The load is followed by 0.125–0.25 mg Qday

Acute monotherapy with β-blockers or CCBs is effective in the majority of the cases, the target ventricular rate in the acute setting being usually 80–110 bpm (ESC). In case of total non-response to one agent, switch to another; in case of partial response to one, combine two agents, then try to wean off the first one. β-Blockers are more effective in hyperadrenergic states (e.g., postoperatively). Avoid digoxin as a sole agent to control the heart rate, except with decompensated heart failure or low blood pressure.
[a] IV diltiazem may be used for a few hours, then oral diltiazem started 3 hours after discontinuation of the IV drip, with a daily oral dose equal to (mg/day): IV drip rate in mg/h x 30 + 30. Short-acting diltiazem may initially be used Q6h.

weight loss). Also, weight loss is synergistic with AF ablation and antiarrhythmic therapy (87% freedom from AF over several years of follow-up after ablation, vs. <40% if no weight loss). This is enhanced by aggressive control of HTN, lipids, diabetes, sleep apnea, and smoking (LEGACY and ARREST-AF studies).[26,27]

IV. Management of a patient who acutely presents with symptomatic AF

1. Direct-current cardioversion (DCCV) is indicated emergently in cases of hypotension, acute severe HF with severe pulmonary edema, or myocardial ischemia attributed to AF. Typically, to attribute hemodynamic compromise to AF and to justify urgent cardioversion, the heart rate must be >150 bpm. **Also, in these cases, look for potential causes of shock that might have triggered both hypotension and AF.**
2. Acute rate control is achieved with β-blockers or CCBs (= first-line agents) in the absence of hypotension or decompensated HF. These agents are given intravenously if AF is severely symptomatic (Table 10.4).
   - *Intravenous digoxin or amiodarone is a first-line option in decompensated systolic HF or borderline low BP (ESC and ACC class I). Amiodarone has the theoretical risk of acutely cardioverting AF in a patient who may have an atrial appendage thrombus, but the short-term likelihood of cardioversion in a patient with HF or critical illness is low. Neither ACC nor ESC guidelines insist on this risk.*
   - *β-Blockers may be used acutely in LV diastolic HF and in LV systolic dysfunction without clinical HF.*
   - *The onset of action of IV drugs is fast (a few minutes), except for digoxin (1–5 hours).*
3. **Acute AF often spontaneously resolves by 24 hours, in ~60% of the cases, even more so in the absence of heart disease**. If it persists beyond 24 hours:
   i. *If a rhythm-control strategy is selected, perform* **acute cardioversion at 24 hours** *(DCCV or drugs), after TEE rules out left atrial appendage thrombus. Alternatively, give 3 weeks of anticoagulation then perform DCCV without TEE. The patient needs to receive acute anticoagulation with heparin or enoxaparin.*
   ii. *May allow the progression to a rate-controlled permanent AF. This depends on the severity of AF-related symptoms, their persistence despite rate control, the age of the patient (young → cardiovert), and the likelihood of AF recurrence.*
4. Hospitalize the patient with severe symptoms, HF, or suspicion of MI or PE. Also, hospitalize if DCCV is planned.
5. Perform an echocardiogram and look for underlying cardiac, systemic, or metabolic diseases: acute HF, MI, acute PE, sepsis, anemia, thyrotoxicosis, electrolyte abnormalities. Correcting these factors (e.g., diuresis and vasodilators for HF) may control the rate and eventually convert AF to sinus rhythm. In fact, DCCV is often ineffective in the presence of uncontrolled triggers or uncontrolled HF, as AF quickly recurs after cardioversion.
   - MI or PE may need to be ruled out if clinically suggested. Stress testing may be performed if CAD is suspected.

V. Peri-cardioversion management and long-term management after the acute presentation

The risk of stroke in the peri-cardioversion period is ~8%, reduced to <0.5% with appropriate anticoagulation. For an AF episode that has lasted *48 hours or more*:

1. TEE or 3 weeks of anticoagulation is required before DCCV.

2. Anticoagulation is required for at least 4 weeks after spontaneous or active cardioversion, regardless of whether the patient's risk factors dictate long-term anticoagulant therapy.[2] AF conversion to sinus rhythm is followed by a few weeks of atrial hypocontractility, during which a thrombus may form then embolize once the atria fully recover their contractility. If the patient does not have an indication for chronic anticoagulant therapy, administer warfarin or another oral anticoagulant for 4 weeks only. If warfarin is initiated, bridging with LMWH is necessary during the critical first few days after cardioversion.

On the other hand, cardioversion of AF that has lasted <48 hours does not mandate, per se, TEE or oral anticoagulation before DCCV, nor oral anticoagulation post-DCCV, in the absence of thromboembolic risk factors; heparin or one dose of LMWH is provided peri-cardioversion (ESC and ACC guidelines suggest forgoing the 4 weeks of anticoagulation when AF <48 hours with no thromboembolic risk factors).[2,28] The issue is, however, that AF may have been asymptomatic for some time before symptoms developed; symptoms may correspond to acceleration of AF rather than its onset. In addition, one study has found that as many as 12% of patients with AF <48 hours have LAA thrombus or dense spontaneous echo contrast, particularly if underlying heart disease is present.[32] Thus, a safe approach may be to perform TEE regardless of the presumed AF duration, especially in case of underlying heart disease, and to give 4 weeks of anticoagulation after DCCV even if AF <48 hours, regardless of the baseline thromboembolic risk (as suggested by ACCP ≠ ESC and ACC).[28,33]

If the initial TEE shows LAA thrombus, anticoagulation should be given for at least 3 weeks, followed by a repeat TEE to document thrombus resolution before cardioversion. If thrombus persists, consider a rate-control strategy.[28]

The recurrence rate is 70–80% at 1 year. Even when antiarrhythmic agents are used, the recurrence rate is ~35–60% at 1 year,[34] this rate being higher in patients with multiple risk factors (Table 10.3).[31,35] Except for lone AF, most patients with paroxysmal AF progress to persistent or permanent AF within a few years. This high failure rate and the lack of clear benefit from a rhythm-control strategy underline why a **rate-control strategy is the most realistic strategy in patients with many risk factors for recurrence or progression**. If a rhythm-control strategy is selected, antiarrhythmic therapy is typically considered after a recurrence, not necessarily after the first episode. The goal of a rhythm-control strategy is symptom control and quality of life improvement; thus, short and infrequent recurrences or mildly symptomatic recurrences of paroxysmal AF are not considered treatment failures in a patient who previously had severely symptomatic paroxysmal or persistent AF. Rate-slowing drugs should be continued throughout the rhythm-control approach to ensure adequate rate control during AF recurrences, unless the baseline sinus rate is slow.

An alternative to antiarrhythmic therapy is catheter radiofrequency isolation of the pulmonary veins, which successfully prevents AF in 70% of the treated cases over 1 year of follow-up.[36] It is indicated for the prevention of recurrent, symptomatic, paroxysmal or persistent AF, especially when the left atrial diameter is <4 cm. It is used as a second-line therapy in a symptomatic patient who failed rate control and rhythm control with at least one antiarrhythmic drug (Appendix 2).[2,12]

In 25% of patients, DCCV fails or AF recurs after a few seconds or minutes of sinus rhythm; in another 25%, AF recurs within 2 weeks. Recurrences may benefit from a second attempt at DCCV after preparation with an antiarrhythmic drug. If DCCV fails or if AF recurs within 2 weeks despite an antiarrhythmic drug, a decision may be made to accept the progression to permanent AF. At this point, if AF is symptomatic, AV nodal ablation with ventricular pacing may be performed; alternatively, catheter isolation of the pulmonary veins or surgical ablation (maze procedure) may be attempted.[2,12]

VI. Decisions about long-term anticoagulation, role of clopidogrel, role of triple therapy

A. Long-term anticoagulation

The annual risk of stroke in patients with AF not receiving any antithrombotic therapy ranges from 1% to 18%, and averages ~5% per year.[37] This risk is similar in those with paroxysmal or permanent AF. Several risk factors help predict the risk; one validated clinical scheme is the CHADS$_2$ score (Table 10.5).[37] Two points are assigned for a history of stroke or transient ischemic attack (TIA), and one point is assigned for each one of the other four features. For any level of CHADS$_2$ score, warfarin *definitely* reduces the risk of stroke by 75% and increases major bleeding ~2.5-fold, whereas aspirin *may*, very questionably, reduce the stroke risk by 21% while increasing major bleeding by 60%.[33] Yet **the absolute stroke reduction with warfarin only overcomes the bleeding risk when the stroke risk is ≥1.7% per year; the equipoise point is 0.9% with the newer oral anticoagulants**.[38] Another risk score, CHA$_2$DS$_2$-VAS, improves the predictive value of CHADS$_2$ and is particularly useful for further classifying a CHADS$_2$ score of 0 or 1.[28,39,40] In fact, some patients with CHADS$_2$ score of 0 or 1 have a high stroke risk (Table 10.5).

In the ESC and ACC guidelines, no antithrombotic therapy (not even aspirin) is recommended for patients with a CHA$_2$DS$_2$-VAS score of 0 (or 1 from female sex), where the absolute stroke reduction with warfarin is marginal (≤0.5%), not justifying the bleeding risk. Anticoagulation is recommended for a score of 2. For a score of 1 (excluding female sex), ESC guidelines suggest oral anticoagulation after assessment of bleeding risk, while the ACC guidelines suggest oral anticoagulation, aspirin, or no antithrombotic therapy.[2,28] In fact, for a CHA$_2$DS$_2$-VAS score of 1, the benefit of anticoagulation is marginal, as the absolute stroke risk is 1.5–2% per year; the stroke reduction with warfarin only balances the bleeding risk. Anticoagulation is likely beneficial if the risk factor is age 65–74 (stroke risk ~3% per year), if the risk factor is severe (uncontrolled diabetes, low-output severe HF), or if a new oral anticoagulant with less intracranial bleeding risk is used.[41]

CHADS$_2$ score does not apply to patients with *valvular AF*, who have a high stroke risk and require anticoagulation with warfarin regardless of the score. Warfarin is used in these patients, rather than the new oral anticoagulants. Also, regardless of CHADS$_2$ score, patients with hypertrophic cardiomyopathy and AF have a high stroke risk that warrants anticoagulation.

Table 10.5 Stroke risk in patients with non-valvular atrial fibrillation not treated with anticoagulation.

CHADS$_2$ score		CHA$_2$DS$_2$-VAS score		Yearly stroke risk according to CHADS$_2$ score[b]	Yearly stroke risk according to CHA$_2$DS$_2$-VAS score[b]
C: Congestive heart failure[a]	1	C: Congestive heart failure	1	0: 1.9%	0: <1%
H: Hypertension	1	H: Hypertension	1	1: 2.8%	1: 1.5–2%
A: Age ≥75	1	A: Age ≥75	2	2: 4.0%	2: 2.5–3%
D: Diabetes	1	D: Diabetes	1	3: 5.9%	3: 3.2%
S: prior stroke or TIA	2	S: prior stroke or TIA	2	4: 8.5%	4: 4%
		V: Vascular disease (CAD, PAD, aortic plaque)	1	5: 12.5%	5: ~7%
		A: Age 65–74	1	6: 18.2%	6–8: ~10%
		S: Sex female	1		9: 15%

[a] "C" mandates either one of the following (ESC): (i) reduced EF, or (ii) documented HF decompensation, whether EF is reduced or normal (i.e., diastolic HF included).
[b] Numbers obtained from references 28 and 37.

Table 10.6 Major bleeding risk associated with HAS-BLED risk score in patients receiving warfarin.

HAS-BLED score	Major bleeding per year
0	1%
1	1%
2	1.9%
3	3.75%
4	8.7%
5	12.5%

Data from Euro Heart Survey.

B. Bleeding risk

Before starting anticoagulation or aspirin, the patient's bleeding risk should be assessed. The HAS-BLED bleeding risk score may be used:[42]

H, hypertension; A, abnormal liver/kidneys; S, stroke; B, history of bleeding; L, labile INR; E, elderly >65; D, drugs (antiplatelet drugs or NSAID) or alcohol

A score ≥3 implies a high bleeding risk and requires frequent evaluations of anticoagulation therapy (Table 10.6). *A high HAS-BLED score warrants the correction of bleeding risk factors rather than the exclusion of anticoagulation*. Five of the seven HAS-BLED risk factors are modifiable: control hypertension, address prior gastrointestinal bleed, switch to the new anticoagulants if labile INR, avoid alcohol and NSAIDs, correct acute renal dysfunction (ESC guidelines).[43] *Patients with a high HAS-BLED score usually have a high CHA$_2$DS$_2$-VAS score and a high stroke risk, the absolute stroke risk increasing more sharply than the bleeding risk. Thus, these patients derive an even greater net clinical benefit from anticoagulation than patients with a low HAS-BLED score and should generally receive anticoagulation.*[43,44] The bleeding risk is not only high with warfarin, but may be as high with aspirin in those patients.[45]

Along the same lines, a patient receiving anticoagulation who develops gastrointestinal bleed must receive optimization of his bleeding risk (PPI, endoscopies, interruption of aspirin and other insults). Data suggest that anticoagulation may be safely resumed beyond the first 7 days of the bleed, without a significant risk of bleeding recurrence, and with a dramatic reduction of thromboembolic risk compared to anticoagulation reinitiation later than 30–90 days.

Note: Patients with AF who develop TIA should be started on effective anticoagulation as soon as possible. Conversely, anticoagulation is postponed 2 weeks in patients with cerebral infarction, given the risk of hemorrhagic transformation (ESC guidelines).

C. Therapy in patients with AF and CAD

Warfarin monotherapy (INR 2.5–3.5) has been shown to reduce mortality and coronary events after MI.[46] In fact, in comparison with aspirin, warfarin monotherapy (INR 2.5–3.5) further reduces recurrent MI at the expense of a counterbalanced increase in bleeding.[47,48] Other data support warfarin monotherapy (INR 2–3) in patients with CAD, beyond 1 year after MI or PCI.[49] Therefore, in a patient with AF and CAD who is beyond 1 year of a PCI, one may use the combination of warfarin (INR 2–2.5) and aspirin 81 mg, or warfarin monotherapy (INR 2–3).[28]

The major bleeding risk is ~1% per year with aspirin, and ~2.5% per year with warfarin. The addition of aspirin to warfarin may increase the yearly bleeding risk by up to 1%, to 3.5% per year.[50] Note that, as opposed to warfarin, the new oral anticoagulants have not shown a reduction in MI, and thus these agents may not be used as monotherapy in CAD.

D. Role of clopidogrel

The ACTIVE W study has shown that in patients with AF and moderate to high thromboembolic risk (CHADS$_2$ score 2 ± 1), warfarin monotherapy is clearly superior to the combination of aspirin and clopidogrel for the reduction of cardiovascular events (yearly rate 3.9% vs. 5.6%, p <0.001), stroke (1.4% vs. 2.4%, p <0.001), and even MI (trend), with a similar major bleeding risk (~2% per year).[51]

The ACTIVE A study has shown that the combination of aspirin and clopidogrel is superior to aspirin monotherapy for stroke prevention in patients with AF (yearly rate 2.4% vs. 3.3%, p <0.001), at the cost of a higher risk of major bleeding (2% per year vs. 1.3% per year, p <0.001).[52] Thus, the combination of aspirin and clopidogrel appears to be an option superior to aspirin but inferior to warfarin. Since this combination has the same bleeding risk as warfarin, it has no definite role in AF therapy, particularly with the availability of newer anticoagulants that facilitate chronic therapy.

E. Triple combination of aspirin, clopidogrel, and oral anticoagulation

Patients who have AF and who undergo stent placement need to be on a triple combination therapy of aspirin, clopidogrel, and warfarin (or alternative anticoagulant) if the bleeding risk is low. The triple combination may significantly improve mortality and cardiovascular outcomes in comparison to the double combination of aspirin and clopidogrel,[53] and the use of warfarin is necessary for stroke reduction. The triple therapy, however, has a 4× higher major bleeding risk than aspirin + warfarin (12% vs. 3–4% yearly bleeding risk).[54] A BMS may be placed in these patients in order that the duration of the mandatory dual antiplatelet therapy is limited to 4 weeks. Afterward, the patient is placed on double therapy with an anticoagulant and aspirin or an anticoagulant and clopidogrel. With the current DESs (Everolimus-eluting stent, Zotaralimus-eluting stent), the discontinuation of one antiplatelet agent at 3–6 months appears safe. Thus, DES may be implanted and triple therapy used for 3 months in stable CAD stenting and 6 months in ACS stenting (ESC), followed by discontinuation of aspirin and the continuation of warfarin + clopidogrel until 12 months (clopidogrel being preferred to aspirin). Beyond 12 months, warfarin monotherapy may be used.[28] Alternatively, if the CHADS$_2$ risk score is 1 (intermediate risk), anticoagulant therapy may be omitted for the first few months then resumed later on.[33] When using triple therapy, aspirin dose should be 81 mg, and INR should be kept 2–2.5 (rather than 3). The adjunctive use of proton pump inhibitors is reasonable.

Patients at a particularly high bleeding risk may not tolerate triple therapy for any duration. A recent trial has shown that, in comparison with upfront triple therapy, upfront therapy with warfarin + clopidogrel (without aspirin) in stable or unstable CAD, after any stent placement, is associated with a reduction in major bleeding (~6% vs. 3% at 1 year) and total death without an increase in MI or revascularization rates (WOEST trial; ~25% of patients had ACS, and 65% received DES).[55] Another trial in patients receiving DES has shown that triple therapy for 6 weeks only followed by double therapy (warfarin + antiplatelet) is as safe from an ischemic standpoint as 6 months of triple therapy (ISAR-TRIPLE; a third of patients had ACS, 18% had MI).[56] Note that therapy with warfarin + aspirin is not equivalent to warfarin + clopidogrel and appears to be associated with a much higher risk of stent thrombosis and MI than warfarin + clopidogrel.[57] The combined inhibition of thrombin generation with anticoagulation and the ADP pathway with clopidogrel may lessen the importance of cyclooxygenase inhibition with aspirin. The early interruption of one antiplatelet agent has also proven to be safe in a patient receiving the oral anticoagulant rivaroxaban (PIONEER trial).

VII. Special situation: atrial fibrillation and heart failure

A. General management

1. If a patient presents with acute severe HF and newly detected AF with a rate >150 bpm, AF may be considered an immediate cause of HF and acute DCCV may be considered to improve LV diastolic filling.

2. If a patient presents with severe HF and AF at a rate of 100–150 bpm, acute DCCV is generally not beneficial. AF may be:

   a. secondary to HF

   b. the cause of the cardiomyopathy and HF (tachycardia-mediated cardiomyopathy)

   c. the major trigger of HF decompensation in a patient with a previously stable cardiomyopathy

It should be assumed that either (b) or (c) is the case, but at the stage of decompensated HF acute DCCV is not helpful.

Pathophysiology – In compensated HF, AF contributes to ~30–40% of cardiac output. Those patients have a large A wave with E/A reversal on echo, confirming the crucial role of atrial contraction. In fast AF, the loss of atrial systole and the reduction of diastolic filling time reduce cardiac output, which increases LA pressure and decompensates HF. However, once HF is decompensated, even if the patient converts back to sinus rhythm, the contribution of atrial systole to cardiac output will be marginal. In fact, decompensated patients have a very small A wave on echo, as the high LV pressure does not allow any filling during atrial contraction (Figure 10.1). At this point, tachycardia of 100–130 bpm may be helpful, as it increases cardiac output and LV emptying by increasing the number of cardiac cycles per minute. In the absence of AF, the patient would probably have sinus tachycardia at a similar rate.

The key here is to treat HF with diuresis and vasodilators. This alone slows down AF and possibly converts it (situation (a) above). Once HF is stabilized and diuresed, the goal becomes to slow down AF to a rate <80 bpm at rest and possibly cardiovert it; at the compensated stage, this reduces HF symptoms and the risk of decompensation, and reverses the possible tachycardia-mediated cardiomyopathy.

In a patient who presents with new HF and a newly detected AF, tachycardia-mediated cardiomyopathy is the diagnosis in 25–50% of the cases (situation (b) above). In a patient who presents with decompensation of a known HF and a new or recurring AF, AF should be considered the trigger for HF decompensation (situation (c) above). In those situations, aggressive rate control should be achieved after acute HF therapy, and elective DCCV should be strongly considered (rhythm-control strategy). *Awaiting HF stabilization increases the success and sustainability of cardioversion.*

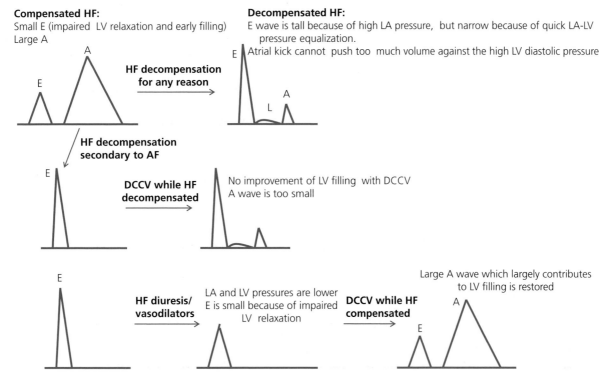

Compensated HF:
Small E (impaired LV relaxation and early filling)
Large A

HF decompensation for any reason →

HF decompensation secondary to AF

DCCV while HF decompensated →

Decompensated HF:
E wave is tall because of high LA pressure, but narrow because of quick LA-LV pressure equalization.
Atrial kick cannot push too much volume against the high LV diastolic pressure

No improvement of LV filling with DCCV
A wave is too small

HF diuresis/vasodilators →

LA and LV pressures are lower
E is small because of impaired LV relaxation

DCCV while HF compensated →

Large A wave which largely contributes to LV filling is restored

Figure 10.1 LV diastolic filling pattern in compensated HF, decompensated HF, decompensated HF secondary to AF, and effects of DCCV.

Table 10.7 Rate control of AF with or without HF.

No HF	β-blocker or CCB or combination
Decompensated HF with low EF	No β-blocker and no CCB Diuresis/HF therapy IV digoxin or amiodarone (class I indication) Once compensated, start β-blocker then uptitrate it
Decompensated HF with normal EF	May use β-blocker or CCB
Compensated HF with low EF	β-blocker (may be uptitrated faster than usually done in HF)

B. Rate control in HF (Table 10.7)

VIII. Special situation: atrial fibrillation with borderline blood pressure

In case of acute AF with borderline BP, work up and treat the cause of reduced BP. In patients with critical illness, a fast rate of 130 bpm may be appropriate and tolerated. Amiodarone IV bolus followed by a drip may be used (ESC), but may precipitate hypotension during fast boluses. Digoxin IV may also be used.

β-Blockers may be cautiously used in the absence of a pre-shock state, in which the patient is dependent on the adrenergic tone and in which β-blockers drop BP precipitously (e.g., severe hypovolemia, sepsis, bleeding). Esmolol IV, being quickly reversible, is the preferred β-blocker in this instance.

AF with clear-cut shock and a rate >150 bpm is often considered contributive to the shock and DC cardioverted emergently, unless a clear cause of hypotension is identified (e.g., massive gastrointestinal bleed).

When there is an active trigger of AF (e.g., sepsis, HF), DCCV is unlikely to be successful (AF will likely recur soon after DCCV). Amiodarone may be the only successful treatment acutely.

Appendix 1. Antiarrhythmic drug therapy (indications and examples)

Antiarrhythmic drugs (AADs) have three main uses. *First*, they are used to prevent AF recurrences if a rhythm-control strategy is selected (this is the most important use of AADs); these drugs are usually given as a long-term therapy after a second episode of AF. *Second*, AADs are used as an adjunctive therapy that increases the effectiveness of DCCV and sustains the sinus rhythm. For that purpose, these drugs are mainly given when AF has been persistent for >3 months, a prior DCCV has failed, or there has been an early recurrence after DCCV. *Third*, AADs may be used to acutely cardiovert AF (this is their least important use).

A. Examples of some AADs and their use in special conditions (Figure 10.2)

β-blockers have shown a moderate but consistent efficacy in preventing AF recurrence and reducing the frequency of paroxysmal AF, comparable to conventional AADs,[58,59] which makes them an appropriate first-line therapy in many instances. However, these agents may potentially aggravate vagally mediated AF.

Class III agents

* **Amiodarone** is a class III AAD that can ***be used in any cardiac condition, including HF or any cardiomyopathy, without an increase in cardiac mortality***. It is the only drug that can be used with substantial LVH. It is also the most effective drug for long-term prevention of AF. In addition, it has a sympatholytic effect that allows rate control.

  It has a fast-onset AF rate-controlling effect and VT/VF antiarrhythmic effect (minutes in case of IV administration, 1 to several hours in case of oral administration), but a slow-onset atrial antiarrhythmic effect (1 to several days). Most of the early amiodarone effect is a β-blocker effect rather than a class III effect, which explains that, at 24 hours, amiodarone is only marginally superior to placebo in cardioverting AF, if at all.

  Being fat-soluble, amiodarone has a large volume of distribution and a very long half-life (60–120 days). The IV form may lead to hypotension in ~15% of patients. Hypotension is related to the rate of administration and is improved by slowing the rate. Hypotension is not seen with oral amiodarone.

  ○ Amiodarone IV dose: 150 mg IV over 10 minutes followed by 1 mg/min infusion for 6 hours, then 0.5 mg/min. When used for VT/VF, amiodarone may be reloaded with 150 mg IV for breakthrough VT/VF, up to 2.2 g/day. Switch to oral amiodarone next day or a few days later.

  ○ Amiodarone oral dose: start with an oral load of 600–800 mg/day for 10 days for a total of ~10 g, then 100–200 mg/day.

> Note also that amiodarone may raise the levels of digoxin and warfarin (the "A–D" and "A–W" interaction). These drugs should routinely be reduced by one-half and levels followed closely when amiodarone is started. Amiodarone also increases the levels of the new oral anticoagulants, particularly rivaroxaban.

* **Sotalol** is an oral class III AAD with a non-selective β-blocker effect. The β-blocker effect starts at low doses and is already half-maximal at 80 mg/day, while the class III effect starts at doses of 160 mg/day. Sotalol is inferior to amiodarone, but is particularly effective for chronic AF prevention in patients with CAD, where it may be as effective as amiodarone.[60] It should not be used for acute cardioversion. Sotalol is associated with a 1.5–2% risk of TdP that is dose-dependent.

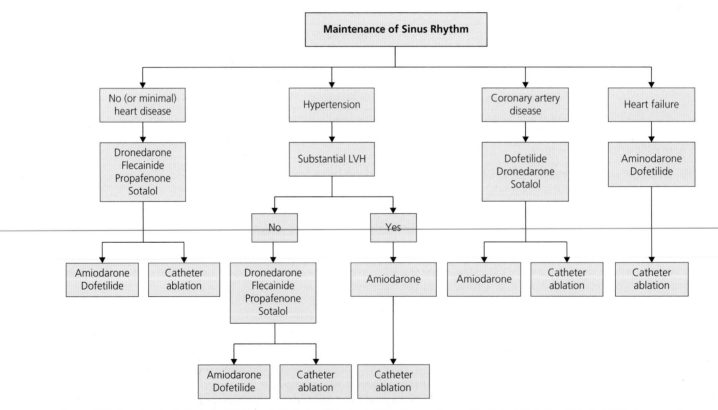

Figure 10.2 Chronic antiarrhythmic drug therapy for the prevention of recurrent paroxysmal or persistent atrial fibrillation. Note that β-blockers are often the first-line antiarrhythmic agents because of their safety in comparison to other anti-arrhythmic drugs. This figure mainly applies to patients who have symptomatic AF recurrences despite rate control. Reproduced with permission of Elsevier from Wann LS, Curtis AB, January CT, et al. 2011 ACCF/AHA/HRS focused update on the management of patients with atrial fibrillation. J Am Coll Cardiol 2011; 57: 223–42.

Use sotalol cautiously in HF and renal failure (↓ dosage to once daily if GFR <60, and avoid if GFR <40). In HF, sotalol may be used slowly but is better avoided, because, in HF, the β-blockers that have demonstrated a positive effect on mortality are preferred.

- **Dronedarone** is a drug similar to amiodarone without the iodine moiety. It lacks the pulmonary and thyroid toxicity of amiodarone, affects QTc less than amiodarone, and has a shorter half-life (1–2 days compared to 2 months). It is less effective than amiodarone in the prevention of AF recurrence, but it is the only AAD that has shown a reduction in hospitalization related to cardiovascular events and a reduction in stroke in **patients without HF** (ATHENA trial); however, it increases mortality in class III or IV HF and in persistent AF, and should be avoided in any HF or LV dysfunction and in persistent AF without a planned DC cardioversion.[61-63] As opposed to class Ic, it **may be used in CAD**.

  Dronedarone has numerous drug interactions. It interacts with digoxin, diltiazem, and the new oral anticoagulants, but not with warfarin.

- **Oral dofetilide** may be used for acute or chronic rhythm control and is relatively safe in HF and CAD (DIAMOND trials). It is associated with a 2–3% risk of TdP. Use it cautiously in renal failure and avoid it with GFR <20.

- **Intravenous ibutilide** may be used for acute rhythm control (1 mg infused over 10 minutes). Ibutilide is the drug with the fastest acute cardioversion effect (10–30 minutes) and is effective in 30% of patients. A second dose can be given 10 minutes later. It also increases the efficacy of DC cardioversion in those who fail the first attempt. It increases QTc by ~60 ms. The risk of TdP is ~3–4%, and this is increased if EF <30%

Class Ic agents (*propafenone, flecainide*) may be used for acute cardioversion and chronic rhythm control, but should be avoided in patients with any heart disease, including CAD, LVH, or HF, in which case they are proarrhythmic and increase mortality (CAST trial).[64] Moreover, they may reduce the atrial rate and reduce the concealed AV conduction of atrial impulses, which may inadvertently increase the full AV conduction and the ventricular rate. In addition, they may organize AF into atrial flutter with 1:1 conduction to the ventricles. Therefore, class Ic agents should be used with AV nodal blocking agents.

Because of their efficacy and limited extracardiac toxicity, class I agents are first-line therapy for patients without any underlying heart disease, including hypertensive patients without substantial LVH. Instead of chronic treatment, they may be used as a "pill in the pocket," as-needed therapy for symptomatic recurrences of paroxysmal AF, as they are the most effective agents in converting AF. Upon recurrence of AF symptoms, the patient is instructed to take one oral dose of flecainide or propafenone, with an expected conversion rate of >60% within 3–6 hours. This approach may be used in selected, highly symptomatic patients with infrequent recurrences of AF (e.g., between once per month and once per year), and this therapy should be tried in the hospital once to ensure safety.

B. Side effects

All AADs can lead to bradyarrhythmias, ventricular arrhythmias, or torsades de pointes. Ventricular arrhythmias are related to an increase in QRS duration with class I agents, and to an increase in QTc interval with class III agents. The QT prolongation and the risk of TdP with class III agents is dose-dependent. Thus, heart rate and QRS and QTc intervals are monitored with these agents. Avoid class Ic drugs if QRS >120 ms at baseline or increases more than 25% with treatment. Avoid class III drugs if QTc >460 ms at baseline, or increases to ≥500 ms or ≥15% with treatment.

Amiodarone has the lowest risk of proarrhythmia (<1%) despite QTc prolongation. It is the safest from the cardiac standpoint but is associated with non-cardiac side effects: pulmonary fibrosis in <3% of patients (reversible if detected early); hyper- or hypothyroidism; hepatitis; photosensitivity; neurologic side effects (ataxia, tremor, neuropathy, rare optic neuropathy). Non-cardiac death may be increased. Pulmonary function testing and chest radiographs should be performed yearly; thyroid and liver profiles every 6 months; and fundoscopic eye exam at baseline, then as needed if symptoms occur. The effect of amiodarone on QTc is not immediate; it begins to appear after the fourth day, and becomes pronounced at 1 to several weeks.

In general, AADs should be initiated in the hospital to monitor QT and QRS intervals and arrhythmia occurrence over 3 days. Class Ic agents and amiodarone can be initiated in the outpatient setting if the patient has normal electrolytes, normal QT/QRS intervals, normal renal function, and does not have any structural heart disease.[2]

Appendix 2. Catheter ablation of atrial fibrillation, surgical ablation, AV nodal ablation

Up to 90% of PACs that trigger AF originate from the pulmonary veins, while the rest originate from other foci, most commonly SVC. Therefore, catheter ablation of AF consists of pulmonary vein isolation. The more complete the pulmonary vein isolation, the better the long-term result. In patients with organic heart disease and left atrial enlargement, additional triggers are possible and ablation of the atrial substrate may be necessary; linear ablation across fractionated electrograms in the LA may be necessary to subdivide the LA into smaller compartments that prevent the propagation of atrial wavelets. Catheter ablation should be reserved for patients with AF who remain symptomatic despite optimal medical therapy, including rate and rhythm control, with failure of at least one antiarrhythmic drug. A recent meta-analysis that included paroxysmal and persistent AF found a 77% success rate for catheter ablation strategies (including patients who received multiple procedures and adjunctive antiarrhythmic drugs) vs. 52% for antiarrhythmic drugs at a mean follow-up of 14 months.[65] At the Cleveland Clinic, a 76% success rate was reported at 1 year, with a 24% recurrence rate (most recurrences were successfully treated with reablation, with >80% success rate at 4.5 years).[66] The success is highest in patients with paroxysmal AF, no or minimal heart disease, no or minimal left atrial enlargement, and no severe lung disease. Ablation of persistent and longstanding persistent AF, or AF with underlying HF, is associated with variable but encouraging success rates and very often requires several attempts. *Weight loss >10% dramatically enhances the long-term success of AF ablation*. After ablation, 24-hour Holter monitoring or event monitoring is recommended every 3–6 months for at least 2 years. While the most common outcome is total resolution of the arrhythmia on monitoring, AF may recur but become responsive to AAD or become asymptomatic. In fact, one study has shown that patients with severely symptomatic AF have additional asymptomatic episodes of AF (52% of episodes are asymptomatic); following ablation, only 58% have total resolution of AF, while 12% continue to have AF that is now totally asymptomatic. AF episodes are more frequently asymptomatic after ablation (79%). Thus, while catheter ablation may not cure AF, it reduces the total AF burden and duration and, as a result, the symptoms related to AF.[67]

Early recurrence (2 days to 2 months) does not imply failure and may be attributed to local irritation and inflammation from ablation; most of these patients will have good long-term result. Patients are often treated with an AAD for 2–3 months to minimize these early recurrences.

Ablation should be performed while the patient is adequately anticoagulated: warfarin is typically continued throughout the procedure with INR 2–3, without a need for LMWH bridging; the new oral anticoagulants are only interrupted for one or two doses before the procedure (new anticoagulants may be associated with a higher bleeding/tamponade risk if uninterrupted). Either way, supplemental doses of heparin are provided during the procedure. Anticoagulation should be continued for at least 3 months after the procedure regardless of CHA_2DS_2-VAS score, as the injured atrial tissue may trigger clot formation.[28] Beyond 3 months, anticoagulation depends on CHA_2DS_2-VAS score. Anticoagulation should not be stopped over the long term, since catheter ablation is not a curative therapy for AF.

Surgical ablation (maze procedure) consists of creating biatrial ablation lines, including lines around the pulmonary veins. The use of radiofrequency energy rather than cutting and sewing allows a faster and less morbid procedure. It is indicated along with mitral valve surgery in a patient with persistent or symptomatic AF (class IIa), or, less strongly, along with other cardiac surgery in a patient with symptomatic AF. Compared with no ablation, surgical ablation is associated with a higher requirement for pacemaker therapy. Excision of the left atrial appendage may also be performed, although the benefit on stroke reduction is unclear. Ligation or stapling of the appendage, rather than excision, is associated with a high residual stroke risk (incomplete appendage ligation may favor clot formation). Even excision may be incomplete and leave a residual stump on TEE/flow on TEE.

In patients with severely symptomatic, fast AF, where the rate cannot be controlled, and where a rhythm-control strategy with antiarrhythmic drugs has failed, AV nodal ablation with RV pacing is indicated. This strategy is safe and markedly effective in improving symptoms. It also improves LV function in patients with reduced EF, where LV dysfunction is fully or partially related to tachycardia-mediated cardiomyopathy.[68,69] However, two additional options are possible *for the management of uncontrolled AF in patients with HF*:

1. AV nodal ablation with biventricular pacing is superior to RV pacing if EF <50%, in regards to HF and LV improvement (APAF and Block-HF trials) (class IIa recommendation, regardless of NYHA class, but guidelines use an EF cutoff of 35%).[70,71]
2. Pulmonary vein isolation may be a better option in HF. The PABA CHF trial has shown that AF ablation is superior to AV nodal ablation and biventricular pacing for symptom and EF improvement in this population.[72]

On the other hand, for patients with *uncontrolled HF who have AF*, biventricular pacing is indicated for HF purposes if the baseline QRS is LBBB ≥150 ms with EF ≤35% and class II–IV symptoms. AV nodal ablation may be performed to ensure consistent biventricular pacing in AF.

Pulmonary vein stenosis is seen in 2–5% of patients after AF ablation. A new diagnosis of HF or worsening of HF after AF ablation is concerning for pulmonary vein stenosis. It is diagnosed by cardiac CT. Right and left heart catheterization show a discrepancy between LVEDP and the much higher PCWP, in the absence of mitral stenosis. PCWP should be measured in the four lung quadrants, as the stenosis may only involve one or two veins.

Appendix 3. INR follow-up in patients receiving warfarin; new anticoagulants

Patients must stay within the intended INR goal for ≥60% of the time to derive the intended benefit from warfarin. While a goal INR 1.5–1.9 has been proposed, cohort studies suggest a striking twofold increase in ischemic stroke risk at INR 1.5–1.9, approximating the risk of no anticoagulation, with a risk of intracranial hemorrhage similar to higher INR; therefore, an INR <2.0 is not recommended. The risk of intracranial hemorrhage remains flat until an INR of 4, beyond which this risk rises sharply (sixfold) and continues to rise exponentially (18-fold for INR >4.5) (Figure 10.3).[73]

Warfarin is usually initiated at 5 mg daily (consider a lower dose in elderly patients). INR reaches a steady state at 7 days, but is initially checked at 3–4 days. At 3–4 days: if INR <1.5, warfarin dose is increased; if INR ≥2, warfarin dose is decreased. An increase in stroke risk has been reported in the early initiation phase, and while bridging with LMWH is not often performed, it may be justified in patients with a prior stroke.

Four new oral anticoagulants have compared favorably to warfarin in AF, with regards to stroke risk, intracranial hemorrhage risk, and mortality (Table 10.8).[74–77] Their onset of action is quick (2–3 hours), their half-lives are 10–15 hours, and no monitoring is necessary (dabigatran prolongs PTT and rivaroxaban/apixaban prolong PT, which may be used to ensure compliance, not to monitor therapy). The selective inhibition of the clotting cascade and the lack of inhibition of the extrinsic pathway (factor VII) explain the reduction of intracranial hemorrhage with all of these agents. The downside includes the increase of mucosal (GI) bleeding with three of these agents and the lack of antidotes, fresh frozen plasma (FFP) being ineffective in reversing their effect. In addition, although approved for GFR 15–30 ml/min, major trials excluded patients with GFR <30 ml/min; therefore, the bleeding risk and the efficacy is unclear in advanced renal failure. Moreover, these drugs have not been studied in valvular AF, i.e., AF with mitral stenosis, valvular prosthesis, or mitral valve repair. Dabigatran has been studied with mechanical prosthetic valves and was associated with a drastic increase in thromboembolic events (5% at 3 months).[78] In fact, an overwhelming activation of the factor VII pathway, after contact with tissue factor expressed at the site of tissue or endothelial injury, may generate more thrombin than dabigatran can inhibit; warfarin may be more effective, as it blocks factor VII activation, in addition to the intrinsic (factor IX) and common pathways (factor X and thrombin).

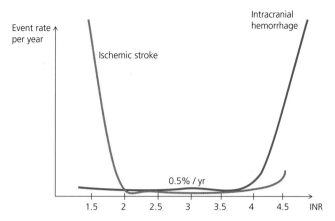

Figure 10.3 Yearly risk of stroke and intracranial hemorrhage with warfarin according to INR. The yearly intracranial hemorrhage risk is reduced from 0.5% per year to ~0.25% with the new anticoagulants. Data from Flaker et al. 2006.[50]

Table 10.8 New oral anticoagulants vs. warfarin.

	Dabigatran 150 mg BID RE-LY trial: median age 71.5, CHADS$_2$ score ≥1 (mean ~2.1)	Rivaroxaban 20 mg QD ROCKET AF: median age 73, CHADS$_2$ score ≥2 (mean 3.5): **higher CHADS$_2$ than other studies Also approved for DVT/PE, acutely and chronically**	Apixaban 5 mg BID ARISTOTLE: median age 70, CHADS$_2$ score ≥1 (mean ~2.1) **Also approved for DVT/PE, acutely and chronically**	Edoxaban 60 mg QD ENGAGE AF-TIMI 48: median age 72, CHADS$_2$ score ≥2 (mean ~2.8)
Mechanism[a]	Thrombin inhibitor	Direct Xa inhibitor	Direct Xa inhibitor	Direct Xa inhibitor
Comparison to warfarin	↓ ischemic stroke ↓ intracranial hemorrhage (~70%) Same overall major bleeding ↓ death (~0.5%/yr) ↑ GI bleeding ? slight ↑ MI (questionable finding in RE-LY)	Same ischemic stroke ↓ intracranial hemorrhage Same overall major bleeding ↓ death trend ↑ GI bleeding No ↑ MI	Same ischemic stroke ↓ intracranial hemorrhage (~50%) ↓ **major bleeding** ↓ death No ↑ GI bleeding No ↑ MI	**↑ ischemic stroke if GFR >95 ml/min (excessive drug clearance),** same ischemic stroke if GFR <95 ml/min ↓ intracranial hemorrhage ↓ major bleeding ↓ death trend ↑ GI bleeding
Renal failure	Renal elimination 80% GFR15–30 → 75 mg BID Avoid if GFR <15	2/3 liver metabolism, 1/3 renal elimination For AF: GFR 15–50: 15 mg QD, and avoid if GFR <15 For DVT/PE therapy: avoid if GFR <30	75% liver metabolism, ~25% renal elimination of unchanged drug (**least affected by renal failure**) Reduce dose to 2.5 mg BID if two of the following: creatinine >1.5 mg/dl, age >80, or weight <60 kg Avoid if GFR <15 but may use in hemodialysis patients	Renal elimination 50% GFR 50–95: 60 mg QD GFR 15–50: 30 mg QD Avoid if GFR <15 or >95
Antidote	FFP not very effective Prothrombin complex may be used (the downstream effect of FFP and prothrombin complex is blocked) **60% dialyzable**	Prothrombin complex may be used	Prothrombin complex improved coagulation tests in one study	
Notable interactions[b]	Not a CYP substrate; P-glycoprotein intestinal efflux Dronedarone doubles dabigatran effect → Avoid combination Amiodarone may increase levels but may be used	CYP3A inhibitors Dronedarone, amiodarone, and diltiazem/verapamil raise rivaroxaban levels → better avoid	CYP3A inhibitors Dronedarone and amiodarone raise apixaban levels → caution, but may be used	Not a CYP substrate; P-glycoprotein intestinal efflux

[a] Warfarin inhibits the recycling of inactive, oxidized vitamin K (it eventually depletes active vitamin K rather than antagonizes its effect). Subsequently, it prevents the synthesis of the vitamin-K-dependent coagulation factors II (thrombin), VII, IX, and X, and regulatory proteins C and S.

[b] **Rivaroxaban is the worst from a drug-interaction standpoint.** Digoxin does not have any significant interaction with any of these three drugs. Specific drug interactions may be more difficult to control with the new agents than with warfarin, where INR allows dose adjustment.

In an analysis of the landmark trials, the switch from a novel oral anticoagulant to warfarin was associated with an early increase in stroke risk, probably because the novel anticoagulant was interrupted immediately upon warfarin initiation and INR was subtherapeutic for several days or weeks. During transition to warfarin, the continuation of the novel anticoagulant alongside warfarin for 3 days or until INR is ≥2 may mitigate the increase in stroke risk. When switching from warfarin to a novel anticoagulant, warfarin is stopped and the novel anticoagulant is started when INR <2 (~2 days).

> Apixaban is likely the safest anticoagulant from a bleeding standpoint, particularly as it is *least affected by renal function*. In AVERROES trial of apixaban versus aspirin in AF (mean $CHADS_2 = 2$), **apixaban was associated with a similar major, minor, and intracranial bleeding risk as aspirin**, with a reduction in mortality and a threefold reduction in ischemic stroke.[79]

A novel alternative to chronic anticoagulation is percutaneous closure of the LA appendage (e.g., Watchman device). Watchman compares favorably with long-term warfarin therapy, but is associated with an early procedural hazard (tamponade) and a short-term requirement for warfarin (6 weeks) and aspirin + clopidogrel (6 months). **It is also noteworthy that 10% of thrombi form in the LA (rather than the appendage, more so in patients with HF or valvular AF).** In light of the safety of the novel anticoagulants, its role is questionable.

Appendix 4. Bridging anticoagulation in patients undergoing procedures and receiving warfarin

The decision to totally withhold anticoagulation for 5 days before a procedure or to bridge depends on the underlying indication for anticoagulation and the $CHADS_2$ score (ACCP guidelines):[33]

a. Low perioperative risk of thromboembolic events if anticoagulation is held for 5–7 days: AF with $CHADS_2$ score of 0–2, DVT/PE >12 months.

b. High risk: AF with $CHADS_2$ score of 5–6, recent stroke/TIA (<3 months), mitral stenosis, mechanical valve, DVT/PE <3 months.

c. The remaining patients have an intermediate risk: AF with $CHADS_2$ score of 3–4; DVT/PE within 3–12 months.

Based on an average annual risk of stroke of 5% with AF, the risk of stroke during 8 days of warfarin interruption should only be 0.1%. However, studies of perioperative interruption of anticoagulation suggest that the risk of arterial thromboembolism in the perioperative period is much higher than mathematically predicted (~0.5–1%). This is likely related to a rebound hypercoagulability that occurs after discontinuation of warfarin, or the procoagulant state of surgery. Therefore, according to ACCP guidelines, bridging with a therapeutic regimen of LMWH or IV heparin may be performed in high- or intermediate- risk patients, while in low-risk patients it is reasonable to interrupt anticoagulation for up to a week without any bridging (grade 1 recommendation for high-risk, grade 2 for intermediate-risk).

Warfarin is stopped 4–5 days before the procedure (4–5 doses). LMWH is started 36 hours after the last dose of warfarin, and is administered until 24 hours before the procedure. For example, for a Monday's surgery (day 0), the last warfarin dose is taken Tuesday evening (day –6), enoxaparin 1 mg/kg SQ BID is given on Thursday, Friday, Saturday, and Sunday morning. Warfarin is resumed on the day of surgery, while therapeutic LMWH is resumed 24 hours after a low-bleeding-risk procedure (endoscopy, skin biopsy) or 48–72 hours after a high-bleeding-risk surgery (e.g., gastrointestinal surgery, orthopedic surgery, pacemaker placement, polyp resection).[33] LMWH is continued for ~5 days, until INR is therapeutic.

Note, however, that **a recent trial (BRIDGE) has not found a benefit of bridging in patients with a mean $CHADS_2$ score of 2.3**. Embolic events were similar with or without bridging, despite the fact that warfarin was interrupted 5 days before the procedure and INR did not become therapeutic until 5 days after the procedure.[80]

In patients requiring minor dental procedures, warfarin interruption for 2 days without bridging or warfarin continuation throughout the procedure with administration of an oral prohemostatic agent is suggested. A *2-day interruption (partial interruption)* allows partial reversal of INR, enough for minor procedures. For patients undergoing a skin procedure or cataract surgery, warfarin continuation throughout the procedure is suggested.[33]

Newer anticoagulants are more easily managed perioperatively. They have a half-life of 10–15 hours. They should be stopped 4 half-lives (~2 days) before major surgery, or 1 day before minor procedures (gastroscopy, colonoscopy without polyp resection). They are resumed 24–72 hours postoperatively, once the bleeding risk is reduced (24 hours after low-bleeding-risk procedures, 48–72 hours after high-bleeding-risk procedures). Renal failure particularly affects the elimination of dabigatran, which should be held for 4 days if GFR <50, and 5 days if GFR <30. Rivaroxaban and apixaban are less dependent on renal function and may be held for 2 days if GFR 30–50, and 3 days if GFR 15–30.

Appendix 5. Management of elevated INR values

In the absence of bleeding (ACCP guidelines)

- INR 4.5–10: Withhold warfarin; it takes ~2.5 days for INR to decline to <4. Grossly, the anticoagulant effect declines by ~50% every 2 days (half-life of warfarin being ~42 hours).
- INR >10: Administer oral vitamin K. The dose of vitamin K is generally a low oral dose of 1–2.5 mg. This dose may also be administered to patients with INR 4.5–10, allowing a faster reversal (~1 day) when warranted for a procedure. Subcutaneous vitamin K is less well absorbed and should be avoided.

In case of bleeding

For any INR elevation, rapid reversal of anticoagulation should be achieved with the use of fresh frozen plasma, or, preferably, prothrombin complex concentrate. The latter is a concentrate of the *non-activated* factors that are reduced by warfarin (IX, X, II ± VII) at a concentration 25 times higher than the normal plasma, presented in a small volume and mixed with heparin to prevent hypercoagulation.

The effect of fresh frozen plasma or prothrombotic complex is short-lived (<24 hours), and thus vitamin K administration is necessary for a sustained reversal of anticoagulation. Except in the case of a metallic valve, the administration of a high dose of vitamin K is generally recommended (10 mg orally, or 5–10 mg by slow IV infusion) and is effective in normalizing the INR by 24 hours, faster than the small doses. High doses should be avoided in patients with metallic valves, as a high dose of vitamin K may lead to a hypercoagulable state; low doses, however, may be used in these patients.

Appendix 6. A common special situation: AF and symptomatic pauses (sinus or AF pauses) or bradycardia

- Some patients have the "tachy–brady syndrome," in which a fast-rate paroxysmal AF alternates with sinus bradycardia or long AF pauses. Sinus bradycardia may be worsened or triggered by the rate-controlling agents used to slow the fast paroxysms of AF. This mainly occurs in patients with "off-and-on" AF, in which the therapy for the "on" episodes is harmful for the "off" sinus periods. ***Particularly risky is the transition from AF to sinus rhythm: the overdrive-suppressed sinus node takes some time to "wake up,"*** leading to a long pause, and possibly syncope, at the junction of AF and sinus rhythm.
- In patients with persistent or permanent AF, an appropriate rate control may be associated with prolonged and symptomatic AF pauses (a symptomatic pause is typically longer than 3 seconds while the patient is awake). An attempt to reduce the dosage of the rate-controlling agents should be made; however, this may lead to an inappropriately fast rate. It is a situation in which it may not be possible to find the fine line between too fast and too slow.

> In the above two situations, attempt rhythm control. If rhythm control fails, place a permanent pacemaker and keep administering the rate-controlling agents. Another option would be to attempt catheter isolation of the pulmonary veins.

- When AF becomes slow and regular, complete AV block with a junctional escape rhythm (usually 40–60 bpm) is diagnosed. Even if asymptomatic, it dictates withdrawing the rate-controlling drugs followed by pacemaker placement if complete AV block persists. Also, AF with pauses >5 seconds during wakefulness dictates pacemaker placement even if asymptomatic, after trying to withdraw drugs (ACC class I indication).

Appendix 7. DC cardioversion in patients with a slow ventricular response

Patients with a slow ventricular response in the absence of rate-controlling drugs probably have AV nodal disease and, along with it, sinus nodal disease. They may develop sinus bradycardia or SA/AV blocks after cardioversion. In these patients, AF is masking and "curing" their sinus node disease and bradyarrhythmia. In addition, AF may overdrive suppress the sinus node, which will take some time to "wake up" after AF cardioversion. Be ready for transcutaneous or transvenous pacing if needed.

This may also occur in patients receiving high doses of rate-controlling agents, and may occur during spontaneous transition from AF to sinus rhythm in patients with off-and-on AF.

Appendix 8. AF occurring post-cardiac surgery and AF related to acute transient triggers

AF occurs postoperatively in 20–40% of patients (more so with valvular surgery, older age, HF, history of AF). It usually occurs between days 1 and 5 and is related to catecholamines and to the pericardial and generalized inflammation. It resolves spontaneously within 2 days in 80% of the patients, and within 6–8 weeks in >95% of the patients. Unless unstable, DCCV is not usually needed as AF will convert spontaneously.

AF should be prevented with β-blockers preoperatively (= first choice) or amiodarone if β-blockers are contraindicated (= second choice; start amiodarone ~600 mg/day 1 week preoperatively and continue it at 200–600 mg/day for the duration of hospital stay). The combination of β-blockers and amiodarone may also be used and may be indicated in the highest-risk patients (i.e., history of AF or mitral valve surgery).[81]

When AF occurs, it is treated similarly to any acute AF. For rate control, β-blockers are primarily used; amiodarone may also be used for rate control in case of borderline blood pressure or acute HF (amiodarone may also accelerate AF conversion). DC cardioversion, amiodarone for the purpose of rhythm control, or any antiarrhythmic drug has a limited role in postoperative AF, as AF will likely recur early on (~45%) then convert spontaneously regardless of these measures.

Even short-term AF is associated with an increased stroke risk; thus, AF lasting more than 24 hours warrants short-term anticoagulation according to the ACCP guidelines (4 weeks of anticoagulation, started a few days postoperatively). If AF does not persist beyond 6–8 weeks, and in the absence of a history of AF, longer-term anticoagulation and antiarrhythmic drug therapy are not warranted.

AF occurring in relation to acute triggers (sepsis, postoperative state, acute lung disease) will likely convert once these issues are treated. Acutely, it is treated like any newly diagnosed AF, with rate control, knowing that a rate of 100–125 bpm may be appropriate in these critical situations. Amiodarone and digoxin may be the only drugs tolerated in patients with borderline or low BP. DC cardioversion may be performed and an antiarrhythmic drug administered only if the rate is >150 bpm and the patient is unstable. Unfortunately, DC cardioversion may not be effective in patients with acute, unresolved triggers; amiodarone may be their only therapeutic option. As in CABG, longer-term anticoagulation and antiarrhythmic therapy may not be warranted in the absence of AF recurrence, severe underlying myocardial/atrial disease or dilatation, or persistence of the trigger (e.g., chronic severe lung disease).

On the other hand, AF that occurs during STEMI or ACS is not simply a transient form of AF as the underlying condition (CAD) is chronic and ischemia may be recurrent. In this context, AF is probably best managed with long-term anticoagulation. Outside the acute triggers discussed above, AF is a recurrent and progressive disorder, even if recurrences seem rare in a particular patient.

Appendix 9. Brief asymptomatic runs of AF seen on telemetry or device interrogation

In one study that analyzed intracardiac electrograms of patients older than 65 years receiving a pacemaker, subclinical atrial tachyarrhythmias lasting over 6 minutes were associated with a 2.5-fold increase in the risk of stroke and an absolute risk of stroke of 1.7% per year, the risk being higher in patients with $CHADS_2$ score ≥3 (~4% per year), albeit lower than the risk associated with clinical AF.[82] Those subclinical episodes were frequent, seen in ~10% of this population during 3 months of monitoring and ~34% during 2.5 years of monitoring, and would account for ~15% of all strokes. Other studies have suggested that AF episodes lasting several hours, rather than minutes, correlate with the stroke risk (TRENDS study).[83,84] The duration of AF episodes may become less important in patients with a high $CHADS_2$ score ≥3, who have a high stroke risk even with brief AF episodes. In the latter patients, AF, by itself, may not be the direct cause of stroke but may be associated with cardioembolic stroke mechanisms (e.g., atrial dysfunction, underlying cardiovascular disease). Anticoagulation seems warranted in patients with subclinical atrial tachyarrhythmias if:[84]

- Duration >6 minutes along with a $CHADS_2$ score ≥3
- Duration of several hours along with a $CHADS_2$ score of 1 or 2

One-year rhythm monitoring using an implantable loop recorder in patients older than 40 with a recent cryptogenic stroke has shown a high incidence of asymptomatic AF episodes lasting ≥30 seconds (12.4%), indirectly implying a relation between brief episodes of AF and stroke and a role of prolonged monitoring in cryptogenic stroke.[85] The median time for AF detection was 84 days, and thus external 30-day event monitoring may not be enough. Yet the latter already detects a significant proportion of AF episodes, particularly in patients older than 55, and is far superior to Holter monitoring.[86]

QUESTIONS AND ANSWERS

Question 1. A 54-year-old man presents with shock (BP 75/50, obtunded). He is found to have atrial fibrillation at a rate of ~125–130 bpm. What is the next step?

Question 2. A 54-year-old man, known to have HF with LVEF of 25%, presents with pulmonary edema. He is found to have AF at a rate of 125 bpm (newly detected AF). How should AF be managed?

Question 3. A 72-year-old man with a history of hypertension is seen in the outpatient setting. He is asymptomatic. An irregular heart rhythm is found on exam; an ECG shows AF at a rate of ~110 bpm. What is the next step?

Question 4. A 69-year-old man is diagnosed with frequent recurrent, symptomatic paroxysmal AF. He has HTN and diabetes, and drinks alcohol daily. He has a history of CAD and underwent stent placement 3 years previously. He has CKD (creatinine 1.4 mg/dl, GFR 48 ml/min/1.73 m²). Echo shows normal EF, LA enlargement (4.3 cm), and mild LVH (septum 12 mm). He has a history of bleeding peptic ulcer 2 months ago, requiring transfusion. His baseline heart rate is 72 bpm. Diltiazem (240 mg QD) did not relieve his symptoms (baseline heart rate is now 58 bpm). What is the next option?
A. Add flecainide or propafenone
B. Add dronedarone
C. Add amiodarone
D. Add sotalol
E. AF ablation

Question 5. Should the patient in Question 4 receive anticoagulation? He is already on aspirin 81 mg for CAD.
A. HAS-BLED score is 5. Anticoagulation should be avoided. Continue aspirin
B. CHA_2DS_2-VAS score is 4. Anticoagulation should be started despite bleeding risk
C. Use dual antiplatelet therapy instead of anticoagulation to mitigate the bleeding risk
D. Ensure the following: proton pump inhibitor (PPI) therapy for peptic ulcer disease, *H. pylori* testing and treatment, hemoglobin stability, alcohol cessation, and HTN control. Avoid NSAIDs. Then stop aspirin and start anticoagulation

Question 6. The patient in Question 4 is placed on dronedarone. Which anticoagulant should he receive?
A. Dabigatran
B. Rivaroxaban
C. Apixaban
D. Warfarin

Question 7. A 62-year-old man presents with palpitations that started several days ago. He has a history of HTN but no significant cardiac history. BP is currently 115/65. He is mildly dyspneic and has bibasilar crackles. An admission ECG shows AF with a ventricular rate of 140 bpm. A bedside echo shows LVEF of 40%. LA is mildly enlarged with LA size of 4 cm. Beside intravenous furosemide, what is the next step?
A. Urgent DC cardioversion
B. IV metoprolol
C. IV diltiazem
D. IV amiodarone or IV digoxin

Question 8. A 62-year-old man presents with palpitations that started several hours ago. He has a history of HTN but no significant cardiac history. BP is currently 115/65. He is mildly dyspneic and has bibasilar crackles. An admission ECG shows AF with a ventricular rate of 140 bpm. A bedside echo shows normal LV systolic function with LVH. LA is mildly enlarged with LA size of 4 cm. What is the next step?

A. Urgent DC cardioversion

B. IV metoprolol or IV diltiazem

C. IV amiodarone or IV digoxin

Question 9. Concerning the patient in Question 8, the AF rate is slowed to 80 bpm, and he becomes asymptomatic. Should DC cardioversion be considered?

A. No. Rate-control strategy is preferred.

B. Yes. TEE with DC cardioversion is not urgent but may be performed the same day if possible

C. Yes. TEE with DC cardioversion should be considered at 24 hours

Question 10. A 78-year-old man had a pacemaker implanted 2 years ago for AV block. He has a well-controlled HTN and no prior history of HF or stroke. The last pacemaker interrogation shows three episodes of asymptomatic AF that lasted 1–4 hours each. What is the next step?

A. Amiodarone

B. Dronedarone or sotalol

C. No need for antiarrhythmic. No need for anticoagulation, as each AF episode lasted <48 hours.

D. Anticoagulation, preferably with apixaban

E. Anticoagulation with warfarin

Question 11. A 62-year-old man has a history of CAD with LVEF of 40%. He presents with persistent, asymptomatic AF. He does not want electrical cardioversion, but accepts pharmacological cardioversion. After 3 weeks of anticoagulation, which of the following drugs may be used for cardioversion of his AF?

A. Dronedarone

B. Sotalol

C. Dofetilide

D. Flecainide

E. IV Amiodarone loading

F. Oral amiodarone loading

Question 12. A 55-year-old man is morbidly obese (BMI 44), has HTN, HFpEF, and AF 1 year ago that was treated with DC cardioversion and sotalol. He presents with palpitations and dyspnea, and is found to have AF, with a ventricular rate of 135 bpm and mild HF. He is rate-controlled with metoprolol and diltiazem. Echo shows LVEF of 60%, LVH (septum 14 mm), LA enlargement (4.7 cm) and mild pulmonary hypertension. Which statement is *incorrect*?

A. The likelihood of successful rhythm control is low. Despite AF-related initial symptoms, allowing AF to persist and adopting a rate-control strategy is appropriate

B. For a rhythm-control strategy to be successful, he has to lose >10% of his weight

C. Obesity and severe LA enlargement are the major predictors of AF recurrence in his case

D. AF ablation has a long-term success rate of 70% in this case

E. If rhythm control is adopted, amiodarone is the only antiarrhythmic drug that can be used

Question 13. If, in the patient of Question 12, rate control cannot be achieved and rhythm control fails (using amiodarone and/or ablation), what is the next and definite treatment strategy for AF?

Question 14. Concerning AF pathophysiology, which of the following is *false*?

A. AF is characterized by the lengthening of the atrial refractory period

B. In AF, the atrial refractory period is heterogeneous

C. The electrical remodeling of AF is characterized by progressive shortening of the atrial refractory period

D. The anatomic remodeling of AF is characterized by progressive LA dilatation and fibrosis

Answer 1. It is likely that AF is secondary to the shock state rather than causing it, especially when heart rate is <150 bpm. Thus, AF may not need to be immediately cardioverted, and one should look for other causes of shock (fever, sources of infection, trauma, bleeding, large MI). In the case of AF + shock, always consider other potential causes of shock before attributing it to AF.

Answer 2. In acute HF, the immediate cardioversion of AF does not usually lead to an immediate improvement, as the contribution of the atrial kick to the cardiac output is minute in decompensated states. Besides, the cardioversion is unlikely to be successful or sustained in this decompensated state. It is only warranted when the heart rate is >150 bpm and the acute HF is severe. HF should be treated with diuresis and vasodilators. AF slows down with appropriate HF therapy, as this reduces the atrial stretch; in fact, AF may convert with HF therapy. *Digoxin*, and if necessary *amiodarone*, may be used to further improve the heart rate. If AF persists after HF therapy, appropriate rate control with β-blockers and digoxin should be instituted to achieve a heart rate <80 bpm at rest. For AF patients in a controlled hospital setting, β-blockers may be titrated faster than usually allowed with HF. A rhythm-control strategy with elective DC cardioversion in the inpatient setting is often selected, particularly when AF is thought to be a major trigger to the current HF decompensation. If DC cardioversion fails or AF recurs early on despite amiodarone therapy in a patient with uncontrolled AF rate, consider AV nodal ablation with biventricular pacing or catheter ablation of AF.

Answer 3. Approximately 21% of patients with a newly diagnosed AF are asymptomatic. AF is diagnosed incidentally on routine pulse exam. Since AF is asymptomatic, there is no indication for DCCV/rhythm control. The rate should be controlled to <100–110 bpm using a β-blocker or diltiazem as first-line therapy. Since the patient's CHA_2DS_2-VAS score is 2, anticoagulation with warfarin or the newer oral anticoagulants is warranted.

Answer 4. B. The patient requires rhythm control in light of the intolerable symptoms during AF recurrences. Class Ic drugs should be avoided in a patient with CAD. In a patient with CAD, dronedarone and sotalol are the first options. Amiodarone is the second option. Since he has CKD, dronedarone is preferred over sotalol. From the HTN/LVH standpoint, LVH is mild and so any of the drugs B–D is acceptable. AF ablation is considered after failure of drug therapy, noting that its success is reduced in a patient with LA enlargement and structural heart disease (LVH).

Answer 5. D. Patients with a high HAS-BLED score usually have a high CHA_2DS_2-VAS score and a high stroke risk, the absolute stroke risk increasing more sharply than the bleeding risk. Thus, these patients derive an even greater net clinical benefit from anticoagulation than patients with a low HAS-BLED score. A high HAS-BLED score warrants the correction of bleeding risk factors rather than the exclusion of anticoagulation. The patient has five factors of the HAS-BLED score, three of which can be addressed as in answer D (prior bleed, HTN, alcohol and antiplatelet use), and one of which, renal dysfunction, can be stabilized (proper hydration, avoid NSAIDs and unnecessary diuretic therapy). This reduces the bleeding risk during anticoagulation. Beyond 1 year after stenting, aspirin may be discontinued if warfarin is used.

Answer 6. C. *From a drug interaction standpoint* – Dabigatran should be avoided in a patient receiving dronedarone. Rivaroxaban should be avoided in a patient receiving dronedarone or diltiazem. Apixaban has fewer interactions with dronedarone. *From a CKD standpoint* – Of the three new oral anticoagulants, dabigatran is the most affected by renal dysfunction, apixaban is the least affected. Apixaban is favored. *From the standpoint of bleeding risk* – In this patient, who has a high bleeding risk, all of the three new oral anticoagulants have the advantage of a lower intracranial bleed than warfarin. However, dabigatran and rivaroxaban are associated with a higher gastric bleeding than warfarin and do not reduce the overall major bleeding risk, whereas apixaban does.

Answer 7. D. The patient has mild HF, which is likely triggered by AF. Since he does not have severe HF, urgent DC cardioversion is not indicated and is unlikely to be immediately beneficial or successful. Rate control is performed, followed by elective DC cardioversion. In case of HF with reduced EF, IV diltiazem is contraindicated and IV metoprolol should be avoided acutely. IV digoxin or amiodarone may be used for rate control. Metoprolol may be used once HF has improved with diuresis. ***TEE with cardioversion is performed, but not urgently; it is left until after initiation of diuresis, to improve the efficacy and the sustainability of the cardioversion.***

Answer 8. B. As opposed to Question 7, this patient has HFpEF. Beside diuresis, diltiazem or metoprolol are appropriate for rate control. AF likely triggered HF decompensation in a patient with underlying LVH and diastolic dysfunction. Yet, unless the patient is in extremis and AF rate is >150 bpm, urgent DC cardioversion is unlikely to be immediately beneficial or successful; the benefit is rather a long-term benefit.

Answer 9. C. The patient has new-onset AF that was severely symptomatic. This favors rhythm control, although he is currently asymptomatic (he may be symptomatic when stressed). The young age <65 favors rhythm control as well. Also, the LA is not severely enlarged, the patient does not have severe underlying heart disease, and AF is recent, all of which predict sustainability of a rhythm-control strategy. Since the patient has 50–60% probability of spontaneous cardioversion at 24 hours, it is best to wait 24 hours before proceeding with DC cardioversion.

Answer 10. D. The patient has a $CHADS_2$ score of 2. If AF had only lasted few minutes, the indication for anticoagulation would be questionable. But since AF lasted several hours, anticoagulation is likely beneficial. While it has classically been taught that it takes over 48 hours of AF to form a thrombus in the left atrial appendage, AF of a much shorter duration, including minutes in patients with $CHADS_2$ ≥3 or hours in patients with $CHADS_2$ score of 1–2, is actually associated with increased stroke risk (may not be a causal effect). Apixaban is associated with a lower intracranial hemorrhage rate than warfarin.

Answer 11. C. Sotalol and dronedarone may be used to maintain sinus rhythm in CAD patients, but are not effective in cardioverting AF. Amiodarone, whether loaded IV or orally, is not effective in cardioverting AF acutely (it takes several days to have an AF-converting effect). Flecainide and dofetilide are effective in cardioverting AF acutely, but only defetilide may be used in CAD and/or LV dysfunction.

Answer 12. D. The extreme obesity is a major predictor of long-term failure of any form of rhythm control, whether drugs or AF ablation. The LA enlargement, the underlying heart disease (LVH, HF), and the prior AF episode further predict failure. Without weight loss, the long-term success of AF ablation is <40% in this patient. If rate control is difficult to achieve, rhythm control may be considered despite its low likelihood of success.

Answer 13. AV nodal abalation with ventricular pacing, including biventricular pacing if EF declines even slightly <50%.

Answer 14. A. Atrial refractory period shortens in AF.

References

1. Go AS, Hylek EM, Phillips KA, et al. Prevalence of diagnosed atrial fibrillation in adults: national implications for rhythm management and stroke prevention: the AnTicoagulation and Risk Factors in Atrial Fibrillation (ATRIA) study. JAMA 2001; 285: 2370–5.
2. January CT, Wann LS, Alpert JS, et al. 2014 AHA/ACC/HRS Guideline for the management of patients with atrial fibrillation: executive summary. J Am Coll Cardiol 2014; 64: 2246–80.
3. Nieuwlaat R, Capucci A, Camm AJ, et al. Atrial fibrillation management: a prospective survey in ESC member countries: the Euro Heart Survey on Atrial Fibrillation. Eur Heart J 2005; 26: 2422–34.

4. Lip GY, Golding DJ, Nazir M, et al. A survey of atrial fibrillation in general practice: the West Birmingham Atrial Fibrillation Project. Br J Gen Pract 1997; 47: 285–9.

5. Levy S, Maarek M, Coumel P, et al. Characterization of different subsets of atrial fibrillation in general practice in France: the ALFA study. The College of French Cardiologists. Circulation 1999; 99: 3028–35.

6. Wachtell K. Atrial fibrillation: maybe it is not so lone? J Am Coll Cardiol 2009; 53: 30–1.

7. Stiles MK, John B, Wong CX, et al. Paroxysmal lone atrial fibrillation is associated with an abnormal atrial substrate: characterizing the "second factor". J Am Coll Cardiol 2009; 53: 1182–91.

8. Parkash R, Green MS, Kerr CR, et al. The association of left atrial size and occurrence of atrial fibrillation: a prospective cohort study from the canadian registry of atrial fibrillation. Am Heart J 2004; 148: 649–54.

9. Tsang TS, Barnes ME, Bailey KR, et al. Left atrial volume: important risk marker of incident atrial fibrillation in 1655 older men and women. Mayo Clin Proc 2001; 76: 467–75.

10. Mattioli AV, Sansoni S, Lucchi GR, et al. Serial evaluation of left atrial dimension after cardioversion for atrial fibrillation and relation to atrial function. Am J Cardiol 2000; 85: 832–6.

11. Hagens VE, Van Veldhuisen DJ, Kamp O, et al. Effect of rate and rhythm control on left ventricular function and cardiac dimensions in patients with persistent atrial fibrillation: results from the rate control versus electrical cardioversion for persistent atrial fibrillation (RACE) study. Heart Rhythm 2005; 2: 19–24.

12. Calkins H, Kuck KH, Cappato R, et al. 2012 HRS/EHRA/ECAS Expert Consensus Statement on Catheter and Surgical Ablation of Atrial Fibrillation: recommendations for patient selection, procedural techniques, patient management and follow-up, definitions, endpoints, and research trial design. Heart Rhythm 2012; 9: 632–96.

13. Kerr C, Boone J, Connolly S, et al. Follow-up of atrial fibrillation: the initial experience of the Canadian Registry of Atrial Fibrillation. Eur Heart J 1996; 17 Suppl C: 48–51.

14. Morgan DE, Tomlinson CW, Qayumi AK, et al. Evaluation of ventricular contractility indexes in the dog with left ventricular dysfunction induced by rapid atrial pacing. J Am Coll Cardiol 1989; 14: 489–95.

15. Page RL, Wilkinson WE, Clair WK, et al. Asymptomatic arrhythmias in patients with symptomatic paroxysmal atrial fibrillation and paroxysmal supraventricular tachycardia. Circulation 1994; 89: 224–7.

16. Sherman DG, Kim SG, Boop BS, et al: National Heart, Lung, and Blood Institute AFFIRM Investigators. Occurrence and characteristics of stroke events in the Atrial Fibrillation Follow-up Investigation of Rhythm Management (AFFIRM) study. Arch Intern Med 2005; 165: 1185–91.

17. Olshansky B, Rosenfeld LE, Warner A, et al. The atrial fibrillation follow-up investigation of rhythm management (AFFIRM) study: approaches to control rate in atrial fibrillation. J Am Coll Cardiol 2004; 43: 1201–8.

18. Gheorghiade M, Fonarow GC, van Veldhuisen DJ, et al. Lack of evidence of increased mortality among patients with atrial fibrillation taking digoxin: findings from post hoc propensity-matched analysis of the AFFIRM trial. Eur Heart J 2013; 34: 1489–97.

19. Van Gelder IC, Groenveld HF, Crijns HJ, et al. Lenient versus strict rate control in patients with atrial fibrillation. N Engl J Med 2010; 362: 1363–73.

20. Wyse DG, Waldo AL, DiMarco JP, et al. A comparison of rate control and rhythm control in patients with atrial fibrillation. N Engl J Med 2000; 347: 1825–33. *AFFIRM trial.*

21. Van Gelder IC, Hagens VE, Bosker HA, et al. A comparison of rate control and rhythm control in patients with recurrent persistent atrial fibrillation. N Engl J Med 2002; 347: 1834–40. *RACE trial.*

22. Roy D, Talajic M, Nattel S, et al. Rhythm control versus rate control for atrial fibrillation and heart failure. N Engl J Med 2008; 358: 2667–77.

23. Corley SD, Epstein AE, DiMarco JP, et al. Relationships between sinus rhythm, treatment, and survival in the Atrial Fibrillation Follow-Up Investigation of Rhythm Management (AFFIRM) Study. Circulation 2004; 109: 1509–13.

24. Saksena S, Slee A, Waldo AL, et al. Cardiovascular outcomes in the AFFIRM Trial: an assessment of individual antiarrhythmic drug therapies compared with rate control with propensity score-matched analyses. J Am Coll Cardiol 2011; 58: 1975–85.

25. Hagens VE, Ranchor AV, Van Sonderen E, et al. Effect of rate or rhythm control on quality of life in persistent atrial fibrillation: results from the Rate Control versus Electrical Cardioversion (RACE) Study. J Am Coll Cardiol 2004; 43: 241–7.

26. Pathak RK, Middeldorp ME, Meredith M, et al. Long-term effect of goal-directed weight management in an atrial fibrillation cohort: a long-term follow-up study (LEGACY). J Am Coll Cardiol 2015; 65: 2159–69.

27. Pathak RK, Middeldorp ME, Lau DH, et al. Aggressive risk factor reduction study for atrial fibrillation and implications for the outcome of ablation: the ARREST-AF cohort study. J Am Coll Cardiol 2014; 64: 2222–31.

28. Camm AJ, Kirchhof P, Lip GYH, et al. ESC Guidelines for the management of atrial fibrillation. Eur Heart J 2010; 31: 2369–429. *Also update in 2012: Eur Heart J 2012; 33, 2719–47.*

29. Haddad F, Doyle R, Murphy DJ, Hunt S. Right ventricular function in cardiovascular disease, part II: pathophysiology, clinical importance, and management of right ventricular failure. Circulation 2008; 117: 1717–31.

30. Chatterjee S, Sardar P, Lichstein E, et al. Pharmacologic rate versus rhythm-control strategies in atrial fibrillation: an updated comprehensive review and meta-analysis. Pacing Clin Electrophysiol 2013; 36: 122–33. *Meta-analysis of randomized trials, not retrospective studies.*

31. de Vos CB, Pisters R, Nieuwlaat R, et al. Progression from paroxysmal to persistent atrial fibrillation clinical correlates and prognosis. J Am Coll Cardiol 2010; 55: 725–31.

32. Kleeman T, Becker T, Strauss M, et al. Prevalence of left atrial thrombus and dense spontaneous echo contrast in patients with short-term atrial fibrillation <48 hours undergoing cardioversion: value of transesophageal echocardiography to guide cardioversion. J Am Soc Echocardiogr 2009; 22: 1403–8.

33. You JJ, Singer DE, Howard PA, et al. Antithrombotic therapy for atrial fibrillation. ACCP practice guidelines. Chest 2012; 141: e 531S–575S.

34. Roy D, Talajic M, Dorian P, et al. Amiodarone to prevent recurrences of atrial fibrillation. N Engl J Med 2000; 342: 913–20.

35. Dittrich HC, Erickson JS, Schneiderman T, et al. Echocardiographic and clinical predictors for outcome of elective cardioversion of atrial fibrillation. Am J Cardiol 1989; 63: 193–7.

36. Wazni OM, Marrouche NF, Martin DO, et al. Radiofrequency ablation vs antiarrhythmic drugs as first-line treatment of symptomatic atrial fibrillation: a randomized trial. JAMA 2005; 293: 2634–40.

37. Gage BF, Waterman AD, Shannon W, et al. Validation of clinical classification schemes for predicting stroke: results from the National Registry of Atrial Fibrillation. JAMA 2001; 285: 2864–70.

38. Friberg L, Skeppholm M, Terént A. Benefit of anticoagulation unlikely in patients with atrial fibrillation and a CHA2DS2-VASc score of 1. J Am Coll Cardiol 2015; 65: 225–32.

39. Lip GY, Nieuwlaat R, Pisters R, Lane DA, Crijns HJ. Refining clinical risk stratification for predicting stroke and thromboembolism in atrial fibrillation using a novel risk factor-based approach: the Euro Heart Survey on atrial fibrillation. Chest 2010; 137: 263–72.

40. Olesen JB, Torp-Pedersen C, Hansen ML,LipGYH. The value of the CHA2DS2-VASc score for refining stroke risk stratification in patients with atrial fibrillation with a CHADS2 score 0–1: a nationwide cohort study. Thomb Haemost 2012; 107: 1172–9.

41. Chao TF, Liu CJ, Wang KL, et al. Should atrial fibrillation patients with 1 additional risk factor of the CHA2DS2-VASc score (beyond sex) receive oral anti-coagulation? J Am Coll Cardiol 2015; 65: 635–42.

42. Lip GY, Frison L, Halperin JL, Lane DA. Comparative validation of a novel risk score for predicting bleeding risk in anticoagulated patients with atrial fibrillation: the HAS-BLED (Hypertension, Abnormal Renal/Liver Function, Stroke, Bleeding History or Predisposition, Labile INR, Elderly, Drugs/Alcohol Concomitantly) score. J Am Coll Cardiol 2011; 57: 173–80.

43. Camm AJ, Lip GYH, De Caterina R, et al. 2012 focused update of the ESC Guidelines for the management of atrial fibrillation. Eur Heart J 2012; 33: 2719–47.

44. Friberg L, Rosenqvist M, Lip G. Net clinical benefit of warfarin in patients with atrial fibrillation: a report from the Swedish Atrial Fibrillation cohort study. Circulation 2012; 125: 2298–307.

45. Friberg L, Rosenqvist M, Lip GY. Evaluation of risk stratification schemes for ischaemic stroke and bleeding in 182 678 patients with atrial fibrillation: the Swedish Atrial Fibrillation Cohort study. Eur Heart J 2012; 33: 1500–10.

46. Smith P, Arnesen H, Holme I. The effect of warfarin on mortality and reinfarction after myocardial infarction. N Engl J Med 1990; 323: 147–52.

47. Hurlen M, Abdelnoor M, Smith P, et al. Warfarin, aspirin, or both after myocardial infarction. N Engl J Med 2002; 347: 969–74. *WARIS 2.*

48. Van Es RF, Jonker JJ, Verheught FW, et al. Aspirin and coumadin after acute coronary syndromes: a randomized, controlled trial. Lancet 2002; 360: 109–13. *ASPECT 2 trial.*

49. Lamberts M, Gislason GM, Lip GYH, et al. Antiplatelet therapy for stable coronary artery disease in atrial fibrillation patients taking an oral anticoagulant: a nationwide cohort study. Circulation 2014; 129: 1577–85.

50. Flaker GC, Gruber M, Connolly SJ, et al. Risks and benefits of combining aspirin with anticoagulant therapy in patients with atrial fibrillation: an explora-tory analysis of stroke prevention using an oral thrombin inhibitor in atrial fibrillation (SPORTIF) trials. Am Heart J 2006; 152: 967–973.

51. Connolly S, Pogue J, Hart R, et al.; ACTIVE Writing Group of the ACTIVE Investigators. Clopidogrel plus aspirin versus oral anticoagulation for atrial fibrilla-tion in the Atrial fibrillation Clopidogrel trial with Irbesartan for prevention of Vascular Events (ACTIVE W): a randomised controlled trial. Lancet 2006; 367: 1903–12. *The majority of the patients in ACTIVE W were receiving oral anticoagulation at the time of study entry. Patients not receiving oral anticoagulation therapy at entry had less major bleeding with the combination of clopidogrel and aspirin than with oral anticoagulation therapy, whereas those already receiving oral anticoagulation therapy at entry had more major bleeding with clopidogrel and aspirin than with oral anticoagulation therapy.*

52. Connolly SJ, Pogue J, Hart RG, et al.; ACTIVE Investigators. Effect of clopidogrel added to aspirin in patients with atrial fibrillation. N Engl J Med 2009; 360: 2066–78.

53. Ruiz-Nodar JM, Marín F, Hurtado JA, et al. Anticoagulant and antiplatelet therapy use in 426 patients with atrial fibrillation undergoing percutaneous coronary intervention and stent implantation: implications for bleeding risk and prognosis. J Am Coll Cardiol 2008; 51: 818–25.

54. Sorensen R, Hansen ML, Abildstrom SZ, et al. Risk of bleeding in patients with acute myocardial infarction treated with different combinations of aspirin, clopidogrel, and vitamin K antagonists in Denmark: a retrospective analysis of nationwide registry data. Lancet 2009; 374: 1967–74.

55. Dewilde WJ, Oirbans T, Verheugt FW, et al. Use of clopidogrel with or without aspirin in patients taking oral anticoagulant therapy and undergoing per-cutaneous coronary intervention: an open-label, randomised, controlled trial. Lancet 2013; 381: 1107–15. *WOEST trial.*

56. Fiedler KA, Maeng M, Mehilli J, et al. Duration of triple therapy in patients requiring oral anticoagulation after drug-eluting stent implantation. J Am Coll Cardiol 2015; 65: 1619–29.

57. Karjalainen PP, Porela P, Ylitalo A, et al. Safety and efficacy of combined antiplatelet–warfarin therapy after coronary stenting. Eur Heart J 2007; 28: 726–32.

58. Plewan A, Lehmann G, Ndrepepa G, et al. Maintenance of sinus rhythm after electrical cardioversion of persistent atrial fibrillation; sotalol vs. bisoprolol. Eur Heart J 2001; 22: 1504–10.

59. Steeds RP, Birchall AS, Smith M, et al. An open label, randomised, crossover study comparing sotalol and atenolol in the treatment of symptomatic par-oxysmal atrial fibrillation. Heart 1999; 82: 170–5.

60. Singh BN, Singh SN, Reda DJ, et al. Amiodarone versus sotalol for atrial fibrillation. N Engl J Med 2005; 352: 1861–72.

61. Hohnloser SH, Crijns HJ, van Eickels M, et al. Dronedarone for maintenance of sinus rhythm in atrial fibrillation or flutter. N Engl J Med 2009; 360: 668–78.

62. Kober L, Torp-Pedersen C, McMurray JJV, et al. Increased mortality after dronaderone therapy for severe heart failure. N Engl J Med 2008: 368: 2678–87.

63. Connolly SJ, Crijns HJ, Torp-Pedersen C, et al. Analysis of stroke in ATHENA: a placebo-controlled, double-blind, parallel-arm trial to assess the efficacy of dronedarone 400 mg BID for the prevention of cardiovascular hospitalization or death from any cause in patients with atrial fibrillation/atrial flutter. Circulation 2009; 120: 1174–80.

64. Echt, DS, Liebson, PR, Mitchell, LB, et al. Mortality and morbidity in patients receiving encainide, flecainide or placebo. The Cardiac Arrhythmia Suppression Trial. N Engl J Med 1991; 324: 781–8.

65. Calkins H, Reynolds MR, Spector P, et al. Treatment of atrial fibrillation with antiarrhythmic drugs or radiofrequency ablation: two systematic literature reviews and meta-analyses. Circ Arrhythm Electrophysiol 2009; 2: 349–61.

66. Hussein AA, Saliba WI, Martin DO, et al. Natural history and long-term outcomes of ablated atrial fibrillation. Circ Arrhythm Electrophysiol 2011; 4: 271–8.

67. Verma A, Champagne J, Sapp J, et al. Discerning the incidence of symptomatic and asymptomatic episodes of atrial fibrillation before and after catheter ablation (DISCERN AF): a prospective, multicenter study. JAMA Intern Med 2013; 173: 149–56.

68. Chattterjee NA, Upadhyay GA, Ellenbogen KA, et al. Atrioventricular nodal ablation in atrial fibrillation: a meta-analysis and systematic review. Circ Arrhythm Electrophysiol 2012; 5: 68–76.

69. Ozcan C, Jahangir A, Friedman PA, et al. Long-term survival after ablation of the atrioventricular node and implantation of a permanent pacemaker in patients with atrial fibrillation. N Engl J Med 2001; 344: 1043–51.

70. Curtis AB, Worley SJ, Adamson PB, et al. Biventricular pacing for atrioventricular block and systolic dysfunction. N Engl J Med 2013; 368: 1585–93.

71. Brignole M, Botto G, Mont L, et al. Cardiac resynchronization therapy in patients undergoing atrioventricular junctional ablation for atrial fibrillation. Eur Heart J 2011; 32: 2420–9.

72. Khan MN, Jais P, Cummings J, et al. Pulmonary-vein isolation for atrial fibrillation in patients with heart failure. NEJM 2008; 359: 1778–85.

73. Hylek EM, Go AS, Chang Y, et al. Effect of the intensity of oral anticoagulation on stroke severity and mortality in atrial fibrillation. N Engl J Med 2003; 349: 1019–26.

74. Connolly SJ, Ezekowitz MD, Yusuf S, et al.; RE-LY Steering Committee and Investigators. Dabigatran versus warfarin in patients with atrial fibrillation. N Engl J Med 2009; 361: 1139–51.

75. Patel MR, Mahaffey KW, Garg J, et al.; ROCKET AF Investigators. Rivaroxaban versus warfarin in nonvalvular atrial fibrillation. N Engl J Med 2011; 365: 883–91.

76. Granger CB, Alexander JH, McMurray JJ, et al.; ARISTOTLE Committees and Investigators. Apixaban versus warfarin in patients with atrial fibrillation. N Engl J Med 2011; 365: 981–92.

77. Giugliano RP, Ruff CT, Braunwald E, et al.; ENGAGE AF-TIMI 48 Investigators. Edoxaban versus warfarin in patients with atrial fibrillation. N Engl J Med 2013; 369: 2093–104.

78. Eikelboom JW, Connolly SJ, Brueckmann M, et al. Dabigatran versus warfarin in patients with mechanical heart valves. N Engl J Med 2013; 369: 1206–14.

79. Connolly SJ, Eikelboom J, Joyner C, et al. Apixaban in patients with atrial fibrillation. N Engl J Med 2011; 364: 806–17.

80. Douketis JD, Spyropulos AC, Kaatz S, et al. Perioperative bridging anticoagulation in patients with atrial fibrillation. N Engl J Med 2015; 373: 823–33.

81. Daoud EG, Strickberger SA, Man KC, et al. Preoperative amiodarone as prophylaxis against atrial fibrillation after heart surgery. N Engl J Med 1997; 337: 1785–91.

82. Healey JS, Connolly SJ, Gold MR, et al. Subclinical atrial fibrillation and the risk of stroke. N Engl J Med 2012; 366: 120–9. *AF >6 min ↑ stroke; no correlation with the number of episodes. Duration >17 hours was most definitely associated with the increase in stroke risk.*

83. Glotzer TV, Daoud EG, Wyse DG, et al. The relationship between daily atrial tachyarrhythmia burden from implantable device diagnostics and stroke risk: the TRENDS study. Circ Arrhythm Electrophysiol 2009; 2: 474–80.

84. Zimetbaum P. Waks JW, Ellis ER, et al. Role of atrial fibrillation burden in assessing thromboembolic risk. Circ Arrhythm Electrophysiol 2014; 7: 1223–9.

85. Sanna T, Diener HC, Passman RS, et al. Cryptogenic stroke and underlying atrial fibrillation. N Engl J Med 2014; 370: 2478–86. *CRYSTAL AF trial. Patients >40 years old; loop recorder detected AF in 12.4% of patients at 1 year.*

86. Gladstone DJ, Spring M, Dorian P, et al. Atrial fibrillation in patients with cryptogenic stroke. N Engl J Med 2014; 370: 2467–77. *EMBRACE trial. Patients >55 years old; 30-day event monitor detected AF in 16% of patients.*

Further reading
Resumption of anticoagulation after a GI bleed

Witt DM, Delate T, Garcia DA, et al. Risk of thromboembolism, recurrent hemorrhage, and death after warfarin therapy interruption for gastrointestinal tract bleeding. Arch Intern Med 2012; 172: 1484–91. *Resuming anticoagulation beyond one week of the bleeding was safe and associated with improved survival, compared to those who do not resume it at 90 days.*

Qureshi W, Mittal C, Patsias I, et al. Restarting anticoagulation and outcomes after major gastrointestinal bleeding in atrial fibrillation. Am J Cardiol 2014; 113: 662–8. *Resuming warfarin after 7 days was not associated with a higher recurrence of bleeding; death and thromboembolism were lower than in patients who resumed warfarin after 30 days.*

11 Atrial Flutter and Atrial Tachycardia

I. Atrial flutter

A. Definition

Typical atrial flutter (Aflutter) is characterized by a macroreentrant RA circuit that runs in a frontal, right-to-left plane, the base of which is a narrow isthmus bordered by the IVC and crista terminalis posteriorly and the tricuspid annulus anteriorly (cavotricuspid isthmus, CTI) (see figures in Chapter 15). The crista terminalis, a fibrous band that separates the anterior and posterior parts of the RA, constitutes the electrical barrier in front of which the Aflutter circuit is sustained.[1]

The typical Aflutter circuit is counterclockwise in >90% of the cases, and clockwise in the remaining cases, where it is also called reverse typical Aflutter (Figure 11.1).

Atypical Aflutter is characterized by a macroreentrant circuit not involving the isthmus. It may involve the left atrium, a right atrial scar, or less commonly a left atrial scar from a prior cardiac surgery (e.g., congenital heart disease surgery, atrial cannulation or incision), or a left atrial scar from pulmonary vein isolation. In these cases, the scar serves as the barrier that allows Aflutter to become sustained. The circuit is smaller than the isthmus-dependent Aflutter, which means the reentrant loop is crossed more quickly, leading to a faster flutter rate and smaller flutter waves on the ECG. Note that CTI-dependent flutter is also common in these patients, and both CTI- and non-CTI-dependent macroreentrant circuits often coexist in the same patient.

B. Electrophysiological features

In order to be sustained, the Aflutter must travel slowly across the CTI, such that the initially excited area recovers its excitability by the time it is reached again, and gets reactivated. This large area of excitability is called the *excitable gap*. This excitable gap allows a premature stimulus or atrial pacing to initiate Aflutter, but also to terminate it. That is how overdrive atrial pacing can penetrate the Aflutter circuit and break it.[2] The excitable gap is larger in patients with a large RA. A small circuit with a small excitable gap eventually leads to collision of impulses inside the circuit and non-sustainability of Aflutter.

Aflutter may, thus, be spontaneously initiated by a PAC. It may also be initiated by transient AF. In the presence of the electrical barrier that acts as a line of conduction block, the microreentrant circuits of AF may eventually organize on one side of this block into a stable Aflutter. *AF is often easier to rate-control than Aflutter.* The high atrial rate of AF leads to partial (concealed) conduction of some atrial beats across the AV node, which makes it refractory to subsequent beats that would otherwise be conducted. The slower atrial rate in Aflutter allows the AV nodal conduction of a higher number of atrial beats (*less concealed conduction*).

On the other hand, Aflutter may trigger AF. Sustained Aflutter results in electrical and anatomical remodeling of the atrial tissue. For instance, the atrial refractory period progressively shortens with Aflutter, and only returns to baseline slowly after conversion of Aflutter. The longer the duration of Aflutter, the slower the recovery of the atrial refractory period. This atrial remodeling may lead to AF.

Drugs that slow the conduction across the CTI increase the excitable gap and allow Aflutter to perpetuate rather than terminate. Therefore, class I drugs (especially Ic) are not helpful for Aflutter therapy. Even worse, by slowing the reentrant circuit, they slow the atrial rate, which allows more atrial impulses to be conducted through the AV node. They convert 2:1 Aflutter into 1:1 Aflutter. They may also organize AF into 1:1 Aflutter. While used as a "pill in the pocket" for acute AF conversion, class Ic antiarrhythmics are generally avoided in Aflutter.

Aflutter tends to be an unstable rhythm, in the sense that it often converts to sinus rhythm or degenerates into AF. However, persistent or permanent Aflutter may be seen. Tachycardia-induced cardiomyopathy may be seen with a slow 2:1 Aflutter that does not attract medical attention early on.

C. Underlying pathology and anatomical substrate

Aflutter may be secondary to LA enlargement/left heart disease. LA disease serves as a substrate for PACs, AF, or atrial runs that enter the RA and initiate the macroreentrant circuit.

Practical Cardiovascular Medicine, First Edition. Elias B. Hanna.
© 2017 John Wiley & Sons Ltd. Published 2017 by John Wiley & Sons Ltd.

Aflutter may also be secondary to RA enlargement, which is often secondary to left heart disease or pulmonary disease. Most patients with left HF develop, at some point, an increase in RA pressure and a degree of RA structural abnormality that elicits Aflutter. Therefore, while right atrial pathology is notoriously an underlying disease (the circuit being a right atrial circuit), left heart disease, through both of the mechanisms explained above, is often the underlying provoker of Aflutter reentry (e.g., hypertension, CAD, valvular disease, any left HF, diabetes).

Aflutter is more commonly seen in men, and in tall patients. These patients have a larger RA and thus a larger excitable gap, which allows the macroreentrant circuit to be sustained.

A large proportion of Aflutter episodes (up to 60%) are triggered by an acute, possibly reversible predisposing event, such as surgery (especially cardiac or thoracic surgery) or acute medical or pulmonary illness (e.g., pneumonia, PE, COPD exacerbation, acute MI).[3] The remaining patients have underlying cardiac or pulmonary disease (HF is most common, COPD is second most common). Lone Aflutter, i.e., Aflutter without any comorbidity, is less common than lone AF. In one study of patients over 50 years old, only 2% of Aflutter cases were lone;[3] however, in other studies of patients undergoing Aflutter ablation, up to 40% of Aflutter cases did not have any underlying structural heart disease.[4,5]

D. ECG

The ECG is characterized by regular sawtooth atrial waves (called *flutter waves*). Look in leads II, III, aVF, and V_1 (Figures 11.1–11.4). Flutter waves are negative in leads II, III, and aVF due to the retrograde activation of the left atrium and are positive in lead V_1. In leads II, III, and aVF, the flutter waves do not return to an isoelectric baseline between the deflections, which gives the sawtooth morphology. In V_1, the positive waves may return to the isoelectric baseline; in fact, since lead V_1 overlies the RA, it mainly "sees" the local RA activity. In clockwise Aflutter, flutter waves are negative in V_1 and positive in the inferior leads.

The typical Aflutter rate is 240–350 per minute. A rate as low as 200 may be consistent with a slow Aflutter and is seen in the case of RA enlargement, wherein the Aflutter circuit is longer, or if drug therapy with class I antiarrhythmic agents or amiodarone is used (slows the conduction across the loop). The atypical Aflutter is usually faster (atrial rate of 350–450), with smaller flutter waves that return to the baseline between waves; the morphology of the flutter waves is similar to the morphology of P waves in atrial tachycardia, and depends on the site of origin of the Aflutter (RA, LA, low atrial).

Aflutter is usually conducted in a 2:1 fashion (two flutter waves for one QRS: ventricular rate ~150 bpm). Conduction may be 4:1 in case of AV nodal disease or rate-slowing drug therapy. Odd conduction ratios (3:1, 5:1) are uncommon, except in the context of variable conduction. Variable conduction (e.g., 2:1, 4:1, and 3:1) usually leads to a regularly irregular rhythm, wherein identical R–R intervals are repeated cyclically. Variable conduction usually represents multilevel block in the AV node (Figure 11.5).

A conduction ratio less than 4:1 suggests a high-grade AV block with a junctional escape rhythm, especially if the QRS complexes are regular and fall erratically over the flutter waves without a constant P–QRS relationship.

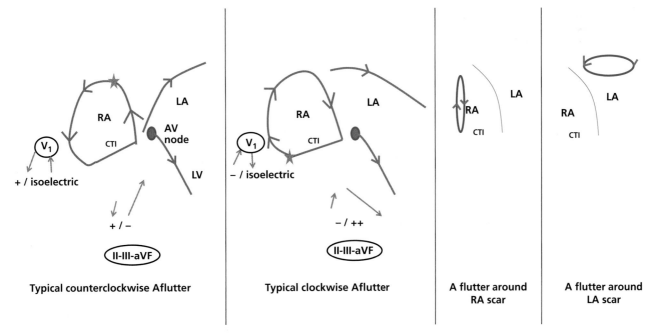

Typical counterclockwise Aflutter   **Typical clockwise Aflutter**   **A flutter around RA scar**   **A flutter around LA scar**

Figure 11.1 Flutter circuit with illustration of the net atrial vectors of depolarization (*gray arrows*) seen by the specific lead and the subsequent morphology of the flutter waves. The *gray star* indicates the starting point of the depolarization vector for illustration purposes. In typical counterclockwise flutter, the negative flutter wave is close to the QRS. Lead V_1 overlies the RA and mainly sees the local current in the RA, hence the positive deflection in V_1, with possible return to isoelectric baseline between deflections.

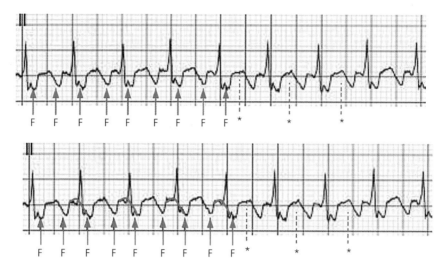

Figure 11.2 Aflutter with flutter waves rate (F wave) ~300 per minute and 2:1 conduction. It is a typical counterclockwise Aflutter, with negative flutter waves in lead II. At first glance, it seems there is ST elevation where the asterisks (*) are placed. This is, in fact, the upslope of the flutter waves. *Bottom image*. One way of diagnosing Aflutter is to imagine that QRS is removed, and then see what the atrial waveform looks like. A typical sawtooth pattern is subsequently seen.

1:1 AV conduction may be seen in patients with accessory pathways or in patients with a slow flutter rate, particularly patients receiving class I antiarrhythmic drugs.

The atrial waves of coarse AF may simulate flutter waves in lead V_1; in fact, V_1 overlies the RA and tends to magnify the RA waves (Figure 11.6). In addition, AF has multiple reentrant circuits, one of which, in the RA close to the isthmus, may be large enough to give a morphology of atrial flutter. These pseudo-flutter waves are slightly irregular and polymorphic and are only seen in lead V_1; in addition, the ventricular rhythm is totally irregular without any cyclical repetition of R–R intervals. This rhythm is sometimes called "AF-Aflutter," but in reality it is AF with one large RA reentrant circuit on top of hundreds of other atrial circuits. The rhythm behaves like AF in response to therapy, and is not cured with isthmus ablation.

E. Management of atrial flutter

1. Acute treatment

Acutely, Aflutter is managed like AF (rate control, anticoagulation). Approximately 55% of Aflutter episodes convert spontaneously, especially in the first 24–48 hours. If not:

- DC cardiovert after performing TEE to rule out LA thrombus. A low current dose (50 J) is usually effective. This is the only treatment necessary in patients with acute, reversible trigger.
- Perform overdrive pacing of the atrium at an atrial rate 60–100 bpm higher than the flutter rate, i.e., an atrial rate of ~400. This is done in the setting of dual-chamber PM, or in the post-cardiac-surgery setting when temporary atrial pacing wires are in place. This effectively converts Aflutter in 80% of the cases. It may induce AF, which is usually easier to rate-control than Aflutter. Similarly to DC cardioversion, overdrive pacing is performed after TEE rules out LA thrombus.
- Continue rate control until catheter ablation of the Aflutter is performed. *Ablation may be performed acutely if Aflutter is not thought to be secondary to a reversible process.*

2. Chronic treatment

When Aflutter occurs in the context of an acute disease process (pneumonia, COPD exacerbation, the first 3 months after cardiac surgery) and in the absence of severe underlying heart or lung disease or prior Aflutter episodes, catheter ablation is not necessary, as Aflutter is unlikely to recur later;[6] DC cardioversion is performed if Aflutter does not revert spontaneously. In the remaining patients, catheter ablation of the CTI is first-line therapy; this has a curative rate >90%, and may be performed in the acute setting, while Aflutter is ongoing. There is no need for antiarrhythmic therapy or long-term anticoagulation after radiofrequency ablation, unless the patient has AF associated with Aflutter. Catheter ablation may be reattempted, with a high success rate, in case of recurrence. Class III antiarrhythmic drugs may be used in patients who refuse ablation, while class Ic drugs are preferably avoided. For an overview of Aflutter ablation, see Chapter 15.

Non-ablated paroxysmal or persistent Aflutter mandates chronic anticoagulation (according to CHA_2DS_2-VAS score), except when it occurs in the context of a clear acute disease process and in the absence of severe underlying heart or lung disease. After curative catheter ablation, and in the absence of concomitant AF, anticoagulation is required for 4 weeks only.

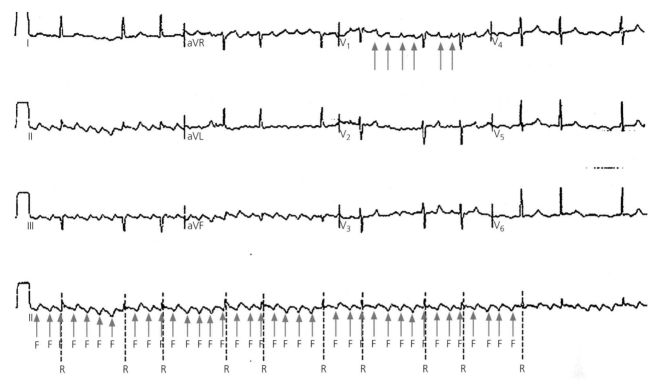

Figure 11.3 Typical counterclockwise Aflutter with variable conduction: 5:1, 4:1, 3:1, 2:1. The rhythm is overall irregular, but there is some repetition of the same R–R intervals. The interval between the 1st and 2nd, the 3rd and 4th, and the 7th and 8th R–R are equal. Typical sawtooth Aflutter waves are seen in lead II. In V$_1$, there are upright P waves with an isoelectric baseline.

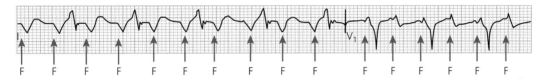

Figure 11.4 Another typical counterclockwise 2:1 Aflutter. See how F is negative in lead II, and positive in lead V$_1$, without return to baseline.

3. The association between Aflutter and AF

Aflutter is seen in 25–35% of AF patients. In some cases, Aflutter waves abut remodeled LA areas with dispersed repolarization, degenerating into multiple small reentries and wavelets (= AF). In others, AF becomes organized along the CTI and triggers Aflutter. In patients whose predominant rhythm is Aflutter, i.e., Aflutter episodes are more often documented on ECGs and Holter monitoring than AF, Aflutter ablation may prevent AF.

In general, AF occurs in ~25% of Aflutter cases at 1–3 years after CTI ablation, more so if LV dysfunction is present or if AF episodes were documented before Aflutter ablation.[4,5] If only Aflutter is documented, the occurrence of AF after CTI ablation is only 8% at 20 ± 14 months. Conversely, for those with a predominant Aflutter but a history of AF, the recurrence rate of AF is 38%, whereas for those with a predominant AF, the recurrence rate of AF is 86%.[5] Thus, Aflutter ablation markedly reduces AF occurrence over the long term only when Aflutter is the dominant arrhythmia.

Occasionally, AF may organize into Aflutter when treated with class Ic drugs (class Ic Aflutter) or with amiodarone. In this subgroup, CTI ablation with continuation of the Ic drug often results in control of both AF and Aflutter.

II. Focal atrial tachycardia

A. Electrophysiological mechanisms

Atrial tachycardia (AT) may be initiated by three different mechanisms: microreentry, automaticity, and triggered activity. The frequency of each of these mechanisms varies according to different studies, with each mechanism probably accounting for a third of atrial tachycardias.[7–9] One study suggested that > 80% of ATs are due to triggered activity. The automatic mechanism is rare in older patients, because automaticity decreases with age.

Reentry and triggered activity can be induced and terminated with programmed electrical stimulation. During EP testing of an ongoing AT, pacing at a slightly faster rate (interval 20–50 ms shorter), called entrainment or incremental pacing, should be performed from the presumed site of origin of the arrhythmia, i.e., site of earliest atrial activation. If pacing does not break the arrhythmia, look at the

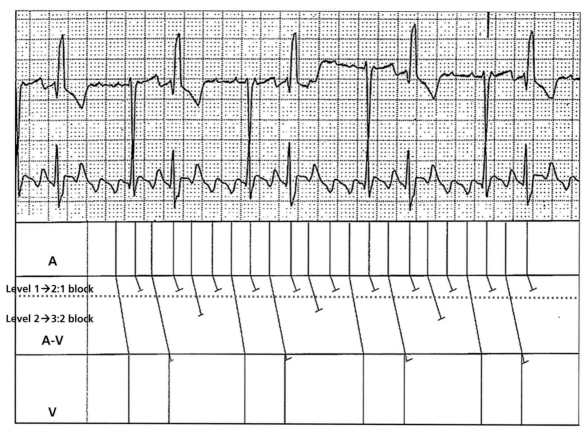

Figure 11.5 Rhythm in lead V₁ (*above*) and lead II (*below*) with a ladder diagram showing how variable AV block occurs. Two levels of second-degree block are present in the AV junction: 2:1 block high in the AV junction and 3:2 type I block low in the AV junction. Flutter waves are indicated by vertical lines in the atrial (A) portion of the diagram. Every other flutter wave is blocked high, at level 1. Of those impulses making it through level 1, one-third are blocked at level 2, and two-thirds are conducted to the ventricles (V). Overall, this translates into an alternation of 2:1 and 4:1 conduction. The QRS complexes following the short R–R intervals are wide because of a functional block in the right bundle branch (Ashman type of aberrancy). Reproduced with permission of Baylor University Medical Center from Glancy DL, Hanna EB. Bigeminal rhythm IV. Proc (Baylor Univ Med Ctr) 2010; 23: 311–12.

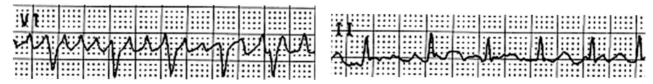

Figure 11.6 Coarse fibrillatory AF waves that simulate Aflutter in lead V1. Note their lack of consistent morphology and timing, and the lack of flutter waves in lead II.

post-pacing interval: a post-pacing interval that is equal to the tachycardia cycle length usually implies that pacing was performed from the actual reentrant focus, and that the mechanism is reentry; the A-wave morphology during pacing is similar to the tachycardia. If the atrium was entrained from outside the reentrant focus, the post-pacing interval will be equal to the tachycardia cycle length plus the distance between the pacing focus and reentry focus. On the other hand, automatic AT cannot be initiated or terminated with pacing or premature stimuli. An automatic focus is overdrive-suppressed during pacing, but "wakes up" after pacing cessation and may be a bit late and slow initially (long post-pacing interval).[8]

The surface ECG may help differentiate automaticity from reentry. In reentry, the PAC that initiates the arrhythmia may have a different P-wave morphology than the arrhythmia. In automatic tachycardia, the P wave that initiates the arrhythmia has a similar morphology to the P wave of the arrhythmia. An automatic mechanism tends to have a warm-up and warm-down phenomenon, but this is not very sensitive or specific.

Through its inhibition of cAMP generation, adenosine terminates atrial tachycardia secondary to triggered activity, and may transiently suppress atrial tachycardia secondary to automaticity by hyperpolarizing the myocardium. It has a variable effect on reentrant atrial tachycardias (some studies suggest no effect,[7] while others suggest a high rate of termination[10]).

Transient atrial tachycardias, lasting < 30 seconds, are very common in patients with or without underlying heart disease, particularly older patients, and are benign and usually asymptomatic.[11] More *sustained* atrial tachycardia is often symptomatic and may be *paroxysmal or persistent (= incessant)*, with a risk of tachycardia-mediated cardiomyopathy (whether persistent or off-and-on paroxysmal).[12] Approximately 40% of patients with sustained AT have an underlying cardiovascular disease, particularly in the case of reentrant AT. In fact, reentrant AT in older patients is frequently associated with AF or Aflutter, and AT may initiate AF or Aflutter. ***Automatic AT and triggered-activity AT are mostly seen in patients < 60–70 years of age who often do not have structural heart disease.[8] The relative frequency of the reentry increases and automaticity decreases beyond the age of 65***. AT, particularly automatic AT, may be related to acute metabolic abnormalities or acute illness (hypoxia, sepsis).

Atrial tachycardia with block (2:1 or, less often, 3:1 or Wenckebach) is usually due to digoxin toxicity or hypokalemia.

> In one systematic review of atrial tachycardia, ~25% of patients with AT had LV dysfunction, and most of those cases (73%) were tachycardia-mediated cardiomyopathy that reversed after tachycardia termination.[12] Therefore, any case of AT and new-onset LV dysfunction should be considered a tachycardia-mediated cardiomyopathy, and an attempt should be made to ablate AT. A similar concept applies to AF or atrial flutter associated with new LV dysfunction.

B. Site of origin

AT most commonly originates from the RA (82%). It typically arises around the tricuspid annulus, the crista terminalis (most common two sites, ~35% each), the venous orifices (pulmonary veins, coronary sinus, IVC, SVC), or less commonly, interatrial septum or mitral annulus. It may also arise around prior scars (e.g., pulmonary vein isolation for AF). Approximately 10% of patients have multiple foci, particularly older patients or those with underlying structural heart disease, where the prevalence of multiple foci increases to ~25%.[12]

C. Natural history

AT may be seen at any age, the mean being 40 years old. Up to 65% of patients have spontaneous remission of AT with time, and a lack of recurrence with cessation of antiarrhythmic therapy. This is more common with automatic AT of young patients, especially those < 25 years of age.[13,14]

D. ECG

- Regular P wave rate, 100–240 per minute (< atrial rate of Aflutter, 200–340 per minute).
- Isoelectric baseline is seen between P waves (different from typical Aflutter).
- The first P wave of the tachycardia is often similar to the subsequent P waves of the tachycardia, particularly in automatic AT. This is different from other forms of SVT.
- Atrioventricular conduction is usually 1:1. *A conduction block (2:1) suggests digoxin toxicity or hypokalemia.*
- PR interval is normal or prolonged, RP interval is long (> half R–R interval). Thus, AT is usually a long RP tachycardia (as opposed to typical AVNRT and AVRT, which are short RP tachycardias).
- As with VT and bypass tract localization, look at the morphology in leads V_1, I-aVL, and II-III-aVF to localize the atrial origin of AT (Figure 11.7):
  - A negative P wave in leads II, III, and aVF implies a *low atrial origin* that simulates a retrograde P wave; a positive P wave in leads II, III, and aVF implies a *high atrial origin*.
  - A P wave that is positive in V_1 (looks to the right) and negative in the left lateral leads I and aVL (looks away from the left) is typical of a *left atrial origin*, with the exception of a right superior pulmonary vein origin (the latter simulates RA origin). Either way, the P axis and morphology are usually different from the sinus P wave in the same patient.

> ### Difference between Aflutter and AT
>
> Aflutter, whether isthmus- or non-isthmus-dependent, is due to macroreentry. Conversely, AT is due to microreentry or other mechanisms. For practical purposes, AT is distinguished from Aflutter by the atrial rate. An atrial rate < 200 per minute is AT, whereas an atrial rate > 200–240 per minute is Aflutter. It is important to differentiate AT from a slow Aflutter, for the following two reasons:
>
> 1. The mechanism is different. Aflutter implies macroreentry and is often isthmus-dependent and easily cured with ablation. AT is less easily mapped and ablated.
> 2. Aflutter is associated with a thromboembolic risk and requires anticoagulation, whereas AT, by itself, may not mandate anticoagulation.[14] However, in older patients, AT is frequently associated with AF/Aflutter, which may necessitate anticoagulant therapy.

> An atrial tachycardia with a low atrial origin resembles PJRT (incessant slow AVRT). In both cases, the P wave is retrograde-like, i.e., negative in leads II/III/aVF, and the RP interval is long.

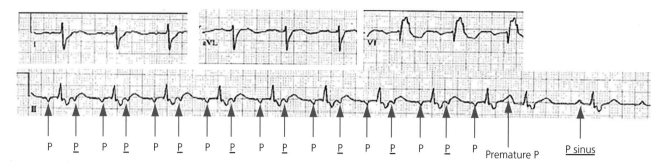

Figure 11.7 2:1 atrial tachycardia, with an atrial rate of ~140 per minute. P wave is negative in the inferior leads, implying a low atrial origin; it is negative in lead V₁ and upright in aVL, implying a right atrial origin. A premature P occurs and breaks the atrial tachycardia at the end of the recording. The change in the T morphology before the premature complex suggests the occurrence of a P wave different from the previous P waves (premature P). The fact that AT breaks with a PAC implies reentrant AT.

E. Treatment

1. Acute treatment

AT, particularly automatic AT, may be secondary to an acute illness that needs to be appropriately treated.

Sustained AT may be terminated with adenosine. Adenosine is mainly effective in triggered activity and its overall efficacy in the termination of AT varies between 10% and 80%.[7-9] Similarly, AT due to triggered activity may be terminated with calcium channel blockers (CCBs) or β-blockers. These drugs have a variable effect on automatic and reentrant AT: adenosine and CCBs may suppress reentrant AT, and β-blockers may suppress automatic AT (in up to 50% of cases).[10] Those three agents should, therefore, be tried first.[6]

When CCBs and β-blockers are not effective in terminating the arrhythmia, they may continue to be used for rate control. However, AT is notoriously very difficult to rate-control, because of the relatively slow atrial rate and the subsequent lack of concealed AV conduction. This allows more atrial beats to conduct through the AV node (in sharp contrast with AF). In fact, in a patient who has a pacemaker, fast atrial pacing may slow down the ventricular rate by blocking the AV node.[1] Therefore, AT may need to be terminated with class I or III drugs (intravenous amiodarone or ibutilide). A better option would be to attempt AT ablation in the acute setting. In fact, once terminated, automatic AT is difficult to induce; in order to localize then ablate the AT focus, AT needs to be ongoing or induced. **Mapping then ablating the AT in the acute setting and avoiding antiarrhythmic drugs may be the preferred approach in patients who are hemodynamically stable.**

In patients with a rate > 150 who are hemodynamically unstable, DC conversion may be contemplated. It is effective in reentrant and triggered-activity AT, but not in automatic AT.

Digoxin is better avoided, as it may initiate AT.

2. Long-term therapy

Regardless of the mechanism of AT, the focus can be ablated by applying radiofrequency energy. In the case of reentry, a critical segment of the reentry loop is ablated. Localization of the focus is performed after inducing AT, by looking for the site of earliest atrial activation during AT. Entrainment is then performed, and a post-pacing interval that is equal to the tachycardia cycle length confirms catheter location within the reentry; this is only helpful in mapping reentrant AT. Catheter ablation has an efficacy of 90%, with an 8% recurrence rate that is partly explained by the occasional presence of multiple foci.[13] Ablation of a left-sided tachycardia is associated with a higher failure rate (~15%). Ablation of foci located near the sinus node or in the low atrial septum, near the AV node, is associated with a higher rate of complications.

Chronic β-blocker or CCB therapy is an acceptable first-line therapy for patients who acutely respond to those two drugs or to adenosine. Catheter ablation is the most appropriate first-line therapy for patients with recurrent or incessant AT, or tachycardia-mediated cardiomyopathy; it is also used in AT refractory to initial drug therapy.[6] If ablation fails or if the patient prefers not to undergo ablation, antiarrhythmic therapy with class Ic or III drugs may be tried.

III. Multifocal atrial tachycardia (MAT) (or chaotic atrial tachycardia)

- MAT is an automatic atrial tachycardia characterized by:
  - Irregularly irregular atrial rhythm with an atrial and ventricular rate usually in the range 100–150 bpm
  - P–P and PR intervals are variable
  - P waves have ≥ 3 different morphologies
- If the atrial rate is < 100 bpm, the rhythm is called *wandering atrial pacemaker* or *multifocal atrial rhythm*.
- Because it is irregular, MAT may mimic AF. Unlike AF, MAT has well-defined P waves.
- MAT is usually associated with acute pulmonary (COPD exacerbation) or cardiac issues (HF), electrolyte disorders, drugs (theophylline, digoxin), or sepsis.
- MAT is frequently preceded or followed by AF or Aflutter. In one series, it was associated with AF in 55% of cases.
- Treatment consists of correcting the underlying disease, in addition to potassium and magnesium repletion. Antiarrhythmic drugs are usually ineffective, but CCBs or β-blockers may help control the rate and cardiovert the arrhythmia.

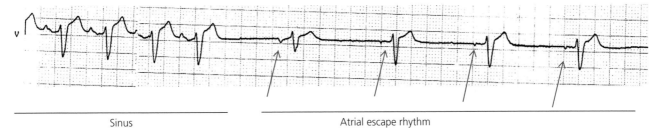

Sinus   Atrial escape rhythm

Figure 11.8 Atrial escape rhythm (rate ~50 bpm) that developed in a patient who had sudden slowing of the sinus rate (e.g., hypervagal situation). The arrows point to the ectopic P waves (morphology different from the sinus P waves).

IV. Ectopic atrial rhythm

An ectopic atrial rhythm is an automatic atrial rhythm characterized by an atrial rate < 100 bpm and a non-sinus P-wave morphology (Figure 11.8). It implies that a quiescent atrial pacemaker is starting to fire at a rate faster than the sinus rate. It may be an escape rhythm/ beat in patients with a slow sinus rate or a sinus pause, or it may be an accelerated automatic rhythm. It is a benign rhythm and may be seen in subjects with or without structural heart disease, including young subjects.

QUESTIONS AND ANSWERS

Question 1. (Questions 1 to 7 refer to the same patient.) A 42-year-old woman, without prior cardiac or hypertension history, presents with palpitations that have been ongoing for the last 2 hours. She has also experienced palpitations over the last 2 months, usually lasting up to 30 minutes. ECG shows atrial tachycardia, 1:1 conduction at a rate of 130 bpm, with a negative P wave in lead V₁, upright P wave in lead aVL, and negative P wave in the inferior leads. The patient is not dizzy and her BP is 125/80 mmHg. How would you ensure this is not 2:1 Aflutter?

Question 2. Adenosine is administered and does not break the AT. Intravenous metoprolol then diltiazem are administered, but they also do not break the AT nor slow the AV conduction. Echo shows a grossly preserved LV function. What is the likely mechanism of this AT?
A. Automaticity
B. Triggered activity
C. Microreentry

Question 3. Where is AT originating from?
A. LA
B. High RA
C. Low RA

Question 4. What is the next step?
A. DC cardioversion
B. Intravenous ibutilide or amiodarone
C. Allow the patient to stay in ongoing AT and attempt AT ablation within the next 24 hours.

Question 5. A few hours later, while the patient is getting ready for the EP mapping and ablation, AT spontaneously converts to sinus rhythm. Attempts to induce AT in the EP laboratory fail, and thus AT cannot be mapped. What is the next step?
A. No further therapy. AT is unlikely to recur
B. Flecainide or propafenone
C. Sotalol
D. Amiodarone
E. Metoprolol or diltiazem

Question 6. If the patient has a breakthrough of persistent AT while receiving antiarrhythmic therapy, what would be the next step?
A. Increase the dose of antiarrhythmic therapy
B. EP study as soon as possible

Question 7. If the patient had a dual-chamber pacemaker, what would be the effect of overdrive atrial pacing on AT (overdrive atrial pacing at an atrial rate of 170 bpm)?
A. Cardioversion of AT, although a risk of degeneration into AF is present
B. No effect

Question 8. (Questions 8 to 10 refer to the same patient.) A 70-year-old man has a history of ischemic cardiomyopathy, with LVEF ~40%, and a dual-chamber ICD. He also has a history of paroxysmal AF. His baseline rhythm is a sinus rhythm with a very long and asymptomatic PR interval of 350 ms and intrinsic AV conduction, without V pacing. In order to avoid AV sequential pacing, his pacing mode has been programmed VVI 40 bpm. Over the last month, his ECG has been showing a persistent, typical Aflutter with 100% ventricular pacing at 40 bpm. Why does he receive ventricular pacing during Aflutter, not during sinus rhythm?

Question 9. The patient's EF appears to have declined to 35% on a repeat echo. He has slightly more fatigue during activity. What is the next step?
A. Keep him in Aflutter. Increase the VVI pacing rate to 60 bpm, with rate response
B. Aflutter ablation
C. Keep him in Aflutter. Upgrade the ICD to a BiV-ICD to prevent further decline of LV function that has occurred with RV pacing

Question 10. Since he has a dual-chamber pacemaker, what specific acute intervention could terminate Aflutter?

Question 11. A 66-year-old man underwent CABG 7 weeks previously. He has a normal EF and no prior history of atrial arrhythmias. He presents with exertional dyspnea; no palpitations are reported. He is found to have a typical Aflutter with 2:1 AV conduction (ventricular rate 140 bpm), and mild pulmonary edema on chest X-ray. He receives diuretic therapy, and Aflutter is rate-controlled with metoprolol (AV conduction ratio becomes 4:1). What is the next step?
A. DC cardioversion followed by 1 month of anticoagulation
B. DC cardioversion followed by long-term anticoagulation
C. Aflutter ablation
D. Keep Aflutter and continue rate-control strategy

Question 12. For the patient in Question 11, was metoprolol appropriate for rate control, considering that he has HF?

Question 13. An 82-year-old man has a history of ischemic cardiomyopathy with prior MI and LVEF of 30%. He presents with mild dyspnea and is found to have a regular SVT at a rate of 135 bpm. He is not in shock but has pulmonary edema. Adenosine is administered and unveils P waves that occur at a rate of 270 per minute. Those P waves are upright in lead V_1 and the inferior leads, and are narrow with an isoelectric line between P waves in V_1 and in the inferior leads. What is the diagnosis?
A. Isthmus-dependent (= typical) Aflutter
B. Non-isthmus-dependent (= atypical) Aflutter arising from the LA
C. Atrial tachycardia arising from the LA

Question 14. The patient in Question 13 receives metoprolol. It does not slow down AV conduction. What is the next step?
A. Aflutter ablation
B. DC cardioversion and chronic amiodarone therapy
C. Chronic rate control

Answer 1. Administer adenosine. Adenosine may break AT, when triggered activity is the mechanism. Otherwise, it may temporarily slow AV conduction and allow visualization of P waves, confirming P rate.

Answer 2. A. Considering the patient's age and the lack of underlying heart disease or potential atrial scars, the most likely mechanism is automaticity. Adenosine does not break automatic AT, but it may break triggered activity or, rarely, reentrant AT.

Answer 3. C.

Answer 4. C. In this young patient with persistent AT and multiple prior episodes, AT ablation is first-line therapy, especially when it originates from the RA (higher success rate with ablation than left AT). In order to ablate the AT focus, AT location has to be mapped with intracardiac recordings while AT is ongoing. Once the patient is in sinus rhythm, it is generally difficult to induce automatic AT. Therefore, it is reasonable to perform ablation within the next few hours, while AT is ongoing, as long as she is hemodynamically stable. In this case, avoid breaking the AT with ibutilide or amiodarone, or class Ic drugs; also, the latter make AT induction more difficult.

Answer 5. B. Since the patient failed ablation, long-term medical therapy is justified. Metoprolol or diltiazem would have been a reasonable long-term therapy if they had been successful acutely. Flecainide and propafenone are likely more effective and less toxic than class III drugs for the long-term treatment of AT (ACC guidelines). Those drugs may be combined with a β-blocker or a CCB to improve efficacy, as per ACC guidelines.

Answer 6. B. Ask the patient to present to the hospital as soon as AT symptoms occur. An EP study should then be performed as soon as possible after presentation, while AT is ongoing, and before it spontaneously converts, so that it can be mapped.

Answer 7. B. Overdrive atrial pacing can break reentrant or triggered-activity AT, but not automatic AT.

Answer 8. The patient has underlying AV nodal disease. Aflutter, by increasing the number of atrial waves "hitting" the AV node, reduces the conduction speed across the AV node and increases its refractory period (the conduction and refractory period were already impaired). The AV node is, in fact, characterized by decremental conduction with fast atrial pacing. In addition, some of these waves partially penetrate the AV node and make it refractory to subsequent waves (concealed conduction). The AV conduction is overall reduced, which triggers VVI back-up pacing.

Answer 9. B. The patient's fatigue is at least partly due to the low ventricular rate of 40 bpm, and thus increasing the VVI pacing rate to 60 bpm will likely improve his symptoms. However, the patient has another issue that needs to be addressed: he has a new, ongoing and harmful RV ventricular pacing with a resulting decline of LV function. One option would be to upgrade the device to a BiV pacemaker. A simpler option consists of ablating the Aflutter and reverting him back to his prior state of intrinsic ventricular conduction after a long PR interval.

Answer 10. Overdrive pacing of the atrium, at a rate faster than the Aflutter rate (e.g., 350–400 bpm), may convert Aflutter into sinus rhythm. Similarly to DC cardioversion, this should only be done if the patient has received 3 weeks of anticoagulation or if TEE rules out LA appendage thrombus. Similarly to DC cardioversion, this is not a definitive therapy of Aflutter in this patient, who has a high likelihood of recurrence.

Answer 11. A. Aflutter that occurs in the first 3 months after CABG, without a prior history of atrial arrhythmia, is likely a transient process that may not recur. Aflutter ablation may not be necessary. DC cardioversion is done, and 1 month of anticoagulation may be reasonable in the absence of further recurrences. If Aflutter recurs, ablation is warranted.

Answer 12. Yes, as his EF was recently normal. Metoprolol may be acutely used in decompensated HFpEF, but not in decompensated systolic HF, where amiodarone may be needed for rate control.

Answer 13. B. The narrow P wave, the presence of an isoelectric segment, and the concordance of P polarity between V_1 and the inferior leads implies AT or atypical Aflutter, not a typical Aflutter. The atrial rate supports Aflutter rather than AT. The upright P wave in V_1 suggests LA origin.

Answer 14. B. Since the Aflutter is non-isthmus-dependent and originating from the LA, ablation is more difficult and less successful than ablation of isthmus-dependent Aflutter. Considering the patient's age, DC cardioversion along with antiarrhythmic therapy is an appropriate strategy. In fact, for atypical Aflutter, first-line catheter ablation is a class IIa recommendation (rather than class I). Standalone rate control is less appropriate, as Aflutter appears to have triggered HF decompensation (poorly tolerated); besides, rate control has not been possible in this case.

References

1. Fogoros N. The electrophysiology study in the evaluation of supraventricular tachyarrhythmias. In: Fogoros N. Electrophysiologic Testing, 4th edn. Oxford: Blackwell, 2006, pp. 103–57.
2. Wellens HJJ. Contemporary management of atrial flutter. Circulation 2002; 106: 649–52.
3. Granada J, Uribe W, Chyou PH, et al. Incidence and predictors of atrial flutter in the general population. J Am Coll Cardiol 2000; 36: 2242–6.
4. Philippon F, Plumb VJ, Epstein A, Kay GN. The risk of atrial fibrillation following radiofrequency catheter ablation of atrial flutter. Circulation 1995; 92: 430–5.
5. Nabar A, Rodriguez LM, Timmermans C, et al. Effect of right atrial isthmus ablation on the occurrence of atrial fibrillation. Circulation 1999; 99: 1441–5.
6. Blomström-Lundqvist C, Scheinman MM, Aliot EM, et al. ACC/AHA/ESC 2003 guidelines for the management of patients with supraventricular arrhythmias. J Am Coll Cardiol 2003; 42: 1493–531.
7. Engelstein ED, Lippman N, Stein KM, Lerman BB. Mechanism-specific effects of adenosine on atrial tachycardia. Circulation 1994; 89: 2645–54.
8. Markowitz SM, Nemirovsky D, Stein KM, et al. Adenosine-insensitive focal atrial tachycardia. J Am Coll Cardiol 2007; 49: 1324–33.
9. Markowitz SM, Stein KM, Mittal S et al. Differential effect of adenosine on focal and macroreentrant atrial tachycardia. J Cardiovasc Electrophysiol 1999; 10: 489–502.
10. Chen SA, Chiang CE, Yang CJ, et al. Sustained atrial tachycardia in adult patients. Electrophysiological characteristics, pharmacological response, possible mechanisms, and effects of radiofrequency ablation. Circulation 1994; 90: 1262–78.
11. Stemple DR, Fitzgerald JW, Winkle RA. Benign slow paroxysmal atrial tachycardia. Ann Intern Med 1977; 87: 44–8.
12. Chen SA, Tai CT, Chiang CE, Ding YA, Chang MS. Focal atrial tachycardia: reanalysis of the clinical and electrophysiologic characteristics and prediction of successful radiofrequency ablation. J Cardiovasc Electrophysiol 1998; 9: 355–65.
13. Poutiainen AM, Koistinen MJ, Airaksinen KE, et al. Prevalence and natural course of ectopic atrial tachycardia. Eur Heart J 1999; 20: 694–700.
14. Roberts-Thomson KC, Kistler PM, Kalman JM. Atrial tachycardias: mechanisms, diagnosis, and management. Curr Probl Cardiol 2005; 30: 529–73.

Further reading

Page RL, Joglar JA, Caldwell MA, et al. 2015 ACC/AHA/HRS guideline for the management of adult patients with supraventricular tachycardia. J Am Coll Cardiol 2016; 67: e27–115.

I. Sinus tachycardia

Sinus tachycardia is not a primary rhythm abnormality. It is secondary to cardiac, pulmonary, septic, or metabolic issues and is often an ominous sign:

- HF, large MI
- Hypovolemia; hypotension of any cause
- Any infectious state/sepsis
- Hypoxia, pulmonary embolism
- Acute bleed, anemia
- Hyperthyroidism; anxiety, pain

Thus, sinus tachycardia is not typically treated with rate-controlling agents. The underlying cause is targeted.

On telemetry monitoring, suspect supraventricular tachyarrhythmia rather than sinus tachycardia in the case of: (1) sharp onset and/or sharp offset of the tachycardia; (2) very steady rate (e.g., 134 bpm). Conversely, in sinus tachycardia, rate variability is seen.

Inappropriate sinus tachycardia (IST) is a non-paroxysmal sinus tachycardia that is present most of the day, at rest and/or mild physical effort, out of proportion to any physiologic need. The mean 24-hour sinus rate on Holter is often >95 bpm. In addition to an early increase in rate during exercise, the rate may increase >30 bpm upon orthostasis without orthostatic hypotension; the latter phenomenon is called POTS (postural orthostatic tachycardia syndrome) and is sometimes associated with IST. IST is due to a dysautonomia that activates the sinus node's I_f current and is mainly seen in young women (<50 years of age). IST is associated with symptoms of palpitations, fatigue, dizziness, and orthostatic intolerance that may be improved with drugs blocking the sinus node. In fact, the use of an I_f current blocker, i.e., a sinus node blocker (ivabradine), eliminated >70% of IST symptoms in one study. β-blockers and CCBs may also be effective, but may not be well tolerated in dysautonomic patients. Sinus node ablation is only temporarily effective, as tachycardia may arise from other sinus sites after ablation, the main issue being autonomic dysfunction.

Conversely, in POTS, sinus tachycardia is useful because it maintains blood pressure and compensate for the significant orthostatic vasodilatation. Thus, β-blocker therapy worsens POTS symptoms, and POTS needs to be ruled out before using β-blockers in these patients.

II. Atrioventricular nodal reentrant tachycardia (AVNRT)

A. Mechanism (see Figure 12.1)

In AVNRT, the AV node has two pathways: fast pathway and slow pathway. Approximately 20% of normal individuals have dual AV node pathways, but most of them do not manifest AVNRT.

Practical Cardiovascular Medicine, First Edition. Elias B. Hanna.

© 2017 John Wiley & Sons Ltd. Published 2017 by John Wiley & Sons Ltd.

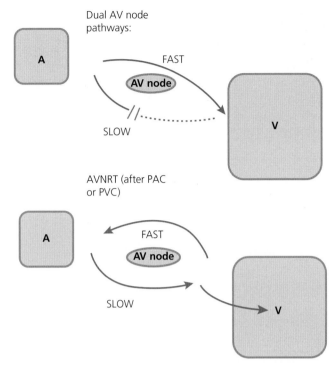

Figure 12.1 AVNRT usually starts with a PAC that has a long PR interval as it goes through the slow pathway. *The slow pathway is slower but has a shorter refractory period than the fast pathway*, allowing conduction of the PAC. If, at the time the impulse reaches the distal slow pathway, the fast pathway is still in its refractory period, the reentrant circuit of AVNRT will not launch. A few subsequent sinus P waves may keep conducting over the slow pathway (Figure 12.5).

If, at the time the impulse reaches the distal slow pathway, the fast pathway has recovered, AVNRT will be initiated. The R–R interval can shorten over the course of the first few beats; it may lengthen during the last few beats before termination with AV nodal blocking agents.

Normally, the AV node conducts impulses through the fast pathway.

The fast pathway conducts faster but has a longer refractory period than the slow pathway. After a PAC, the fast pathway may still be in its refractory period, whereas the slow pathway, having the short refractory period, has already recovered and conducts forward. The impulse then conducts retrogradely through the fast pathway if it has recovered; this leads to a typical ***"slow-then-fast" ("SF")*** AVNRT. If the fast pathway has not recovered its refractory period, the impulse will lead to one QRS having a longer PR interval; arrhythmia is not initiated.

Other, less common forms of AVNRT are the fast-then-slow AVNRT, and the slow-then-slow AVNRT. In the fast-then-slow AVNRT, the slow pathway has a longer refractory period than the fast pathway.

AVNRT usually occurs in patients without underlying heart disease.

B. ECG

AVNRT typically manifests as a regular, narrow QRS complex tachycardia, with a ventricular rate of ~150–250 bpm (most often ~180 bpm).

P waves are retrograde and are usually hidden inside the QRS or at the terminal portion of the QRS (Figure 12.2). These P waves manifest as terminal r' in V_1 and pseudo-S in the inferior leads, with a short RP (often < 90 ms). P waves are often simultaneous to the QRS and therefore are clearly visible in only ~1/2 of the cases (Figures 12.2, 12.3). Rarely, P waves may precede QRS, with a short PR interval < 110 ms (Figure 12.4). If P waves cannot be identified in patients presenting with a regular narrow complex tachycardia, AVNRT is the most likely diagnosis.

The tachycardia being initiated by an ectopic atrial beat that goes down the slow pathway, the PR interval of this initial beat is longer than the sinus PR interval. As opposed to automatic atrial tachycardia, this initial ectopic P wave usually differs from the subsequent (retrograde) P waves and does not march out with them.

The atypical forms of AVNRT (fast–slow or slow–slow AVNRT) have a long RP interval, longer than 1/2 RR interval, and may thus simulate atrial tachycardia. The loop is overall slower than in typical AVNRT; thus, the atypical forms tend to be incessant tachycardias.

Occasionally, dual AV nodal pathways manifest on the baseline sinus rhythm. In this case, two different PR intervals are seen in sinus rhythm (Figure 12.5).

C. Treatment

1. Acute therapy

- Adenosine 6 mg IV (followed by 12 mg IV if the 6 mg dose is ineffective). Adenosine breaks AVNRT and AVRT by blocking the AV node. AVNRT and AVRT are the main arrhythmias that break rather than simply slow down with adenosine; atrial tachycardia can sometimes break with adenosine.
- Diltiazem IV or β-blocker IV is also effective.

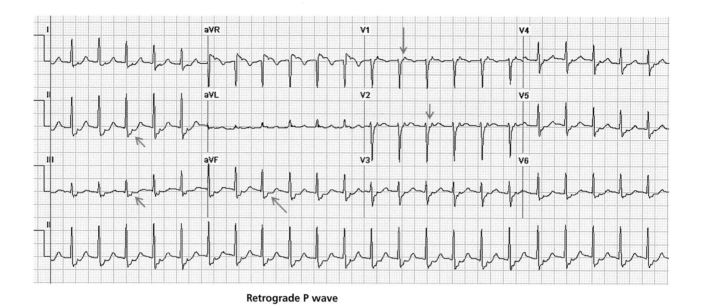

Retrograde P wave

↓

Pseudo-r′ in V1 + Pseudo S in inferior leads

(a)

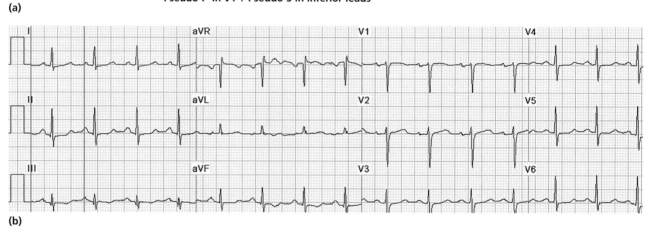

(b)

Figure 12.2 (a) Arrows point to the retrograde P wave that is superimposed on the ST segment, appearing as a notch on the ST segment. (b) An ECG of the same patient in sinus rhythm after adenosine therapy: note the difference in V_1–V_2 and in the inferior leads (no "pseudo-r′" or "pseudo S").

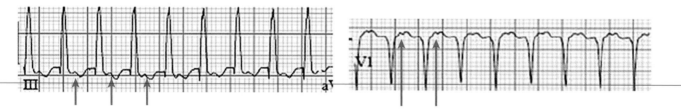

Figure 12.3 Narrow complex tachycardia with retrograde P waves (*arrows*) seen in leads III and V_1. RP is short, < 1/2 RR interval; hence, atrial tachycardia is unlikely. In AVNRT, P wave typically falls within or immediately after QRS (RP interval < 90 ms), giving a pseudo-S shape in the inferior leads and pseudo-r′ shape in V_1. In this case, P wave falls a bit further away and RP is > 90 ms; thus, the arrhythmia could be either AVNRT or AVRT.

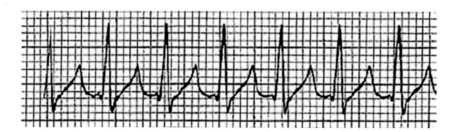

Figure 12.4 P waves are seen just before the QRS, with a PR interval < 110 ms. In a narrow complex tachycardia, this suggests AVNRT, although it is only seen in 4% of AVNRTs.

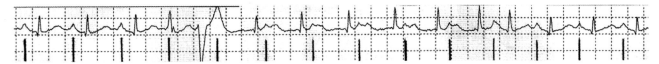

Figure 12.5 Sinus rhythm is present throughout the tracing. Vertical lines indicate P waves. Initially, the PR interval is normal (0.20 s), but after a couplet of PVCs (4th and 5th QRS complexes), the PR interval lengthens markedly. The AV conduction shifts from the fast pathway to the slow pathway. With the 7th sinus P wave after the couplet, the PR returns to normal. Reproduced with permission from Glancy DL, Hanna EB, Jain N. Long P-R intervals following certain ventricular premature complexes. J La State Med Soc 2010; 162: 185–6.

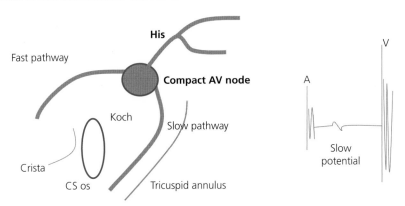

Figure 12.6 Anatomy of the slow pathway, fast pathway, and compact AV node. Note their potential relationship with a His catheter and coronary sinus catheter. The Koch triangle, where the slow pathway lies, is bordered by the His, the coronary sinus, and the tricuspid annulus. The crista terminalis is behind the Koch triangle. A slow potential recorded across the slow pathway is shown. CS, coronary sinus.

2. Long-term treatment is required in case of frequent recurrences of sustained episodes
There are two options:

- Chronic β-blockers or CCBs. When AVNRT is infrequent, one dose of these drugs may be used intermittently upon each recurrence (e.g., rapid-release diltiazem 120 mg) (pill-in-the pocket strategy).
- Radiofrequency ablation of the AV node's slow pathway is a second-line therapy after failure of drug therapy. It is a first- line therapy in poorly tolerated AVNRT, recurrent AVNRT, or even one or infrequent episodes of well-tolerated AVNRT if the patient wishes complete control of the arrhythmia (class I recommendation).

Anatomically, the slow pathway is located inferiorly, along the tricuspid annulus in front of the coronary sinus os, whereas the fast pathway is located superior to the coronary sinus os. They both coalesce more distally to form the compact AV node then His, which is located anteriorly (Figure 12.6). The slow pathway is located anatomically using a His catheter and coronary sinus catheter, and electrically by searching for an area where both A and V deflections are recorded, along with a slow potential in between, not a His potential.

D. Termination
Spontaneous termination may occur if a PAC occurs at a time when it can enter the slow-pathway arm of the reentrant circuit without fully penetrating it. This PAC gets blocked and stops the reentry (Figure 12.7). Spontaneous termination may also occur when the vagal tone blocks the slow pathway.

Vagal tone and AV nodal blocking agents block the slow pathway, usually in a Wenckebach pattern. They terminate the AVNRT after a few cycles, when an impulse that has conducted retrogradely fails to reenter the slow pathway (Wenckebach block). The tachycardia ends with a P wave.

In AVNRT, the atria and ventricles are not required for AV nodal reentry. Thus, if a PAC, a PVC, or atrial or ventricular pacing does not penetrate the AV nodal reentry, AVNRT will not be disrupted. On ECG, AVNRT appears to resume at the same rate after the PAC or PVC; in fact, the reentry circuit has not been affected at any time by this premature beat.

III. Atrioventricular reciprocating tachycardia (AVRT) and Wolff–Parkinson–White (WPW) syndrome
A. Pathophysiology
AVRT and WPW syndrome are characterized by an accessory pathway (AP), also called bypass tract, that connects one atrium to one ventricle.
1. Approximately 30% of diagnosed *APs are concealed pathways, meaning they can only conduct retrogradely from the ventricle to the atrium.* A concealed AP is silent when the patient is in sinus rhythm and only manifests itself during a tachycardia that involves its retrograde conduction (orthodromic AVRT).
2. *Most diagnosed APs are manifest pathways, meaning that they conduct from the atrium to the ventricle on a regular basis,* bypassing the slower AV nodal conduction. The manifest AP conducts faster than the AV node. The normal sinus impulse conducts through both the AV node and the AP. The relative contributions of the AP and the AV node depend on the conduction speed across the AP vs. AV node and how far left/laterally the AP originates. The conduction over the pathway leads to a delta wave and PR shortening, more evident when relatively more ventricle is stimulated through the AP.

This pathway conducts from the atrium to the ventricle and can conduct from the ventricle to the atrium. There are four possible AP locations: (1) left lateral, free wall (the most common, ~50% of APs); (2) right free wall (10–20%); (3) posteroseptal (20–30%); (4) anteroseptal (least common, ~5%). Approximately 5–10% of patients have multiple APs.

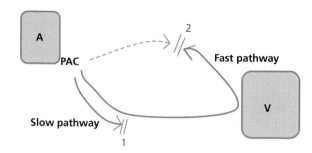

Figure 12.7 An appropriately timed PAC conducts down the slow pathway but cannot go deep enough as the distal parts of this pathway (1) or the fast pathway (2) are in the refractory period. Eventually, the reentrant cycle is broken and the next P wave is a sinus P wave. Depending on where the block occurs:

- There is no conduction to the ventricles or the atria (block 1), the tachycardia ends with the premature P wave.
- There is conduction downstream to the ventricle but no retrograde conduction to the atria (block 2); the tachycardia ends with a QRS.

A PAC may not penetrate the reentrant circuit at all if the whole slow and fast pathways are in the refractory period; in this case, the PAC does not affect the AVNRT, which continues unaffected. The tachycardia also ends with a P wave when the spontaneous vagal tone or AV nodal agents interrupt the tachycardia (they block the slow pathway).

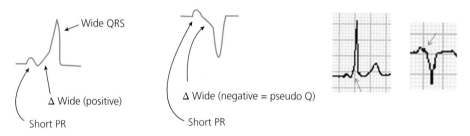

Figure 12.8 Electrocardiographic features of pre-excitation. Arrows point to the positive and negative delta waves.

This AP "pre-excites" the ventricles and the phenomenon is called pre-excitation. *WPW pattern* is used to describe the baseline pre-excitation, while *WPW syndrome* is used when arrhythmias occur as a result of the manifest AP. WPW pattern is seen in ~0.2% of the population. It has a higher prevalence in Ebstein's anomaly and HOCM.

B. Baseline ECG is not affected by a concealed accessory pathway

C. Baseline ECG is affected by a manifest accessory pathway (pre-excitation or WPW pattern) (see Figures 12.8, 12.9, 12.10)
1. The baseline ECG is characterized by:
   - Short PR interval (< 120 ms). The pre-excited PR is shorter than the AV nodal conduction but may not be short in the absolute sense.
   - Delta wave, which corresponds to the early onset of ventricular activation through the AP. Delta wave is a slur on the initial portion of QRS, *usually riding the P wave*. This slur may be negative, mimicking a Q wave.
   - Wide QRS > 120 ms, with secondary ST–T abnormalities (directed opposite to QRS). As opposed to RBBB and LBBB, QRS is slurred and delayed in its initial rather than terminal portion. QRS may be narrower than 120 ms in up to half of pre-excitation cases, whenever the ventricular excitation spreading down the AP does not occur long enough before the excitation spreading down the AV node.
2. The degree of pre-excitation depends on (Figure 12.9):
   - *The relative amount of ventricular tissue stimulated through the AP versus the AV node, which depends on the relative conduction speed through the AP versus the AV node.* PR may be normal and delta wave may be absent in patients who have a fast AV nodal conduction and a left lateral AP. In the latter case, it takes a long time for the atrial impulse to reach the atrial insertion of the AP, by which time a slick AV node would have stimulated most of the myocardium: an increasing amount of ventricular muscle is excited through the normal AV pathway and a decreasing amount is excited through the anomalous pathway, which results in a less pre-excited QRS complex.
   - *The refractory period of the AP*, which is longer than the refractory period of the AV node. An AP with a long refractory period is more likely to block at a relatively slow heart rate (e.g., 100 bpm).

Always distinguish refractory period from conduction speed. AP can conduct very fast and lead to a very wide delta wave, yet have a long refractory period and thus block at a relatively slow heart rate. In this case, AP conducts the atrial waves *fast*, but *cannot conduct too many* atrial waves back-to-back. The A-to-V interval is short, but the V-to-V interval is not.

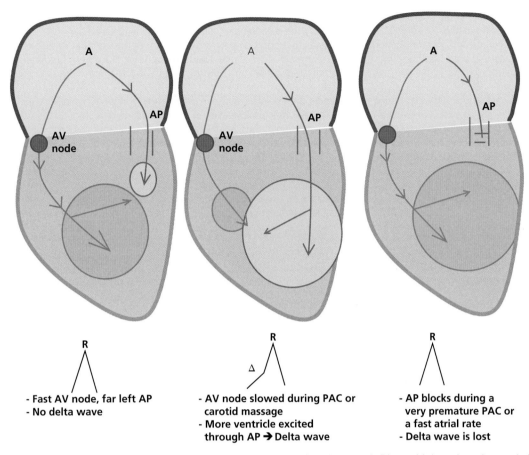

- Fast AV node, far left AP
- No delta wave

- AV node slowed during PAC or carotid massage
- More ventricle excited through AP ➔ Delta wave

- AP blocks during a very premature PAC or a fast atrial rate
- Delta wave is lost

Figure 12.9 Amount of myocardium depolarized by the accessory pathway (gray circle) vs. the AV node (blue circle) depends on the speed of AV conduction, how far laterally the AP originates, and the refractory period of the AP. A PAC is slowly conducted through the AV node, which allows more ventricular mass to be depolarized through the AP. However, a very premature PAC may get blocked across the AP which, although faster than the AV node, has a longer refractory period and is more likely to block its conduction.

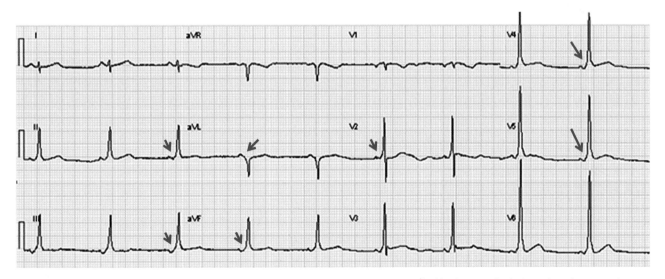

Figure 12.10 A slur is seen on the upslope of the QRS complex (e.g., leads II, III, aVF, V_2–V_6, as marked by the *arrows*). Also, note how the P wave is very close to the QRS complex (almost abuts it). The QRS seems negative in V_1 but the initial deflection, i.e., delta wave, is positive. The accessory pathway is left-sided, as delta is positive in V_1–V_2; it is left lateral, as delta wave is negative (pseudo-Q wave) in aVL.

3. When antegrade AP conduction and delta wave only manifest intermittently, or when the ECG criteria of pre-excitation are not completely fulfilled (PR slightly > 120 ms, QRS 100–120 ms), pre-excitation and delta wave may be unveiled by:

- *Slowing the conduction over the AV node*, which leads to proportionally larger amount of myocardium stimulated through the AP (adenosine, carotid sinus massage). This leads to a shorter PR interval and a wider delta wave. Since sinus bradycardia is many times associated with slowing of the AV nodal conduction (high vagal tone, drugs), delta wave is often more prominent during sinus bradycardia.
- *PAC*. Delta wave is typically wider during a PAC, and a progressive increase in prematurity of the PAC usually results in a progressive increase in the pre-excitation of the QRS complex. PAC results in prolongation of the conduction time through the AV node (increased AH interval), whereas the AP keeps a constant conduction time; thus, relatively more ventricular muscle gets excited through the AP. However, with a further increase in prematurity, the refractory period of the anomalous pathway is reached, and conduction is achieved through the AV node without any pre-excitation; this actually allows estimation of the refractory period of the AP (Figure 12.9). A similar phenomenon may be seen with progressively faster atrial pacing, wherein AV nodal conduction slows down allowing delta wave to become more prominent, until the AP refractory period is reached.
- In exertional sinus tachycardia, delta wave may diminish as a result of: (1) increased AV conduction; or (2) long AP refractory period leading to a block of conduction in AP. A consistent lack of delta wave during tachycardia suggests the latter alternative.
- As opposed to aberrancy, the pre-excitation/delta wave is more likely to manifest after a long R–R interval.

If, despite those maneuvers, the only abnormality seen on the ECG is a short PR interval, the patient simply has accelerated AV nodal conduction rather than pre-excitation, i.e., a short AV delay that is within the spectrum of normal AV delays. It was suggested previously that this may be due to an atriofascicular bypass tract, especially if the patient develops SVT (Long–Ganong–Levine syndrome). However, this is very rarely the case.

D. Localization of the accessory pathway according to the baseline ECG

In order to localize the AP, it is key to identify the leads with negative delta waves. Delta is negative in the leads surrounding the origin of the AP, as AP will be pointing away from those leads. Analyze the right-sided lead V_1, the inferior leads, and the left lateral leads I and aVL:

- Lead V_1 provides an assessment of right vs. left pathway. A negative delta in lead V_1 (QS pattern) implies that AP is pointing away from the right side, and thus the pathway is right-sided. A positive delta wave in lead V_1 (R, RS, or RSr' pattern) implies a left-sided pathway.
- The inferior leads provide an assessment of anterior vs. inferior pathway. A negative delta in the inferior leads implies an AP that points away from the inferior wall, often a posteroseptal pathway.
- The lateral leads provide an assessment of left lateral vs. septal or RV pathway. A negative delta wave in the left lateral leads I and aVL often implies a left lateral pathway (Table 12.1).

The same rules apply to localizing the origin of VT. The orientation of QRS is analyzed in those same leads. There is one additional rule in VT: negative QRS concordance in all precordial leads V_1–V_6 implies an apical origin, a pattern not seen with delta wave or pre-excited SVT.

E. Types of tachyarrhythmias: mechanisms and initiation

1. Concealed accessory pathway (see Figure 12.11)

The pathway cannot conduct antegradely, and therefore it does not conduct during sinus rhythm; no delta wave is seen. However, partial, concealed penetration of the AP occurs at baseline and puts it in a refractory period, so that retrograde impulses coming from the ventricle cannot get conducted and cannot initiate reentry. This is called concealed conduction into the AP.

The AP has a longer refractory period than the AV node; thus, when a very premature PAC occurs, it cannot penetrate the AP to any degree, allowing the AP to rest. When the electrical activation reaches the ventricle, it can conduct retrogradely through the AP for two reasons: (1) the AP is capable of conducting retrogradely; (2) the AP has had time to rest and recover from the refractory period, since the PAC did not penetrate it at all. This initiates a reentry called **orthodromic AVRT**. As opposed to AVNRT, in orthodromic AVRT the atria and the ventricles are depolarized sequentially rather than simultaneously and distinct P waves are almost always seen, with a short RP interval < 1/2 RR, but not too short (> 90 ms). The ventricular rate is ~150–250 bpm.

Also, a PVC can initiate retrograde AP conduction and reentry because it occurs after the sinus-originating ventricular stimulation, at a time when the AP has recovered from the refractory period.

2. Manifest accessory pathway (see Figure 12.12)

The AP can conduct both antegradely and retrogradely.

Table 12.1 Electrocardiographic localization of the AP.

	V_1		II/III/aVF	I, aVL
Left lateral	(+)		(+)	(–)
Right free wall	(–)		(±) (e.g., + in II, – in III)	(+)
Posteroseptal (near the coronary sinus)	(–) with sharp transition to (+) in V_2 if right posteroseptal	(+) if left posteroseptal	(–)	(+)
Anteroseptal (right)	(–), isoelectric, or biphasic		(+)	(+)

Those rules may apply to localizing the origin of PVC or VT based on the voltage of QRS in those leads. Lead I is more important than aVL in AP localization. Since the AP is basal, i.e., not close to the apex in any form, the QRS cannot be negative in leads V_4–V_6.

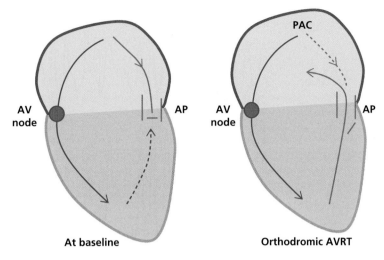

Figure 12.11 Concealed accessory pathway (AP).

The pathway cannot fully conduct antegradely; thus, it does not conduct during sinus rhythm and no delta wave is seen. Yet, partial penetration of the AP occurs at baseline and puts it in a refractory period, so that retrograde impulses coming from the ventricle get blocked and cannot initiate reentry. This is called concealed conduction into the AP. The AP has a longer refractory period than the AV node; thus, when a very early PAC occurs (*right*), it cannot penetrate the AP to any degree, allowing the AP to rest. When the electrical activation reaches the ventricle, it can conduct retrogradely through the AP, which has had time to rest and recover from the refractory period, since the PAC did not penetrate it at all. This initiates reentry (orthodromic AVRT).

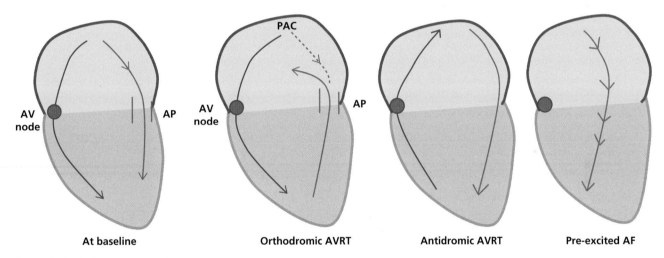

Figure 12.12 Manifest accessory pathway.

The AP can conduct both antegradely and retrogradely. The normal sinus impulse conducts through both the AV node and the AP. The conduction over AP leads to delta wave and PR shortening, more evident when relatively more ventricle is stimulated through the AP. The AP conducts faster than the AV node but has a longer refractory period than the AV node. Thus, when a very premature PAC occurs, the PAC conducts solely through the AV node without any delta wave and initiates reentry (orthodromic AVRT). *The larger the difference in refractory period between the AV node and the AP, the more likely it is for a PAC to get blocked in the AP and initiate AVRT.* Occasionally, the PAC conducts down the AP and leads to antidromic AVRT. AF or atrial flutter may conduct rapidly and antegradely over the accessory pathway.

a. The AP is a myocardial structure that **conducts faster than the AV node; however, it has a longer refractory period than the AV node**. When a very early PAC occurs, **orthodromic AVRT** may occur (similar mechanism to the concealed AP). PVC can also propagate up the AP and initiate reentry.

b. It is rare for the PAC to solely conduct down the AP and not the AV node, because the AP usually has a longer refractory period than the AV node. However, the refractory period of the AP is occasionally very short, shorter than the AV node's refractory period; in this case, the impulse of a PAC can conduct down through the AP then up through the AV node (**antidromic AVRT**). Since the ventricle is stimulated through a ventricular focus rather than the His bundle, the tachycardia is a wide complex tachycardia that has VT morphology. As opposed to VT, the pre-excited QRS complex cannot be negative in leads V_4–V_6, as the pre-excitation is usually basal rather than apical

c. Pre-excited AF or atrial flutter: in this case, AF or atrial flutter conducts very quickly from A to V over the accessory pathway (Figure 12.13). This leads to very fast (> 200 bpm), very wide, bizarre-looking QRS complexes, without a typical bundle branch block morphology.

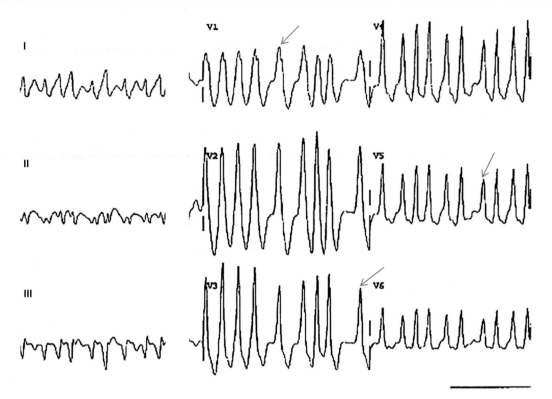

Figure 12.13 Irregular tachycardia with wide, polymorphic, bizarre-looking QRS, with VT rather than SVT features (positive QRS concordance in V1–V6, QRS morphology not consistent with RBBB or LBBB). This is a pre-excited AF in a patient with WPW. Note that, as opposed to aberrancy, QRS becomes wider after a longer R–R interval (*arrows*). AP is likely left posteroseptal (delta wave is negative in the inferior leads).

By using the SVT/VT differentiation algorithm, pre-excited SVT typically has morphological VT features, yet the irregularity and the variable QRS morphology (variable pre-excitation) point to a pre-excited AF. This is the most dangerous tachycardia associated with the accessory pathway. Sudden death is, fortunately, rare, seen in < 1% of patients with WPW pattern over the course of 10 years.

Patients with WPW are prone to develop AF, possibly because of reentry around the atrial insertion of the AP (prevalence of AF in young patients with WPW ~15–30%). Also, any AVRT can trigger AF and become poorly tolerated.

- "Irregular VT" is often AF with pre-excitation.
- As opposed to AF with Ashman aberrancy, AF with pre-excitation may be characterized by a QRS that gets wider after a long R–R interval. The long R–R interval allows the AP to recover from its refractory period.

Note that the AP behaves like atrial or ventricular myocardium during stimulation, not like the AV node; thus, the faster the tract is stimulated, the faster it conducts. The lack of AV interval prolongation with incremental pacing is a hint to the presence of AP. However, depending on its refractory period, the AP may block at fast rates if it is a benign AP; it blocks in a Mobitz II fashion, rather than a Wenckebach fashion. In the particular case of AVRT, the occurrence of block ends the reentry.

Concealed pathway tachycardias are all orthodromic AVRT. Of tachycardias occurring with a manifest pathway (WPW syndrome), 75% are orthodromic AVRTs, 5% are antidromic AVRTs, and ~20% are pre-excited AF or atrial flutter (5% atrial flutter).

F. More electrophysiological mechanisms

A PAC or a PVC may occur at a particular time when it can partially penetrate the reentrant AVRT circuit but encounters a refractory period deep in the circuit and, therefore gets blocked inside it; this terminates AVRT.

On the other hand, a PAC, PVC, or extrastimulus that does not block the arrhythmia resets the tachycardia. The atrium and the ventricle being parts of the reentrant circuit, if a premature complex depolarizes the atrium or the ventricle, the reentrant circuit cannot keep looping independently. It either gets blocked by the premature complex, or gets entrained by it (Figure 12.14). Similarly, any block of the atrial or ventricular impulse leads to cessation of the arrhythmia, as the reentry cannot continue without both atrial and ventricular excitations; 2:1 conduction cannot be seen with AVRT (conversely, 2:1 conduction may occasionally be seen with AVNRT if a block occurs in the AV node beyond the small reentrant circuit).

In orthodromic AVRT, if a functional BBB occurs on the same side as the accessory pathway, the reentrant circuit lengthens, and thus the cycle length of the tachycardia increases (Figures 12.15, 12.16). In contrast, the occurrence of BBB does not affect the AVNRT rate, and in fact BBB is usually seen with faster rates.

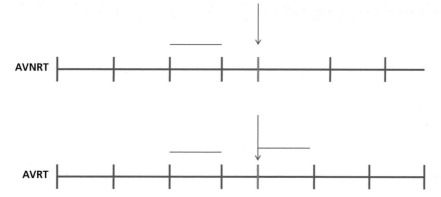

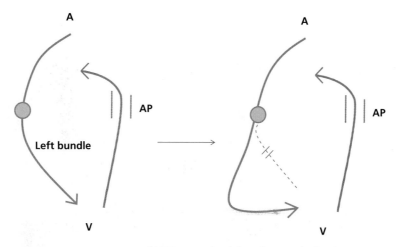

Figure 12.14 In AVNRT, the occurrence of a PAC or PVC (*gray bar*) either blocks the tachycardia, or, as in this case, gets conducted to the atria or ventricles but does not change the reentry, which keeps looping at its own rate. The interval between the QRS preceding the premature beat and that following it is double the R–R interval of the tachycardia.

In AVRT, PAC or PVC either blocks the tachycardia, or, as in this case, gets conducted through the tachycardia and resets its cycle. The R–R interval that follows the premature beat is equal to the R–R interval of the tachycardia.

If LBBB occurs in a left pathway orthodromic AVRT, the length of the macroreentry↑→ tachycardia becomes slower

Figure 12.15 Bundle branch block during orthodromic AVRT.

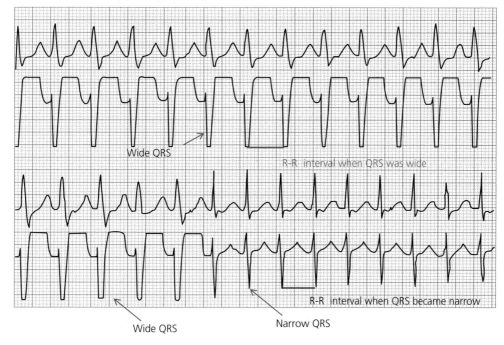

Figure 12.16 When the wide complex tachycardia becomes narrow, the R–R interval becomes shorter (the rate becomes faster). This implies orthodromic AVRT with transient block of the bundle branch ipsilateral to the AP (the bundle branch involved in the reentry).

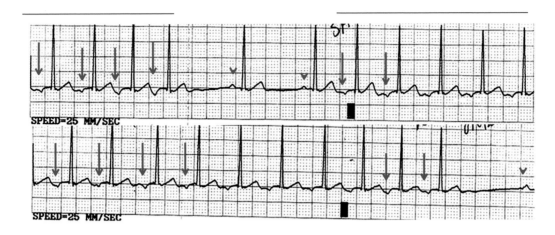

Figure 12.17 A 22-year-old woman with no prior cardiac history presents with runs of SVT interspersed with sinus beats. The SVT rate is ~105 bpm. Two types of P waves are seen: sinus P waves (*arrowheads*) and P waves related to SVT (*arrows*). RP interval is long (long RP tachycardia). The differential diagnosis of this SVT includes:

- Atrial tachycardia, with the focus being low in the RA or LA, near the AV node.
- Incessant AVRT (PJRT) with retrograde P waves, negative in lead II.

The recurrent runs interspersed with sinus beats indicate that the tachycardia is easy to initiate, which is consistent with PJRT. Each run starts with a PAC and seems to end with a QRS rather than the typical P wave of the run: this may be consistent with atrial tachycardia or PJRT (intermittent block of the slow retrograde AP).

> A tachycardia that becomes slower when it becomes wider is orthodromic AVRT.

The retrograde conduction across the AP may be slow and decremental, which increases the cycle length of the tachycardia. AVRT ends up being slow (100–150 bpm) with a long RP interval. The cycle of the tachycardia is so long that, as the stimulation is spreading retrogradely through the AP, the AV node recovers from its refractory period. As opposed to the fast AVRT, at any particular point in time, most of the reentrant circuit is not in a refractory period. Thus, a PAC is unlikely to only partially penetrate the circuit and block the tachycardia; it is likely to get conducted through the reentry and reset the tachycardia. This is the large "excitable gap" concept seen with very slow reentry, which explains why this atypical AVRT is unlikely to break spontaneously and tends to be incessant and persistent for weeks, leading to a tachycardia-mediated cardiomyopathy. The tachycardia is called ***permanent junctional reciprocating tachycardia (PJRT)***. Even when this arrhythmia breaks, it is easy to reinitiate it. Owing to the slow retrograde conduction, any PAC or PVC easily conducts retrogradely all the way up the AP, as the AP is given time to recover from its refractory period (Figure 12.11). Similarly to other AVRTs, PJRT can be seen at any age, including in young patients without heart disease (Figure 12.17). In PJRT, the AP is usually a concealed posteroseptal pathway that only conducts retrogradely.

G. Treatment

1. Acute treatment

- Orthodromic AVRT, whether related to a concealed AP or WPW, is benign. Acute treatment is similar to AVNRT.
- Antidromic AVRT and pre-excited AF/atrial flutter are wide QRS-complex tachycardias with QRS features of VT. They should be treated like VT. In a hemodynamically stable patient, intravenous class I or class III drugs (procainamide or ibutilide) may be used as they increase the AP's antegrade refractory period. In contrast to the ESC guidelines, intravenous amiodarone is contraindicated in the ACC guidelines, as acute amiodarone has a β-blocker effect and may block the AV node more than the AP (conversely, chronic amiodarone may be used, as it increases the AP's refractory period).

Avoid AV nodal blocking agents in wide complex tachycardia, particularly calcium channel blockers and digoxin, because these drugs reduce the antegrade refractory period of the accessory pathway, allowing more back-to-back conduction of atrial waves over this pathway. Also, while adenosine does not reduce the refractory period of the accessory pathway, it can trigger transient AF in up to 12% of patients, which will decompensate a patient with WPW.

2. Chronic preventive treatment

a. Orthodromic AVRT with concealed AP, i.e., no WPW pattern on the resting ECG: prevention and treatment are similar to AVNRT:
   - Chronic or "pill-in-the pocket" CCB or β-blocker (50% preventive efficacy)
   or
   - Ablation of the accessory pathway, which is preferred when AVRT is poorly tolerated
b. Any tachyarrhythmia, including orthodromic AVRT, with WPW pattern on the resting ECG:
   - Ablation of the accessory pathway (class I recommendation).
   - AV nodal blocking agents reduce the occurrence of orthodromic AVRT but have drawbacks: they may reduce the AP refractory period. Should AF occur, AP will conduct more readily. Digoxin should be totally avoided in WPW syndrome, even if the original manifestation was orthodromic AVRT (ACC class III recommendation); β-blockers or CCBs may be used in selective cases, especially in combination with antiarrhythmic drugs or if it is established that AP has a long antegrade refractory period (class IIb recommendation).

- Antiarrhythmic drugs class I (flecainide or propafenone), amiodarone, and sotalol increase the antegrade and retrograde refractory periods across the accessory pathway. However, by increasing the antegrade refractory period, they increase the difference in refractory period between the AV node and AP, making it easier for a PAC to initiate orthodromic AVRT (Figure 12.12). Combining a β-blocker with the antiarrhythmic drug may circumvent this phenomenon. This is also less likely to occur with antiarrhythmic agents that have an AV nodal blocking effect (amiodarone or sotalol). Antiarrhythmic drugs (class Ic, amiodarone, sotalol) are given a class IIa recommendation for WPW syndrome in a patient who is not a candidate for, or prefers not to undergo, catheter ablation. Class Ic drugs are particularly effective. Conversely, antiarrhythmic drugs are ineffective in PJRT, which is an orthodromic AVRT, and may aggravate it.

3. Asymptomatic pre-excitation/WPW diagnosed on a resting ECG

The risk of sudden death is low (0.05%–0.1% per year, < 1% per 10 years), but may be higher, up to 0.5% per year in some subgroups. Sudden death is related to the antegrade rapid conduction of AF, and depends on how short the antegrade refractory period of the AP is. About 30% of adults lose the capacity for antegrade conduction over 5 years of follow-up, and their risk of sudden death becomes negligible.

The risk of sudden death *does not depend on how fast* the AP conducts the atrial waves, as by definition the AP has a fast conduction; what is more important is *how many* back-to-back atrial waves the AP can conduct, which depends on the AP refractory period. The best predictor of sudden death is the assessment of the shortest pre-excited R–R interval during AF. An interval of ≤ 250 ms, i.e. ≤ 1.25 large box on standard ECG, implies an increased risk of cardiac arrest.

- Risk stratification on the baseline ECG:
  - Intermittent pre-excitation, particularly when intermittent on the same ECG, implies that the antegrade refractory period of the AP is long (Figure 12.20). Intermittent pre-excitation at disparate points in time may be related to intermittent increase in AV conduction in a patient with a left lateral pathway, rather than a short AP refractory period.
  - The presence of multiple APs, i.e., multiple delta morphologies on serial ECGs, implies a higher risk.
- Every asymptomatic patient should undergo either **an invasive or a non-invasive assessment of the refractory period of the AP** (especially if young, < 30–40 years old) (class I indication for exercise testing, class IIa for EP testing, ACC guidelines 2015).
  - During exercise testing, an accessory pathway with a long refractory period will not be able to antegradely conduct. Thus, the loss of pre-excitation during exercise implies a long AP refractory period. However, delta wave may be lost because of increased AV nodal conduction during exercise rather than a block in the AP, and therefore only a *complete* and *abrupt* loss of pre-excitation during exercise testing confirms a long AP refractory period.
  - EP testing consists of inducing AF and measuring the shortest pre-excited R–R interval. If this interval is ≤ 250 ms (rate ≥ 240 bpm), it is reasonable to ablate the asymptomatic pathway (class IIa). Instead of inducing AF, rapid atrial pacing may be used as a surrogate. The mortality risk associated with ablation is low (< 0.05%) and lower than the yearly risk of sudden cardiac death, which may justify AP ablation in these asymptomatic patients.

As opposed to the intermittent loss of delta wave on a resting ECG, the intermittent loss of delta wave during exercise is not definitely reassuring and does not necessarily imply a long refractory period (positive predictive value of only 40%); an invasive assessment is indicated at this point.

AF is the most common supraventricular tachyarrhythmia, followed by atrial flutter, then paroxysmal supraventricular tachycardias. Of the paroxysmal supraventricular tachycardias:

- 60% are AVNRT.
- 30% are AVRT (AVNRT and AVRT are also called paroxysmal junctional tachycardias).
- 10% are atrial tachycardia or sinus node reentrant tachycardia (SNRT). SNRT is secondary to a reentrant circuit inside the sinus node and is usually slower than AVNRT and AVRT (rate 100–200, often 130–140 bpm). SNRT looks identical to sinus tachycardia, except for having a very steady rate and an abrupt onset and termination, unrelated to any physiological trigger; it often resolves with carotid message or adenosine. As compared to AVNRT/AVRT, there is a slightly higher incidence of underlying heart disease.

H. Additional WPW examples (Figures 12.18–12.21)

IV. Junctional escape rhythm and accelerated junctional rhythm (or non-paroxysmal junctional tachycardia)

A. Junctional escape beats or rhythm

The AV junction (= AV node and His bundle) has the property of "automaticity" which allows it to function as a latent pacemaker. This latent pacemaker is normally suppressed by the more rapid sinus activity but can become manifest if: (a) the sinus node is slow or suppressed, in which case the AV junction assumes the pacemaker function by default (junctional escape); (b) the AV junction's automaticity increases, allowing it to compete with the sinus node (accelerated junctional rhythm). The junctional escape has a rate of 30–60 bpm, and may be associated with retrograde P waves or may compete with a slow sinus rhythm (isorhythmic AV dissociation).

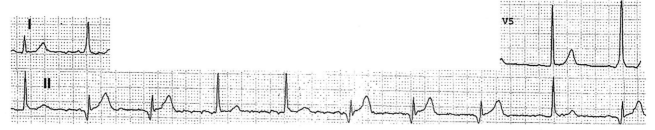

Figure 12.18 Two types of QRS complex are seen. This intermittent widening of the QRS may represent intermittent bundle branch block (BBB) or intermittent pre-excitation. Intermittent BBB usually occurs with an increase in rate, but that is not the case here. Moreover, the morphology of the wide QRS favors pre-excitation. A positive delta wave with a short PR interval is seen on the wide complexes in leads I and V_5, while a negative delta wave (pseudo-Q wave) is seen in the inferior lead. This intermittent conduction across the accessory pathway implies a long refractory period and an inability to consistently conduct even at a normal rate (good prognosis). The AP is likely posteroseptal.

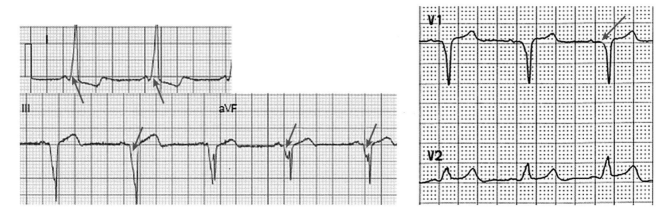

Figure 12.19 Another WPW pattern on a baseline ECG. Note the short PR, with P almost attached to R. There is a positive delta slur on the upslope of R wave in lead I, and a negative delta slur manifested as Q wave in leads III and aVF (delta marked by arrows). Delta wave is negative in the inferior leads, implying that the AP is posteroseptal, with the electrical depolarization going away from the inferior wall. The delta wave is positive in lead I, meaning that the impulse propagates towards the left lateral wall. Delta wave is negative in lead V_1, implying that the AP is right-sided, and thus the AP is right posteroseptal. The sharp delta transition in lead V_2 is consistent with a posteroseptal pathway.

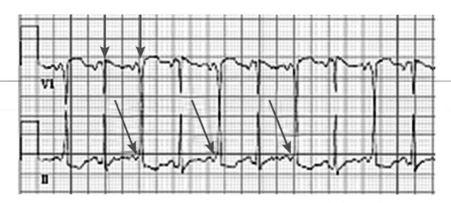

Figure 12.20 Alternation of a narrow and an equidistant wide QRS (*vertical arrows*). Ventricular bigeminy is unlikely, since QRSs are equidistant. PR interval shortens and a delta wave is seen on the wider beats (*oblique arrows*). This is intermittent pre-excitation. Every other QRS conducts antegradely over an accessory pathway with a delta wave and a short PR interval (WPW). The next beat proceeds down the AV node rather than the accessory pathway, the accessory pathway being in a refractory period. This is 2:1 conduction over the accessory pathway at a high sinus rate. This alternation in pre-excitation on the same ECG is likely secondary to a long AP refractory period, which blocks every other beat. Intermittent pre-excitation on separate ECGs is less reassuring, as it may be due to increased AV nodal conduction, rather than AP block. Intermittent pre-excitation during exercise is also less reassuring. The pathway is likely a left lateral pathway (QRS is negative but delta is positive in V_1).

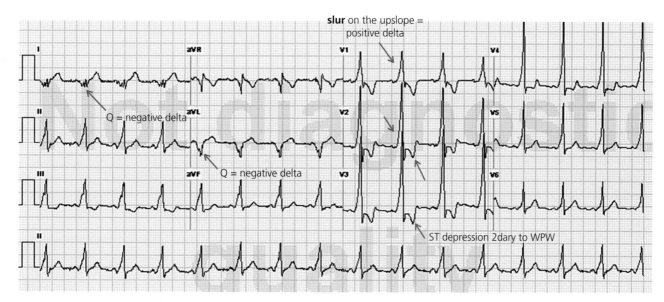

Figure 12.21 At first glance, this ECG shows a wide and tall R wave in V$_1$, Q wave in leads I and aVL, and ST-segment depression localized to leads V$_1$–V$_3$. This may suggest posterior and lateral Q-wave MI, and the ST depression suggests this MI is acute. On further ECG analysis:
1. PR is short, ~100 ms.
2. QRS is wide with delta wave: the P wave is "riding" the upslope of the R wave in leads V$_1$–V$_6$ and the downslope of Q in leads I and aVL. The upslope of QRS is slurred.
3. ST–T depression in V$_1$–V$_3$ is opposite in direction to the large QRS and likely secondary to the wide QRS.

The presence of the first two features defines a pre-excitation pattern. Pre-excitation may masquerade as MI: the Q waves are actually negative delta waves, and ST depressions or elevations are secondary to the wide QRS.

Localization of the pathway: look at leads V$_1$, I–aVL, and the inferior leads. Delta wave is negative in leads I and aVL, which is consistent with a left lateral pathway. The positive delta in V$_1$ and in the inferior leads is consistent with this. Left lateral pathway frequently leads to this positive QRS morphology in all precordial leads V$_1$–V$_6$.

B. Accelerated junctional rhythm

Accelerated junctional rhythm is an automatic rhythm arising from the AV node or the His bundle at a rate of 60–130 bpm, in contrast to the junctional escape rhythm that fires at a rate of 30–60 bpm. The rhythm is regular but may have a warm-up phase like any automatic rhythm.

Being relatively slow, the junctional rhythm competes with the sinus rhythm. Some sinus P waves fall distantly from the junctional QRS complexes and get conducted, whereas other P waves fall too close to the junctional QRS complexes and do not get conducted. There is dissociation between the sinus P waves and the junctional rhythm. This is isorhythmic (= competitive) AV dissociation.

On the other hand, the junctional rhythm may lead to retrograde P waves that inhibit the initiation and propagation of sinus P waves. These retrograde P waves may precede or follow QRS. When they precede QRS, the PR interval is usually <0.12 seconds.

The QRS is narrow but may be wide if a bundle branch block pre-existed. If it is wide, the rhythm simulates accelerated idioventricular rhythm (AIVR). The rhythm is considered junctional rather than ventricular if the wide QRS morphology is similar to the sinus-originating complexes or the baseline ECG. Otherwise, the rhythm is considered ventricular; the interposition of sinus-originating complexes that are narrow rules out a baseline bundle branch block and implies that the wide rhythm is ventricular.

This rhythm is generally due to underlying heart disease: acute MI (most commonly inferior MI, where it is a benign finding), digoxin toxicity, myocarditis, and post cardiac surgery. Occasionally, it occurs without underlying heart disease or represents a form of accelerated junctional escape in patients with sinus node disease or AV block.

QUESTIONS AND ANSWERS

Question 1. The accessory pathway:
A. Conducts faster than the AV node
B. Has a shorter refractory period than the AV node
C. Antegrade conduction of atrial fibrillation depends on how fast the accessory pathway conduction is
D. Antegrade conduction of atrial fibrillation depends on how short the refractory period of the accessory pathway is

Question 2. Delta wave is exaggerated:
A. During a premature atrial complex
B. After a premature atrial complex
C. During carotid massage
D. During exertional sinus tachycardia

Question 3. A negative delta wave in the left lateral leads often implies:
A. Left lateral accessory pathway
B. Right free wall accessory pathway

Question 4. Concerning the arrhythmias that may occur with accessory pathways:
A. Orthodromic AVRT can occur with both concealed and manifest APs
B. Antidromic AVRT can only occur with manifest AP
C. Only a PAC can initiate AVRT

Question 5. Features that differentiate a pre-excited tachyarrhythmia from ventricular tachycardia:
A. Both tachyarrhythmias have a QRS morphology that is not consistent with bundle branch block aberrancy
B. As opposed to ventricular tachycardia, a pre-excited atrial fibrillation is irregular and polymorphic
C. The pre-excited QRS complex cannot be negative throughout all of the precordial leads (negative concordance)

Question 6. A 35-year-old man presents with orthodromic AVRT. After the administration of adenosine, he converts to sinus rhythm with pre-excitation (Figure 12.19). Catheter ablation is considered, but he prefers medical therapy. What is the best regimen?
A. Metoprolol
B. Diltiazem
C. Flecainide or propafenone
D. Amiodarone, sotalol, or dofetilide

Question 7. A 30-year-old asymptomatic patient is found to have pre-excitation on an ECG performed before orthopedic surgery. What is the next step?
A. Ablation of the AP
B. Risk stratification using exercise ECG or looking for intermittent loss of pre-excitation on resting ECG
C. Risk stratification using EP study, measuring the shortest pre-excited R–R interval
D. No further workup, as he is asymptomatic
E. B or C

Question 8. In the asymptomatic patient with pre-excitation, which of the following implies a low-risk AP?
A. Intermittent loss of delta waves on ambulatory ECGs
B. Intermittent loss of delta waves on exercise ECG
C. Complete and abrupt loss of delta wave on exercise ECG
D. A and C

Question 9. Typical AVNRT is characterized by:
A. Slow pathway-then-fast pathway conduction (slow–fast), with a VA interval < 70 ms on intracardiac recording and RP interval < 90 ms on the surface ECG
B. Fast–slow conduction with RP interval < 70 ms on ECG

Answer 1. A, D.

Answer 2. A, C.

Answer 3. A.

Answer 4. A, B.

Answer 5. A, B, C.

Answer 6. C. Class Ic and III drugs increase the AP's antegrade and retrograde refractory period. Class Ic are likely more effective than class III, with more data supporting their use. Metoprolol and diltiazem are best avoided, in case the patient goes into pre-excited AF (yet, ACC guidelines allow their use in WPW patients whose only arrhythmia is orthodromic AVRT [grade IIb recommendation]).

Answer 7. E (B is given a class I recommendation, C is given a class IIa recommendation in asymptomatic pre-excitation).

Answer 8. D. If delta wave does not completely disappear during exercise testing, invasive assessment of the AP's refractory period is warranted.

Answer 9. A. Typical AVNRT is slow–fast AVNRT ("SF"). Fast–slow AVNRT is atypical with a long RP interval and a generally slower rate (even the fast pathway is a bit slow).

Further reading

Blomström-Lundqvist C, Scheinman MM, Aliot EM, et al. ACC/AHA/ESC 2003 guidelines for the management of patients with supraventricular arrhythmias. J Am Coll Cardiol 2003; 42: 1493–531.
Page RL, Joglar JA, Caldwell MA, et al. 2015 ACC/AHA/HRS guideline for the management of adult patients with supraventricular tachycardia. J Am Coll Cardiol 2016; 67: e27–115.

IST

Cappato R, Castelvecchio S, Ricci C, et al. Clinical efficacy of ivabradine in patients with inappropriate sinus tachycardia. J Am Coll Cardiol 2012; 60: 1323–9.

AVNRT and AVRT pictures and mechanisms

Fogoros N. The electrophysiology study in the evaluation of supraventricular tachyarrhythmias. In: Fogoros N. Electrophysiologic Testing, 4th edn. Oxford: Blackwell, 2006, pp. 103–57.

Effect of pacing on AVNRT vs. AVRT

Michaud GF, Tada H, Chough S, et al. Differentiation of atypical atrioventricular node re-entrant tachycardia from orthodromic reciprocating tachycardia using a septal accessory pathway by the response to ventricular pacing. J Am Coll Cardiol 2001; 38: 1163–7.

Prognosis of WPW

Munger TM, Packer DL, Hammill SC, et al. A population study of the natural history of Wolff–Parkinson–White syndrome in Olmsted County, Minnesota, 1953–1989. Circulation 1993; 87: 866–73.

Assessment of asymptomatic WPW

Cohen MI, Triedman JK, Cannon BC, et al. PACES/HRS expert consensus statement on the management of the asymptomatic young patient with a Wolff–Parkinson–White (WPW, ventricular preexcitation) electrocardiographic pattern. Heart Rhythm 2012; 9: 1006–24.

13 Bradyarrhythmias

I. AV block

A. Types of AV block

1. First-degree AV block = PR interval >200 ms (may be as long as 1000 ms).
2. Second-degree AV block. Types (Figures 13.1–13.5):
   i. Mobitz type I (Wenckebach type): PR interval progressively prolongs until QRS drops, i.e., until a regularly occurring P wave is not followed by a QRS. This is in contrast to SA block, where both P and QRS drop. To make the diagnosis, compare the PR that follows the blocked P wave (the shortest PR) with the PR that immediately precedes the blocked P wave (the longest PR).
   ii. Mobitz type II: QRS suddenly drops without a preceding PR change. *The baseline QRS is usually wide*. It may present as intermittently non-conducted P waves or as one non-conducted P wave that is not preceded by progressive PR prolongation and not followed by PR shortening. It is more ominous than Mobitz type I and is almost always a distal infranodal AV block. It progresses to a complete infranodal AV block commonly and suddenly.
   iii. 2:1 AV block (alternative drop of one QRS) could be equivalent to Mobitz I or Mobitz II AV block. If QRS is wide, the block is likely a Mobitz II equivalent. If QRS is narrow, the block is likely a Mobitz I equivalent. Also, look for periods of 3:2 conduction on a rhythm strip, as this may elucidate the Mobitz type of block.

Notes

3:2 AV block means that two consecutive P waves conduct while the third P wave gets blocked (i.e., three P waves with two QRS complexes). 4:3 block means three consecutive P waves conduct while the fourth P wave gets blocked. These blocks could be Mobitz I or II depending on the occurrence of progressive PR prolongation.

3:1 block means only one of three consecutive P waves is conducted (three P waves with one QRS). This is also called *high-grade AV block* or advanced second-degree AV block and has the same implication as complete AV block. Unlike Mobitz II AV block, however, it can be a less ominous nodal or vagal AV block.

Second-degree AV block is characterized by group beating, in which a group of P–QRS complexes is followed by a pause, then the cycle repeats (Figures 13.2–13.5). The cycle length may be variable (2:1 alternating with 3:2, 4:3, 8:7, etc.). Think of second-degree AV block whenever there is a repetition of groups of beats.

In patients with a long Wenckebach cycle (e.g., 8:7), PR only slightly prolongs between the last beats, making PR prolongation unnoticeable. **PR prolongation is most easily addressed by comparing the PR immediately following the pause (the shortest) to the one immediately preceding it (the longest)**. Also, R–R progressively shortens before the pause, and the R–R interval containing the blocked P wave is shorter than the sum of the shortest two R–R intervals (Figure 13.2).

Frequently, however, in case of a long Wenckebach period (e.g., 7:6), the R–R cycles preceding the block lengthen after the initial shortening.

3. Third-degree or complete AV block (Figures 13.6, 13.7). No P wave is conducted.

   A junctional or ventricular escape rhythm takes over. The ventricular rate is regular and unrelated to P waves (AV dissociation). **The PR distance is variable yet the R–R interval is regular**, providing evidence that none of these P waves is conducted. The number of P waves is larger than the number of QRS complexes.

   High-grade or advanced second-degree AV block is a block in which the AV conduction ratio is 3:1 or worse. In one form, P waves and the escape QRS complexes are dissociated but P wave occasionally conducts: R–R intervals are mostly regular, with occasional R–R intervals that are shorter as they relate to the few conducted P waves.

   In patients with AF, a long AF pause, >3 seconds, generally implies high-grade AV block.

Practical Cardiovascular Medicine, First Edition. Elias B. Hanna.

© 2017 John Wiley & Sons Ltd. Published 2017 by John Wiley & Sons Ltd.

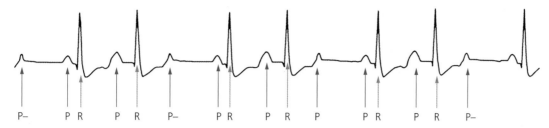

Figure 13.1 Wenckebach 3:2 AV block. P–P intervals are typically regular. P–, non-conducted P wave.

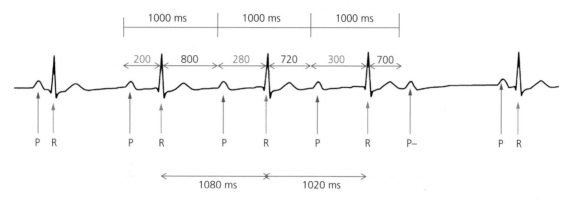

Figure 13.2 Wenckebach 5:4 AV block. P–P intervals are regular. **PR progressively lengthens, whereas R–R progressively shortens.** This is due to the fact that the absolute PR interval increases less with each cycle, not compensating for the larger reduction of the preceding RP interval, P–P interval being stable (e.g., PR 200 → 280 → 300).

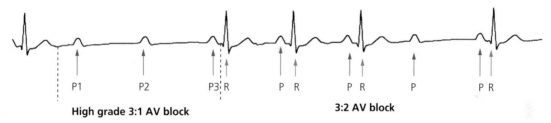

Figure 13.3 High-grade AV block.

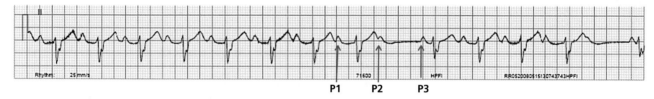

Figure 13.4 Wenckebach AV block. Two groups of beats are seen, which raises the suspicion of a second-degree AV block. P2 is not conducted: this could be AV block or a block of a very premature PAC. Since P2 is not premature, the diagnosis is AV block. The clue to Wenckebach is the progressive PR prolongation, especially manifest when comparing P3R to P1R (P3R <P1R) and the progressive R–R shortening before the block.

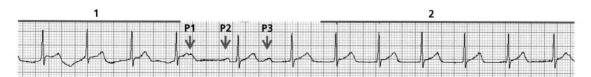

Figure 13.5 ECG of a patient presenting with palpitations. Looking at parts 1 and 2 of this ECG, no P wave is seen and one might think the patient has a junctional rhythm. **Sinus rhythm with a very long PR interval should be considered in any case of presumed junctional rhythm.** The pause between 1 and 2 unveils the diagnosis. P waves are seen: P1 is a blocked P wave, P2 and P3 are conducted with a progressively longer PR interval. Thus, the patient has a Mobitz type 1 AV block with a very long cycle. Outside P2 and P3, PR interval is very long with P waves falling onto T waves (fusion of P and T). Palpitations are due to simultaneous atrial and ventricular contractions.

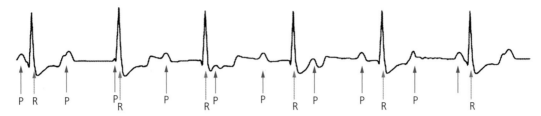

Figure 13.6 Third-degree AV block with regular P rate and regular QRS rate, unrelated to each other. Many P waves fall onto the QRS–T complexes and appear as notches over QRS or T. **PR interval is variable but R–R interval is regular, which implies AV dissociation and, in this case, complete AV block.**

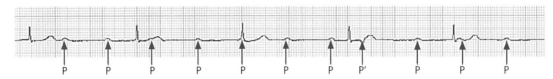

Figure 13.7 Regular, slow QRS rate of ~33 bpm. P rate is mainly regular at ~75 bpm. There is AV dissociation, with no evidence of any P-wave conduction (as also evidenced by the regular QRS escape rhythm). This is complete AV block. P′ could be a PAC or a retrogradely conducted P wave (patients with abnormal AV conduction may have a preserved VA retrograde conduction).

The escape is ventricular with a wide QRS complex if the block is infranodal (rate 20–40 bpm). The escape is junctional with a narrow QRS complex if the block is at the nodal level (rate 40–60 bpm); the junctional escape may be wide if a bundle branch block is present on the baseline ECG. Patients with complete AV block at the infranodal level may have preserved VA conduction, and retrograde P waves may be seen.

Look carefully for 2:1 AV block in any case of sinus bradycardia. 2:1 AV block may mimic sinus bradycardia when the blocked P waves fall on the preceding T waves and go unnoticed or get mistaken for U waves. Conversely, in patients with sinus bradycardia, U waves may be misinterpreted as blocked P waves, causing a false diagnosis of AV block. Blocked P waves are distinguished from U waves by the fact that they march out almost equidistantly with the P waves that precede the QRS complexes, whereas U waves do not. Also, P waves are often more peaked than U waves (Figure 13.8).

AV dissociation is present in all cases of AV block, but AV dissociation does not imply AV block. A competing accelerated junctional or ventricular rhythm that is equal in rate to the sinus rhythm, or faster than it, may lead to AV dissociation. The latter is a competing form of AV dissociation, rather than an AV block form of AV dissociation. One form of competing AV dissociation is *isorhythmic AV dissociation*, in which the junctional or ventricular rhythm almost has the same rate as the sinus rhythm, allowing intermittent conduction of sinus P waves that are falling far enough from the QRS complexes (e.g., AIVR, accelerated junctional rhythm). One beat may be a sinus beat preceded by a P wave, the other may be a junctional beat dissociated from P wave and showing up at any deceleration of the sinus rate. **AV block is implied when a P wave falls far enough from the QRS complex but does not get conducted** (Figure 13.9).

B. Causes of a pause on the rhythm strip
Outside the pause that follows an obvious PAC or PVC, a pause on a rhythm strip may be secondary to:

1. Sinus pause: no P wave is seen within the pause.
2. Second-degree AV block (Mobitz I or Mobitz II): a blocked P wave is seen within the pause. The blocked P wave marches out with the regularly occurring sinus P wave. Occasionally, however, if sinus arrhythmia is present, the blocked P wave of the AV block may not perfectly march out with the other P waves. A particular form of sinus arrhythmia seen with AV block (especially 2:1 AV block) is *ventriculophasic sinus arrhythmia*, in which the P–P interval containing a QRS is shorter than the P–P interval not containing a QRS (the QRS complex leads to a stroke volume which leads to reflex slowing of the P–P interval).
3. Blocked PAC (the most benign pause): the blocked P wave is a very premature P wave that falls in the AV nodal refractory period and does not get conducted. As opposed to AV block, the blocked P wave does not march out with the sinus P waves and often has a different morphology.
4. Concealed premature junctional complex (less common): a premature junctional complex (His complex) is rare, much less common than a PAC or a PVC. A blocked premature junctional complex prevents the conduction of the next sinus impulse through the His (still in refractory period), creating the impression of a Mobitz II AV block. The presence of conducted premature junctional complexes elsewhere on the rhythm monitor is a hint to this phenomenon.

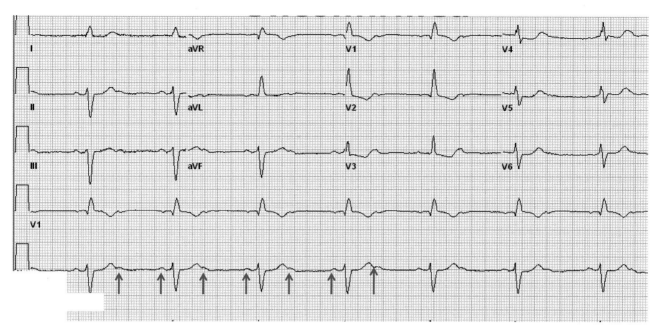

Figure 13.8 At first glance, the rhythm seems to be sinus bradycardia, ~40bpm, and the waves that follow QRS complexes seem to be U waves. However, ***in any sinus bradycardia of 40–50bpm, one must verify whether the true rhythm is, in fact, a sinus rhythm of 80–100bpm with 2:1 AV block.*** The presumed U waves are actually P waves as they march out with P waves preceding the QRS complexes (*arrows*).Thus, the rhythm is a sinus rhythm with 2:1 AV block. In 2:1 AV block, one cannot tell if the dropped QRS is preceded by progressive PR prolongation or not, i.e., Mobitz I or II. In order to say Mobitz I or II in 2:1 AV block, analyze the following:

1. QRS width. If QRS is wide, the block is usually an infranodal block, i.e., Mobitz II; if QRS is narrow, the block is usually Mobitz I. The 2:1 AV block on the current ECG is, therefore, a Mobitz II AV block.
2. PR interval of the conducted beats. PR interval is normal in this case (~200ms), implying that the block is unlikely to be at the level of the AV node.

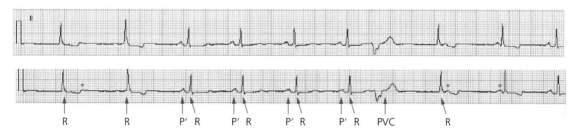

Figure 13.9 Outside the PVC, the rhythm seems regular. But on further analysis, there is some R–R irregularity.

Analyze the P–QRS relationship. Some QRS complexes seem to be preceded by P waves, with a consistent PR relationship (conducted P wave, noted as P'). On the other hand, some QRS complexes are not preceded by any P wave and are junctional QRS complexes. This suggests that a sinus rhythm and a junctional rhythm are competing at a rate of ~60bpm. When the sinus rhythm slows a bit, the junctional rhythm takes over. This is isorhythmic AV dissociation. Note that during the junctional rhythm sinus P waves occur regularly, dissociated from QRS and falling around it (marked by*). This is not AV block, as P waves get conducted when the competing junctional rhythm does not kick in. Note also that QRS of the junctional rhythm is a bit wider, suggesting a low junctional or fascicular origin.

Group beating on ECG (repetition of a series of beats followed by a pause) may be:
- Type I or II second-degree AV block or SA block
- Frequent PVCs or PACs, blocked or conducted, followed by a pause

In particular, a bigeminal rhythm, characterized by a repetition of two beats followed by a pause, may be due to:
- 3:2 AV block (type I or II): drop of every third QRS
- 3:2 SA block: drop of every third P–QRS
- PACs or PVCs occurring in a bigeminal pattern
- Non-conducted PACs occurring in a trigeminal pattern (after every second QRS)
- Atrial flutter with alternating 4:1 and 2:1 conduction (see Chapter 11, Figure 11.5)

On a rhythm strip, a *single blocked P wave* that is not premature and not preceded by progressive PR prolongation is likely a Mobitz II AV block, particularly when it occurs outside a vagal situation (Figure 13.10). However, it may also be a Mobitz I block with small overlooked changes in PR interval or a vagotonic AV block secondary to a sudden increase in vagal tone; in the latter case, the sinus rate typically slows down before the blocked P wave, even if PR does not appear to prolong (Figure 13.11). Another possibility is a concealed His premature complex.

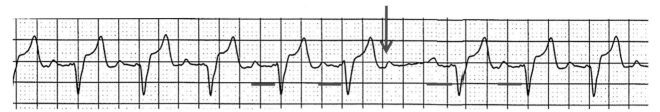

Figure 13.10 P blocks (*arrow*) without being premature and without progressive PR prolongation before the dropped beat, or PR shortening after the dropped beat. This implies Mobitz II AV block, *further suggested by the wide QRS*. The rate is ~60 bpm and the patient is asymptomatic, which may falsely suggest that the block is innocuous. In fact, this block is ominous because it is likely Mobitz II not Mobitz I, with a class I indication for pacemaker placement. **That is why it is important to carefully analyze every small pause. A benign Mobitz I or a blocked PAC may simulate the malignant Mobitz II block.**

In Mobitz II, the first PR interval that follows the pause may be shorter than the steady-state PR interval seen prior to the pause and the subsequent PR intervals, and may lead to a misdiagnosis of Mobitz I. Two explanations: (1) the first QRS after the pause may actually be an escape beat falling over the P wave, simulating a short PR interval; (2) the first QRS may be narrow, as the bundles are given time to recover from their refractory period; PR may seem shorter if it includes less isoelectric QRS.

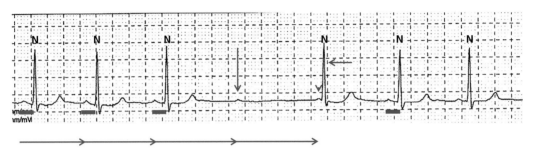

Figure 13.11 Note the block of a P wave (*vertical arrow*). This blocked P wave is not premature, and therefore the diagnosis is AV block. This blocked P wave is not preceded by any change in PR interval, even when PR intervals before and after the blocked P wave are compared (*bars*), which is concerning for a Mobitz II AV block. However, note that the P–P interval preceding the pause is lengthening progressively, a hint to an increase in vagal tone causing the AV block (*line of arrows*). Therefore, this is an AV nodal block, an equivalent of Mobitz I AV block. Also, the narrow QRS argues against Mobitz II AV block. Note that a junctional escape complex is seen after the pause (*horizontal arrow*), and coincides with the subsequent sinus P wave (*arrowhead*), preventing it from getting conducted: this is isorhythmic AV dissociation over one beat.

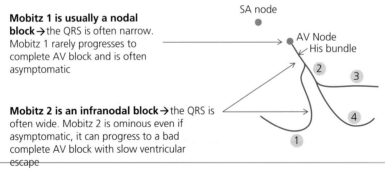

Mobitz 1 is usually a nodal block → the QRS is often narrow. Mobitz 1 rarely progresses to complete AV block and is often asymptomatic

Mobitz 2 is an infranodal block → the QRS is often wide. Mobitz 2 is ominous even if asymptomatic, it can progress to a bad complete AV block with slow ventricular escape

Figure 13.12 Mobitz I vs. Mobitz II AV block. (1) is the right bundle, (2) is the left bundle, (3) is the left anterior fascicle, (4) is the left posterior fascicle.

C. Location of the AV block

AV block may occur at the level of the AV node or at the infranodal level, i.e., at the His or the infra-His/Purkinje level (Figure 13.12). Infranodal AV block is ominous and leads to a slow ventricular escape rhythm. Usually, in infranodal AV block, the baseline QRS is wide as the fascicles have abnormal baseline conduction. Occasionally, the block is at the His level and the baseline QRS may not be wide.

Nodal AV block is less ominous and leads to a faster, junctional, narrow escape rhythm.

Location of the block in each type of AV block:

a. First-degree AV block is usually a nodal block, particularly if QRS is narrow. A PR interval >250 ms with a narrow QRS ~always implies a nodal block.

b. Mobitz I is often a nodal block, especially when QRS is narrow. When the QRS is wide, 75% of Mobitz I blocks are still nodal blocks, while 25% are infranodal blocks. A wide-QRS Mobitz I block with a maximal PR change of <50 ms is likely an infranodal Mobitz I block.

c. Mobitz II is an infranodal block, with a QRS that is often wide on the baseline ECG. If the baseline QRS is narrow, the block is likely infranodal at the level of the His bundle (~20% of Mobitz II block). Occasionally, what seems to be a narrow-QRS Mobitz II can be an overlooked Mobitz I with small overlooked increments in PR intervals, or can result from a sudden burst of vagal tone blocking one or several consecutive P waves.

d. 2:1 AV block: analyze the QRS width and the PR interval to define the site of the block:

   i.   if QRS is wide, the block is likely infranodal; if QRS is narrow, the block is likely nodal.

   ii. PR interval has two components: nodal component (AH interval, normally <125 ms) and infranodal component (HV interval, normally <55 ms and shorter than the AH component). A PR interval >250–300 ms more likely results from a delay of the nodal component, i.e., an increase in AH interval; however, the block may very well result from an infranodal delay, wherein HV severely prolongs to >200 ms (in this case, QRS must be wide). On the other hand, a PR interval that is <200–250 ms implies that the block is unlikely to be at the AV nodal level.

Two additional modalities help elucidate the type of 2:1 AV block: *exercise testing* (Table 13.1) or *prolonged rhythm monitoring (Holter).*

e. Third-degree AV block or high-grade AV block (e.g., 3:1, 4:1) is most often infranodal, but can be nodal. Determine the location of the AV block by the width and the rate of the escape. An escape rhythm that is wide usually implies an infranodal block; the rate is usually, but not necessarily, <40 bpm (Figure 13.13). VA conduction (retrograde P waves) implies an infranodal block as well.

> Sometimes, a block is present at both levels: very prolonged PR interval with Mobitz II, very prolonged PR interval or Mobitz I AV block with bundle branch block, complete nodal AV block in a patient with an underlying bundle branch block.[1]

D. Causes

1. Idiopathic degenerative disease is the most common cause of AV block: Lev disease in the elderly (fibrosis of the left cardiac skeleton, with involvement of the mitral annulus and aortic valve), and Lenegre disease in the young (rapidly progressive sclerodegenerative disease).

2. AV block may result from acute anterior or inferior ischemia, or chronic ischemic cardiomyopathy with diffuse myocardial fibrosis.

Table 13.1 Effect of atropine and exercise on AV block.

AV nodal block	Conduction ratio improves (AV node has rich autonomic innervations and is affected by cholinergic and sympathetic effects)
Infranodal block	Conduction ratio remains unchanged or worsens
	His and Purkinje conduction is not directly affected by the cholinergic or sympathetic system. On the other hand, the increase in sinus rate leads to more atrial depolarizations reaching the infranodal area. Many of these atrial depolarizations partially penetrate the infranodal area *without getting conducted all the way*, thus preventing subsequent beats from getting conducted (extended refractory period). This is *concealed conduction* = blocked, partial conduction that does not show up on the ECG yet modifies the expected behavior of subsequent beats (*blocked P waves prevent the conduction of subsequent P waves*). A slower atrial rate is more likely to get conducted

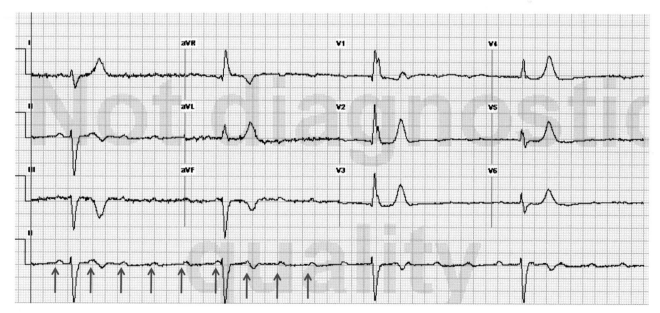

Figure 13.13 Complete AV block, with underlying sinus tachycardia (*arrows* point to sinus P waves), and a wide QRS escape of ~25 bpm. The escape has the morphology of pseudo-RBBB + LAFB. It may be a junctional escape with RBBB + LAFB; however, short of a baseline ECG showing RBBB + LAFB, the escape should be considered ventricular. The RBBB morphology suggests a left ventricular origin, while the LAFB morphology suggests a posterior origin. Overall, the block is infranodal and the escape originates from the LV posterior wall close to the posterior fascicle. The underlying sinus tachycardia indicates that the complete AV block is due to an intrinsic conduction disease, rather than a high vagal tone or drugs.

AV block occurring in association with acute inferior MI is usually secondary to increased vagal tone (first 24 hours) or to AV nodal stunning and edema (first few days), and is reversible within 1–2 weeks. AV block occurring with anterior MI is due to extensive infranodal myocardial stunning ± necrosis and is usually reversible but may become irreversible.

Only AV block that accompanies ACS with ongoing ischemic ST changes is expected to reverse with revascularization. Unless it is purely exertional, advanced AV block associated with angina, incidental CAD, or ischemic cardiomyopathy is not expected to reverse with revascularization and dictates pacemaker implantation.

3. Calcific valvular disease.

4. Any cardiomyopathy can affect the conduction system. Varying degrees of AV blocks are seen in up to 15% of dilated cardiomyopathies, particularly acute myocarditis and Chagas disease; in infiltrative cardiomyopathies, particularly sarcoidosis of the young; and in some connective tissue disorders (lupus, ankylosing spondylitis).

5. Drugs (β-blockers, calcium antagonists, digoxin, antiarrhythmic drugs), electrolytes (hypo- or hyperkalemia, hypermagnesemia).

6. High vagal tone (sleep, vomiting, cough, athlete's heart) may lead to AV block at the nodal level. This includes sleep apnea. Also, athletes may have AV Wenckebach, especially at night.

7. AV block after cardiac surgery (mainly congenital heart disease surgery, in which AV block resolves in 2/3 of the cases; or, less commonly, valvular surgery). AV block usually resolves within 7 days, if at all.

8. Lyme disease leads to a reversible AV nodal block. This AV block may take months to resolve and is a form of nodal AV block that paradoxically worsens with exercise, leading to significant exercise limitation.

Causes of AV block in the young
- Sarcoidosis
- Lenegre disease
- Congenital AV block: this is a nodal AV block that most often occurs without any other congenital abnormality. It may be hereditary or may occur in patients born to a mother with lupus. It starts in the neonatal period but may remain asymptomatic for many years.

On Holter or telemetry monitoring, sinus pauses or AV block at night, including complete or high-grade AV block, suggest sleep apnea. Hypoxia increases vagal tone, leading to nodal AV block.

E. Treatment

1. Place a **permanent pacemaker** in the following AV block situations, *after withdrawing rate-slowing drugs and ruling out reversible causes, such as a high vagal tone state:*[2]

- Symptomatic bradycardia (<50 bpm) or pauses (≥3 seconds while awake). This means that any of following occurs **concomitantly** to bradycardia or pauses: syncope/near-syncope, severe fatigue, or decompensated heart failure (regardless of the type or location of AV block).
- Mobitz type II second-degree AV block, even if the patient is asymptomatic.
- High-grade or third-degree AV block, even if the patient is asymptomatic (class I recommendation if symptomatic or if the escape is ventricular or slow <40 bpm ; class IIa otherwise). In patients with AF, AF pause >5 seconds indicates PM, even if asymptomatic, as long as it occurs during wakefulness and without a reversible cause.
- First-degree AV block or Mobitz type I second-degree AV block associated with symptomatic bradycardia or "pacemaker syndrome"–like symptoms: this occurs with a very prolonged PR interval (≥300 ms), which makes the P wave very close to the precedent QRS. AV synchrony is lost, and the atria sometimes contract against closed valves (Figure 13.5). On echo, E and A waves are fused, the diastolic filling time is reduced, and there is diastolic MR. Consequently, cardiac output is reduced and LA pressure is increased, which leads to fatigue, dyspnea, and syncope.
- In the case of Mobitz type I AV block or 2:1 AV block with uncertain effects, exercise testing may be performed. A second- or third-degree AV block during exercise signifies that the AV block is infranodal and worsens with increasing atrial activity; or AV block is ischemic.[3] It dictates PM placement after ruling out ischemia. EP study may also be performed to record the His–ventricle interval (>100 ms signifies severe infra-Hisian block), and to see whether infranodal block occurs with incremental pacing.
  An EP study is, in fact, indicated to further assess the AV block in the following two situations: (i) 2:1 AV block of unclear location. EP study, by measuring the HV interval and the HV response to atrial pacing, establishes the definite site of block. (ii) Mobitz I AV block with a wide QRS complex. An infranodal AV block mandates PM placement.

If the rate-controlling drug(s) is necessary (i.e., off-and-on AF or SVT), it may be reasonable to continue the drug(s) and place a permanent PM.

Also, an infranodal AV block is not much affected by β-blocker, CCB, or digoxin withdrawal, and therefore a PM may be indicated regardless of drug interruption.

2. Temporary transvenous pacemaker (placed through a transvenous sheath and used for a few days): for an advanced AV block associated with persistent hemodynamic changes, a temporary transvenous PM is placed while awaiting permanent PM placement. Atropine may be administered, but atropine does not improve infranodal block and may worsen it by increasing the ineffective impulses reaching the infranodal zone (this extends the time the infranodal zone is refractory); atropine is avoided in infranodal blocks. Isoproterenol (given temporarily) may help with AV block at any level and may be used en route to the transvenous PM placement. Isoproterenol is risky in patients with CAD as it may trigger ischemia and VT. Transcutaneous pacing may also be used en route to the transvenous PM placement; however, it does not reliably capture the ventricles and is painful. When transcutaneous pacing is used, large and wide pacing spikes are seen on the ECG, which precludes adequate assessment of capture; thus, capture can only be ensured by checking the pulse, usually brachial or femoral pulse away from muscle twitches, a pulse oximeter, or seeing true T waves after the spikes.

In the case of asymptomatic, advanced AV block, and while awaiting a permanent PM placement, a temporary PM is required if the AV block is infranodal, but it is not required if the AV block is nodal.

In reversible cases of AV block, a temporary PM is placed without the eventual need for a permanent PM: inferior MI, electrolyte disorders, drug effect/overdose, hypervagotonic states.

F. Other ECG examples of AV block (see Figures 13.14–13.17)

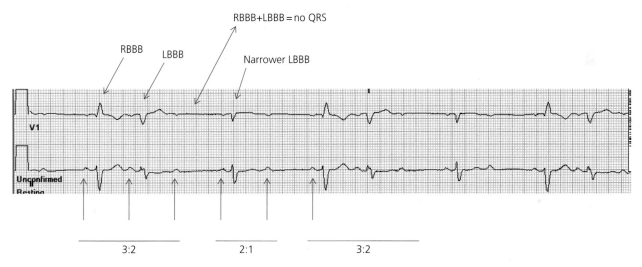

Figure 13.14 Second-degree Mobitz II AV block, with 3:2 block alternating with 2:1 block (*arrows* point to P waves). In lead V₁, one can see that on the conducted beats, RBBB alternates with LBBB. Beside Mobitz II, the alternation of RBBB and LBBB is indicative of infranodal AV block. In fact, QRS is dropped when both bundles simultaneously block in a patient with underlying RBBB, LBBB, or alternating RBBB and LBBB.

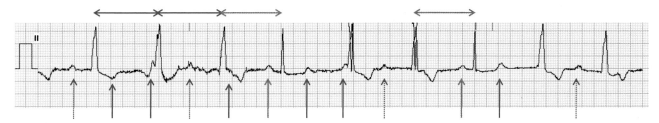

Figure 13.15 P waves and QRS complexes are dissociated on most beats, with most P waves not conducted to the ventricles (*blue arrows, solid and dashed*). One knows that these P waves are not conducted by the fact that: (1) they fall too close to the QRS complexes or there are ≥2 P waves for every QRS; (2) **the R–R interval is steady despite varying PR distance**; if some P waves were to conduct at various PR intervals, the R–R interval would vary as well. Two P waves are conducted (*gray arrows*), and this is indicated by the fact that their R–R interval (*gray double-arrows*) is shorter than the remaining, dominant, R–R interval (*blue double-arrows*); and by the fact that QRS following these P waves is narrow (ventricular capture from a sinus-originating stimulation).

This AV dissociation could be due to: (1) AV block, or (2) competitive (interference) AV dissociation. AV block is the diagnosis here as enough time is provided for a P wave after one QRS and before the next QRS to conduct, yet it does not conduct (*dashed arrows*). Therefore, this is a high-grade AV block with a fast ventricular escape rhythm (~55 bpm). The fact that one or more P waves are conducted precludes calling this rhythm complete AV block.

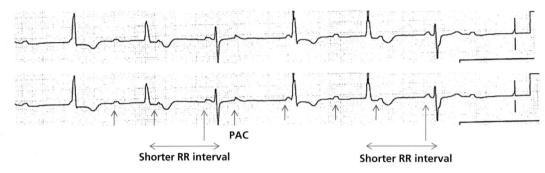

Figure 13.16 Another example of a high-grade AV block. Most P waves are not conducted (*blue arrows*) and a wide ventricular escape rhythm is seen. Occasionally, P wave conducts (*gray arrows*), and this manifests as a shorter R–R interval (*double-arrows*) and a narrow QRS complex. Note that the P–P interval containing a QRS is shorter than the P–P interval that does not contain a QRS (ventriculophasic sinus arrhythmia). The PR interval of the conducted P waves is ~200 ms (not significantly prolonged), which, along with the wide escape, indicates an infranodal block.

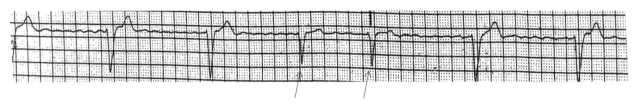

Figure 13.17 AF with a ventricular rate that is slow and mostly regular. This is AF with an almost complete AV block and a wide, regular escape rhythm that is ventricular in origin. Two narrower QRS complexes occur at a shorter R–R distance and signify occasional AV conduction. This is AF with a high-grade rather than a complete AV block.

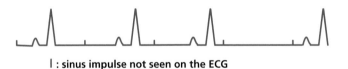

I : sinus impulse not seen on the ECG

Figure 13.18 4:3 Mobitz I SA block. Progressive lenghtening of the sinus impulse-to-P-wave interval, with shortening of the P–P interval, before the drop of one full P–QRS complex. It mimics a sinus pause.

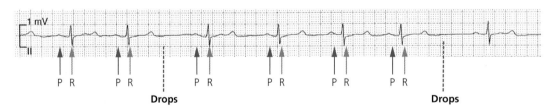

Figure 13.19 A whole P–QRS drops, which may be consistent with a sinus pause. On looking more carefully, group beating is seen. In addition, the P–P as well as the R–R intervals progressively shorten before the P–QRS drops. This is a 5:4 SA Wenckebach block; it is not AV Wenckebach, as PR interval is constant and the whole P–QRS drops. This is not sinus arrhythmia, as in the latter, P–P interval progressively, rather than abruptly, lengthens (not an abrupt jump from the shortest P–P to the longest P–P).

II. Sinus bradyarrhythmias

A. Types

1. Sinus bradycardia: sinus rhythm slower than 60 bpm.
2. Sinoatrial (SA) exit block.
   - Second-degree SA block, Mobitz type I: progressive increase in the interval between the sinus node and the P wave (this interval is not seen on ECG), progressive shortening of the P–P and R–R intervals, then drop of one whole P–QRS. As opposed to Mobitz I AV block, P wave drops as well (Figures 13.18, 13.19).
   - Second-degree SA block, Mobitz type II: sudden drop of one whole P–QRS complex (Figure 13.20). As opposed to AV block, P wave drops as well.
   - Third-degree SA block: drop of multiple P–QRS complexes. It is similar to a sinus pause, except that in SA block, P–P interval of the pause is a multiple of the baseline P–P interval.

   Clinically significant pauses are usually >3 seconds in an awake situation.

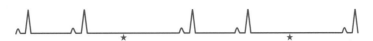

Figure 13.20 3:2 type II SA block. Both P and QRS intermittently drop (stars).

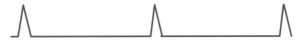

Figure 13.21 Sinus arrest or third-degree SA block with a ventricular escape rhythm. The fact that the escape is ventricular (wide and slow, originating from below the AV node), proves that there is AV infranodal disease in addition to the SA nodal block.

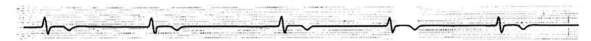

Figure 13.22 No P wave is seen → complete SA block vs. AF with small fibrillatory waves. The rhythm is a slow, wide complex rhythm at a rate of 30 bpm, suggesting a ventricular escape rhythm (slow and wide). This means that, in addition to the SA block, there is an infranodal, high-grade AV block. In fact, in the absence of AV infranodal disease, SA block should lead to a junctional rather than ventricular escape rhythm.

A prolonged SA block or sinus pause leads to a junctional escape rhythm (a slow rhythm with no P waves). A prolonged sinus pause is called *sinus arrest* (Figures 13.21, 13.22).

3. Tachy–brady syndrome: sinus bradyarrhythmia interspersed with episodes of AF or atrial tachyarrhythmia. Atrial tachyarrhythmia may be fast or slow, as AV nodal disease may coexist.

4. Chronotropic incompetence: inability to increase the heart rate to 80% of the maximal predicted heart rate during exercise (which equals 220 minus age).

> The most common differential of a sinus pause is a PAC that is not conducted and that is followed by a pause (in this case, a P wave is seen soon after QRS and may be within the T wave). Hint: T-wave morphology changes before the pause. The most important differential is Mobitz I or Mobitz II AV block causing a blocked P wave.

5. Sinus arrhythmia: phasic changes in P–P interval, often related to respiration. The sinus rate gradually increases with inspiration as the left output decreases; thus, P–P interval gets shorter with inspiration. The difference between the smallest and the longest P–P intervals is >120 ms or >10% of the smallest interval.

Sinus arrhythmia may be a sign of a healthy heart with good heart rate variability and a high vagal tone (especially in young patients). It is more common at slower heart rates. In the elderly patient, sinus arrhythmia is more often due to sinus node disease.

Also, the phasic P–P changes may not be related to respiration, in which case sinus arrhythmia is a sign of sinus node disease.

Ventriculophasic sinus arrhythmia may occur in complete AV block or 2: 1 AV block. P–P interval containing a QRS is shorter than the P–P interval not containing QRS (i.e., P–P interval varies). The cardiac output is higher when there is QRS, which reduces the adrenergic tone and the subsequent sinus P rate.

Sick sinus syndrome is any of the preceding disorders (1–5) due to an intrinsic sinus node disease, often degenerative in nature. Tachy–brady syndrome occurs in 55–75% of cases of sick sinus syndrome. In particular, 40–70% of patients requiring pacemaker implantation for sinus node disease have or develop AF. Patients with sinus node disease may have AV conduction disease as well (AV block is seen in ~15% of patients initially, then develops at a rate of 2% per year).

> *Notes*
> Any severe sinus bradyarrhythmia may lead to a junctional escape rhythm, typically at a rate of 40–60 bpm. The patient may not have P waves or may have slow sinus P waves that are dissociated from the narrow escape rhythm (Tables 13.2, 13.3).
>
> In the case of a junctional or ventricular accelerated rhythm (60–120 bpm), or escape rhythm (<60 bpm), the junctional/ventricular rhythm may compete with the sinus rhythm at a similar rate. One beat may be sinus preceded by a P wave, the other may be junctional showing up at any deceleration of the sinus rate. This is *isorhythmic AV dissociation* (two competing rhythms) (Figure 13.23). This illustrates the fact that AV dissociation does not necessarily mean complete AV block; it may be that P wave does not get a chance to conduct, in the presence of a competing "isorhythmic" or faster junctional or ventricular rhythm. However, AV dissociation with a P wave that does not conduct despite a long pause signifies complete or high-grade AV block.

B. Causes
- Idiopathic degenerative, age-related sinus node disease (most common cause of sinus node disease)
- Acute ischemia may lead to transient SA block
- Any chronic cardiomyopathy (e.g., ischemic, hypertensive, dilated) may lead to scarring of the SA node

Table 13.2 Differential diagnosis of a regular, non-tachycardic (<100 bpm) narrow complex rhythm without P waves.

- Complete SA block with junctional escape rhythm or accelerated junctional rhythm
- AF with AV block and junctional escape or accelerated junctional rhythm (the small atrial fibrillatory waves may not be seen)
- Hyperkalemia

Either way, it is a junctional rhythm. Make sure it is not a sinus rhythm with a very long PR interval and a P wave hidden atop T wave

Table 13.3 Differential diagnosis of a regular, non-tachycardic wide complex rhythm without P waves.

- Complete SA block + AV block with ventricular escape rhythm or accelerated idioventricular rhythm
- AF with complete AV block and ventricular escape rhythm or accelerated idioventricular rhythm
- Hyperkalemia
- Junctional escape rhythm with a pre-existing BBB. In order to differentiate it from a ventricular rhythm, a supraventricular capture complex needs to be seen. A review of a baseline ECG or ECG performed after the arrhythmia resolves is also helpful.

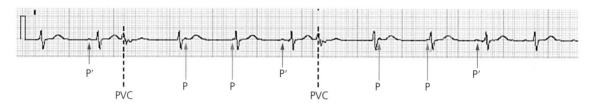

Figure 13.23 Outside PVCs, the rhythm seems regular, but, on further analysis, there is some R–R irregularity. Analyze the P–QRS relationship: some QRS complexes seem to be preceded by P waves with a consistent PR relationship (conducted P waves, called P' and marked by *blue arrows*). On the other hand, some QRS complexes are not preceded by any P wave (junctional QRS). This suggests a sinus rhythm and a junctional rhythm competing at a rate of ~60 bpm. When the sinus rhythm slows a bit, the junctional rhythm takes over. Note that during the junctional rhythm, sinus P waves occur regularly, dissociated from the QRS complexes and falling around them, marked by the *gray arrows*. There is no AV block, as P wave gets conducted whenever it occurs long enough after the QRS and whenever the junctional rhythm does not kick in close to it.

- Drugs
- Hyper- or hypokalemia, hypothyroidism, obstructive jaundice
- High vagal tone (athlete, acute gastric illness)
- Severe HTN may stimulate the carotid sinus receptors and lead to a reflex bradycardia (the converse of hypotension and reflex tachycardia)

C. Treatment

Hold the offending drugs if the patient is symptomatic. A permanent PM is indicated in the following cases (the first three are class I recommendations, the last two are class IIa):[2]

- Symptomatic sinus pauses or sinus bradyarrhythmia <50 bpm occurring during wakefulness, manifesting as syncope/near-syncope, severe fatigue, or HF, outside of a drug effect, a vagal state, acute ischemia, or a metabolic effect (hypothyroidism).
- If the drug is necessary (β-blocker for episodes of paroxysmal AF or SVT), a case can be made to continue the drug and place a permanent PM.
- Chronotropic incompetence: fatigue with exertion related to the inability to appropriately increase heart rate during exertion, documented on stress testing.
- Unexplained syncope associated with cardioinhibitory carotid sinus hypersensitivity, in which a carotid massage induces SA and/or AV block with a pause >3 seconds, even if syncope does not occur in a circumstance of spontaneous carotid sinus stimulation. In this case, carotid sinus massage unveils significant sinus node or AV node disease which is the likely mechanism of syncope. Syncope may not be directly related to carotid sinus stimulation.

  The full "carotid sinus syndrome," wherein syncope occurs in a context of spontaneous carotid sinus stimulation, is much less common than carotid sinus hypersensitivity (class I indication for PM).
- Unexplained syncope with severe sinus node dysfunction on EP study (prolonged sinus node recovery time). However, ***EP study is not highly sensitive or specific for the diagnosis of sinus node disease; monitoring is the best diagnostic modality for sinus node disease.***

Important clinical tips

1. A bradycardia <50 bpm is considered a contributor to syncope or severe fatigue when it is documented to occur *concomitantly* to symptoms (Holter monitoring or pulse exam). Short of that, a heart rate <40 bpm or pauses >3 seconds occurring during wakefulness, in a patient who had these symptoms at one point, are considered enough evidence to diagnose "symptomatic bradycardia." On the other hand, the occurrence of these symptoms while the rate is documented to be over 50 bpm without pauses or advanced AV block is a proof that these symptoms are not due to bradyarrhythmia, even if bradyarrhythmia incidentally occurs at some point. PM is not indicated in the latter case.
2. *Whenever the symptomatic effect of a bradycardia is unclear, stress testing should be performed. A heart rate of 40 bpm at rest may be appropriate, as long it has the capacity to appropriately rise with exercise* (to 80% of maximal predicted heart rate).

3. Sinus pauses without symptoms, including sinus pauses >3 seconds or AF pauses >3 seconds (especially nocturnal pauses), do not dictate PM placement. These prolonged pauses do, however, dictate a reduction of the offending drugs.

4. *Before making the diagnosis of a sinus pause, make sure that the pause is not an advanced AV block or Mobitz II AV block with blocked P wave(s) – in which case a pacemaker is indicated even if the patient is asymptomatic.*

5. Severely decompensated HF is typically associated with a compensatory increase in heart rate that attempts to maintain cardiac output and ventricular emptying. A relative bradycardia (even 50–60 bpm) during the decompensated stage is a sign of chronotropic incompetence and may be the major trigger of decompensation. It may warrant down-titration of the rate-slowing drugs, or PM therapy if the patient was not receiving those drugs.

6. Similarly, a mild or relative bradycardia (50–70 bpm) in a patient with symptomatic hypotension, who should otherwise be tachycardic, indicates that bradycardia is a major contributor to hypotension and is diagnostic of chronotropic incompetence, unless both bradycardia and hypotension are due to the same cause (such as a high vagal state, hypothyroidism, or adrenal crisis).

III. Bundle branch blocks, bifascicular and trifascicular block
A. Definitions
The His bundle branches into the right bundle and left bundle, which branches into the left anterior fascicle and the left posterior fascicle (Figure 13.24). A bifascicular block implies a block in two of the three conduction fascicles, such as:

- LBBB
- Or RBBB + LAFB (~ RBBB with left axis)
- Or RBBB + LPFB (~ RBBB with right axis, which may also be RBBB + RVH)

A trifascicular block implies that all three fascicles have a conduction block. The block is incomplete in at least one fascicle, explaining the lack of a complete AV block. Trifascicular block may manifest as:

- Bifascicular block + increased PR interval: this is often a trifascicular block, but may also be a bifascicular block with a first-degree AV block.
- Alternating RBBB and LBBB, i.e., RBBB and LBBBB alternate on the same ECG or on different ECGs obtained up to several years apart.
- RBBB with alternating LAFB and LPFB.

B. Causes and workup
The right bundle and the anterior fascicle are long and slender and have a single blood supply (LAD); this makes these structures vulnerable to injury or to the aging process earlier than the left bundle. The main left bundle and the posterior fascicle are short and thick, and both have dual blood supply (LAD and RCA); this makes those structures less vulnerable to injury. After cardiac contusion or cardiac compressions, transient RBBB is the most common block.

LAFB is common in the general population and often occurs without any underlying heart disease. RBBB is also common, and in patients without a clinical history of CAD or HF, RBBB is usually unrelated to any underlying heart disease. It is seen in otherwise healthy individuals and, in most long-term follow-up studies of patients with isolated RBBB and unsuspected CAD or HF at baseline, RBBB has not been associated with an adverse prognosis.[4–7] Only in one recent Danish study of older individuals (mean 64 years of age), complete RBBB has been associated with a 1.3 hazard ratio of long-term mortality and MI, suggesting that RBBB may be a marker of subclinical CAD in some patients.[8]

On the other hand, because the left bundle and the left posterior fascicle are thick and more diffcult to injure, LPFB and LBBB often appear in patients with underlying heart disease, typically a chronic myocardial process, ischemic or non-ischemic, with a dilated or hypertrophied myocardium. About a third of patients with LBBB have CAD, while only 11% have no apparent heart disease.[9] Even in the absence of obvious heart disease during the initial evaluation, an isolated LBBB is associated with cardiac disease during follow-up. LBBB is associated with an increase in the long-term mortality, MI, coronary and sudden death, even in relatively young (45–55 years) and asymptomatic patients without obvious underlying cardiac disease.[4,5] This increase in risk occurs over 20–30 years of follow-up. In addition, LBBB, per se, may induce dyssynchrony, abnormal diastolic function, and reduced LV ejection fraction.

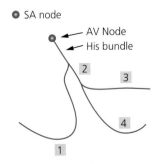

Figure 13.24 1, right bundle; 2, left bundle; 3, left anterior fascicle; 4, left posterior fascicle.

RBBB that occurs without underlying heart disease results from a benign focal degeneration of the slender right bundle. Conversely, RBBB that occurs in LV systolic dysfunction is at least as malignant as LBBB and is more frequently associated with ischemic cardiomyopathy and a large scar burden than LBBB, more specifically a large anteroseptal scar.[10–14] The right bundle is supplied by the first septal branch, and thus RBBB may result from proximal LAD occlusion; the left bundle has dual supply, and thus LBBB does not usually result from an ischemic scar but from LV dilatation or hypertrophy. The increased wall stress and the patchy myocardial fibrosis lead to strain, fibrosis, and calcification of the left bundle. LBBB is associated with extensive CAD, but not disease in any particular coronary segment.[15] A new LBBB is more frequently the result of non-ischemic than ischemic cardiomyopathy (30% ischemic cardiomyopathy). LBBB rarely results from acute infarction, and if it does, it is usually a large infarction involving both the LAD and RCA territories.[10,11]

In light of this pathophysiology, LBBB, RBBB, bi- and trifascicular block can be due to:

a. *Degeneration of the conduction system, particularly in the case of RBBB*. In this setting, RBBB is twice as common as LBBB, and the prevalence of both increases with age and male sex. The prevalences of LBBB and RBBB are ~0.4% and 1%, respectively, at age 50 vs. 6% and 10%, respectively, at age 80.

b. *Underlying heart disease such as ischemic cardiomyopathy, hypertensive cardiomyopathy, or any cardiomyopathy (valvular, dilated, hypertrophic, infiltrative)*. In these cases, a bundle branch block (BBB) is a sign of diffuse myocardial disease, with scarring and slowing of conduction through a dilated or hypertrophied myocardium rather than a discrete bundle branch delay. It is often preceded by LVH, RVH, or incomplete blocks on ECG, has more left or right axis deviations and *may be >150 ms, which is unusual with a discrete bundle block*. It is associated with a worse cardiomyopathy prognosis and a reduced long-term survival. It suggests a more extensive underlying disease and a more severe left ventricular dysfunction (vs. no BBB). RBBB and LBBB have the same adverse independent prognostic value in patients with underlying systolic HF, with RBBB being a worse mortality predictor in several studies.[12,13] In patients with severe HF who qualify for CRT, RBBB is associated with a poor response to CRT, and thus a worse prognosis and a higher mortality than LBBB.[14]

Beside their established prognostic value in acute MI, both RBBB and LBBB are independent prognostic markers in patients with underlying chronic stable CAD and imply more extensive CAD and worse LV function.[15]

Although innocent congenital aberration of the conduction system is possible, ***isolated right heart pathologies or subclinical myocardial disease should be sought in a young patient (<50) with RBBB:*** ASD, ARVD, sarcoidosis, Chagas disease.

c. While LBBB or RBBB may be solely due to disease of the bundle branch rather than myocardial disease, a non-specific intraventricular conduction delay (IVCD) >110 ms often signifies underlying myocardial disease with intramyocardial slowing of conduction. The disease may be subclinical and the echocardiogram may be normal. Baseline IVCD was associated with higher mortality than LBBB over the long-term follow-up of relatively young individuals with unsuspected heart disease (45–55 years of age).[5]

Perform an echocardiogram to evaluate RBBB or LBBB. If there is no evidence of a cardiomyopathy and no clinical suggestion of CAD, the bundle branch block is most likely isolated and related to a degeneration of the conduction system and, in the case of RBBB, does not usually portend an impaired prognosis. Perfom ischemic evaluation with stress testing for any possible angina equivalent (fatigue, dyspnea), especially in LBBB.

RBBB is not usually associated with right-axis deviation. Frank right-axis deviation implies an associated RVH or LPFB.

LBBB that is due strictly to conduction disease usually has a normal or slightly leftward axis. A left axis is often seen when the LV is dilated or when LV activation spreads from the distal septum to the base. A right axis implies a dilated cardiomyopathy with RV and LV dilatation.

The wider the QRS (especially >150 ms), the more likely it is for LV function to be impaired and cardiomyopathy to be present.

C. Treatment

PM placement is not indicated in asymptomatic RBBB, LBBB, or bi- or trifascicular block, except when associated with episodes of third-degree AV block, high-grade AV block, Mobitz type II AV block, or alternating RBBB+LBBB. The rate of progression of RBBB or LBBB to high-degree AV block is 1–4% per year.[4]

LBBB, IVCD, and possibly RBBB in older individuals are associated with increased cardiac events and mortality over the very long term. Therefore, these individuals are categorized as higher-risk patients who require aggressive risk-factor modification and a low threshold for CAD screening upon initial diagnosis or during follow-up.

An unexplained, non-neurally mediated syncope that occurs in a patient with RBBB or LBBB is most likely due to AV block and often dictates PM placement. One study addressed patients with BBB (RBBB 60%, LBBB 40%) who had unexplained syncope, negative carotid sinus massage, and negative EP study (no inducible VT, infranodal block, or sinus node disease). After placement of a loop recorder, 42% of these patients had recurrence of syncope (median 48 days), mainly attributable to complete AV block. Overall, 54% had significant bradyarrhythmic events.[16] Thus, pacemaker placement is reasonable in patients with unexplained syncope and RBBB or LBBB. Consider performing EP study prior to PM placement, not so much to diagnose infranodal disease, as EP study was not sensitive enough to detect it in the above study, but to rule out VT inducibility (ACC class IIa recommendation). In fact, VT is inducible in ~14% of patients with BBB and syncope.[17,18]

D. Tachycardia or acceleration-dependent bundle branch block

Aberration may be induced in normal individuals when tachycardia occurs beyond a certain rate or premature excitation occurs at a very short R–R interval, particularly when the preceding R–R interval is long (Ashman's phenomenon). This physiologic aberration is more likely

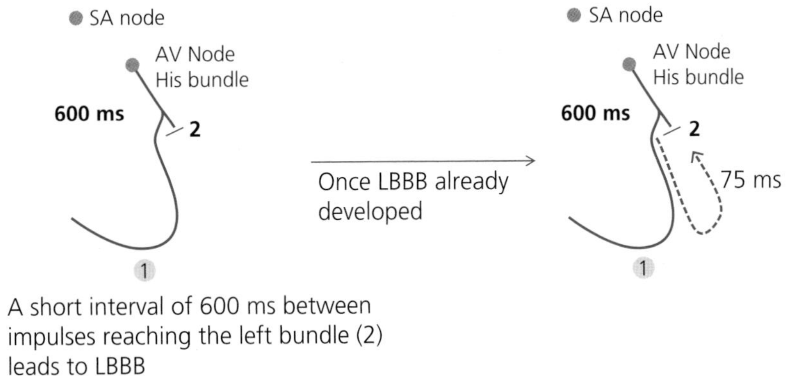

A short interval of 600 ms between
impulses reaching the left bundle (2)
leads to LBBB

Figure 13.25 Suppose that a tachycardia-mediated LBBB has developed at a rate of 100 bpm (R–R interval = 600 ms). When the heart rate slows back down to 100 bpm, the LBBB persists. For a 600 ms interval between impulses reaching the AV node, it takes the left bundle that is now blocked an extra 75 ms to be depolarized, so that the interval between the left bundle depolarization and the next impulse is 600 − 75 = 525 ms. This perpetuates the LBBB even at a rate <100 bpm. The left bundle may recover once the cycle length is 675 ms (HR = 88).

to affect the right bundle, which has a longer refractory period than the left bundle. It may be seen with extreme heart rates (e.g., SVT with rate >150–180 bpm), or may be initiated by a very premature beat having a long–short sequence.

On the other hand, rate-related BBB occurring at lower rates (<130 bpm) or longer R–R cycles is often pathologic and implies an underlying bundle branch disease; it may very well be seen at rates <100 bpm and is less dependent on a long–short sequence. In these patients the aberration may be LBBB or RBBB (more commonly LBBB), and it has the same diagnostic and prognostic value as BBB seen at rest.[19,20] During tachycardia, the diseased bundle has less time to recover from its long refractory period and subsequently blocks.

Let us suppose that LBBB occurs in a particular patient after the heart rate reaches 100 bpm (R–R cycle length of 600 ms). Once it occurs, the aberrancy may not resolve until the rate is much lower than 100 bpm. In fact, once LBBB has occurred, the supraventricular impulse travels down the right bundle, traverses the septum, and depolarizes the blocked left bundle retrogradely. The very early part of the left bundle depolarizes late, such that the time between left bundle depolarization and the next impulse is much shorter than the 600 ms cycle length that perpetuates the aberrancy (Figure 13.25). It is this *delay of "trans-septal activation"* that perpetuates aberrancy at lower rates. A similar phenomenon explains the perpetuation of Ashman's aberrancy even after the R–R interval lengthens; only the first R–R interval of the wide complex rhythm may be short.

The concept of bundle "fatigue" during tachycardia may also explain why it takes a slower rate to resolve it than to initiate it. BBB may reverse in a cyclic pattern, wherein it intermittently occurs every few beats before fully reversing.

E. Bradycardia or deceleration-dependent bundle branch block

With bradycardia, spontaneous diastolic (phase 4) depolarization of one bundle may occur. This depolarization may create a concealed action potential that prevents propagation of supraventricular impulses. Deceleration block implies significant underlying bundle branch disease and infranodal disease. In addition, these patients usually have tachycardia-dependent BBB, and the heart-rate range of normal conduction is inversely related to the amount of bundle injury. It may be extremely narrow (e.g., 55–75 bpm).

Deceleration AV block may be seen; this suggests infranodal AV block.

F. Alternating bundle branch block

This is an alternation of RBBB and LBBB on the same ECG or, much more commonly, on several ECGs obtained several days, months, or years apart. This usually implies an incomplete block of one bundle, e.g., left bundle (even if QRS >120 ms) and intermittent complete block of the other bundle, e.g., right bundle: the baseline ECG shows LBBB, but during deceleration or acceleration, RBBB develops and conduction occurs over the slow, but not completely blocked, left bundle.[21,22] Depending on the refractory period of the right bundle, conduction may resume over the right bundle intermittently on the same ECG, or may resume once the trans-septal activation is delayed enough to allow the right bundle to recover. In other patients, the baseline QRS is narrow, some ECGs show RBBB, while others show LBBB; this pattern is more concerning, as complete BBB is developing alternately over each bundle, and it may be a stronger incentive for pacemaker implantation. In asymptomatic patients, the risk of progression to complete AV block is higher than with unilateral BBB. Pacemaker implantation is warranted even in asymptomatic patients, although most of these patients do not develop complete AV block over several months or 1 year of follow-up.[22]

QUESTIONS AND ANSWERS

Question 1. A 65-year-old man has occasional episodes of vague fatigue, and an event monitoring is performed. It shows the tracing of Figure 13.10. The patient was asymptomatic during this tracing. Should a PM be placed?

Question 2. A 65-year-old man has occasional episodes of vague fatigue, and a Holter monitoring is performed. It shows the tracing of Figure 13.11 during sleep. He is asleep and asymptomatic during the tracing. Should a PM be placed?

Question 3. A 65-year-old man has occasional episodes of vague fatigue. He is mostly bothered by palpitations. An ECG is performed (Figure 13.15). Should a PM be placed?

Question 4. A 65-year-old man had one episode of near-syncope after working in his yard, in a hot environment. His ECG shows AF with a spontaneously slow ventricular response of 55 bpm. The patient is not taking any rate-slowing drugs. A Holter monitor is performed. It shows a 3.5 seconds AF pause during sleep. Should a PM be placed?

Question 5. A 65-year-old man has severe nausea and vomiting. He has deep fatigue. He is known to have chronic AF. The emergency room monitor shows a pause of 4 seconds while the patient is awake. He has not had syncope, but is gagging. He receives chronic metoprolol for AF. What is the next step?

Question 6. A 65-year-old man had one episode of near-syncope after working in his yard in a hot environment. His ECG shows AF with a spontaneously slow ventricular response of 55 bpm. The patient is not taking any rate-slowing drugs. A Holter monitor is performed. It shows the rhythm strip of Figure 13.17 during sleep. Should a PM be placed?

Question 7. A 65-year old man complains of occasional episodes of dizziness. Rhythm monitoring is performed and shows the rhythm strip of Figure 13.9, during wakefulness. He had mild palpitations during the recording. Should a PM be placed?

Question 8. A 50-year-old woman presents with a syncope that occurred after prolonged standing. She has no prior cardiac history and does not take any medication. She still has malaise and feels tired and nauseated. ECG shows sinus bradycardia at a rate of 42 bpm. Should a PM be placed?

Question 9. A 65-year-old man has occasional episodes of dizziness at rest. His pulse at rest is consistently slow, ~45–50 bpm. ECG shows sinus bradycardia. What is the next step?
A. PM placement
B. Prolonged rhythm monitoring (event monitor)
C. Stress testing
D. EP study
E. B or C

Question 10. A 58-year-old man is found to have LBBB of 125 ms on his ECG. He is hypertensive and asymptomatic. Which of the following statement(s) are true?
A. Compared with RBBB, LBBB is more likely to be associated with underlying heart disease (cardiomyopathy, CAD) upon diagnosis or follow-up
B. Even in the absence of obvious underlying heart disease, LBBB is still associated with increased long-term mortality, HF and MI, which is not the case with RBBB
C. In the presence of underlying myocardial or coronary disease, both LBBB and RBBB have the same adverse prognostic implication. RBBB may have worse implication in ischemic cardiomyopathy.
D. In patients with cardiomyopathy, RBBB is often due to a large ischemic scar, while LBBB is most often due to ischemic or non-ischemic LV dilatation or hypertrophy.
E. Echo is indicated to look for subclinical myocardial disease. In this case, hypertensive LV hypertrophy is the likely myocardial disease.

Question 11. A patient has mild dizziness. He is not hypotensive. An ECG is performed (Figure 13.23). Which statement is correct?
A. There is intermittent AV dissociation. AV dissociation implies AV block. He needs PM
B. There is intermittent AV dissociation without AV block. His AV dissociation is a competitive type of AV dissociation. No need for PM

Answer 1. Yes. This is Mobitz type II AV block. It requires PM placement, even if asymptomatic and even if only one beat appears to drop.

Answer 2. No. This is a benign finding of increased vagal tone. Consider sleep study. No need for PM based on this tracing.

Answer 3. Yes. This is a high-grade AV block with a wide, ventricular escape. Even if he is asymptomatic (no syncope/near-syncope), a PM is definitely warranted. Palpitations are explained by AV dissociation and the simultaneous atrial and ventricular contractions at times, leading to cannon A waves.

Answer 4. No. AF pauses are common during sleep, and even pauses >3 seconds do not have therapeutic or diagnostic implications, per se. AF pause >3 seconds during wakefulness indicates PM placement in a patient who had near-syncope at one point, even if the documented pause is not symptomatic per se. AF pause >5 seconds during wakefulness indicates PM placement even in the absence of prior symptoms (a marker of high-grade AV block). All of this assumes that a high vagal tone state has been ruled out and offending drugs have been removed.

Answer 5. This long AF pause occurred during wakefulness but was triggered by a high vagal tone (gagging, nausea), a transient cause. It does not indicate PM placement. Even metoprolol dose may not need to be reduced.

Answer 6. Yes. The rhythm strip shows a rate of ~40 bpm, which is acceptable and common at night. However, in this case, the 40 bpm rate is mostly a regular, ventricular escape rhythm, with a high-grade AV block. High-grade AV block with ventricular escape dictates PM placement, especially in a patient with prior near-syncope, even if it occurs at night.

Answer 7. No. The patient has episodes of accelerated junctional rhythm with isorhythmic AV dissociation. This is a competitive form of AV dissociation, without AV block. PM is not indicated based on this tracing. Palpitations are due to the simultaneous atrial and ventricular contractions.

Answer 8. No. The patient has severe sinus bradycardia that may initially seem symptomatic (malaise, recent syncope). However, considering the context of her syncope and the tiredness/nausea, it is likely that the patient has had vasovagal syncope and lingering vasovagal symptoms along with sinus bradycardia. Rather than being the cause of syncope, sinus bradycardia is secondary to the vasovagal state. To prove that, this patient was monitored for 24 hours. Symptoms progressively resolved, and sinus bradycardia improved to 55 bpm. To further prove that her bradycardia was innocuous, a stress testing was performed. Her sinus rate appropriately increased to 165 bpm at peak exercise.

Answer 9. E. Sinus bradycardia of 40–50 bpm at rest may be a normal, innocuous finding. Unless the dizziness actually coincides with the sinus bradycardia, or unless the sinus bradycardia is severe (<40 bpm while awake or pause >3 seconds while awake), dizziness is not necessarily related to the bradycardia, and most likely is not. In order to prove the effect of a sinus bradycardia, stress testing is the best testing modality. ***Sinus bradycardia is innocuous if the sinus rate increases appropriately when needed most, during stress.*** Rhythm monitoring is also useful, seeking more severe bradycardia or pauses during wakefulness. EP study is not sensitive enough for the diagnosis of bradyarrhythmias, particularly sinus node disorders.

Answer 10. All are true.

Answer 11. B. AV dissociation may be due to: (i) AV block, or (ii) competitive AV dissociation. Complete AV block is always associated with AV dissociation, but the reverse is not true.

References

1. Dhingra RC, Whyndham C, Armat-y-Leon F, et al. Significance of AH interval in patients with chronic bundle branch blocks. Clinical, electrophysiologic, and follow-up observations. Am J Cardiol 1976: 37: 231–6.
2. Epstein AE, DiMarco JP, Ellenbogen KA, et al. ACC/AHA/HRS 2008 guidelines for device-based therapy of cardiac rhythm abnormalities: a report of the American College of Cardiology/American Heart Association Task Force on Practice Guidelines. J Am Coll Cardiol 2008; 51: e1–62.
3. Woelfel AK, Simpson RJ, Gettes RS, Foster JR. Exercise-induced distal atrioventricular block. J Am Coll Cardiol 1983: 2: 578–81.
4. Eriksson P, Wilhelmsen L, Rosengren A. Bundle-branch block in middle-aged men: risk of complications and death over 28 years. The Primary Prevention Study in Goteborg, Sweden. Eur Heart J 2005; 26: 2300–6.
5. Aro AL, Anttonen O, Tikkanen JT, et al. Intraventricular conduction delay in a standard 12-lead electrocardiogram as a predictor of mortality in general population. Circ Arrhythm Electrophysiol 2011; 4: 704–10.
6. Smith RF, Jackson DH, Harthorne JW, Sanders CA. Acquired bundle branch block in a healthy population. Am Heart J 1970; 80: 746–51.
7. Fleg JL, Das DN, Lakatta EG. Right bundle branch block: long-term prognosis in apparently healthy men. J Am Coll Cardiol 1983; 1: 887–92.
8. Bussink BR, Holst AG, Jespersen L, et al. Right bundle branch block: prevalence, risk factors, and outcome in the general population: results from the Copenhagen City Heart Study. Eur Heart J 2013; 34: 138–46.
9. Schneider JP, Thomas HE, Kreger BE, et al. Newly acquired left bundle branch block: the Framingham study. Ann Intern Med 1979; 90: 303–10.
10. Strauss DG, Loring Z, Selvester RH, et al. Right, but not left, bundle branch block is associated with large anteroseptal scar. J Am Coll Cardiol 2013; 62: 959–67.
11. Zareba W, Klein H, Cygankiewicz I, et al. Effectiveness of cardiac resynchronization therapy by QRS morphology in the Multicenter Automatic Defibrillator Implantation Trial-Cardiac Resynchronization Therapy (MADIT-CRT). Circulation 2011; 123: 1061–72.
12. Wang NC, Maggioni AP, Konstam MA, et al. Clinical implications of QRS duration in patients hospitalized with worsening heart failure and reduced left ventricular ejection fraction. JAMA 2008; 299: 2656–66.
13. Barsheshet A, Goldenberg I, Garty M, et al. Relation of bundle branch block to long-term (four-year) mortality in hospitalized patients with systolic heart failure. Am J Cardiol 2011; 107: 540–4.
14. Gervais R, Leclercq C, Shankar A, et al. Surface electrocardiogram to predict outcomes in candidates of cardiac resynchronization therapy: a sub-analysis of the CARE-HF trial. Eur Heart J 2009; 11: 699–705.
15. Freedman RA, Alderman EL, Sheffield LT, et al. Bundle branch block in patients with chronic coronary artery disease: angiographic correlates and prognostic significance. J Am Coll Cardiol 1987; 10: 73–80. *Both RBBB and LBBB are independent prognostic markers in patients with underlying chronic stable CAD, with LBBB being a worse finding in this setting.*
16. Brignole M, Menozzi C, Moya A, et al. Mechanisms of syncope in patients with bundle branch block and negative electrophysiological test. Circulation 2001; 104: 2045–50.
17. Ezri M, Lerman BB, Marchlinski FE, Buxton AE, Josephson ME. Electrophysiologic evaluation of syncope in patients with bifascicular block. Am Heart J 1983; 106: 693–7.
18. Morady F, Higgins J, Peters RW, ct al. Electrophysiologic testing in bundle branch block and unexplained syncope. Am J Cardiol 1984; 54: 587–9.
19. Fisch C, Zipes DP, McHenry PL. Rate dependent aberrancy. Circulation 1973; 48: 714–24.
20. Rosenbaum MB, Elizari MV, Lazzari JO, et al. The mechanism of intermittent bundle branch block: relationship to prolonged recovery, hypopolarization and spontaneous diastolic depolarization. Chest 1973; 63: 666–77.
21. Wu D, Denes P, Dhingra RC, et al. Electrophysiological and clinical observations of patients with alternating bundle branch block. Circulation 1976; 53: 456–64.
22. Simpson RJ, Rosenthal HM, Rimmer MH, Foster JR. Alternating bundle branch block. Chest 1978; 74: 447–8.

14 Permanent Pacemaker and Implantable Cardioverter Defibrillator

I. Indications for permanent pacemaker implantation[1]

1. Any symptomatic sinus bradyarrhythmia or AV block (symptomatic means near-syncope/syncope, severe fatigue, or active HF concomitant to bradycardia).

2. AV block (see Chapter 13, Table 13.2):

   a. Mobitz II AV block even if it is asymptomatic

   b. High-grade or third-degree AV block, even if it is asymptomatic

   c. Asymptomatic, severely prolonged HV interval (His-ventricle) >100 ms or infra-His block during incremental pacing on EP study

   d. Any AV block (including Mobitz I) with associated symptomatic bradycardia (e.g., symptomatic rate <40–50 bpm) or symptomatic pauses

   e. Mobitz I or first-degree AV block leading to "pacemaker syndrome"-like symptoms.

3. Syncope with periods of sinus pauses or AF pauses >3 seconds or heart rate <40 bpm while awake, as evidenced by Holter or telemetry monitoring, even when a clear association between the syncope and the bradycardia is not documented.

4. All this in the absence of a reversible cause, such as drugs, electrolytes, high vagal tone, acute ischemia, or the immediate post-cardiac surgery state, in which a temporary transvenous PM may be indicated for temporary support.

   If the bradyarrhythmia does not resolve after treatment of these causes, especially in the case of an acute anterior MI, a permanent PM is indicated. Also, if rate-slowing drugs are necessary to control frequent paroxysms of SVT, a PM is indicated.

II. Types of cardiac rhythm devices

Pacemakers (PMs) are designated by a three- or four-letter code: e.g., AAI, VVI or DDD.

- 1st letter = chamber paced: A (right atrium), V (right ventricle), or D (dual, both chambers)
- 2nd letter = chamber sensed: A, V, or D
- 3rd letter = action taken by the PM when it senses an event: I (inhibits pacing), T (triggers pacing, like pacing V after sensing A), or D
- There is often a 4th letter, R, which indicates a rate-response mode. A rate response means the device has accelerometer or ventilatory sensors that increase the rate with activity.

A. VVI = ventricular demand pacing

A VVI PM has a single sensing and pacing lead in the right ventricle. It paces the ventricle when it sees that the interval between two QRS complexes is longer than the back-up limit, called the *lower rate interval*; a limit of 1 second, for example, corresponds to a heart rate (HR) of 60 bpm.

   It does not see or pace the atrium, and does not make the ventricle track the atrium. In patients with sinus rhythm, VVI may lead to AV dissociation and loss of the atrial contribution to the cardiac output.

Practical Cardiovascular Medicine, First Edition. Elias B. Hanna.
© 2017 John Wiley & Sons Ltd. Published 2017 by John Wiley & Sons Ltd.

VVI pacing is mainly used in chronic AF, wherein the atrium cannot be paced or tracked. It may also be an acceptable option in older sedentary patients with AV block.

VVI pacing may lead to a *pacemaker syndrome*. This is a syndrome of fatigue, dyspnea, and pre-syncope that results from: (i) loss of the atrial contribution to the cardiac output; (ii) some of the asynchronous atrial contractions occur during ventricular systole while the AV valve is closed, leading to increased atrial pressure. Moreover, ventricular pacing may lead to retrograde P waves; those retrograde P waves are an additional cause of atrial contraction during ventricular systole and may be a major contributor to the pacemaker syndrome.

B. DDD = AAI + VAT + VVI
DDD is a dual-chamber PM, with sensing and pacing leads placed in both the right atrium and the right ventricle.

- PM tracks the P wave and paces the ventricle whenever a P wave is not followed by a ventricular activity. After a P wave, PM waits a certain time before pacing the ventricle; this time is the *programmed AV interval*. This function is the VAT function or AV sequential pacing: PM sees the atrium ("A") then triggers ("T") the ventricle ("V"). It will appropriately track sinus tachycardia up to a certain rate (upper tracking rate).
- PM paces the atrium if P wave is absent (sinus node disease) and lets it spontaneously conduct to the ventricle (AAI function).
- PM sequentially paces the atrium then the ventricle in case of severe sinus node disease combined with severe AV block (AAI + VAT functions).

Notes
i. In patients requiring ventricular pacing, DDD is a more physiologic pacing mode than VVI. DDD preserves AV synchrony and the atrial contribution to the cardiac output, which may decrease left atrial pressure and augment cardiac output by 20–30% in comparison with VVI. It improves symptoms and quality of life in comparison with VVI and reduces the incidence of AF.

DDD pacing is indicated for sinus node disease and AV nodal disease. If the patient develops AF, DDD senses the excessive atrial activity and switches the pacing mode to VVI or DDI (mode-switch function).

ii. In pure sinus node disease, AAI PM may be placed. AAI senses the atrium and paces it when the atrial rate is slower than a certain limit; it does not sense or pace the ventricles. However, some of these patients have AV nodal disease as well (~15%), or progress to AV nodal disease (~2% per year), thus requiring V pacing at some point. When DDD pacing is performed in patients without AV nodal disease, ensure that only the atrium is paced with the DDD pacemaker, and let it normally conduct to the ventricles, thus minimizing RV pacing. The programmed AV interval should be long (250 ms if tolerated). RV pacing leads to dyssynchronous contractions within the LV and between the RV and LV, which may decrease LV function, especially in patients with pre-existing LV dysfunction. The avoidance of RV pacing reduces the risk of AF, stroke, and HF (post-hoc data from MOST and DAVID trials).[2,3]

iii. RV pacing leads to a wide QRS complex, with typically LBBB morphology as the electrical activity spreads from the RV to the LV. Usually, the axis is deviated to the left, except in the case of RV outflow tract pacing, in which the axis is vertical (depolarization goes up to down). QRS should be negative in V_1–V_3 as in LBBB. However, a positive QRS may be seen in V_1–V_2 (in up to 10%), but never in V_3. A positive QRS in V_3 signifies LV pacing, and thus BiV pacing or septal perforation of the RV lead. Rarely, there are q or Q waves in leads I–aVL, but, as in LBBB, there should not be qR or QR in the precordial leads V_1–V_6 or the inferior leads (if present, these q waves are very specific for an anterolateral or inferior infarct).[4]

C. Biventricular pacemaker
A biventricular pacemaker (BiV PM, also called cardiac resynchronization therapy, CRT), is a pacemaker that typically has three leads: RA lead, RV lead, and LV epicardial lead placed via the coronary sinus. In a way, it is a DDD PM with an additional LV lead. This PM is indicated for HF (functional class III or IV) with an EF ≤35% and LBBB or RV-paced rhythm that delays the LV excitation and contraction. A wide QRS, particularly LBBB, is seen in 20–30% of patients with systolic HF. LBBB is associated with dyssynchronous LV contraction, i.e., the RV contracts before the LV (interventricular conduction delay) and the septal wall contracts before the posterolateral wall (intraventricular conduction delay). This leads to ineffective systolic function, as one wall contracts while the other stretches in the opposite direction, a reduction in stroke volume, a larger LV volume in systole, and subsequently, a maladaptive LV dilatation.

Typically, BiV PM is used in patients who are not bradycardic. On the other hand, when patients with HF and low EF (≤35%) require PM placement for bradycardia, and when the ventricle is expected to be frequently paced (>40%), the implantation of a BiV PM rather than a right ventricular PM seems to be the best option regardless of NYHA symptoms (class IIa recommendation).

The purpose of the BiV PM is to allow simultaneous contraction of the LV septal and posterolateral walls, as well as the RV and LV, to improve cardiac function. To be beneficial, it has to track the atrial rate and pace both ventricles ~100% of the time. It cannot be in a standby mode. The AV tracking interval needs to be programmed shorter than the intrinsic PR interval to ensure ventricular tracking. AV delay is also optimized to ensure appropriate diastolic filling (a long AV delay reduces diastolic filling and leads to fusion of E–A waves on echo; a very short AV delay leads to atrial contraction near systole and A truncation).

In AF, the BiV PM is programmed in VVI mode (no A tracking). The AV conduction has to be aggressively slowed so that the intrinsic QRS rate is slow, and the BiV pacing would pace the ventricles at a rate faster than the spontaneous ventricular rate. AV nodal ablation may need to be performed to ensure consistent BiV pacing in patients with AF and an indication for BiV pacing.

The QRS of a BiV-initiated complex is typically narrower than the RV pacemaker-initiated complex and the baseline non-paced QRS, even though the QRS often remains wide. The morphology is not an LBBB morphology, and the QRS has at least one of the following two features: (i) prominent negativity in lead I, or (ii) prominent positivity in lead V1. If not negative, the QRS in lead I needs to have at least a q or Q wave. If the LV lead is positioned close to the LV apex, QRS may be negative in all precordial leads V_1–V_6, simulating RV apical pacing in those leads (Figure 14.1).

Examples of pacemaker ECGs are provided in Figures 14.2–14.6.

D. Implantable cardioverter defibrillator (ICD)
An ICD has one (V) or two (A + V) leads. In addition to antitachycardia capacity provided by the special RV lead, it has single- or dual-chamber sensing and pacing capacities (VVI or DDD).

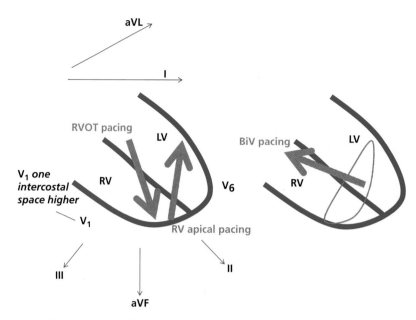

Figure 14.1 The paced QRS morphology varies according to the vector of depolarization. Analyze the QRS morphology in lead I, the inferior leads, and the precordial leads V$_1$–V$_6$.

In RV apical pacing, the QRS is characterized by a left axis and by being negative in the inferior leads II, III, and aVF. It has an LBBB morphology, and similarly to LBBB, QRS may be negative in V$_1$–V$_3$ and upright in V$_4$–V$_6$, I, and aVL. However, the vector of depolarization may also be looking away from all precordial leads, leading to a deep negative QS in V$_1$–V$_6$, and may be looking away to the right, leading to a negative QRS in lead I. If the vector is looking to the right, the QRS may paradoxically be upright in leads V$_1$ and V$_2$, simulating LV or BiV pacing (especially if V$_1$ is high in relation to the heart).

In RVOT pacing, the depolarization looks towards the inferior leads (vertical or right axis). QRS may be positive or negative in lead I. In the precordial leads, QRS simulates an LBBB morphology and, as opposed to RV apical pacing, cannot be negative all the way from V$_1$ through V$_6$.

In BiV pacing, the QRS: (1) is predominantly negative in lead I with a Q wave (QR or qR pattern), and (2) has a positive QRS or at least a prominent R wave in the precordial lead V$_1$. This is different from RV pacing, which occasionally has either one of these two features. If the LV lead is close to the apex, QRS may be negative in all precordial leads V$_1$–V$_6$, similar to RV pacing.

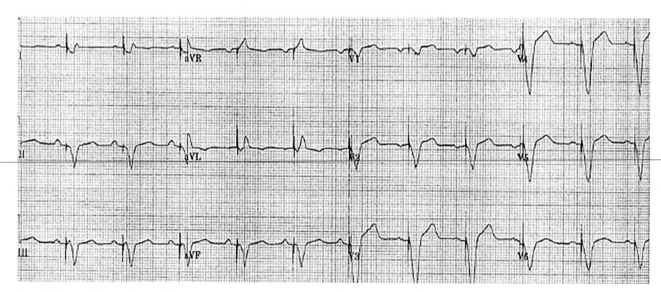

Figure 14.2 Ventricular pacing regularly tracking the sinus P activity (DDD PM, VAT action). The paced ventricular complexes have an LBBB morphology with QS or rS pattern that extends further to the left (V$_1$–V$_6$) than in a typical LBBB (in which QRS often transitions to positive in lead V$_4$). The large Q wave in lead I is not typical of RV apical pacing but may be seen if the vector of depolarization is turned a bit rightward. BiV pacing is unlikely, because of the negative QRS in V$_1$–V$_2$. This is not RVOT pacing, because in RVOT pacing the depolarization vector is directed up to down, and the QRS is consequently [+] in the inferior leads.

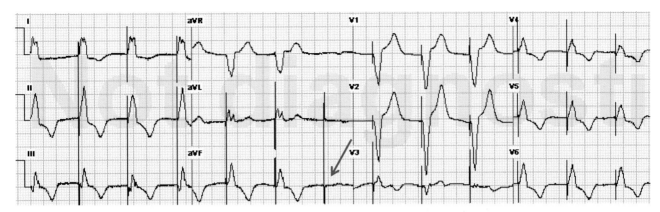

Figure 14.3 VVI pacing in a patient with no P wave (sinus arrest or subtle AF). RV lead is in the RVOT (QRS is positive in the inferior leads). Off/on failure to capture is noted (*arrow*, failure to capture). This is actually a temporary pacemaker. ***RVOT is an unstable position for a temporary pacemaker.***

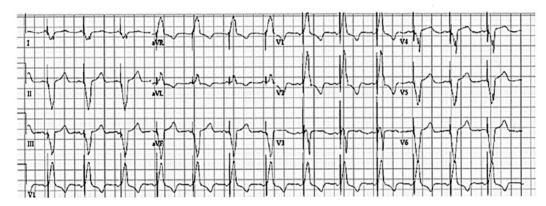

Figure 14.4 Ventricular pacing that consistently tracks a preceding sinus P wave. This is AV sequential pacing (probable DDD mode). Note that QRS is negative in lead I and starts with a Q wave, and QRS is positive in V_1: this is typical of BiV pacing. Also, PR is very short to ensure ~100% pacing, which is characteristic of BiV programming. Q or qR in lead I is rare in RV pacing, but is often present with BiV pacing (90%). If initially present with BiV pacing, the loss of Q wave in lead I is 100% predictive of loss of LV capture.

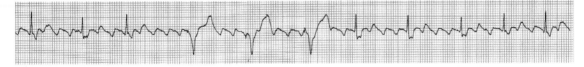

Figure 14.5 Atrial flutter with variable conduction. Note that when the R–R interval increases to >1200 ms (which corresponds to 6 large boxes, or a rate of 50 bpm), V pacing kicks in at an interval of 1000 ms (60 bpm). This is called *hysteresis*, wherein V pacing is initiated only when the heart rate drops well below the programmed pacing rate, allowing a reduction of V pacing.

The V lead has one (RV) or two coils (RV + SVC) that allow the delivery of the shock energy. The vector of shock goes between the battery can and the coil; in patients with two coils, the vector may be modified to provide superior efficacy (e.g., can-to-RV, or can + SVC-to-RV). The ICD is best placed on the left side to allow the vector of shock to be orthogonal to the heart, fully traversing the myocardium.

ICD patients often do not require pacing. The pacing function is a standby function that should only be initiated at very low ventricular rates (e.g., 34–40 bpm). Harmful ventricular pacing should be prevented.

The sensing function is what detects VF/VT. Typically, a certain ventricular rate is considered VT, regardless of its true origin. Many ICDs are programmed into two detection zones: VT and VF. Those two zones are differentiated by their rate (e.g., VT zone encompasses any ventricular rate of 170–220; VF zone encompasses ventricular rates >220). The ICD may have, on the other hand, SVT–VT discrimination algorithms, particularly the dual-chamber ICD, wherein the atrial lead can see the atrial activity:

i. Irregularity of ventricular activity during tachycardia → AF
ii. Progressive onset → sinus tachycardia
iii. More atrial activity than ventricular activity → SVT; more ventricular activity than atrial activity → VT
iv. No significant change in the morphology of the ventricular electrogram as compared to baseline → SVT

These discrimination algorithms are applied only for the VT zone. Any tachycardia in the VF zone is considered VF. Moreover, these discrimination algorithms *may* have a time out. For example, ICD may be programmed in such a way that if the tachycardia persists more than 5 minutes it is treated as VT regardless of the initial diagnosis.

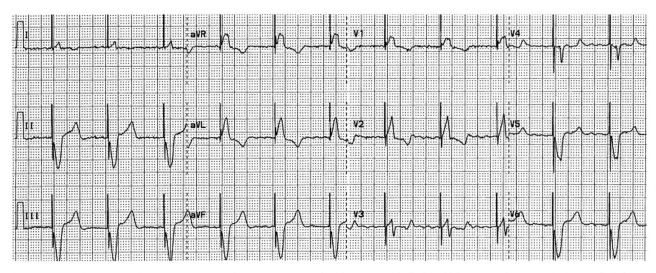

Figure 14.6 Prominent R wave in V₁–V₂ may suggest BiV pacing. However, there is no Q wave in lead I, which suggests that RV pacing is more likely (RV apical pacing by the fact that QRS is negative in the inferior leads and in V₄–V₆). **V₁ may be placed one intercostal space lower and the ECG repeated; QRS of V₁ should become negative in RV apical pacing.**

Typically, VT is initially treated with multiple cycles of antitachycardia pacing (ATP: overdrive ventricular pacing at a cycle length ~85% the tachycardia cycle length). If these fail, the ICD delivers a shock. If the tachycardia is fast enough to fall in the programmed VF zone, ICD immediately delivers a maximal shock. ATP enters the VT reentry cycle and breaks it in many patients; however, if the excitable gap of the reentry is wide, ATP may entrain the reentry at a faster rate, and may trigger further reentries that lead to VF. In fact, the most important ICD primary prevention trial (SCD-HeFT) recommended against ATP therapy and used a single-chamber rather than dual-chamber ICD, with shock therapy for tachycardia >187 bpm.[5]

III. Pacemaker intervals

A. VVI

A VVI pacemaker is characterized by two basic intervals: (i) *lower rate interval* (the basic pacing rate), and (ii) *ventricular refractory period*, during which the pacemaker cannot sense any signal or reset its timing based on signals.

Even if the lower rate interval is 1 second, the pacemaker may not initiate pacing until a 1.5 second pause occurs. In other words, the pacemaker may not start pacing until the ventricular rate falls to 40 bpm, after which it will start pacing at 60 bpm. This is the hysteresis function of a pacemaker, meant to reduce the burden of ventricular pacing.

> Note that "interval" terminology, rather than "rate," is used in PM programming. The rate corresponding to a particular interval is equal to 60,000 divided by this interval. For example, if the lower rate interval is 1500 ms, the lower rate is 40 bpm.

B. DDD pacemaker's four basic intervals (Figure 14.7)

A DDD pacemaker is characterized by four basic intervals:[4,6]

a. *Lower rate interval* is the basic interval between paced P waves (the basic pacing rate). A hysteresis function may be established to delay the onset of atrial pacing.

b. *Ventricular refractory period* occurs after a sensed or paced ventricular event. This prevents the ventricular lead from sensing the residual energy from its own ventricular spike and from seeing and double-counting the QRS or the T wave.

c. *Post-ventricular atrial refractory period* (PVARP) begins immediately after the start of a ventricular event. An atrial activity falling in PVARP cannot initiate P-synchronous pacing. PVARP is meant to prevent: (i) sensing the ventricular activity by the atrial channel and tracking it (far-field), (ii) sensing and tracking a very premature PAC or a retrograde P wave occurring after a PVC. If the PM tracks those early P waves, pacemaker-mediated tachycardia (PMT) is initiated; a long PVARP protects against PMT. PVARP is initiated after a sensed or paced ventricular event.

d. *Programmed AV delay* from a sensed P wave (sAV) or a paced P wave (pAV) (A = atrial, V = ventricular). As opposed to the paced P wave, the PM senses an intrinsic P wave only after the atrial activity has spread for some time; therefore, the sensed AV interval is programmed shorter than the paced AV interval by ~30 ms.

C. Two other intervals are derived from the four basic intervals

a. *Atrial escape interval*, which is the V-to-A interval. After an intrinsic QRS or a PVC occurs, the pacemaker is reset. How long does it take for the pacemaker to pace the atrium? Atrial escape interval is the answer. After a sensed QRS, the PM initiates a new atrial escape interval. It is equal to (lower rate interval – AV interval)

b. *Total atrial refractory period* (TARP) = AV interval + PVARP

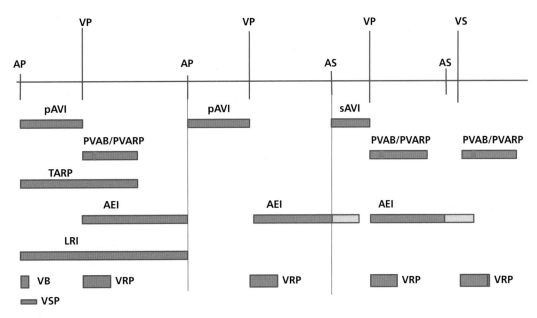

Figure 14.7 DDD pacemaker timing intervals.

AP, atrial paced event; AS, atrial sensed event; VP, ventricular paced event; VS, ventricular sensed event.

AEI, atrial escape interval after any ventricular sensed or paced activity (the occurrence of an atrial sensed event aborts AEI); LRI, lower rate interval; pAVI, paced atrioventricular interval; PVARP, post-ventricular atrial refractory period; PVAB, post-ventricular atrial blanking period; sAVI, sensed atrioventricular interval; VB, ventricular blanking (post-atrial); VSP, ventricular safety pacing.

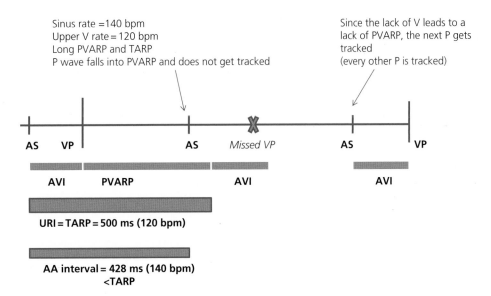

Figure 14.8 Sinus/atrial tachycardia with atrial rate > upper rate. Case where TARP (total atrial refractory period)=URI (upper rate interval), which leads to 2:1 ventricular pacing pattern. Other abbreviations as in Figure 14.7.

D. Upper rate behavior (see Figures 14.8, 14.9)

In the case of sinus tachycardia, the pacemaker senses the intrinsic sinus P waves and tracks them, leading to fast ventricular pacing. However, the pacemaker can only track the P waves up to a certain upper rate, called the *upper rate limit (e.g., 500ms=120bpm)*. If the atrial rate is faster than this upper rate, the PM will only track some of the P waves. If this upper rate limit is equal to the TARP and if the atrial rate exceeds 120bpm, the P wave that follows the paced QRS will fall into PVARP, which means that only every other P wave gets conducted; the patient's rate suddenly falls from 120 to 60bpm (Figure 14.9). However, if PVARP is reduced in such a way that TARP is shorter than the upper rate interval (e.g., TARP=400ms, TARP rate 150bpm), the ventricular rate will remain steady at 120bpm even if the atrial rate exceeds 120bpm. P waves will be conducted with progressively longer PR intervals. One P will drop every few cycles in a pseudo-Wenckebach fashion. When the atrial rate reaches 150bpm (TARP), every other P wave gets conducted. Shortening the TARP, however, allowed a delay in onset of the 2:1 atrial conduction. PM can also be programmed to have an adaptive PVARP and AV delay that decrease with exercise, allowing a reduction in TARP and in the onset of sudden rate drop.

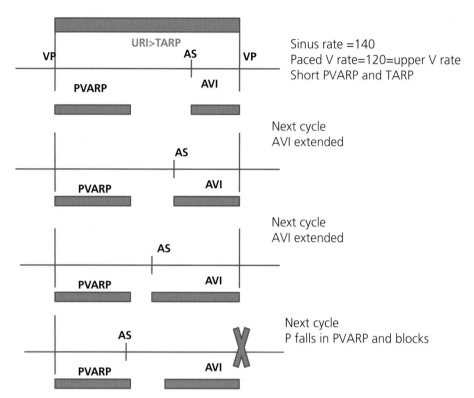

Figure 14.9 Sinus tachycardia with pseudo-Wenckebach ventricular pacing pattern. In contrast to Figure 14.8, PVARP is short with TARP <URI. This shortened PVARP allows AS to fall outside PVARP and get tracked. AVI extends after every cycle, until one beat drops. It is a pseudo-Wenckebach rather than a true Wenckebach pattern, as the R–R interval remains steady rather than shortens.

Unlike patients with a dual-chamber PM, patients with BiV often need a higher upper rate limit (e.g., 140 bpm) to ensure consistent biventricular pacing at upper rates and prevent Wenckebach from occurring, particularly since higher sinus rates are seen in decompensated HF at rest and with activity. The prolongation of the paced AV delay (Wenckebach) that occurs as the atrial rate reaches the upper rate may allow an undesirable intrinsic AV conduction. A short PVARP is necessary to allow an increase in the upper rate, and a rate-adaptive PVARP that automatically decrements at higher rates may be programmed.

E. Prevention of crosstalk[4,6]
Atrial-initiated ventricular blanking period
The pacer spike has a high voltage (measured in volts), much higher than the voltage of the intrinsic cardiac activity (millivolts). If the ventricular lead senses the atrial spike, ventricular pacing will be inhibited after atrial pacing. Therefore, atrial pacing automatically initiates a short interval called the *ventricular blanking period*, during which the ventricular sensing is totally blind to any signal. This only occurs after a paced atrial event (not an intrinsic atrial event).

A ventricular activity that is detected early after the atrial activity (<110 ms) but beyond the ventricular blanking period may be a far-field artifact or a PVC. The PM tends to immediately pace over it. As opposed to the blanking period, this activity cannot be ignored; in fact, if it turns out to be a PVC that is ignored, the ventricular pacing that follows the end of the AV delay would fall on the PVC's T wave and trigger VF. Conversely, it cannot be automatically considered PVC and allowed to reset ventricular pacing, as there is a high rate of atrial output artifacts within this zone (called afterpotentials). That is why, during this interval, any sensed activity by the V channel triggers immediate V pacing (*ventricular safety pacing*). **On ECG, a spike in the middle of a PVC with a short PR interval implies safety pacing rather than undersensing.**

Ventricular-initiated atrial refractory period
The PVARP is meant to prevent the PM from tracking retrograde or premature P waves. The PM sees the atrial activity during most of the PVARP and counts it for mode-switch purposes, but does not track it with V pacing. However, the PVARP, whether initiated by a sensed or a paced QRS, contains a small interval called PVAB (post-ventricular atrial blanking), where the atrial channel does not even see any electrical activity. In fact, in order to detect the small electrograms of atrial tachyarrhythmias, atrial sensitivity is programmed high, and may erroneously detect ventricular activity. PVAB prevents it from sensing ventricular activity and counting it as a P wave. PVAB and PVARP are initiated after both paced and intrinsic ventricular events (the atrial channel may sense the ventricular pacing spike but also the QRS ventricular complex, which is much louder than the atrial complex). Overcounting P waves, including those falling in a refractory period, leads to a harmful mode switch (to VVI).

F. Upper rate intervals (see Figure 14.10)
In a DDD pacemaker, the **upper rate limit** (or maximal tracking rate) designates the maximal ventricular pacing in response to an **intrinsic/ sensed atrial rate** (e.g., tracking intrinsic sinus tachycardia in a patient with complete AV block).

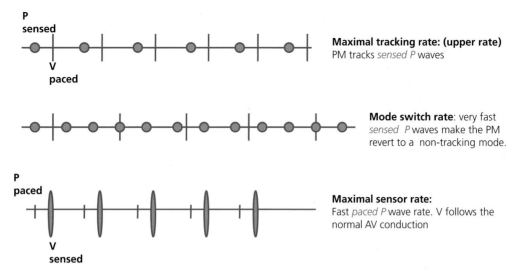

Figure 14.10 Difference between maximal tracking rate, mode-switch rate, and maximal sensor rate.

The ***mode-switch rate*** is the maximal ***intrinsic/sensed*** atrial rate at which the pacemaker continues to track some of the atrial rate and pace the ventricle. Beyond the mode-switch rate, the pacemaker calls the atrial rhythm atrial tachyarrhythmia and reverts to a non-tracking mode (VVI-R). The mode-switch rate is higher, sometimes much higher, than the upper rate limit (e.g., the PM remains in DDD mode and continues to track some of the atrial rate up to 170 bpm, while only pacing the ventricle at 120 bpm).

In a DDD-R pacemaker, the ***upper sensor rate*** is the maximal ***paced*** atrial rate of a sensor-driven pacemaker. This is different from the maximal tracking rate, which refers to the tracking of intrinsic atrial activity.*

G. Magnet mode

Magnet mode is the pacemaker behavior when a magnet is applied over it. A magnet closes a reed switch in the generator and makes it convert to an asynchronous ventricular and/or dual pacing mode (VOO or DOO). This mode is useful as a means of breaking PMT (pacemaker-mediated tachycardia). Furthermore, the magnet rate is programmed in a way that indicates the status of the battery (e.g., a lower magnet rate indicates that the battery is close to end of life). A magnet is part of the modem used in pacemaker transtelephonic follow-up.

A magnet may be present in programmer heads, and this temporarily closes the reed switch, ending a PMT. However, after the programmer is turned on, the magnet effect is functional for only a short period of time.

In contrast to a PM, the application of a magnet on an ICD does not affect the pacing mode or the sensing function, i.e., the DDD pacing function of an ICD keeps its DDD pacing function. It does not affect arrhythmia detection either. It only inhibits antitachycardia therapy and shock.

IV. Leads (see Figure 14.11)

Leads detect electrical activity between two electrodes (anode and cathode) and deliver the output current between these two electrodes. A unipolar lead has one electrode at the distal tip, the metal of the can constituting the other electrode. The pacing current flows through a large circuit and may cause stimulation of the chest muscle and a large pacing spike on the ECG. Also, the sensing current is large and is prone to sensing myopotentials.

A bipolar lead has two electrodes on its distal end (ring and tip electrodes) creating a smaller sensing and pacing circuit. However, it has to contain two wires to conduct signals to and from both electrodes and needs to be slightly thicker. If the ring wire breaks, the lead converts to a unipolar mode.

A bipolar defibrillator lead contains two pacing electrodes and one or two defibrillator coils: one at the distal end (RV coil) ± one more proximal (SVC coil). After VT is sensed, the defibrillation circuit occurs between the can, which functions as an electrode, and the RV coil. Various configurations are possible (e.g., energy can be delivered between the can and the SVC coil as one pole, and the RV coil as second pole). Generator placement on the left side allows delivery of energy that is orthogonal to the heart and traverses it more effectively.

The current that flows through the lead and is delivered to the myocardium depends on both the battery voltage delivered and the lead resistance/impedance. In fact: current (mA) = voltage/resistance. The battery voltage is typically 2.8 volts. The lead itself needs to have a high impedance to reduce the current that is being drained. The lead tip needs to have a low resistance to allow electrical flow to the myocardium.

Upon new PM implantation, the pacing threshold rises over the first few weeks then goes down to a chronic baseline 8 weeks later. This is due to the initial inflammation at the lead tip and mandates programming of high pacing thresholds initially, followed by reprogramming 8 weeks later. A steroid-eluting lead prevents this phenomenon and allows chronically lower pacing thresholds.

Pacing leads are insulated, meaning they are covered with material that does not conduct electricity and prevents loss of current from the lead, allowing current to travel all the way to the myocardium.

---

* The upper sensor rate of patients with preserved AV conduction may exceed the maximal tracking rate. In fact, in patients with preserved AV conduction, a high atrial sensor rate, higher than the tracking rate, will lead to a correspondingly high ventricular activity through the native AV conduction.

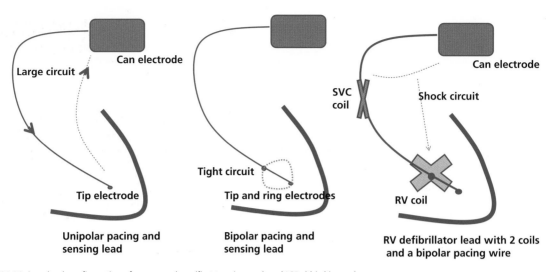

Figure 14.11 Various lead configurations for pacemakers (first two images) and ICD (third image).

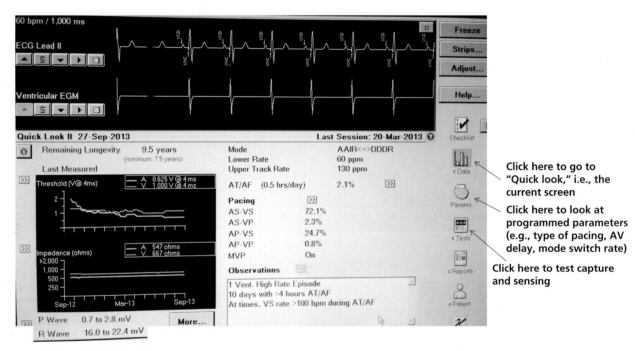

Figure 14.12 Example of a "quick look" or "summary" screen of pacemaker/ICD interrogation. On the right, the three most important icons are indicated (data, parameters, and tests).

On top of the screen, three types of live recordings are shown: (1) surface ECG (uppermost recording), (2) intracardiac electrograms (EGM), which capture the actual signals occurring in each cardiac chamber (in this case, ventricular EGM is shown), and (3) marker representation, which indicates how the pacemaker sees and interprets these signals. AS and VS are sensed intrinsic atrial and ventricular activities, while AP and VP are paced atrial and ventricular activities. The pacemaker may interpret a signal as VS on the marker channel, while in fact it is a T wave oversensing, false signal, or far-field atrial sensing. *Looking at the EGMs allows one to understand what the issue is; looking at the markers allows one to see how the pacemaker interprets or misinterprets signals*.

At the bottom left, capture thresholds, impedance, and the sensed amplitudes of A and V are shown.

V. Systematic PM/ICD interrogation using the programmer

A. Summary screen

Under summary/quick look/diagnostics (Figure 14.12), look at the following:

- Battery longevity: end of life (EOL) means the battery is depleted and can no longer consistently support PM functions. ERI (elective replacement indicator) means the battery voltage is reduced but will be able to support basic functions for up to 3 months.
- Pacing mode and percentage of ventricular pacing. The latter should be as limited as possible in patients without complete, chronic AV block. Conversely, ventricular pacing should be close to 100% in patients with a CRT device.

- Episodes of high atrial rate and episodes of automatic mode switch, indicative of atrial tachyarrhythmias. These may dictate rate-control therapies. Also, atrial tachyarrhythmias lasting >6 minutes have been associated with an increased risk of stroke. Frequent or prolonged periods of high atrial rate >120–140 bpm may be indicative of atrial tachyarrhythmias, sometimes below the mode-switch rate. A high atrial rate beyond a certain point (e.g., 140–150 bpm) should be programmed as a trigger for electrogram (EGM) recording. The EGMs of these atrial activities should be reviewed. The sudden onset and steady rate distinguish atrial arrhythmia from sinus tachycardia. If atrial arrhythmia is confirmed, the mode-switch rate may need to be reduced.
- Episodes of high ventricular rates (whether in the monitoring or treatment zone).
- Review stored EGMs, if any (arrhythmias).
- Check the programmed parameters:
  - Lower rate interval and AV delay. AV delay should be programmed long enough to promote intrinsic AV conduction.
  - PVARP.
  - Maximal tracking rate and mode-switch rate of sensed P waves.
  - Sensor-driven paced P wave rate, and sensor-driven rate histogram. If a sedentary patient is having frequent sensor-driven rates, the rate-adaptive slope and the maximal rate may need to be reduced. The opposite may be necessary in a young active patient.

B. Lead impedance
Check impedances and impedance trends of A and V leads. Any significant change (>200 ohms) in lead impedance can indicate lead failure.

C. Capture testing
- *Test A capture in a DDD pacemaker*: in a patient with sinus rhythm, increase the atrial rate beyond the patient's intrinsic sinus rate. A high pacing output (in volts) is initially selected then reduced in small decrements until atrial capture is lost. The lowest value before loss of capture is the capture threshold.
  Testing is performed in DDD mode. In patients with intrinsic V activation, the loss of atrial capture is seen as a loss of ventricular sensed events; make sure the AV delay is long enough to allow intrinsic V activation for this test (if possible).
- *Test V capture in DDD pacemaker*: increase the atrial rate and set a short AV delay to ensure ventricular pacing during this test. Alternatively, testing may be performed in VVI mode. Gradual step-down of ventricular output is performed until V capture is lost.
- The output energy is determined by the *output voltage* as well as the *pulse duration*. Increasing the pulse duration increases the output; beyond 0.3 ms, increasing the pulse duration does not affect the output by much. Testing may be performed by varying the voltage at a constant pulse duration of 0.3–0.5 ms. The programmed output should be double the pacing threshold. Typically, the pacing thresholds for A and V are <2.5 volts at 0.5 ms, particularly with steroid-eluting leads.
- In temporary PMs, one typically programs the output in terms of generator current (milliamperes) rather than voltage. The temporary PM is usually a VVI PM, so testing is similar to the capture testing in VVI PM: increase the pacing rate and start pacing at a high output with small decrements until V capture is lost.

D. Sensing assessment
Sensitivity is the programmed wall below which the PM cannot detect electrical activity. The higher the wall is in millivolts, the less sensitive the PM is, and the more likely it is to dismiss noise but also, on occasions, native complexes. To test sensing of the V channel, set the PM in VVI mode and reduce the pacing rate below the patient's intrinsic rate (if the patient has a tolerable intrinsic rate). Start at a low millivolt sensitivity then slowly increase until the PM stops sensing intrinsic activity and starts pacing at the low set rate. Sensitivity should be set below that value. *Note that testing for sensing involves maneuvers opposite to those used in testing for capture (low rate and starting with the lowest setting).*

In addition, current PMs measure the *sensed amplitude* of the intrinsic A and V activities. The sensed RV amplitude is typically >5 mV, while the sensed A amplitude is typically >2 mV. The sensitivity should be a half or a third this value. A very low sensitivity may detect myopotential noise or oversense T wave.

VI. Pacemaker troubleshooting
A. Undersensing or failure to sense
Ventricular undersensing is a situation in which the pacemaker does not see intrinsic QRS and thus does not get inhibited by it. This leads to overpacing, with pacing spikes occurring regularly, including early after intrinsic QRS complexes and unrelated to them.

Causes of undersensing:

- Lead damage: lead fracture, insulation break, or loose connection of the lead to the generator (loose set screw, mainly seen early after PM implantation).
- Inappropriate programming (low sensitivity).
- Undersensing of a PVC is possible and is not considered abnormal, especially when the PVC occurs shortly after QRS, within the ventricular refractory period. PVC may not reset the atrial escape interval, and the next P wave may fall close to the PVC.
- Undersensing of atrial activity may be seen in AF, where many of the small-amplitude atrial waves are not sensed by the device. This precludes mode switching and allows tracking of the waves that are sensed, an inappropriately fast tracking. This is treated by increasing the atrial sensitivity if AF is paroxysmal, or reprogramming the PM to a VVI mode if AF is permanent.

  Undersensing may also be seen in atrial flutter, where every other P wave falls in the blanking portion of PVARP and is not sensed. This precludes mode switching and allows tracking of the sensed P waves (e.g., atrial rate of 280 bpm, every other P is sensed and tracked at a fast rate of 140 bpm). It is treated by shortening the blanking period.

B. Oversensing
Ventricular oversensing is a situation in which the pacemaker senses electrical activity that is not QRS and considers it V, therefore inhibiting the ventricular output. It does not pace the ventricle when it should. This leads to underpacing and a paucity of pacer spikes.

Causes of oversensing:

- Lead fracture or insulation break creating false signals.
- Inappropriate programming.
- The ventricular lead senses from a distance the atrial spike and considers it a ventricular event (far-field crosstalk). This is reduced by creating a post-atrial ventricular blanking period.
- Oversensing of a tall T wave and considering it QRS.
- Oversensing of myopotentials (diaphragmatic contractions, especially with unipolar leads) and electromagnetic interference.

Undersensing leads to overpacing, and oversensing leads to underpacing.

C. Failure to capture
In this case, the pacer spike occurs appropriately but is not followed by any paced activity (a paced QRS is not seen).
Causes of failure to capture:

- Lead fracture or insulation break.
- Inappropriate programming.
- Battery depletion.
- An increase in capture threshold due to drugs (class Ic overdose), MI, hyperkalemia, hypoxia, acidosis.
- Atrial failure to capture may be due to unsuspected AF. Many of the fibrillatory waves are unseen/undersensed by the PM, which leads to undersensing and pacing over AF without capture.
- Failure to capture may also occur in case of undersensing a premature complex, with subsequent pacing very close to it, in the refractory phase. The latter case may occur normally (functional non-capture).

D. Manifestations of lead fracture and insulation defect
Lead fracture can cause undersensing and loss of capture, but also oversensing when both fractured ends abut each other, creating signals (false signals or "make-break artifacts").

The insulation material protects and conceals signals within the lead. An insulation break results in loss of current along the lead path and, consequently, loss of capture. This break also results in loss of sensed signals and, consequently, undersensing. Oversensing may also be seen, as signals coming from the surrounding structures easily penetrate the unshielded lead (Figure 14.13).

Oversensing, by itself, can lead to undersensing. For example, oversensing false signals puts the respective channel in a refractory period, during which an intrinsic complex may occur and be missed. *A pattern of oversensing, undersensing, and intermittent loss of capture may occur with lead problems and progress to a chaotic pattern of pauses and overpacing*.

Lead fracture or insulation break is suspected from analysis of the lead impedance (a recent ↑ >200 ohms in case of fracture or ↓ >200 ohms in case of insulation break). Lead or insulation breaks may be intermittent, and may be associated with a normal impedance, sensing, and capture at the time of interrogation. If an intermittent break is suspected, review stored EGMs looking for oversensed false signals, or perform Holter monitoring if the EGMs are unrevealing (PM may not store EGMs as it does not recognize that there is a problem). Also, perform maneuvers: move the generator in its pocket, move the ipsilateral arm (up and behind the back), perform a pulling maneuver with the ipsilateral arm, and assess capture during deep inspiration and after cough. CXR should be performed, but it does not always detect a lead fracture.

Some causes of lead problems: subclavian crush syndrome (the lead is crushed against the clavicle as it passes through the subclavian vein), twiddler syndrome (the lead twists on itself if the pocket is loose, especially in old patients), loose connector screws.

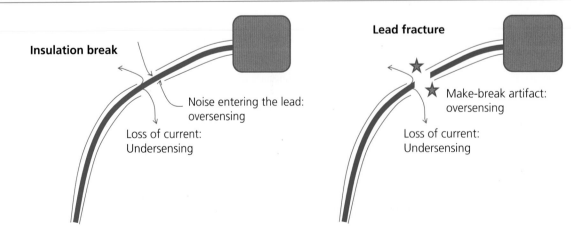

Figure 14.13 Insulation break and lead fracture.

E. Absence of a pacemaker spike (or spikes) when there should be one

This is caused by oversensing, failure to capture with small overlooked pacer spikes, or total battery failure. Differentiate by magnet application, which solves oversensing but not the other two issues.

F. Pacemaker syndrome

This syndrome is seen in 10–20% of patients with VVI pacemakers. It results from the lack of atrial contribution to cardiac output *and/or* from atrial contraction against closed AV valves. It may also be seen in patients with P-synchronous DDD pacing if the AV delay is very long, such that P wave abuts the preceding QRS, particularly during exercise. Also, a long AV delay facilitates retrograde VA conduction: a long AV delay gives enough time for the atria to recover from their refractory period by the time the ventricular activity occurs. Retrograde P waves lead to atrial contraction against closed AV valves with a subsequent increase in atrial pressure and a reduction in cardiac output, i.e., pacemaker syndrome. While PVARP prevents retrograde P waves from inducing PMT, retrograde P waves remain harmful by inducing a pacemaker syndrome.

G. Pacemaker-mediated tachycardia (PMT) (see Figure 14.14)

PMT is a complication of DDD pacing. After a paced QRS or a PVC, retrograde atrial activation (VA conduction) may occur if the atria are not in their refractory period. Many (but not all) patients are capable of retrograde VA conduction; this is more likely in patients with intact AV conduction but may interestingly be seen in those with complete AV block. The retrograde P wave may be tracked by the ventricular channel, leading to a short R–R interval close to the upper tracking rate of the pacemaker (usually 110–130 paced beats per minute). This cycle continues, leading to PMT.

In order for retrograde atrial activation to occur, the preceding atrial activity must be far (no atrial refractory period). *In order to be seen and tracked by the pacemaker, the retrograde P wave must also fall beyond the PVARP.* In *patients whose atrial activity is paced*, PMT may be triggered by: (a) a PVC, wherein the atrium gets enough time to recover from its refractory period; (b) a preceding atrial non-capture, wherein the atrium does not get depolarized and thus is easy to stimulate retrogradely; (c) atrial undersensing with subsequent atrial overpacing and functional non-capture; (d) atrial oversensing of far-field QRS with initiation of AV delay without any atrial activity (Figure 14.14). In addition, whether atrial activity is intrinsic or paced, a very long AV interval may propitiate VA conduction by giving the atria time to recover from their refractory period.

PMT is prevented by prolonging the PVARP (e.g., 300 ms) and further automatic prolongation of PVARP after a PVC. PVARP may be made dynamic: it prolongs after a PVC but shortens with tachycardia to allow upper rate behavior. When the ventricle is paced at a rate close to the upper rate, the differential diagnosis includes PMT or tracking of atrial tachycardia; in this case, a "PMT algorithm" allows the pacemaker to omit ventricular pacing once so that PMT, if present, will break. Acutely, a magnet inhibits any sensing, including P sensing, and stops PMT.

H. Differential diagnosis of a tachycardia occurring in a patient who has a DDD PM

- PMT, where the pacemaker tracks retrograde P waves.
- Atrial arrhythmia is getting tracked by the pacemaker for one of the following reasons:
  - The atrial rate is slower than the mode-switch rate.
  - The arrhythmia is atrial flutter with sensing and tracking of every other flutter wave, or AF with sensing of many, but not all, of the atrial waves; this alternate sensing prevents sensing the high rate and mode switching. Pacemakers usually allow for a refractory sense during PVARP, except when some of the AF or flutter waves fall in the blanking portion of PVARP.

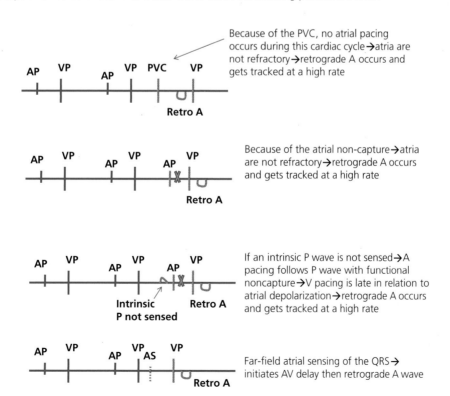

Figure 14.14 Triggers and mechanisms of PMT.

○ AF waves and some atrial tachycardia waves have a small amplitude and may, consequently, fall below the programmed atrial sensitivity wall; therefore, many of them are not sensed by the device and do not trigger a mode switch.

In all of these cases, P waves are getting tracked by the pacemaker. Differentiate from PMT by pacemaker interrogation and by placing a magnet. The P waves persist in the case of atrial arrhythmia, whereas the rhythm goes back to sinus in the case of PMT.

The inappropriate P-wave tracking is treated by reducing the rate at which mode switch occurs, by increasing atrial sensitivity, or by reducing the PVAB so that alternate atrial waves do not fall in the blanking period.

- Oversensing myopotentials and tracking them.
- Any VT or SVT/AF that is being spontaneously conducted, independently of the pacemaker. In contrast to the above three diagnoses, the ventricular activity is intrinsic rather than paced (no V pacing spike).

PM and ICD magnet effect

Placing a magnet over a PM makes it lose its sensing functions. It turns to a VOO or DOO mode – that is, ventricular ± atrial asynchronous pacing – at a particular magnet rate. This can stop tracking retrograde P waves and PMT. The same magnet effect occurs in the first few seconds after placement of some programmer heads over the PM.

The magnet rate correlates with the battery life; the transtelephonic checkup assesses the PM response to magnet placement and the magnet rate.

A magnet over an ICD eliminates its antitachycardia and defibrillation function, but does not affect its pacing/sensing function (a DDD function remains DDD). Therefore, it does not stop PMT.

I. Fusion and pseudofusion

A pacemaker spike may be seen within a QRS that is intrinsically conducted through the AV node, or just before or after it. A pacer spike may also be seen just before, just after, or within a PVC. This does not imply undersensing, as it takes time for the V channel to sense the intrinsic V activity. Even a pacing spike falling as far as the T wave may not mean undersensing. A ventricular pacing spike falling just before the intrinsic complex may lead to a fusion beat, i.e., fusion between the pacing complex and the intrinsic complex. A ventricular pacing spike falling too close to the intrinsic complex may not lead to any conduction of pacer activity, a phenomenon called pseudofusion. In this case, the lack of capture is called functional non-capture (Figures 14.15, 14.16).

On the other hand, in a patient receiving both atrial and ventricular pacing, a PVC may fall over the atrial spike. The ventricular activity will be perceived as a ventricular activity occurring within the early period after atrial pacing and will trigger ventricular safety pacing. Thus, in addition to the A pacing spike, a V pacing spike is seen within the QRS or ST–T at a very short AV delay (Figure 14.15). The ventricular safety pacing should not be perceived as undersensing.

A PVC that falls too close to the intrinsic or paced ventricular complex, within the ventricular refractory period, may not be sensed and thus may not reset the atrial escape interval.

J. Diaphragmatic stimulation

Diaphragmatic stimulation may occur when the atrial lead is laterally placed in the RA, which stimulates the right phrenic nerve. It may also occur with a coronary sinus lead that stimulates the left phrenic nerve (BiV PM). Left diaphragmatic stimulation may also be seen with the RV lead, but more so if it perforates into the LV. That is why perforation must be excluded whenever diaphragmatic pacing is observed.

Diaphragmatic stimulation may occur late after device placement, in which case it is usually related to an insulation break with loss of current into the surrounding muscles (diaphragm, deltopectoral muscles). Deltopectoral muscle stimulation is due either to the use of unipolar leads or to insulation break.

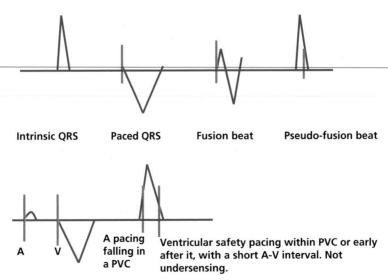

Figure 14.15 Fusion, pseudofusion, and ventricular safety pacing.

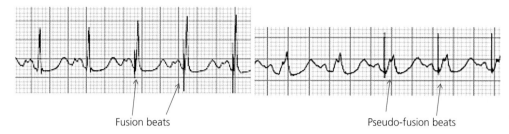

Fusion beats   Pseudo-fusion beats

Figure 14.16 In fusion beats, the native conduction reaches the ventricle around the same time as the expected pacemaker spike, leading to a fusion between the native and paced QRS complex. In pseudofusion, the QRS seen is purely the result of the native conduction, the pacemaker spike does not result in any ventricular stimulation; the resulting QRS is similar in morphology to the intrinsic QRS.

VII. Perioperative management of PM and ICD (during any surgery)

Electrocautery may lead to oversensing of electrical noise and inhibition of the PM output. Oversensing may also result in ICD shock.

Other possible complications: PM resets to a VOO mode, i.e., noise reversion mode; permanent damage to the pulse generator; or myocardial thermal injury at the lead tip, changing the sensing and pacing thresholds.

Preoperatively, cardiac rhythm devices are managed as follows:

1. PM: for pacer-dependent patients, as evidenced by the baseline ECG and by the device interrogation, program the PM to VOO or DOO mode preoperatively (asynchronous uninhibited pacing) or place a magnet over it.

2. ICD: placing a magnet will inhibit the antitachycardia therapies, but will not lead to asynchronous pacing. Thus, if the patient has an ICD and is pacer-dependent, a magnet is not enough. The pacing function is programmed preoperatively to VOO or DOO, and the VT therapies are turned off.

Either way, postoperatively, the PM or ICD needs to be interrogated to assess sensing and capture thresholds, to ensure there is no "phantom" reprogramming of the device (noise reversion mode), and to turn the ICD therapies on.

For external cardioversion or defibrillation in a patient who has a PM, place the paddles in the anteroposterior position and at least 4 inches (10 cm) away from the pulse generator (right parasternal, left paraspinal). The anteroposterior position ensures that the shock vector is not coaxial with the leads. Interrogate the PM after the procedure.

VIII. Differential diagnosis and management of the patient who presents with ICD shock(s)

The differential diagnosis of an ICD shock includes:

1. Appropriate shock for VT/VF: clinically, the patient often feels palpitations, malaise, or dizziness before the shock occurs. In the case of sudden and repeated episodes of VT (VT storm), look for triggers: active ischemia, decompensated HF, electrolyte imbalance, TdP (long QT due to drugs). In a patient with chronic cardiomyopathy, sudden back-to-back episodes of VT/VF may not have any particular trigger.

Manage the triggers, and, if necessary, place the patient on amiodarone + β-blocker, or sotalol.

2. Inappropriate shock for a supraventricular arrhythmia: the ICD considers any tachycardia above a certain programmed rate (e.g., 170 bpm) as VT and treats it as such, with antitachycardia overdrive pacing initially, then a shock if it persists. This may occur with AF, atrial flutter, AVNRT/AVRT, or sinus tachycardia during strenuous activity (clue to the latter: shock during strenuous activity).

The ICD may use SVT–VT discrimination algorithms to withhold on treating SVT.

3. Inappropriate shock due to oversensing:
   a. Oversensing T wave.
   b. Far-field sensing of the atrial spike.
   c. Myopotentials: oversensing myopotentials may be reproduced by asking the patient to exercise (move arms across shoulder, compress hands together).
   d. Electromagnetic interference (e.g., welding).
   e. Lead fracture or insulation break may also lead to oversensing of false signals (shock during repetitive shoulder movements). Hints: lead impedance changes with time, sometimes intermittently; interrogation shows extra spikes on the ventricular channel, particularly when performed during deep inspiration or during arm or can movement. Also, the situation in which the shock occurs helps with the diagnosis of lead issues, myopotentials, and electromagnetic interference.

4. In the MADIT II and SCD-HeFT trials, ~33% of patients experienced a shock by 2 years of therapy. A third of shocks were inappropriate (AF 44%, SVT 36%, oversensing 20%). In both those trials, the occurrence of any shock, appropriate or inappropriate, was associated with a two- to fourfold increase in mortality from progressive HF.[7,8] A shock, whether appropriate (VT) or inappropriate (AF, SVT), implies a more severe underlying HF and thus a higher mortality by association. However, shock or even ATP may be directly harmful. In fact, the MADIT-RIT trial suggests that reducing VT therapies, whether ATP or shock, through alternative programming reduces mortality by 55%, which implies a direct role of unnecessary ICD therapies, including ATP, in speeding death.[9] Even what is considered appropriate therapy for VT is not always clinically appropriate, as many of these VTs are not sustained and spontaneously convert. An example of alternative programming used in MADIT-RIT consists of a higher rate requirement of at least 200 bpm for initiation of therapy, and a longer delay to therapy (e.g., 12 seconds or 40 beats in the VT zone 200–250 bpm, and 2.5 seconds in the VF zone ≥250 bpm). This restrictive strategy is used in primary prevention and may not apply to secondary prevention, where a lower threshold for intervention is applied, guided by the rate of prior VTs.

5. Management. An ED visit is usually required after an ICD shock, especially if the clinical status changes or multiple shocks occur. Interrogate the device to distinguish between situations 1, 2, and 3 above.[10] Look for triggers, assess HF status, and perform ECG and chest

X-ray. In the absence of a reversible cause, institute an antiarrhythmic agent. Because amiodarone may increase the defibrillation threshold and VF detection threshold, the ICD defibrillation threshold may need to be retested after amiodarone institution. Also, amiodarone may slow VT below the detection zone; thus, a new, lower-limit VT monitoring zone should be instituted to see if this phenomenon happens.

In case of SVT, make sure SVT–VT discrimination algorithms are on (only applies to VT zone, not VF zone) and consider using a higher rate threshold for the institution of VT therapies. SVT may be treated with antiarrhythmic drugs.

IX. Evidence and guidelines supporting various pacing devices

A. DDD or AAI vs. VVI pacing

The Danish randomized trial of patients with sick sinus syndrome has shown that VVI pacing increases mortality (~1.5 times) in comparison to AAI pacing, and doubles the risk of AF and stroke. This is due to the deleterious effect of unnecessary ventricular pacing in a patient with sinus node disease.[11]

Other trials that included an exclusive (UKPACE) or predominant AV nodal disease population (CTOPP) have overall shown that DDD vs. VVI pacing reduces the incidence of AF and improves quality of life, through preservation of AV synchrony and LA pressure, without affecting mortality.[12,13]

The MOST trial of DDD vs. VVI pacing has shown that regardless of the type of pacemaker used, ventricular pacing >40% of the time increased the risk of AF and HF. A similar result was obtained when AV sequential pacing at 70 bpm was compared with stand-by ventricular pacing in ICD patients in the DAVID trial (>40% V pacing worsens outcomes); and in a MADIT II analysis (>50% V pacing worsens outcomes).[2,3] Overall, V pacing >40% of the time vs. < 40% is associated with a 3–4.5 times higher risk of HF hospitalization. However, while the highest risk is associated with >40% ventricular pacing, there is a linear and continuous increase in risk between 0% and 40% of ventricular pacing in the DAVID trial, and even more so in the MOST trial.

The main lesson learned from these trials is that it is most important to reduce ventricular pacing. If ventricular pacing is necessary (AV block), the main advantage of DDD over VVI pacing is better symptom control and a reduction of AF incidence. Therefore, DDD pacing is recommended for patients with AV nodal disease, except if permanent AF is present. Minimal ventricular pacing should be ensured; for example, program the AV interval as long as 250 ms after a sensed P wave to promote intrinsic ventricular activation.[14] PR may be programmed long but rate-adaptive, wherein it is allowed to shorten when the atrial rate increases, to reduce potential symptoms from a long PR interval and improve upper rate behavior. VVI is an acceptable therapy in elderly sedentary patients or those with multiple comorbidities.

Owing to the progressive risk of AV nodal disease over time, a DDD pacemaker is preferred over AAI pacemaker in patients with sinus node disease, with a long AV interval programmed (class I recommendation).

B. Mechanism of action of biventricular pacing (cardiac resynchronization therapy), evidence supporting its use, and clinical subsets

Patients with LBBB, particularly >150 ms, have mechanical dyssynchrony, wherein the right and left ventricles and various left ventricular walls contract at different times. Depolarization and contraction of the LV free wall and LV base is significantly delayed compared to that of the RV, the interventricular septum, and the apex (inter- and intraventricular dyssynchrony) (Figure 14.17).[15] This leads to inefficient LV contraction, as one wall contracts while the other is stretched in the opposite direction, which increases LV systolic volume and reduces stroke volume. LV further dilates with time as a result of reduced LV ejection. Moreover, the overall systolic time is ineffectively increased, which reduces the time provided for LV diastolic filling and thus increases LA pressure; dyssynchrony is thus detrimental to the diastolic function as well.

Dyssynchronous papillary muscle contraction and functional MR also occur with LBBB. If the posteromedial LV wall contracts before the anterolateral LV wall, the posterior leaflet is pushed up before the anterior leaflet, which precipitates or exaggerates leaflet non-coaptation; also, the posteromedial muscle relaxes while the anterolateral muscle is still contracting, which sustains leaflet non-coaptation.

Several trials, particularly MIRACLE, have shown that CRT improves symptoms and quality of life, reverses remodeling, reduces functional MR, and improves EF by ~5–7% in patients with EF ≤35%, QRS ≥130 ms, and functional class III or ambulatory class IV.[16] Two trials have established a benefit of CRT on hard outcomes in this population (COMPANION and CARE-HF).[17,18] In the COMPANION trial, CRT vs. no CRT was associated with a 34% reduction in HF hospitalization or HF death and a trend towards a 25% reduction in mortality; the combination of CRT and ICD was associated with the greatest reduction in mortality.[17] In the CARE-HF trial, CRT vs. no CRT was associated with a 36% relative reduction in mortality (20% vs. 30% mortality at 2.5 years). Note that COMPANION and CARE-HF only included a small proportion of class IV patients (<15%). Patients with refractory class IV HF who cannot tolerate chronic HF drugs or who have refractory volume overload are usually not good candidates for CRT, as CRT is generally not a good last-resort therapy.

Two trials addressed the use of CRT in patients with EF ≤35%, QRS ≥130 ms, and functional class II (MADIT-CRT and RAFT).[19,20] In the MADIT-CRT trial, CRT-ICD vs. ICD was associated with a reduction of HF hospitalizations and reverse remodeling in patients with low EF and functional class I or II, but no reduction in mortality. In the RAFT trial, CRT-ICD vs. ICD only was associated with a reduction in mortality of ~1.5% per year in patients with class II or III (80% of patients had class II). While the relative reduction in mortality may be similar in class II as in class III or IV, the absolute reduction is inherently lower in the lower-risk class II patients.

Beside the functional class, two other factors hamper the benefit from CRT in HF patients: QRS duration of <150 ms, and QRS prolongation from RBBB or non-specific delay as opposed to LBBB.

(a) QRS < 130 ms and QRS 130–150 ms

CRT in HF patients who have echocardiographic signs of dyssynchrony but a QRS <130 ms has not shown any clinical benefit, with a potential for harm (RethinQ and EchoCRT trials).[21] QRS prolongation >150 ms implies electrical and often mechanical dyssynchrony, hence the benefit of CRT in these patients. While it was thought at one point that QRS <130 ms might be associated with mechanical dyssynchrony that can be detected by echocardiography and reversed with CRT, hard outcome data did not support the use of CRT in this population. In

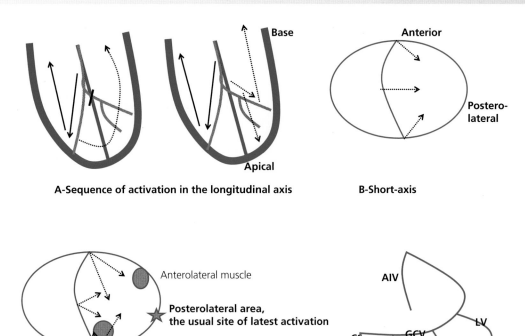

A-Sequence of activation in the longitudinal axis

B-Short-axis

Anterolateral muscle

Posterolateral area, the usual site of latest activation

Posteromedial muscle

C

AIV

LV

CS into RA   GCV

MCV   PV

D

Figure 14.17 Various patterns of LV activation in LBBB. *Black arrows* indicate the spread of electrical activation across the conduction system, *dashed arrows* indicate the spread of activation across the LV.

(A) In most LBBB patterns, on the longitudinal axis, the LV is slowly depolarized from mid-level or apex to base. This is also the case in RV apical pacing, including RV pacing that is performed as part of BiV pacing.

(B) In LBBB, on the short-axis view, the LV is depolarized from the septum to the lateral wall. The depolarization starts at the anterior, mid, or posterior septum, and spreads towards the anterior wall and then the lateral wall. Combining both longitudinal and short-axis views, the *posterolateral basal* site is seen as the site of latest activation, but any *basal* site, including *anterior basal*, is relatively late.

(C) The pattern of activation of the papillary muscles is shown on a short-axis view. The posteromedial papillary muscle is activated sooner than the anterolateral papillary muscle; this is less prominent in the case of a more anterior trans-septal breakthrough of activation.

(D) Coronary venous anatomy. The lead should be placed in the posterior vein (PV) or, best, the lateral marginal vein (LV). The middle cardiac vein (MCV) runs adjacent to the PDA, and the anterior interventricular vein (AIV) runs parallel to the LAD. The lead should not be placed in those veins. Before reaching the RA, the coronary sinus (CS) is called the great cardiac vein (GCV).

fact, LV wall motion heterogeneities in these patients may be related to akinesia rather than dyssynchronous, delayed contraction. Akinesia is not a marker for CRT response; echocardiographic methods differ in their ability to discriminate truly delayed contraction from abnormal contraction.

Only 30–40% of patients with QRS 130–150 ms are responders to CRT. On subgroup analyses of three of the above trials (COMPANION, MADIT-CRT, and RAFT), the benefit from CRT was seen only in patients with QRS >150 ms; no benefit was seen in patients with QRS 130–150 ms.[22] The use of echocardiographic parameters of dyssynchrony may be most useful in selecting the subgroup of patients with QRS of 130–150 ms in whom electrical dyssynchrony implies mechanical dyssynchrony. In fact, in the CARE-HF trial, two out of three echocardiographic parameters of dyssynchrony were required to qualify for CRT in patients with QRS <150 ms. CARE-HF is the only major trial where this subgroup of patients had a strong trend towards clinical benefit.

Guidelines: As a result of this, CRT implantation is given a class I indication in patients with sinus rhythm, EF ≤35%, QRS ≥150 ms, LBBB morphology, and functional class II, III, or ambulatory IV. On the other hand, QRS 130–150 ms with LBBB morphology and functional class II–IV or QRS >150 ms with RBBB morphology is given a class IIa recommendation.[23] Before CRT implantation, it is recommended to provide maximal medical therapy and wait >40 days after MI, > 3 months after revascularization of chronic ischemia, and >3 months in non-ischemic cardiomyopathy (similar to the waiting times before ICD placement).

(b) RBBB and non-specific intraventricular conduction delay

About 70% of HF patients with QRS >120 ms have LBBB; the remaining patients have RBBB or non-specific delay. While it seems, intuitively, that RBBB is not associated with left-sided mechanical dyssynchrony and that the use of CRT in patients with right bundle delay would not improve outcomes, RBBB in patients with HF actually means generalized conduction and electromechanical delay rather than discrete right bundle delay. Patients with RBBB may have delayed conduction in the left bundle as well, the ECG showing RBBB because of a longer right bundle delay.

Therefore, non-LBBB patterns were included in all major trials. However, subgroup analyses of COMPANION, MADIT-CRT, and RAFT, as well as a large meta-analysis, have shown that a non-LBBB pattern does not derive a benefit from CRT.[24–26] This may not apply to the very wide non-LBBB (>150 ms). RBBB, per se, is associated with a higher risk of mortality than LBBB in HF registries and in the CARE-HF study, partly because the prognosis cannot be improved with CRT.[25,27] CRT is still reasonable in non-LBBB with QRS >150 ms and functional class III/IV in light of the pathophysiology described above and some clinical evidence (class IIa recommendation).[28] CRT is less reasonable for non-LBBB pattern with QRS 130–150 ms (class IIb recommendation). Echocardiographic assessment of left-sided activation delays and dyssynchrony may help fine-tune the CRT indication in these patients.

(c) Atrial fibrillation

i. CRT for HF purposes. CRT is recommended in AF patients with HF, a low EF, and a wide QRS, similarly to patients in sinus rhythm (class IIa), as long as the rate is controlled enough to allow 100% ventricular pacing.

ii. CRT for AF purposes. If AV nodal ablation and pacing are performed to control the AF rate in a patient with EF ≤35%, CRT is preferred to RV pacing as it prevents pacing-induced dyssynchrony and is given a class IIa recommendation, regardless of the functional class. One may, however, choose RV pacing early on, followed by CRT at a later time if EF does not simply improve with AV nodal ablation.

(d) Paced ventricular rhythm

Similarly to LBBB, RV pacing induces inter- and intraventricular dyssynchrony, which may worsen LVEF and increase LV volume. CRT prevents this deleterious negative remodeling and is associated with better symptom control in patients with normal or low EF, as has been shown in patients with permanent AF requiring AV nodal ablation.[29,30] Therefore, CRT is recommended in patients with EF ≤35% requiring ventricular pacing >40% of the time for AV block, regardless of the functional class (class IIa recommendation); this also applies to AF patients requiring AV nodal ablation. While the guidelines use a 35% EF cutoff, one randomized study (BLOCK HF) addressed patients with EF ≤50% and HF functional class I–III requiring ventricular pacing for AV block, and showed that CRT reduces HF hospitalization and LV remodeling in comparison to RV pacing.[31] In fact, even in patients with normal EF, RV pacing is associated with a ~7% reduction in EF vs. CRT; ~9% of patients with normal EF have EF reduction to <45% within 1 year of RV pacing.[32] Therefore, RV pacing induces deleterious mechanical dyssynchrony even in patients with normal EF. This effect is only expected to be more prominent in patients with reduced EF. The application of CRT to patients with normal EF requiring ventricular pacing is premature, but those patients require echo follow-up to check for any ventricular deterioration. The use of alternative RV pacing sites, such as RVOT or RV septal pacing, may induce less dyssynchrony by pacing close to the His bundle, i.e., the normal path of activation.[33,34] However, this is not always technically feasible and the benefit varies with the actual level of septal pacing.[35]

(e) Wide QRS and severe functional MR

Moderate or severe functional MR improves by at least one grade in 50% of CRT patients.[36] However, it persists in about 20–25% of CRT patients and, in an additional 10–15%, it may actually worsen after CRT. MR reversal parallels the degree of reverse remodeling achieved with CRT.[37]

(f) RV failure

RV failure is a powerful negative prognostic marker, but did not diminish the benefit from CRT in the CARE-HF trial.[38]

C. Response to CRT and LV lead position

Approximately 30% of patients receiving CRT do not have a beneficial response. A response to CRT therapy has been defined as an improvement of NYHA functional class or a reduction of LV end-systolic volume ≥15%, called reverse remodeling.[39] Several mechanisms explain the lack of response:

a. Treatment of patients with QRS 130–150 ms or RBBB, in whom electrical dyssynchrony does not necessarily imply mechanical dyssynchrony. This is the most common mechanism of non-response. Echocardiography may be used in these patients to determine mechanical dyssynchrony but is subject to inter-observer variability. No dyssynchrony parameter was able to meaningfully distinguish responders from non-responders in the PROSPECT trial.[40]

b. Lack of appropriate AV optimization (seen in 10% of CRT patients).

c. LV lead placement in a scarred region (pre-assessment with MRI may be useful).

d. Large amount of scarred myocardium (e.g., patients with ischemic cardiomyopathy and scarring of >50% of the myocardium are unlikely to benefit).[39,41]

e. LV lead positioning outside the area of latest activation on echocardiography.[39] The echocardiographic assessment of the site of latest activation before CRT implantation may allow targeted lead placement and significant improvement of LV response and clinical outcomes.[42]

f. LV lead positioned in the anterior or apical position rather than the lateral position. Lead position should be analyzed in a short-axis plane (anterior vs. posterolateral) and in a longitudinal plane (basal vs. apical). In most patients, the *posterolateral basal wall* is the site of latest activation; however, lateral LV lead position should be avoided in patients with a lateral scar. In the longitudinal plane, the *basal wall* is the site of latest activation (vs. the apex) (Figure 14.17). While one study suggests that the anterior wall is the site of latest activation in only ~10–25% of patients,[43] another study shows that an *anterior basal* position is acceptable, the apical LV position being the one to avoid.[44] This is particularly the case because the patient is also simultaneously paced from the RV apex, further making the LV base a late site of activation.

Unfortunately, patients with ischemic cardiomyopathy are less likely to have a left marginal vein for lateral LV lead implantation. Besides, lead placement is limited by constraints of left phrenic nerve pacing, lead stability, and pacing threshold.

In the absence of randomized data, if an optimal lateral vein is not accessible for LV pacing or if the lead is not stable in this position, it would be acceptable to implant the LV lead at a suboptimal site. If the patient does not respond adequately, a surgical approach may be performed in a subsequent procedure.[43] A **lateral CXR** displays the location of the LV lead.

In general, in responders, an immediate hemodynamic improvement is seen with CRT: improvement of LV filling, reduction of LA pressure, and improvement of LV dP/dt, MR, and cardiac output. Reverse remodeling, LVEF improvement, and further MR reduction are progressively seen over 3–12 months.

Conversely, up to 25% of patients are super-responders, i.e., experience 15–20% improvement of LVEF (EF almost normalizes) in 6–12 months. A very wide LBBB, non-ischemic cardiomyopathy, female sex, and LA volume <40 ml/m² correlate with super-response.[37] In those patients, dyssynchrony may be the direct cause of LV dysfunction.

D. Optimization of AV delay in patients with CRT

CRT improves diastolic function by reducing systolic time, thus allowing more time for diastolic filling. However, an appropriate AV delay needs to be programmed to improve this diastolic filling. *First*, AV delay should be shorter than the intrinsic PR interval to allow consistent biventricular pacing. *Second*, the AV delay should not be too short; a very short PR makes A wave abut the ventricular systole (simultaneous AV contraction with interruption of A contribution to the diastolic filling). *Third*, a long AV delay leads to fusion of A wave with E wave and induces diastolic MR. The best AV delay is the one that allows clear E/A separation, with A wave ending at 40 ms after the QRS onset, corresponding to the exact onset of ventricular systole (Figure 14.18). This is achieved by setting the AV delay as long as possible while maintaining BiV pacing, then reducing it by 20 ms decrements until the optimal shape is achieved. Approximately 10% of patients will have improved diastolic filling profiles after optimization, which may convert a non-responder to a responder.[45,46] Some may also aim for the AV delay that leads to the highest LVOT or aortic valve VTI (the latter corresponding to the stroke volume).

E. Echocardiographic dyssynchrony parameters

Based on the RethinQ and EchoCRT trials, CRT should not be used and echo parameters of dyssynchrony should not be sought in patients with QRS <130 ms. Those parameters are subjective and have not been shown to correlate with CRT response in patients with QRS >130 ms either (PROSPECT trial).[40] However, they are probably still useful for two purposes:

a. The site of latest activation that is not akinetic or scarred may be targeted for appropriate lead positioning.

b. Select patients with QRS of 130–150 ms who are likely to respond to CRT. The only large trial where QRS of 130–150 ms appeared to derive a benefit close to QRS >150 ms is CARE-HF,[25] in which patients with QRS <150 ms required the fulfillment of two out of the following three criteria:

- Aortic pre-ejection delay of >140 ms: this is the delay between the onset of QRS and the onset of aortic flow (on the three- or five-chamber view)
- Interventricular delay of >40 ms: this is the difference between the left and right pre-ejection delay
- Septal-to-posterior wall motion delay >130 ms (on M-mode of parasternal views)

In addition, myocardial tissue Doppler or tissue speckle-tracking may be used in the short-axis and apical views to see the site of latest activation, and to see the difference in peak tissue velocity between the septal and lateral walls. While the PROSPECT trial showed a low predictive yield of individual dyssynchrony parameters (in patients with QRS mostly >140 ms), one study suggested that dyssynchrony parameters are, in fact, useful in predicting which patients with QRS of 130–150 ms benefit from CRT.[47]

F. Importance of the change of QRS width after CRT

Several studies have shown that a reduction in QRS width after CRT implantation is associated with a positive response to CRT. On average, QRS shortens by 20–40 ms with CRT. This QRS shortening is mostly seen in patients with a baseline QRS >150 ms, in whom the QRS reduction is largest. Typically, non-responders do not exhibit any reduction of QRS or experience QRS widening.[48,49]

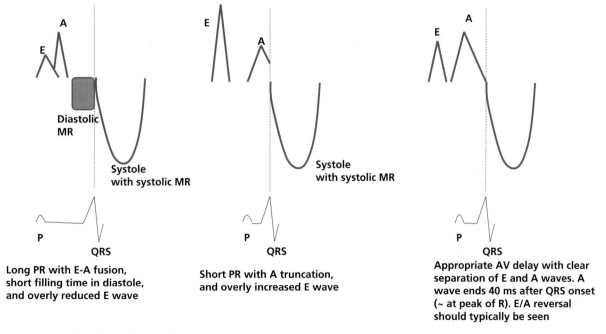

Long PR with E-A fusion, short filling time in diastole, and overly reduced E wave

Short PR with A truncation, and overly increased E wave

Appropriate AV delay with clear separation of E and A waves. A wave ends 40 ms after QRS onset (~ at peak of R). E/A reversal should typically be seen

Figure 14.18 CRT: echocardiographic AV synchronization

G. Arrhythmic death in patients with ICD

While ICD reduces arrhythmic death, patients with advanced HF eventually die of pump failure or recurrent MI, explaining how ICD may not affect the overall mortality in the early post-MI setting or in class IV HF (reduction of arrhythmic death with a relative increase in non-arrhythmic death). Moreover, while ICD drastically reduces arrhythmic death, it does not fully eliminate it for the following reasons (in order of frequency): (1) in patients with severe or decompensated HF, the sudden death may be pulseless electrical activity (PEA) rather than VF; also, *VF may evolve into PEA after defibrillation*, this being the most common cause of sudden death in patients with ICD; (2) failure to terminate VF with multiple shocks (ICD delivers a shock for a certain number of times, usually 6–8, then times out); (3) incessantly recurrent VT/VF, i.e., VT/VF that recurs immediately after successful therapy, over and over; (4) the ICD may undersense the VF fibrillatory waves, because of a low sensitivity setting or because of lead dysfunction.[50] Reasons (2) and (4) may justify defibrillation testing at the time of ICD implant, during which VF is induced, appropriate sensing ensured, and successful internal defibrillation achieved (with up to 35 J). An ineffective ICD shock may justify changing the lead position to create a different, more effective, shock vector; or changing the shock vector between the can and the coils. However, this defibrillation testing has not been shown to improve outcomes in SAFE-ICD study, and thus may not be necessary in the primary prevention setting, when experienced operators appropriately place ICD leads.

QUESTIONS AND ANSWERS: Cases of PM troubleshooting

On a pacemaker ECG, always assess the type of pacemaker by looking at A and V spontaneous activity, A and V pacing, and the A–V relationship; then assess for capture and sensing of the A and V chambers (Figures 14.19–14.34). Occasionally, the ECG or telemetry software places a pacer spike whenever it senses a high-frequency signal, such as artifact, AF wave, or QRS notching, even in the absence of pacing, which creates a false impression of PM malfunction.

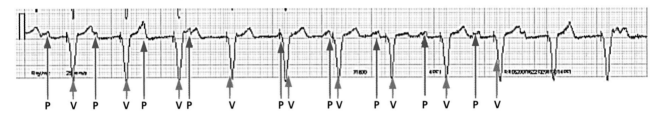

Figure 14.19 Regular V pacing without any spontaneous ventricular activity. Regular P waves are seen but are dissociated from the paced QRS complexes and not tracked by the PM. Thus, there is complete AV block but the PM is functioning in a VVI mode, in which it just senses and paces the ventricle and ignores P waves.

Assess capture and sensing. V capture is appropriate. V undersensing is assessed by the reaction of the PM to a spontaneous complex. Since there is no spontaneous QRS complex, it is not possible to comment on ventricular undersensing. There is no ventricular oversensing (which would lead to underpacing).

If the PM is programmed in a DDD mode but is behaving as VVI, the differential diagnosis would include: phantom reprogramming; end-of-life changes with mode conversion to VVI; atrial oversensing, making the PM "think" there is a fast atrial arrhythmia and switch to VVI mode; or atrial undersensing and subsequent lack of atrial tracking (lead problem). However, in case of atrial undersensing, atrial overpacing should be seen, which is not the case here.

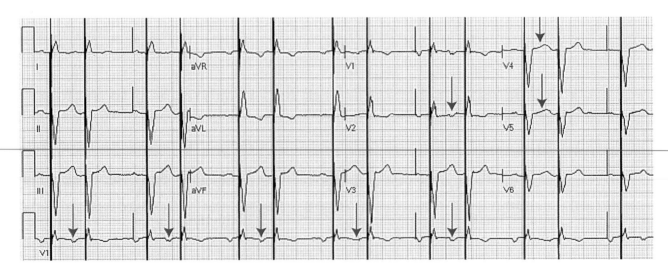

Figure 14.20 DDD pacemaker with atrial pacing and AV sequential pacing.

Intermittently, the ventricle is paced at a short interval (fast). As this is AV sequential pacing, there must be a premature P hidden in this short interval that gets tracked by the pacemaker, rather than inappropriate fast pacing. Atrial bigeminy is, in fact, present and evidenced by the alternation of two different T morphologies (P hidden in T) (*arrows* indicate the premature P waves in leads V_1, V_2, V_4, V_5). The PAC falls on the T wave after PVARP ends, and so gets appropriately tracked by the ventricular channel at an interval close to the upper rate limit. PVARP is an interval after QRS during which P wave is not tracked.

Is this RV or BiV PM? QRS is positive in V_1; however, QRS is also positive in lead I with no Q wave. Thus, this is RV pacing. In ~10% of RV pacing, QRS may be positive in lead V_1; however, QRS should always become negative by lead V_3. Also, moving the V_1 electrode one intercostal space lower should make QRS negative.

Summary: Atrial bigeminy, normally functioning AV sequential pacemaker.

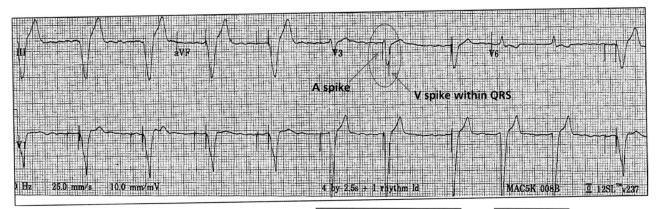

Intrinsic QRSs occurring after atrial spike, at an interval shorter than AV delay

Intrinsic QRSs occuring before atrial pacing, at intervals shorter than AEI

Figure 14.21 Atrial and ventricular pacing spikes are seen. The underlying rhythm is AF and is undersensed by the atrial lead, leading to inappropriate atrial pacing (the pacemaker should mode switch to VVI). The PM paces the ventricle at an AV delay that is appropriately timed to the atrial spike. Intrinsic QRS complexes are seen. They occur after an atrial spike at an interval shorter than the pacing AV delay; or before atrial pacing occurs, at an interval shorter than the atrial escape interval. In the latter case, the atria do not get paced because the intrinsic QRS resets the atrial escape interval (AEI). One pseudofusion complex is seen, wherein a V spike falls within the intrinsic QRS. In this case, the intrinsic QRS falls too close to the atrial spike, in the ventricular safety period, which makes the pacemaker immediately deliver a V spike at an interval shorter than the regular AV delay.

Final diagnosis: AF with atrial undersensing, normal AV sequential pacing (V pacing normally follows the abnormal atrial spike), pseudofusion complex with ventricular safety pacing.

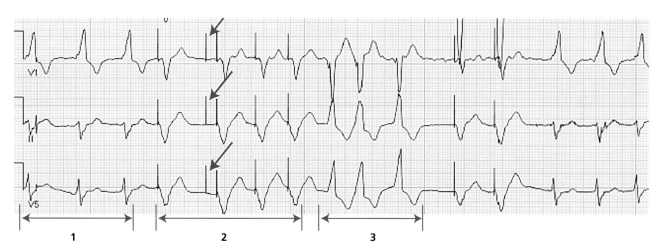

Figure 14.22 Ventricular pacing occurs at irregular intervals and one atrial pacing spike is seen (*arrow*). This is most likely a DDD pacemaker with AV sequential pacing. The pacemaker is tracking an underlying irregular atrial rate.

- The baseline rhythm appears to be AF. The pacemaker should sense the very fast atrial activity and mode-switch to a non-tracking mode (VVI) and pace at a regular rate. In this case, it seems that there is atrial undersensing, so that the pacemaker senses many of the atrial waves and tracks them irregularly at a fast rate (close to the upper rate interval of the pacemaker); however, it does not sense enough of these waves to mode-switch. The non-paced QRS complexes (sequence 3) are QRS complexes that are spontaneously conducted at the fast AF rate, inhibiting any V pacing.
- On one occasion, AF is not sensed for a longer time, which triggers an atrial pacing spike (*arrows*) at the atrial escape interval. However, the atrium is not captured because of AF (this is non-capture related to undersensing).
- Is it BiV or RV pacing? Three different QRS morphologies are seen. The morphology of beats 4–7 (*2*) fits with RV pacing. The first 3 beats (*1*) are not preceded by any spike, but may very well represent BiV pacing (QRS positive in V_1). Beats 8–10 (*3*) are different, fast, and may represent the native QRS complexes (LBBB morphology).
- The alternation between RV and BiV pacing morphologies means that LV capture is intermittently lost.

Summary: AV sequential BiV pacemaker with underlying AF rhythm. Atrial undersensing and lack of mode switch, with pacemaker tracking AF activity. Intermittent LV non-capture.

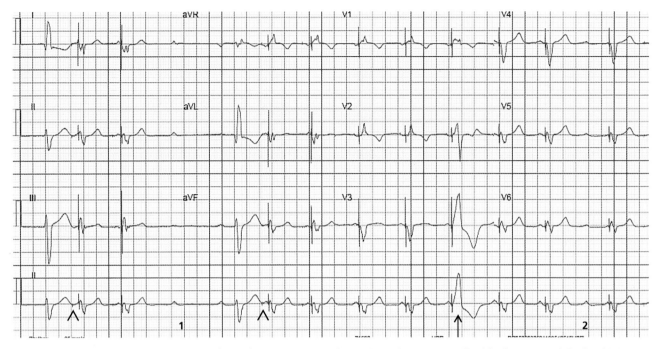

Figure 14.23 Ventricular pacing spikes are seen. They track sinus P waves at a short PR interval. At times, small atrial spikes are seen in lead II. This is a dual-chamber PM, likely DDD mode. Three issues are seen:

1. There is a long (*1*) and a short (*2*) pause (AV block) during which the ventricle is not paced, implying ventricular oversensing. P waves are not tracked during these pauses. ***Ventricular oversensing explains the lack of tracking of sinus P waves, rather than atrial undersensing; atrial undersensing affects AV synchrony but does not lead to ventricular pauses***.
2. Ventricular undersensing is also present at times, as the A and V are paced too soon after an intrinsic QRS, implying that the intrinsic QRS is not sensed (*arrowheads* point to A pacing after the intrinsic QRS).
3. The paced QRS morphology is variable. The baseline paced morphology is positive in V_1–V_2, and negative (Q) in lead I, which means that the baseline pacing is BiV pacing. The very short PR interval supports this. One QRS is wider and is more positive in V_1–V_3 than the BiV-paced QRS, implying LV pacing and thus an intermittent loss of RV capture (*arrow*).

Conclusion: V oversensing and undersensing, intermittent loss of RV capture. The patient may have fracture of the RV lead, or loose connector set screws.

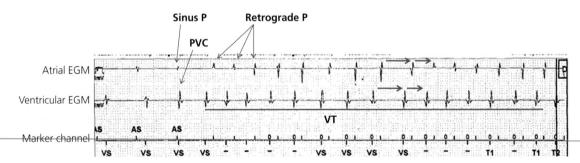

Figure 14.24 Intracardiac electrograms (EGMs) of VT. The atrial and ventricular EGMs are intracardiac ECGs capturing intracardiac activity; the atrial EGM captures the atrial activity A, while the ventricular EGM captures the ventricular activity V. The marker channel indicates how the PM interprets or misinterprets these activities. The tachycardia starts with a PVC falling over the sinus P wave, and is characterized by a number of V deflections = number of A deflections. The V activity drives the A activity; in fact, the tachycardia starts with a V, then A keeps tracking V. Whenever there is a change in the tachycardia interval, the V–V interval changes first, the A–A interval changes afterward (*arrows*). This indicates that the tachycardia is VT with 1:1 VA conduction.

During pacemaker interrogation of arrhythmias, two types of tracing are available: (1) intracardiac electrograms (EGMs), which record the actual signals from each cardiac chamber (A and V), and (2) the marker representation, which indicates how the pacemaker sees and interprets these signals; AS and VS mean sensed intrinsic atrial and ventricular activities, while AP and VP mean paced atrial and ventricular activities. The pacemaker may interpret a signal as VS on the marker channel, while it is in fact T-wave oversensing, false signal, or far-field sensing of an atrial spike. It calls a pacing attempt VP even if the pacemaker does not eventually capture the ventricle. **Looking at the EGMs allows one to understand what the issue is, while looking at the marker channel allows one to see how the pacemaker is interpreting or misinterpreting signals.**

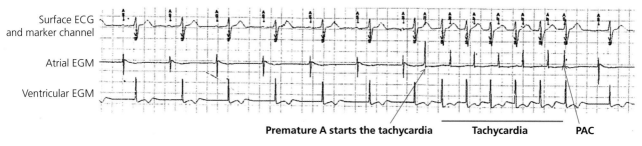

Surface ECG and marker channel

Atrial EGM

Ventricular EGM

Premature A starts the tachycardia   **Tachycardia**   **PAC**

Figure 14.25 Electrograms of a tachycardia that starts with a premature A wave and ends with a PAC.

- *SVT vs. VT:* a tachycardia that starts with a PAC is often SVT, but a PAC may initiate VT as well. The tachycardia breaks with a PAC that does not conduct to the ventricles, implying SVT. The morphology of the V electrogram does not change after the onset of the tachycardia, also indicating SVT.
- *Type of SVT:* this is a short run of AVNRT, AVRT, or reentrant AT that breaks with a PAC. In contrast, automatic AT does not break with a PAC and is usually initiated by a PAC that has a morphology similar to subsequent A waves (not the case here).

The surface ECG may be a true surface ECG obtained with surface electrodes during PM interrogation; in patients with ICD, the vector between the SVC and RV coils may be used as an continuous internal ECG lead.

Conducted sinus Ps   **PVCs with retrograde Ps**

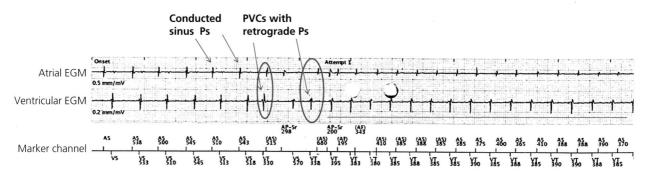

Atrial EGM

Ventricular EGM

Marker channel

Figure 14.26 Tachycardia with number of V waves = number of A waves→ could be SVT or VT. It is unclear whether A drives V or V drives A, but since the tachycardia starts with a PVC it is more likely VT (it could also be AVRT, or less likely AVNRT or reentrant AT). Moreover, the morphology of the ventricular activity is different from the sinus-originating ventricular activity on the ventricular EGM, and similar to the second PVC, which suggests VT.

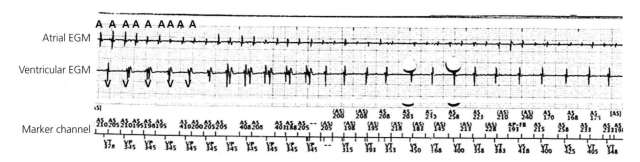

A A A A A AAA A

Atrial EGM

Ventricular EGM

Marker channel

Figure 14.27 The analysis of the atrial and ventricular EGMs reveals more atrial waves than ventricular waves, implying SVT. Furthermore, A activity is irregular, which implies AF. The PM senses that the ventricular rate is in the VT zone (>150 bpm), and the marker channel calls the ventricular activity "VT" rather than "VS." Typically, to avoid unnecessary shocks, a higher rate is used for VT zone (>180–200 bpm), and SVT–VT algorithm is used.

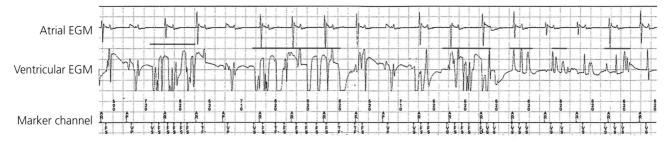

Atrial EGM

Ventricular EGM

Marker channel

Figure 14.28 The patient presents with multiple shocks. The marker channel shows that the PM calls the ventricular activity "FS" (VF zone). On analysis of the ventricular EGM, the ventricular activity is of large amplitude (which is different from VF) and "noisy," with a V–V interval that is non-physiologic (some V–V intervals are <100 ms, even shorter than VF can generate) (*bars*). This is indicative of ventricular lead fracture with "make–break" false potentials.

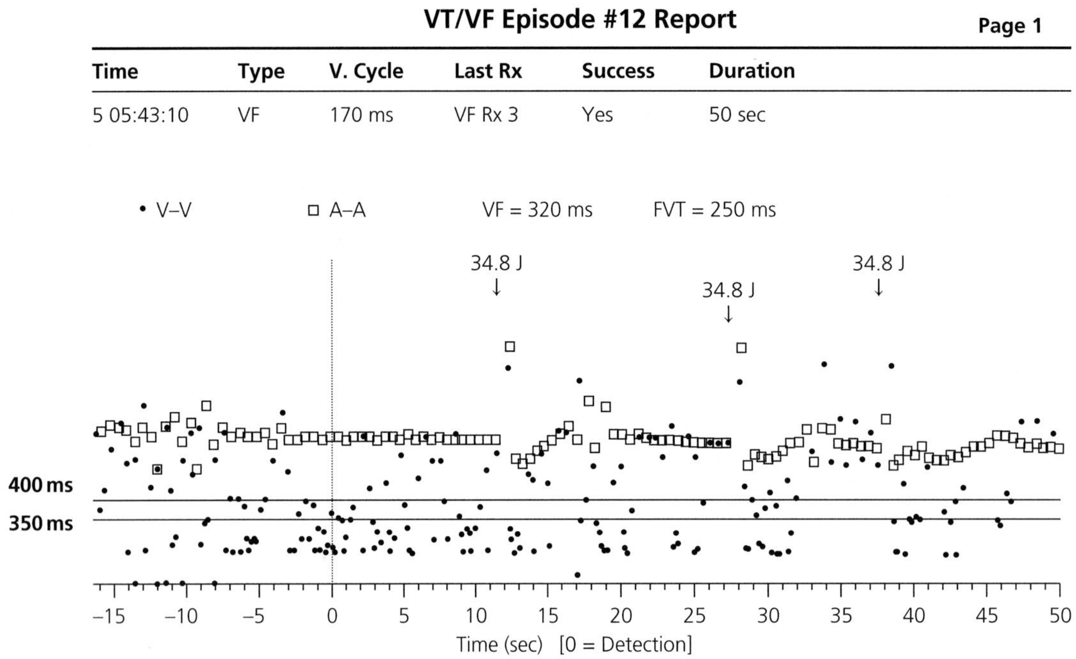

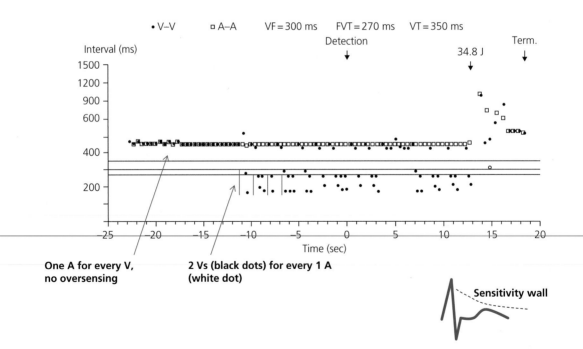

VT/VF Episode #12 Report   Page 1

Time	Type	V. Cycle	Last Rx	Success	Duration
5 05:43:10	VF	170 ms	VF Rx 3	Yes	50 sec

• V–V   ☐ A–A   VF = 320 ms   FVT = 250 ms

Figure 14.29 Electrogram interval plot (same patient as Figure 14.28). It represents the A–A interval of every A wave (*white squares*) and the V–V interval of every presumed V wave (*black dots*). Normally, the squares and the dots should be at the same horizontal level (same rate). Having a higher number of V waves at a shorter interval than the A waves implies VT, or, in this case, oversensing. The V–V intervals fall in the programmed VF zone (<350 ms). The V–V interval is too short (~100 ms).

• V–V   ☐ A–A   VF = 300 ms   FVT = 270 ms   VT = 350 ms

One A for every V, no oversensing

2 Vs (black dots) for every 1 A (white dot)

Sensitivity wall

Figure 14.30 Interval plot showing at one point two V waves (*black dots*) for every A wave (*white dot*). The two V waves are lower than the A waves, correlating with the faster rate. The V waves are at two different levels, implying a V–V interval that alternates between two values. This gives the black dots (V–V interval) the morphology of a railroad. Railroad tracking usually implies double counting of the V waves during every cardiac cycle. This may be due to oversensing the T wave and calling it ventricular signal, far-field sensing of the atrial spike, or sensing the LV pacing activity by the RV lead if the RV–LV time interval is very long (unusual).

In ICD, as opposed to PM, the ventricular sensitivity wall progressively decrements after QRS to allow sensing of the low-amplitude VF waves. In order to prevent T-wave sensing, the decrement is progressive. T-wave oversensing may remain an issue, particularly in sinus tachycardia wherein T-wave amplitude increases, and particularly if the RV lead is positioned such that the vector between its two poles catches a small R wave with a large T wave. One may reduce V sensitivity or reprogram the decrement of sensitivity wall. One may also reprogram the sensing vector: instead of bipolar tip-to-ring sensing, program sensing between the tip and the RV coil (at the risk of increasing far-field sensing).

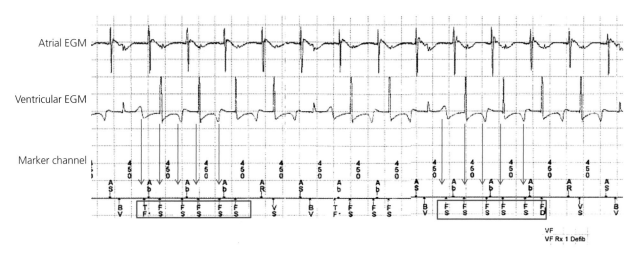

Figure 14.31 Electrograms and marker channel from the case shown in Figure 14.30. Note that the T wave is large on the ventricular EGM and is intermittently read as ventricular signal by the ICD on the marker channel (*arrows*). "VS" implies a sensed ventricular beat, "FS" implies a sensed ventricular beat that is falling at a very short R–R interval (VF rate zone). The ICD senses the T waves as QRS complexes and thus "thinks" that the rhythm is VF. One can understand what the PM "thinks" by looking at the marker channel. This ICD was programmed in such a way that, if 12 of the last 16 beats fell in the VF zone, it would deliver a shock. A shock was eventually delivered in this case. The reason the last 16 beats do not all have to be in the VF zone is that the VF waves are of small amplitude and may be intermittently undersensed.

Concerning atrial sensing, on the marker channel, Ab describes an atrial beat that falls in the PVAB and is completely ignored by the device; AR describes an atrial beat that falls in the PVARP and does not get tracked. T wave being considered V complex, it initiates additional PVAB and PVARP intervals, far away from the true V complex. Therefore, *those atrial waves do not get tracked in a patient who needs BiV pacing, which is another untoward result of T-wave oversensing.* BiV pacing ("BV" on the marker channel) only occurs in the zones where T wave is not oversensed.

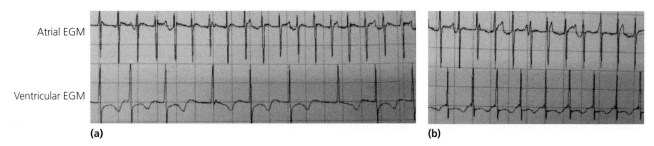

Figure 14.32 EGM of a tachycardia. **(a)** The number of A deflections is larger than the number of V deflections, which implies SVT. Atrial activity is regular with a regular A–A interval of ~200 ms (300 bpm), which implies atrial flutter with variable AV conduction. **(b)** A few minutes later, the patient developed a faster ventricular rate. The atrial activity and A–A interval are unchanged; the ventricular activity has become regular and faster, with a V–V interval of 270 ms. The regular V–V interval that is not a multiple of the A–A interval suggests AV dissociation and implies the unusual presence of two arrhythmias: atrial flutter and VT. The V deflection and its T wave have changed in morphology between **(a)** and **(b)**, which also suggests VT. VT reentry may have been triggered by the supraventricular tachycardia or by a drug-induced pause.

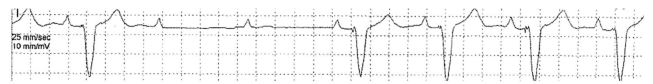

Figure 14.33 Patient with DDD PM has two non-tracked P waves with a pause and symptoms of dizziness. The lack of V pacing implies: (1) V oversensing; (2) lack of V capture (in which case V pacing spikes should be seen, but may be small and overlooked on a Holter monitor). Atrial undersensing that prevents tracking of P waves is not a possibility; the latter should lead to atrial overpacing that is subsequently tracked by V pacing. ***Atrial issues do not lead to a pause in V pacing.***

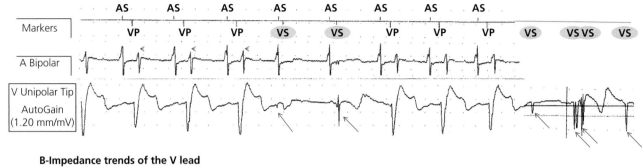

A-Intracardiac electrograms

B-Impedance trends of the V lead

Figure 14.34 PM interrogation of the same patient as Figure 14.33.

(A) The intracardiac electrogram shows noise on the ventricular channel (*arrows*). The PM calls this noise intrinsic ventricular activity ("VS" on the marker channel). This is oversensing related to a lead issue. This oversensing prevents ventricular pacing. The "VS" is ventricular noise rather than true ventricular activity, as the morphology and timing are too erratic. However, if a simultaneous surface ECG is not performed, this noise may be confused with intrinsic V activity and the diagnosis may be missed. This is a case where the PM may not recognize and store the abnormality, and where external Holter monitoring may be necessary to make the diagnosis. On a different note, see that the atrial channel is capturing the far-field ventricular activity (*arrowheads*); however, the PM is not marking these signals on the marker channel, suggesting that they are falling in the PVAB period.

(B) The impedance trend graph of the V lead shows intermittent drop in impedance, suggestive of a lead insulation defect. This defect is intermittent, explaining that oversensing is intermittent. It may be exaggerated by shoulder movements. While awaiting placement of a new lead, the PM should be programmed in an asynchronous, non-sensing pacing mode to allow consistent pacing (VOO).

References

1. Tracy CM, Epstein AE, Darbar D, et al. 2012 ACCF/AHA/HRS focused update incorporated into the ACCF/AHA/HRS 2008 guidelines for device-based therapy of cardiac rhythm abnormalities. J Am Coll Cardiol 201361: e6–75
2. Sweeney MO, Hellkamp AS, Ellenbogen KA, et al. Adverse effect of ventricular pacing on heart failure and atrial fibrillation among patients with normal baseline QRS duration in a clinical trial of pacemaker therapy for sinus node dysfunction. Circulation 2003; 107: 2932–7.
3. Sharma AD, Rizo-Patron C, Hallstrom AP, et al. Percent right ventricular pacing predicts outcomes in the DAVID trial. Heart Rhythm 2005; 2: 830–4.
4. Kenny T. Dual chamber pacing and troubleshooting and diagnostics. In: Kenny T. The Nuts and Bolts of Cardiac Pacing. Oxford: Blackwell, 2005, pp. 129–34.
5. Kadish A, Dyer A, Daubert JP, et al. Prophylactic defibrillator implantation in patients with nonischemic dilated cardiomyopathy. N Engl J Med 2004; 350: 2151–8. *SCD-HeFT trial*.
6. Barold SS, Stroobandt RX, Sinnaeve AF. Cardiac Pacemakers Step by Step. Oxford: Blackwell, 2004, pp. 291–328.
7. Daubert J, Zareba W, Cannom DS, et al. Inappropriate cardioverter-defibrillator shocks in MADIT II. J Am Coll Cardiol 2008; 51: 1357–65.
8. Poole JE, Johnson GW, Hellkamp AS, et al. Prognostic importance of defibrillator shocks in patients with heart failure. N Engl J Med 2008; 359: 1009–17. *From SCD-HeFT*.
9. Moss A, Schuger C, Beck CA, et al. Reduction of inappropriate therapy and mortality through ICD programming. N Engl J Med 2012; 367: 2275–83.
10. Gehi AK, Mehta D, Gomes JA. Evaluation and management of patients after implantable cardioverter-defibrillator shock. JAMA 2006; 296: 2839–47.
11. Andersen HR, Nielsen JC, Thomsen PE, et al. Long-term follow-up of patients from a randomised trial of atrial versus ventricular pacing for sick-sinus syndrome. Lancet 1997; 350: 1210–16.
12. Connolly SJ, Kerr CR, Gent M, et al. Effects of physiologic pacing versus ventricular pacing on the risk of stroke and death due to cardiovascular causes. Canadian Trial of Physiologic Pacing Investigators. N Engl J Med 2000; 342: 1385–91.
13. Toff WD, Camm AJ, Skehan JD. Single-chamber versus dual-chamber pacing for high-grade atrioventricular block. N Engl J Med 2005; 353: 145–55.
14. Gillis AM, Russo AM, Ellenbogen KA, et al. HRS/ACCF expert consensus statement on pacemaker device and mode selection. J Am Coll Cardiol 2012; 60: 682–703.
15. Rodriguez LM, Timmermans C, Nabar A, Beatty G, Wellens HJ. Variable patterns of septal activation in patients with left bundle branch block and heart failure. J Cardiovasc Electrophysiol 2003; 14: 135–41.
16. Abraham WT, Fisher WG, Smith AL, et al. Cardiac resynchronization in chronic heart failure. N Engl J Med 2002; 346: 1845–53.
17. Bristow MR, Saxon LA, Boehmer J, et al. Cardiac-resynchronization therapy with or without an implantable defibrillator in advanced chronic heart failure. N Engl J Med 2004; 350: 2140–50. *COMPANION*.

18. Cleland JGF, Dauber JC, Erdmann E, et al. The effect of cardiac resynchronization on mortality and morbidity in heart failure. N Engl J Med 2005; 352: 1539–49. *CARE-HF.*
19. Moss AJ, Hall WJ, Cannom DS, et al. Cardiac-resynchronization therapy for the prevention of heart-failure events, N Engl J Med 2009; 361: 1329–38. *MADIT-CRT.*
20. Tang ASL, Wells GA, Talajic M, et al. Cardiac resynchronization for mild-to-moderate heart failure. N Engl J Med 2010; 363: 2385–95. *RAFT.*
21. Ruschitzka F, Abraham WT, Singh JP, et al.Cardiac-resynchronization therapy in heart failure with a narrow QRS complex. N Engl J Med 2013; 369: 1395–405 *EchoCRT.*
22. Sipahi I, Carrigan TP, Rowland DY, et al. Impact of QRS duration on clinical event reduction with cardiac resynchronization therapy: meta-analysis of randomized controlled trials. Arch Intern Med 2011; 171: 1454–62.
23. Tracy CM, Epstein AE, Darbar D, et al. 2012 ACCF/AHA/HRS focused update of the 2008 guidelines for device-based therapy of cardiac rhythm abnormalities. J Am Coll Cardiol 2012; 60: 1297–313.
24. Zareba W, Klein H, Cygankiewicz I, et al. Effectiveness of cardiac resynchronization therapy by QRS morphology in the Multicenter Automatic Defibrillator Implantation Trial-Cardiac Resynchronization Therapy (MADIT-CRT). Circulation 2011; 123: 1061–72.
25. Gervais R, Leclercq C, Shankar A, et al. Surface electrocardiogram to predict outcomes in candidates of cardiac resynchronization therapy: a sub-analysis of the CARE-HF trial. Eur Heart J 2009; 11: 699–705.
26. Sipahi I, Chou JC, Hyden M, et al. Effect of QRS morphology on clinical event reduction with cardiac resynchronization therapy: meta-analysis of randomized controlled trials. Am Heart J 2012; 163: 260–7.
27. Bilchick KC, Kamath S, DiMarco JP, et al. Bundle branch block morphology and other predictors of outcomes after cardiac resynchronization therapy in Medicare patients. Circulation 2010; 122: 2022–30.
28. Rickard J, Bassiouny M, Cronin EM, et al. Predictors of response to cardiac resynchronization therapy in patients with a non–left bundle branch block morphology. Am J Cardiol 2011; 108: 1576–80.
29. Doshi RN, Daoud EG, Fellows C, et al. Left ventricular-based cardiac stimulation post AV nodal ablation evaluation (the PAVE study). J Cardiovasc Electrophysiol 2005; 16: 1160–5.
30. Brignole M, Botto G, Mont L, et al. Cardiac resynchronization therapy in patients undergoing atrio-ventricular junctional ablation for atrial fibrillation. Eur Heart J 2011; 32: 2420–9. *Randomized trial of CRT vs. RV pacing after AV nodal ablation.*
31. Curtis AB, Worley SJ, Adamson PB, et al. Biventricular pacing for atrioventricular block and systolic dysfunction. N Engl J Med 2013; 368: 1585–93. *BLOCK HF.*
32. Yu CM, Chan JY, Zhang Q, et al. Biventricular pacing in patients with bradycardia and normal ejection fraction. N Engl J Med 2009; 361: 2123–34.
33. Tse HF, Yu C, Wong KK, et al. Functional abnormalities in patients with permanent right ventricular pacing: the effect of sites of electrical stimulation. J Am Coll Cardiol 2002; 40: 1451–8.
34. Victor F, Mabo P, Mansour H, et al. A randomised comparison of permanent septal versus apical right ventricular pacing: short-term results. J Cardiovasc Electrophysiol 2006; 17: 238–42.
35. Ng AC, Aliman C, Vidaic J, et al. Long-term impact of right ventricular septal versus apical pacing on left ventricular synchrony and function in patients with second- or third-degree heart block. Am J Cardiol 2009; 103: 1096–101.
36. van Bommel RJ, Marsan NA, Delgado V, et al. Cardiac resynchronization therapy as a therapeutic option in patients with moderate-severe functional mitral regurgitation and high operative risk. Circulation. 2011; 124: 912–19.
37. Hsu JC, Solomon SD, Bourgoun M, et al. Predictors of super-response to cardiac resynchronization therapy and associated improvement in clinical outcome: the MADIT-CRT study. J Am Coll Cardiol 2012; 59: 2366–73.
38. Damy T, Ghio F, Rigby AS, et al. Interplay between right ventricular function and cardiac resynchronization therapy. J Am Col Cardiol 2013; 61: 2153–60.
39. Bax JJ, Gorcsan J. Echocardiography and non-invasive imaging in cardiac resynchronization therapy. J Am Coll Cardiol 2009; 53: 1933–43.
40. Chung ES, Leon AR, Tavazzi L, et al. Results of the Predictors of Response to CRT (PROSPECT) trial. Circulation 2008; 117: 2608–16.
41. Ypenburg C, Schalij MJ, Bleeker GB, et al. Impact of viability and scar tissue on response to cardiac resynchronization therapy in ischaemic heart failure patients. Eur Heart J 2007; 28: 33–41.
42. Khan FZ, Virdee MS, Palmer CR, et al. Targeted left ventricular lead placement to guide cardiac resynchronization therapy. J Am Coll Cardiol 2012; 59: 1509–18.
43. Macias A, Gavira JJ, Castano S, et al. Left ventricular pacing site in cardiac resynchronization therapy: clinical follow-up and predictors of failed lateral implant. Eur J Heart Fail 2008; 10: 421–7.
44. Singh JP, Klein HU, Huang DT, et al. Left ventricular lead position and clinical outcome in the Multicenter Automatic Defibrillator Implantation Trial–Cardiac Resynchronization Therapy (MADIT-CRT) Trial. Circulation 2011; 123: 1159–66.
45. Kedia N, Ng K, Apperson-Hansen C, et al. Usefulness of atrioventricular delay optimization using Doppler assessment of mitral inflow in patients undergoing cardiac resynchronization therapy. Am J Cardiol 2006; 98: 780–5.
46. Mullens W, Tang WH. Optimizing cardiac resynchronization therapy in advanced heart failure. Congest Heart Fail 2011; 17: 147–51.
47. Gorcsan J, Oyenuga O, Habib PJ, et al. Relationship of echocardiographic dyssynchrony to long-term survival after cardiac resynchronization therapy. Circulation 2010; 122: 1910–18.
48. Lecoq G, Leclercq C, Leray E, et al. Clinical and electrocardiographic predictors of a positive response to cardiac resynchronization therapy in advanced heart failure. Eur Heart J 2005; 26: 1094–100.
49. Molhoek SG, Van Erven L, Bootsma M, et al. QRS duration and shortening to predict clinical response to cardiac resynchronization therapy in patients with end-stage heart failure. Pacing Clin Electrophysiol 2004; 27: 308–13.
50. Mitchell LB, Pineda EA, Titus JL, et al. Sudden death in patients with implantable cardioverter defibrillator. J Am Coll Cardiol 2002; 39: 1323–8.

15 Basic Electrophysiologic Study

I. General concepts; intracardiac electrograms

Four main catheters are used: RA catheter, RV catheter, His catheter, and coronary sinus (CS) catheter. These catheters record electrograms (EGMs) and may also be used for pacing. The His and CS catheters typically have multiple recording electrodes (e.g., proximal, mid, and distal).

- **RA recording** is characterized by A wave (atrial activity).
- **RV recording** is characterized by V wave (ventricular activity).
- **His recording** is characterized by three waves: A, H (His activity), and V (Figures 15.1, 15.2). The A wave on His recording normally occurs slightly later than the A wave on RA recording, due to the delayed transmission of the atrial activity to the His catheter. The His spike is typically narrower and of smaller amplitude than the A and V waves, and looks like a narrow bar.
- **CS recording** mainly shows A wave; it may show a far-field, low-amplitude V wave (Figure 15.2).

In order to identify the deflections on any channel, always correlate them with the surface ECG. This should always be the first step in analyzing intracardiac EGMs. The A wave coincides with the P wave, the V wave coincides with the QRS complex (~superimposed with QRS), and H is between A and V. **Regardless of the channel, V waves line up with the QRS complexes.**

The AH interval corresponds to AV nodal conduction, while the HV interval corresponds to the infra-Hisian conduction. AH is measured from the onset of A on His recording to the onset of H, while HV is measured from the onset of H to the onset of the earliest ventricular activation, which is usually the onset of QRS on the ECG. The HV interval is the only interval where the surface ECG is needed not just for identification but for measurement as well; in fact, the electrocardiographic QRS often starts earlier than the His V wave, and is closer to the RV V wave, as the ventricular stimulation starts at the mid-ventricular wall then spreads up to His. The normal AH interval is 60–120 ms, while the normal HV interval is 35–55 ms; HV is severely increased if >100 ms.

In the EP lab, programmed stimulation may be performed using two pacing techniques: (i) *extrastimulus*, where a progressively more premature extrastimulus S2 is introduced after a baseline pacing sequence S1 (~8-beat train S1, at a fixed cycle length of ~600 ms); (ii) *incremental pacing*, where a steady pacing sequence, faster than the baseline rate, is introduced; progressively faster pacing sequences are then introduced.

II. AV conduction abnormalities

AH prolongation or, worse, A wave that is not followed by H and V waves, indicates AV block at the nodal level.

HV prolongation, or A wave that is followed by H but not V wave, indicates infra-Hisian block and thus is more ominous and more readily dictates pacemaker placement, in a symptomatic or even asymptomatic patient (Figure 15.3).

In the EP lab, the AV conduction may be stressed using the *incremental pacing* or the *extrastimulus technique*.

Incremental pacing. The AV node is characterized by decremental conduction and longer refractory period with faster atrial pacing, which is opposite to the myocardial tissue. With progressively faster atrial pacing trains, the AH interval normally increases, and a conduction block may normally be seen at the AV nodal level, which manifests as a drop of both H and V complexes in a Wenckebach pattern. The pacing interval at which this occurs is the Wenckebach cycle length, normally ≤450 ms (≥130 bpm). Wenckebach AV block occurring at a slower rate implies AV nodal disease. The HV interval should not change with pacing; an increase in HV interval (especially >100 ms) or a drop of V wave with fast atrial pacing indicates infra-Hisian block.

Practical Cardiovascular Medicine, First Edition. Elias B. Hanna.
© 2017 John Wiley & Sons Ltd. Published 2017 by John Wiley & Sons Ltd.

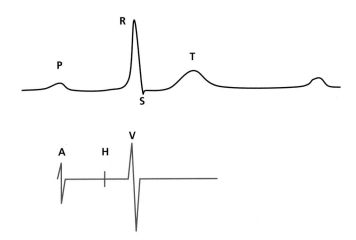

Figure 15.1 Normal His recording.

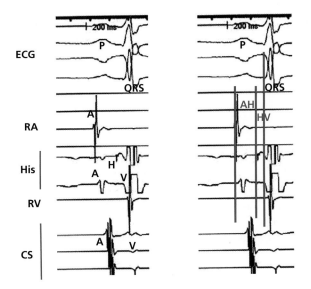

Figure 15.2 Example of a typical A, V, His, and CS recording. AH and HV intervals are shown. When looking at an intracardiac tracing, **always start by identifying the V wave, which corresponds to the electrocardiographic QRS**. The remaining intracardiac waves are mainly A waves. H wave is a small wave that is only seen on the His recording and may be overlooked. The CS recording mainly shows A waves (LA A waves), but low-amplitude, far-field V waves may also be seen.

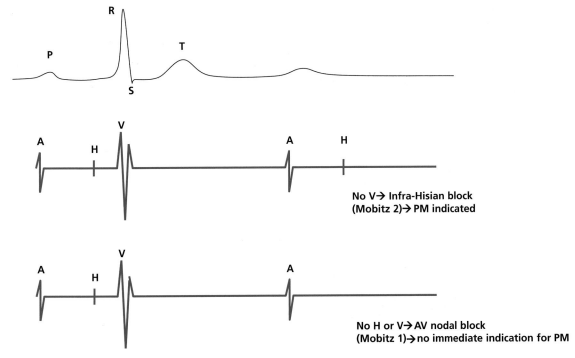

No V→ Infra-Hisian block
(Mobitz 2)→ PM indicated

No H or V→ AV nodal block
(Mobitz 1)→no immediate indication for PM

Figure 15.3 Types of AV block.

Extrastimulus technique. Progressively more premature atrial extrastimuli are inserted until A fails to conduct to His. The earliest A–A interval at which A stops leading to H complex is the AV nodal effective refractory period. On the other hand, the earliest interval at which the premature extrastimulus does not lead to A complex is the atrial effective refractory period. Beside having slower conduction than the atrial and ventricular tissues, the AV node normally has a longer refractory period. An AV node effective refractory period >425 ms is abnormal.

III. Sinus node assessment

During fast overdrive atrial pacing (~30 seconds), and similarly to atrial fibrillation, the sinus node activity is inhibited. Upon cessation of atrial pacing, the sinus node needs time to recover its electrical activity. The duration of the pause between the last paced A complex and the recovery A complex is called the sinus node recovery time (SNRT). A diseased sinus node has a prolonged SNRT. The corrected SNRT is equal to SNRT minus basic cycle length, basic cycle length being the A–A interval prior to atrial pacing (e.g., SNRT 1100 ms, basic cycle length 700 ms, corrected SNRT =400 ms). The corrected SNRT is normally <550 ms.

Also, a blunted sinus node response to atropine + propranolol (i.e., to the removal of the autonomic tone) implies sinus node disease.

Note, however, that rhythm monitoring (e.g., event monitor), which correlates symptoms with paroxysmal conduction blocks/sinus pauses, has the highest yield in establishing that AV or sinus nodal conduction blocks are the cause of the patient's symptoms. Invasive EP evaluation of the AV or sinus node does not have a high sensitivity or specificity for conduction abnormalities. For example, the presence of sinus nodal disease or AV nodal block does not imply that the conduction abnormality underlies the patient's symptoms. ***Only the finding of HV infra-Hisian block (a drop of V wave or HV interval >100 ms) is highly specific for a serious conduction disorder and usually mandates pacemaker placement regardless of symptoms.***

IV. Ventricular vs. supraventricular tachycardia

AV dissociation is easily characterized on EGM. *Identify V deflections, which line up with QRS complexes on the ECG; then identify the other deflections, seen on the atrial and His channels, which correspond to the A deflections.* VT is diagnosed if V deflections are more numerous than A deflections. SVT is diagnosed if A deflections are more numerous than V deflections. If A deflections are equal in number to V deflections, the tachycardia could be SVT or VT with 1:1 VA conduction. Assess the onset of the tachycardia (V or A) *and* which interval changes first (A–A or V–V). In VT, the tachycardia starts with a V deflection and the A–A interval's length tracks the V–V interval's length, meaning a change in A–A interval follows, rather than precedes, a similar change in V–V interval.

In VT, V deflections are typically more numerous than A deflections and are dissociated from them. However, V and A could be associated in a 1:1 fashion (1:1 VA conduction), or a 2:1 or 3:1 fashion (2:1 or 3:1 VA conduction). In VT with AV dissociation, His spikes are typically absent. In VT with AV association, His spikes may result from retrograde VA conduction.

V. Dual AV nodal pathways

Normally, after a premature atrial extrastimulus, the AV nodal conduction slows and AH interval increases (relative refractory period). With progressively more premature atrial extrastimuli, AH interval progressively increases, and at some point H and V may drop. If, however, with a small decrement of A–A interval (e.g., 340 ms to 330 ms), AH interval disproportionately increases, by >50 ms (as opposed to a slight increase or a block), it is implied that the AV node has a fast and a slow pathway. While the fast pathway conducts the normal, sinus-initiated beats and the atrial extrastimuli, a very early extrastimulus falls in the absolute refractory period of the fast pathway and fails to conduct through it. Subsequently, this extrastimulus conducts over the slow pathway, leading to an AH jump (Figure 15.4). **The slow pathway has a slower conduction but a shorter refractory period**, hence the slow pathway conducts when the fast pathway is blocked. This may initiate AVNRT, if the fast pathway recovers quickly enough to allow retrograde conduction (slow–fast reentry).

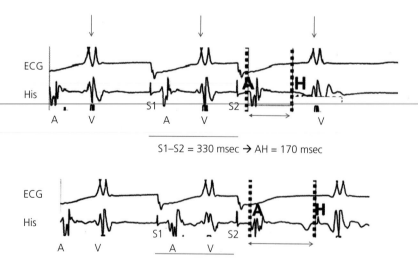

S1–S2 = 330 msec → AH = 170 msec

S1–S2 = 320 msec → AH = 250 msec

Figure 15.4 Arrows point to QRS complexes on the ECG, which are the starting point in intracardiac electrogram interpretation. S1 is a baseline pacing train, S2 is a premature pacing stimulus. A slightly earlier pacing stimulus (10 ms earlier) leads to a large jump in AH conduction interval >50 ms, indicative of the presence of dual AV nodal pathways. The latter conduction occurs over the slower pathway. This phenomenon is called **AH jump** after progressively premature atrial extrastimuli.

VI. AVNRT

During AVNRT, A conducts down the AV node's slow pathway, which then conducts to V and A quickly and almost simultaneously (Figures 15.5, 15.6). The conduction to A occurs retrogradely through the fast pathway. **A tachycardia with almost simultaneous V and A deflections is usually AVNRT.**

VII. Accessory pathway, orthodromic AVRT, antidromic AVRT

An accessory pathway connects the A and the V. The accessory pathway may conduct from the atrium all the way to the ventricle at baseline (manifest pathway = WPW pattern), or may only partially conduct and not reach the ventricle (concealed pathway).

The accessory pathway has a faster conduction than the AV node but a longer refractory period. Thus, a PAC is more likely to conduct through the AV node than the accessory pathway. By the time the electrical activity reaches the ventricle, the accessory pathway may have recovered, and thus fast retrograde conduction may occur and lead to orthodromic AVRT (= AVRT with retrograde conduction through the accessory pathway). In this case, A conducts to V through His, then V rapidly conducts to A retrogradely through the fast-conducting accessory pathway (Figure 15.7). **In contrast to AVNRT, A and V activities are not as close**.

Antidromic AVRT is a reentrant AV tachycardia which conducts antegradely over the accessory pathway. It is unusual for a PAC to initiate antidromic AVRT, as it blocks through the accessory pathway before it blocks through the AV node (the accessory pathway has a longer refractory period than the AV node). Antidromic AVRT may occur in rare cases where the accessory pathway has a shorter refractory period than the AV node. In this case, A conducts to V through the accessory pathway, then V conducts back to A through His (Figure 15.7).

A CS catheter helps further differentiate AVNRT from AVRT and localizes the site of the accessory pathway (Figure 15.8). Analyze the His, CS, and RA channels and see the site of earliest A activity during the tachycardia: in AVNRT the earliest A activity is in His, followed by the proximal part of the CS catheter, whereas in AVRT the earliest A activity is in the distal CS catheter (left-sided pathway), proximal CS catheter (posteroseptal pathway), or the RA (right-sided pathway). The site of earliest A activity in the CS (proximal, mid, or distal) allows the localization of the accessory pathway site.

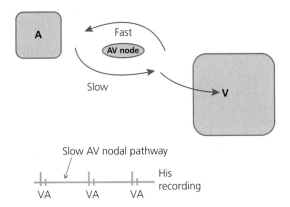

Figure 15.5 AVNRT. V and A almost coincide, with a VA interval <70 ms. On ECG, this corresponds to RP interval <90 ms.

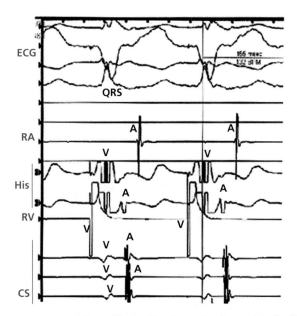

Figure 15.6 AVNRT. After V, the site of earliest A activation is located in the His catheter, then it spreads to the RA and LA (CS catheter). VA interval is very short; in fact, V and A almost coincide.

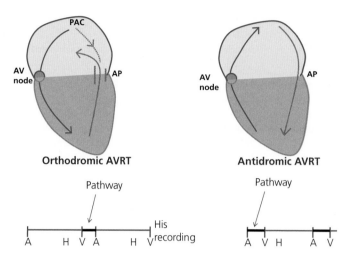

Figure 15.7 Activation sequence in orthodromic AVRT and antidromic AVRT. As opposed to AVNRT, in orthodromic AVRT the site of earliest A activation after V is either CS or RA, depending on the site of the accessory pathway, but not His (usually).

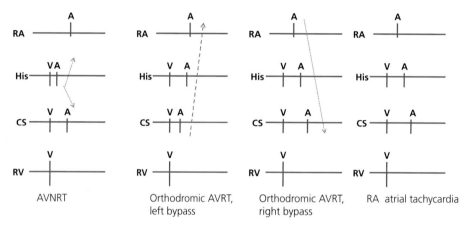

Figure 15.8 Earliest site of atrial activation during AVNRT, AVRT, and atrial tachycardia.
- In AVNRT, retrograde A is seen first in His, then proximal CS, then RA. Importantly, the VA interval is very short.
- In left-sided bypass tract AVRT, the earliest A activation is in the CS catheter (LA).
- In right-sided bypass tract AVRT, the earliest A activation is in the RA, followed by His (atrial septum) and LA.
- In atrial tachycardia, the earliest A activation is in the RA (RA AT) or the CS (LA), which may simulate AVRT. In AT, as opposed to AVRT and AVNRT, when one paces the ventricle and entrains the atrium then stops pacing, the junction between pacing and the AT rhythm is characterized by V–A–A–V. Also, V pacing may not capture the atrium at all, which keeps beating at its own rhythm and dissociates from the ventricle, which is different from AVRT, where the A and V cannot be dissociated.

During a baseline study, before arrhythmia induction, the accessory pathway may be diagnosed and localized through ventricular pacing and mapping of the retrograde atrial activation. Normally, retrograde atrial activation spreads through the AV node and the earliest atrial activation is in the His, followed by concentric spread to both atria (*concentric atrial activation* through His). If an accessory pathway is present, retrograde atrial activation will spread through this pathway into one of the atria first, then spread contralaterally (*eccentric atrial activation*). The earliest atrial activation is right, left, or posteroseptal (coronary sinus). Occasionally, the retrograde activation may appear normal if the pathway is anteroseptal.

In patients with antegrade accessory pathway, progressively earlier atrial extrastimuli do not lengthen the AV interval, which remains *flat* until a block occurs in the accessory pathway and conduction shifts to the AV node. This is different from the response of the AV node to extrastimuli and is a hint to the presence of an accessory pathway.

In the EP analysis of tachyarrhythmias and accessory pathways, induce the tachyarrhythmia with pacing and extrastimuli (e.g., atrial extrastimuli for SVT) then look for the site of earliest activation to localize the ectopic focus or the pathway (Figure 15.8). In the EP lab, rhythms are described in terms of their cycle length rather than rate, i.e., the length of time between two waves (cycle length =60,000/rate).

Reentrant supraventricular arrhythmias can be induced with atrial extrastimuli that fall into the refractory period of one arm of the reentry loop (e.g., refractory period of the fast pathway in AVNRT, refractory period of the accessory pathway in AVRT, and refractory period of some atrial cells in AF or Aflutter). AVRT can be initiated with both ventricular or atrial extrastimuli. Automatic tachycardia, such as automatic AT, cannot be induced by pacing but may be induced with catecholamines (isoproterenol).

VIII. Atrial flutter

Atrial flutter is characterized by a macroreentrant RA circuit that runs in a frontal, right-to-left plane, the base of which is a narrow isthmus bordered by the IVC and crista terminalis posteriorly and the tricuspid annulus anteriorly (cavotricuspid isthmus, CTI) (Figures 15.9–15.12). The crista terminalis, a fibrous band that separates the anterior (tricuspid annulus) and posterior (IVC) parts of the RA, constitutes the electrical barrier that allows the atrial flutter circuit to be sustained.

A *halo mapping catheter* with 10–20 electrodes is placed in the RA, crossing the isthmus and overlapping with the atrial flutter circuit (almost in the same plane). These electrodes are activated sequentially in a counterclockwise fashion, leading to a "zigzag" shape of A deflections, with activation spreading from the proximal into the distal tip electrodes (Figures 15.13, 15.14). The *ablation catheter* is introduced through the IVC and advanced across the tricuspid valve, and its tip is torqued so that it is inferior to the coronary sinus catheter. The catheter is then withdrawn to the tricuspid annulus. Pacing through the ablation catheter is performed at this level while atrial flutter is ongoing; an adequate isthmus position is confirmed if the post-pacing interval is equal to the tachycardia cycle length. Radiofrequency

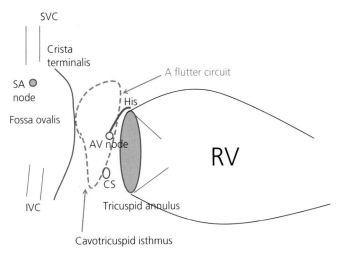

Figure 15.9 RAO view (side view) of the RA. The crista terminalis is a structure that separates the anterior and posterior parts of the RA. The cavotricuspid isthmus (CTI) is a narrow tunnel in front of the crista terminalis. The atrial flutter circuit loops anterior to the IVC and crista terminalis, parallel to the tricuspid annulus. Note that both AV node and His bundle are located in the interatrial septum. The His bundle is at the anterior tip of the interatrial septum, just behind the aortic valve; it extends to the membranous interventricular septum and gives the bundle branches. CS, coronary sinus ostium.

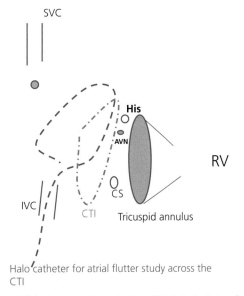

Figure 15.10 RAO view of the RA. Note the position of the halo mapping catheter, which is typically in a frontal plane, parallel to the tricuspid annulus and the atrial flutter circuit. AVN, AV node; CTI, cavotricuspid isthmus.

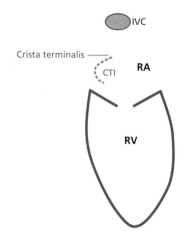

Figure 15.11 Axial view of the RA, RV, and tricuspid valve.

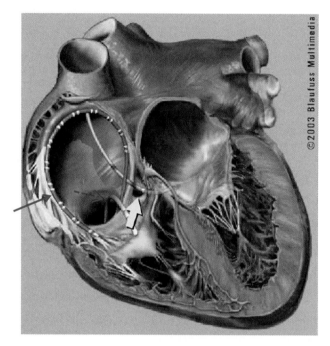

Figure 15.12 Note the *halo catheter* (*solid blue arrow*), positioned in the RA parallel to the tricuspid annulus and overlapping with the atrial flutter circuit. Note the *ablation catheter* (*dashed arrow*) positioned across the cavotricuspid isthmus. The *white arrow* points to the coronary sinus and the *coronary sinus catheter*. Reproduced from Blaufuss Multimedia.

energy is subsequently used while the catheter is very slowly pulled back into the IVC; the CTI is thus ablated. To ensure complete CTI interruption, pacing through the coronary sinus catheter is performed after ablation. Normally, pacing through the coronary catheter spreads into both the lower and upper parts of the RA, leading to ~simultaneous activation of proximal and distal halo catheter electrodes, with the latest activation being somewhere around the middle electrodes. However, when CTI ablation is successful, there is a block of conduction across the lower RA, leading to a unidirectional spread of conduction (Figure 15.15).

IX. Inducible VT

In patients with structural heart disease and unexplained syncope, one should attempt to induce VT. If inducible, the study is specific for ventricular arrhythmia as the underlying trigger of syncope and is a class I indication for ICD placement. If not, it does not necessarily rule out an underlying VT.

VT is induced by rapid ventricular pacing (at a V–V interval of 400 ms, for example) followed by inserting a single premature extrastimulus at a progressively tighter coupling interval (e.g., premature V stimulus at 320 ms, then 280 ms, then 240 ms). If VT is not induced, pace and insert double extrastimuli then triple extrastimuli. If arrhythmia is not induced from the RV apex, these same steps may be repeated from the RVOT.

An abnormal response is defined as the induction of **sustained monomorphic VT** >30 seconds with up to three extrastimuli, or sustained polymorphic VT/VF with up to double extrastimuli. Polymorphic VT/VF induced with triple extrastimuli is a non-specific response that may be seen in normal individuals. Some operators consider the induction of polymorphic VT with any type of stimulation a non-specific response; some operators accept non-sustained VT >10 beats as a positive study. The use of polymorphic VT or

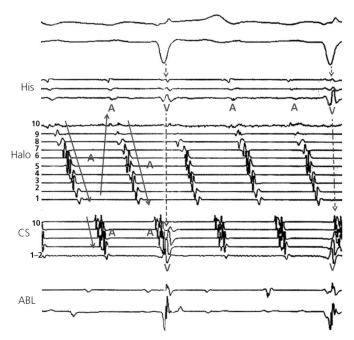

Figure 15.13 Atrial flutter mapping. Note the atrial activation along the halo catheter (10 to 1) with the zigzag shape (*solid arrows*). Electrodes 1, 2 are the distal tip electrodes, whereas electrodes 9, 10 are the proximal electrodes (see Figure 15.12). Note how the activation spreads in a counterclockwise fashion from 10 to 1, then reaches the coronary sinus and His bundle and reaches back to electrode 10. *The RA is constantly activated throughout the recording, with no quiescent isoelectric phase.*

   As always, identify complexes on all channels by correlating with the QRS on ECG. On any channel, V is the complex that aligns with QRS (dashed arrows); the rest are A complexes.

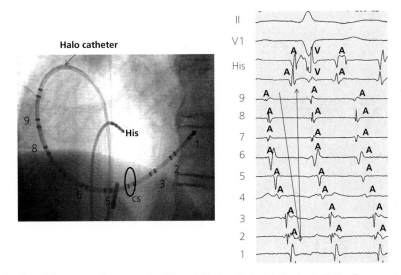

Figure 15.14 Another example of atrial flutter mapping across the right atrial halo catheter (electrodes 1–9). The fluoroscopic view is an LAO view of the RA, which looks at the plane of the halo catheter and splays it (as opposed to RAO view, which is aligned with the halo catheter plane, Figure 15.10). Note how the atrial activity spreads from 9 to 1 and His in a counterclockwise fashion. Courtesy of Paul Lelorier, MD.

non-sustained VT as a positive endpoint lessens the specificity of the study. Only a sustained monomorphic VT <220 bpm can be mapped and potentially ablated.

X. Mapping for ablation

Typically, in order to be mapped, an arrhythmia must be induced. Reentrant arrhythmias are induced and terminated with programmed electrical stimulation. Pacing at short cycle lengths (from A or V, depending on what arrhythmia one is trying to induce) decreases the refractory period of normal myocardial tissue and increases the conduction speed. This allows premature impulses to reach the reentrant circuit earlier, which increases the chance of initiating the reentrant arrhythmia. Pacing is performed at a fast and fixed cycle length for a number of beats, e.g., eight beats (***incremental pacing train, called S1***). Then, one, two, or three extrastiumuli may be introduced at the end of pacing, at a short interval called the "coupling interval," shorter than the pacing cycle length (***extrastimulus technique, S2–S3–S4***). It is

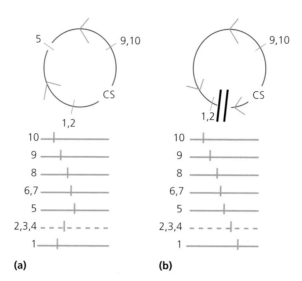

Figure 15.15 (a) Normal atrial activity along the halo catheter when one paces from the CS catheter (*in the absence of ongoing atrial flutter*). Note the bidirectional conduction into the upper and lower RA. **(b)** After ablation of the CTI, a conduction block occurs along the CTI, hence the unidirectional conduction and the sequential activation from 10 to 1.

easier to induce reentry when the difference in refractory period between the two arms of the reentry is large (*tachycardia zone*) and when the conduction velocity is very slow across part of the reentry (*excitable gap*). Also, **the closer the catheter is to the reentrant circuit, the easier it is to induce or interrupt reentry with extrastimuli**. This is similar to quickly throwing a ball through a revolving door. The ball is the extrastimulus, the revolving door is the reentry. The closer one is to the door, the more likely it is for the ball to enter and entrain the revolving door. Furthermore, the slower the revolving door, the more likely it is for the ball to enter it. In fact, *the ability to induce an arrhythmia from one site often implies that the reentrant circuit is close to that site; this is a useful first step in mapping*. Pacing from various locations may be attempted to induce the arrhythmia, as this increases the likelihood of being close to the reentry. *SVT that is readily induced or interrupted with ventricular pacing is likely AVRT (AVNRT or AT are much less likely to be induced with ventricular pacing)*.

> Being able to entrain an arrhythmia from one site often implies that this site is part of the reentry loop or close to it. For example, if AVRT is more easily induced from LA than RA, a left-sided bypass is probable; inducing AT with LA pacing often implies left atrial origin.

In general, the functional reentry of AVNRT and atrial flutter is more difficult to induce than anatomical reentry, such as scar reentry or AVRT. Automatic arrhythmias (such as a subset of ATs) cannot be induced by programmed stimulation.

After inducing the arrhythmia, or if the arrhythmia is spontaneously present, the first step is to diagnose the type of arrhythmia. Tips described under Sections IV–VII allow the diagnosis. Furthermore, one may use A or V pacing to see how it affects the arrhythmia, and thus see if the atrial or ventricular myocardium is required for reentry.

Afterwards, several types of mapping are performed to fine-tune the type and exact origin of the arrhythmia.

Pacing for the differential diagnosis of SVT

A short RP tachycardia (V–A interval) may be AVNRT, AVRT, or atrial tachycardia with a long AV conduction. The site of earliest A activity helps distinguish those tachycardias (Figure 15.8). Additionally, one may pace the ventricle then pace the atrium and see how this affects the tachycardia:

i. When ventricular pacing does not disrupt A activity, i.e., when A activity continues at the same rate, unaffected by V pacing, the reentry cycle of the SVT is not dependent on the ventricles → it is either AVNRT (nodal reentry) or atrial tachycardia. It is not AVRT.

ii. When atrial pacing does not disrupt V activity and the tachycardia, the reentry cycle is not dependent on the atria → it is AVNRT.

iii. As per (i) and (ii), when pacing dissociates A and V, a diagnosis is implied. When pacing terminates a tachycardia, a diagnosis is implied as well: the reentry usually involves the paced chamber. However, when pacing one chamber entrains the other chamber, a specific diagnosis is not implied, and additional features are used. Pacing the ventricle may entrain the atria in AVNRT without affecting the small AVNRT loop; upon cessation of pacing, the tachycardia resumes. In this case, the junction between pacing and the tachycardia helps make the diagnosis. In AVNRT, the junction is a V–A–V–A junction, the first V and A being related to pacing. The V–V interval at this junction is longer than the V–V interval during AVNRT (long post-pacing interval) (Figure 15.16).

In AVRT, the atria may get entrained during V pacing, but through the AVRT loop, with the same pattern and sequence of atrial activation as during AVRT. The junction between pacing and the tachycardia is a V–A–V–A junction, but the V–V interval at the junction approximates the V–V interval of the AVRT (resetting of the tachycardia).

In atrial tachycardia, the atrium may get entrained with V pacing without affecting the atrial focus or loop. Upon cessation of pacing, the tachycardia resumes with a long post-pacing V–V interval and a V–A–A–V junction.

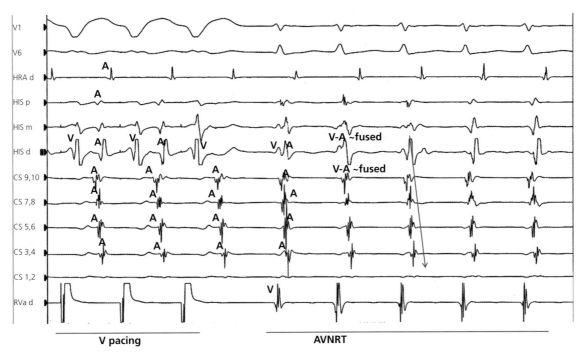

Figure 15.16 Ventricular pacing in a patient with AVNRT. Always start by aligning QRS complexes on the ECG with V complexes on all channels. The remaining complexes are, by default, A complexes. During RV pacing, the ventricle captures the atria retrogradely. Meanwhile, the reentrant circuit continues to loop independently so that, when pacing is stopped, the tachycardia resumes at its prior rate. The junction between pacing and the tachycardia is V–A–V–A, and the V–V interval at the junction (post-pacing V-V interval) is longer than the tachycardia cycle length (vs. equal to it or within 115 ms of it in AVRT).

Outside pacing, note how the V and A almost occur simultaneously, with the earliest A being in the His, followed by CS then RA (direction of the arrow). V and A are almost fused together when V and A activations are initiated through the AVNRT loop, which is different from when RV is paced, where a clear interval is seen between V and A.

Activation mapping

This addresses the *site of earliest activation* in relation to various RA, RV, His, and CS catheter electrodes, ± LA and LV catheters, after inducing the arrhythmia. The site of earliest activation during the arrhythmia corresponds to the location of the reentrant circuit. For example:

- In atrial tachycardia, the localized atrial electrogram at the site of earliest activation just precedes the ECG P wave.
- In VT, the localized ventricular electrogram at the site of earliest activation just precedes QRS.
- In mapping accessory pathways during orthodromic AVRT, look for the site of earliest A activation, i.e. see which part of the RA catheter or CS catheter (posterior septum, LA) is activated soonest after QRS. *This may also be performed without inducing AVRT*:
  - Pace the ventricle and look for the site of earliest retrograde atrial activation (concentric vs. eccentric atrial activation).
  - In antegrade accessory pathway, one may pace the atrium during sinus rhythm and see which part of the CS or RV catheter is activated first after A wave.
  - With atrial pacing at the site of the bypass tract, the A–V interval is very short, typically <60 ms. Also, the closer A pacing is to the bypass tract, the more pre-excited the electrocardiographic QRS is.
  - When the baseline QRS is pre-excited, V recording at the bypass tract shows a V wave occurring earlier than the electrocardiographic QRS.
  - A small sharp bypass potential may also be recorded at the site of the bypass tract.
  - In addition to the standard catheters, a catheter positioned across the tricuspid annulus and capturing both the A and V deflections may be used for mapping when a right-sided bypass tract is suspected (the shortest AV interval corresponds to the location of the bypass tract).

Entrainment mapping and post-pacing interval (see Figures 15.17, 15.18)

Let us take the example of an ongoing reentrant atrial tachycardia. After localizing the site of earliest activation, the atrium is paced from the electrode positioned at that site at a cycle length 20–50 ms faster than the tachycardia cycle length (*entrainment pacing*). The pacing is then interrupted. An interval between the last paced A wave and the post-pacing A wave that is equal to the tachycardia cycle length, as measured through the pacing electrode, confirms that pacing was performed from the reentrant circuit. If the atrium was entrained from outside the reentrant circuit, the post-pacing interval will be equal to the tachycardia cycle length plus the distance between the pacing focus and reentry focus (Figure 15.17).

Additional features: (1) the morphology of the paced A wave and the tachycardia A wave are compared; if pacing was performed from the reentrant circuit, the morphologies are often similar; (2) pacing from within the reentrant circuit produces the same pattern of atrial activation as the tachycardia; for example, in typical atrial flutter, overdrive pacing from the isthmus will produce the same zigzag sequence of activation as spontaneous atrial flutter.

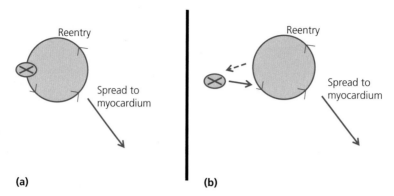

Figure 15.17 The reentry circuit is shown as a circle, the pacing point is shown as an X. **(a)** Entrainment pacing from inside the reentry circuit. After cessation of pacing, the reentry cycle continues at its own, slightly slower speed, and cycles back to the pacing point at about the same speed as the baseline reentry speed. **(b)** Entrainment pacing from outside the reentry. After interruption of pacing, the reentry cycle continues at its own speed, and reaches the pacing point at a duration that equals baseline reentry time + time to the pacing site (*dashed arrow*). The post-pacing interval is longer than the tachycardia (reentry) cycle length.

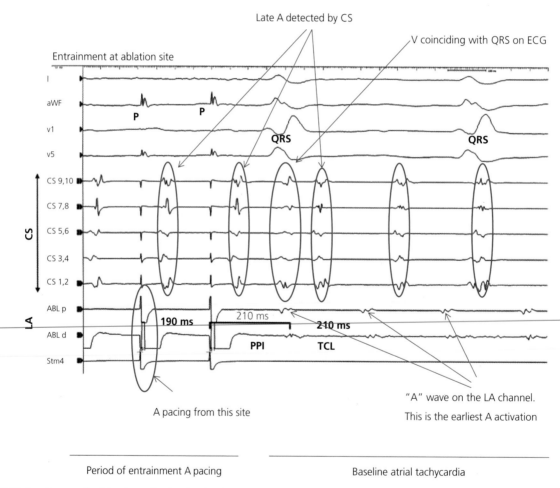

Figure 15.18 Entrainment of atrial tachycardia. The site of earliest A activation was identified to be in the LA, at the level of the LA electrode (non-paced tracings in the second half of the figure). Pacing from this early site accelerates the tachycardia and the post-pacing interval (PPI) approximates the tachycardia cycle length (TCL). In addition, pacing from this site reproduces the same sequence of atrial and late CS activation as the spontaneous tachycardia. Reproduced with permission of Elsevier from Markowitz SM, Nemirovsky D, Stein KM, et al. Adenosine-insensitive focal atrial tachycardia. J Am Coll Cardiol 2007; 49: 1324–33.

This technique is useful for localizing the reentrant focus in AT and VT. It is also useful for atrial flutter, whether it appears isthmus-dependent on the halo and CS catheters recording (pace from the isthmus), or non-isthmus-dependent (pace from the presumed RA or LA site of earliest activation).

Pace mapping

For mapping of VT, pace the appropriate ventricle from various locations, seeking the location that exactly reproduces the QRS morphology of the VT. This location would be very close to the reentrant circuit.

Fractionated electrogram mapping

A portion of the reentrant circuit has a slow conduction, a prerequisite for reentry. This site of slow conduction is identified by a low amplitude, fractionated signal. This mapping can be performed during sinus rhythm.

Note that fractionated electrograms have a different significance in different arrhythmias. In VT, fractionated electrograms are seen over the area of slow conduction, i.e., the area that is critical to the maintenance of reentry; this is the area that should be ablated. In AF, fractionated electrograms signify continuous electrical activity and are actually microreentrant circuits.

Further reading

Knight BP, Ebinger M, Oral H, et al. Diagnostic value of tachycardia features and pacing maneuvers during paroxysmal supraventricular tachycardia. J Am Coll Cardiol 2000; 36: 574–82.

Michaud GF, Tada H, Chough S, et al. Differentiation of atypical atrioventricular node re-entrant tachycardia from orthodromic reciprocating tachycardia using a septal accessory pathway by the response to ventricular pacing. J Am Coll Cardiol 2001; 38: 1163–7. *In AVNRT, as opposed to AVRT, post-pacing interval is longer than tachycardia cycle length.*

Fogoros N. The electrophysiology study in the evaluation and treatment of ventricular arrhythmias; *and* Transcatheter ablation: therapeutic electrophysiology. In: Fogoros N. Electrophysiologic Testing, 4th edn. Oxford: Blackwell, 2006, pp. 158–210 *and* 211–52.

Markowitz SM, Nemirovsky D, Stein KM, et al. Adenosine-insensitive focal atrial tachycardia. J Am Coll Cardiol 2007; 49: 1324–33.

Kaneko Y, Nakajima T, Irie T, et al. Differential diagnosis of supraventricular tachycardia with ventriculoatrial dissociation during ventricular overdrive pacing. Pacing Clin Electrophysiol 2011; 34: 1028–30.

I. Action potential (see Figures 16.1, 16.2)

II. Action potential propagation and mechanisms of arrhythmias

Two features characterize the propagation of the action potential: (1) how fast it propagates, i.e., conduction velocity; and (2) how fast it recovers and accepts new impulses, i.e., refractory period. Some tissues, like the slow AV nodal pathway, have a slow conduction yet a fast refractory period (in comparison to the fast AV nodal pathway). Other tissues, like the accessory pathway, have a fast conduction but a slow refractory period (in comparison to the AV node).

An arrhythmia may result from the following mechanisms:

1. *Reentry* (the most common mechanism, shown in Figures 16.3–16.6).
2. *Increased automaticity*. In this case, atrial or ventricular myocardial cells develop abnormal pacing capacity with spontaneous diastolic depolarization (e.g., accelerated idioventricular rhythm). Alternatively, after a pause, latent pacemaker cells may start firing in phase 4 (e.g., ventricular escape rhythm). Like sinus tachycardia, which is an automatic rhythm, an automatic arrhythmia generally displays a warm-up phenomenon at onset and warm-down phenomenon at offset.
3. *Triggered activity secondary to afterdepolarizations*. Afterdepolarizations are depolarizing oscillations in membrane potential that occur during the late part of phase 3 repolarization (early afterdepolarization, EAD) or during phase 4 (delayed afterdepolarization, DAD). If the afterdepolarization reaches a threshold potential, arrhythmia may be initiated (Figure 16.7). Afterdepolarization, whether EAD or DAD, is related to excessive intracellular accumulation of calcium. EADs are mainly seen during a very prolonged repolarization that allows spontaneous calcium release from the sarcoplasmic reticulum (e.g., after a pause or bradycardia). DADs, on the other hand, are promoted by a fast heart rate rather than a pause; the fast heart rate impedes reuptake of calcium into the sarcoplasmic reticulum, which increases intracytosolic calcium accumulation and thus the amplitude of DADs.

EAD-triggered activity may be due to a congenital or acquired long QT syndrome, electrolyte disturbances, or antiarrhythmic drugs. Automaticity and DAD-triggered activity are generally due to ischemia, catecholamine excess, hypoxia, acid–base disorders, or calcium overload from digoxin toxicity. Automaticity may also be due to cavity stretch.

A premature ventricular or atrial complex results from the same three mechanisms. In patients with heart disease, a change in sinus rate may create a ventricular reentry around the abnormal myocardial tissue, which could be isolated (PVC) or could become sustained into VT. PVC may also result from triggered activity arising from the abnormal tissue, which is a tissue prone to spontaneous depolarization, or fractionated late diastolic potential (a form of automaticity). Overall, the morphologies of the PVC and VT are frequently similar. Idiopathic PVCs arising from the RVOT are generally due to triggered activity.

All arrhythmias can exhibit a warm-up phenomenon, wherein the rate quickly accelerates upon initiation, but this is most characteristic of automatic tachycardias (such as automatic atrial tachycardia).

Induction of arrhythmias in the EP lab- *Reentry* can be initiated by pacing or by premature impulses. Reentry can be terminated by overdrive pacing or by premature impulses that enter the reentrant circuit and get blocked inside it, breaking it.

Conversely, pacing and premature impulses are not effective in initiating or terminating *automatic tachycardias*, which are thus difficult to induce in the EP lab. *In fact, in the EP lab, automatic tachycardia is defined as a tachycardia that cannot be initiated or terminated with*

Practical Cardiovascular Medicine, First Edition. Elias B. Hanna.
© 2017 John Wiley & Sons Ltd. Published 2017 by John Wiley & Sons Ltd.

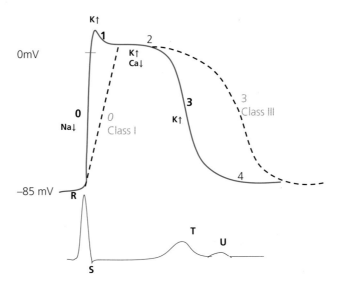

Figure 16.1 Action potential of atrial and ventricular myocardium. Phase 0 corresponds to myocardial depolarization and QRS on ECG, phases 1 and 2 (plateau) correspond to the ST segment, phase 3 corresponds to the T wave, and phase 4 corresponds to the TP segment. Phases 1–3 correspond to repolarization, during which the cells are refractory to a new depolarization (refractory period). All myocardial cells reach the same phase 2 plateau level around the same time, and thus the ST segment is normally a flat isoelectric segment without intramyocardial gradient. Conversely, the T wave is like the bell curve of the repolarization of all myocardial cells, some of which repolarize early, and some late. The width of T and the length of QT indicate, in a way, how heterogeneous and dispersed the repolarization is, and thus the risk of arrhythmia. The normal U wave is a diastolic wave related to the mechanical stretch of the myocardium in phase 4 (diastole). The abnormal U wave could be part of phase 4 (delayed afterdepolarization, DAD), or part of phase 3 in patients with prolonged repolarization (early afterdepolarization [EAD] seen in patients with prolonged QT). In the latter patients, the U wave is actually a T2 repolarization wave; their QT is a QTU interval, and the distinction between T and U may not be very relevant in these patients.

The depolarization of one cell causes the sodium channels of adjacent cells to open and depolarize. There are two properties of electrical propagation: **(1) conduction velocity**, which depends on phase 0; **(2) refractory period**, which depends on the duration of phases 2–3. A reduction in the steepness of phase 0 (dashed phase 0, class I AAD) leads to slower velocity and wide QRS, while a prolonged phase 3 (dashed phase 3, class III AAD) leads to a prolonged QT interval.

Phase 1 uses I_{Kto} (transient outward K channel), phases 2 and 3 use I_{Kr} and $I_{Ks,}$ and phase 4 depends on I_{K1} (the cell potential is close to the equilibrium potential of K)

The action potential duration is increased at lower heart rates, and is reduced with tachycardia or β-adrenergic stimulation. It is mainly the duration of phase 3 that is affected with changes in heart rate.

↓ indicates the entry of the ion inside the cell; ↑ indicates the exit of the ion.

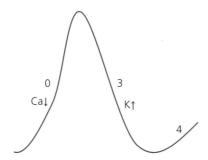

Figure 16.2 Action potential of the SA and AV nodes is characterized by a spontaneous depolarization in phase 4. In addition, phase 0 is characterized by calcium rather than sodium entry, explaining the effect of calcium channel blockers on slowing the SA and AV node. Phase 0 is also slower than phase 0 of the atrial and ventricular cells, thus explaining the slower conduction through the AV node. Phase 4 depends on the funny K and Na channel (If). Spontaneous phase 4 depolarization may be seen in ischemic atrial or ventricular cells (increased automaticity).

programmed electrical stimulation. Also, as opposed to reentry, automatic tachycardias do not respond well to DC cardioversion, as the automatic focus keeps firing independently of the surrounding electrical stimuli.

Triggered activity can be spontaneous like automaticity, resulting from leakage of positive ions into the myocardial cell, but can also be induced with a premature beat or with a pause, particularly a pause introduced after fast pacing. Similarly to reentry, it may get entrained with pacing or terminated. Thus, during EP study, triggered activity resembles reentry. Since it depends on calcium channels, triggered activity may respond to calcium channel blockers (Table 16.1).

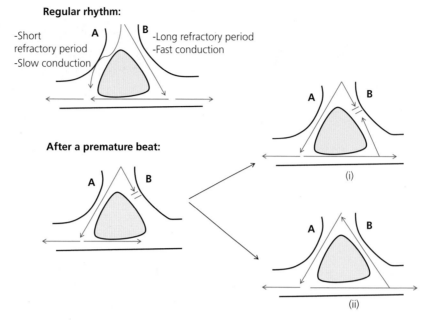

Regular rhythm:

-Short
refractory period
-Slow conduction

A   **B**
-Long refractory period
-Fast conduction

After a premature beat:

A   **B**

(i)

(ii)

Figure 16.3 Illustration of reentry as a mechanism of tachyarrhythmia. In order to have reentry, adjacent myocardial areas (A and B) need to have **different refractory periods *and* different conduction velocities, separated by an anatomical or functional barrier. The pathway with the shorter refractory period needs to have a slower conduction.** The larger the difference in refractory period between A and B, the easier it is to initiate an arrhythmia; this difference between refractory periods is called the ***tachycardia zone***. The slower the conduction velocity in A, the more likely it is to sustain the arrhythmia (slow conduction leads to a large ***excitable gap***, Figure 16.4).

When the rhythm is regular, the electrical activity spreads through both areas simultaneously (*top*). After a **premature beat**, region B is still in its long refractory period, but region A has recovered (*lower left*). The electrical activity spreads through region A, then meets the tail end of region B; at that time, if region B has not recovered from its refractory period, arrhythmia does not occur (i). Since A conducts slowly, region B may well recover from its refractory period, allowing conduction to spread retrogradely through region B (ii). Eventually, this retrograde impulse reaches A faster than the electrical activity originating from the sinus node reaches A. Since A has a short refractory period, the impulse may propagate through A and stimulate the whole cardiac chamber again. Thus, this circle keeps repeating itself, stimulating the myocardial tissue at a rate faster than normal: this is the reentrant tachyarrhythmia.

These areas of slow conduction and different refractory period are seen around a scar (prior infarct, fibrosis, cardiomyopathy), an ischemic area, or a functionally slow area (crista terminalis for atrial flutter, slow pathway of AVNRT) or fast area (accessory pathway of AVRT). Scarred myocardium is an anatomic barrier for reentry. **The peri-scar myocardium has a slow conduction, but shorter action potential and shorter repolarization than the surrounding tissue.** An area is functionally slow when fibers in that area are organized transversally rather than longitudinally; electrical activity spreads more slowly transversally than longitudinally through gap junctions.

PVC or ventricular pacing may have three effects on a reentry that involves the ventricle (VT, AVRT) (Figure 16.5):

- The PVC or ventricular pacing may conduct into the reentry and block it.
- The PVC or ventricular pacing may enter the reentrant circuit and become part of it. Pacing at a rate faster than the tachycardia cycle length may actually entrain the tachycardia, if the *refractory period is short enough and the excitable gap large enough to prevent pacing from being blocked in the reentry circuit*. This is evident on the ECG by the fact that the interval between the last paced beat (or PVC) and the next QRS, i.e., post-pacing interval, is equal to the R–R interval of the tachycardia (if pacing is close enough to the reentrant zone, which is usually the case if one can engage the reentry). This is called *resetting of the tachycardia*. Since fast pacing may shorten the cycle length of the tachycardia and accelerate it, antitachycardia pacing may be risky.
- In the case of VT microreentry, the ectopic or pacing focus may be far from the reentry, so that it conducts to the ventricles and prevents most or all of the ventricular myocardium from being activated through the reentry. The reentry, however, keeps looping independently, unaffected by the faraway pacing, with a post-pacing interval longer than the tachycardia cycle length. This does not usually happen with AVRT, where the reentry involves a large part of the ventricular myocardium; pacing either conducts through the AVRT or breaks it.

AVNRT and atrial tachycardia may break with PVC or ventricular pacing if it conducts retrogradely and enters the reentrant circuit. This is unlikely to happen, as the loops of AVNRT and atrial tachycardia are far from the ventricle. Usually, their cycle will not be affected, they keep looping independently of the QRS at their own pre-existing rate (post-PVC or immediate post-pacing interval >tachycardia cycle length, with V–A–V–A junction in AVNRT, and V–A–A–V junction in atrial tachycardia) (Figure 16.8).

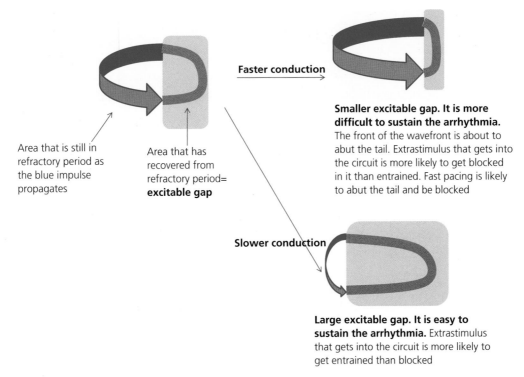

Faster conduction

Smaller excitable gap. It is more difficult to sustain the arrhythmia. The front of the wavefront is about to abut the tail. Extrastimulus that gets into the circuit is more likely to get blocked in it than entrained. Fast pacing is likely to abut the tail and be blocked

Area that is still in refractory period as the blue impulse propagates

Area that has recovered from refractory period= **excitable gap**

Slower conduction

Large excitable gap. It is easy to sustain the arrhythmia. Extrastimulus that gets into the circuit is more likely to get entrained than blocked

Figure 16.4 Slowing the conduction across the reentrant cycle reduces the area that is refractory per unit of time, i.e., increases the area that is excitable per unit of time, and allows the reentry to be sustained. The maintenance of the arrhythmia relies on (i) slow conduction, (ii) short refractory period, and (iii) large circuit (e.g., large scar, large RA in atrial flutter). A fast conduction combined with a long refractory period makes the two ends of the propagating wavefront (*blue arrow*) abut, meaning that the fast propagating wavefront reaches an area that is still in refractory period, which terminates the reentry. *This may happen when fast pacing engages the reentry loop and abuts the tail of the propagating wavefront.*

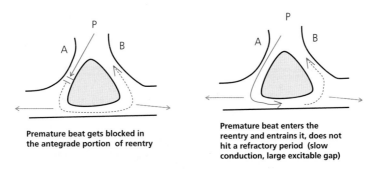

Premature beat gets blocked in the antegrade portion of reentry

Premature beat enters the reentry and entrains it, does not hit a refractory period (slow conduction, large excitable gap)

Figure 16.5 Termination of reentrant arrhythmias. The *dashed arrows* represent the wavefront of reentry that is in refractory period, the *straight blue arrows* represent propagation of a premature complex or pacing (P). In a patient with sustained reentrant arrhythmia, appropriately timed pacing penetrates path A but gets blocked in it as the distal part of A is in refractory period. The wavefront of reentry will then get blocked as path A is now refractory. The reentrant cycle is thus broken. If this is AVNRT, it may end with QRS if A is fully penetrated before the block.

If pacing goes down A and progressively encounters tissue that has fully recovered (slow conduction), it will get conducted through the reentry cycle without breaking it.

Pacing may not be able to enter a refractory reentrant loop, which then keeps looping independently of its surroundings. Those surroundings may be activated through pacing (e.g., pacing the ventricle during VT), but the loop continues independently; when pacing is stopped, the loop restarts, activating the whole cardiac chamber.

III. General mechanism of action of antiarrhythmic agents

Antiarrhythmic agents act either by slowing the conduction across a reentry loop (particularly class I agents), or by increasing the refractory period (particularly class III agents):

1. Slowing the conduction is effective in suppressing the arrhythmia only when it creates an almost complete block across the reentry, allowing supraventricular activity to take over. Conversely, slowing the conduction without producing a block or lengthening the refractory period may, in fact, be arrhythmogenic by itself, as the myocardium becomes more frequently "free" from the refractory period and thus excitable. This increased excitable gap allows the arrhythmia to be sustained (Figure 16.4). Therefore, classes Ia and Ic agents should not be used in patients prone to ventricular arrhythmias (low EF, CAD).

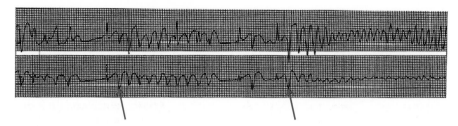

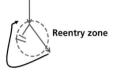

Reentry occurs when PVC hits a heterogeneous myocardium:

Figure 16.6 VF initiated by R-on-T phenomenon. In a patient with myocardial scar, myocardial disease, or ischemia, there is a **heterogeneity of refractory periods across various myocardial areas.** A PVC that occurs during T wave will encounter the refractory period of one area, but will conduct through another area, which initiates reentry.

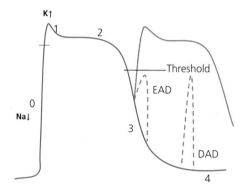

Figure 16.7 Once the EAD (early afterdepolarization) or DAD (delayed afterdepolarization) reaches a threshold, the sodium channels get activated and a second action potential is initiated.

Table 16.1 Differentiation of various mechanisms of arrhythmias.

	Reentry	Automaticity	Triggered activity
Induction and termination with pacing (= programmed electrical stimulation)	+	−	+
Catecholamine facilitation (isoproterenol)	+/−	+	+
After entrainment with pacing then interruption of pacing: post-pacing interval = tachycardia cycle length	+ if paced from the actual site of reentry (reentry resumes at its own speed)	−	+/−
Response to calcium channel blockers			+
Adenosine suppression of atrial arrhythmias	+/−	−	+

2. Increasing the refractory period halts reentry, as the propagating wavefront abuts an area that is refractory (Figure 16.4). Increasing the refractory period occurs through prolonging the repolarization; *prolonging the repolarization* often exaggerates the *dispersion of repolarization*, which can initiate reentry cycles. In fact, the refractory period of some zones gets more prolonged than others, which widens the tachycardia zone, i.e., widens the difference in refractory periods between arms A and B in Figure 16.3. A prolonged repolarization may also trigger early afterdepolarizations. This proarrhythmic effect is seen with class III drugs, but less so with amiodarone, since the latter prolongs repolarization without exaggerating the dispersion of repolarization.

Class III antiarrhythmic drugs are K channel blockers (I_{Kr} channel). They block phase 3 of the action potential and thus increase the action potential duration and the refractory period and prolong QT (Figure 16.1).

Class Ic antiarrhythmic drugs are Na channel blockers (I_{Na} channel). They depress phase 0 and thus slow the conduction and may prolong the QRS but usually not the total action potential duration. *Class Ia* drugs slow the conduction through Na channel blockade but also prolong the action potential duration through some K channel blockade. *Class Ib* drugs shorten (rather than slow) phase 0 and subsequently shorten the repolarization and the refractory period; by shortening the refractory period across arm B, they narrow the difference

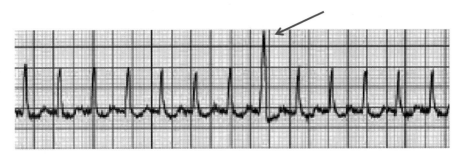

Figure 16.8 Narrow complex tachycardia. A wide complex is seen, likely PVC or aberrant PAC. The distance from the QRS that precedes this wide complex to the QRS that follows it is double the distance of the baseline R–R interval, implying that this complex does not interrupt the underlying tachycardia rhythm. Suppose the wide complex is an aberrant PAC. The fact that PAC does not affect the reentry implies that the atrium is not part of the reentry cycle. This implies that the tachyarrhythmia is not AVRT. It can be AVNRT, wherein the nodal reentry continues independently of the atrial or ventricular activity, or atrial tachycardia, wherein the atrial microreentry or automaticity continues independently of ectopic atrial activity.

In AVNRT, the reentry is in the AV node, and thus the atrial and ventricular myocardium are not required for reentry. Thus, PAC, PVC, or atrial or ventricular pacing does not necessarily disrupt the AV nodal reentry. Only if the atrial or ventricular extrastimulus propagates to the AV node at a particular time might the reentry cycle and the arrhythmia break. Also, in AVNRT, an occasional P or QRS may be dropped (antegrade or retrograde Wenckebach) but the tachycardia does not stop, indicating that the atria and ventricles are not required to maintain the tachycardia (≠ AVRT)

in refractory periods between arms A and B, thus narrowing the tachycardia zone, so critical for the initiation of reentry. Class Ib drugs also reduce automaticity, EAD, and DAD. They are mainly useful in acute ischemia; they minimally affect the normal tissue and have minimal effect on QRS and QT.

Class II drugs are β-blockers: they slow the conduction through the SA node and AV node without affecting the refractory period. In addition, they reduce automatic atrial and ventricular arrhythmias that are induced by ischemia or catecholamine excess (ACS, postoperative state, or sepsis). Catecholamine excess can lead to increased automaticity, triggered activity, and premature beats that initiate reentry in abnormal tissues.

Class IV drugs are calcium channel blockers. They slow the conduction through the SA node and AV node. They are also effective in triggered-activity atrial tachycardia and idiopathic VT.

> β-Blockers and calcium channel blockers do not affect the Hisian and infra-Hisian conduction. Conversely, class I drugs do not affect the AV nodal conduction (except propafenone).

Digoxin inhibits the Na/K-ATPase, leading to increased intracellular Na and subsequent increase of intracellular Ca through the Ca/Na sarcoplasmic passive exchange, leading to its inotropic effect. It also increases vagal tone, leading to SA and AV nodal blocking effect. At toxic levels, calcium overload has a direct effect on the atrial, ventricular, and AV nodal tissue, leading to increased automaticity and delayed afterdepolarization.

Adenosine effects:

- Adenosine activates an outward potassium current ($I_{K,ADO}$), which leads to hyperpolarization of the *sinus node and AV node*, causing them to block conduction, thus terminating AVNRT, AVRT, and SNRT.
- Adenosine antagonizes the cardiac effect of catecholamines by inhibiting adenylcyclase, the enzyme that generates cAMP; thus, adenosine may terminate atrial or ventricular arrhythmias secondary to *catecholamine-triggered activity*.
- In the atrial tissue, the outward potassium current reduces the action potential duration, thus facilitating the induction of *reentrant* arrhythmias, such as AF, atrial flutter, or reentrant atrial tachycardia, in up to 12% of patients. Conversely, it may variably suppress reentrant atrial arrhythmias.
- Automatic atrial tachycardia may be transiently suppressed by the hyperpolarizing effect of adenosine, but owing to its incessant nature the tachycardia quickly resumes.

IV. Modulated receptor hypothesis and use dependence

Na and K channels go through various states: (i) resting state during phase 4, (ii) active/open state during the depolarization phase (Na channel) or the repolarization phase (K channels), and (iii) inactive state during the repolarization phase (Na channel). Antiarrhythmic drugs have different binding capacity to these receptors depending on their state.

Drugs that mainly bind to the active or inactive state are more effective at fast heart rates (use-dependent), while drugs that bind to the resting state are more effective at slow heart rates (reverse use-dependent). **Class I drugs are use-dependent and are more effective when the patient is actively having the tachyarrhythmia, while class III drugs are reverse use-dependent and are more effective in preventing the arrhythmia when the patient is in sinus rhythm**. Thus, class I agents are more effective in cardioverting than preventing AF, while class III agents may be more effective at preventing AF. Furthermore, the use dependency implies that the toxic effect of class I drugs, such as QRS widening and ventricular arrhythmia, is more likely seen during tachycardia; that's why stress testing is used to unveil toxicity after initiating class I therapy.

V. Concept of concealed conduction

Concealed conduction is a concept wherein blocked, non-conducted impulses that do not get recorded on the ECG (= concealed) manage to change the behavior of subsequent impulses. Concealed conduction is seen in the following situations:

- *Atrial fibrillation:* a relatively small proportion of AF waves fully conduct through the AV node, yet the non-conducted AF waves partially penetrate the AV node and make it refractory to subsequent waves. An increase in the number of AF waves leads to more frequent AV nodal penetration and refractoriness and a slowing of the ventricular rate. This explains why the ventricular rate in AF is generally slower and easier to control than the ventricular rate in atrial flutter (the faster atrial rate in AF leads to more concealed conduction across the AV node). This also explains why slowing the rate of the fibrillatory or flutter waves with class I antiarrhythmic drugs paradoxically increases the ventricular rate.

  The instantaneous rate in AF is inversely proportional to the instantaneous number of AF waves hitting the AV node.
- *Infranodal AV block:* an increase in the atrial rate with atropine worsens the infranodal conduction ratio.
- *A blocked premature His complex* does not leave any trace on the ECG, yet it prevents the conduction of the next sinus impulse through the His (still in refractory period), creating the impression of a Mobitz II AV block.
- *Deceleration-dependent bundle branch block*
- In patients with first-degree AV block, a PVC may retrogradely depolarize the AV node prematurely, allowing early repolarization and full AV nodal recovery during the compensatory pause. The next sinus impulse conducts with a shorter PR interval. This is called "peeling back of the AV nodal refractory period" by the PVC.

VI. Specific examples of drugs (see also Chapter 10)

A. Class I

Class Ic drugs (flecainide, propafenone) are the class I drugs most commonly used in clinical practice. They are used for the treatment and prevention of atrial arrhythmias (AF, atrial tachycardia) in patients without any underlying structural heart disease. Class Ia drugs (quinidine, procainamide, disopyramide) are rarely used; disopyramide may be used as an antiarrhythmic and a negative inotrope in HOCM, while IV procainamide may be used in acute VT or pre-excited AF. All class I drugs are preferably avoided in patients with a baseline QRS >120 ms, as they further impair infranodal conduction; they should be discontinued if QRS prolongs >25% after initiation of therapy. A stress test may be performed a week after therapy initiation to unveil QRS prolongation or arrhythmia with exercise/tachycardia. Note that all class I drugs have a *negative inotropic effect*.

Lidocaine is an intravenous class Ib that is only useful in ventricular arrhythmia, particularly VT secondary to acute ischemia.

In the CAST trial, the use of class Ic agents to suppress PVCs in patients with a history of MI and normal or low EF resulted in tripling of cardiac death secondary to arrhythmias and tripling of cardiac death secondary to MI and shock (~8% cardiac death at 10 months). This is related to their proarrhythmic effect (slowing conduction facilitates reentry), which increases sustained arrhythmias at baseline and even more so during MI. They raise defibrillation thresholds and may make VT/VF refractory to shock. The negative inotropic effect also contributes to the increased mortality and shock during MI.

- Class Ia and Ic agents slow the reentrant circuits, thereby reducing the rate of the fibrillatory AF impulses. The non-conducted atrial impulses partially penetrate the AV node and make it partially refractory to subsequent impulses (concealed conduction); thus, a reduction in the rate of atrial impulses allows more impulses to conduct through the AV node, which paradoxically increases the ventricular rate. Also, class I agents may organize AF into a slow atrial flutter with 1:1 conduction, again increasing the ventricular rate. Class I agents are ineffective in cardioverting atrial flutter and may actually allow it to sustain, as they slow the conduction across the large macroreentry, widening its excitable gap.
- Proarrhythmia should be considered whenever a patient on antiarrhythmic drugs presents with a new arrhythmia or even worsening of a pre-existing arrhythmia.

B. Class III (amiodarone, dronedarone, sotalol, ibutilide, dofetilide)

These drugs are proven efficacious for the treatment of atrial arrhythmias. Amiodarone and sotalol can be used for ventricular arrhythmias as well. Class III drugs prolong QT and are associated with a dose-dependent risk of TdP (~2% with sotalol or dofetilide, less so with amiodarone). They should be avoided in patients with QTc >460 ms at baseline (or >500 ms when QRS >120 ms), or if QTc increases by >15% or to >500 ms with therapy. The QT prolongation and risk of TdP are dose-dependent.

After initiating therapy with one of these drugs, patients should be hospitalized and monitored for 3 days with twice-daily ECGs (except amiodarone, where monitoring is often not necessary).

Specific examples of these drugs:

- *Amiodarone* mainly has class III and sympatholytic effects, but also class I and vasodilator effects. Acutely, amiodarone mostly causes a sympatholytic and class I effect; class III effect occurs later. Thus, the effect of amiodarone on ventricular repolarization is slow, with QT prolongation appearing at 4–10 days of therapy and peaking several weeks later. Also, in AF, the early effect is rate slowing (the effect on AF conversion being late).

  Amiodarone reduced total and arrhythmic mortality and progressive HF mortality in patients with ischemic or non-ischemic HF in the older GESICA trial, most of whom had NSVT. Amiodarone reduced arrhythmic death (but not total death) in the EMIAT trial of post-MI patients with LV dysfunction. This was not shown in modern trials (SCD-HeFT), but as opposed to class I agents, amiodarone is a proven safe therapy in HF. Conversely, amiodarone appeared to increase non-cardiac death in the AFFIRM trial, with a similar trend in the EMIAT and AVID trials.

Amiodarone prevents and treats atrial and ventricular arrhythmias in patients with or without underlying heart disease. It is available intravenously and orally.

- *Dronedarone* has a structure similar to amiodarone without the iodine moiety, and thus has reduced extracardiac side effects and a shorter half-life (1–2 days compared to 2 months). However, it is less effective than amiodarone in preventing AF.
- *Sotalol* has both class III and β-blocker effects; the β-blocker effect starts at low doses and is already half-maximal at 80 mg/d, while the class III effect starts at doses of 160 mg/d. Sotalol prevents AF, less effectively than amiodarone, and is mainly effective in AF associated with CAD (SAFE-T trial). Sotalol is also effective in preventing VT and shocks in patients with ICD.
- *Ibutilide* is an intravenous drug that acutely cardioverts AF.
- *Dofetilide* is efficacious in AF prevention. It has proven to be safe in HF and CAD (DIAMOND-CHF and DIAMOND-MI trials).

VII. Amiodarone toxicity

Thyroid toxicity
Amiodarone contains iodine and has the following effects on the thyroid system:

1. It inhibits the T4-to-T3 deiodinase. This leads to increased free T4, reduced T3, and increased TSH early on (first 3–6 months). This is a benign, normal phenomenon.

2. If the patient has a subclinical hypothyroidism, the excessive iodine delivered by amiodarone inhibits thyroid hormone synthesis. This is the Wolff–Chaikoff effect; normal individuals escape from the Wolff–Chaikoff effect, but not patients with thyroid abnormalities.

3. If the patient has an autonomous nodule or subclinical Graves disease, the thyroid autoregulation is disturbed and thus the excess of iodine leads to excessive thyroid hormone synthesis.

4. Amiodarone may lead to an inflammatory thyroiditis, with early hyperthyroidism, followed by normalization of the thyroid function in a few months. Radioiodine uptake study is not very helpful as it shows reduction of iodine uptake in thyroiditis but also in any patient taking amiodarone. It is suggested by elevated inflammatory markers (IL-6) and by thyroid ultrasound showing hyperemia.

If hypothyroidism is present at baseline or develops with therapy, amiodarone may still be used as long as levothyroxine therapy is provided and the thyroid function is closely monitored.

If hyperthyroidism develops, amiodarone should often be stopped. Due to the long half-life of amiodarone, the thyroid function will not improve for a few months. That is why it is acceptable to continue amiodarone for a few more days if necessary (e.g., VT). Hyperthyroidism is treated with β-blockers and thionamides; radioiodine therapy has no role in iodine overload states, and thyroidectomy may be necessary if thyrotoxicosis cannot be controlled. If thyroiditis is suspected, prednisone therapy is given for 1 month with subsequent taper; amiodarone therapy may be continued in this case.

Lung toxicity
Interstitial lung disease occurs at a rate of 0.5–1% per year. It may develop acutely in the first few days (rare), subacutely (weeks), or chronically. Acute and subacute presentations are febrile pneumonitis. The risk is likely higher if underlying lung disease, including COPD, is present, and if doses higher than 200 mg/d are used. Amiodarone lung toxicity often simulates pulmonary edema/heart failure progression. **Amiodarone toxicity should therefore be sought in any patient receiving amiodarone whose pulmonary function is not improving with diuresis and/or antibiotic therapy.** The earliest and most sensitive abnormality is a reduction of diffusion capacity (DL_{CO}). Therefore, it is important to perform a lung function study before initiation of therapy. This study should then be repeated every year.

No diagnostic test is specific for amiodarone lung toxicity. Mononuclear cells on bronchoalveolar lavage are consistent with amiodarone therapy and do not necessary imply toxicity. The clinical context, a refractory pulmonary process, and DL_{CO} are most useful for diagnosis. The lung toxicity is reversible only if diagnosed early, and sometimes improves with steroids.

Neuropathy, ataxia (dose-dependent), blue skin discoloration

VIII. Effect on pacing thresholds and defibrillation thresholds
Class I agents and amiodarone increase defibrillation threshold, i.e., increase the energy requirement for defibrillation of VT/VF. Class I agents also increase pacing threshold, which may lead to a loss of capture, particularly in case of toxicity (e.g., propafenone toxicity).

Further reading
Chen SA, Chiang CE, Yang CJ, et al. Sustained atrial tachycardia in adult patients. Electrophysiological characteristics, pharmacological response, possible mechanisms, and effects of radiofrequency ablation. Circulation 1994; 90: 1262–78.

Engelstein ED, Lippman N, Stein KM, Lerman BB. Mechanism-specific effects of adenosine on atrial tachycardia. Circulation 1994; 89: 2645–54.

Roberts-Thomson KC, Kistler PM, Kalman JM. Atrial tachycardias: mechanisms, diagnosis, and management. Curr Probl Cardiol 2005; 30: 529–73.

Fogoros RN. Abnormal heart rhythms; *and* Treatment of arrhythmias. In: Fogoros RN. Electrophysiologic Testing, 4th edn. Oxford: Blackwell, 2006, pp. 12–22 and 22–34.

Markowitz SM, Nemirovsky D, Stein KM, et al. Adenosine-insensitive focal atrial tachycardia. J Am Coll Cardiol 2007; 49: 1324–33.

Part 6   PERICARDIAL DISORDERS

17   Pericardial Disorders

Practical Cardiovascular Medicine, First Edition. Elias B. Hanna.
© 2017 John Wiley & Sons Ltd. Published 2017 by John Wiley & Sons Ltd.

1. ACUTE PERICARDITIS

I. Causes of acute pericarditis
The four most common causes are:

1. *Viral or idiopathic pericarditis* is the most common form of acute pericarditis (80–90%).
2. *Metastatic cancer*, where a moderate or large effusion is usually seen.
3. *Connective tissue disease* (lupus, rheumatoid arthritis, scleroderma).
4. *Infections* (HIV, tuberculosis, bacterial, fungal, Lyme disease). In patients with HIV infection, pericarditis may be secondary to HIV itself or to a concomitant infection, particularly tuberculosis.

Other common causes of pericarditis, occurring in specific contexts:

1. *Uremia*: an effusion is seen in >50% of patients with uremic pericarditis.
2. *Radiation*: acute pericarditis, with or without effusion, may develop soon after radiation.
3. *Post-MI*: pericarditis can occur early post-MI or late (Dressler syndrome).
4. *Post-cardiac surgery*: pericarditis may occur early (in the first few days) or late (between 2 weeks and 2 months, similarly to Dressler syndrome and called *post-pericardiotomy syndrome*).
5. *Trauma* (blunt or penetrating).

II. History and physical findings
A. Chest pain
- Chest pain is sharp, pleuritic, usually not constricting. It usually has a rapid, sometimes abrupt, onset. It radiates to the trapezius ridge (a typical radiation of pericarditis) and/or the left arm.
- Positional feature: pain is relieved by leaning forward and worsens with lying down, swallowing, or moving (including exertion).
- Concomitant systemic findings may suggest a neoplastic, tuberculous, or autoimmune disease.

B. Friction rub
- The rub is due to the friction of the inflamed visceral and parietal pericardial layers. It is heard during systole, early diastolic filling, and atrial contraction (three components). It is best heard at the left lower sternal border with the patient leaning forward. A sound with a single component is less specific for pericarditis as it may actually represent a murmur.
- The rub is dynamic (it comes and goes), and all three components may not be evident all the time, hence the importance of frequent examinations when pericarditis is suspected.
- A rub may be heard with pericardial effusion when concomitant inflammatory pericarditis is present.

III. ECG findings
(For the differential diagnosis of STEMI vs. pericarditis, see Chapter 31)

A. Diffuse concave ST elevation in all leads except aVR and V₁
The axis of the subepicardial injury being the axis of the heart (~+45°), the ST elevation is most prominent in lead II and in the anterolateral leads, while the ST segment is often depressed in lead aVR, and sometimes V_1 (and occasionally V_2, III, or aVL, which are close to orthogonal to +45°).[1]

The ST segment is elevated at some point in >90% of patients, but normalizes in 1–5 days, often within 7 days. Thus, the ECG of pericarditis can look normal within a few days, at the time the patient presents.

The return of ST segment to baseline is followed, sometimes, by T-wave inversion that may last weeks or months. T wave may become biphasic before ST normalization, mimicking ischemia.

B. PR depression
The PR segment is depressed in 82% of patients, and this may be the earliest change. It is seen in all leads except lead aVR, where reciprocal PR elevation is always seen. While it commonly coexists with ST elevation, it can be an isolated change in ~25% of patients.

ST elevation and PR depression are mainly seen in idiopathic pericarditis, post-cardiac surgery pericarditis, and traumatic and hemorrhagic pericarditis.[2] They are rarely seen in uremic, malignant, or tuberculous pericarditis, probably because of associated processes masking the pericarditis pattern.

C. Low QRS voltage and QRS alternans
If an effusion is present, the ECG may show low QRS voltage and sometimes QRS electrical alternans (which means an every-other-beat alternation of two different QRS morphologies). P- and T-wave alternans, in which two different P- and T-wave morphologies alternate, increases the likelihood of a pericardial effusion. Sinus tachycardia associated with a low QRS voltage or QRS alternans suggests tamponade.

IV. Echocardiography
- **Echocardiography is usually normal, and most often no effusion is appreciated ("dry" pericarditis).** A small effusion is seen in 40% of pericarditis cases.
- **Moderate or large effusions are uncommon, seen in 5% of acute pericarditis cases.** Idiopathic pericarditis is a less likely diagnosis in a patient with a moderate/large effusion but remains the most likely diagnosis; 25–50% of moderate or large pericardial effusions are idiopathic, whereas 80–90% of pericarditis cases with no or small effusions are idiopathic. An effusion increases the likelihood of a specific cause, such as malignancy, infection, or connective tissue disorder.
- LV dysfunction, sometimes segmental, suggests an associated severe myocarditis.

The diagnosis of pericarditis requires two of the following four features:[3]

(1) chest pain; (2) rub; (3) typical ECG findings (widespread ST-segment elevation and/or PR depression); (4) pericardial effusion

- Pericardial effusion is not necessary but confirms the diagnosis when present.
- CRP is a confirmatory finding. CRP is required by some authors for the diagnosis of pericarditis and is a useful monitoring marker.
- ESR may be used but is less specific and rises and falls later than CRP. Conversely, a severely elevated ESR has a valuable diagnostic value and suggests tuberculosis or autoimmune disease.
- A low-titer ANA is very common in idiopathic pericarditis (~40%) and often does not have any clinical significance. ANA testing may be useful in high-risk pericarditis (see below).

V. Myopericarditis and perimyocarditis

Various degrees of myocardial inflammation are seen in patients with pericarditis. In fact, the ST-segment elevation implies subepicardial myocardial involvement rather than just pericardial involvement, the pericardium being electrically silent. Therefore, a troponin rise is common in pericarditis. *Myopericarditis* implies mild myocardial involvement, as evidenced by an elevated troponin, with a normal EF and no wall motion abnormalities. Myopericarditis has a good prognosis, with normalization of the ECG within 12 months and persistence of a normal EF.[3–5] Troponin may be strikingly elevated (median 7 ng/ml, interquartile range 0.5–35 in one study).[5] Unlike in ACS, this elevated troponin does not portend an increase in long-term complications. However, a reduction of the NSAID dose is considered (e.g., aspirin 500 mg TID), exercise is restricted for 4–6 weeks, and return to athletic activity is considered only after 6 months and after normalization of ECG and LV, and in the absence of arrhythmias on Holter and stress test.

When the process predominantly involves the myocardium, it is termed *perimyocarditis* or pure *myocarditis* and manifests as clinical HF or significant LV dysfunction, sometimes segmental. This predominant myocarditis may have ST changes of pericarditis or, more commonly, focal ST changes or Q waves mimicking STEMI. Coronary angiography is done to rule out ACS. Perimyocarditis with mild LV dysfunction (EF 40–50%) is associated with a good long-term prognosis and persistence of LV dysfunction in only 15% of patients.[5] Perimyocarditis with severe LV dysfunction portends an altered long-term prognosis with persistent LV dysfunction in up to 60% of patients.

VI. Treatment

Pericarditis is a self-limiting disease with no complication or recurrence in >70% of patients.

A. Initial therapy

1. A full anti-inflammatory dose of NSAID or aspirin is administered for 1–2 weeks. One dose is usually associated with a dramatic symptomatic effect. Some authors suggest the continuation of therapy until CRP normalizes. One regimen consists of the administration of a full-dose NSAID for a week (e.g., ibuprofen 600 mg TID, aspirin 750–1000 mg TID), followed by gradual tapering over 3 weeks, rather than abrupt cessation (e.g., taper ibuprofen by 200–400 mg per dose every week).[3–6]

2. The systematic use of colchicine (for 3 months) as an adjunct to NSAID during the first episode of pericarditis strikingly reduces the recurrence of pericarditis by 70% (COPE trial).[6] Colchicine therapy may thus be considered systematically and is given a class I in ESC guidelines (1 mg BID the first day, followed by 0.5 mg BID; a lower dose of 0.5 mg BID the first day followed by 0.5 mg once daily is given to patients weighing <70 kg).[4]

3. In the absence of a response to NSAID, reconsider the possibility of specific etiologies. The NSAID dose may need to be increased, as inappropriately low doses may explain some therapeutic failures. Colchicine should be added. Glucocorticoids are generally avoided, as they increase the risk of recurrence, probably through the exacerbation of viral proliferation. Yet, glucocorticoids may be used in refractory cases.

4. Exercise restriction is warranted until clinical, ECG, and CRP resolution of acute pericarditis, more so in athletes (3 months). In myopericarditis or perimyocarditis, exercise restriction of 4–6 weeks is suggested in non-athletes, and at least 6 months in athletes. A normalization of the ECG, LV function, and CRP is required before return to athletic activity.[3,4]

5. The following high-risk features increase the likelihood of a specific diagnosis (i.e., neoplastic, autoimmune, infectious) and the likelihood of complications, and therefore warrant hospitalization and a specific etiologic workup:[3,4,7]

    a. No response to 1 week of NSAID therapy

    b. Moderate or large effusion

    c. Subacute onset over days to weeks

    d. Fever >38 °C

    e. Clinical suspicion of a specific etiology

    The specific etiologic workup consists of: HIV testing, PPD, ANA/rheumatoid factor, screening for specific cancers.

    Also, myocarditis warrants hospitalization.

B. Recurrent pericarditis

Between 15% and 30% of patients with idiopathic or autoimmune pericarditis develop recurrent pericarditis within 20 months after the initial episode, and pericarditis may keep relapsing for several years.[8] It is due to an autoimmune process initiated by the initial viral infection, although persistent or recurrent infection is possible. A recurrence within 6 weeks of the initial episode is usually considered a persistence of the initial pericarditis and is called "incessant" rather than recurrent pericarditis.

In the absence of high-risk features, recurrent pericarditis is usually idiopathic and does not warrant specific workup.[3] Moreover, recurrent idiopathic pericarditis is usually milder than the initial pericarditis and is not associated with pericardial constriction; in fact, the risk of constrictive pericarditis is lower after a recurrence than after the initial episode of pericarditis.[9] One-third of patients have pleuropericardial involvement during these recurrences.

For each recurrence, repeat the course of NSAID for a longer duration (2–4 weeks) with slow tapering over an additional 3–4 weeks, and give a course of colchicine for ≥6 months.[10] Avoid glucocorticoids, except for refractory pericarditis.

C. If an effusion is present, look for a specific etiology (see Section 3, *Pericardial effusion*, below) and perform serial echocardiographic exams. Echo is repeated during the hospital stay to ensure stability of the effusion, then serial outpatient echo exams are performed to ensure resolution of the effusion within a few months.

D. The occurrence of constrictive pericarditis after acute idiopathic pericarditis is uncommon (<1%), and even less common after recurrent pericarditis. Approximately 9% of patients may have a transient constrictive physiology that resolves in a few months (mean 2.1 months).[3,11]

2. TAMPONADE

I. Definition

Cardiac tamponade is defined as a pericardial effusion compressing one or more cardiac chambers and leading to hemodynamic compromise.

In tamponade, the pericardial fluid distends the pericardium and raises the intrapericardial pressure to ~10–25 mmHg, compressing one or more cardiac chambers. In typical, circumferential tamponade, *this high intrapericardial pressure compresses all cardiac chambers in diastole until the pressure inside the four cardiac chambers equalizes with the intrapericardial pressure.* This leads to equalization of the diastolic pressures of the four cardiac chambers. Since the right-sided chambers have thin walls, they tend to collapse when the intrapericardial pressure is equal to or larger than their intracavitary pressure.

In acute conditions, the pericardium cannot distend and its pressure rises markedly with small volume changes. This explains how tamponade develops with a small acute effusion (~200 ml). This also explains how the pericardium gets stretched in acute RV dilatation, leading to a "functional" constrictive pericarditis. Conversely, a slowly developing pericardial effusion induces tamponade only after a large volume of fluid has accumulated.

II. Pathophysiology and hemodynamics

The equalization of diastolic pressures is similar to what is observed in constrictive pericarditis. As opposed to constrictive pericarditis, however, the respiratory changes of intrathoracic pressure are transmitted to the cardiac chambers.[12,13] This explains why RA pressure decreases with inspiration, and thus venous flow from outside the thorax to the RA increases during inspiration (jugular venous pressure decreases, explaining the absence of Kussmaul's sign). Left-sided flow does not increase because both pulmonary veins and LV are exposed to the negative intrathoracic pressure. The increased venous flow to the right cavities makes the RV "push" against the LV in diastole, rather than "push" against the pericardium, since the high pericardial pressure prevents that (*ventricular interdependence*). This reduces LV filling in normal inspiration and explains the reduction of systolic arterial pressure by more than 10 mmHg with *normal* inspiration (pulsus paradoxus, which is an extreme form of RV–LV discordant filling).[14]

Also, as opposed to constrictive pericarditis, where the heart briefly expands in early diastole before getting constrained, the heart is compressed throughout all diastole in tamponade, including early diastole. Thus, there is no deep Y on the RA tracing and no diastolic dip on the RV tracing. There is a deep X in early systole as the RV annulus moves down and stretches out the compressed RA.[14]

In summary, tamponade is characterized by the following three hemodynamic findings:

1. Elevation and equalization of diastolic pressures of the four cardiac chambers, similarly to constrictive pericarditis: **CVP = PCWP** = diastolic PA pressure = RVEDP = LVEDP. This equalization of diastolic pressures may also be seen in severe RV failure that creates a functional pericardial constriction.

2. Elevated RA pressure with a **deep X descent** (mainly during inspiration), and a **flat Y descent**. The elevated RA pressure is equalized with the intrapericardial pressure on simultaneous RA–pericardial recording, particularly in expiration (Figure 17.1).

3. While the systolic aortic pressure is initially normal or even elevated as a result of the adrenergic release, **pulsus paradoxus** is present and pulse pressure is abnormal early on. On any arterial or aortic tracing, pulsus paradoxus means that systolic pressure decreases >10 mmHg

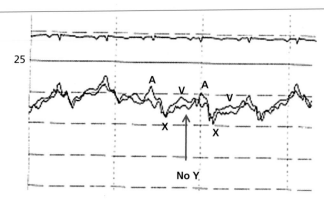

Figure 17.1 Simultaneous pericardial and RA pressures are recorded in tamponade, before pericardiocentesis. The RA and pericardial pressures are elevated and equalized (~20 mmHg); this defines tamponade. The two tracings are actually superimposed, particularly in expiration; the pericardial pressure falls a bit more than the RA pressure in inspiration. Furthermore, X descent is seen, but Y descent is flat (**mnemonic: Flat Y Tamponade = FYT**).

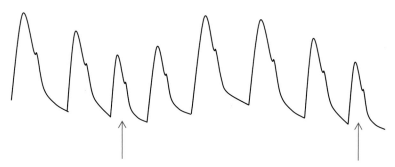

Figure 17.2 Pulsus paradoxus. Note the drop of systolic and pulse pressure during *normal* inspiration (*arrows*). The arterial waveform also becomes narrower.

with *normal* inspiration. In addition, the arterial waveform is narrow and the pulse pressure is reduced (arterial tracing is "short" and narrow) (Figure 17.2).

III. Diagnosis: tamponade is a clinical diagnosis, not an echocardiographic diagnosis
Tamponade is diagnosed when a *large pericardial effusion* is associated with *hemodynamic compromise*, i.e., any one of the following clinical findings:

1. Elevated JVP.

2. Pulsus paradoxus, which is a decrease of SBP of >10 mmHg during *normal, quiet inspiration*. Example: when using the BP cuff, the Korotkoff sounds are heard intermittently at a systolic pressure of 150 mmHg and consistently (with each cardiac cycle) at a pressure of 120; therefore, the pulsus paradoxus is 30 mmHg. Avoid deep breathing during this measurement, as deep breathing is normally associated with an inspiratory drop of aortic pressure.

The blood pressure is normal or elevated early on. Ultimately, the blood pressure declines. An increase in systolic pressure up to 150–210 mmHg and diastolic blood pressure up to 100–130 mmHg is frequent in tamponade and occurred in up to one-third of tamponade cases in one report, particularly in patients with a history of hypertension who are sensitive to the catecholamine surge.[15] Hypertension does not imply preserved cardiac output; in fact, cardiac output is as low as in cases of normal arterial pressure, but increased peripheral vascular resistance preserves arterial pressure (pressure = flow × resistance). Patients with tamponade and hypertension have a reduction in blood pressure, reduction in systemic vascular resistance, and increase in cardiac output following pericardiocentesis.[15]

3. Sinus tachycardia that attempts to compensate for the low stroke volume. Tachycardia may be absent in hypothyroidism and sometimes uremia (sinus node disease).

4. Dyspnea/tachypnea/orthopnea with clear lungs. PCWP is increased up to 30 mmHg but the intracardiac and pulmonary venous volume is low, hence the *lack of pulmonary edema and lack of significant hypoxemia despite severe dyspnea*.

A decrease in heart sounds is characteristic of a large effusion but not necessarily tamponade. Even when an effusion is large, a friction rub may still be heard with inflammatory etiologies.

IV. Echocardiographic findings supporting the hemodynamic compromise of tamponade
(See also Chapter 32, Section VI)

1. RV collapse in diastole. This is the most specific echo finding in tamponade. Sometimes, just an early diastolic indentation of the RVOT is seen on the parasternal long-axis M mode.

2. RA collapse in ventricular systole. RA collapse lasting over one-third of systole is specific for tamponade. RA collapse is generally more sensitive but less specific for tamponade than RV collapse.

3. Inspiratory changes of transmitral and transtricuspid flow. An inspiratory decrease of left-sided transmitral flow by >25%, or an inspiratory increase of right-sided transtricuspid flow, during *normal breathing*, suggests tamponade (this is equivalent to the pulsus paradoxus). This is the earliest echo sign of tamponade.

4. IVC dilatation with poor inspiratory collapse. IVC abnormality has a sensitivity of 97% and a specificity of 40% for tamponade. IVC is rarely normal in tamponade (the so-called low-pressure tamponade).

Findings on **hepatic venous Doppler**: the flat Y descent on the RA tracing corresponds to a *flat D wave on the hepatic venous Doppler. This contrasts with constriction, where both S and D are prominent. Inspiratory rise of these waves may be seen in both conditions.*

5. Other findings

- A rapid change in the effusion size suggests a threatened tamponade.
- An abnormal septal motion may be seen as a result of ventricular interdependence.
- A swinging heart, i.e., a heart that changes position in a phasic manner, may be seen with a large effusion and corresponds to the electrical alternans seen on ECG. It does not necessarily imply tamponade.
- Strands in the pericardial fluid imply inflammation or bleeding and can be seen with most effusions, except transudative effusions.

TEE, CT, or MRI may be performed when a loculated effusion with a regional tamponade is suspected.

V. Role of hemodynamic evaluation

The diagnosis of tamponade is established on clinical and echo grounds, and right heart catheterization is not usually necessary. However, if a Swan catheter is in place (e.g., post cardiac surgery), the following findings suggest tamponade: (i) an elevated CVP that approximates PCWP and PA diastolic pressure; (ii) a flat Y descent on RA tracing.

Also, right heart catheterization may be performed before and particularly after pericardiocentesis to document the hemodynamic improvement. Pericardial pressure is measured before drainage, in which case it is elevated (>0 mmHg) and equal to the RA pressure. ***Normalization of the pericardial pressure (to ≤0 mmHg) and the RA pressure must be documented after drainage. In fact, the normal pericardial pressure is ≤0 mmHg. The lack of full hemodynamic improvement suggests effusive–constrictive pericarditis.***

VI. Special circumstances: low-pressure tamponade, tamponade with absent pulsus paradoxus, regional tamponade

A. Low-pressure tamponade

In patients who are hypovolemic, compression of intracardiac chambers (i.e., tamponade), particularly right-sided chambers, may occur at a lower intrapericardial pressure of 6–12 mmHg. In this case, there will be equalization of intrapericardial pressure and RA pressure at 6–12 mmHg. Thus, tamponade with pulsus paradoxus or hypotension occurs with a high-normal or mildly increased right-sided filling pressure and jugular venous pressure.[14] Were it not for hypovolemia and the low right-sided filling pressure, this pericardial effusion would not yet be hemodynamically significant. Fluid administration may correct the pulsus paradoxus; however, excessive fluid administration may sometimes increase the right-sided volume, which further stretches the already distended pericardium and elevates its pressure, leading to a full-blown tamponade picture.[16,17] That is why fluids are helpful in hypovolemic patients with tamponade but may harm euvolemic or hypervolemic patients. In order to maintain a proper transmural pressure of the cardiac chambers, it is important to maintain a higher level of intracardiac pressure without excessive volume resuscitation (transmural pressure = intracavitary pressure minus pericardial pressure). Ultimately, patients with a low-pressure tamponade require pericardiocentesis since even at 6–12 mmHg, the intrapericardial pressure is at a steep portion of the pressure–volume relationship and is liable to rise with any change in pericardial volume (Figure 17.3).

B. Underlying RV or LV failure and causes of absent pulsus paradoxus

While it is easy to induce tamponade in case of hypovolemia, it is difficult to induce tamponade physiology in patients with severely increased right-sided or left-sided diastolic pressure.[14] In fact, it is harder for the pericardial pressure to compress both ventricles, and tamponade develops when pericardial pressure equilibrates with the lower-pressure ventricle. Moreover, the respiratory variation in venous return does not significantly change the cardiac output and the systolic pressure of the failing ventricle (flat portion of the Frank–Starling curve). The latter two conditions, that is, the lack of biventricular compression (and therefore lack of interdependence) and the lack of respiratory variation in ventricular output explain the lack of pulsus paradoxus. This situation may be seen in patients with cor pulmonale and in patients with end-stage renal disease and underlying left heart failure.

In addition, pulsus paradoxus may not be seen in: (1) ASD, where the increase in right-sided flow during inspiration is balanced by an increase in right-to-left shunt or reduction in left-to-right shunt, leading to less ventricular interdependence; (2) local tamponade (e.g., localized compression of one ventricle or atrium by a clot after cardiac surgery, leading to a localized increase in pressure); (3) AI, where the diastolic regurgitant flow damps down respiratory fluctuations of flow. In addition, pulsus paradoxus is difficult to detect in case of an irregular rhythm such as atrial fibrillation.

C. Regional tamponade

This occurs when only one cardiac chamber, a pulmonary vein, or the SVC or IVC is compressed by a loculated effusion (e.g., anterior loculation compressing the RV or RA, posterior loculation compressing the LV or LA). Since there is no uniform compression of the four chambers, there is no equalization of diastolic pressures and no ventricular interdependence/pulsus paradoxus. There is increased pressure of the compressed chamber, e.g., increased RA pressure or PCWP, and hypotension, which in the right context suggest tamponade (e.g., after cardiac surgery). However, loculation can also produce classic tamponade, presumably by tightening the uninvolved pericardium.

TEE or cardiac CT or MRI should be performed when a regional tamponade is suspected.

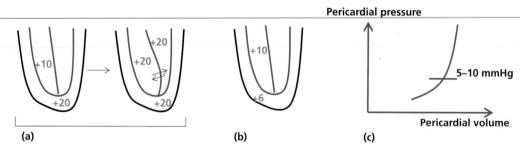

Figure 17.3 The normal pericardial pressure is negative and reaches 0 mmHg at end-expiration (–10 to 0 mmHg). **(a)** Tamponade occurs when the pericardial pressure exceeds the pressure of a cardiac chamber (e.g., RV), thus compressing it and making it equalize with it. Typically, both ventricles get constrained by the pericardial shell, such that their pressure rises and equalizes with the pericardial pressure. They expand at the expense of each other (*arrows*). **(b)** Even before the RV gets compressed by the pericardial pressure, the transmural pressure of the RV and the RV expansion are affected (RV diastolic pressure = 10, pericardial pressure = 6 → the RV transmural, expansile pressure is reduced to +4). **(c)** Compliance curve of the pericardium, showing how the pericardial pressure rises quickly beyond a certain pressure point, even before tamponade occurs (threatened tamponade). This curve is more leftward in sudden acute effusions, wherein the pericardium is not compliant.

D. COPD and other causes of pulsus paradoxus and RV–LV respiratory discordance

Because of large intrathoracic pressure swings, COPD, asthma, morbid obesity, or positive-pressure ventilation may lead to discordance in RV and LV filling and pulsus paradoxus.

VII. Effusive–constrictive pericarditis

Some patients have a pericardial effusion with the hemodynamics of tamponade, i.e., pulsus paradoxus with elevated and equalized right- and left-sided filling pressures. However, upon drainage of the pericardial fluid, the hemodynamic compromise does not fully resolve. RV and LV diastolic pressures remain equalized, RA pressure remains elevated (RA pressure declines by <50%), and the pericardial pressure declines but remains high. A flat RA Y descent (tamponade) may become deep (constriction) after drainage of the pericardial fluid. Effusive–constrictive pericarditis is an effusion that occurs on a background of constrictive pericarditis. In patients with a non-compliant pericardium, tamponade may occur with relatively little accumulation of fluid.

Effusive–constrictive pericarditis may be seen with constrictive pericarditis of any origin, particularly idiopathic or radiation-induced constrictive pericarditis, and is usually seen early in the disease course. In fact, up to 24% of constrictive pericarditis cases and 7% of tamponade cases have an effusive–constrictive pathophysiology.[18,19] When idiopathic, effusive–constrictive pericarditis is often an inflammatory constrictive pericarditis that is transient in 50% of the cases and resolves with anti-inflammatory therapy; this is not the case with radiation-induced effusive– constrictive pericarditis.[18]

VIII. Treatment of tamponade

Tamponade is initially temporized with fluid resuscitation. For example, administer one 500 ml fluid bolus at a time. Avoid excessive fluid resuscitation, as it may worsen pericardial distension and ventricular interdependence.

Similarly, avoid preload reduction (nitrates, diuretics).

Pericardiocentesis is urgently indicated, and the catheter is allowed to drain for ~3 days. Pericardiocentesis is often a definitive treatment of idiopathic effusions and late postoperative effusions, and at least a temporary treatment of malignant effusions.

A pericardial window is particularly useful for recurrences or loculated effusions (see below).

3. PERICARDIAL EFFUSION

A pericardial effusion without tamponade is not associated with hemodynamic compromise but may be associated with a dull ache and sometimes a pericarditic chest pain, particularly in the case of an inflammatory effusion. Dyspnea on exertion may occur and is, in fact, a manifestation of early tamponade. In order to be well tolerated and asymptomatic, a large effusion must be chronic. A large effusion is defined as an effusion larger than 2 cm; moderate and small effusions are 1–2 cm and <1 cm wide, respectively. The effusion is measured as the summation of the anterior and posterior echo-free spaces in *diastole*.[20,21] This measurement is smaller in diastole than systole, but the diastolic measurement is what accounts for the diastolic compression and for the ability to tap (must be >2–3 cm to allow a safe pericardiocentesis).

I. Causes of a pericardial effusion with or without tamponade

Several series of moderate to large pericardial effusions have reported a lower prevalence of idiopathic causes compared with acute pericarditis. *Similarly to acute pericarditis,* the five most common causes of a moderate or large effusion are: [3,20,22,23]

1. *Viral/idiopathic.* Viral/idiopathic pericarditis rarely leads to a large effusion or tamponade, yet is still the most common cause of effusion and tamponade. Approximately 30–50% of large pericardial effusions are viral/idiopathic. While most HIV effusions are small, a large HIV effusion has a high rate of progression to tamponade (PRECIA study).[24]

2. *Neoplastic (lung, breast, lymphoma, melanoma).* Malignancy causes 20–30% of pericardial effusions. Approximately 20% of patients with tamponade of unsuspected etiology are diagnosed with malignant effusion, this being their first cancer manifestation. Tamponade is a greater predictor of malignancy than an asymptomatic effusion.

3. *Metabolic (uremia or hypothyroidism).*

4. *Connective tissue diseases.*

5. *Specific bacterial infection or tuberculosis.* Bacterial infections can spread from contiguous sites (pneumonia, empyema, ruptured valvular abscess, thoracic surgery) or hematogenously.

Other causes are seen in specific contexts:

1. *Post-cardiac surgery.* The effusion may be an early hemorrhagic effusion, occurring in the first postoperative week. The effusion may also occur late, > 1 week postoperatively, secondarily to a post-pericardiotomy syndrome; it usually resolves within weeks.

2. *Post-MI.* The effusion may occur early (resolves slowly over months) or late (along with Dressler syndrome). An early small effusion is often not worrisome, per se, and may accompany post-MI pericarditis or HF. Conversely, an early moderate or large effusion suggests a threatening free wall rupture.

3. *Radiation therapy.* An early effusion (<1 year) may occur as part of an acute pericarditis and is sometimes recurrent. A late effusion (>1 year) is part of an effusive–constrictive pericarditis.

4. *HF or volume overload states (nephrotic syndrome, cirrhosis).* Pericardial effusion is usually small or moderate in size, transudative, and only develops when right heart failure is present, as the pericardial veins drain in the coronary sinus. Isolated left heart failure does not lead to a pericardial effusion. A large pericardial effusion is rare but possible.[21]

5. *Hemorrhagic pericardial effusion,* from a penetrating or blunt trauma, free wall rupture post-MI, complication of PCI (coronary perforation) or complication of device implantation (RA or RV rupture). Outside these traumatic/rupture contexts, a bloody effusion may be seen with a broad range of etiologies, such as *malignant, viral, or infectious,* with a prognosis that depends on the underlying etiology.

6. *Drugs* (mainly *minoxidil* and drug-induced lupus: *hydralazine,* izoniazide).

A large idiopathic pericardial effusion has a relatively low risk of progression to tamponade. Conversely, neoplastic, bacterial/tuberculous/HIV, and postoperative large effusions have a high risk of progression to tamponade. Hemorrhagic effusions have an imminent risk of tamponade.

II. Management of asymptomatic effusions and role of pericardiocentesis

A. General approach to a large asymptomatic effusion (Figure 17.4)

Two main concerns dictate the management of asymptomatic effusions: (i) etiology and (ii) risk of progression to tamponade. Up to 60% of patients with moderate/large pericardial effusions have a known medical condition, such as cancer, uremia, previous cardiac surgery, or connective tissue disease, which points toward a specific diagnosis.[20] The following strategy is suggested:

1. In the absence of a known medical condition that could cause a pericardial effusion, screen for some cancers, HIV/tuberculosis, and metabolic disorders using clinical findings and: CXR, mammography, chest CT; PPD, HIV; TSH, renal function, rheumatoid factor, ANA.

2. Check markers of inflammation (CRP, ESR), which, if elevated without any cancer/infection/autoimmune disease, suggest a pericarditic process (viral/idiopathic).[1]

3. If a *malignant* or *bacterial (including tuberculous)* etiology is suspected, pericardiocentesis is indicated both for its diagnostic and staging value and because of the high risk of progression to tamponade ("threatened tamponade").[3] Only 50% of effusions in cancer patients are due to malignant metastasis, the remaining being induced by inflammation, obstruction of lymphatic drainage, or radiation; hence the additional diagnostic importance of pericardiocentesis in these patients.[25]

If a *hemorrhagic pericardial effusion* is suspected (traumatic, iatrogenic), pericardiocentesis is indicated because of the imminent risk of tamponade.

If an effusion is increasing in size, pericardiocentesis is warranted because of the risk of tamponade.

4. Ensure the patient is truly asymptomatic. Even when the intrapericardial pressure is lower than the right-sided pressures, the RV or RA transmural pressure (RV pressure minus intrapericardial pressure) is reduced, which impairs RV outward expansion and filling. For example, if the pericardial pressure is 6 mmHg and the RV diastolic pressure is 10 mmHg, the RV does not collapse towards the LV, but it cannot appropriately expand and the cardiac output is already reduced. Also, at this point, pericardial pressure is at a steep slope and there is at least a threatened tamponade (Figure 17.3).[26] In fact, one study has shown that almost all patients with a large asymptomatic effusion who underwent pericardiocentesis had a high intrapericardial pressure and a reduced RA transmural pressure.[21,25] Thus, vague symptoms of fatigue or dyspnea on exertion often represent early hemodynamic compromise and warrant pericardiocentesis. The same applies to the echo signs of pre-tamponade.

5. If all of the above is ruled out, the asymptomatic effusion is likely isolated, i.e., idiopathic. If the inflammatory markers are increased or if inflammatory signs are present (characteristic chest pain, friction rub, fever, or typical ECG changes), a pericarditic process is suspected and may be treated with NSAID and colchicine (class I indication).[3,4,25] Echo follow-up is warranted to detect improvement of the effusion (or lack thereof), on a weekly basis initially.[25] An autoimmune process is managed similarly.

6. A chronic, large idiopathic effusion that persists for >3 months has a significant risk of progression to tamponade of 33%.[3,4,21] Tamponade may develop unexpectedly and suddenly in patients who have had a chronic stable effusion for several years.[21] The remaining patients remain stable; the effusion may regress at least partially, and a specific cause does not usually emerge with time.[21] Thus, close echo surveillance is warranted. Alternatively, pericardial drainage may be considered for effusions persisting >3 months because of the 33% risk of tamponade.[3,25]

A pericardiocentesis has a therapeutic but also a diagnostic value. The overall diagnostic yield of a pericardiocentesis is ~30%,[27] but it is higher in neoplastic or bacterial effusions. The yield in neoplastic effusions is >50% (50%[28] to 80%[21,23]). The pericardial fluid should be sent for cytology, cell count, bacterial and mycobacterial culture, and polymerase chain reaction of *Mycobacterium tuberculosis* (the latter is highly sensitive for tuberculous pericarditis).

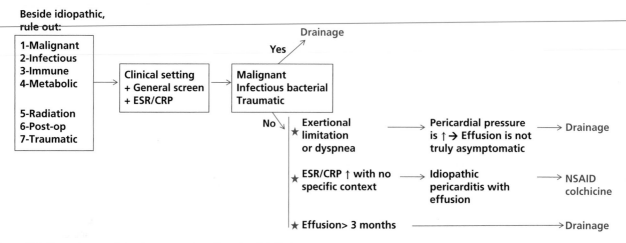

Figure 17.4 General approach to a large, asymptomatic pericardial effusion.

B. Pericardiocentesis and open pericardiotomy (pericardial window)

Pericardiocentesis alone is often a definitive treatment of idiopathic pericardial effusion; in one series, recurrences only occurred in 8% of patients over long-term follow-up.[3,29] However, another series suggested that recurrences are common and occur in 65% of patients with idiopathic large effusions.[21] The duration of catheter drainage may explain the discrepancy. This recurrence rate is higher in malignant effusions, although pericardiocentesis may still be tried as a first-line therapy or as a temporizing measure in the unstable patient. Since fluid reaccumulation most commonly occurs in the first 48 hours after drainage, pericardiocentesis with prolonged catheter drainage is associated with an acceptable risk of recurrence of malignant effusions (<20%), particularly in view of the fact that patients with malignant effusions have a median survival of 3.5 months only.[28] Hence, some authors recommend pericardiocentesis as a first and effective therapy in malignant effusions.[25]

A catheter should be left in the pericardial space at least until the drainage is <25 ml/24 hours. Prolonged catheter drainage for several days (e.g., 3–5 days), even after the drainage ceases, is preferred, as it provokes inflammation that obliterates the pericardial space and reduces the risk of recurrence to <20–25%.[25,28,29]

Echo-guided pericardiocentesis may be performed through a *left subxiphoid* approach. The needle accesses the *inferior (diaphragmatic)* aspect of the pericardial space, *not the posterior/lateral* aspect. In a supine position, a free-flowing effusion accumulates on the posterior/lateral aspect; thus, the patient should be placed in an upright position to allow a free-flowing pericardial effusion to collect over the diaphragmatic aspect (Figures 17.5, 17.6). An effusion loculated at the posterior (lateral) aspect of the LV is not accessible; the same applies to an effusion loculated over the anterior aspect of the heart (RV free wall). An apical approach for the former and a parasternal approach for the latter may allow drainage. An apical approach is also simpler in obese patients, where it is difficult for the subxiphoid needle to cross the abdominal fat and get underneath the ribs. Right heart catheterization is typically performed after pericardiocentesis, to document the hemodynamic improvement.

Open pericardiotomy consists of cutting a "window" in the parietal pericardium to allow it to chronically drain in the mediastinum, which prevents recurrences. This is also known as a "pericardial window" and is usually performed through a subxiphoid access. Pericardial tissue and biopsies obtained through this procedure should be sent for analysis. A pericardial window is considered in the following cases: (i) recurrence of a large effusion, (ii) loculation, (iii) recurrence expected (malignant effusion), or (iv) a surgical biopsy is required for diagnosis (malignant effusion). Pericardiocentesis is still warranted for acute tamponade while awaiting surgery. After a pericardial window, the open parietal pericardium may adhere to the visceral pericardium or the sternum, in which case the effusion may recur (<5%). Even after a window procedure, prolonged drainage may reduce recurrences.

III. Note on postoperative pericardial effusions (after cardiac surgery)

Postoperative pericardial effusions may occur early, in the first postoperative week, in which case they are hemorrhagic with a high risk of tamponade; they usually require urgent drainage.

Outside these early bleeding complications, inflammatory postoperative effusions are common and typically appear or progress over the first 8–10 days, then tend to spontaneously regress thereafter (called late postoperative effusions). In fact, by postoperative day 8, ~40% of patients have a small effusion, ~20% have a moderate effusion, and 1% have a large effusion. By postoperative day 20–30, most of these effusions resolve or improve (by 5–10 mm on average), but ~10% of patients still have a moderate effusion.[30-32] Large effusions have at least a 25% risk of progressing to tamponade within 30 days, while the risk with moderate effusions is ~10%; the risk may even be higher when these effusions persist longer.

These late effusions may be due to slow blood oozing in the pericardium or to a post-pericardiotomy syndrome, which is a pericardial and pleural inflammatory process occurring later than a week after surgery. In fact, half of these late effusions are hemorrhagic, while the other half are serosanguinous.

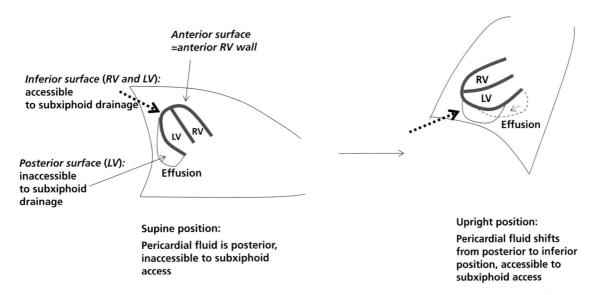

Figure 17.5 Heart surfaces in relation to the subxiphoid pericardiocentesis, in both supine and upright positions. On echo, the long-axis view and the apical four-chamber view show the posterior part of the effusion, not the one that will be accessed by pericardiocentesis. The subcostal view best shows the inferior part of the effusion, next to the inferior diaphragmatic wall of the RV (next to the liver).

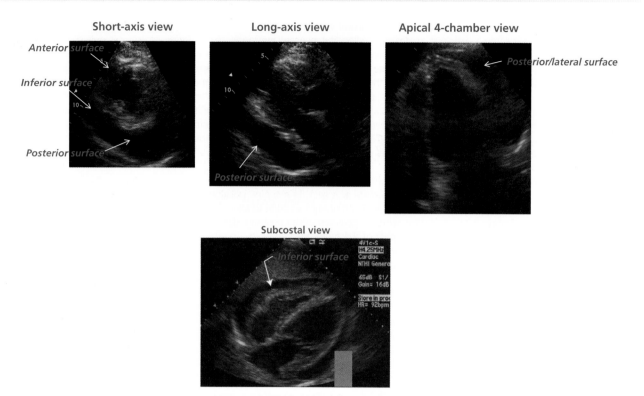

Figure 17.6 Various echo views showing the various heart surfaces in a patient with pericardial effusion. The long-axis and four-chamber views show the posterolateral aspect of the effusion. The subcostal view shows the inferior aspect of the effusion next to the liver and is the one used to guide the left subxiphoid access.

During cardiac surgery, the pericardium is opened and left open, which may seem protective against the development of a pericardial effusion. In reality, the edges of the cut pericardium may adhere to the sternum and create a new pericardial space, which is bound by the sternum anteriorly and the pericardium posterolaterally and superiorly. Moreover, the parietal pericardium may adhere to the visceral pericardium, thus closing the pericardial space. Hence, half of the postoperative pericardial effusions are circumferential, more so in case of tamponade, while the other half are loculated. Most loculated effusions are either anterior (meaning, over the RV) or posterolateral. Isolated loculation over the RA is less common (LA much less common).

Management

Moderate pericardial effusions warrant close echo follow-up (1–2 weeks) to document regression, especially if the patient is receiving anticoagulation. Small effusions may also require follow-up, especially if they develop early on (<7 days) or if the patient is receiving anticoagulants.[30–33]

Asymptomatic large pericardial effusions typically need to be drained, particularly if the patient is receiving anticoagulants.[30,33] Early drainage or close surveillance followed by drainage (in the absence of a quick improvement within a week) are both acceptable strategies in patients not receiving anticoagulants.

Echo-guided pericardiocentesis is a safe and effective treatment of late postoperative effusions requiring drainage. In two major series, most postoperative effusions were drained percutaneously, with a low recurrence rate of only 4%.[33] Subxiphoid pericardial window is another alternative, and is particularly useful for loculated effusions inaccessible percutaneously (posterior effusions), recurrent effusions, and possibly effusions occurring in patients receiving anticoagulants (higher recurrence risk).

NSAIDs have not been shown to significantly change the natural history of asymptomatic postoperative effusions (POPE trial), even though the mechanism of these effusions is thought to be inflammatory.[31] Nonetheless, NSAIDs may be useful in patients with increased CRP.

IV. Note on uremic pericardial effusion

Two forms of renal pericarditis are seen. One form occurs in acute or advanced chronic renal failure not undergoing dialysis (classic uremic pericarditis), while the second form occurs in patients undergoing adequate chronic dialysis with normal BUN and creatinine (dialysis-associated pericarditis).

Uremic pericardial effusion usually resolves after several weeks of intensive hemodialysis (heparin should be used cautiously during dialysis); unless tamponade is present, watchful management is appropriate.[2] The effusion occurring in patients adequately receiving chronic dialysis inconsistently responds to dialysis intensification. A pericardial window may be required.

4. CONSTRICTIVE PERICARDITIS

Constrictive pericarditis is due to pericardial scarring that takes years to develop, but in some instances it only takes a few months. The pericardium becomes a stiff "shell" that surrounds the right and left cardiac chambers and impairs their filling, leading to signs of right heart failure and symptoms of left heart failure. A transient constrictive physiology without pericardial scarring may be seen after any pericardial inflammation (such as 9% of acute idiopathic pericarditis).[34]

I. Causes

The three most common causes of constrictive pericarditis are, in order of frequency: idiopathic, post-cardiac surgery, and post-mediastinal irradiation.[35,36]

Other, less common causes, are: autoimmune (especially rheumatoid arthritis), post-infectious, traumatic, malignant.

Postoperative constrictive pericarditis may appear as early as 2 weeks or as late as 25 years after cardiac surgery, the majority of cases appearing 3–24 months postoperatively. The constrictive process has an incidence of ~0.1% and may be related to the post-pericardiotomy syndrome. Constrictive pericarditis occurring within 2 months postoperatively warrants medical therapy with anti-inflammatory agents, as this early process is often an inflammatory, transient constrictive process with limited fibrosis.

Constrictive pericarditis typically develops years after radiation therapy (range 1–40 years, median 13 years).

II. Pathophysiology and hemodynamics

The stiff pericardial shell results in three effects:

1. Early during diastole, the pressures of all four cardiac chambers increase enough to equalize with the pressure exerted by the stretched "shell", i.e., *a high pressure* of 15–25 mmHg.
2. The shell prevents the transmission of intrathoracic pressure to the cardiac chambers (dissociation between intracardiac and intrathoracic pressures).
3. Both LV and RV are constricted within this shell, so that a change in volume of one chamber reflects upon the other (ventricular interdependence).

These three effects explain the following pathophysiology:

- ***Diastolic pressure of all four cardiac chambers, diastolic PA pressure, and diastolic PCWP (~mean PCWP) all become high and equal to the pressure of the stretched pericardium (high equalization of diastolic pressures)****. Thus, mean RA pressure = mean PCWP and RVEDP = diastolic PA pressure = LVEDP.*
- ***Ventricular dip–plateau pattern and deep atrial X and Y descents (high RA pressure with M or W shape)*** (Figure 17.7).
- ***During inspiration*** (Figure 17.8):[37–40]

  ○ In the absence of constriction, there is an inspiratory decrease in pulmonary venous pressure and an inspiratory decrease in LA pressure and LV pressure, such that the driving gradient between the pulmonary veins and the LV remains grossly unchanged, and the flow only minimally changes. In constriction, there is an inspiratory decrease in pulmonary venous pressure, but the LA and LV pressures are

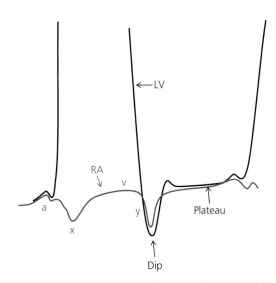

Figure 17.7 Simultaneous RA and LV pressure recordings in constrictive pericarditis. These demonstrate a dip–plateau pattern on the LV tracing, deep X and Y descents on the RA tracing, and equalization of diastolic pressures of LV and RA. In early diastole, upon ventricular relaxation, there is a sharp decrease of ventricular pressure with subsequent "sucking" from the atria in early diastole. However, due to constriction, the pressure in the ventricles quickly rises and equalizes with the pericardial pressure. This explains the *dip–plateau (square root)* shape of the RV and LV tracings in diastole and the *deep and rapid Y descent* on the RA and LA tracings during the early diastolic "sucking." Y descent and the ventricular dip are superimposed.

In early systole, upon downward movement of the valvular annulus, RA and LA pressures sharply decrease before they again promptly equalize with the pericardial pressure; this explains the *deep and rapid X descent*. X and Y descents are mainly deep in inspiration. Reproduced with permission of Demos Medical from Hanna (2012).[37]

unchanged, so that the driving gradient between the pulmonary veins and the LV is reduced. This reduces flow towards the LV (manifested as reduced transmitral E velocity on Doppler). Owing to ventricular interdependence, the reduced LV volume "sucks" the RV during inspiration; thus, the RV "sucks" flow from the RA and the flow between the RA and RV increases (transtricuspid E velocity increases on Doppler). This explains the **ventricular systolic discordance** (RV systolic pressure increases whereas LV systolic pressure decreases during inspiration).

- The flow between RA and RV is mainly increased for a short period of time that corresponds to the deep Y descent (the deep diastolic Y descent on the RA tracing is mainly seen during inspiration).
- Constriction prevents a decrease in RA pressure. Thus, the flow between SVC and RA decreases with inspiration, which ultimately leads to increased SVC pressure, hence the increased jugular venous pressure with inspiration (Kussmaul's sign).
- IVC pressure, on the other hand, is not subject to the negative intrathoracic pressure changes. Thus, since RV-to-RA sucking is increased with inspiration in early diastole and early systole, this "sucks" flow from the IVC and increases IVC-to-RA flow, which manifests as increased hepatic forward flow on Doppler echocardiography. Also, the positive intra-abdominal pressure during inspiration augments the IVC flow. The hepatic antegrade S and D velocities increase with inspiration, then become reduced and even partially reversed with expiration (S corresponds to the systolic flow, i.e., X descent, while D corresponds to the diastolic flow, i.e., Y descent). Thus, *SVC and IVC pressures and flow patterns are divergent in constrictive pericarditis.*

While ventricular interdependence is present in both constriction and tamponade, a different mechanism is incriminated in each case: during inspiration, RV "pushes" LV in tamponade, whereas RV is "sucked" by LV in constrictive pericarditis. As opposed to constrictive pericarditis, LV flow is reduced in tamponade because of RV compression, not because of a lack of transmission of the negative intrathoracic pressure to the LV. In addition, because of the uniform pericardial fluid, the constraint is more uniform across both the LV and the RV in tamponade. **Thus, ventricular interdependence is more prominent in tamponade and leads to pulsus paradoxus, which is only present in one-third of cases of constriction. Also, the cardiac chambers are compressed throughout diastole in tamponade, including early diastole, making Y descent flat in tamponade (vs. deep in constriction).**

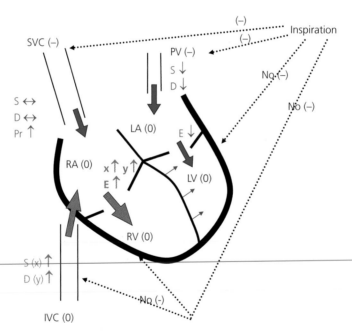

Figure 17.8 Sequence of events occurring during inspiration in constrictive pericarditis. *(–)* sign adjacent to a structure signifies there is transmission of the negative intrathoracic pressure to this structure, whereas *(0)* corresponds to the lack of transmission of the intrathoracic pressure to this structure. *Gray block arrows* signify increased flow between two chambers, while the *blue block arrows* signify reduced flow between two chambers. ↔ indicates lack of change.

During inspiration, the negative pressure is transmitted to PV and SVC but not to the intracardiac chambers or the IVC. This reduces blood flow between PV and LA, and thus between LA and LV, which "sucks" the ventricular septum to the left. This increases RV volume, which "sucks" blood from RA and IVC. It cannot suck blood from the SVC because the SVC pressure is initially reduced by the negative inspiratory effect. The flow between SVC and RA is unchanged while the flow between IVC and RA is increased. SVC pressure ultimately increases (Kussmaul's sign) and RA pressure remains unchanged or increases slightly because of increased IVC flow.

D, diastolic flow wave of IVC, SVC, and PV on Doppler, corresponds to Y descent; E, mitral inflow Doppler wave; S, systolic flow wave of IVC, SVC, and PV on Doppler, corresponds to X descent; Pr, pressure change that ultimately occurs in the SVC; PV, pulmonary veins. **D on echo is Y on pressure tracing, S is X (DY--SX)**. Reproduced with permission of Demos Medical from Hanna (2012).[37]

In pericardial processes, there are marked respiratory variations of flow, and thus **marked and discordant variations of RV and LV *systolic* pressures, without marked variation of *diastolic* pressures and atrial pressures** (shielding effect of the shell). The respiratory variations of flow, manifesting as discordant RV–LV systolic pressures and respiratory variations of S and D, are key diagnostic features of constriction.

III. Hemodynamic findings in constrictive pericarditis and differential diagnosis of constrictive pericarditis: restrictive cardiomyopathy, decompensated RV failure, COPD (Table 17.1)

A. Restrictive cardiomyopathy is characterized by poor relaxation and poor compliance of the RV and LV myocardium. As opposed to dilated cardiomyopathy, systolic function is relatively preserved (or mildly impaired) and the LV cavity is not dilated. The myocardial thickness is normal in idiopathic restrictive cardiomyopathy but is increased in infiltrative restrictive cardiomyopathies, such as amyloidosis or sarcoidosis, and may reach levels seen with hypertrophic cardiomyopathy (>20 mm). As opposed to hypertrophic or hypertensive cardiomyopathy, the increase in thickness is due to myocardial infiltration rather than myocardial hypertrophy, explaining the discrepancy between the low voltage and the Q waves on the ECG on the one hand and a thick myocardium on echocardiography on the other hand. As in any decompensated ventricular failure, LA and RA are markedly dilated, and functional TR and MR, sometimes severe, may be seen. The RV may dilate at an advanced stage, and such a dilatation is a poor prognostic sign.[41]

Hemodynamically, restrictive cardiomyopathy has similar features to any decompensated ventricular failure. The stiff non-compliant myocardium acts as a "shell" explaining the following three restrictive findings: (1) elevated left and right ventricular diastolic pressures, (2) ventricular dip–plateau pattern, and (3) deep/rapid atrial X and Y descents. A prominent V wave and prominent X and Y descents are seen as a result of the poor atrial and ventricular compliances (atrial pressure goes sharply down then up in early diastole and early systole).

As opposed to constrictive pericarditis, in restrictive cardiomyopathy the intrathoracic pressure is transmitted to the cardiac chambers, there is no ventricular interdependence, and the intracavitary pressures are not all forced to equalize with the pericardial pressure.

B. Severe ventricular failure (particularly RV failure)

The three restrictive findings may be seen in the right-sided cavities with any decompensated RV failure and in the left-sided cavities with any decompensated LV failure, and they are explained by the severely reduced ventricular compliance. In addition, the pericardium is stretched by the dilated ventricle(s) and becomes functionally constrictive, forcing the ventricles to expand at the expense of each other and to equalize their diastolic pressures. In fact, if the RV or LV develops *severe or rapid* volume overload, the pericardium does not have time to expand and accommodate the increased intracavitary volume. Thus, a fourth finding, the equalization of right- and left-sided end-diastolic pressures, may be seen with severe ventricular failure.[42] The four findings may also be seen in severe TR or acute severe AI or MR, and are more readily seen with RV failure as the latter is thin and more readily dilates than the LV. In a way, the pericardium prevents further ventricular dilatation and afterload rise at the expense of "functional constriction."

Table 17.1 Comparison of hemodynamic findings in constrictive pericarditis, restrictive cardiomyopathy, and severe ventricular failure.

Features shared by constrictive pericarditis, restrictive cardiomyopathy, and ventricular failure

1. Elevated right- and left-sided filling pressures (elevated RA pressure and PCWP)
2. Ventricular dip–plateau pattern
3. Deep atrial X and Y descents with an atrial M morphology (V wave may be large with flattened X descent in restrictive cardiomyopathy or ventricular failure, particularly in severe TR)

Constrictive pericarditis	Restrictive cardiomyopathy or any decompensated LV failure	Decompensated RV failure
1. Equalization of RV and LV end-diastolic pressures (**RV = LV** in inspiration, **RV < LV** in expiration)	LV diastolic pressure often > RV diastolic pressure by > 5 mmHg	Equalization of RV and LV end-diastolic pressure (**RV = LV** in expiration, **RV > LV** in inspiration)[a]
2. No or minimal inspiratory decrease of RA pressure (X and Y become deeper and RA pressure may *increase* with inspiration)	Inspiratory *decrease* of RA pressure	Inspiratory *increase* of RA pressure
3. Early diastolic gradient between PCWP and LV varies with respiration > 5 mmHg[b]	No significant change of PCWP–LV early diastolic gradient[b]	No significant change of PCWP–LV early diastolic gradient[b]
4. During respiration, there is a discordant change of the systolic peaks of LV and RV (when RV pressure ↑, LV pressure ↓)	During respiration, there is a concordant change of the systolic peaks of LV and RV	During respiration, there is a concordant change of the systolic peaks of LV and RV
5. Systolic PA pressure < 55 mmHg	Systolic PA pressure may be > 55 mmHg	

[a] Severe RV failure or TR has an inspiratory increase in RA pressure and V wave. Also, mean RA pressure may be > mean PCWP. In fact, RVEDP is higher than LVEDP in inspiration, whereas in constriction RVEDP increases only to become equal to LVEDP during inspiration. In RV failure, the severely impaired RA/RV compliance leads to an inspiratory rise in diastolic pressure with the rise in preload, overcoming the direct negative respiratory pressure.

[b] In constriction, the LV diastolic pressure varies minimally with respiration whereas the PCWP varies markedly, which explains the significant respiratory change of the early diastolic PCWP–LV gradient (lowest during inspiration). In other disease states, the LV diastolic pressure changes as much as the PCWP with respiration, hence the lack of significant change of the PCWP–LV early diastolic gradient.

In RV failure, the ventricular interdependence is not markedly affected by respiration, as the RV is already markedly distended and may not further distend with inspiration. In addition, the RV is at a flat portion of the Frank–Starling curve, and cannot significantly increase its flow with the inspiratory rise in preload. Thus, the systolic discordance of RV and LV pressures is not as often or as markedly seen.

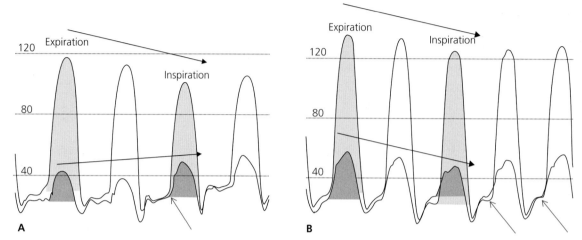

Figure 17.9 Simultaneous RV and LV pressure tracings in two different patients. **Analyze three elements on the RV–LV simultaneous tracing:** (1) in diastole, dip–plateau pattern of the LV and the RV; (2) in diastole, elevation and equalization of RV and LV end-diastolic pressures; (3) in systole, concordance vs. discordance of RV–LV systolic peaks. Both patients A and B have the dip–plateau pattern and the elevation and equalization of RV and LV end-diastolic pressures (in inspiration, *blue arrows*). Patient A has constrictive pericarditis: note the discordance of the systolic peaks of RV and LV with respiration. Also, the LV and RV areas change discordantly (*light and dark shaded areas*, respectively). Patient B has a restrictive myocardial disease: note the concordance of the LV and RV systolic peaks.

Concordance pattern is analyzed by choosing the *peak inspiratory beat*, which is the beat preceded by the lowest diastolic dip, and the *peak expiratory beat*, which is the beat preceded by the highest diastolic dip. Thus diastole helps determine which beats are selected for systolic analysis. Reproduced with permission from Elsevier from Talreja et al. (2008).[39]

Only the discordance between LV and RV systolic pressures is highly sensitive and highly specific (>90%) for the diagnosis of constrictive pericarditis (Figure 17.9).[39] The second most specific feature is the respiratory change in the early diastolic gradient between PCWP and LV. The other features are useful but have low sensitivity, specificity, and predictive values in the range of 50–70% for constrictive pericarditis. The discordance and the respiratory changes are best evaluated during *deep respiration*. This contrasts with the clinical evaluation of discordance by pulsus paradoxus, and the Doppler evaluation of discordance by transmitral analysis, performed during *normal respiration*.

Some of the abnormalities of constrictive pericarditis are made more evident by hypovolemia, while others are made more evident with volume loading (500–1000 ml over 10 minutes in the cath lab):

- The dip–plateau pattern and the deep and rapid X and Y descents, which are signs of severely reduced compliance, are better shown with volume loading and are masked with hypovolemia. In fact, RA pressure may be normal and may have a normal pulse morphology in hypovolemia (occult constrictive pericarditis).[43]
- The equalization of diastolic pressures is better shown with volume loading.
- The discordant respiratory changes of LV and RV systolic pressures are better seen in hypovolemia (similar to the accentuation of pulsus paradoxus with hypovolemia). **While a volume load creates more ventricular interdependence, the respiratory changes of ventricular interdependence become attenuated.**[44]

C. COPD and other causes of RV–LV respiratory discordance

While RV failure may lead to four-chamber diastolic pressure equalization and abnormal RV and RA pressure tracings mimicking constriction, COPD may mimic another aspect of constriction. Because of large intrathoracic pressure swings, COPD or asthma may lead to discordant RV and LV filling and pulsus paradoxus. This may also be seen in patients receiving mechanical ventilation and in sedated patients breathing deeply, as in many routine cardiac catheterization procedures. With the deep negative intrathoracic pressure, right-sided filling increases because a large volume is driven from outside the thorax to inside the thorax, which does not happen on the left side. RV and LV will have opposite phasic changes in volume and discordant systolic pressures. These discordant changes in RV–LV filling that lead to pulsus paradoxus may also be seen in normal subjects who are hypovolemic, i.e., are on the steep portion of the cardiac output–preload curve (Frank–Starling curve), and breathing deeply; they are often absent in hypervolemic patients (non-preload-dependent). That is why discordant RV–LV filling is unusual in restrictive cardiomyopathy and severe heart failure.

The phasic changes in RV and LV filling are also present in normal subjects breathing quietly, but are very subtle. In normal subjects, right-sided flow increases during inspiration but RV and LV systolic pressures both concordantly and mildly decrease during inspiration, due predominantly to the direct effect of the negative intrathoracic pressure on the measured cardiac or vascular pressures, the effect of RV–LV filling discordance being minimal. The same concordance phenomenon is seen in non-constriction and non-COPD disease states, such as restriction and RV failure. The filling discordance overwhelms the direct negative inspiratory pressure effect in cases of constrictive pericarditis, COPD, or large respiratory swings in hypovolemic patients.

In COPD, as opposed to constriction:

1. The end-diastolic pressures of the four cardiac chambers are not equalized (RA pressure and RVEDP<PCWP and LVEDP).
2. The respiratory pressure is transmitted to the cardiac chambers, and thus Kussmaul's sign is not seen (i.e., SVC and RA pressures are reduced with inspiration).
3. There is no dip–plateau pattern on the RV or LV tracing. RA pressure does not have a deep X and deep Y pattern and is usually normal.

On echocardiography, SVC flow may be used to differentiate COPD from constriction. In constriction, SVC flow does not increase during inspiration (Kussmaul's sign), while in COPD, SVC flow increases during inspiration. Thus, in constriction, the SVC Doppler velocities (S and D) show little change from inspiration to expiration, whereas in COPD, S and D velocities markedly increase in inspiration (S velocity in particular).[45] IVC and hepatic flow increases during inspiration and is reduced and partially reversed in expiration in both COPD and constriction.

IV. Practical performance of a hemodynamic study when constrictive pericarditis is suspected (see Table 17.2)

Table 17.2 The three most important recordings in the hemodynamic assessment of constriction.

- **RA pressure tracing:** look for deep X and deep Y descents and the lack of inspiratory decrease in pressure
- **LV and RV simultaneous recording:**
  1. Analyze *diastole* for dip–plateau pattern
  2. Analyze *diastole* for equalization of LV and RV end-diastolic pressures. See if LVEDP>RVEDP at one point (vs. RVEDP>LVEDP, which would suggest RV failure)
  3. Analyze *systole* during *deep breathing* to assess discordance vs. concordance of LV and RV systolic pressure peaks
- **LV and PCWP simultaneous recording:** in constrictive pericarditis, the gradient between PCWP and early diastolic LV dip changes with respiration

When constriction is suspected clinically and the mean RA pressure is<8mmHg or mildly elevated (8–15mmHg) but without the typical constrictive pericarditis contour, one may use volume loading to unveil the deep X and deep Y pattern and the elevation and equalization of LV/RV diastolic pressures (*occult constrictive pericarditis*).

V. Echocardiographic features of constrictive pericarditis, and differentiation between constrictive pericarditis and restrictive cardiomyopathy (see Table 17.3)

In both constrictive pericarditis and restrictive cardiomyopathy:

1. The transmitral and transtricuspid E-wave velocities are increased, reflecting elevated filling pressures (E/A>1.5)
2. The right and left ventricular systolic function is preserved, ventricular size is normal, and the atria are enlarged.

However, in restrictive cardiomyopathy, there is no ventricular interdependence and the intrathoracic pressures are transmitted to the cardiac chambers. This explains the lack of significant respiratory variation of the transmitral and the transtricuspid flows and the lack of significant respiratory variation of the hepatic and the pulmonary venous flows (in contrast to constrictive pericarditis, where E velocity varies by >25%

Table 17.3 Echocardiographic differentiation between constrictive pericarditis and restrictive cardiomyopathy.

	Constrictive pericarditis	Restrictive cardiomyopathy
Similarities		
E/A	>1.5	>1.5
E deceleration time	Reduced<160ms	Reduced<160ms
Ventricular size/systolic function	Normal	Normal
Atria	Mildly dilated	More markedly dilated
IVC	Dilated	Dilated
Differences		
Respiratory E variation (*during normal respiration*)	>25%	<25%
Medial annular E′ velocity	>10cm/s	<10cm/s
Hepatic venous pattern	S>D	S<D
Hepatic venous flow respiratory variation	↑ S and D with inspiration ↓ S and D with partial reversal of flow in expiration	Minimal variation
Pulmonary venous flow respiratory variation	↑ S and D with expiration	Minimal variation
Color M-mode mitral valve velocity of propagation (Vp)	Normal (>55cm/s) (implies normal diastolic recoil, like medial E′)	Reduced
Septal motion on M-mode and 2D echo	Abnormal (septal bounce in diastole due to competitive filling of RV and LV)	Normal
Posterior wall motion in diastole on M mode	Dip–plateau (after early expansion, posterior wall remains flat in diastole)	Normal
Pulmonary hypertension	<55mmHg	May be>55mmHg
TR and MR	Infrequent	Frequent, may be severe

Reproduced with permission of Demos Medical from Hanna (2012).[37]

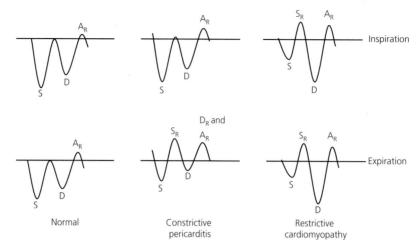

Figure 17.10 Respiratory variations of hepatic venous flow velocities. S flow corresponds to the X descent on RA and IVC pressure tracing, D flow corresponds to the Y descent (S = X, D = Y), and Ar flow corresponds to A wave. In constrictive pericarditis, S and D increase with inspiration (i.e., increase in X and Y descent); S and D decrease with expiration along with a terminal S reversal (S_R) and a terminal D reversal (D_R). Minimal respiratory variations are seen in normal individuals and in restrictive cardiomyopathy. In the latter case, there is a reduction of S velocity (= X descent) with terminal S reversal (= V wave), and an increase of D velocity (= Y descent) and A reversal. Reproduced with permission of Demos Medical from Hanna (2012).[37]

during normal breathing) (Figure 17.10).[46] In restrictive cardiomyopathy, the intrathoracic pressure is transmitted to the LA and LV so that, with respiration, there is respiratory tracking of the pulmonary vein-to-LA gradient and, consequently, no change in pulmonary venous flow with respiration. On the right side, the negative intrathoracic pressure tries to draw flow from the IVC and SVC branches; however, the RA and RV being poorly compliant, the venous flow does not change much with normal inspiration (IVC does not collapse on echo). In constriction, there are respiratory variations of transmitral, pulmonary venous, and hepatic venous flow regardless of the patient's rhythm. The respiratory variation may be absent in up to 12% of patients with constrictive pericarditis, particularly those with severe hypervolemia; the respiratory variation is unmasked by preload reduction, e.g., head-up tilting or sitting.[44] In AF, the respiratory variations are more subtle, and manifest as a paradoxical increase of E velocity after a short R–R cycle in expiration and a paradoxical decrease of E velocity and pulmonary venous S and D velocities after a long R–R cycle in inspiration; the analysis of venous flow reversal is often more helpful than the analysis of transmitral flow in AF.[47]

Furthermore, in restrictive cardiomyopathy as in any LV failure, the tissue Doppler velocity of the mitral annulus is reduced in diastole signifying reduced relaxation/recoil (E' < 10 cm/s). In constriction, the medial annular velocity is preserved or elevated. In fact, the pericardial constraint limits the lateral expansion of the heart which reduces the lateral recoil E'; the medial recoil E' tries to compensate for the lateral constriction and becomes exaggerated despite elevated filling pressures.

Three septal motion abnormalities occur in constrictive pericarditis and are best identified on M-mode. These septal motion abnormalities may also be seen in tamponade (see Chapter 32, Figure 32.17):

1. Similarly to RV failure, the septum collapses towards the LV in diastole and paradoxically moves towards the RV in systole.
2. This septal collapse varies with the respiratory cycle, more than seen with RV failure. It increases with inspiration.
3. Even within the same diastole and the same respiratory cycle, an instantaneous change in the RV-to-LV push is seen (septal bounce). This signifies that the two chambers are constantly competing for space within the stiff pericardium.

VI. Physical exam, ECG findings, BNP, pericardial thickness (CT/MRI)
A. Physical exam

1. *Signs of right heart failure,* sometimes isolated right heart failure. Constrictive pericarditis should always be considered in the differential diagnosis of isolated right heart failure:
  • Increased JVP with the following features:
    a. Kussmaul's sign (i.e., increased JVP with inspiration, which may also be seen with severe RV failure)
    b. Deep X and Y descents on JVP exam
  • Peripheral edema
  • Ascites, hepatic congestion with jaundice (differentiate from cirrhosis by the elevated JVP and the hepatomegaly, vs. atrophic liver in cirrhosis).
2. *Symptoms of elevated LA pressure* (dyspnea, orthopnea). Similarly to tamponade, dyspnea occurs but pulmonary edema and hypoxemia do not usually occur because of the low volume reaching the left heart.
3. *Low-output signs* (fatigue).
4. *Pulsus paradoxus* in one-third of patients. Pulsus paradoxus is more common in tamponade than constriction, because of the more potent and uniform compression of both ventricles in tamponade (more extreme RV–LV discordance). Pericardial knock may be heard in diastole (occurs at the end of the ventricular dip, sounds like a high-pitched S_3).

B. ECG
The ECG is almost always abnormal: low QRS voltage (very commonly), and non-specific T-wave abnormalities (flat, inverted).

C. BNP

In restrictive cardiomyopathy, BNP is~always >200 pg/ml, whereas in idiopathic constrictive pericarditis, it is <200 pg/ml. BNP may be >200 pg/ml in other forms of constrictive pericarditis (e.g., post-radiation).

Severe right HF with a normal BNP suggests constrictive pericarditis.

D. Pericardial thickness

Pericardial thickness is usually increased (≥3 mm) in constrictive pericarditis and may be assessed by echo, CT or MRI. However, a study using operative specimens has shown that 18% of patients with constrictive pericarditis have normal pericardial thickness, and those patients are as likely as patients with a thickened pericardium to benefit from pericardiectomy.[48] On the other hand, a thickened pericardium does not necessarily lead to constriction.

A thickened pericardium with severe late gadolinium hyperenhancement of the pericardium itself suggests a reversible, inflammatory constrictive process.

E. Endomyocardial biopsy

A biopsy is useful to diagnose infiltrative forms of restrictive cardiomyopathy (amyloidosis; the yield for sarcoidosis is low).

VII. Transient constrictive pericarditis

Up to 17% of patients with constrictive pericarditis may have a transient (reversible) constrictive pericarditis. This may be seen with idiopathic, post-surgical, traumatic, infectious, or collagen vascular disease-associated constrictive pericarditis, particularly when the onset of symptoms is recent. In this case, inflammation and edema lead to pericardial thickening and stiffening without fibrosis. *Radiation-induced constrictive pericarditis cannot be transient.* A pericardial effusion is often present (67%), sometimes large, and 50% of cases of *idiopathic* effusive–constrictive pericarditis are transient. Constrictive physiology resolves with observation and anti-inflammatory therapy within 6 months (mean 2.1 months).[11,34] NSAIDs, steroids, and colchicine have been used.

The following markers have been shown to identify a reversible (vs. persistent) constrictive pericarditis with a high specificity:[49]

a. On cardiac MRI; thick (≥3 mm) late gadolinium hyperenhancement of the pericardium. The normal pericardium and the fibrotic pericardium are poorly vascularized, and thus do not enhance with gadolinium; the fibrotic pericardium may mildly enhance. Conversely, severe gadolinium enhancement implies a predominantly inflamed, hyperemic rather than fibrotic pericardium.
b. Elevated markers of inflammation: CRP > 2.1 mg/dl, ESR > 41 mm/h.

VIII. Treatment
A. Survival and symptomatic improvement after pericardiectomy

Unless transient constrictive pericarditis is suspected, in which initial observation and anti-inflammatory therapy are warranted, constrictive pericarditis is treated with pericardiectomy. Complete pericardiectomy consists of removing the pericardium from phrenic nerve to phrenic nerve and removing the diaphragmatic pericardium. The perioperative mortality is 6%, and varies with the etiology (~3% for idiopathic, ~20% for radiation-induced constrictive pericarditis). Similarly, long-term survival is excellent for idiopathic constriction, good for postoperative constriction, and poor for radiation-induced constriction (7-year survival 88% vs. 66% vs. 27%, respectively).[35,36] NYHA class IV, age >55, and especially radiation etiology are predictors of poorer long-term outcomes. Post-radiation pericarditis is often associated with myocardial, valvular, and coronary disease and mediastinal scarring that partially explain the mortality, the residual symptomatology, and the inability to completely resect the pericardium.

Symptomatic improvement is seen in ~80% of survivors.

B. Persistent diastolic dysfunction

Echocardiographic normalization of diastolic filling pattern occurs slowly over several months and is seen in ~40% of patients at 3 months and 60% at 6 months.[50] One-third of patients are left with a residual restrictive pattern while 10% have a residual constrictive pattern. The diastolic filling pattern normalizes in only ~25% of radiation pericarditis. Patients with a longer duration of symptoms are more likely to have residual diastolic dysfunction and symptoms at later follow-up. This is presumably due to:

a. Extension of the fibrotic process to the myocardium in longstanding constriction. In fact, a residual restrictive rather than constrictive process is responsible for the residual postoperative symptoms in most patients and may slowly improve with time.
b. Inability to fully resect the pericardium in patients with extensive scarring (residual constriction).

C. Systolic function

As a result of longstanding underfilling, LV myocardial atrophy occurs in patients with longstanding constrictive pericarditis. The sudden "flooding" of the LV that occurs postoperatively may lead to a transient LV systolic dysfunction with pulmonary edema and a low output syndrome, responsible for some of the early fatalities. In survivors, LV systolic function improves with time.

Summary

Constrictive pericarditis clinically manifests as HF, particularly right HF, with elevated right- and left-sided filling pressures on echo, biatrial enlargement, yet normal right and left ventricular systolic function and size and normal LV wall thickness, simulating diastolic HF.

Keys to diagnosis: On echo → *Respiratory* variations of mitral/tricuspid inflow and pulmonary/hepatic venous flow. On invasive hemodynamics → *respiratory* discordance of RV–LV systolic peaks. BNP is typically normal.

QUESTIONS AND ANSWERS

Question 1. A 58-year-old woman presents with atypical non-exertional and non-positional chest pain. She has no significant functional limitation. She is a smoker and hypertensive. Echo shows large circumferential pericardial effusion (2.5 cm sum diastolic diameter). JVP is normal, pulse is 80 bpm, and there is no pulsus paradoxus. All of the following are appropriate, *except for which one*?

A. Screen for breast cancer (mammogram) and lung cancer (chest CT)

B. Perform PPD, TSH, creatinine, and HIV testing, and assess joints and skin for rheumatologic disorders

C. Perform ESR and CRP

D. Drain the effusion for diagnostic purpose and to prevent tamponade

E. If CRP is elevated without a suspected malignant or immune process, treat with NSAID and colchicine

Question 2. A 65-year-old man, smoker, presents with severe dyspnea, progressive over several days. BP is 145/105 mmHg, pulse is 110 bpm, JVP is 14 cm H_2O, peripheral O_2 saturation 95%. Chest X-ray shows clear lungs but cardiomegaly. Echo shows a large pericardial effusion. Which one of the following additional findings is likely to be true?

A. On catheterization, RA pressure shows a deep Y descent and a flat X

B. RA pressure and RVEDP exceed PCWP and LVEDP

C. Tamponade is unlikely as the patient is hypertensive.

D. Tamponade is unlikely as the patient has normal O_2 saturation

E. Pulsus paradoxus is likely to be present on exam

F. Pulsus alternans is likely to be present on exam, and electrical alternans may be present on ECG

Question 3. The patient in Question 2 undergoes pericardiocentesis. 1200 ml of blood-tinged fluid is removed. Which of the following is *incorrect*?

A. The likelihood of malignant effusion is ~30%

B. A subxiphoid approach targets the posterior aspect of the pericardial space, while an apical acess targets the lateral pericardial space

C. Pericardiocentesis followed by 3 days of drainage is often a definitive treatment of idiopathic effusions

D. Pericardiocentesis followed by 3 days of drainage is associated with a low effusion recurrence rate, even if the effusion is malignant (<25%)

E. The overall diagnostic yield of pericardiocentesis is ~30%, and exceeds 50% in case of malignant effusion.

Question 4. A 34-year-old man presents with chest pain and diffuse ST elevation and PR depression on the ECG. No rub is heard on exam. Echo is normal and CRP is elevated. Troponin is elevated at 0.6 ng/ml. Which of the following is *false*?

A. Diffuse ST elevation and PR depression without reciprocal ST changes may be consistent with anteroapical MI

B. ECG is consistent with pericarditis if all five of the following features are present: no Q waves, no tall or inverted T waves, no reciprocal ST depression except in aVR and V_1, ST elevation <5 mm and smaller than QRS, concave ST elevation

C. The troponin rise implies myopericarditis and impaired long-term prognosis

D. The risk of recurrent idiopathic pericarditis is 15–30%

Question 5. The patient in Question 4 is placed on NSAID. Which of the following is *incorrect*?

A. The patient needs to undergo routine workup for pericarditis: HIV, PPD, ANA/rheumatic factor

B. A reduced dose of NSAID is suggested

C. Adding colchicine to the initial therapy reduces recurrence

D. Exercise restriction is warranted for 4–6 weeks

Question 6. A 64-year-old woman with a history of radiation for left breast cancer 6 years previously presents with progressive dyspnea on exertion. JVP is elevated at 12 cm and pulsus paradoxus is present. Echo shows a 2.5 mm pericardial effusion with evidence of right-sided chamber compression. Pericardiocentesis is performed, after which RA pressure declines from 15 mmHg to 10 mmHg, and pericardial pressure improves but remains elevated at 10 mmHg. Which statement is *incorrect*?

A. Upon pericardial drainage of this patient, the flat Y descent gives place to an abnormally deep Y descent

B. Before pericardial drainage, RA pressure was not significantly declining during inspiration (as opposed to classic tamponade)

C. Before and after pericardial drainage, RV and LV end-diastolic pressures are equal

D. Before and after pericardial drainage, RV and LV systolic pressures are discordant

E. This condition is often transient and reversible

Question 7. A 52-year-old man presents with dyspnea on exertion. He has a distant history of tuberculosis while living in India. Echo shows normal-size LV and RV with normal systolic function yet abnormal septal motion (without any LBBB). The atria are mildly dilated. The IVC is mildly dilated but collapses properly (RA pressure of 5–10 mmHg). The respiratory variations of the mitral inflow and the hepatic venous flow (S and D) are exaggerated, with prominent S and D velocities in inspiration. During catheterization, the RA pressure is normal. Which of the following is *incorrect*?

A. Volume loading should be performed to show the typical RA waveform and RA pressure elevation

B. Volume loading attenuates RV–LV systolic discordance

C. The following two findings are highly specific for constrictive pericarditis: deep X and deep Y descents on RA tracing, and equalization of RV and LV end-diastolic pressures

D. Systolic discordance is the most sensitive and specific finding in constrictive pericarditis

Question 8. Concerning the prior case, which statement is true?
A. A normal BNP excludes constrictive pericarditis
B. The pericardial thickness is normal in 18% of patients with constrictive pericarditis (applies to MRI imaging)
C. Late gadolinium hyperenhancement of the pericardium on MRI implies a scarred pericardium
D. The operative mortality of pericardiectomy is 3%

Question 9. Concerning constrictive pericarditis, which statement is *incorrect*?
A. Restrictive cardiomyopathy and RV failure may mimic three classic features of constriction: (i) deep X and Y on RA tracing; (ii) dip–plateau pattern on RV and LV tracings; (iii) equalized RV and LV end-diastolic pressures
B. Respiratory discordance of RV–LV systolic peaks best differentiates constriction from restrictive cardiomyopathy and RV failure
C. Respiratory discordance of constriction may be mimicked by COPD
D. In both constriction and RV failure, RA pressure may paradoxically increase with inspiration
E. On echo: severe pulmonary hypertension, severe MR or TR, or a reduced medial E′ are more consistent with constrictive pericarditis than restrictive cardiomyopathy

Question 10. As compared to constrictive pericarditis, in tamponade (multiple possible answers):
A. More ventricular compression occurs with more ventricular interdependence → Y descent is flat (vs. deep in constriction) and pulsus paradoxus is more common
B. Inspiratory pressure gets transmitted to the RA → RA pressure and JVP decline with inspiration (as opposed to constriction, where JVP increases and RA pressure remains unchanged or increases)
C. The hepatic venous flow shows a flat D wave (= Y descent), as opposed to the large D wave of constriction
D. The hepatic venous flow shows inspiratory rise of S and D in both constriction and tamponade

Question 11. Which statement concerning tamponade is *incorrect*?
A. RV failure and elevated RV diastolic pressure protect against tamponade
B. In RV failure and elevated RV diastolic pressure, an isolated LV compression with isolated LV tamponade may occur
C. In patients with RV failure who develop tamponade, pulsus paradoxus may be absent (isolated LV tamponade without pulsus paradoxus)
D. Pulmonary hypertension, per se, even in the absence of RV failure, is protective against tamponade

Question 12. In order of frequency, what are the causes of acute pericarditis and what are the causes of pericardial effusion?
A. Idiopathic
B. Specific infections (tuberculosis, HIV)
C. Neoplastic
D. Autoimmune/collagen vascular disease

Question 13. A 25-year-old, previously healthy woman presents with acute onset of severe chest pain, worse with supine position and with inspiration. ECG shows sinus tachycardia of 110 bpm with diffuse ST elevation. CRP is elevated. Echo shows a moderate-size 1 cm pericardial effusion. The patient has low-grade fever. Which of the following is *incorrect*?
A. Admit to hospital and perform HIV–PPD–ANA testing
B. Treat with ibuprofen 600 mg 4× daily until CRP normalizes, then taper ibuprofen over the ensuing 3 weeks. Symptoms typically resolve within 1 week of therapy
C. Start colchicine therapy only if symptoms persist or recur
D. Use corticosteroids only for pericarditis refractory to NSAID and colchicine
E. Restrict exercise until symptom resolution (restrict athletic activity for 3 months)

Answer 1. D. If asymptomatic without a suspected malignant etiology, the effusion is followed by echo for 6–12 weeks. It may be treated with NSAID and colchicine if CRP is elevated. Only a persistent effusion >12 weeks is associated with a substantial risk of tamponade (~33%) and may be drained.

Answer 2. E. The patient has an effusion with evidence of hemodynamic compromise (tachycardia, elevated JVP); thus, he has tamponade. RA pressure is characterized by a flat Y descent, i.e., flat diastolic filling (mnemonic: **Flat Y Tamponade = FYT**). Y becomes progressively more flat as more fluid cumulates. RA, RVEDP, PCWP, and LVEDP are typically equalized to the pericardial pressure. Early on, in tamponade, the patient may be hypertensive. Importantly, even when hypertensive, the pulse pressure is relatively narrow and there is pulsus paradoxus on exam. Tamponade may lead to severe orthopnea yet the lungs are usually clear and O_2 saturation is normal. While electrical alternans is seen on ECG, pulsus paradoxus rather than pulsus alternans is found on exam. Pulsus alternans is a sign of severe HF.

Answer 3. B. A subxiphoid approach targets the inferior, not posterior, pericardial space. An apical approach may target the posterior/lateral pericardial space (Figures 17.5, 17.6).

Answer 4. C. The patient has two features of pericarditis (chest pain and consistent ECG), and an additional confirmatory finding (CRP). The elevated troponin implies myopericarditis. As long as EF is normal, the long-term prognosis of myopericarditis is good regardless of the rise in troponin.

Answer 5. A. Immune or infectious workup is only performed if symptoms persist despite NSAID, symptoms are subacute, severe constitutional symptoms/fever are present, or moderate effusion is present (in the latter case, also perform cancer screen). The elevated troponin, i.e., myopericarditis, warrants exercise restriction for 4–6 weeks in non-athletes, and 6 months in athletes (ESC guidelines).

Answer 6. E. The patient has effusive constrictive pericarditis related to radiation injury. The RA and pericardial pressures improve but do not normalize after drainage, Y descent becomes abnormally deep. Features of constrictive pericarditis are present before drainage (answer B). Answers C and D are seen with tamponade (before drainage) and constriction (after drainage). Effusive–constrictive pericarditis is often transient in idiopathic cases, but not in radiation-induced cases.

Answer 7. C. The patient likely has occult constrictive pericarditis with subtle suggestive signs on echo, particularly signs of excessive respiratory variation of hepatic flow, mitral flow, and septal position. The RA pressure is not increased as the patient is likely hypovolemic. Mild volume loading will unveil abnormalities of RA pressure. As opposed to the abnormalities of RA tracing, the systolic discordance of RV–LV is unveiled by hypovolemia or upright positioning rather than volume loading. Findings under answer C are not specific for constriction, and are commonly seen in patients with restrictive cardiomyopathy or isolated RV failure; yet, in the right context such as this case, they are strongly suggestive of constriction.

Answer 8. B. A normal BNP is the rule in idiopathic constrictive pericarditis. Late gadolinium enhancement of the pericardium usually implies an inflammatory pericardial process, often reversible with anti-inflammatory therapy. The operative mortality of pericardiectomy is ~6% (may be lower in idiopathic, low-risk cases).

Answer 9. E. The findings described in E are more consistent with restrictive cardiomyopathy than constriction.

Answer 10. All are correct.

Answer 11. D. Elevated RV diastolic pressure makes it hard for the pericardial pressure to equalize with the RV diastolic pressure, and is thus protective against RV compression and RV tamponade. In this case, tamponade occurs when pericardial pressure exceeds LV pressure. Since RV and LV are not compressed together, they are not interdependent; thus, pulsus paradoxus may be absent.

Answer 12. Acute pericarditis: A>C~D>B. In a study of 453 patients with acute pericarditis, 83% of cases were idiopathic, 5% were neoplastic, 7% were autoimmune, 3.5% were due to tuberculosis, and 0.7% were purulent.[7]
Pericardial effusion: A>B=C>D. In a study of 204 patients with pericardial effusion, 48% of cases were labeled as idiopathic, 16% were infectious, 15% were malignant, and 8% were due to collagen vascular disease (lupus, rheumatoid arthritis, and scleroderma).[22]

Answer 13. C. Colchicine is recommended along with NSAID as initial combination therapy for pericarditis (class I, ESC guidelines). Colchicine is used for 3 months. The significant effusion dictates initial inpatient monitoring.

References
Acute pericarditis
1. Surawicz B, Lassiter KC. Electrocardiogram in pericarditis. Am J Cardiol 1970; 26: 471–4.
2. Bailey GL, Hampers CL, Hager EB, et al. Uremic pericarditis: clinical features and management. Circulation 1968; 38: 582–91.
3. Imazio M, Spodick DH, Brucato A, et al. Controversial issues in the management of pericardial diseases. Circulation 2010; 121: 916–28.
4. Adler Y, Charron P, Imazio M, et al. 2015 ESC guidelines for the diagnosis and management of pericardial diseases. Eur Heart J 2015; 36: 2921–64.
5. Imazio M, Brucato A, Barbieri A, et al. Good prognosis for pericarditis with and without myocardial involvement: results from a multicenter, prospective cohort study. Circulation 2013; 128: 42–9.
6. Imazio M, Bobbio M, Cecchi E, et al. Colchicine in addition to conventional therapy for acute pericarditis. Circulation 2005; 112: 2012–16.
7. Imazio M, Cecchi E, Demichelis B, et al. Indicators of poor prognosis of acute pericarditis. Circulation 2007; 115: 2739–44.
8. Imazio M, Trinchero R, Shabetai R. Pathogenesis, management, and prevention of recurrent pericarditis. J Cardiovasc Med 2007; 8: 404–10.
9. Imazio M, Brucato A, Adler Y, et al. Prognosis of idiopathic recurrent pericarditis as determined from previously published reports. Am J Cardiol 2007; 100: 1026–8.
10. Imazio M, Belli R, Brucato A, et al. Efficacy and safety of colchicine for treatment of multiple recurrences of pericarditis (CORP–2): a multicentre, double-blind, placebo-controlled, randomised trial. Lancet 2014; 383: 2232–7.
11. Sagrista-Sauleda J, Permanyer-Miralda G, Candell-Riera J, et al. Transient cardiac constriction. an unrecognized pattern of evolution in effusive acute idiopathic pericarditis. Am J Cardiol 1987; 59: 961–6.

Tamponade
12. LeWinter MM. Pericardial diseases. In: Libby P, Bonow RO, Mann DL, Zipes DP, eds. Braunwald's Heart Disease, 8th edn. Philadelphia, PA: Saunders Elsevier, 2008, pp. 1829–54.
13. Robb JF, Laham RJ. Profiles in pericardial disease. In: Baim DS, ed. Grossman's Cardiac Catheterization, Angiography, and Intervention, 7th edn. Philadelphia, PA: Lippincott Williams & Wilkins, 2006, pp. 725–43.
14. Hanna EB. Tamponade. In: Hanna EB, Glancy DL. Practical Cardiovascular Hemodynamics. New York, NY: Demos Medical, 2012.
15. Brown J, MacKinnon D, King A, Vanderbush E. Elevated arterial blood pressure in cardiac tamponade. N Engl J Med 1992; 327: 463–6.
16. Spodick DH. Threshold of pericardial constraint: the pericardial reserve volume and auxiliary pericardial functions. J Am Coll Cardiol 1985; 6: 296–7.
17. Hashim R, Frankel H, Tandon M, Rabinovici R. Fluid resuscitation-induced cardiac tamponade. Trauma 2002; 53: 1183–4.
18. Sagrista-Sauleda J, Angel J, Sanchez A, et al. Effusive–constrictive pericarditis. N Engl J Med 2004; 350: 469–75.
19. Cameron J, Oesterle SN, Baldwin JC, Hancock EW. The etiologic spectrum of constrictive pericarditis. Am Heart J 1987; 113: 354–60.

Pericardial effusion
20. Sagrista-Sauleda J, Merce J, Permanyer-Miralda G, Soler-Soler J. Clinical clues to the causes of large pericardial effusions. Am J Med 2000; 109: 95–101.
21. Sagrista-Sauleda J, Angel J, Permanyer-Miralda G, Soler-Soler J. Long-term follow-up of idiopathic chronic pericardial effusion. N Engl J Med 1999; 341: 2054–9.
22. Levy PY, Corey R, Berger P, et al. Etiologic diagnosis of 204 pericardial effusions. Medicine (Baltimore) 2003; 82: 385–91.

23. Corey GR, Campbell PT, Van Trigt P, et al. Etiology of large pericardial effusions. Am J Med 1993; 95: 209–13.
24. Heindenrish PA, Eisenberg MJ, Kee LL. Pericardial effusion in AIDS. Circulation 1995; 92: 3229–34.
25. Sagrista-Sauleda J, Merce AS, Soler-Soler J. Diagnosis and management of pericardial effusion. World J Cardiol 2011; 3: 135–43.
26. Spodick DH. Acute cardiac tamponade. N Engl J Med 2003; 349: 684–90.
27. Permanyer-Miralda G, Sagristá-Sauleda J, Soler-Soler J. Primary acute pericardial disease: a prospective series of 231 consecutive patients. Am J Cardiol 1985; 56: 623–30.
28. Tsang TS, Seward JB, Barnes ME, et al. Outcomes of primary and secondary treatment of pericardial effusion in patients with malignancy. Mayo Clin Proc 2000; 75: 248–53.
29. Tsang TS, Barnes ME, Gersh BJ, et al. Outcomes of clinically significant idiopathic pericardial effusion requiring intervention. Am J Cardiol 2003; 91: 704–7.
30. Pepi M, Muratori M, Barbier P, et al. Pericardial effusion after cardiac surgery: incidence, site, size and haemodynamic consequences. Br Heart J 1994; 72: 327–31.
31. Meurin P, Tabet JY, Thabut G, et al. NSAID treatment for postoperative pericardial effusion. A multicenter randomized double-blind trial. Ann Intern Med 2010; 152: 137–43. *POPE trial.*
32. Meurin P, Wever H, Renaud N, et al. Evolution of the postoperative pericardial effusion after day 15: the problem of the late tamponade. Chest 2004; 125: 2182–7.
33. Ashikhmina EA, Schaff HV, Sinak LJ, et al. Pericardial effusion after cardiac surgery: risk factors, patient profiles, and contemporary management. Ann Thorac Surg 2010; 89: 112–18.

Constrictive pericarditis

34. Haley JH, Tajik AJ, Danielson GK, et al. Transient constrictive pericarditis: causes and natural history. J Am Coll Cardiol 2004; 43: 271–5.
35. Ling LH, Oh JK, Schaff HV, et al. Constrictive pericarditis in the modern era. Evolving clinical spectrum and impact on outcome after pericardiectomy. Circulation 1999; 100: 1380–6.
36. Bertog SC, Thambidorai SK, Parakh K, et al. Constrictive pericarditis: etiology and cause-specific survival after pericardiectomy. J Am Coll Cardiol 2004; 43: 1445–52.
37. Hanna EB. Constrictive pericarditis. In: Hanna EB, Glancy DL. Practical Cardiovascular Hemodynamics. New York, NY: Demos Medical, 2012.
38. Hurrell DG, Nishimura RA, Higano ST, et al. Value of respiratory changes in left and right ventricular pressures for the diagnosis of constrictive pericarditis. Circulation 1996; 93: 2007–13.
39. Talreja DR, Nishimura RA, Oh JK, Holmes DR. Constrictive pericarditis in the modern era: novel criteria for diagnosis in the cardiac catheterization laboratory. J Am Coll Cardiol 2008; 51: 315–19.
40. Tabata T, Kabbani SS, Murray DR, et al. Difference in the respiratory variations between pulmonary venous and mitral inflow Doppler velocities in patients with constrictive pericarditis with and without atrial fibrillation. J Am Coll Cardiol 2001; 37; 1936–42.
41. Patel AR, Dubrey SW, Mendes LA, et al. Right ventricular dilation in primary amyloidosis: an independent predictor of survival. Am J Cardiol 1997; 80: 486–92.
42. Jaber WA, Sorajja P, Borlaug BA, Nishimura RA. Differentiation of tricuspid regurgitation from constrictive pericarditis: novel criteria for diagnosis in the cardiac catheterization laboratory. Heart 2009; 95: 1449–54.
43. Bush CA, Stang JM, Wooley CF, Kilman JW. Occult constrictive pericardial disease diagnosis by rapid volume expansion and correction by pericardiectomy. Circulation 1977; 56: 924–30.
44. Oh JK, Tajik AJ, Appleton CP, et al. Preload reduction to unmask the characteristic Doppler features of constrictive pericarditis: a new observation. Circulation 1997; 95: 796–9.
45. Boonyaratavej S, Oh JK, Tajik AJ, et al. Comparison of mitral inflow and superior vena cava Doppler velocities in chronic obstructive pulmonary disease and constrictive pericarditis. J Am Coll Cardiol 1998; 32: 2043–8.
46. Klein AL, Cohen GI, Pietrolungo GF, et al. Differentiation of constrictive pericarditis from restrictive cardiomyopathy by Doppler echocardiographic measurements of respiratory variations in pulmonary venous flows. J Am Coll Cardiol 1993; 22: 1935–43.
47. Tabata T, Kabbani SS, Murray DR, et al. Difference in the respiratory variations between pulmonary venous and mitral inflow Doppler velocities in patients with constrictive pericarditis with and without atrial fibrillation. J Am Coll Cardiol 2001; 37; 1936–42.
48. Talreja DR, Edwards WD, Danielson GK, et al. Constrictive pericarditis in 26 patients with histologically normal pericardial thickness. Circulation 2003; 108: 1852–7.
49. Feng D, Glockner J, Kim K, et al. Cardiac magnetic resonance imaging pericardial late gadolinium enhancement and elevated inflammatory markers can predict the reversibility of constrictive pericarditis after antiinflammatory medical therapy. Circulation 2011; 124: 1830–7.
50. Senni M, Redfield MM, Ling LH, et al. Left ventricular systolic and diastolic function after pericardiectomy in patients with constrictive pericarditis. J Am Coll Cardiol 1999; 33: 1182–8.

Further reading

Atar S, Chiu J, Forrester JS, et al. Bloody pericardial effusion in patients with cardiac tamponade: is the cause cancerous, tuberculous, or iatrogenic in the 1990s? Chest 1999; 116: 564–9.

Part 7 CONGENITAL HEART DISEASE

18 Congenital Heart Disease

1. ACYANOTIC CONGENITAL HEART DISEASE

I. Atrial septal defect (ASD)

A. Embryology (see Figure 18.1)

The interatrial septum has two parts:

- A lower part connected to the endocardial cushions at the valvular level and called **septum primum**. The septum primum is **thin and membranous**.
- An upper part called **septum secundum**. The septum secundum is **thick and muscular**.

These two septa meet and overlap. The overlap area is called *fossa ovalis*.[1,2]

In the fetus, the overlap area is not sealed, leaving a tunnel that allows blood to flow from right to left. This tunnel is called *foramen ovale*. In the fetus, oxygenated blood flowing from the IVC is directed towards the left heart through the septum secundum and foramen ovale, and is ejected into the ascending aorta, the brain, and upper body. Deoxygenated blood flowing from the SVC continues into the RV and is ejected into the high-resistance pulmonary circulation, then the descending aorta through the ductus arteriosus. Overall, the RV provides ~55% of the systemic cardiac output (lower body), while the LV provides ~45% of the systemic output (upper body). The pulmonary vascular resistance is elevated in the fetus, as a reaction to the poorly oxygenated lung, and the pulmonary arterial pressure is higher than the systemic pressure; at birth, the pulmonary resistance and pressure dramatically drop.

Practical Cardiovascular Medicine, First Edition. Elias B. Hanna.

© 2017 John Wiley & Sons Ltd. Published 2017 by John Wiley & Sons Ltd.

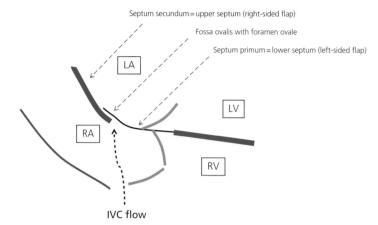

Figure 18.1 Interatrial septum. Embryologically, blood coming from the IVC is directed into the LA by the right-sided, septum secundum flap. The septum primum acts like a one-way door that opens when the RA pressure rises, and closes when the LA pressure supersedes the RA pressure, closing the foramen ovale. The prominent, septum secundum boundary of the fossa ovalis is called limbus (on the side of the RA).

The septum primum was initially localized at the upper portion of the RA. It grew down and touched the endocardial cushions, then developed a defect in its middle and top portions (ostium secundum) to allow blood shunting. This defect got covered by a growing muscular septum secundum, which eventually met the septum primum.

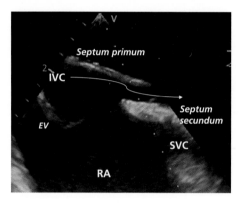

Figure 18.2 Bicaval TEE view showing a PFO between the septum primum (thin, at bottom) and the septum secundum (thick, on top). EV, Eustachian valve.

B. Pathology (see Figures 18.2, 18.3, 18.4)

1. At birth, the PA pressure significantly drops and the pulmonary arterial and venous flow significantly increase. As a result, the LA pressure rises and pushes the septum primum to seal the overlap area.[1] **If it does not seal, a *patent foramen ovale* (PFO) persists. PFO is a persistent tunnel or flap; this is different from the gap of an ASD.**[2]

2. If the two septa do not meet and overlap, a wide, open gap will exist between the two septa in the middle of the interatrial septum: this is called *ostium secundum ASD* (70% of ASDs).

3. If the septum primum does not connect with the endocardial cushions, a gap will be present at the lower level of the interatrial septum: this is *ostium primum ASD* (15–20% of ASDs). *No atrial septal tissue is seen above the base of the atrioventricular valves.*

Ostium primum ASD may be continuous with a defect of the membranous ventricular septum, in which case the defect is called *complete atrioventricular (AV) canal defect*, or *endocardial cushion defect*. The endocardial cushions are central embryonic structures that develop into the AV valves and the membranous ventricular septum. In complete AV canal defect, no tissue separates the AV valves; the AV valves are actually one valve at one horizontal plane, with an atrial and ventricular septal defect in the middle.

An ostium primum ASD without VSD is called *partial AV canal defect*. In the partial AV defect, the ventricular septum is closed by the endocardial cushions or by the septal tricuspid leaflet early in life, so that only a primum ASD is present. In another form called *transitional AV canal defect*, most of the ventricular defect is closed by the septal leaflets of the AV valve, so that only a small residual inlet VSD is seen and two AV valves are present. Thirty-five percent of patients with AV canal defect have Down syndrome, especially those with complete AV canal defects.

Whereas normally the tricuspid valve is a bit lower (more apical) than the mitral valve, the tricuspid and mitral valves are at the same level in AV canal defect, as the mitral valve plane is pulled down. The down-pulling of the mitral valve elongates the LVOT, creating a "goose neck" narrowing of the LVOT with potential LVOT obstruction (Figure 18.5). Mitral valve defects (cleft valve) are frequently seen and result in eccentric MR; tricuspid defects may also be seen.

4. Sinus venosus defect is a gap at the upper posterior part of the septum at the SVC–RA connection. It is almost always associated with some degree of anomalous pulmonary venous return, in which the right upper pulmonary vein, and sometimes a right middle or inferior pulmonary vein, drain into the RA.

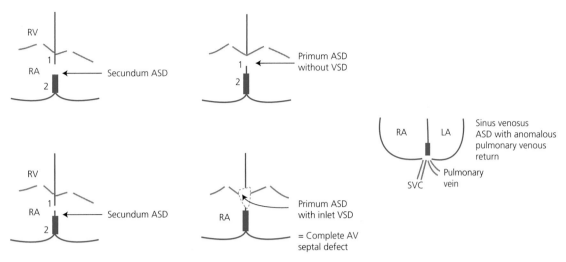

Figure 18.3 Types of ASD. Secundum ASD results from excessive involution of the top portion of the septum primum (→ does not meet the septum secundum). Primum ASD results from failure of the septum primum to reach the endocardial cushions. **Thus, beside primum ASD, secundum ASD is also a defect of the septum primum.** Septum primum is the thinner septum, marked by *1*; septum secundum is marked by *2*.

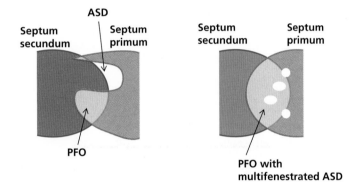

Figure 18.4 En face view of the interatrial septum. Occasionally, both a PFO and a small ASD may be present: ASD in one plane where the septum primum has excessively involuted, PFO in the other planes where the two septa continue to overlap. Alternatively, PFO may be present with multiple small ASD holes.

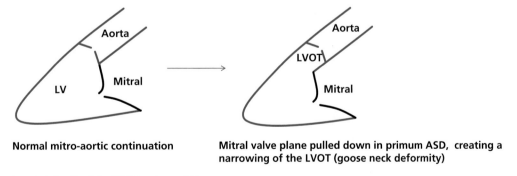

Figure 18.5 Goose-neck deformity of the LVOT in primum ASD.

Partial anomalous pulmonary venous return may also be seen with secundum ASD. A right upper pulmonary vein draining into the RA or SVC is the most common anomaly, accounting for >90% of the anomalous venous return; a left pulmonary vein draining into the innominate vein may also be seen. If only one pulmonary vein is involved, the amount of shunting induced by the anomalous vein is, per se, mild. However, in conjunction with an ASD, the anomalous vein may significantly add to the shunt burden.

C. Consequences

1. A significant ASD is an ASD with a prominent left-to-right shunt leading to a pulmonary flow (Qp) 1.5 times larger than the systemic flow (Qs): Qp/Qs ≥1.5/1.0.

A large ASD is characterized by a Qp/Qs ≥2.

2. A significant ASD causes RA/RV volume overload, dilatation, and failure. This may, rarely, occur in childhood if the ASD is large. Most patients are minimally symptomatic in the first three decades; exercise intolerance and hemodynamic compromise occur later in adulthood (30s to 40s), and most patients are symptomatic by the age of 50. AF and right heart failure develop by the age of 40 in ~10% of patients, then become more prevalent with age. In fact, for the same ASD size, left-to-right shunting may become more severe with age, as LV diastolic dysfunction occurs and LA pressure rises. Also, LA enlargement that occurs with age stretches and widens the ASD. ASD does not, by itself, lead to LA enlargement unless AF occurs.

A complete AV canal defect, on the other hand, leads to a severe shunt and Eisenmenger syndrome early in infancy if not corrected. Paradoxical embolism may be seen.

3. *Pulmonary hypertension (PH) may occur but is rarely severe, because the RV usually fails before severe PH develops. In a way, the failing RV constitutes a barrier that protects the pulmonary arteries from volume overload.* If PH is severe, a second causative diagnosis should be considered, especially if ASD<2 cm. Under 10% of ASDs develop significant pulmonary vascular disease with PVR >5 Wood units.[3] Cyanosis and reversal of the shunt to a right-to-left shunt often result from RV failure and the consequent rise of RA pressure, even without any PH.

D. Diagnosis

1. Exam:
- Fixed split S_2
- Scratchy systolic ejectional murmur at the pulmonic area (left upper sternal border) due to the increased right-sided flow. Systolic TR murmur may also be heard.
- RV heave
- Increased JVP with a large V wave indicative of RV failure ± TR

> RV heave is more prominent in RV volume-overload states, such as ASD, than in pressure-overload states (cor pulmonale, pulmonic stenosis).

2. ECG:
- Ostium secundum ASD: RBBB (usually incomplete), right axis deviation, R-wave notching in the inferior leads (crochetage), right atrial enlargement
- Ostium primum ASD: RBBB + left axis deviation ± prolonged PR interval (primum ASD damages the infra-Hisian conduction system)
- Sinus venosus ASD: ectopic atrial rhythm (non-sinus P waves)
- AF or atrial flutter may be present

3. CXR features: enlarged RV, enlarged central PA knob, and pulmonary plethora from increased flow.

4. Echo:
- TTE often establishes the diagnosis by visualizing the defect and the Doppler flow across it. The defect is usually >8 mm, as smaller defects usually close spontaneously in infancy and do not usually cause hemodynamic compromise. TTE can calculate Qp/Qs ratio (pulmonary to systemic flow ratio), which is equal to:

$$(velocity\ [VTI] \times diameter)\ at\ the\ RVOT,\ divided\ by\ (velocity\ [VTI] \times diameter)\ at\ the\ LVOT$$

  TTE also shows RA and RV enlargement, consequences of any significant ASD.
- The subcostal view is orthogonal to the interatrial septum and is the best diagnostic view for ASD. Over 90% of secundum ASDs are seen in this view, which is also the best view for the sinus venosus defect and for assessment of shunt direction by spectral Doppler. However, the sinus venosus defect, or, rarely, other defects, may be missed by TTE. SVC view (right parasternal view) or superior angulation in a subcostal view may allow the diagnosis of sinus venosus defect. TEE permits better visualization if the diagnosis is suspected but not clearly established in a patient with RA/RV enlargement. Also, intravenous bubble injection may suggest the diagnosis of ASD in these patients. In PFO or secundum ASD, the bubbles fill the RA then the LA; in sinus venosus ASD, the bubbles simultaneously fill both the RA and LA.

> RA and RV enlargement without any obvious cause (such as left HF) in an otherwise healthy adult should prompt a search for an overlooked ASD, especially sinus venosus ASD.

5. Right heart catheterization: catheterization permits the hemodynamic diagnosis of ASD (O_2 saturation step-up ≥8% between SVC and RA), and permits Qp/Qs quantification.

E. Treatment

1. Up to 62% of secundum ASDs may spontaneously close in the first year of life, especially ASD < 3–8 mm.

2. Closure of ASD is indicated in the following cases:
- Qp/Qs ≥1.5 in patients older than 1 year, including asymptomatic patients, as soon as possible. In infants < 1 year old, wait to see if spontaneous closure occurs.
- Right-sided enlargement or failure with a persistent left-to-right shunt. The calculation of Qp/Qs is not usually necessary in this case (except when ASD seems anatomically small and needs to be confirmed as the cause of RV failure, or when the shunt is bidirectional).
- Pulmonary hypertension that is not severe, or, if severe, is still associated with a left-to-right shunt and a reversible pulmonary vascular resistance (reversible with a vasodilator challenge).

Closure is performed percutaneously or surgically (direct surgical closure or patch closure).

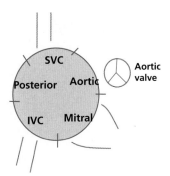

Figure 18.6 Interatrial septum viewed from the side. Various rims are identified. **The three best TEE views to visualize the interatrial septum are:**
- 0° four-chamber view with a clockwise torque to the right (mitral and posterior rims)
- 30–50° aortic view with a clockwise torque to the right (aortic and posterior rims)
- Bicaval 90° view: from the 0° view torqued towards the right-sided structures, a 90° rotation allows visualization of the SVC and IVC (bicaval view) (SVC and IVC rims).

The mitral and IVC rims are septum primum, while the aortic and SVC rims are septum secundum; the two septa meet in the middle. An ostium primum ASD is characterized by an absent mitral rim, while a sinus venosus ASD is characterized by an absent SVC rim.

3. Percutaneous closure can be used for secundum ASD that is ≤ 38 mm in diameter with 5 mm rims and without severe TR or anomalous pulmonary venous return (Figure 18.6). TEE assessment of the rims and of the pulmonary veins, especially the right upper pulmonary vein, is critical in determining if the patient qualifies for percutaneous closure.

Primum ASD and sinus venosus ASD are only treated surgically, as the lack of rims prevents device apposition.

4. ASD closure improves survival and functional status, especially when performed at an early age. Closure before the age of 25 establishes a normal longevity (Mayo registry).[3] Closure after the age of 40 in patients with right heart failure or Qp/Qs >1.5 does not re-establish normal longevity but still reduces long-term mortality by 70% and improves functional status.[4] The reduction of right heart volume starts early after closure, within 24 hours, and may continue for over a year. This reverse remodeling is more complete in younger patients.

While improving survival and functional status, closure in patients >40 years of age does not prevent AF or stroke.

5. Secundum ASD does not require endocarditis prophylaxis. After correction and in the absence of a residual shunt, patients require endocarditis prophylaxis for 6 months only (i.e., until the surgical site endothelializes). If a residual defect persists, endocarditis prophylaxis is indicated lifelong.

II. Patent foramen ovale (PFO)

A cryptogenic stroke is a stroke that is unexplained by carotid disease, cardiac disease such as AF or LV thrombus, or prothrombotic coagulopathies (mainly antiphospholipid syndrome). Moreover, to make the diagnosis of a cryptogenic stroke, a lacunar stroke must be excluded (lacunar stroke being a small, deep white-matter stroke < 15 mm in a patient with HTN, diabetes, or age >50). There is an association between PFO and cryptogenic stroke, patients with cryptogenic stroke having a higher prevalence of PFO than the normal population (~40–50% prevalence). This association is particularly established in patients < 55 years old and is uncertain in older patients.[5,6] PFO patients may have paradoxical embolization of a DVT or an in situ thrombosis formed at the PFO level, especially if the interatrial septum is hypermobile and ejects it.

PFO is common in the normal population (prevalence ~25%), and thus a causal relationship with a stroke is, at best, a diagnosis of exclusion. In some, but not all studies, a large shunt or the coexistence of an atrial septal aneurysm had a clearer association with stroke.[5,7] A large shunt is defined as >10–30 microbubbles or PFO tunnel width ≥2–4 mm, meaning that the separation between secundum septum and primum septum is ≥2–4 mm. An atrial septal aneurysm, defined as hypermobility of the thin septum primum >1 cm from midline, is less clearly associated with an increased stroke risk when isolated,[7] although one meta-analysis suggests it is.[6] The combination of the following three patient characteristics increases the probability that the stroke is PFO-related: age < 55, cortical location of the stroke (as opposed to deep white matter or periventricular), and the lack of uncontrolled HTN, uncontrolled diabetes, and smoking.

Importantly, despite the association between PFO and cryptogenic stroke, evidence suggests that PFO is not a predictor of stroke recurrence in patients receiving antiplatelet therapy, regardless of PFO size and regardless of the presence of atrial septal aneurysm.[5]

PFO is diagnosed by TTE or TEE performed with microbubbles/agitated saline injected during Valsalva (bubble study). In case of PFO, these bubbles will go from the RA to the LA within 3–5 cardiac cycles during the Valsalva release phase. Even the shunting of one bubble to the LA indicates the presence of a right-to-left shunt. If it takes >3–5 cycles for the bubbles to appear on the left side, the shunt is at the pulmonary level (e.g., AV malformation). Normally, during quiet breathing, the LA pressure is larger than the RA pressure, thereby closing the septum primum towards the septum secundum and preventing any significant shunting, except very briefly. A physiologic right-to-left shunt occurs when the RA volume suddenly and largely increases at a time when the LA volume does not, which reverses the LA–RA pressure differential; this is seen during deep inspiration or during the release phase of the Valsalva maneuver. Conversely, the strain phase of Valsalva may reduce right venous return and right-to-left shunting.

Treatment of a cryptogenic stroke presumably due to PFO
- Aspirin or warfarin. The PICSS trial, a large trial that compared aspirin to warfarin in patients with cryptogenic stroke, did not find any difference in stroke recurrence between the two therapies in patients with PFO.[5]

- In patients who had one or more prior strokes/TIAs, PFO closure has not shown superiority to medical therapy in reducing stroke recurrence, according to three randomized trials (in one trial, 37% of patients had more than one prior TIA/stroke). In fact, the risk of stroke recurrence after a cryptogenic stroke is relatively low, ~4–5% at 4 years under antiplatelet therapy (as seen in all three PFO trials), with a potentially higher risk in combined PFO and atrial septal aneurysm.[7–10] While low, this risk is cumulative over time and may be particularly consequential in young patients over the long term. PFO closure showed a trend toward stroke reduction, which may become more significant upon long-term follow-up. PFO closure may be considered in young patients with cortical stroke and no smoking, diabetes, or HTN.

A PFO can lead to mild and insignificant degree of left-to-right (L–R) or right-to-left (R–L) shunting, depending on instantaneous RA–LA pressure differential and breathing cycle. PFO, per se, does not lead to a hemodynamically significant shunting or cavitary dilatation. Conversely, severe RA dilatation/pressure elevation may lead to a significant shunting across the PFO. *In fact, R–L shunting through a PFO in patients with RV failure is a compensatory, secondary process that relieves RV failure, and PFO is an innocent bystander rather than a primary shunt process.* For example, in severe primary pulmonary hypertension, R–L shunt may be seen through a PFO or a small ASD. This shunt is secondary to pulmonary hypertension rather than a cause of pulmonary hypertension, and is associated with improved survival in primary pulmonary hypertension. *Rarely,* significant R–L shunting occurs across a PFO despite a normal RA/RV; this shunt occurs in the upright position (platypnea–orthodeoxia syndrome) or during exertion. The diagnosis is made by documenting orthostatic or exertional O_2 desaturation that is otherwise unexplained.

While the higher LA pressure serves to appose the septum primum over the septum secundum and close the PFO tunnel, preventing any shunt, a severely increased LA pressure may lead to a L–R shunt.[11,12]

III. Ventricular septal defect (VSD)

A. Types (see Figure 18.7)

The interventricular septum has a small membranous portion and a large muscular portion. The muscular portion is divided into three zones (inlet between the atrioventricular valves, outlet beneath the great arteries, and trabecular). A VSD is either perimembranous or muscular:[13]

1. Perimembranous VSD is the most common VSD (70–80% of VSDs). It involves the membranous septum and extends a *bit* into one of the three muscular regions (inlet, trabecular, or outlet). An entirely membranous VSD is rare, as the membranous septum is a small fibrous center.

2. Muscular trabecular VSD is the next most common VSD.

3. Inlet VSD. The inlet septum separates the septal cusps of the mitral and tricuspid valves. Inlet VSD is mainly a defect of the muscular inlet septum, but the membranous septum is frequently involved. A gross deficiency of the inlet septum is associated with AV canal defect. Conversely, a small inlet VSD is not usually associated with AV canal defect.[13]

4. Outlet VSD (subarterial or infundibular VSD). Outlet VSD is mainly a defect of the muscular outlet septum, but the membranous septum is frequently involved. When outlet VSD is very high and abuts both arterial valves, it is called supracristal VSD or doubly committed VSD (the crista supraterminalis being a muscular ridge in the RV outflow).

B. Consequences and associations

- A large VSD leads to a left-to-right shunt, with progressive pulmonary hypertension and progressively large volume circulating back to the LV and leading to LV failure from volume overload. As pulmonary hypertension becomes more severe, Eisenmenger syndrome and cyanosis occur.

A hemodynamically significant VSD leads to LV and LA dilatation and LV failure from volume overload. Since the LV-to-RV shunt is systolic, the RV does not get overloaded in diastole and therefore *RV failure does not occur. Even when pulmonary hypertension develops, right-sided enlargement and tricuspid regurgitation are very unusual because the VSD allows decompression of the RV.* This is in contrast to ASD, which leads to RV diastolic volume overload, RV dilatation and failure, and tricuspid regurgitation; in ASD, the LV is protected by the unloading that occurs at the LA level.[14]

- A VSD, especially an outlet VSD, may be associated with aortic insufficiency. This results from high-velocity jet lesions, similarly to what occurs with subaortic membranous stenosis; also, the outlet defect diminishes the cuspal support and may lead to aortic cusp(s) prolapse. Outlet VSD may be associated with subpulmonic or subaortic stenosis; the subpulmonic stenosis may lead to a right-to-left shunt but protects from Eisenmenger syndrome.
  Any VSD may also be associated with a bicuspid aortic valve and coarctation of the aorta.
- The membranous septum has an interventricular portion but also a more proximal (posterior) portion that separates the LV from the RA. A Gerbode defect is a perimembranous VSD extending more proximal to the tricuspid insertion, leading to a high-velocity LV-to-RA shunt and RV failure, in addition to the LV-to-RV shunt (Figure 18.8).

C. Exam and natural history

With the exception of bicuspid aortic valve, VSD is the most common congenital defect in children. A small VSD leads to a loud, harsh pansystolic murmur at the left lower sternal border, sometimes with a thrill, whereas a large VSD has a softer murmur. *Thus, a loud murmur implies a more benign VSD than a soft murmur.* Small VSDs are called restrictive because they allow only limited shunting.

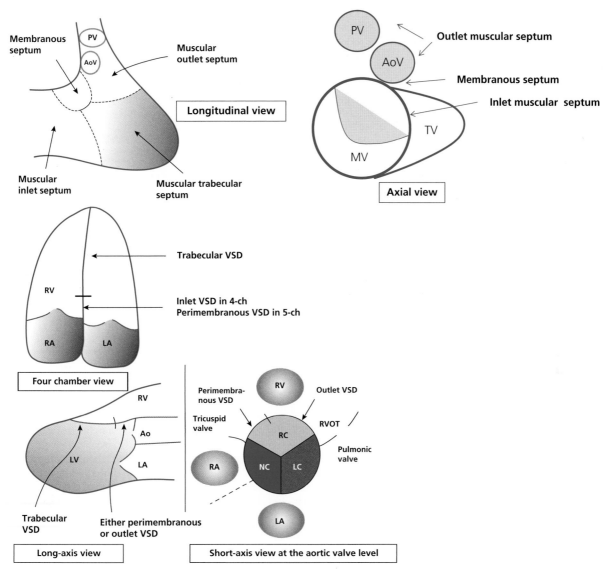

Figure 18.7 Anatomic and echocardiographic localization of VSD. The *membranous septum* is bordered by the septal tricuspid leaflet on the right and the subaortic area on the left; it is superior to the mitral valve. Perimembranous VSD is actually a superior/anterior form of VSD, and therefore it is seen on the long-axis echo view. *Inlet VSD* is bordered by the tricuspid valve on the right and the mitral valve on the left and is the one that continues with an atrial septal defect to form the AV canal defect.

Note that the pulmonic valve (PV) is higher and more anterior than the aortic valve (AoV), and the outlet septum is larger on the right than the left side. An outlet VSD that extends all the way to the PV is called supracristal VSD.

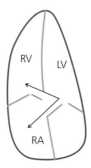

Figure 18.8 Gerbode defect on an **apical five-chamber view**. Perimembranous VSD extends more proximal to the tricuspid valve and leads to LV–RA shunt, in addition to the LV–RV shunt. Being a perimembranous defect, it may not be seen on the four-chamber view. The defect may have an inlet extension.

Small perimembranous or trabecular VSDs have a high closure rate (50–80%) by 2–10 years of age. A perimembranous VSD may close by the apposition of the septal tricuspid leaflet, which sometimes forms a pouch at the level of the sealed defect.[15] A small VSD is hemo-dynamically insignificant, but is associated with a risk of endocarditis.

Large VSDs (*non-restrictive*, Qp/Qs >2) have a low spontaneous closure rate and lead to left HF, then Eisenmenger syndrome in infancy or childhood. They are typically corrected early on, before 1 year of age. Moderately large VSDs (Qp/Qs 1.4–2) may be tolerated for years before leading to hemodynamic compromise later on, in adulthood.

Adults presenting with VSD usually have a small VSD that did not close spontaneously and is not leading to any hemodynamic com-promise. Other possibilities are: VSD that persisted after surgical repair; moderate VSD that is leading to hemodynamic compromise in adulthood (unusual); or large, non-corrected VSD that led to Eisenmenger syndrome long before adulthood.

D. Diagnosis, location, and shunt fraction Qp/Qs are established by TTE

TTE allows estimation of the VSD size: a small VSD has a diameter smaller than 1/3 of the aortic root diameter, a large VSD is a VSD larger than the aortic root. A large VSD typically has a large Qp/Qs ratio (>2), a small velocity, and a small pressure gradient across it because of the high RV systolic pressure (non-restrictive VSD).

TTE may miss a small trabecular VSD but very rarely misses other types of VSD.

E. Treatment

Surgical closure (direct closure or patch closure) is indicated as soon as possible for:

- Significant VSD (moderately restrictive or large non-restrictive) with a Qp/Qs ≥1.5.
- Pulmonary hypertension that is not severe or, if severe, is responsive to vasodilator challenge. The improvement of pulmonary hyperten-sion with vasodilator challenge means it is reversible, as opposed to Eisenmenger syndrome's pulmonary hypertension.
- Large VSD with LV or LA dilatation or LV dysfunction.
- Outlet VSD, regardless of its size, because of the risk of progressive AI.

Perform the surgery soon in infancy if needed (at the age of 3–6 months). Postoperative patch leaks may be seen but rarely require reopera-tion. Occasionally, if VSD closure cannot be immediately performed, *PA banding* is performed to reduce the pulmonary flow and the risk of Eisenmenger syndrome before definitive surgery.

IV. Patent ductus arteriosus (PDA)

A. Definition and consequences

PDA is a persistent communication between the left pulmonary artery and the descending aorta just distal (~1 cm) to the left subclavian artery. It leads to left-to-right shunt and massive LV volume overload from the shunt volume that circulates back to the LV. LV failure, which is initially a high-output failure, subsequently ensues (left HF being the most common complication).

It can also lead to progressive pulmonary hypertension and Eisenmenger syndrome with shunt reversal to a right-to-left shunt. In this case, a differential rather than a generalized cyanosis is seen (cyanosis of the feet only). The right-to-left shunt occurs distal to the innomi-nate artery, so that the O_2 saturation in the upper extremities is preserved whereas the O_2 saturation in the lower extremities is low, explain-ing the differential cyanosis and clubbing, i.e., cyanosis that is much more prominent in the lower extremities. The origin of the left subclavian artery may be close enough to the ductus to receive unoxygenated blood, and therefore cyanosis and clubbing of the left hand may be seen. The right hand remains normal until a severely reduced cardiac output leads to generalized cyanosis.

Infectious endarteritis at the shunt level may also be seen.

B. Severity and presentation

Spontaneous closure of a PDA is unlikely in term infants older than 3 months or pre-term infants older than 12 months. A large shunt (Qp/Qs >2) is symptomatic in infancy and leads to Eisenmenger syndrome early on, as early as 8 months, if untreated.

A moderate shunt (Qp/Qs 1.5–2) may lead to hemodynamic compromise at a later age (childhood or adulthood, up to the third decade). A small shunt (Qp/Qs <1.5) presents as an isolated murmur.

A loud, continuous "machinery" murmur is heard at the first or second left intercostal space. As a result of the large stroke volume, the pulse pressure is wide with bounding pulses.

The continuous murmur of PDA is different from a systolic–diastolic murmur; the former has only one peak that occurs at S_2 or just before it, whereas the latter has two peaks. The continuous murmur of PDA is loudest at the left upper sternal border; if it is louder anywhere else, it suggests the diagnosis of a fistula, such as coronary fistula, or sinus of Valsalva aneurysm ruptured in the RV or the RA.

Remember that in both VSD and PDA, LV failure generally precedes Eisenmenger syndrome. LV failure is generally present by the time the patient develops Eisenmenger syndrome.

C. Diagnosis

Two TTE views allow the diagnosis of PDA: the suprasternal notch view *and* the parasternal short-axis view (pulmonary artery level). These views show a flow extending from the aorta to the left PA and establish the diagnosis in 42% of the patients. TEE establishes the diagnosis in 97% of the patients.[16] For echo shunt calculation, the flow across the RVOT is proximal to the shunt and corresponds to Qs, whereas the flow across the LVOT corresponds to Qp (the reverse is true in ASD and VSD).

D. Treatment

Intervention is indicated for the hemodynamically significant PDA (class I recommendation), but also for any audible PDA, which includes the small PDA with Qp/Qs <1.5, because of the risk of endarteritis (class IIa). Only the tiny, silent PDA does not warrant intervention. Transcatheter closure is the preferred therapy for PDA.

V. Coarctation of the aorta

Coarctation is a narrowing of the aorta around the level of the ductus arteriosus, and may be discrete or long and tubular. The site of coarctation is usually less than 1–5 cm distal to the left subclavian origin. In addition to the pre-stenotic dilatation, most patients with significant aortic coarctation have post-stenotic aortic dilatation, sometimes aneurysmal. Aortic coarctation is associated with a high prevalence and a wide variety of congenital cardiovascular anomalies (>50%). Approximately 75% of these patients have bicuspid aortic valves. Also, there is an increased prevalence of mitral valvular disease, VSD, PDA, and intracranial berry aneurysm (10%). Aortic coarctation is usually diagnosed in an infant or child, but may remain asymptomatic until the young adult age, when the patient succumbs to severe HTN, HF, premature CAD, or intracranial hemorrhage (average survival of untreated coarctation is 34 years).

A. Diagnosis

1. *Clinical:* the patient presents with hypertension, a murmur, and a blood pressure discrepancy of >20 mmHg between the upper and lower extremities with a radial-to-femoral pulse delay. The blood pressure discrepancy may attenuate and become unnoticeable as more collaterals develop with age. The murmur is mid-systolic, heard best over the left upper sternal border, radiates to the back and spine, and may become continuous if the stenosis is severe enough to produce a diastolic pressure gradient.

CXR shows rib notching and a figure of 3, which is a double bubble of the descending aorta (pre- and post-stenotic dilatation).

2. *Hemodynamic:* a 20 mmHg peak-to-peak gradient defines significant aortic coarctation. In patients with collaterals, the aortic gradient may be reduced to 10–20 mmHg; acquired aortic ectasia, significant collateral flow, or left ventricular hypertrophy would define significant coarctation in this case.

The diastolic gradient is usually mild; in fact, collateral flow prevents a drop in distal aortic pressure during diastole but is not enough to prevent the systolic drop in pressure.

3. *Echo* (suprasternal view), *and CT or MRI* are useful imaging modalities.

B. Treatment

The coarctation may be treated surgically: excision followed by end-to-end anastomosis with or without patch repair, or excision with placement of an interposition graft. This treatment may be performed in infancy in very severe cases, or in the first 5 years of life in less severe cases. The aorta reaches 50% of its eventual size at 3–5 years of age, such that, when surgery is performed at this age, a lack of growth of the surgical site does not translate into severe stenosis. A younger age at the time of initial repair translates into better long-term outcomes (less irreversible damage of the aortic wall and less LV hypertrophy). The best survivorship was observed in patients operated at 9 years of age or less.[17]

Coarctation may be treated percutaneously with angioplasty in patients older than 1 year. At less than 1 year of age, there is a high risk of recurrence and aneurysm formation after angioplasty. Stenting is the percutaneous treatment of choice in patients >30 kg, while angioplasty is the treatment of choice for patients >1 year and <30 kg, where the use of a stent is limited by aortic growth issues.[18]

C. Long-term sequelae

Residual hypertension is seen in a third of patients and may be related to residual coarctation or to the fact that longstanding hypertension permanently remodels the aortic wall.[19]

Residual coarctation or recurrent coarctation is seen in ~10–20% of patients after surgical repair. If focal, recoarctation is best treated with balloon angioplasty.

After surgical or percutaneous repair, patients have a long-term risk of aneurysm formation at the site of surgical repair, and late dissection, as the aorta itself is diseased. This warrants surveillance with MRI or CT every few years.

Late mortality is related to coronary artery disease (most common cause of late death), residual hypertension, associated valvular disease, and cerebral berry aneurysms

VI. Other anomalies

Subvalvular aortic stenosis, supravalvular aortic stenosis, and pulmonic stenosis are discussed in Chapter 6. Additional anomalies:

A. Sinus of Valsalva aneurysm

Sinus of Valsalva aneurysm is a congenital localized dilatation of a single sinus of Valsalva (usually). It is different from the aortopathy of bicuspid aortic valve or Marfan disease, wherein all sinuses are enlarged, usually along with dilatation of the sinotubular junction and ascending aorta. The latter conditions may, however, have this localized form of sinus dilatation.

The sinus of Valsalva aneurysm often involves the right sinus and usually ruptures in the RV, at the age of 15–45. Less frequently, it may arise from the non-coronary sinus and rupture in the RA. It usually comes to attention after rupture and manifests as a continuous murmur, predominantly at the right sternal border, and a large left-to-right shunt with left HF from the volume overload circulating back to the LV (like VSD), but also right HF from the diastolic shunting into the RV. It may also lead to coronary compression and myocardial ischemia. Not infrequently, it may remain asymptomatic. It is frequently associated with VSD (~50%) and AI (~50%).

B. Scimitar syndrome

The pulmonary veins of the right upper lobe and most of the right lower lobe empty into the IVC just below the RA. The anomalous right pulmonary vein descending to connect with the IVC has the shape of a scimitar and may get compressed as it emerges through the lung. Similar to ASD, the scimitar shunt occurs proximal to the tricuspid valve, is usually small, and does not, by itself, lead to pulmonary hypertension. However, patients with scimitar syndrome have associated anomalies that explain most of the untoward effects and pulmonary hypertension:

- Hypoplasia of the right lung with hypolasia of the right pulmonary artery.
- Branches of the upper abdominal aorta (e.g., celiac artery) or the lower thoracic aorta supply part of the right lung and may lead to pulmonary hypertension and significant left-to-right shunting at the PA level.
- Associated congenital heart disease in 20–25% of the cases (ASD, PDA, coarctation of the aorta).

C. Persistent left SVC

Persistent left SVC is a condition wherein the left innominate vein drains directly into the coronary sinus, leading to the isolated finding of a dilated coronary sinus. Bubbles injected through a left arm vein briskly fill the coronary sinus (which does not normally fill). It is a benign condition per se, found in <0.5% of the population. It has a higher prevalence in patients with other congenital heart diseases (5–10%).

2. CYANOTIC CONGENITAL HEART DISEASE

I. Pulmonary hypertension secondary to shunt

A. Definition and mechanisms

Eisenmenger syndrome is defined as severe, irreversible pulmonary hypertension that results from left-to-right shunting. The high PA flow leads to a reactional increase in pulmonary vascular resistance, which eventually exceeds the systemic vascular resistance and leads to shunt reversal (the left-to-right shunt becomes a right-to-left shunt with cyanosis). Usually, in Eisenmenger syndrome, the systemic and pulmonary pressures are nearly equal, but more importantly, the **pulmonary vascular resistance (PVR) exceeds the systemic vascular resistance (SVR)**. The shunt is purely a right-to-left shunt in the majority of the cases, but may be bidirectional (right-to-left and left-to-right).

At an early stage of left-to-right shunting, the pulmonary pressure may be elevated solely from the increased pulmonary flow. Pressure being equal to flow multiplied by vascular resistance, an increase in pulmonary flow (e.g., Qp/Qs=4) leads to a severe increase in pulmonary pressure even if PVR is normal. For example, a large VSD may lead to a large left-to-right shunting and an almost equalization of LV and RV systolic pressures and aortic and pulmonary pressures. However, early on, this increase in pulmonary pressure is due mainly to the increase in flow (not Eisenmenger syndrome). Later on, PVR progressively increases, eventually exceeding SVR: Eisenmenger syndrome with shunt reversal occurs. Thus, in the evaluation of a shunt associated with severe pulmonary hypertension, the calculation of PVR is the most important next evaluation step. Pulmonary vasoreactivity is assessed by using 100% O_2 and pulmonary vasodilators in the following cases:

- Pulmonary pressure that is >2/3 the systemic pressure, particularly when the PVR is severely increased, >6 Wood units or >2/3 the SVR
- Left-to-right shunt that has become bidirectional with significant right-to-left shunting and hypoxemia

A significant response is characterized by a reduction of the mean PA pressure by >10 mmHg to <40 mmHg and PVR by >20% to <5 Wood units; also, the left-to-right shunt typically increases and Qp/Qs rises to >1.5. In the absence of a significant response, the pulmonary arterial remodeling is at an advanced and irreversible stage and the shunt should not be closed. If the shunt is closed at this stage, the right-sided volume overload and the pulmonary hypertension worsen postoperatively. In case of a significant response, the patient is treated with pulmonary vasodilators until the PA pressure declines to an operable range, then the shunt is closed.[20]

Eisenmenger syndrome is usually due to VSD (most common cause), PDA, or, less commonly, ASD. More specifically in ASD, shunt reversal and cyanosis may be seen without pulmonary hypertension. RV volume overload leads to RV failure, which leads to an increase in RA pressure, at times exceeding LA pressure. **In ASD, the right-to-left shunt is often determined by RV failure rather than PA pressure, and hypoxemia may be seen without severe pulmonary hypertension**.[20]

In cases of ASD with elevated PVR and/or bidirectional shunting, *balloon occlusion testing* may be performed. Temporary balloon occlusion of the ASD is performed, and RA pressure, PA pressure, and PCWP are measured through a Swan catheter. A significant increase in right-sided pressures or a drop in CO indicates a significant risk of right-sided failure associated with ASD closure. On the other hand, a significant increase in LA pressure measured through the balloon occlusion catheter indicates that the patient has significant LV dysfunction (e.g., LVH with diastolic failure) and was getting relieved by the left-to-right shunting, i.e., the preload reduction. LV may not be able to cope with the acute increase in preload following ASD closure, which may lead to acute pulmonary edema. This is mainly seen when ASD is closed in an older population. ASD closure should be postponed and the patient appropriately treated with antihypertensive agents and diuretics before attempting closure.[21]

B. Clinical presentation of Eisenmenger syndrome

Eisenmenger syndrome that is secondary to VSD or PDA typically develops before the age of 2 years. Eisenmenger patients have a good functional capacity up until their 20s, then develop a progressive functional decline, cyanosis, atrial and ventricular arrhythmias (common), and hemoptysis. Hemoptysis results from the systemic arterial collaterals to the lung; it may be severe and is the cause of death in ~15% of patients. Right heart failure develops later. Stroke and brain abscess from paradoxical emboli may occur; polycythemia is also a factor.

Similarly to pulmonic stenosis, the RV does not fail and TR does not occur until late in the course of disease (age 40s). On the one hand, the congenital RV tolerates pressure overload more than the adult RV, and on the other hand, the right-to-left shunt allows RV or PA decompression, therefore delaying failure. This explains why Eisenmenger is much better tolerated than idiopathic pulmonary hypertension. RV heave is present but the RV is not dilated; on JVP exam, A wave is large but V wave and mean JVP are normal.

On exam, Eisenmenger is characteristically a *silent cyanotic heart disease*, i.e., no murmur is heard. The equalization of pressures across chambers makes the right-to-left shunt a low-gradient, silent shunt. In fact, the presence of a VSD or a PDA murmur makes the diagnosis of irreversible pulmonary hypertension unlikely.

CXR is characterized by an enlarged central PA with rapid tapering and lung oligemia. The PA is sometimes calcified, which is not the case in idiopathic pulmonary arterial hypertension, where pulmonary hypertension is not as longstanding.

C. Treatment

The causal shunt should not be closed at this point, as the right-to-left shunt relieves the severity of pulmonary hypertension and prevents RV failure. Treatment consists of avoiding exacerbating factors, such as dehydration, systemic vasodilators (which increase right-to-left shunt), and excessive physical activity. Pulmonary vasodilators may be used (bosentan, sildenafil, IV prostacyclin) and have been shown to improve symptoms. Beware that pulmonary vasodilators may increase pulmonary flow and lead to pulmonary edema, in which case diuretics may be required. They may also have an untoward systemic vasodilatory effect. In advanced cases, lung transplant with repair of the cardiac defect may be performed.

> In all cases of right-to-left shunt, hot conditions, systemic vasodilators, and sedation/anesthesia are risky and should be avoided as much as possible. They reduce SVR and thus increase the right-to-left shunt and may lead to hemodynamic collapse. Dehydration may also reduce the marginal right-sided flow and lead to hemodynamic collapse.
>
> If a patient presents with a hyperviscosity syndrome (neurological symptoms accompanying polycythemia, usually hematocrit>65%), first rule out dehydration as a cause of polycythemia. If symptoms persist, phlebotomy with adequate fluid replacement may be considered. Also, search for microcytosis and iron deficiency even in patients with polycythemia, as iron-deficient red blood cells are less deformable and more prone to sludging. Polycythemic patients are prone to both thrombosis and bleeding.

II. Tetralogy of Fallot

A. Pathology and consequences

Tetralogy of Fallot has four components (Figure 18.9):

a. Outlet VSD with right-to-left shunt and cyanosis
b. RV outflow obstruction: the major site of obstruction is usually at the subvalvular, infundibular level. In addition, there is often a stenotic, bicuspid pulmonic valve with supravalvular hypoplasia. There may also be a distal pulmonary arterial stenosis, i.e., pulmonary stenosis may be present at multiple levels. Occasionally, there is an outflow tract atresia (this is a more complex form of tetralogy).
c. Overriding of the aorta over the interventricular septum (<50% of patients). In addition, a right aortic arch is seen in 25% of patients. In the absence of an overriding aorta, the disorder is called *partial tetralogy*.
d. RV hypertrophy.
e. A fifth component, ASD (secundum ASD or primum ASD/AV canal defect), is seen in 15% of patients (pentalogy of Fallot).

The severity of this malformation and of the right-to-left shunt and cyanosis depends on the degree of RV outflow obstruction. A mild RV outflow obstruction may not lead to significant right-to-left shunting and the cyanosis may be mild or absent, in which case the entity is termed "pink tetralogy" or "acyanotic tetralogy." Pink tetralogy may become blue as the RV obstruction progresses with age.

A tetralogy spell is an acute fall in O_2 saturation that occurs when the pulmonary blood flow further declines because of reduced preload (e.g., dehydration), or increased right-to-left shunt (e.g., systemic vasodilatation [exercise]). It is relieved with systemic vasoconstriction or squatting, which reduces the right-to-left shunting, hydration, O_2 therapy, and propranolol (↓ RV outflow contractility and narrowing).

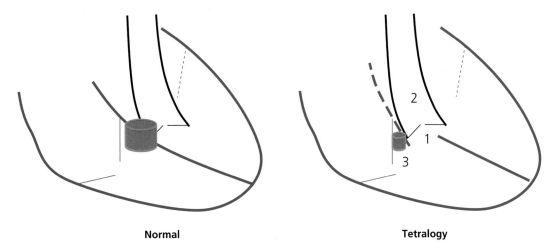

Normal   **Tetralogy**

Figure 18.9 Anatomy in normal patients and in tetralogy of Falllot. In tetralogy, the outlet septum is not only defected but malaligned with the trabecular septum and displaced towards the RV. The aortic origin is rightward and overrides the VSD. The RV outflow tract (gray cylinder) is narrowed, partly from the septal deviation and partly from the fact that the aorta occupies the RV outflow, allowing right-sided blood to be directly ejected in the aorta. The VSD is different from non-tetralogy VSD in that the aorta overrides the VSD. 1, VSD; 2, overriding aorta; 3, RV outflow obstruction.

CXR shows a boot-shaped heart. The apex points upward because of RV enlargement, and the region of the left pulmonary artery (left hilum) has a sharp inward concavity. This is opposite to isolated PS, wherein the left PA area is enlarged from post-stenotic dilatation (Figure 18.10). Moreover, a decreased pulmonary vascularity, and sometimes, a right aortic knob with an absent left knob are seen (Figure 18.11).

> As opposed to Eisenmenger, which is characterized by a silent cyanosis, tetralogy is characterized by a cyanosis and a systolic murmur that is secondary to RV outflow obstruction. The more severe the obstruction, the less flow goes through the RV outflow and the milder the murmur.

B. Treatment

1. *Palliation with a Blalock–Taussig shunt (subclavian artery to pulmonary artery shunt) or Glenn shunt (SVC to PA shunt).* These shunts increase pulmonary flow and serve as a bridge to a more complete correction. They are used when complete correction is not possible in the neonatal period or when PA is small and underdeveloped from underfilling. The systemic-to-PA shunt (e.g., Blalock–Taussig shunt) should not be kept too long, as it may lead to pulmonary hypertension and high-output LV failure, similarly to PDA.

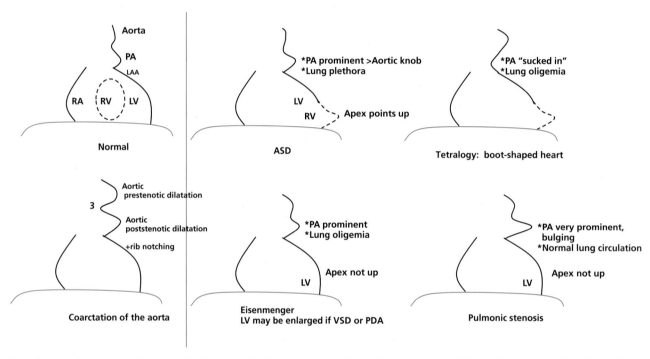

Figure 18.10 Radiographic cardiac and mediastinal silhouettes in various congenital heart diseases. In congenital heart disease, assess the following four features: (1) shape of the heart and apex; (2) proximal PA; (3) lung circulation; (4) normal vs. right-sided aortic arch.

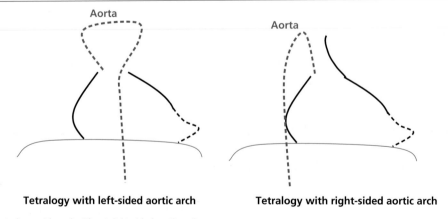

Figure 18.11 CXR in tetralogy with and without right-sided aortic arch

2. *Surgical correction*. The VSD is closed with a patch. The infundibular muscular stenosis is resected and the RV outflow tract enlarged and patched all the way up to the pulmonic valve. Pulmonic valvotomy is performed in the case of pulmonic stenosis. This can be performed at any age, including the first few months of life. Freedom from late reintervention and normal exercise tolerance are expected in up to 90% of patients.[22]

3. Patients may present in adulthood with the following complications:
   - Severe pulmonary regurgitation is very common and leads to progressive RV enlargement 10–20 years postoperatively. In fact, during surgical repair of tetralogy, the RV outflow is enlarged and patched all the way up to the pulmonic valve, which dilates the valvular annulus and disrupts the valve, making it incompetent; occasionally, the valve is even removed during surgical repair. Pulmonic valve replacement is required whenever severe RV dilatation, RV systolic dysfunction, or exercise limitation occurs.
   - Persistent RVOT obstruction.
   - Residual VSD with significant left-to-right shunt (this and the preceding two complications require surgical repair).
   - Persistent RV dysfunction.
   - Dilated aortic root, progressive AI secondary to VSD
   - VT, SVT, and sudden cardiac death, especially in the case of a persistent RV dysfunction or a very wide QRS >180 ms. One-third of late deaths are sudden. ICD is indicated in case of syncope or sustained VT.

The late occurrence of arrhythmia or QRS widening warrants a search for pulmonary regurgitation or other complications.

RV outflow obstruction protects from pulmonary hypertension, and thus patients with tetralogy do not usually develop this complication over the long term. Pulmonary hypertension in a patient with tetralogy may imply peripheral pulmonic stenosis, a mild RV outflow obstruction (before correction) that allowed for a left-to-right shunt, or a Blalock–Taussig shunt that produced pulmonary hypertension.

III. Ebstein anomaly

The insertion of one or two of the tricuspid valve leaflets (the septal ± posterior leaflets) is displaced toward the apex, which puts part of the RV in the atrium ("atrialization" of the RV and reduction of the "functional RV" mass, which reduces RV output). While the tricuspid valve is normally more apical than the mitral valve, in Ebstein, the distance between the septal tricuspid leaflet and the mitral annulus is excessive, i.e., >8 mm/m^2 of BSA. *The anterior tricuspid leaflet is never displaced but is elongated and tries to catch the low septal leaflet.*

Because of the tricuspid abnormality, patients with severe Ebstein anomaly may have severe TR. This is often the biggest issue, as TR leads to progressive RA enlargement, RV failure, and RV volume overload, worsened by the loss of parts of the functional RV. These patients end up with severe right heart failure. They typically present in young adulthood.

Fifty percent of patients have an associated ASD, with right-to-left shunting and cyanosis at some point. This shunt occurs when the RV fails and RA pressure increases, and early on it may only be exertional.

Twenty-five percent of patients have accessory pathways and SVT.

A. Natural history and exam

The natural history varies widely and depends on *three factors*: degree of atrialization of the RV, degree of TR, and presence of right-to-left ASD shunt. Some patients develop symptoms as newborns or infants, while some occasionally remain asymptomatic until their 50s or 60s. Patients present with reduced exercise tolerance (reduced cardiac output), right heart failure, and sometimes right-to-left shunt with cyanosis, which may only be exertional early on.

Exam findings: TR murmur that increases with inspiration, loud and split S$_1$ secondary to the loud closure of the tricuspid valve, and split S$_2$ secondary to ASD. Pectus excavatum may be associated with this anomaly.

B. ECG and CXR

ECG is characterized by a Himalayan P wave, which is a gigantic, peaked P wave in lead II, as large as the QRS. RBBB may be present and is characteristically splintered, with RSR'S' pattern. PR may be short, consistent with WPW.

CXR shows an enlarged cardiac silhouette (gigantic RA). The lung vasculature is normal or reduced.

C. Treatment

Ebstein anomaly may be mild. It does not require surgery when the tricuspid displacement and the TR are mild. Surgical intervention, which mainly consists of tricuspid valve repair (rather than replacement) to correct the harmful severe TR, is indicated in cases of deteriorating functional capacity, progressive RV dilatation or RV systolic dysfunction, even if asymptomatic, or any cyanosis (class I indication). Cyanosis is associated with an increased risk of paradoxical embolization.

3. MORE COMPLEX CYANOTIC CONGENITAL HEART DISEASE AND SHUNT PROCEDURES

I. Functionally single ventricle and Fontan procedure

A. Fontan procedure

The Fontan procedure is a palliative surgery that redirects the systemic venous return directly to the pulmonary artery without passing through the RV (= atriopulmonary connection) (Figure 18.12). It is performed in patients who have a "functionally single ventricle," usually associated with cyanosis. This procedure relieves the chronic volume load on the systemic ventricle that is pumping to both the pulmonary

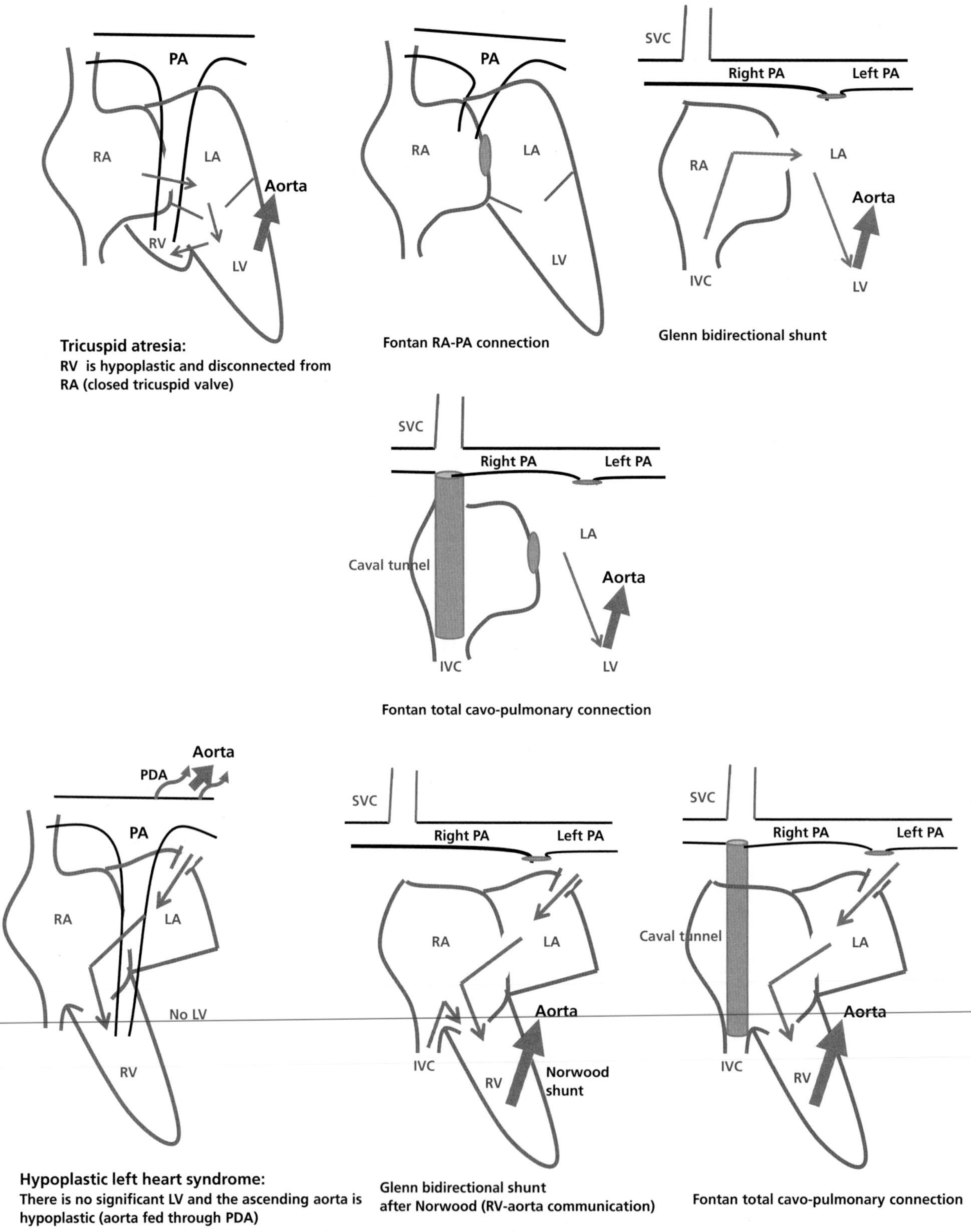

Tricuspid atresia:
RV is hypoplastic and disconnected from RA (closed tricuspid valve)

Fontan RA-PA connection

Glenn bidirectional shunt

Fontan total cavo-pulmonary connection

Hypoplastic left heart syndrome:
There is no significant LV and the ascending aorta is hypoplastic (aorta fed through PDA)

Glenn bidirectional shunt after Norwood (RV-aorta communication)

Fontan total cavo-pulmonary connection

Figure 18.12 Tricuspid atresia and Fontan procedure (top 2 rows). Hypoplastic left heart syndrome and Fontan procedure (bottom row). Note: a Glenn bidirectional shunt is half of a total cavopulmonary connection: the SVC is disconnected from the RA, then connected to the right PA, while the common PA is tied up; the IVC continues to flow into the RA then the single ventricle (all of the IVC flow is right-to-left shunted). Later on, an IVC-to-PA tunnel is created, which converts Glenn into a Fontan procedure. When Fontan is done for tricuspid atresia, the pre-existing ASD is typically closed.

and systemic circulations. *What is interesting is that blood flows passively to the PA without an interposed RV, as long as the PA pressure is not increased. In a way, humans who have a normal PA pressure may live without RV for many years or decades; the RV may be forgone for a passive conduit in patients with **a normal PA pressure***. The venous pressure must be high enough, higher than the pulmonary pressure, to let blood flow towards the pulmonary artery. The systemic venous pressure is, therefore, elevated chronically and allows forward flow. The RA is chronically and severely enlarged. The procedure cannot be performed in patients with pulmonary hypertension.[23,24]

B. Indications for Fontan

The Fontan procedure is indicated for:

- *Tricuspid atresia*: RV is hypoplastic and not connected to the RA (tricuspid valve is closed). Blood flows from the RA to the LA through an ASD, then the LV pumps to the PA through a VSD and to the aorta (Figure 18.12). Initially, these patients temporarily receive a Blalock–Taussig shunt to increase PA flow, then a bidirectional Glenn procedure, then Fontan.
- *Hypoplastic left heart syndrome*: the left heart and the proximal aorta are underdeveloped. The RV pumps to the PA and then the aorta through a PDA.
- *Double-inlet single ventricle*: double atria and AV valves drain into a single ventricle.

In all those complex anomalies, both right-to-left and left-to-right shunts are present.

C. Variations of Fontan: the three surgeries required in single-ventricle syndromes

One variation of Fontan consists of connecting the SVC to the right PA, and creating a tunnel that connects the IVC to the right PA; this variation reduces blood turbulence and the ensuing waste of blood-flow energy. Another variation consists of creating fenestrations of the conduit into the RA (and leaving a small ASD), which allows decompression of the venous circulation in case of pulmonary hypertension, so that blood still flows to the left heart and prevents collapse; this allows the performance of the Fontan procedure in patients with pulmonary hypertension.

Note that the Fontan procedure is not performed upfront in newborns and infants. Patients < 2 years of age have a high pulmonary resistance that may lead to Fontan failure. That is why patients with a single ventricle often require a three-step procedure (Figure 18.12):[17]

1. In tricuspid atresia, a systemic-to-PA shunt is initially performed in newborns with poor pulmonary flow (***Blalock–Taussig shunt***). In patients with large VSD and high pulmonary flow, PA banding is performed.

Hypoplastic left heart syndrome is initially corrected with a ***Norwood procedure***. The main PA is disconnected from the its base and from the RV. A direct communication is then created between the RV and the aorta, using the PA base as a conduit. A systemic artery-to-PA shunt, like a *Blalock–Taussig shunt*, is created for the pulmonary circulation. PDA is closed, while a large ASD is kept open for the pulmonary venous return.

2. As a second step, the systemic-to-PA shunt is taken down, and a ***Glenn bidirectional shunt**, which is a **hemi-Fontan***, is performed at 3–6 months of age. It consists of disconnecting the SVC from the RA and connecting it to the right PA, while the common PA is tied. SVC blood flows to the lungs, while IVC blood goes to the left side and recirculates (residual cyanosis); this avoids the risk of failure of full Fontan as pulmonary resistance is still increased in these very young patients, and is also useful in borderline cases with increased PA pressure.

3. At 2–5 years of age, the ***full Fontan*** is completed by connecting the IVC to the right PA through a tunnel or a conduit.

The first two steps improve pulmonary blood flow and hypoxemia, but the patients continue to have right-to-left shunting and some degree of cyanosis.

D. Exam and long-term complications

Fontan patients have a quiet auscultation without any significant murmur; a murmur suggests associated abnormalities. They survive until early adulthood (20s) before they develop failure of their single ventricle and arrhythmias.

Long-term complications:

- Anastomotic obstruction (leads to increased venous pressure and reduced functional capacity).
- AF or atrial flutter is common.
- Ventricular failure.
- Thrombus formation in the RA, the venous system, or the Fontan circuit. Fontan patients frequently receive aspirin or warfarin prophylaxis to prevent thrombotic events.
- Protein-losing enteropathy, from the chronically elevated venous pressure, develops in 10% of patients and carries a poor prognosis (50% mortality at 5 years)

Eventually, patients with Fontan complications require cardiac transplantation.

A functionally single ventricle is the only congenital heart disease with cyanosis yet isolated LVH on ECG, rather than RVH.

II. Transposition of great arteries (TGA)

A. D-TGA

In d-TGA, the aorta originates from the morphological RV (RA–RV–aorta connection), and the pulmonary artery originates from the morphological LV (LA–LV–PA connection) (Figure 18.13). Some communication must exist between the two systems (ASD usually, sometimes VSD or PDA). These patients are cyanotic and die within the first year if untreated. Complex TGA is d-TGA associated with other major congenital abnormalities (PS, VSD).

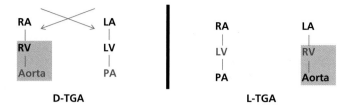

Figure 18.13 D-TGA is characterized by RV–aorta on the right, while l-TGA is characterized by RV–aorta on the left. The transposed chambers are named in blue. The arrows on d-TGA describe the tunnels (baffles).

The following surgeries may be performed in d-TGA:

- *Atrial switch (Mustard or Senning procedures)* consists of creating a baffle (tunnel) that redirects SVC/IVC flow to the LA/mitral valve, and a second baffle that redirects the pulmonary venous flow to the tricuspid valve. The problem is that the morphological RV behaves as the systemic ventricle and may ultimately fail after 20–30 years. TR and atrial arrhythmias may develop. Baffle leak may occur and lead to L–R or R–L shunt. Baffle obstruction may lead to pulmonary hypertension or peripheral venous hypertension. Baffle issues may be treated percutaneously. Severe failure of the systemic ventricle may warrant cardiac transplantation or two-step arterial switch (banding the PA to allow hypertrophy of the anatomic LV, followed by arterial switch later on).
- *Arterial switch (Jatene procedure)* consists of transposing the PA and aorta to their respective ventricles. The aorta is transposed above its base, i.e., above the valve and the coronary level, and thus the coronaries need to be separately transposed and sutured to the new aortic base, previously left-sided PA. There is a long-term risk of ostial coronary stenosis, regurgitation of the neoaortic valve (actually a pulmonic valve), and supravalvular stenosis of the PA and aorta at the anastomotic sites (may be treated percutaneously).
- *Rastelli procedure* is performed in patients with TGA + VSD + subvalvular PS. The LV is connected to the aorta with a patch passing through the VSD, and the RV is connected to the transected PA through a valved conduit.

B. L-TGA

In l-TGA, or congenitally corrected TGA, the LV and RV with their respective valves are transposed (RA–LV–PA circuit on the right, and LA–RV–aorta circuit on the left). The circulation is physiologically corrected but the morphological RV supports the systemic circulation. L-TGA, when isolated, is well tolerated until late adulthood. However, it is most commonly associated with other congenital anomalies, such as progressive regurgiation of the systemic (tricuspid) valve or VSD.

The letter "d" or "l" corresponds to the *location of the RV and aorta, which are always connected in TGA*. In d-TGA (dextro), the RV and aorta are on the right, the arteries are transposed; in l-TGA (left), the RV and aorta are on the left, the ventricles are transposed.

III. Other anomalies

A. Truncus arteriosus

In this case, only one trunk leaves the heart and branches into PA and aorta. This trunk usually sits over both the RV and LV, which also communicate through a VSD. It is corrected early on by separating the pulmonary artery and connecting it to the RV.

B. Total anomalous pulmonary venous return

As opposed to the partial anomalous venous return that occurs with ASD, in which one or two pulmonary veins drain into the RA, in total anomalous venous return all four veins drain as a trunk into the RA, SVC, coronary sinus, or IVC, leading to a very large left-to-right shunt. Some degree of right-to-left shunting must be present to create a circulation. This anomaly must be corrected in infancy.

A murmur in an infant usually means:

- Ventricular outflow obstruction, such as congenital PS, AS, subvalvular obstruction, or tetralogy.
- A left-to-right shunt (such as VSD, PDA) before the equalization of right and left pressures, i.e., before the Eisenmenger stage, and without a right-sided obstruction that reverses the shunt (in tetralogy or PS, the VSD, by itself, may be silent).

A murmur at birth usually implies PS or AS. The murmur of VSD and PDA is not usually present at birth, as the right-sided pressures are still elevated at birth. VSD and PDA murmurs develop over the course of the first week.
Eisenmenger and Fontan patients are typically silent.

QUESTIONS AND ANSWERS

Question 1. A 20-year-old man presents with dyspnea on exertion and mild cyanosis on exertion. His exam reveals a split S_2 and a systolic murmur at the left sternal border. CXR shows cardiomegaly, enlarged PA, and lung plethora. Incomplete RBBB is seen on ECG. What is the most likely diagnosis?

A. ASD with large L–R shunt and some R–L shunt

B. Eisenmenger syndrome

C. Ebstein anomaly

Question 2. On echo, the patient in Question 1 has a large secundum ASD with bidirectional shunting, severe right-sided enlargement, and systolic PA pressure of 75 mmHg (systemic pressure 100 mmHg). He undergoes right heart catheterization: SVC O_2 sat 72%, PA sat 80%, PV O_2 sat 96%, arterial O_2 sat 90%. His PA pressure is 75/40 mmHg, and PVR is 7.5 Wood units. What is the Qp/Qs and what is the next step?

A. Qp/Qs is only 1.1. The shunt is now balanced bidirectional and should not be closed

B. Qp/Qs is 1.1. Perform vasoreactivity testing and see if PVR declines and the shunt becomes mostly left-to-right with vasodilators, with Qp/Qs becoming >1.5

C. Qp/Qs is 1.5. The patient qualifies for ASD closure

D. Regardless of Qp/Qs, the presence of right-sided enlargement indicates a need for ASD closure

Question 3. A 20-year-old man presents with dyspnea on exertion. He has a fixed split S_2, a systolic murmur, and RV heave. JVP is elevated. He is not hypoxic or cyanotic. Echo shows enlarged RV, secundum ASD of 1 cm with left-to-right shunting. Qp/Qs is calculated at 1.3. What is the next step?

A. Patient does not qualify for closure as Qp/Qs < 1.5

B. Perform catheterization to better assess Qp/Qs and decide about the need for ASD closure

C. Patient qualifies for ASD closure. Perform TEE and catheterization before closure

Question 4. A 15-year-old Fontan patient presents with cyanosis. What is the differential diagnosis?

A. Development of veno-venous collaterals (systemic veins communicate with pulmonary veins)

B. Fontan fenestration

C. Pulmonary arteriovenous malformations

D. Failing single ventricle

E. A + B + C + D

F. B + D

Question 5. A 32-year-old woman presents with progressive dyspnea on exertion and cyanosis. Arterial O_2 saturation is 86% at rest and drops to 78% with exercise. Exam shows elevated JVP and a loud, fixed split S_2. CXR shows cardiomegaly and lung oligemia. She denies a history of heart murmur during childhood. What is the most likely diagnosis?

A. ASD with Eisenmenger

B. Ebstein anomaly

C. Tetralogy of Fallot

D. VSD with Eisenmenger syndrome

Question 6. A 32-year-old woman presents with progressive dyspnea on exertion and cyanosis. Arterial O_2 saturation is 86% at rest and drops to 78% with exercise. Exam shows elevated JVP, a loud, fixed split S_2, and a systolic murmur at the left sternal border. CXR shows cardiomegaly and lung oligemia. What is the most likely diagnosis?

A. ASD with Eisenmenger

B. Ebstein anomaly

C. Tetralogy of Fallot

D. VSD with Eisenmenger syndrome

Question 7. Which of the following is *not true* of d-TGA?

A. RV and aorta are on the right, LV and PA are on the left

B. Mustard procedure is associated with a late risk of baffle leak, with R–L or L–R shunt

C. Mustard procedure is associated with a late risk of baffle obstruction, with a subsequent pulmonary hypertension (obstruction of the pulmonary venous baffle) or high RA pressure (SVC/IVC baffle)

D. Rastelli procedure is not useful in d-TGA (only l-TGA)

E. In arterial switch, the original pulmonic valve serves as a neoaortic valve and has a risk of regurgitation

F. In arterial switch, the coronary arteries are separately moved and sutured to the base of the PA (now aorta), with a risk of late obstruction

Question 8. A 20-year-old man presents with dyspnea on exertion. He has a prior history of murmur during infancy but his parents were not compliant with follow-up. On exam, a holosystolic murmur is heard at the left lower sternal border. His LV is enlarged, S_3 is present, and he has crackles on pulmonary exam. Echo shows a moderate-size VSD with enlarged LV and normal RV. What is the next step?

A. Closure of VSD

B. Right heart catheterization to ensure VSD is hemodynamically significant. A small RV suggests VSD is not significant

C. Right heart catheterization to ensure the lack of severe pulmonary hypertension, followed by referral for closure

D. TEE

Question 9. A 25-year-old man with a prior history of tetralogy of Fallot corrected surgically presents with progressive dyspnea on exertion. His echo shows a dilated RV with increased velocity across the RVOT (2.5 m/s). What is the most likely diagnosis?

A. RVOT obstruction

B. Severe PR

C. Residual large VSD

Question 10. A 30-year-old woman presents with exertional chest pain. She has a short stature, a web neck, and increased distance between the eye corners. On exam, a 3/6 harsh mid-systolic murmur is heard at the left upper sternal border. Blood pressure checked in both arms is normal. What is the diagnosis?
A. Turner syndrome and coarctation of the aorta
B. Noonan syndrome and pulmonic stenosis
C. Down syndrome and complete AV canal defect
D. Williams syndrome and supravalvular AS

Question 11. A 20-year-old man has a history of a surgically treated coarctation of the aorta. What is the most common long-term sequela?
A. Recurrent coarctation
B. Aortic dissection or aneurysm
C. Hemorrhagic stroke (berry aneurysms) or ischemic stroke
D. CAD

Question 12. A 40-year-old man presents with new onset of dyspnea for the last month. He is not hypoxic. A continuous murmur is heard all over the precordial area. Echo shows severe pulmonary hypertension and pulmonic regurgitation but could not delineate a shunt. What is the diagnosis?
A. Patent ductus arteriosus
B. Sinus of Valsalva aneurysm ruptured in the RV (most common location) or RA
C. Sinus of Valsalva aneurysm ruptured in the RA (most common location) or RV
D. Severe primary PH with systolic flow murmur and diastolic murmur of pulmonic regurgitation

Question 13. Match each description (A–D) with the corresponding procedure (1–4):
A. Common PA is tied, SVC is connected to right PA, IVC continues to flow into the systemic ventricle
B. Common PA is tied, SVC is connected to the right PA, IVC is connected to the right PA through a tunnel
C. Disconnect PA from RV, connect aorta to RV using the PA base as a conduit, feed PA through a Blalock–Taussig shunt
D. Subclavian artery-to-PA shunt

1. Glenn bidirectional shunt
2. Blalock–Taussig shunt
3. Fontan procedure
4. Norwood procedure

Question 14. Select true or false for each statement
A. In the newborn, before performing a Blalock–Taussig shunt, use prostacyclin to keep the PDA open and allow an increase in pulmonary flow (tricuspid atresia) or systemic flow (hypoplastic left heart syndrome)
B. The three surgical steps in tricuspid atresia are: (1) subclavian artery-to-PA shunting if low PA flow, or PA banding if high PA flow through the VSD, (2) Glenn bidirectional shunt, (3) Fontan
C. In d-TGA, or congenitally corrected TGA, RV and aorta are on the left

Answer 1. A. Eisenmenger syndrome is typically silent on exam, and is associated with lung oligemia rather than plethora on CXR. Cyanosis, exam, and ECG are consistent with Ebstein; however, in Ebstein, CXR usually shows lung oligemia. Thus, the most likely diagnosis is ASD with a degree of shunt reversal and cyanosis, particularly with exercise.

Answer 2. B. There is significant O_2 step-up on the right side (SVC to PA), implying a significant left-to-right shunt, and O_2 step-down on the left side (pulmonary vein to aorta), implying a significant right-to-left shunt.

$$Qp/Qs \quad = \text{systemic saturations/pulmonary saturations}$$
$$= (\text{arterial } O_2 - \text{SVC } O_2)/(\text{pulmonary venous } O_2 - \text{PA } O_2) = 1.1 \text{ (see Chapter 36)}$$

The shunt is bidirectional and almost balanced. However, the large O_2 step-up on the right side implies that a large residual left-to-right shunt is present, which may benefit from closure. In order to proceed with closure: (i) a residual left-to-right shunt must be present, (ii) PVR must be < 2/3 SVR and < 6 Wood units or must be reversible with pulmonary vasodilators. In a suitable patient, pulmonary vasodilators reduce PVR and increase the left-to-right shunting, leading to a post-vasodilator Qp/Qs > 1.5 (usually).

Answer 3. C. The patient has RV failure on exam and RV enlargement on echo. This implies that ASD is causing hemodynamic compromise. A hemodynamically significant ASD qualifies for closure regardless of the calculated Qp/Qs, as long as no evidence of R–L shunt or severe pulmonary hypertension is present. Qp/Qs is likely miscalculated echocardiographically. In addition, the patient may have anomalous pulmonary venous return contributing to his shunt; this warrants TEE before closure (an anomalous pulmonary vein mandates surgical closure).

Answer 4. E.

Answer 5. A. The patient has cyanosis and no significant murmur on exam. She likely has Eisenmenger syndrome. Lung oligemia is consistent with this diagnosis. While VSD more commonly leads to Eisenmenger syndrome than ASD, VSD's Eisenmenger typically occurs early, in childhood. At the stage of Eisenmenger syndrome, VSD becomes silent on exam; however, the patient typically has a prior history of loud murmur – which is not the case here. Ebstein anomaly leads to similar findings, except for an additional TR murmur.

Answer 6. B. Patients with Ebstein anomaly may present at a late age, depending on the severity of TR, degree of atrialization of the RV, and the presence of ASD shunting.

Answer 7. D. The Rastelli procedure is used in d-TGA with VSD and subpulmonic stenosis.

Answer 8. C. VSD is hemodynamically significant and has led to LV enlargement and left HF. VSD typically leads to left HF rather than right HF; RV does not enlarge in VSD (unlike ASD). The patient does not seem to have Eisenmenger clinically, as he is not hypoxic and a murmur is still heard, implying large left-to-right shunting. Yet, in this older patient with longstanding VSD, catheterization is warranted to rule out severe and irreversible pulmonary hypertension.

Answer 9. B. All three diagnoses are possible causes of exercise limitation and elevated velocity across the RVOT, but PR is the most common long-term sequela following the surgical correction of the tetralogy of Fallot. RVOT obstruction leads to higher velocities and less RV dilatation than PR. Severe PR is common and may be tolerated for years; pulmonic valve replacement is recommended in case of exertional limitation, RV enlargement, or RV dysfunction, to prevent irreversible RV failure and VT.

Answer 10. B. The syndrome associations described in A, C, and D are accurate but do not correlate with the patient's exam. In most of those anomalies, facial features are present, such as increased distance between eye corners, elfin facies (Williams syndrome), and facial hypoplasia.

Answer 11. A. Recurrent or persistent coarctation occurs in 10–20% of patients. Options B–D are also possible complications.

Answer 12. B. A PDA that leads to severe pulmonary hypertension is a large PDA that manifests in infancy or childhood, usually along with shunt reversal (right-to-left shunt) and hypoxemia. Thus, PDA is unlikely to be the cause of dyspnea and pulmonary hypertension at this age. Also, the continuous murmur of PDA predominates at the left upper sternal area. Conversely, sinus of Valsalva aneurysm often remains asymptomatic for years, until it ruptures in the RV (right coronary cusp aneurysm) or RA (non-coronary cusp aneurysm), at an age between 15 and 45. The pulmonary hypertension is secondary to the increased right-sided flow. Option D is associated with a combined systolic and diastolic murmur with two peaks, rather than a continuous murmur. TEE, cardiac CT, or cardiac MRI usually allows the diagnosis of PDA or another shunt not seen on TTE.

Answer 13. A–1, B–3, C–4, D–2.

Answer 14. A true; B true; C false (l-TGA is the congenitally corrected TGA).

References

1. Kutty S, Sengupta PP, Khandheria BK. Patent foramen ovale: the known and the to be known. J Am Coll Cardiol 2012; 59: 1665–71.
2. Rana BS, Shapiro LM, McCarthy KP, et al. Three-dimensional imaging of the atrial septum and patent foramen ovale anatomy: defining the morphological phenotypes of patent foramen ovale. Eur J Echocardiogr 2010; 11: i19–25.
3. Konstantinides S, Geibel A, Olschewski M, et al. A comparison of surgical and medical therapy for atrial septal defect in adults. N Engl J Med 1995; 333: 469–73.
4. Murphy JG, Gersh BJ, McGoon MD, et al. Long-term outcome after surgical repair of isolated atrial septal defect: follow-up at 27 to 32 years. N Engl J Med 1990; 323: 1645–50.
5. Homma S, Sacco RL, Di Tullio MR, et al. Effect of medical treatment in stroke patients with patent foramen ovale. Patent foramen ovale in Cryptogenic Stroke Study. Circulation 2002; 105: 2625–31.
6. Overell JR, Bone I, Lees KR. Interatrial septal abnormalities and stroke: a meta-analysis of case–control studies. Neurology 2000; 55: 1172–9.
7. Mas JL, Arquizan C, Lamy C, et al. Recurrent cerebrovascular events associated with patent foramen ovale, atrial septal aneurysm, or both. N Engl J Med 2001;345: 1740–6.
8. Meier B, Kalesan B, Mattle HP, et al. Percutaneous closure of patent foramen ovale in cryptogenic embolism. N Engl J Med 2013; 368: 1083–91.
9. Carroll JD, Saver JL, Thaler DE, et al. Closure of patent foramen ovale versus medical therapy after cryptogenic stroke. N Engl J Med 2013; 368: 1092–100.
10. Furlan AJ, Reisman M, Massaro J,et al. Closure or medical therapy for cryptogenic stroke with patent foramen ovale. N Engl J Med 2012; 366: 991–9.
11. Wu CC, Chen WJ, Chen MF, et al. Left-to-right shunt through patent foramen ovale in adult patients with left-sided cardiac lesions: a transesophageal echocardiographic study. Am Heart J 1993; 125: 1369–74.
12. Sommer RJ, Hijazi ZM, Rhodes JF. Pathophysiology of Congenital Heart Disease in the Adult. Part I: Shunt Lesions. Circulation 2008; 117: 1090–9.
13. Soto B, Becker AE, Moulaert AJ, Lie JT, Anderson RH. Classification of ventricular septal defects. Br Heart J 1980; 43: 332–43.
14. Hanna EB, Glancy DL. Long cases: self-assessment problems. In: Hanna EB, Glancy DL. Practical Cardiovascular Hemodynamics. New York, NY: Demos Medical, 2012, pp. 291–300.
15. Gabriel HM, Heger M, Innerhofer, et al. Long-term outcomes of patients with ventricular septal defect considered not to require surgical closure during childhood. J Am Coll Cardiol 2002; 39: 1066–71.
16. Shyu KG, Lai LP, Lin SC, et al. Diagnostic accuracy of transesophageal echocardiography for detecting patent ductus arteriosus in adolescents and adults. Chest 1995; 108: 1201–5.
17. Cohen M, Fuster V, Steele PM, et al. Coarctation of the aorta. Long-term follow-up and prediction of outcome after surgical correction. Circulation 1989; 80: 840–5.
18. Forbes T, Turner DR. Complications encountered in intravascular stent placement for native and recurrent coarctation of the aorta. In: Hijazi ZM, Feldman T, Cheatham JP, et al. Complications During Percutaneous Interventions for Congenital and Structural Heart Disease. London: Informa Healthcare, 2009: pp. 125–30.
19. Glancy DL, Morrow AG, Simon AL, Roberts WC. Juxtaductal aortic coarctation. Am J Cardiol 1983; 51: 537–51.

20. Hanna EB. Evaluation of right-to-left and left-to-right shunts and calculation of shunt ratio. In: Hanna EB, Glancy DL. Practical Cardiovascular Hemodynamics. New York, NY: Demos Medical, 2012, pp. 53–8.

21. Kenny D, Cao Q, Hijazi ZM. Fenestration of a Gore Helex septal occlude device in a patient with diastolic dysfunction of the left ventricle. Catheter Cardiovasc Interv 2011; 78: 594–8.

22. Nollert G, Fischlein T, Bouterwek S, et al. Long-term results of total repair of tetralogy of Fallot in adulthood: 35 years of follow-up in 104 patients corrected at the age of 18 or older. Thorac Cardiovasc Surg 1997; 45: 178–81.

23. Fontan operation homepage. http://www.fontanoperation.com/fontan.htm (accessed June 30, 2016).

24. Gersony WM. Fontan operation after 3 decades: what we have learned. Circulation 2008; 117: 13–15.

Part 8 PERIPHERAL ARTERIAL DISEASE

19   Peripheral Arterial Disease

1. LOWER EXTREMITY PERIPHERAL ARTERIAL DISEASE

Most patients with lower extremity PAD are asymptomatic. Approximately 30–50% have intermittent claudication or atypical leg symptoms.[1–3] Patients may be asymptomatic because PAD is either mild, or moderate-to-severe but collaterals are well developed. Patients may also be inactive because of comorbidities that prevent them from experiencing claudication.

    Claudication usually remains stable or improves with conservative management. At 5 years, only 20% of patients have progressive claudication, and only 4% progress to critical limb ischemia (CLI).[1,4,5] **This explains why, in the absence of critical limb ischemia, revascularization is only justified for very severe claudication.** On the other hand, diabetic patients, patients who continue to smoke, and patients with severely reduced ankle–brachial index (ABI) <0.5 have a particularly aggressive course, with CLI of 10–20% at 5 years.[5–7] In addition, progressive functional decline frequently occurs in these patients and may conceal disease progression.[7] Some studies suggest that patients <50 years of age may have a more aggressive course (~40% have unstable, progressive disease with multiple revascularizations and frequent progression to CLI).[8,9]

Practical Cardiovascular Medicine, First Edition. Elias B. Hanna.

© 2017 John Wiley & Sons Ltd. Published 2017 by John Wiley & Sons Ltd.

As opposed to the relatively benign course from a limb ischemia perspective, patients with PAD have a high rate of cardiovascular events and mortality, that is at least equal to patients with CAD (5–7% yearly risk of cardiovascular death/MI/stroke with 3–5% yearly mortality risk).[10,11] The mortality drastically increases in subgroups of moderate PAD (ABI <0.7), and, even more so, severe PAD (ABI <0.5).[12] Patients with CLI have a 25% mortality risk at 1 year.

In comparison to isolated CAD, the mortality and event rate is doubled in patients with combined CAD and PAD. Aggressive risk-factor modification and CAD therapy is expected to improve cardiovascular events in PAD. **Except for CLI, peripheral revascularization does not clearly reduce mortality or the long-term risk of limb loss.**

> Two-thirds of patients with PAD have obstructive CAD of at least one vessel, with a high prevalence of three-vessel CAD. One-fourth of patients have significant carotid disease.[13,14] This partly explains the high risk of cardiovascular events in these patients. Even in the absence of obstructive CAD, PAD patients usually have diffuse, sometimes heavy and calcified coronary atherosclerosis and are at a risk of MI, albeit a lower risk than patients with obstructive CAD.[10]

I. Clinical tips

Typical claudication is described as lower extremity discomfort, fatigue, or weakness initiated with exertion and resolving within 10 minutes of rest. Claudication is consistently reproduced by almost the same walking distance and is worse uphill. It does not occur with prolonged standing per se; it does not occur at rest or at night unless there is also a severe exertional component and signs of CLI on exam. Isolated nocturnal leg cramps without exertional limitation are neuromuscular in origin.

Leg pain is considered **atypical** when it occurs on exertion but also at rest without signs of rest ischemia. Other atypical symptoms include leg pain that starts with exertion but does not make the patient stop or does not quickly resolve upon cessation of activity. In patients with PAD, those atypical symptoms frequently represent mixed arterial and non-arterial, comorbid pain (PAD combined with neuropathy, spinal stenosis, or arthritis). PAD may not be the primary driver of symptoms (Table 19.1).

Claudication involves the buttocks, hips, and thighs in aortoiliac disease, simulating hip or spinal disease; the thighs in common femoral disease; and the calves in superficial femoral or popliteal disease. Patients with aortoiliac disease sometimes report weakness with walking rather than pain. While isolated internal iliac disease does not usually cause claudication, bilateral internal iliac disease may lead to buttock/hip claudication and erectile dysfunction with a normal ABI; the internal iliac arteries provide gluteal branches that may suffer in case of bilateral disease, depending on the degree of collateralization from the external iliac and common femoral circumflex branches.

Rarely, patients with isolated severe infrapopliteal disease develop foot claudication, which often simulates plantar fasciitis or vasculitic pain (thromboangiitis obliterans). More commonly, these patients present with ischemic, painful distal ulceration.

Isolated superficial femoral artery (SFA) disease with intact common femoral, profunda, and popliteal arteries is less symptomatic than disease in other segments. The profunda femoris, which is rarely diseased, usually provides robust collaterals to the popliteal artery, bypassing the diseased SFA. A diseased profunda particularly increases the risk of progression to CLI.

On physical exam, a normal posterior tibial (PT) pulse or dorsalis pedis (DP) pulse rules out significant PAD with 96% and 92% accuracy, respectively. A normal femoral pulse without bruit rules out aortoiliac PAD with over 90% accuracy. Thus, physical exam is highly accurate in ruling out significantly obstructive PAD. Conversely, only 50% of patients with abnormal femoral pulse or distal pulses have significant

Table 19.1 Differential diagnosis: arterial claudication, neurologic claudication (spinal stenosis), diabetic neuropathy, venous insufficiency.

	Arterial claudication	Neurologic claudication	Diabetic neuropathy	Venous insufficiency
Pain type	Cramp, tightness, or tiredness; anywhere from buttocks to feet "Difficulty walking" Weakness	Paresthesia, sharp or shooting pain bilaterally History of back pain	Paresthesia, burning or shooting pain Starts distally bilaterally and progresses proximally	Heaviness
Walking distance	Constant Worse uphill Pain not triggered by standing still	Variable Improves with walking uphill Pain may be triggered by standing still	Pain unrelated to exertion Occurs at night, at rest	Variable Pain worse at the end of the day rather than after a particular walk
Disturbance with standing	No	Yes	Not necessarily	Yes
Relief	Walking cessation	Sitting, leaning forward	Spontaneous	Leg elevation
Exam findings	Abnormal pulses, femoral bruits In advanced cases: • Pallor that worsens with leg elevation and slowly becomes blue with feet dangling (rubor cyanosis) • Cold feet, capillary refill >3 seconds • Loss of distal hair, nail dystrophy, skin atrophy • Disuse muscle atrophy	Abnormal sense and deep tendon reflexes	Hyperkeratosis of the skin and nails Abnormal sense and deep tendon reflexes	History of DVT Brown stasis dermatitis, varicose veins

PAD; the combination of multiple pulse abnormalities more accurately predicts PAD.[3,15] Femoral pulse may be reduced because of body habitus or a deep femoral course. Owing to anatomical variation, DP is absent unilaterally or bilaterally in up to 10% of the population (the anterior tibial artery may quickly taper at the ankle level, giving only a lateral tarsal artery; also, a peroneal perforating branch may be supplying the dorsum of the foot). DP palpation is improved by dorsiflexion of the foot, which prevents DP compression by tendons. PT is absent in 2% of the normal population.

II. Clinical classification of PAD: critical limb ischemia, acute limb ischemia, atheroembolization

Grossly, there are three clinical forms of PAD: asymptomatic PAD, claudication, and CLI.

A. Rutherford classification

The Rutherford classification is commonly used and incorporates all these clinical forms of PAD into six categories: 0=asymptomatic; 1–3=claudication; 4–6=critical limb ischemia, with 4=rest pain; 5=minor tissue loss/skin loss at the digits; 6=major tissue loss with gangrene.

B. Critical limb ischemia (CLI)

CLI is defined as one of the following (in order of increasing severity): ischemic rest pain, non-healing ulcer, or extensive ulceration with gangrene. *CLI is a chronic process that progresses over weeks or months and should be distinguished from acute limb ischemia* (Table 19.2). CLI most commonly occurs in patients with ABI≤0.4, ankle pressure <50 mmHg, or toe pressure <30 mmHg. The latter three features correlate with poor flow that can spontaneously initiate an ulcer and prevent it from healing. However, an ulcer that is initiated by a non-ischemic process (e.g., insect bite, injury, venous or neuropathic ulcer) may not heal in the presence of even moderate PAD, such as ABI 0.7. Revascularization is required to allow the ulcer to heal.

Ischemic rest pain is typically a nocturnal pain that forces the patient to wake up and dangle his legs. On physical exam, CLI is characterized by a cool, dry, and fissured skin, lack of hair, dystrophic thick toenails, lack of superficial veins (flat skin), calf atrophy, and dependent rubor cyanosis. Ulcers often occur distally at the toe level and at pressure and friction points (between toes), or at the lateral malleolus level (Table 19.3). As noted above, an ulcer occurring at another location for another reason may not heal if ischemia is present (mixed ulcer). Dependent rubor is an important marker of rest ischemia. To test for dependent rubor, raise the leg for 30–60 seconds, observe for pallor, then let it down and see how it slowly fills with a dusky red color suggestive of CLI, rather than quickly fills with a normal pink color.

In CLI, PAD is typically extensive with either one of the following:

i. Multilevel involvement (e.g., iliac and SFA, SFA and popliteal, SFA and profunda, SFA and infrapopliteal). Isolated SFA disease does not generally cause CLI, as robust collaterals develop through the profunda and "bypass" the SFA disease into the popliteal artery; additional disease should be sought in a patient with CLI and SFA disease. Conversely, isolated common femoral or popliteal disease may affect flow similarly to a combination of SFA and profunda disease and may cause CLI.

ii. Isolated three-vessel infrapopliteal involvement. In general, patients with isolated infrapopliteal disease do not develop CLI or significant claudication *unless both the anterior and posterior tibial arteries are involved or the common infrapopliteal inflow, i.e., distal popliteal artery, is severely diseased*. A single non-obstructed tibial vessel generally provides enough flow to prevent ulceration or claudication and to allow ulcer healing.

Table 19.2 Acute limb ischemia vs. critical limb ischemia.

Acute limb ischemia	Critical limb ischemia
Persistent rest pain	**Intermittent** rest pain (nocturnal) or non-healing ulcer
More severe pallor (marble); darker, more mottled cyanosis	
Sudden onset, progresses over hours or days	Progresses over weeks/months
Distal pulses inaudible on Doppler exam	**Distal pulses audible on Doppler exam**
Caused by acute embolization or acute thrombosis, with multiple distal emboli	Severe progressive atherosclerosis±some thrombus
Emergent revascularization required	Non-urgent revascularization is required

Table 19.3 Types of lower extremity ulcers.

Ischemic ulcers	Neuropathic ulcers	Venous ulcers
Painful	Painless	Achy discomfort
Location: lateral malleolus, tip of toes, friction areas (between toes)	Plantar foot, metatarsal heads	Medial malleolus
Shape: black, white/pale, or blue, does not bleed	Red with increased blood flow	Shallow ulcer with red granulating exudative base
Ischemic signs (pallor, cold, cyanosis, capillary refill >3 seconds)	Presence of calluses, bone deformities	Stasis dermatitis: reddish-brown edematous skin
Absent pulses	Neuropathic signs on examination	
ABI≤0.5		

Some ulcers have mixed neuropathic and ischemic features. Any ulcer or gangrene, whether neuropathic or ischemic, can become infected (wet gangrene). Also, consider the possibility of osteomyelitis with any ulcer.

In patients with CLI, it is important to provide *one straight line of normal, unobstructed flow all the way to the plantar arch*; this is achieved by revascularizing all involved levels, checking pressure gradients across moderate iliac disease, and revascularizing at least one infrapopliteal vessel in patients with three-vessel infrapopliteal disease. This is generally performed in one session. The treated infrapopliteal vessel is preferably the one that supplies the ulcerated area (each artery supplies a vascular territory called angiosome). However, as a first step, one may opt to revascularize the vessel that is easiest to percutaneously treat. Most often, this allows the ulcer to heal. If the ulcer does not heal, the patient is brought back for revascularization of the appropriate angiosome, according to the *angiosome concept*. In general, after appropriate revascularization, *ulcers heal slowly, by ~1 cm² per month*; hence therapy should be provided early, before extensive ulceration occurs. A superficial dry gangrene requires debridement and local care but often heals well after revascularization (amputation is not usually required).

This concept of aggressively achieving "one line of normal flow" only applies to CLI. *A more perfect flow is needed to heal ulcers than to prevent them from occurring.* In the absence of CLI, severe PAD may be observed and treated conservatively, as CLI infrequently develops; yet once a small ulcer occurs, revascularization becomes urgent.

In patients with severe claudication, revascularization of the inflow disease (e.g., iliac, SFA) provides enough symptom relief; infrapopliteal disease is not usually treated.

CLI is associated with a 25% mortality risk at 1 year and a 25% amputation rate, with only 50% amputation-free survival at 1 year. Amputation is required in patients who cannot be revascularized or who present at a stage of deep necrosis. Amputation is associated with the highest mortality (40% at 2 years).

C. Acute limb ischemia (ALI) and acute compartment syndrome

Acute limb ischemia is rest ischemia that develops over hours, sometimes days (occasionally weeks, generally <14 days), and is usually due to: (i) acute embolization from a cardiac or aortic origin (30% of cases), (ii) acute thrombosis of an underlying atherosclerotic stenosis or popliteal aneurysm (60% of cases), (iii) thrombosis in situ from a hypercoagulable state or traumatic injury/dissection, or (iv) graft thrombosis, which mainly occurs when there is obstructive disease at the inflow or outflow of the graft (e.g., disease progression in the common femoral or profunda past an aortofemoral graft; early or late anastomotic stenosis). *Regardless of the underlying process, multiple distal emboli are characteristic of ALI.* Acute thrombosis generally manifests less severely and less abruptly than acute embolization (days or weeks), as it occurs on top of chronic disease and pre-existing collaterals.

As opposed to ALI, CLI and non-healing ulcers are due to severe progressive atherosclerosis, frequently with some amount of thrombus, and develop over weeks or months (Table 19.2). CLI generally requires revascularization soon (days or 1 week), but not emergently. In ALI, the abrupt occlusion does not allow for the development of robust collaterals, which explains how ALI can lead to limb loss within a few hours (6 hours), dictating emergent reperfusion. In addition, distal embolization is universal in ALI and further accelerates tissue loss. *Distal pulses are usually audible on Doppler exam in CLI, but often not in ALI.*

CLI progresses at a much slower rate than ALI yet provokes tissue loss and ischemic ulcers at a relatively earlier stage. ALI has the following progression:

Stage 1. Rest pain with audible, monophasic distal pulses by Doppler.
Stage 2. Very distal sensory loss with inaudible distal pulses by Doppler ("limb threatened"). The skin is initially "marble" white, then becomes dark purple and mottled as it fills with deoxygenated, stagnant blood.
Stage 3. Sensory loss beyond toe level or moderate motor loss ("limb immediately threatened").
Stage 4. Profound paralysis and/or major tissue loss (irreversible necrosis of muscles and skin).
Stage 1 dictates urgent revascularization, while stages 2 and 3 dictate emergent revascularization. Stage 4 requires early amputation, followed by revascularization to allow healing of the wound and the remaining viable tissue, limiting the need for a more extensive amputation in the future.

In ALI, stages 1 and 2 may be treated with a local thrombolytic infusion (12–48 hours) delivered through an endovascular approach. After the extensive thrombus burden and emboli are attenuated with thrombolysis, attention is turned towards the endovascular or surgical therapy of underlying/residual stenoses. For stage 3 ALI (motor loss or extensive sensory loss), ischemia needs to be emergently improved and one cannot wait 12–24 hours for thrombolysis to be effective. Surgical revascularization, if feasible, may need to be emergently performed at stage 3; moreover, at this stage, patients have a high risk of reperfusion injury and compartment syndrome and often need prophylactic fasciotomy during surgical revascularization.

Carefully monitor for reperfusion injury whenever ALI is reperfused and whenever any severe limb ischemia, whether ALI or CLI, is reperfused at or beyond the stage of motor loss (stages 3 or 4). This entails monitoring for systemic reperfusion syndrome (renal function, potassium) *and* local reperfusion syndrome. The latter manifests as calf swelling and induration, followed by impaired neurological and muscular functions. Early on, the patient has calf pain with passive stretching of the involved compartment; later on, paresthesias occur as a result of nerve injury, and finally, muscle weakness occurs (late sign that often implies permanent muscle damage). Anterior compartment syndrome being most common, the patient initially manifests tenderness on plantar flexion, followed by impaired dorsiflexion. The distal foot perfusion, capillary refill, and pulses are initially preserved despite the severe calf pain and muscular necrosis (this distinguishes compartment syndrome from ALI).

D. Atheroembolization

Atheroembolization is embolization of atheromatous cholesterol debris rather than thrombi, and is therefore different from ALI. It typically occurs after angiography or aortic surgery that sloughs off aortic atherosclerotic debris and leads to cholesterol embolization in the small vessels of the kidneys, dermis, lower extremities, and gastrointestinal tract. Yet, ~50% of the cases are spontaneous. Atheroembolism often induces progressive renal failure that develops a week or more after the procedure and is frequently irreversible. It leads to livedo reticularis, "blue toes," and distal cyanosis or gangrene despite preserved distal pulses, as the ischemia is due to small vessel occlusion. Obstructive PAD may, however, be present and may reduce distal pulses, yet *the ischemic findings are generally disproportionate to PAD and ABI*. No specific therapy is provided; limb ischemia often improves spontaneously in patients without a severely obstructive underlying PAD. Revascularization may be required in patients with severe PAD to allow healing, but invasive manipulations are better avoided in patients with only mild PAD, as these manipulations may induce further embolization. The role of anticoagulation is unclear (some data suggest benefit while other data suggest harm).

III. Diagnosis of PAD

A. Ankle–brachial index (ABI)

ABI has two purposes: (i) diagnosis of obstructive PAD and its severity; (ii) cardiovascular prognosis (the risk of death/MI of patients with a low ABI approximates or exceeds the risk of patients with CAD) (Table 19.4). If PAD is suspected in a symptomatic patient with an abnormal pulse exam, ABI is first performed, followed by a lower extremity arterial Doppler study if revascularization is considered.

Asymptomatic patients at a high risk of PAD need to be screened with ABI only, particularly if the pulse exam is abnormal (age >65, age 50–70 with diabetes or smoking). A low ABI correlates with increased mortality and dictates more aggressive medical therapy, but not further workup and revascularization, per se.

To calculate ABI, posterior tibial (PT) and anterior tibial (AT) pressures are measured using a well-sized BP cuff and a Doppler stethoscope, then the highest of these pressures is divided by the highest arm pressure.[1] ABI testing is ~85% sensitive and 100% specific for angiographically confirmed PAD.[1] ABI has the following three pitfalls: (i) ABI may be falsely elevated in calcified, poorly compressible vessels; these vessels are not compressible even if the pressure and flow inside them are low (elderly, longstanding diabetes, or CKD); (ii) ABI may be normal at rest if sufficient collaterals are present; (iii) ABI may also be normal at rest in symptomatic patients with moderate aortoiliac stenoses.

Thus, when ABI is normal at rest but pitfall (ii) or (iii) is suspected, exercise ABI or an arterial Doppler study should be obtained. During exercise, peripheral vasodilatation occurs; a flow-limiting stenosis prevents blood flow from increasing enough to fill the dilated distal vascular space, and thus the distal pressure paradoxically decreases. This process translates into a low exertional ABI (ABI drops ≥ 20%, or >0.2) and explains how DP and PT pulses that are weak but palpable before exercise may become non-palpable after exercise. In fact, post-exertional pulse exam is valuable in the assessment of the PAD patient with only mild pulse abnormality.

Note: elevated ABI

When arterial non-compressibility is suspected in patients with a normal ABI or elevated ABI ≥ 1.4 (pitfall [i]), arterial Doppler should be done or, alternatively, toe pressure and toe–brachial index (TBI) should be measured using a special small plethysmograph. Medial calcinosis does not typically involve digital arteries, and thus digital arteries remain compressible when pedal arteries are not. TBI <0.6 indicates significant PAD. Also, patients with significant PAD have pulseless pedal pulses despite the high measured pedal pressure (*high pressure yet pulseless*). In patients evaluated for leg symptoms, an elevated ABI is associated with significant PAD in 60–70% and CLI in up to 37% of patients; this prevalence may be lower in asymptomatic patients.[16,17] An elevated ABI has the same negative prognostic implication as a low ABI, more so in the presence of obstructive PAD.[16] Even without obstructive PAD, an elevated ABI implies a heavy amount of calcified atherosclerosis and predicts increased cardiovascular mortality.

Note: use of the higher ankle pressure (the higher of the AT and PT pressures) vs. the lower pressure in ABI calculation

The higher pressure correlates with the pressure through the arterial inflow into the best infrapopliteal vessel, and may best correlate with symptoms. A low ABI through only one of AT or PT, with a normal ABI through the other vessel, indicates single-vessel infrapopliteal disease with no significant inflow or femoral disease; this is unlikely to cause symptoms, since only one-vessel runoff to the foot is usually enough to prevent severe symptoms or CLI. However, one study has shown that the use of the lower ABI better correlates with the risk of cardiovascular events, and therefore both numbers should be reported and accounted for.[18]

B. Doppler study

A Doppler study is over 95% sensitive and specific for the diagnosis of obstructive stenoses. It is only indicated in patients with severe symptoms who qualify for angiography and revascularization (class I indication). It allows localization of the disease and planning for a potential peripheral intervention. A stenosis is characterized by a focal increase in velocity (>250 cm/s, or >2.5:1 in comparison to the proximal segment), and by a monophasic flow distal to the stenosis (Figure 19.1).

C. CT angiography (CTA)

CTA is particularly helpful when aortoiliac disease is suspected with absent femoral pulses, in which case CTA delineates the disease and allows the planning of a peripheral intervention. CTA has several pitfalls: (i) it may not properly delineate infrapopliteal disease; (ii) heavy calcifications may preclude accurate assessment of the severity of disease; (iii) additional radiation and contrast is used before the eventual angiography or intervention. While a Doppler study has a class I indication before performing angiography, CTA has a class IIb indication.

D. Peripheral angiography is only performed when revascularization is indicated.

Table 19.4 Classification of PAD severity based on ABI.

1–1.3: normal	0.7–0.9: mild PAD	>1.3: non-compressible pedal vessels[a]
0.9–0.99: borderline	0.4–0.7: moderate PAD	
	<0.4: severe PAD	

[a] A high ABI is often associated with significant PAD, particularly in patients with claudication. A high ABI is associated with the same increase in cardiovascular mortality as a low ABI.

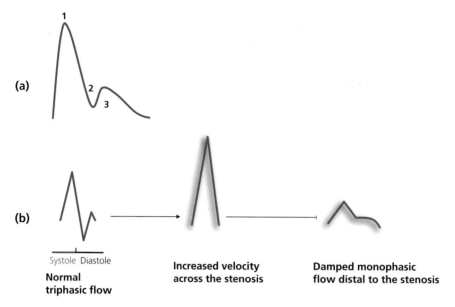

Figure 19.1 (a) The peripheral arterial pressure has three phases (1, 2, 3). The second phase corresponds to a brief reversal of flow in early diastole before the artery recoils and maintains its pressure. Phases 2 and 3 correspond to an exaggerated and "spread-out" dicrotic notch. **(b)** The triphasic pressure waveform translates into a triphasic Doppler velocity waveform (sometimes biphasic, with a systolic spike and a diastolic reversal). *Distal to an arterial stenosis, the peripheral pressure loses its dicrotic notch and the Doppler loses the early diastolic flow reversal and becomes monophasic.* In this case, the arterial volume is reduced past the stenosis and does not allow a backflow in diastole, but rather requires a persistent forward flow throughout diastole. Beside stenosis, this lack of flow reversal may be seen in peripheral vasodilatation.

Across a stenosis, the velocity increases and the flow becomes monophasic, turbulent, with spectral thickening of the waveform (turbulent flow). Beyond the stenosis, the flow is damped and monophasic, with a persistent flow in diastole. Flow may also be monophasic just proximal to the stenosis (e.g., monophasic common femoral velocity when the proximal SFA is occluded).

IV. Medical therapy of PAD

Medical therapy consists of:

a. Smoking cessation, which reduces the amputation risk 10-fold and the mortality risk by 50%.[19] Over 85% of patients who quit smoking have an improvement in symptoms. Bypass graft failure is twice as high in smokers as in non-smokers.
b. Walking program (30 minutes a day for at least 3 days a week), which improves the walking distance twofold to fourfold within 3 months. Early benefits are seen at 4 weeks.
c. Aspirin or clopidogrel. In the absence of percutaneous revascularization or prior MI, the combination is not clearly superior to aspirin or clopidogrel monotherapy for the prevention of cardiovascular events.[20]
d. Secondary prevention measures that reduce cardiovascular and coronary events: statin and aggressive therapy of hypertension and diabetes.
e. Cilostazol is a phosphodiesterase inhibitor that increases cAMP levels and induces vasodilatation. It effectively improves walking distance by ~50% and is useful in reducing in-stent restenosis and thrombosis (antiplatelet and antiproliferative effects). It has milrinone-like cardiac effects and is thus contraindicated in HF or recent MI (<6 months).

V. Revascularization for PAD

A. Indications

Revascularization is indicated for:

- CLI (absolute indication).
- Lifestyle-limiting claudication despite a 3-month exercise program, e.g., claudication upon walking <1 block or performing activities of daily living (relative indication).

PAD has a benign course from a limb's perspective, and, outside CLI, revascularization does not clearly alter the natural history of limb ischemia. Therefore, severe PAD with ABI≤0.4 but without symptoms or ulcers is not an indication for revascularization per se. These asymptomatic patients may be debilitated and often have comorbidities that prevent them from walking and experiencing claudication; they do not have an immediate limb threat. They have, however, an increased risk of limb loss with any minor skin injury and need to be routinely examined for the early occurrence of ulcers, which would dictate revascularization. *While tissue integrity may be preserved for several years in a patient with severe PAD, once tissue loss occurs, complete revascularization and a straight line of flow are required to allow the ulcer to heal, as soon as possible.*

B. Revascularization modalities: surgical bypass vs. percutaneous therapy

Lower extremity arteries are divided into three segments: aortoiliac, femoropopliteal, and infrapopliteal. The more distal the disease is, the lower the long-term patency is for any revascularization modality (Figure 19.2).

Surgical patency is *slightly* superior to that achieved with percutaneous revascularization at all levels, particularly for TASC C and D lesions at the femoropopliteal level (e.g., long SFA occlusion). A synthetic graft anastomosed to the popliteal artery below the knee or to a tibial artery is the only exception, as it has a very poor long-term patency, but its short-term patency may still serve to resolve CLI in a patient with no possibility for percutaneous intervention. A poor or small distal runoff reduces the long-term success of both strategies, particularly bypass surgery.

While having a superior long-term patency, historical comparisons show that surgery is associated with a much higher postoperative mortality than percutaneous revascularization (3–5% vs. 0.5%). In addition, surgery has a much higher risk of major periprocedural complications that include cardiovascular, renal, pulmonary, and bleeding complications (8–10% vs. 1–3%).[21–23] One randomized comparison of bypass surgery vs. percutaneous revascularization in patients with CLI and infra-inguinal disease has shown that percutaneous revascularization is associated with lower post-procedural complications, morbidity, and costs (BASIL trial). Yet, patients who survived over 2 years had a lower amputation rate with surgery, which suggests that CLI patients who are less sick with fewer comorbidities may benefit from surgery early on. Interestingly, most CLI patients who were screened for this study were either not eligible for surgery because of comorbidities or not eligible for percutaneous therapy because of technical complexity, and ~50% were not eligible for any therapy (with a subsequent high amputation rate).[24]

In sum, percutaneous revascularization has the advantage of lower periprocedural mortality and complications, is the only option in patients with significant cardiovascular comorbidities or lack of venous conduits, and has a lower but acceptable long-term patency, particularly for TASC A, B, ± C lesions. It is recommended as a first-line therapy for TASC A and B lesions and is an acceptable first-line alternative for TASC C lesions, while TASC D lesions are generally treated surgically if the patient is an appropriate surgical candidate (Table 19.5).[1,25] A restenosis may be retreated with angioplasty if possible. After a second restenosis, surgery is considered. A failed angioplasty does not usually compromise future surgical therapy. Importantly, hybrid therapy is frequently used, especially in patients with CLI and multisegmental disease; for example, the iliac artery is stented while endarterectomy is performed for common femoral disease or femoropopliteal bypass is performed for SFA disease.

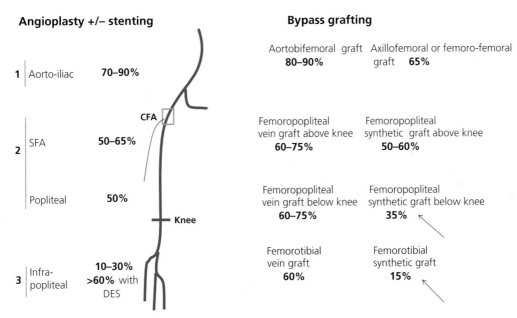

Figure 19.2 Three-year patency of percutaneous therapy and 5-year patency of bypass surgery. The long-term patency rate of percutaneous therapy for long, totally occlusive SFA disease >15 cm is ≤50%. Surgical patency rates obtained from the ACC guidelines document[1] and from Gray & Sullivan (1997).[19]

Table 19.5 Highlights of the TransAtlantic InterSociety Consensus (TASC) classification of angiographic extent and complexity.

Iliac disease

TASC C is a long total EIA occlusion, bilateral CIA occlusions, or extensive stenoses involving two segments, part of which may be occlusive (EIA and CIA, EIA and CFA, or both EIAs)

TASC D is a more *extensive total occlusion involving two major segments* (e.g., distal aorta and CIA, EIA and CIA, or bilateral EIAs); *or* non-occlusive but long disease involving all three segments: CIA, EIA and CFA

Femoropopliteal disease

TASC C is SFA and/or popliteal disease or occlusion >15 cm, with or without calcification, but not total occlusion of both SFA and popliteal artery

TASC D is total occlusion that *involves two major segments* (e.g., total occlusion of the SFA that also involves the common femoral artery or popliteal artery, or total occlusion of the popliteal artery that extends into the infrapopliteal trifurcation)

More limited disease or occlusion is TASC A or B (for example, short CIA occlusion or SFA occlusion <15 cm is TASC B). TASC A and B lesions are generally treated with percutaneous therapy (as initial therapy). TASC C lesions can receive percutaneous or surgical therapy. TASC D lesions are generally treated surgically.
CFA, common femoral artery; CIA, common iliac artery; EIA, external iliac artery; SFA, superficial femoral artery.

VI. Notes on the technical aspects of surgical and percutaneous therapies

A. Technical aspects of surgical therapy

1. Aortobifemoral grafting, femorofemoral and axillofemoral grafting

Aorotobifemoral bypass surgery consists of clamping the infrarenal aorta, suturing a synthetic graft to the aorta then the iliac arteries, followed by stapling of the distal aorta. This cuts the native flow through the aorta and diverts all of it through the graft into the common femoral arteries and retrogradely into the internal iliac arteries (Figure 19.3). This end-to-end anastomosis at the aortic level prevents competitive flow with the native iliac vessels and improves long-term patency. The native aorta is left patent in a few cases (end-to-side anastomosis at the aortic level), e.g., when the inferior mesenteric artery or a low accessory renal artery needs to be preserved or when no retrograde flow is expected into any internal iliac artery, as in patients with occluded external iliac arteries.

When the patient has severe complex disease on one side (e.g., right) and less complex disease on the other side (e.g., left), iliac stenting may be performed on the left and femorofemoral bypass graft used from the left femoral artery to the right femoral artery. Alternatively, an axillofemoral graft may be used for the right femoral artery. Those extra-anatomic bypass surgeries (femorofemoral, axillofemoral) are less complex than aortobifemoral surgeries and are particularly useful in high-surgical-risk patients; the long-term patency is, however, reduced.

When the common femoral artery (CFA) is not diseased, the distal anastomosis is performed at the common femoral level. However, when the disease extends into the CFA, the anastomosis is performed at the profunda level or, in a bifurcating fashion, to the profunda and SFA (if SFA is patent). SFA is a vessel subject to major motion stress and frequently occludes; thus, it is not a robust outflow for aortofemoral grafting, which should always involve the common femoral or the profunda (the graft provides robust flow to the profunda, which provides robust flow to the popliteal artery should SFA occlude).

2. Femoropopliteal or femorotibial bypass

A saphenous vein or a synthetic graft may be used. A venous graft is preferred, even more so for below-knee bypass. Even when the disease is distal, the proximal anastomosis is performed at the CFA level; endarterectomy of the CFA is performed if the CFA is diseased. Rarely, in patients with infrapopliteal disease yet intact femoropopliteal segments, a graft between the popliteal and a tibial artery may be performed.

B. Technical aspects of percutaneous revascularization

Femoral and infrapopliteal stenoses are usually treated through a *contralateral femoral access with a crossover sheath*. The same applies to external iliac disease. Conversely, isolated common iliac disease is usually treated through an ipsilateral femoral access. Even in the latter case, however, a contralateral access is required for imaging, mapping the ipsilateral access, and wire protection. Thus, *contralateral femoral access is commonly the starting point of peripheral interventions*.

1. Iliac level

An excellent long-term result is achieved with iliac stenting, stenting being superior to plain balloon angioplasty at this level, both for immediate and for long-term patency.[26–28] A less successful but still acceptable long-term patency is achieved in TASC C or D lesions.[27,28] Balloon-expandable stents are generally preferred for common iliac disease because of a superior radial strength and an accurate positioning. In case of bilateral ostial iliac or aortoiliac disease, kissing stents may be positioned across both common iliac arteries. Both balloon-expandable and self-expanding flexible nitinol stents may be used for the external iliac arteries.

2. SFA and popliteal level

The SFA is subject to tremendous stress (bending, torsion, flexion, extension), which explains its frequent atherosclerotic involvement. When diseased, it frequently becomes totally occluded (up to 75% of significant SFA disease is totally occlusive). This stress at the SFA level explains the poor long-term result with percutaneous therapy of long occlusions >15 cm (TASC C lesions), where the long-term patency may not exceed 50%. As opposed to plain balloon angioplasty, the use of self-expanding nitinol stents has improved the long-term SFA patency, particularly for lesions of medium complexity and length 6–15 cm (Figure 19.4).[29,30] These stents are flexible and crush-recoverable, yet still have ~5–15% risk of fracture; fracture increases the risk of restenosis and, more particularly, reocclusion (50% reocclusion risk when

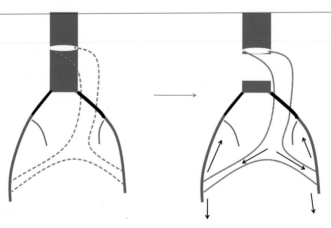

Figure 19.3 Aortobifemoral bypass grafting.

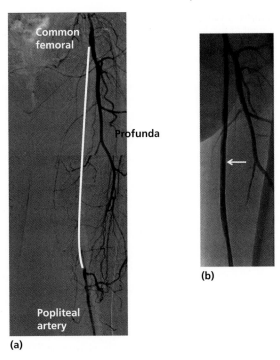

(a)

(b)

Figure 19.4 (a) SFA is totally occluded all the way from the ostium to the popliteal artery (the path of the occluded SFA is marked in *white*, TASC C lesion). It reconstitutes at the popliteal level through collaterals from the profunda, as is usually the case. **(b)** SFA after stenting (*arrow*).

a circumferential fracture occurs).[31] Fracture is particularly increased with the length of the stented area (>16 cm) and with distal stenting around the popliteal level. Beside fracture, long stenting over 15 cm is associated with a high risk of restenosis (50%) and is not clearly superior to a strategy of **balloon angioplasty or atherectomy followed by drug-coated angioplasty and a more limited, focal stenting of segments achieving a suboptimal angioplasty result.**

Self-expanding drug-eluting (paclitaxel) stents are available and have a moderately higher patency than bare self-expanding stents. *Drug-coated balloons* deliver paclitaxel to the arterial wall upon inflation; paclitaxel, an anti-proliferative drug, is maintained in the arterial wall for several months, leading to a higher 1-year patency than standard balloons.

SFA restenosis may be retreated percutaneously with balloon angioplasty or atherectomy, especially when restenosis is not occlusive. The long-term patency is, however, reduced to ~50%. This patency may be improved by two modalities: drug-coated balloons and laser atherectomy.

The popliteal artery may be stented if needed; in general, it is treated with atherectomy or balloon angioplasty as a first-line therapy. Stenting is initially avoided to elude the fracture risk and to preserve a landing zone for a future bypass. Note that the proximal popliteal artery, at the level of the adductor hiatus (about where it intersects with the femoral bone), is more subject to the stress of flexion and torsion than the mid-popliteal artery at the joint-space level. Stenting the popliteal artery exposes not only to a risk of stent fracture but also to a risk of excessive trauma at the edge of the stent (the stiff stent bends less than the adjacent artery). Yet, recent data suggests that stenting the popliteal artery is safe when necessary.[32]

3. Infrapopliteal level

As explained above, infrapopliteal disease does not lead to severe claudication or CLI unless the popliteal inflow or all three infrapopliteal vessels are involved. Moreover, the proximal portions of all those vessels need to be involved to have calf claudication (usually distal calf). Infrapopliteal revascularization of at least one vessel is indicated in patients with three-vessel involvement and:

- Ischemic ulcer (with or without multilevel disease, as part of establishment of a normal, straight line of flow to the foot)
  or
- Claudication with isolated proximal three-vessel infrapopliteal disease. In the case of concomitant iliac or SFA disease, only revascularization of the iliac or SFA is initially performed; infrapopliteal revascularization may be secondarily performed if claudication remains severe.

The infrapopliteal vessels are treated with balloon angioplasty or atherectomy. While long-term patency is low, restenosis occurs after tissue has healed, and thus limb salvage rates exceed 80–90% after successful recanalization. *A healed tissue requires less flow to maintain its integrity than an ulcerated tissue.* Thus, restenosis does not usually result in recurrent CLI.

In addition, excellent long-term results have been achieved with coronary DESs.[33,34] The three arteries run deep in the muscular compartments of the leg and are well protected from trauma and fracture (anterior compartment for AT, posterior compartment for PT and peroneal). However, there are several pitfalls of stenting: (i) coronary DESs are short and several stents are often required to cover the typical, long disease; (ii) the genu of the AT is subject to compression and torsion; (iii) distally, at the ankle joint and below, the arteries are unprotected and subject to torque and extravascular compressive forces that will crush the stent.

C. Special case of the common femoral artery (CFA)

The CFA is located at the hip joint, and a stent at this location is subject to fracture. In addition, a CFA stent prevents the use of the CFA for future arterial access (e.g., coronary interventions) and may jail the profunda, which is the major supplier of collaterals to the SFA. A CFA stent may also preclude future femoropopliteal bypass. While plain angioplasty or atherectomy may circumvent these problems, a dissection or a poor angiographic result mandates stenting, and thus one cannot pre-emptively rule out the requirement for CFA stenting.

Conversely, the surgical therapy of CFA is relatively simple and consists of performing femoral endarterectomy and patch angioplasty through a small incision. The femoral plaque is removed followed by enlargement of the CFA and the ostia of the SFA and profunda with patch placement. It is a local and relatively quick surgery that may be performed under regional anesthesia with excellent long-term patency of up to 90% at 5 years.[35] If the disease extends distally into the femoral bifurcation and if the SFA is occluded, endarterectomy is extended to the profunda with a patch that sometimes covers the SFA (pitfall: this precludes future percutaneous therapy of the SFA).

Percutaneous therapy, particularly atherectomy, is an acceptable alternative when CFA stenosis has the following features:[36] short (≤2 cm), no heavy calcifications, and no extension to the femoral bifurcation. The lack of calcifications predicts the success of plain balloon angioplasty and atherectomy and a lower risk of dissection. If stenting is needed, a short stent that does not involve the whole CFA and does not jail the profunda leaves room for future arterial access.

VII. Management of acute limb ischemia

ALI is characterized by a large amount of thrombus and distal embolization. Whether due to native artery or graft thrombosis, stages 1 and 2 ALI are typically treated by percutaneous wiring of the thrombotic area, followed by positioning of an infusion catheter that allows local, intra-clot, slow delivery of thrombolytic therapy for 12–48 hours (e.g., r-tPA 1.5 mg/h for a few hours then 1 mg/h). Local thrombolysis achieves recanalization in 80% of patients and full thrombus dissolution in 70% of patients, and is as effective in saving the limb as immediate surgical recanalization.[37] Additional reduction of the thrombus burden may be achieved early on with a thrombectomy system (such as Angiojet rheolytic thrombectomy), but is plagued by a low efficacy in case of adherent, organized thrombus and a high rate of distal embolization. Thrombectomy may be used in selective cases of small and localized thrombus burden without evidence of distal embolization, and with the use of distal embolic protection. Angioplasty should not be performed early on, as it worsens embolization and distal perfusion.

Angiography is repeated after the thrombolytic infusion, and the underlying cause of thrombosis identified, such as severe atherosclerotic disease. The underlying disease is then revascularized percutaneously or surgically, depending on the anatomical complexity.

In case of a graft thrombosis, disease proximal to the graft, distal to the graft, or at the anastomosis is addressed after thrombolysis and treated surgically or with angioplasty/stenting.[37–39]

Patients with stage 3 ALI (motor loss or extensive sensory loss) cannot afford the long waiting period of thrombolytic therapy and often require immediate surgical thromboembolectomy with additional bypass surgery as appropriate.[1] The risk of reperfusion syndrome is increased at this stage and usually dictates adjunctive, prophylactic fasciotomy, which my further justify surgical therapy.

Patients with ALI have a high amputation risk of ~30% at 6 months, a mortality risk of ~15% at 6 months, and a high bleeding risk of ~12.5% when receiving thrombolytic therapy.[37] After acute therapy, these patients need to be assessed for a source of embolus (echo, CT of the thoracic and abdominal aorta looking for aneurysm, popliteal ultrasound looking for aneurysm).

VIII. Management of lower extremity ulcers (Table 19.6)

Table 19.6 Management of lower extremity ulcers.

---

1. Look for ischemia. Quickly revascularize an ischemic ulcer (days to 1–2 weeks)
2. Antibiotic therapy whenever there are infectious signs: red/warm borders, deep ulcer, pus, fever, elevated CRP/white cell count
3. Debride the necrotic tissue
4. Unload the limb by using a cane ± perform Achilles tendon lengthening in case of a neuropathic ulcer
5. Rule out osteomyelitis
   Clinically:
   • A deep ulcer that can be probed to the bone (= the bone can be palpated at the ulcer base) highly suggests osteomyelitis
   • An ulcer that is large and deep (>2 cm² in size or >3 mm in depth) suggests osteomyelitis
   Perform X-ray, which shows bone destruction in osteomyelitis (late finding, occurring several weeks later)
   ± *Perform MRI* (sensitive and specific, useful if the diagnosis is not established clinically)
   Osteomyelitis dictates bone debridement or limited amputation, along with longer antibiotic therapy

---

2. CAROTID DISEASE

Asymptomatic carotid stenosis >70% is associated with a 1.5–2% yearly risk of ipsilateral stroke, *much lower than the common perception*.[40,41] Moreover, this risk is only slightly higher for asymptomatic carotid stenosis >90% (~2.5% yearly stroke risk) and for progressive disease.[42] In fact, a recent analysis has shown that even the progression to complete occlusion is usually asymptomatic and is associated with a rather low stroke risk of <1% (this risk is 10% in other series, still relatively low).[43]

Symptomatic carotid stenosis >50% is associated with ~30% risk of stroke at 2 years, most of which occurs in the first 3 months (~15% at 30 days, 20–30% at 3 months) (NASCET, ECST trials).[44–46] The risk decreases with time from the event. The risk is higher, 35% per year, for symptomatic carotid stenosis >90%.[47]

I. Assessment of carotid stenosis

In old trials, invasive angiography has provided the gold-standard assessment of carotid stenosis. Two angiographic methods have been used to calculate stenosis severity, the NASCET and ECST methods (Figure 19.5). NASCET provides a more conservative estimate of the stenosis; it is the most widely used method and is adopted by the ACC guidelines to define treatment cutoffs.

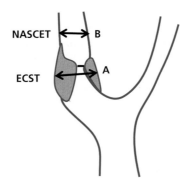

Figure 19.5 In the ECST method, the stenosis is measured in reference to the original carotid bulb diameter **(A)**. In the NASCET method, the stenosis is measured in reference to the distal internal carotid diameter **(B)**. A 50% stenosis by NASCET corresponds to ~65% stenosis by ECST.

Doppler ultrasound indirectly estimates the severity of a carotid stenosis by measuring the rise in velocity across the stenosis (severe stenosis >70% is suggested by systolic velocity across the bulb or internal carotid artery >230 cm/s). It may overestimate the severity of a stenosis and therefore, when the stenosis range is equivocal (70–80% range), confirmation with another modality, CTA or MRA, is recommended. In general, after Doppler ultrasound suggests a severe stenosis, CTA or MRA is performed to confirm the finding, define the exact location of the disease, and look for intracranial disease in preparation for CEA. MRA may be performed without gadolinium contrast, although the latter improves arterial delineation. Unlike CTA, MRA is not affected by calcifications and is a better imaging modality in patients with heavy carotid calcifications. Invasive angiography is not usually needed, unless non-invasive studies yield discordant results or the plan is to perform carotid stenting. CEA may be performed based solely on the result of non-invasive studies.

II. Medical therapy of carotid stenosis
Medical therapy of carotid stenosis consists of:

- Aspirin or clopidogrel monotherapy.
- Aggressive treatment of HTN; statin therapy.
- In patients with prior stroke:
  - The combination aspirin–dipyridamole (Aggrenox) may be used, but did not prove superior to clopidogrel monotherapy.[48] The MATCH trial did not show any advantage of long-term aspirin–clopidogrel combination vs. clopidogrel monotherapy in patients with a recent stroke (<3 months), with a significant increase in the rates of major and intracranial bleeding.[49] However, more recently, the CHANCE trial and a meta-analysis have shown that, in comparison with aspirin monotherapy, the very early initiation of aspirin–clopidogrel in the first 24 hours of a transient ischemic attack (TIA) or a minor stroke, and its continuation for 3 weeks only rather than long-term, reduces the risk of stroke within 3 months. This combination therapy, when administered early and for a brief period, proved useful because the highest risk of stroke is in the first 3 months, especially the first few days, after a TIA or a minor stroke (10–20%). Later and more prolonged therapy becomes less beneficial, and the benefit is counterbalanced by the bleeding risk. [50]
  - Warfarin is not superior to aspirin in case of stroke related to carotid disease and is associated with a higher bleeding risk.[51,52]

III. Revascularization of asymptomatic carotid stenosis
Two trials, ACAS and ACST, have shown that carotid endarterectomy (CEA) reduces the 5-year stroke risk in patients with asymptomatic carotid stenosis >60%, with a reduction of the yearly stroke risk from 2% to 0.5%, at the expense of an early periprocedural stroke hazard of 2%.[40,41] However, the benefit of CEA is not dramatic in asymptomatic patients, whose risk of stroke is relatively low despite a severe stenosis. Furthermore, medical therapy has improved since these trials (statin therapy, better HTN control), such that the benefit of CEA over contemporary medical therapy is unclear.

CEA is assigned a class IIa recommendation in patients with asymptomatic carotid stenosis >70% if the surgical risk of death or stroke is <3% (class IIa).[53] A 70–80% stenosis by ultrasound must be confirmed using another modality. Patients with cardiopulmonary comorbidities placing them at a high surgical risk and those with unfavorable neck anatomy may undergo carotid stenting. The SAPPHIRE trial has shown that stenting is equivalent to CEA in high-operative-risk patients, most of whom had asymptomatic carotid stenosis.[54] However, as opposed to CEA, no head-to-head comparison of stenting and medical therapy is available. Stenting asymptomatic patients is thus a class IIb recommendation.

IV. Revascularization of symptomatic carotid stenosis
Two major trials, NASCET and ECST, have shown that CEA reduces the 2- and 3-year stroke risk in patients with symptomatic carotid stenosis of 50–99%, more particularly patients with a stenosis of 70–99% (2-year stroke risk 9% vs. 26%). CEA or carotid stenting is given as a class I indication for recently symptomatic carotid stenosis, meaning carotid stenosis with a prior TIA or non-disabling stroke *in the prior 6 months*, if the periprocedural risk of death or stroke is <6%.

The recurrence risk being highest in the first 3 months (20–30% recurrence), surgery is most effective when performed within 2 weeks of the index event, and still very effective when performed 2 weeks to 3 months after the index event. The further away the clinical event is (>3 months), the less beneficial surgery is. While there has been a concern about hemorrhagic transformation when surgery is performed within 2 weeks of a stroke, several studies have shown that revascularization is relatively safe and protective from the much higher risk of ischemic stroke recurrence during this period.[55–57] Thus, when indicated, the intervention should be done as soon as possible after the event, within 2 weeks (ACC guidelines).[53]

In symptomatic patients, the carotid stenosis must be >70% by non-invasive studies, or >50% by angiography to qualify for revascularization. Invasive angiography may be needed in symptomatic patients with carotid stenosis of 50–70% on non-invasive imaging to prove the severity of the stenosis, as non-invasive imaging frequently overestimates the true severity of a stenosis in this range.

V. Main risks of CEA and carotid stenting

Risk of perioperative stroke after CEA or carotid stenting:

- 1–2% when performed for asymptomatic carotid stenosis
- 3–4% when performed for symptomatic carotid stenosis

The risk of minor stroke is slightly higher with carotid stenting than with CEA. The perioperative stroke risk is followed by a 0.5%–1% stroke risk per year (0.5% for asymptomatic and 1% for symptomatic carotid stenosis). There is also a restenosis risk of 5–10%, mainly in the first 18 months (neointimal hyperplasia early on, recurrent atherosclerosis later on). To assess for restenosis, carotid Doppler is performed at 1 month and 6 months, then annually.

VI. CEA versus carotid stenting

The SAPPHIRE trial has shown that in high-surgical-risk patients with symptomatic or asymptomatic carotid stenosis, carotid stenting provides a non-inferior alternative to CEA.[54]

The CREST trial enrolled average-risk surgical patients with symptomatic or asymptomatic carotid stenosis (stenosis was symptomatic in ~50% of patients). There was no difference between CEA and stenting for the combined risk of death/MI/stroke up to 4 years (~7%). CEA was associated with a higher risk of periprocedural MI, while carotid stenting was associated with a higher risk of minor strokes, mainly in patients older than 70 years. CEA was associated with ~5% risk of cranial nerve palsy.[58] When carotid stenting is performed, the use of embolic protection is mandatory. The procedure should be aborted if difficult anatomy precludes the use of embolic protection.

Decisions to perform CEA vs. carotid stenting may be individualized based on the patient's age, difficult angiographic anatomy (favors CEA), cardiopulmonary or neck comorbidities (favor stenting), and patient's preference, keeping in mind the higher risk of minor stroke with stenting and the higher risk of MI with CEA (Table 19.7).[53]

The combination of aspirin and clopidogrel is mandatory for 1 month after stenting, followed by aspirin monotherapy. A 2-week duration of dual antiplatelet therapy may be acceptable if necessary (SAPPHIRE trial).[54]

VII. Carotid disease in a patient undergoing CABG

Observational studies have consistently reported that the risk of stroke associated with CABG is ~2% in patients with no significant carotid stenosis and 3% in patients with asymptomatic severe carotid stenosis.[59–61] These figures, however, increase to ≥5% in those with bilateral carotid stenoses or a history of stroke or TIA. No clear evidence supports prophylactic CEA in CABG patients with unilateral (>80%) asymptomatic carotid stenosis. Most postoperative strokes occur in patients without any carotid disease (76%) or in patients with carotid disease receiving synchronous CEA–CABG.[61] In addition, primary carotid disease alone is responsible for less than 40% of postoperative strokes, the rest being due to aortic atheroembolization, postoperative hypercoagulable state, and atrial fibrillation.[59] However, there is agreement that prophylactic carotid intervention is still justified in CABG patients with a carotid stenosis >80% and a history of stroke or TIA in the last 6 months (class IIa),[53] and probably in patients with asymptomatic severe (>80%) bilateral carotid stenoses.

The timing of CABG and CEA is controversial. A systematic review has shown that death is highest for synchronous CEA–CABG, stroke is highest for staged CABG first–CEA second, and MI is highest for staged CEA first–CABG second.[59] A registry analysis suggests that the risk of stroke is higher in patients undergoing synchronous CEA–CABG as opposed to staged CEA first–CABG second.[61] *Concomitant CEA–CABG seems to be the least favored revascularization approach.* CABG alone is reasonable for patients with asymptomatic carotid stenosis and critical left main disease, refractory acute coronary syndrome, or other indications for urgent CABG. In contrast, patients with recent (<2 weeks) TIA and carotid stenosis >80% should be considered for urgent CEA if CABG can be safely deferred for several days.

Carotid stenting followed by CABG 3 weeks later is another alternative (clopidogrel is provided for 2 weeks after carotid stenting, then is interrupted for 5–7 days before CABG). Stenting pre-CABG, as opposed to CEA pre-CABG, is associated with lower periprocedural MI and complications in those patients with advanced CAD.[62–64]

VIII. Subtotal and total carotid occlusions

While the yearly risk of ipsilateral stroke is ~10% in patients with symptomatic carotid stenosis of 70–89%, the risk increases to 35% in those with a stenosis 90–95%, but is actually lower, at 10% (or 2% in ECST trial), in those with *symptomatic subtotal carotid occlusion,*

Table 19.7 High-risk features for CEA and carotid stenting.

Features increasing CEA risk (carotid stenting may be preferred [SAPPHIRE criteria])	Features increasing the risk of carotid stenting (CEA is preferred)
High surgical risk from comorbidities:	- Age >70, much more if >80
- Major cardiac or pulmonary disease	**Technical reasons:**
High surgical risk for anatomical reasons:	- Circumferential, heavy carotid calcifications
- Prior neck surgery, prior neck radiation	- Tortuosity
- Postsurgical restenosis	- Type 3 aortic arch
- ±Contralateral occlusion	- Heavy aortic arch atherosclerosis
- High lesions above C2 or low lesions below the clavicle	- Visible thrombus

where the carotid artery fills antegradely but faintly and is reduced in size (string sign).[47,65] A similar, reduced yearly risk of ipsilateral stroke of 2–10% is found in patients with symptomatic *total carotid occlusion*.[66] The reduced antegrade flow in subtotal and total occlusions lessens arterial emboli. However, recurrent ipsilateral stroke may still occur and is related to reduced perfusion, depending on the robustness of collaterals; the risk is highest, ~8%, within 30 days of an ischemic event.[66] *Note that the stroke risk is very low with asymptomatic carotid occlusion.*

The NASCET trial included patients with *subtotal carotid occlusion* and found that the benefit of CEA in those patients was similar to that in patients with lesser stenosis.[47] Carotid stenting is risky in those patients, as the string sign often implies a large thrombus burden, which is a strong negative predictor of outcomes with carotid stenting, making CEA the preferred approach.

Total carotid occlusion, on the other hand, while associated with a risk of stroke that approximates that of subtotal occlusion, is technically challenging for both CEA and percutaneous recanalization.[67] Medical therapy is therefore the standard therapy for total carotid occlusion.

3. RENAL ARTERY STENOSIS

I. Forms of renal artery stenosis

There are two major forms of renal artery stenosis (RAS):

a. Atherosclerotic RAS, which typically involves the ostia of renal arteries. It is frequently accompanied by parenchymal renal disease, often secondary to hypertension or diabetes rather than RAS, which attenuates any potential benefit from renal artery revascularization. In a subgroup of patients with RAS, renal failure is secondary to renal ischemia and may be improved with revascularization (even CKD stages 4 and 5).

According to old data, atherosclerotic RAS is progressive, with 50% of significant lesions progressing over 2–3 years, and 5–10% progressing to a total occlusion. Occlusion leads to renal atrophy and irreversible loss of renal function.[68] Aggressive control of blood pressure and risk factors reduces this risk.

b. Fibromuscular dysplasia (FMD) is characterized by intimal *or* medial constriction without any intimal thickening on IVUS. The intima is thin but is rigid and constricted, a form of negative remodeling (fibroplasia). This may lead to serial areas of constriction (string of beads) or to one focally constricted area. The process often involves the mid- to distal parts of the renal artery. It typically occurs in women 15–50 years old (female/male ratio = 8:1) and tends to progress. Progressive renal failure and renal atrophy are, however, unusual.[68]

Because of vasoconstriction, RAS-induced hypertension usually affects both the systolic and diastolic components of blood pressure and is not usually an isolated systolic hypertension.

II. Screening and indications to revascularize renal artery stenosis

A. Screen with renal arterial Doppler and consider renal revascularization for the following three groups:

- Recurrent, unexplained flash pulmonary edema/acute HF
- Refractory HTN (on ≥ 3–4 drugs at optimal dose, including a diuretic)
- Progressive azotemia, seen with bilateral RAS or unilateral RAS of a solitary kidney

B. Once RAS is diagnosed in one of the three scenarios above, assess non-invasively and invasively for:[69,70]

1. Lack of renal parenchymal disease
2. Functional significance of a stenosis (a lesion >50–70% is not necessarily significant hemodynamically)

Patients most likely to benefit are those with no intrinsic parenchymal renal disease *and* a functionally significant stenosis, rather than just an anatomically significant stenosis (Table 19.8, Figure 19.6). This combination proves that HTN and the decline in GFR result from reduced perfusion rather than severe intrinsic nephron damage (from diabetes, hypertension, or glomerulopathy). Only after assessment of these two features non-invasively, then invasively if needed, is stenting appropriate. *Invasively*, a lack of cortical blush and a lack of cortical vascularity

Table 19.8 Signs of advanced renal parenchymal disease and signs of functional significance of a renal artery stenosis.

Signs suggestive of advanced parenchymal disease
- Proteinuria >1 g/24 h
- Renal atrophy (renal size <8 cm)
- Renal resistive index >0.8, which indicates a high intrarenal microvascular resistance
- On renal angiography: poor cortical blood flow, cortical vascular pruning (no cortical ramifications)

Signs suggestive of functional significance of renal artery stenosis
- Renal asymmetry >1.5 cm without atrophy (conversely, atrophy implies advanced intrinsic damage)
- Creatinine rise >20% with ACE inhibitors, along with bilateral RAS
- Invasively: Translesional systolic pressure gradient under maximal hyperemia (papaverine) >21 mmHg[a]
                FFR <0.9[a]

---

[a] Measurements should be made with a pressure wire similar to the one used for coronary assessment, with the guide catheter disengaged into the aorta to allow measurement of simultaneous aortic pressure and post-stenotic pressure. Avoid gradient measurement using pull-back of the bulky catheter across the stenosis, as this may create a false obstruction. **Adenosine is a renal vasoconstrictor** and is not suitable to induce renal hyperemia; an intrarenal bolus of papaverine is used.

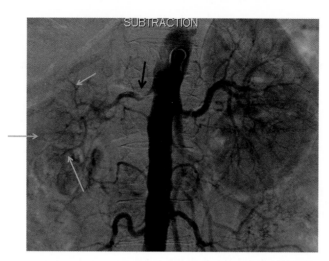

Figure 19.6 Compare the right and left kidneys. Note the right renal atrophy, the poor cortical blood flow (*horizontal blue arrow*) and the vascular pruning without distal ramification (*oblique blue arrows*), all of which are suggestive of severe parenchymal disease. The 90% renal artery stenosis (*black arrow*) should not be stented at this stage.

are surrogates of nephropathy, while a high translesional pressure gradient is a surrogate of functional significance.

III. Notes

A. Benefit of percutaneous intervention in FMD vs. atherosclerotic RAS

The success rate of percutaneous intervention is higher for FMD than for atherosclerotic RAS. Also, RAS is more likely the sole cause of hypertension in FMD than in atherosclerotic RAS. In the latter, RAS may just be one factor or an incidental finding, the majority of these patients having pre-existing HTN or renal failure. Hence, there is a lower threshold for renal angioplasty in FMD. Also, in this case, angioplasty alone without stenting is often successful and is often curative of hypertension. High-pressure angioplasty is required to allow the stiff intima or media to yield.

B. ASTRAL and CORAL trials

These two trials randomized patients with unilateral or bilateral renal artery stenosis, hypertension, and moderate renal disease (mean GFR 40 ml/min in ASTRAL, 58 ml/min in CORAL) to stenting vs. medical therapy. Stenting did not improve blood pressure control or renal function.[71,72] Both trials had the following pitfalls:

- In most patients, renal failure was disproportionate to the degree of RAS. In fact, the majority of patients had renal failure yet RAS was mostly unilateral. This indicates intrinsic parenchymal disease rather than renal ischemia, a process not affected by renal stenting (potentially aggravated by atheroemboli and contrast).
- ~40–50% of patients had RAS <70% obstructive, which may not be functionally significant.
- Most patients in ASTRAL had normal diastolic blood pressure (whereas RAS-induced HTN typically has a diastolic component).
- HTN was not very severe (SBP ~150 mmHg on 2–3 drugs), and was properly controlled by adding one more drug.

These trials indicate that the widespread application of renal stenting in hypertensive patients with RAS is not effective. Conversely, in other studies, appropriate stenting of carefully selected patients has dramatically improved blood pressure control, in over 85% of treated patients, and renal function.[70,73,74]

C. Role of ACE inhibitors or ARBs

ACE-Is may be used in patients with unilateral RAS. Since renal flow of the stenotic kidney may depend on the renin–angiotensin system, ACE-Is may worsen ischemia of the involved kidney. However, ACE-Is are the most effective antihypertensive agents in RAS, reduce the damage to the uninvolved kidney, and reduce the atherosclerotic progression in the involved renal artery. Thus, they may be used in unilateral RAS.[68]

In bilateral *significant* RAS, ACE-Is almost always lead to deterioration of the renal function, with over 20% creatinine rise within 4–14 days.[75] While the creatinine rise with ACE-Is is frequently due to other processes, such as low-output HF, hypovolemia, or underlying hypertensive nephropathy with microvascular obstruction, its occurrence in patients with bilateral RAS strongly suggests that RAS is hemodynamically significant and is appropriate for stenting (if hypertension is refractory). In a way, ACE-I therapy is a diagnostic test, and renal deterioration is reversible upon interruption of ACE-I therapy. Thus, in patients with hemodynamically significant bilateral RAS, ACE-Is are contraindicated. However, in the general population of bilateral RAS, ACE-Is are not absolutely contraindicated, as RAS may not be hemodynamically significant; they may be used with close follow-up of creatinine levels. A rise in creatinine would lead to cessation of ACE-I therapy.

QUESTIONS AND ANSWERS

Question 1. A 55-year-old man, smoker, presents with severe right calf and foot pain that has been progressive for the last 3 weeks. The pain is present at rest, persists throughout most of the day, and is worse at night. On exam, his great toe is mottled, purple, and distal pulses cannot be heard on Doppler. Motor exam is intact but sensing is impaired at the tip of the great toe. Which of the following is correct?

A. This is critical limb ischemia by duration. Revascularization is warranted within a few days

B. The lack of pulses on Doppler, the persistent pain, and the severe cyanosis suggest acute limb ischemia rather than critical limb ischemia. Revascularization is urgent

C. The lack of pulses on Doppler and severe cyanosis suggest acute limb ischemia rather than critical limb ischemia. Revascularization is emergent

D. The progression suggests acute limb ischemia from an embolic phenomenon

Question 2. A 70-year-old man with no known history of CAD has right calf pain when he walks one block. This is not lifestyle-limiting for him. He does not have any tissue loss. ABI is 0.5 on the right and 0.8 on the left. Which statement is correct?

A. Angiography and revascularization should be considered in light of the severity of right lower extremity PAD

B. His likelihood of CLI is >20% at 5 years

C. His claudication is likely to progress over the next few years

D. Peripheral revascularization would reduce his risk of limb loss

E. His risk of cardiovascular events and mortality is >5% per year

Question 3. A 58-year-old man, active, former smoker, complains of bilateral calf pain (right>left) after walking one block. This is impeding his daily walks. ABI is 0.6 on the right, 0.7 on the left. He tried a daily walking routine to improve his symptoms, without success. Angiography shows a totally occluded right SFA, ~15–20 cm in length, calcified, with reconstitution at the popliteal level. What is the next step?

A. Add cilostazol, recommend daily walking program, for 3 months

B. Percutaneous revascularization is not acceptable, as this is a TASC D lesion

C. Percutaneous revascularization is acceptable, as this is a TASC C lesion. The 1-year patency is ≤60%

D. Percutaneous revascularization is acceptable, as this is a TASC C lesion. The 1-year patency is >60%

Question 4. A patient presents with left great toe ulcer and dorsum of the foot ulcer. He has non-compressible left tibial vessels with ABI >1.5. His left distal pulses are not palpable. Which statement is *incorrect*?

A. The elevated ABI does not rule out significant PAD but rules out critical PAD

B. The elevated ABI has at least the same negative cardiovascular implication as a low ABI, especially in symptomatic patients

C. A toe–brachial index or arterial Doppler may be used to confirm the severity of PAD

D. Abdominal aortic angiography with bilateral femoropopliteal runoff is warranted

Question 5. The patient in Question 4 is found to have a severely diseased left external iliac, a heavily calcified, totally occluded left SFA, and severely diseased but patent AT, with a patent, non-obstructed PT. AT feeds the ulcerated area. What is the next step?

A. Perform stenting of the left iliac. If the ulcer does not heal, bring back for angioplasty/stenting of the SFA

B. Perform percutaneous therapy of both the iliac and the SFA

C. Perform percutaneous therapy of the iliac, SFA, and AT

D. Perform iliac stenting and femoropopliteal bypass

Question 6. A patient has severe left lower extremity claudication (Rutherford category 3). He has severe disease of the left external iliac, a totally occluded SFA, and infrapopliteal disease across the AT. What is the next step?

A. Perform stenting of the left iliac. If severe claudication persists, bring back for angioplasty/stenting of the SFA

B. Perform percutaneous therapy of both the iliac and the SFA

C. Perform percutaneous therapy of the iliac, SFA and AT

D. Perform iliac stenting and femoropopliteal bypass

Question 7. Which statement is *incorrect*?

A. Surgical bypass has higher patency than percutaneous therapy for all lower extremity segments (aortofemoral graft, femoropopliteal graft, femorotibial graft) except when a synthetic graft is used for below-knee femoropopliteal grafting or femorotibial grafting

B. For initial revascularization, percutaneous therapy is generally preferred to surgical bypass because of the lower perioperative morbidity, mortality, and convalescence period

C. For infrapopliteal disease, femorotibial grafting is preferred to percutaneous therapy, as it allows better ulcer healing

D. For common femoral disease, femoral endarterectomy is the preferred therapy and is a relatively low-risk vascular surgery

Question 8. A patient has lifestyle-limiting claudication while walking one block, mostly involving the thighs. Distal pulses are palpable and femoral pulses are normal. Which statement is correct?

A. The patient likely has pseudo-claudication from hip osteoarthritis or spinal stenosis

B. Arterial claudication is possible. The patient may have moderate iliac or distal aortic disease, with normal flow and pulses at rest but insufficient flow and reduced pulses with exercise.

C. Perform ABI

D. Perform ABI at rest and with exercise

E. B + D

F. B + C

Question 9. A patient presents with severe right foot pain, persistent for the last 2 days. His foot is mottled blue. What is the most important immediate step?

A. Emergent angiography and revascularization

B. Doppler the distal pulses and perform sensory and motor exam of the right lower extremity

C. CTA

Question 10. A 72-year-old man, heavy smoker, presents with pain, mottling, and cyanosis of his right great toe, which has been progressive over the last week. He has purple patches on his calf. The femoral pulse is mildly reduced (1+). The PT and DP are not palpable but have a good Doppler signal. The right ABI is 0.75; on Doppler, the flow is monophasic throughout the right lower extremity. CTA shows a heavy atherosclerotic aorta and iliac arteries, with 80% right iliac stenosis. The femoral, popliteal, and infrapopliteal arteries are patent. Creatinine is 1.7 mg/dl. What is the next step?

A. Heparin and urgent stenting of the right iliac
B. Conservative management

Question 11. A 71-year-old smoker with a history of CAD has a right carotid bruit. He has no history of stroke or TIA. A carotid Doppler reveals a 260 cm/s velocity across the right internal carotid. Which statement is *incorrect*?

A. The yearly risk of stroke is 2%
B. CT or MRA may be needed to confirm the severity of the stenosis before an intervention
C. CEA is recommended but only has a marginal benefit in an asymptomatic patient
D. Revascularization with either CEA or stenting is recommended; stenting has the same level of recommendation as CEA
E. Invasive angiography is not necessary before CEA
F. Before deciding whether stenting is an acceptable alternative, the carotid anatomy needs to be defined by invasive angiography

Question 12. A 64-year-old man, smoker, diabetic, has uncontrolled HTN (BP 160/80, on optimal doses of chlorthalidone, amlodipine, and lisinopril). Creatinine is 1.6 mg/dl (GFR 45). Renal Doppler suggests severe right renal artery stenosis. The renal resistive index is 0.85. Invasive angiography shows 80% right renal artery stenosis. What is the next step?

A. Renal artery stenting is unlikely to improve BP control or renal function
B. Renal stenting is warranted for refractory HTN

Answer 1. C. The patient has acute rather than critical limb ischemia, as evidenced by the absent pulses on Doppler, the constant (rather than intermittent) rest pain, and the degree of cyanosis. In this context, the distal sensory loss implies an emergent need for revascularization. This acute limb ischemia is, in fact, subacute and suggestive of in-situ thrombosis (on top of severe atherosclerosis), rather than an abrupt embolic event.

Answer 2. E. The patient has claudication, without CLI (Rutherford 1–3). The risk of symptom progression over the next 5 years is 20% and the risk of progression to CLI is 4%, particularly if he quits smoking. Revascularization, at this point, can only improve symptoms, not the risk of limb loss. Since his symptoms are not severe, revascularization is not indicated. In contrast to the benign limb outcomes, the patient has a high risk of MI, stroke, and cardiac death.

Answer 3. C. The occlusion is a TASC C occlusion, as it is >15 cm (> TASC B), but does not extend to the popliteal or common femoral artery (which would make it TASC D). Percutaneous revascularization is an acceptable strategy for TASC C occlusions, albeit at a high risk of restenosis. Surgical bypass should be considered for restenosis. A is a wrong answer as the patient has already tried the conservative strategy of daily walking.

Answer 4. A. An elevated ABI with claudication or ulcer often corresponds to significant, obstructive PAD, sometimes critical (37% of symptomatic patients with elevated ABI have CLI). Also, a "pulseless" elevated ABI often implies obstructive PAD.

Answer 5. C. In case of critical limb ischemia, one unobstructed straight line of flow should be achieved. All diseased segments should be treated. At the infrapopliteal level, at least one artery should be unobstructed, preferably the artery supplying the ulcer if its recanalization is technically feasible (angiosome concept). In this case, the AT supplies the ulcer and should be treated.

Answer 6. A. In case of claudication, the goal is symptom control. When disease involves multiple segments, the inflow disease (iliac) may be treated first. Percutaneous therapy of the SFA may be performed in the same session but is not necessary. The patient may be brought back if symptoms persist. As opposed to CLI, in claudication, infrapopliteal disease does not need to be treated unless it is the only diseased segment.

Answer 7. C. The long-term patency of femorotibial graft, even venous graft, is not much higher than contemporary tibial percutaneous angioplasty/DES. Moreover, percutaneous therapy is good enough over the short and intermediate term to allow ulcer healing. Restenosis usually occurs after the ulcer has healed; much less flow is required to prevent an ulcer than to heal an ulcer. Restenosis does not usually result in recurrent CLI.

Answer 8. E. Pulses may be palpable and only mildly reduced in patients with true arterial claudication that is related to moderate aortoiliac disease. The lesion allows normal flow at rest, but cannot accommodate the dramatic increase in flow required from the iliac artery with exertion. During exercise, the required increase in flow across the iliac is far larger than that across the SFA, as the iliac supplies a much larger territory. ABI and pulses may be normal or mildly reduced at rest but drastically drop with exercise.

Answer 9. B. The patient's persistent foot pain and severe cyanosis are suggestive of acute limb ischemia. He typically requires emergent revascularization. However, a thorough exam is required to classify the stage of ALI. Pulses are typically absent on Doppler exam. In the absence of motor loss, percutaneous recanalization with local, prolonged r-tPA infusion is appropriate. If motor loss is present, surgical revascularization with fasciotomy is often more appropriate. Profound paralysis or acute tissue gangrene dictates amputation. CTA is a useful test later on (looks for aortic or popliteal aneurysm, as a source of emboli).

Answer 10. B. The patient has atheroembolization from the aortoiliac segments. This is evidenced by the discrepancy between the severity of foot ischemia and the rather mild impairment of pulses (good pulse signals) and the mild ABI reduction. In fact, *the patient has foot ischemia with much less ankle ischemia, implying very distal atheroemboli.* Stenting the right iliac may lead to more atheroembolization and may aggravate the foot ischemia. Conservative management and foot care is warranted; foot ischemia improves in most of these cases.

Answer 11. D. The yearly risk of stroke with asymptomatic stenosis is low. CEA is a class IIa recommendation (based on ACAS and ACST trials), while stenting is class IIb (based on the carotid stenting trials, such as CREST, which included asymptomatic patients). In addition, before finalizing the decision to stent, the patient must have appropriate anatomical features (heavy calcium, tortuosity, type 3 arch).

Answer 12. A. The patient has unilateral RAS yet significant CKD, implying that CKD is related to intrinsic renal disease (from diabetes, HTN) rather than renal ischemia. The high renal resistive index implies intrarenal microvascular disease, i.e., intrinsic renal disease. Renal disease is likely the mechanism of severe HTN. Renal artery stenting is unlikely to improve outcomes in this patient.

References
Lower extremity peripheral arterial disease

1. Hirsch AT, Haskal ZJ, Hertzer NR, et al. ACC/AHA 2005 guidelines for the management of patients with peripheral arterial disease (lower extremity, renal, mesenteric, and abdominal aortic). J Am Coll Cardiol 2006; 47: 1239–312.
2. McDermott MM, Greenland P, Liu K, et al. Leg symptoms in peripheral arterial disease. JAMA 2001; 286: 1599–606.
3. Criqui MH, Fronek A, Barrett-Connor E, et al. The prevalence of peripheral arterial disease in a defined population. Circulation 1985; 71: 510–15.
4. McAllister FF. The fate of patients with intermittent claudication managed non-operatively. Am J Surg 1976; 132: 593–5.
5. Jelnes R, Gaardstring O, Hougaard Jensen K, et al. Fate of intermittent claudication: outcome and risk factors. Br Med J 1986; 293: 1137–40.
6. Aquino R, Johnnides C, Makaroun M, et al. Natural history of claudication: long-term serial follow-up study of 1244 claudicants. J Vasc Surg 2001; 34: 962–70.
7. McDermott MM, Liu K, Greenland P, et al. Functional decline in peripheral arterial disease: associations with the ankle brachial index and leg symptoms. JAMA 2004; 292: 453–61.
8. Harris LM, Peer R, Curl GR, et al. Long-term follow-up of patients with early atherosclerosis. J Vasc Surg 1996; 23; 576–81.
9. Valentine RJ, Jackson MR, Modrall JG, et al. The progressive nature of peripheral arterial disease in young adults: a prospective analysis of white men referred to a vascular surgery service. J Vasc Surg 1999; 30: 436–45.
10. Steg G, Bhatt DL, Wilson PWF, et al. One-year cardiovascular event rates in outpatients with atherothrombosis. JAMA 2007; 297: 1197–206.
11. Diehm C, Lange S, Darius H. et al. Association of low ankle brachial index with high mortality in primary care. Eur Heart J 2006; 27: 1743–9.
12. Diehm C, Allenberg JR, Pittrow D, et al. Mortality and vascular morbidity in older adults with asymptomatic versus symptomatic peripheral arterial disease. Circulation 2009; 120: 2053–61.
13. Aronow WS, Ahn C. Prevalence of coexistence of coronary artery disease, peripheral arterial disease, and atherothrombotic brain infarction in men and women ≥ 62 years of age. Am J Cardiol 1994; 74: 64–5.
14. Valentine RJ, Grayburn PA, Eichhorn EJ, Myers SI, Clagett GP. Coronary artery disease is highly prevalent among patients with premature peripheral vascular disease. J Vasc Surg 1994; 19: 668–74.
15. Criqui MH, Fronek A, Klauber MR, et al. The sensitivity, specificity, and predictive value of traditional clinical evaluation of peripheral arterial disease: results from noninvasive testing in a defined population. Circulation 1985; 71: 516–22.
16. Suomen V, Rantanen T, Venermo M, et al. Prevalence and risk factors of PAD among patients with elevated ABI. Eur J Vasc Endovasc Surg 2008; 35: 709–14.
17. Arain FA, Ye Z, Bailey KR, et al. Survival in patients with poorly compressible leg arteries. J Am Coll Cardiol 2012; 59: 400–7.
18. Espinola-Klein C, Rupprecht HJ, Bickel C, et al. Different calculations of ankle-brachial index and their impact on cardiovascular risk prediction Circulation 2008; 118: 961–7.
19. Gray BH, Sullivan TM. Claudication: how to individualize treatment. Clev Clin J Med 1997; 64: 429–36.
20. Bhatt DL, Fox KAA, Hacke W, et al. Clopidogrel and aspirin versus aspirin alone for the prevention of atherothrombotic events. N Engl J Med 2006; 354: 1706–17.
21. Hunink MG, Wong JB, Donaldson MC, et al. Revascularization for femoropopliteal disease: a decision and cost-effectiveness analysis. JAMA 1995; 274: 165–71.
22. de Vries SO, Hunink MGM. Results of aortic bifurcation grafts form aorto-iliac occlusive disease: a meta-analysis. J Vasc Surg 1997; 26: 558–69. *Perioperative mortality 3%, morbidity 8%.*
23. McFalls EO, Ward HB, Moritz TE, et al. Coronary-artery revascularization before elective major vascular surgery. N Engl J Med 2004; 351: 2795–804. *CARP trial.*
24. Adam DJ, Beard JD, Cleveland T, et al. Bypass versus angioplasty in severe ischaemia of the leg (BASIL): multicentre, randomised controlled trial. Lancet 2005; 366: 1925–34.
25. Norgren L, Hiatt WR, Dormandy JA, et al. Intersociety Consensus for the management of peripheral arterial disease (TASC II). Eur J Vasc Endovasc Surg 2007; 33 Suppl 1: S1–75.
26. Tetteroo E, van deer Graaf Y, Bosch JL, et al. Randomised comparison of primary stent placement versus primary angioplasty followed by selective stent placement in patients with iliac-artery occlusive disease. Dutch Iliac Stent Trial Study Group. Lancet 1998; 351: 1153–9.
27. Scheinert D, Schroder M, Ludwig J, et al. Stent-supported recanalization of chronic iliac occlusions. Am J Med 2001; 110: 708–715.
28. Mwipatayi BP, Thomas S, Wong J, et al. A comparison of covered versus bare expandable stents for the treatment of aortoiliac occlusive disease. J Vasc Surg 2011; 54: 1561–70.
29. Schillinger M, Sabeti S, Loewe C, et al. Balloon angioplasty versus implantation of nitinol stents in the superficial femoral artery. N Engl J Med 2006; 354: 1879–88.
30. Laird JR, Katzen BT, Scheinert DT, et al. Nitinol stent implantation versus balloon angioplasty for lesions in the superficial femoral artery and proximal popliteal artery. Twelve-month results from the RESILIENT randomized trial. Circ Cardiovasc Interv 2010; 3: 267–76.
31. Scheinert D, Scheinert S, Sax J, et al. Prevalence and clinical impact of stent fractures after femoropolpliteal stenting. J Am Coll Cardiol 2005; 45: 312–15.

32. Rastan A, Krankenberg H, Baumgartner I, et al. Stent placement versus balloon angioplasty for the treatment of obstructive lesions of the popliteal artery: a prospective, multicenter, randomized trial. Circulation 2013; 127: 2535–41.

33. Bosiers M. DESTINY trial: 12 months clinical and angiographic findings. Presented at the Leipzig Interventional Course. Leipzig, Germany, 19 January 2011.

34. Scheinert D, Ulrich M, Scheinert S, et al. Comparison of sirolimus-eluting vs. bare-metal stents for the treatment of infrapopliteal obstructions. EuroIntervention 2006; 2: 169–74.

35. Ballotta E, Gruppo M, Mazzalai F, Da Giau G. Common femoral artery endarterectomy for occlusive disease: an 8-year single-center prospective study. Surgery 2010; 147: 268–74.

36. Bonvini RF. Rastan A, Sixt S. Endovascular treatment of common femoral artery disease: medium-term outcomes of 360 consecutive procedures. J Am Coll Cardiol 2011; 58: 792–8.

37. Ouriel K, Veith FJ, Sasahara AA. A comparison of recombinant urokinase with vascular surgery as initial treatment for acute arterial occlusion of the legs. Thrombolysis or peripheral arterial surgery (TOPAS) investigators. N Engl J Med 1998; 338: 1105–11.

38. Browse DJ, Torrie EP, Galland RB. Low-dose intra-arterial thrombolysis in the treatment of occluded vascular grafts. Br J Surg 1992; 79: 86–8.

39. Gardiner GA, Harrington DP, Koltum W, et al. Salvage of occluded arterial bypass grafts by means of thrombolysis. J Vasc Surg 1989; 9: 426–31.

Carotid disease

40. Executive Committee for the Asymptomatic Carotid Atherosclerosis Study. Endarterectomy for asymptomatic carotid artery stenosis. JAMA 1995; 273: 1421–8. *ACAS trial*.

41. Halliday A, Mansfield A, Marro J, et al. Prevention of disabling and fatal strokes by successful carotid endarterectomy in patients without recent neurological symptoms: randomised controlled trial. Lancet 2004; 363: 1491–502. *ACST trial*.

42. Nicolaides AN, Kakkos SK, Griffin M, et al. Severity of asymptomatic carotid stenosis and risk of ipsilateral hemispheric ischaemic events: results from ACSRS. Eur J Vasc Endovasc Surg 2005; 30: 275–84.

43. Yang C, Bogiatzi C, Spence D. Risk of stroke at the time of carotid occlusion. JAMA Neurol 2015; 72: 1261–7.

44. North American Symptomatic Carotid Endarterectomy Trial Collaborators. Beneficial effect of carotid endarterectomy in symptomatic patients with high-grade carotid stenosis. N Engl J Med 1991; 325: 445–53. *NASCET trial*.

45. Randomised trial of endarterectomy for recently symptomatic carotid stenosis: final results of the MRC European Carotid Surgery Trial (ECST). Lancet 1998; 351: 1379–87.

46. White CJ. Carotid artery stent placement. J Am Coll Cardiol 2010; 3: 467–74.

47. Morgenstern LB, Fox AJ, Sharpe BL, et al, for the North American Symptomatic Carotid Endarterectomy Trial (NASCET) Group. The risks and benefits of carotid endarterectomy in patients with near occlusion of the carotid artery. Neurology 1997; 48: 911–15.

48. Diener HC, Bogousslavsky J, Brass LM, et al. Aspirin and clopidogrel compared with clopidogrel alone after recent ischaemic stroke or transient ischaemic attack in high-risk patients (MATCH): randomised, double-blind, placebo-controlled trial. Lancet 2004; 364: 331–7.

49. Sacco RL, Diener HC, Yusuf S, et al. Aspirin and extended-release dipyridamole versus clopidogrel for recurrent stroke. N Engl J Med 2008; 359: 1238–51.

50. Wang Y, Wang Y, Zhao X, et al. CHANCE Investigators. Clopidogrel with aspirin in acute minor stroke or transient ischemic attack. N Engl J Med 2013; 369: 11–19.

51. Mohr JP, Thompson JLP, Lazar RM, et al. A comparison of warfarin and aspirin for the prevention of recurrent ischemic stroke. N Engl J Med 2001; 345: 1444–51.

52. Chimowitz MI, Lynn MJ, Howlett-Smith H, et al. Comparison of warfarin and aspirin for symptomatic intracranial arterial stenosis. N Engl J Med 2005; 352: 1305–16.

53. Brott TG, Halperin JL, Abbara S, et al. 2011 ASA/ACCF/AHA/AANN/AANS/ACR/ASNR/CNS/SAIP/SCAI/SIR/SNIS/SVM/SVS Guideline on the management of patients with extracranial carotid and vertebral artery disease. J Am Coll Cardiol 2011; 57: e16–94.

54. Yadav JS, Wholey MH, Kuntz RE. Protected carotid-artery stenting versus endarterectomy in high-risk patients. N Engl J Med 2004; 351: 1493–501. *SAPPHIRE trial*.

55. Ballotta E, Da GG, Baracchini C, et al. Early versus delayed carotid endarterectomy after a nondisabling ischemic stroke: a prospective randomized study. Surgery 2002; 131: 287–93.

56. Eckstein HH, Ringleb P, Dorfler A, et al. The Carotid Surgery for Ischemic Stroke trial: a prospective observational study on carotid endarterectomy in the early period after ischemic stroke. J Vasc Surg 2002; 36: 997–1004.

57. Ricco JB, Illuminati G, Bouin-Pineau MH, et al. Early carotid endarterectomy after a nondisabling stroke: a prospective study. Ann Vasc Surg 2000; 14: 89–94.

58. Brott TG, Hobson RW, Howard G, et al. Stenting versus endarterectomy for treatment of carotid-artery stenosis. N Engl J Med 2010; 363: 11–23. *CREST trial*.

59. Naylor AR, Mehta Z, Rothwell PM, Bell PR. Carotid artery disease and stroke during coronary artery bypass: a critical review of the literature. Eur J Vasc Endovasc Surg 2002; 23: 283–94.

60. Naylor AR, Cuffe RL, Rothwell PM, Bell PRF. A systematic review of outcomes following staged and synchronous carotid endarterectomy and coronary artery bypass. Eur J Vasc Endovasc Surg 2003; 25: 380–9.

61. Li Y, Walicki D, Mathiesen C, et al. Strokes after cardiac surgery and relationship to carotid stenosis. Arch Neurol 2009; 66: 1091–6.

62. Ziada KM, Yadav JS, Mukherjee D, et al. Comparison of results of carotid stenting followed by open heart surgery versus combined carotid endarterectomy and open heart surgery (coronary bypass with or without another procedure). Am J Cardiol 2005; 96: 519–23.

63. Van der Heyden J, Suttorp MJ, Bal ET, et al. Staged carotid angioplasty and stenting followed by cardiac surgery in patients with severe asymptomatic carotid artery stenosis: Early and long-term results. Circulation 2007; 116: 2036–42.

64. Hanna EB, Abu-Fadel MS. Management of severe bilateral carotid artery stenosis concomitant to severely symptomatic coronary arterial disease requiring coronary artery bypass grafting: a case-based review. J Invasive Cardiol 2010; 22: E192–6.

65. Rothwell PM, Gutnikov SA, Warlow CP; European Carotid Surgery Trialist's Collaboration. Reanalysis of the final results of the European Carotid Surgery Trial. Stroke 2003; 34: 514 –23.

66. Flaherty ML, Flemming KD, McClelland R et al. Population-based study of symptomatic internal carotid artery occlusion: incidence and long-term follow-up. Stroke 2004; 35: 349–52.

67. Paty PSK, Adeniyi JA, Mehta M, et al. Surgical treatment of internal carotid artery occlusion. J Vasc Surg 2003; 37: 785–8.

Renal artery stenosis

68. Main J. Atherosclerotic renal artery stenosis, ACE inhibitors, and avoiding cardiovascular death. Heart 2005; 91: 548–52.

69. Safian RD, Madder RD. Refining the approach to renal artery revascularization. JACC Cardiovasc Interv 2009; 2: 161–74.

70. Leesar MA, Varma J, Shapira A, et al. Prediction of hypertension improvement after stenting of renal artery stenosis: comparative accuracy of translesional pressure gradients, intravascular ultrasound, and angiography. J Am Coll Cardiol 2009; 53: 2363–71.

71. ASTRAL Investigators, Wheatley K, Ives N, et al. Revascularization versus medical therapy for renal artery stenosis. N Engl J Med 2009; 361: 1953–62.

72. Cooper CJ, Murphy TP, Cutlip DE, et al; CORAL Investigators. Stenting and medical therapy for atherosclerotic renal-artery stenosis. N Engl J Med 2014; 370: 13–22.

73. Mitchell JA, Subramanian R, White CJ, et al. Predicting blood pressure improvement in hypertensive patients after renal artery stent placement. Catheter Cardiovasc Interv 2007; 69: 685–9.

74. Kalra PA, Chrysochou C, Green D, et al. The benefit of renal artery stenting in patients with atheromatous renovascular disease and advanced chronic kidney disease. Cath Cardiovasc Interv 2010; 75: 1–10.

75. Van de Ven PJ, Beutler JJ, Kaatee R, et al. Angiotensin converting enzyme inhibitor-induced renal dysfunction in atherosclerotic renovascular disease. Kidney Int 1998; 53: 986–93.

20 Aortic Diseases

I. Aortic dissection

A. Two types of aortic dissection

- Type A dissection involves the ascending aorta, with or without any other part of the aorta. Type A dissection is the most common type of aortic dissection (>65% of aortic dissections), and generally requires emergent surgical correction.
- Type B dissection involves the descending aorta and/or the aortic arch, without extension to the ascending aorta. Involvement of the aortic arch without the ascending aorta is labeled as type B dissection (ACC guidelines). Non-surgical treatment is generally recommended, with surgery reserved for vital branch compromise.

Aortic dissection, whether type A or B, can be acute (onset within the last 2 weeks) or chronic.

B. Causes

The media of the ascending aorta is rich in elastic fibers. Medial degeneration consists of a loss of elastic fibers and predisposes to ascending aortic aneurysm and dissection. Medial degeneration may be seen with repetitive injury (HTN) and aging; in fact, the combination of age and HTN is responsible for aortic dissection in most patients.

More severe medial degeneration, called cystic medial necrosis, may occur in the contexts of bicuspid aortic valve, Marfan syndrome, or coarctation of the aorta.

The aortic wall stress drastically increases with aortic size. Thus, the risk of aortic dissection and progressive aortic dilatation is drastically increased in patients whose aorta is already dilated. The yearly risk of aortic dissection or rupture is 2% if the aortic diameter is 4–5 cm, and ≥7% if the aortic diameter is >5.5–6 cm. However, since a normal-size aorta is much more common than a dilated aorta, only 40% of aortic dissections occur in patients with an aortic diameter of 5.5 cm or more, while 10–20% occur in patients with an aortic diameter of 4 cm or less.[1]

C. Mechanisms of acute and chronic aortic dissection

The typical aortic dissection consists of an intimal tear that allows blood to penetrate a diseased medial layer and cleave this media longitudinally. The blood-filled space within the media is the false lumen. Distention of the false lumen with blood may cause the intimal flap to bow into the true lumen and obstruct the lumen or the branches causing ischemia (e.g., carotid, mesenteric, or renal artery). The false lumen may also extend into the branches and cause ischemia. Most intimal tears occur in the ascending aorta, within a few centimeters of the aortic valve, or in the descending aorta just distal to the left subclavian artery.

In chronic aortic dissection, one or more *spontaneous fenestrations* occur in the intimal flap, which allows the false lumen to decompress and allows blood to flow through it. The false lumen becomes a functional lumen. Flow to vital branches supplied by the false lumen is improved, and organ ischemia improves (Figure 20.1). In fact, one of the endovascular therapies of aortic dissection consists of creating fenestrations in the intimal layer.

D. Other acute aortic syndromes: intramural hematoma and penetrating atherosclerotic ulcer

Intramural hematoma is characterized by bleeding within the media from rupture of vasa vasorum vessels without any obvious intimal tear, and thus without communication with the true lumen. This can usually be distinguished by CT: the intramural hematoma does not enhance with contrast. Invasive angiography misses intramural hematoma, owing to the lack of communication between the true and false lumens. However, the management is identical to the classical type A or B aortic dissection (intramural hematoma is more often distal, i.e., type B, than A). The prognosis and complications are similar to aortic dissection, and intramural hematoma often progresses to dissection, aneurysm, or rupture.[2,3]

Penetrating atherosclerotic ulcer is an ulceration of an atherosclerotic lesion of the aorta, usually the descending aorta, that penetrates into the media and results in a localized hematoma. There is a focal aortic outpouching rather than a false lumen. However, this ulcer may progress to a typical aortic dissection or aortic perforation, and, over time, it often leads to the late formation of aortic aneurysm or contained aortic perforation, i.e., pseudoaneurysm. Atherosclerotic ulcer is often seen in elderly patients with a heavily atherosclerotic and

Practical Cardiovascular Medicine, First Edition. Elias B. Hanna.

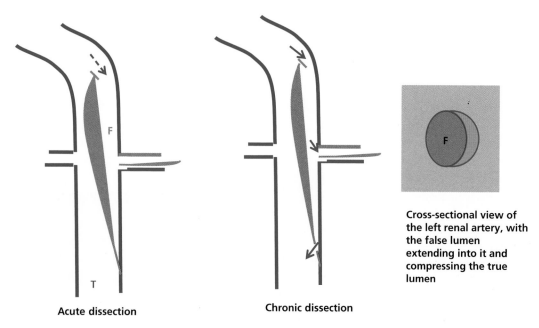

Figure 20.1 In acute aortic dissection, the false lumen (*F*) is tense with sluggish flow and becomes larger than the true lumen (*dashed arrow*). In chronic dissection, multiple tears occur in the intimal flap and allow the false lumen to decompress and blood to flow through it (*arrows*).

In this illustration, the dissection extends into the left renal artery rather than around it. Thus, the left renal artery is now practically supplied by the false lumen. There is no flow through the renal artery acutely, but once the false lumen decompresses, some flow is re-established through the false lumen of the renal artery, which becomes a functional lumen.

ulcerated *descending aorta*, many of whom already have a descending or abdominal aortic aneurysm. CT can distinguish it from a typical dissection. A penetrating ulcer is generally treated conservatively with surveillance. The treatment is surgical in case of persistent or recurrent pain, transmural extension with pseudoaneurysm, or progressive aneurysmal dilatation.

E. Clinical suspicion
Three clinical features suggest the possibility of aortic dissection:[4]

- Predisposing condition (aortic valve disease, known aortic aneurysm, Marfan, or family history of dissection).
- Suggestive symptoms: chest, back, or abdominal pain that is very abrupt (within seconds), severe, or tearing. Contrary to common belief, the pain of aortic dissection is commonly sharp rather than tearing.
- Suggestive exam findings: AI murmur (in 25–45%), pulse deficit or blood pressure differential between both arms (~20%), neurologic deficit concomitant to chest pain (5%).

The presence of two or three features makes aortic dissection highly probable. In the presence of one feature, the probability is intermediate and aortic imaging is warranted if the patient's symptoms are not clearly explained on chest X-ray or ECG. Up to 5% of aortic dissections have none of these features, but may be suspected by a widened mediastinum on chest X-ray.[4]

> Aortic dissection should be suspected in any patient with chest pain and concomitant stroke, mental status changes, or peripheral ischemia.

F. Diagnosis
Chest X-ray shows widening of the aorta and mediastinal silhouette and widening of the aortic knob in 80–90% of patients (Figures 20.2, 20.3). The "calcium sign" may be seen (outer displacement of the aortic knob calcium by more than 1 cm).

Perform any of the following three gold-standard studies to establish the diagnosis and define the type of dissection:

- CT angiogram.
- MR angiogram.
- TEE. This has the additional potential of assessing acute AI and the coronary ostia. It is also advantageous if the patient is unstable, because TEE can be performed at the bedside.
- Invasive aortography used to be the gold standard. It is still useful if the ECG shows acute STEMI but the clinical picture suggests aortic dissection. In the latter case, aortography may be performed, followed by coronary angiography once dissection is ruled out.

Typically, the false lumen is larger than the true lumen because of its slower emptying (or lack of emptying). On a TEE short-axis cut: (i) the true lumen is compressed and crescentic, while the false lumen is oval; (ii) the false lumen has "smoke" and no flow, or less flow, on Doppler imaging (Figure 20.4).

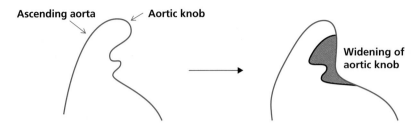

Figure 20.2 Chest X-ray in aortic dissection or dilatation.

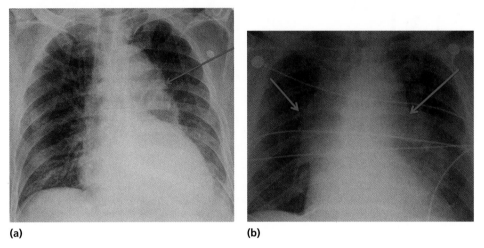

(a)   **(b)**

Figure 20.3 (a) Widening of aortic knob (*arrow*) indicative of descending aortic dissection or aneurysm. **(b)** Widening of the ascending aortic shadow (*right arrow*) and the descending aortic knob (*left arrow*). This patient has ascending and descending aortic dilatation and dissection.

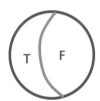

Figure 20.4 Axial cut across aortic dissection. True lumen (*T*) and false lumen (*F*) are shown.

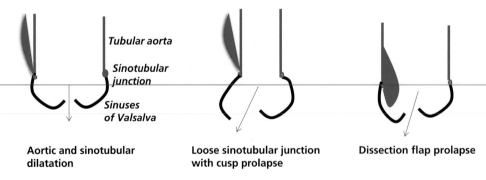

Aortic and sinotubular   **Loose sinotubular junction**   **Dissection flap prolapse**
dilatation   **with cusp prolapse**

Figure 20.5 Mechanisms of aortic insufficiency (AI) with aortic dissection: (i) dissection dilates the sinotubular junction, preventing leaflet coaptation; (ii) dissection extends into the sinotubular junction, where the sinuses of Valsalva insert, resulting in leaflet prolapse and eccentric AI; (iii) dissection flap prolapses through the aortic orifice and prevents leaflet coaptation. AI may also be pre-existent, secondary to a bicuspid aortic valve. Note that the valvular leaflets (cusps) are attached to the *sinuses of Valsalva*.

G. Complications
- Aortic regurgitation (Figure 20.5).
- Aortic rupture into the pericardium, leading to tamponade.
- Stroke is seen in 6% of type A aortic dissections. It is due to carotid obstruction by an aortic flap or extension of the dissection into a carotid artery.

- STEMI is seen in 4% of type A aortic dissections. It is easier for the dissection to extend on the outer curve of the aorta into the RCA, explaining why two-thirds of MIs are inferior MIs (IRAD registry).[2] MI may be due to the false lumen compressing the coronary ostium or extending into it. In addition, ST depression or T inversion occurs in up to 50% of patients with type A aortic dissection, as a result of demand/supply mismatch or catecholamine-induced ST–T abnormalities.[5] Those ST–T abnormalities may mimic ACS and delay the diagnosis of aortic dissection.
- Hemorrhagic, large pleural effusion may be seen with descending aortic dissection. It results from aortic leakage into the mediastinal pleural space.
- Peripheral and mesenteric ischemia.

H. Treatment

1. Administer IV β-blockers to decrease the aortic wall stress dP/dt

- Aggressively control blood pressure with β-blockers ± vasodilators. IV labetalol or the combination of IV esmolol + IV nitroprusside may be used. β-Blockers reduce the stroke volume and thus reduce the pulse pressure (dP), the slope of aortic pressure rise in systole (dP/dt), and the frequency of aortic exposure to the pulse pressure. The aortic pressure rises gradually rather than sharply (↓ dP/dt). Diltiazem IV may be used if β-blockers are contraindicated. Morphine may be used for pain control.
- Goal: Mean BP 60–70 mm Hg, SBP <120 mm Hg, heart rate <60 bpm.[6]

2. Type A aortic dissection

Emergent surgery should be performed and consists of excising the dissected segment of the aorta and interposing a prosthetic graft. If the sinuses of Valsalva are dilated, the graft needs to extend to the aortic valve. If moderate or severe AI is present, the aortic valve is repaired (resuspend the leaflets); it may need to be replaced if severe intrinsic valvular disease is present. A composite graft consisting of an aortic graft and valvular prosthesis is used whenever the aortic valve needs replacement.

> Except in a patient with PEA arrest, avoid preoperative pericardiocentesis for aortic dissection-induced tamponade. Pericardiocentesis may, in this context, reopen a clotted communication between the aorta and the pericardial space and precipitate hemodynamic collapse.

3. Type B aortic dissection

Aggressive blood pressure control is the initial therapy. Surgery is indicated for: (i) impending aortic rupture, such as aneurysmal dilatation of the false lumen; or (ii) peripheral ischemia, such as carotid, mesenteric, renal, spinal cord, or lower extremity ischemia.

Surgery may simply involve revascularization of the ischemic territories rather than extensive, laborious aortic repair.

Surgery is not typically indicated solely for persistent pain (pain being secondary to a distended false lumen).

4. If surgery is not performed, the mortality risk with type A dissection is 1% per hour for the first 48 hours (~50% at 48 hours) and 85% at 2 weeks.

> One study has shown that medially treated type B aortic dissection has the lowest 30-day mortality (10%), considerably lower than type B aortic dissection that requires surgical therapy (31%) or type A aortic dissection treated surgically (26%) or medically (>60%).[2]

> Hypotension in a patient with aortic dissection may be:
>
> - Pseudo-hypotension resulting from the obstruction of flow to one limb. Measuring blood pressure in all limbs may unveil this phenomenon.
> - True hypotension resulting from tamponade or acute AI. A clinical shock with impaired mental status occurs. Patients with a truly severe hypotension are stabilized with fluid resuscitation and vasopressors if needed, until surgery is performed.

5. In survivors, there is a long-term risk of AI, recurrence of dissection, and secondary aneurysm formation, especially during the first 2 years. This mandates frequent CT/MRI monitoring every 3–6 months for the first 2 years then every 6–12 months afterward.

6. Chronic dissection (= dissection that occurred >2 weeks prior)

Whether it is type A or B, chronic medical therapy without surgical intervention is the initial treatment of choice at this point. Medical therapy consists of aggressive BP control (SBP <130 mmHg) with regular monitoring for aneurysm formation and size, extension of the dissection, and development of severe AI. *Aneurysmal dilatation of the aorta, particularly the false lumen, occurs frequently and dictates surgery.*

I. Notes on surgical techniques

1. Ascending aortic dissection

Cardiopulmonary bypass is initiated through a femoral vein–femoral arterial access, then deep hypothermic circulatory arrest is initiated for <30 minutes. This circulatory standstill allows suturing the graft distally, at the junction with the aortic arch; the distal ascending aorta is sewn and the suture strengthened with Teflon felt. The distal extent of the dissection into the arch or the descending aorta does not need

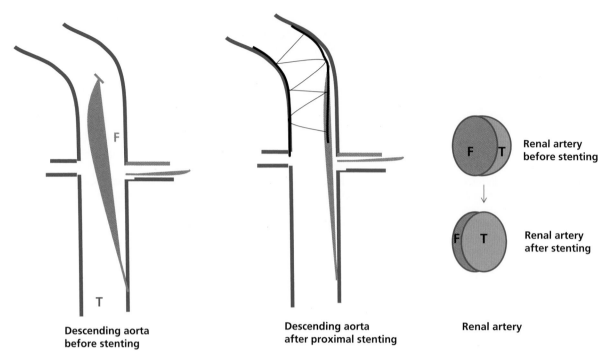

Figure 20.6 Descending aortic dissection with false lumen extending into the renal artery. A stent graft covering the proximal part of the dissection impedes flow through the false lumen. This makes the false lumen collapse and allows the true lumen to expand. If this does not re-establish flow across the renal artery or worsens flow across it (e.g., chronic dissection with functional false lumen flow), the true lumen of the renal artery may be stented, which allows it to expand and provide flow.

to be replaced as long as the false lumen is sealed proximally; sealing of the false lumen in the ascending aorta prevents it from expanding and allows it to collapse. After performing the distal graft anastomosis, the graft is clamped, the patient is rewarmed, and cardiopulmonary bypass is reinitiated through a peripheral artery. The proximal dissection tear is then localized and the aorta is removed proximally to the tear, followed by proximal suturing of the graft.

If the dissection extends to the sinuses, or if the sinuses are dilated, the graft may be extended to the aortic valve, and the valve and coronaries reimplanted and sutured to the graft (David reimplantation). An abnormal valve may require the use of a composite aorta–valve graft.

2. Dissection extending into the aortic arch with malperfusion
If the dissection extends into the branches of the aortic arch with malperfusion, the involved branches may be debranched and bypassed from the ascending aortic graft (or ascending aorta if only the arch is involved).

3. Acute type B aortic dissection that requires therapy (peripheral ischemia)
Stenting the entry point may be all that is needed. Percutaneous stenting of the entry point with a stent graft prevents the expansion of the false lumen and leads to its thrombosis (class I recommendation). The false lumen shrinks, and even if it was extending into visceral arteries, this shrinking allows the expansion of the true lumen of these organs. In fact, stenting re-establishes flow to ischemic organs supplied or compressed by the false lumen and relieves ischemia in 76% of the obstructed branches (Figure 20.6).[7]

Other percutaneous procedures are alternatively performed: (i) distal fenestration of the intimal flap may be performed to decompress the false lumen and allow flow through it into the distal organs; (ii) the affected branch(es) may be stented through the true lumen to allow true luminal flow. Alternatively, bypass surgery of the ischemic territories (mesenteric, iliac) may be performed.

Chronic type B dissection may not benefit from the use of aortic stent graft as much as acute type B dissection. Because of spontaneous distal fenestration, the false lumen may have flow and may supply vital organs. The use of a thoracic stent graft is, however, necessary in case of aneurysmal dilatation of the aorta; in this case, arterial branches distal to the graft may need to be stented through the true lumen if ischemia develops (Figure 20.6).

II. Thoracic aortic aneurysm
While the ascending aorta is richer in elastic fibers than the descending aorta, the descending aorta is much more likely to become heavily atherosclerotic than the ascending aorta. This explains the differences in etiology of ascending vs. descending thoracic aneurysms. ***Ascending aortic aneurysm or dissection is caused by cystic medial degeneration, while descending aortic aneurysm is caused by atherosclerosis***. Only rarely, cystic medial necrosis extends to the descending aorta and leads to aneurysmal dilatation of the entire thoracic aorta. On a similar note, atherosclerosis infrequently leads to aneurysmal dilatation of the ascending aorta. *Arch aneurysms* are related to either medial degeneration or atherosclerosis, and are often an extension of an adjacent ascending or descending aneurysm.

Cystic medial degeneration may result from repetitive aortic injury occurring with age and HTN, or from connective tissue disorders (Marfan), or may be associated with bicuspid aortic valve or a history of aortic coarctation.

AI induces a large stroke volume and a high shear stress on the aortic wall, which worsens the aortic dilatation. However, severe aortic dilatation is not fully caused by AI. Rather, aortic dilatation is usually the cause of AI or is associated with the same connective tissue disorder as AI (e.g., bicuspid aortic valve). AS may also lead to some aortic enlargement as the high-velocity stenotic jet hits the aorta (post-stenotic dilatation).

Chronic aortic dissection may lead to progressive aortic dilatation and aneurysm formation because of the weakened media or the progressive enlargement of the false lumen.

A. Ascending thoracic aortic aneurysm (TAA)

Three levels of TAA must be distinguished (sinuses of Valsalva, sinotubular junction, and tubular aorta). Ascending TAA may involve the sinuses of Valsalva or may be limited to the tubular portion of the aorta, above the sinuses, as in many elderly hypertensive patients with TAA (Figure 20.7). Typically, aortic dilatation associated with bicuspid aortic valve or connective tissue disorders involves both the sinuses and the tubular aorta and may involve the annulus (in the latter case, it is called annuloaortic ectasia). Approximately 40–50% of patients with bicuspid aortic valve have aortic dilatation by the age of 30, most often involving the mid-tubular aorta but frequently involving the sinuses and the sinotubular junction as well.[8] In one study of all comers with bicuspid aortic valve (mean age of 43 years), the overall prevalence of aortic dilatation >37 mm was 79% at the mid-tubular aorta and 58% at the sinuses of Valsalva (aortic root). It is usually mild, <45 mm. The prevalence and severity of aortic dilatation increases with age.[8,9]

Dilatation that involves the sinuses or the sinotubular junction is the most common cause of severe AI requiring surgery.

1. Diagnosis

TTE provides good images for measurement of the aortic root at the sinuses of Valsalva, sinotubular junction, and early tubular aorta, but may totally miss the mid-ascending aorta. TEE allows more extensive aortic measurements, but cannot accurately assess the distal ascending aorta and the aortic arch; also, the cut may be oblique rather than central.

CT provides excellent diagnostic value for the whole extent of the aorta. However, axial measurements overestimate the true diameter of the aorta, especially in patients with an elongated, widely curved rather than vertical aorta. Also, axial cuts may miss an aneurysm at the level of the sinuses. Three-dimensional reconstruction overcomes these pitfalls (Figure 20.8).

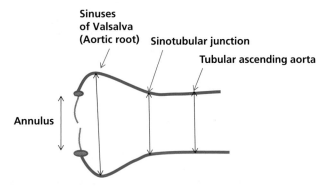

Figure 20.7 Various aortic measurements. The annulus is a stable structure that is part of the ventricle/outflow tract and infrequently dilates, but may dilate in connective tissue disorders (bicuspid aortic valve, Marfan). The aortic diameter at the sinuses of Valsalva level (i.e., the aortic dilatations where the aortic cusps insert, also called aortic root) is normally up to 3.7 cm, while the diameter of the proximal ascending aorta and of the sinotubular junction (junction of the tubular ascending aorta with the sinuses of Valsalva) is normally up to 3.2 cm (must be adjusted for height).

Aortic dilatation may occur at the level of the ascending aorta and sinotubular junction (e.g., HTN), or may involve the sinuses of Valsalva. Aortic dilatation associated with bicuspid aortic valve and cystic medial necrosis (Marfan disease) often involves the sinuses as well as the aorta more distally. HTN often affects the aorta distal to the sinuses with less effect on the sinuses (e.g., in HTN, the sinotubular junction and distal ascending aorta are dilated with normal diameter at the sinuses).

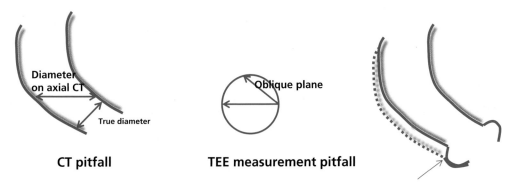

Figure 20.8 Pitfalls of aortic measurements by axial CT and TEE. On TEE or TTE, the aorta may be cut in an oblique plane and miss the major dimension, potentially underestimating the true aortic diameter. Beside the size, the loss of indentation at the sinotubular junction (on CT or invasive angiography, *arrow*) suggests aortic dilatation.

2. Prognosis and surgical indications

Ascending TAA is associated with a yearly risk of aortic dissection and rupture of ≥7% when the aortic diameter exceeds 5.5–6 cm (in one study, the risk of dissection/rupture sharply increased to 34% at 6 cm); this yearly risk is 2% when the aortic diameter is <5 cm.[10,11] Since the surgical mortality approximates 5%, 5.5 cm is considered an appropriate surgical cutoff. Conversely, patients with Marfan have a 40% lifetime risk of aortic dissection or rupture, explaining the earlier need for surgical therapy in these patients. The ascending aorta of patients with bicuspid aortic valve grows more quickly and tends to dissect and rupture at a younger age than degenerative TAA; 25% of these patients require aortic surgery at 25-year follow-up, mainly for aortic dilatation or in conjunction with aortic valve surgery (the risk of aortic dissection in properly followed patients is actually low, ~1% at 25-year follow-up).[12]

While the aorta at the level of the sinuses of Valsalva is normally larger than the supracoronary tubular aorta, the same cutoffs are used for both levels to decide on the need for aortic surgery:[6]

- Aorta or sinuses ≥5.5 cm
- Aortic growth ≥0.5 cm/year (the growth is usually 0.1 cm/year)
- Aorta or sinuses ≥4.5 cm in patients undergoing aortic valve surgery
- Aorta or sinuses ≥5 cm in case of Marfan syndrome, familial thoracic aortic disease, other connective tissue disorders (Turner, aortic coarctation), or bicuspid aortic valve with a family history of aortic dissection. For bicuspid aortic valve without a family history of dissection or rapid growth, 5.5 cm is the aortic cutoff that indicates surgery. The cutoff may be altered depending on the patient's height, and surgery is indicated for a smaller aorta of 4.5–5 cm if aortic area/height >10 cm²/m (aortic area being equal to 0.785 × diameter²). Patients with the genetic Loeys–Dietz syndrome have a surgical indication at a cutoff of 4.4 cm.
- Chronic, unexplained, chest or back pain. Pain results from impingement on adjacent structures and may predict a risk of aortic rupture. In acute rupture, acute severe pain, collapse, or rupture into an adjacent structure (pleura, bronchus) occurs.

3. Surgical treatment

There are three forms of TAA repair:

I. If the sinuses are not dilated and the aortic valve is not significantly affected (no moderate or severe AS or AI), the ascending aorta is replaced and the graft sutured proximally at the sinotubular junction.

II. If the sinuses are dilated and the valve has significant regurgitation secondary to the aortic dilatation but is not significantly calcified or fibrotic, the native aorta and sinuses are removed (after freeing the coronary buttons), but the valvular leaflets are left in place and the aortic graft is extended all the way to the aortic valve. The graft is sutured to the aortic annulus and the aortic leaflets are resuspended if prolapsed. The coronary buttons are then sutured to the graft (David procedure, which may be performed even if the valve is bicuspid) (Figure 20.9).

III. If the sinuses are dilated and the valve has severe intrinsic abnormality, a composite graft (aorta and aortic valve) is used to replace both the aorta and aortic valve. The coronary buttons are sutured to the aortic graft (Bentall procedure), sometimes with the use of interposition graft (Cabrol procedure).

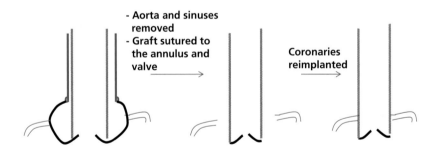

Aortic graft with valve sparing/resuspension

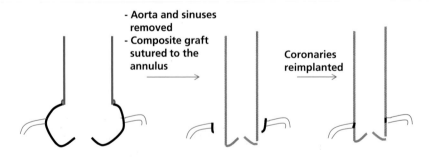

Composite graft of the aorta and aortic valve

Figure 20.9 Ascending aortic repair with valve sparing (top) and with composite graft (bottom).

Hypothermic circulatory arrest may be needed for the distal anastomosis if aortic replacement is extended up to the aortic arch, without a good landing zone for aortic clamping and cardiopulmonary bypass. Hypothermic arrest is also needed if the aortic arch is additionally replaced.

4. Perioperative complications
Mortality (3–5%), MI (5–7%), stroke (2–5%).

5. Surveillance schedule when surgery is not indicated
A yearly CT is indicated when the aorta is 3.5–4.4 cm. CT is indicated every 6 months when the aorta is 4.5–5.4 cm. On average, the thoracic aneurysm grows by 0.1 cm per year.[10] The tensile wall stress increases with the aortic radius, and thus the larger the aorta, the faster it grows (Laplace law).

It is reasonable for patients with bicuspid aortic valve to undergo, at least once, a screening with CT to assess for dilatation throughout the ascending aorta. Those with aortic diameter >4 cm should undergo yearly surveillance with echo, CT, or MRI. Echo is appropriate if the dilatation predominantly involves the sinuses, sinotubular junction, or proximal tubular aorta, with the condition that these segments are adequately visualized by echo.

B. Descending TAA
Two forms of treatment are available for descending TAA: (i) open replacement of the aorta with a graft, and (ii) percutaneous endograft placement (stent graft). Endograft placement has the potential advantage of being much less invasive with lower postoperative morbidity and mortality and is of particular value in poor surgical candidates. In fact, the postoperative mortality is 5–14% with open repair and is probably lower with endograft placement (~5%).[13,14] Both open repair and endograft repair of the descending TAA are associated with a loss of intercostal branches and a risk of spinal cord ischemia and paraplegia. This currently occurs in 5–6% of open repairs, and is probably as likely to happen with endograft procedures. This risk is higher if the repaired aorta is long or if the patient has already had abdominal aortic aneurysm repair.

In patients with extensive thoracoabdominal aneurysms, the endograft may have to extend into the distal aorta and cover branches, such as celiac, renal, or superior mesenteric artery. In those cases, in addition to the endograft, the covered branches need to be bypassed from the distal aorta or from branches distal to the endograft (e.g., mesenteric to celiac bypass, iliac to renal bypass) (Figure 20.10).[15] If an open repair is performed, these branches are reimplanted into the graft.

The cutoff for descending aortic repair is 5.5 cm in patients who can undergo endograft placement. In patients with a high surgical risk and no endograft option, the cutoff for open repair is 6 cm. In patients with chronic type B dissection, endograft may worsen distal organ perfusion provided by the false lumen and is given a class IIb recommendation; open repair is preferred in the ACC guidelines and is given a class I recommendation for chronic dissection.[6]

C. Aortic arch aneurysm
Treatment of aortic arch aneurysm is indicated when the aortic diameter is ≥5.5 cm. In low-risk patients, classic surgical correction is done; this involves removal of the brachiocephalic arteries en bloc at their common base, followed by replacement of the aortic arch with a graft and reimplantation of the brachiocephalic bloc (deep hypothermic arrest required). Alternatively, in patients with comorbidities, a stent

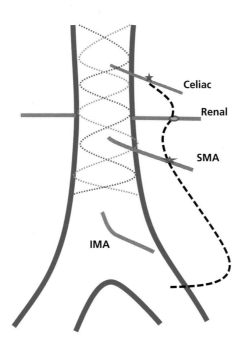

Figure 20.10 Throracoabdominal endograft covering the renal arteries, celiac trunk, and superior mesenteric artery (SMA). The latter branches are ligated and bypassed from the left iliac artery using a sequential graft. IMA, inferior mesenteric artery.

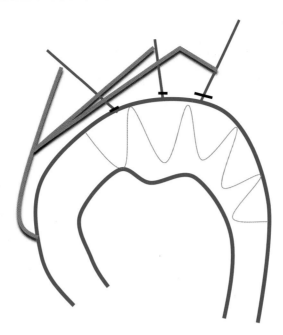

Figure 20.11 Debranching of the brachiocephalic vessels followed by antegrade placement of a stent graft into the arch and descending aorta through the ascending aorta. If the ascending aorta is dilated >4–4.5 cm, it may need to be replaced to allow a good proximal seal of the stent graft. The ascending aorta is replaced first, with hypothermic arrest for the distal anastomosis and cardiopulmonary bypass for the proximal anastomosis. If the ascending aorta does not need replacement, cardiopulmonary bypass may not be needed.

graft may be positioned in an open antegrade fashion to cover the arch (and the descending aorta if needed), after debranching the brachiocephalic arteries and attaching them to the ascending aorta (hybrid procedure) (ACC guidelines) (Figure 20.11).[6] This is done without hypothermic arrest, and sometimes without a need for cardiopulmonary bypass, using a partial aortic clamp. Aortic arch procedures are associated with a high mortality that approaches 10% and a stroke risk of ~8–10%.

When aortic arch aneurysm is associated with ascending aortic aneurysm, the ascending aorta is replaced, the brachiocephalic vessels are then debranched and attached to the ascending aortic graft, and a stent graft is antegradely placed to cover the arch.

In patients with aneurysm involving the ascending aorta, arch, and descending aorta, a complex surgery called elephant trunk may be performed (replacement of the ascending aorta and arch, with part of the graft protruding into the descending aorta; this is followed by placement of an endograft in the descending aorta, attached to the protruded graft). Alternatively, an ascending aortic graft is placed, followed by debranching of the brachiocephalic vessels then endograft placement over the arch and descending aorta.

D. Traumatic transection of the aorta
Deceleration trauma leads to aortic transection, most commonly at the level of the isthmus, immediately past the left subclavian artery. Most of these individuals die immediately. The remaining patients form a pseudoaneurysm and may be treated surgically or with an endograft (class I indication). Stable patients may not need to be treated urgently.

Some undiagnosed patients go on to develop a chronic aortic pseudoaneurysm, which, as opposed to an aneurysm, is usually eccentric and saccular rather than fusiform. A pseudoaneurysm may also be postoperative or spontaneous (penetrating aortic ulcer). Since it implies a contained aortic rupture, it is appropriately treated with an endograft, regardless of size.

E. Medical therapy of TAA
β-Blocker therapy reduces stroke volume and thus reduces pulse pressure and ejectional wall stress (dP/dt or sharpness of pressure rise). However, only one small randomized trial supports its specific use in Marfan TAA.[16] Some evidence suggests that ARB reduces the progression of aortic dilatation in Marfan.[17] Overall, in patients with TAA from any cause and no surgical indication, β-blocker therapy and aggressive blood pressure reduction with a β-blocker and an ARB are recommended (ACC guidelines recommend blood pressure reduction to the lowest point tolerated).

III. Abdominal aortic aneurysm
An arterial aneurysm is defined as a focal arterial dilatation over 1.5 times the normal baseline diameter or the expected normal diameter. Abdominal aortic aneurysm (AAA) is generally defined as an abdominal aorta >3 cm. AAA is often infrarenal, but may extend above the renal arteries and may be thoracoabdominal. Similarly to descending TAA, AAA is related to atherosclerotic weakening of the aortic wall, smoking being the primary risk factor for AAA. Genetics contribute to the occurrence of AAA, and AAA occurs in up to 30% of siblings of patients with AAA.[18]

Approximately 10% of patients with AAA have popliteal aneurysms, usually bilateral aneurysms, which should always be sought. On the other hand, ~40% of patients with popliteal aneurysms have AAA. The main risks of popliteal aneurysms are thrombosis, embolization, and limb ischemia rather than rupture.

Table 20.1 Types of endoleaks.

Type 1	Poor sealing at the proximal or distal end of the graft.
Type 2	Retrograde endoleak from collateral flow. Leak from lumbar, inferior mesenteric, internal iliac or middle sacral artery that are covered by the endograft but receive retrograde flow through collaterals[a]
Type 3	Fabric tear or stent frame fracture or separation

[a] Type 2 endoleak may be followed with serial CT scans and treated selectively if the aneurysmal sac grows.

A. Diagnosis

Ultrasound is the best screening tool, but CT generally provides more accurate sizing and better defines the extent of AAA and its relation with branch vessels (e.g., renal arteries). CT is a better modality in patients whose AAA is close to surgical cutoffs (>4 cm). MRI may alternatively be used.

The wall of AAA being usually laminated with thrombus, invasive angiography underestimates the true size of AAA.

AAA usually grows by 0.4 cm/year (faster than TAA, as the aortic pressure further amplifies distally).[13]

B. Surgical treatment of AAA, iliac aneurysm, popliteal aneurysm

In men, the yearly risk of rupture is 1.5% for AAA <5.5 cm, ~10% for AAA 5.5–7 cm, and 35% for AAA ≥7 cm.[19–21] Two studies have shown that in men with AAA <5.5 cm, surgical repair is associated with the same survival as surveillance and later repair.[19,20] However, AAA ruptures earlier in women (mean 5 cm in women vs. 6 cm in men) and 3 times more frequently; thus, earlier repair may be warranted in women.[13] In conclusion, surgical repair is indicated for AAA ≥5.5 cm in men and 4.5–5 cm in women, AAA expanding >1 cm/year or 0.5 cm/6 months, or symptomatic AAA regardless of size. AAA is considered symptomatic when associated with atheroembolization or with prolonged episodes of hypogastric or back pain, lasting hours. A vague and non-specific abdominal pain may be attributed to AAA if no other explanation is found.

Surgical mortality is ~5% in elective cases (2% in low-risk patients); ~50% in emergent cases of aortic rupture.

Surgical treatment consists of opening the aneurysm longitudinally with clot removal, followed by transecting the aneurysmal pocket proximally and distally, then suturing a graft proximally and distally to the iliac arteries. The open aneurysmal sac is left in place and wrapped around the graft for support and protection from the bowels.

Common and internal iliac aneurysms are rarely isolated and frequently accompany AAA (up to 40% of AAAs). Rupture may occur when the aneurysm exceeds 3–3.5 cm in diameter, this being used as a threshold for repair. A popliteal aneurysm is treated when it exceeds 2 cm, preferably before limb ischemia occurs; when the latter occurs, the risk of limb loss is high.

C. Percutaneous endovascular aortic repair (EVAR)

EVAR involves stent graft placement at the level of the aneurysm, excluding the AAA from the circulation. It leads to a lower perioperative mortality than open repair. Endoleaks, however, frequently occur. An endoleak means that the aneurysm is not fully excluded from the circulation; it is identified by a persistent flow of contrast into the aneurysm (Table 20.1). Because of endoleaks, endovascular repair is mainly indicated for patients at intermediate or high operative risk.

The EVAR-1 and DREAM trials have shown that, in comparison with open repair, EVAR is associated with a lower early mortality (1.8% vs. 4.3%), but a higher late mortality, such that the survival curves merge at 2 years.[22,23] There is a slightly higher risk of graft rupture with EVAR (up to 2% per year), and a significantly higher need for reinterventions for endoleaks (~20–30% at 6 years). In the particular case of AAA >6.5 cm, EVAR is associated with a high risk of late complications, because of inappropriate seal and inability to fully exclude AAA. Types 1 and 3 endoleaks have, however, been recently reduced with the newer generation of devices.

In patients unsuitable for open repair, EVAR is performed, but in those high-risk patients even EVAR has a high early mortality (8%) and most patients die from comorbidities within 5 years, without a clear benefit of EVAR in terms of overall survival (EVAR-2 trial).[24]

The technical requirements for EVAR are: at least 1.5 cm of normal aorta (diameter <3 cm) between the renal arteries and the AAA to allow proximal anchoring of the device, minimal angulation of the AAA, patency of the superior mesenteric/celiac side branches (as the inferior mesenteric branch is covered by the endograft), and patent distal iliac vessels ≥7 mm in diameter. The endograft is a bifurcating endograft that covers the aorta and both iliacs. It has two parts: (i) a body and a right limb landing into the right iliac (deployed through a right femoral access), and (ii) a left limb landing into the left iliac (deployed through a left femoral access).

D. Surveillance for smaller aneurysms (3.0–5.5 cm)

CT or ultrasound is performed every 1–2 years for AAA <4 cm, every 6 months for AAA 4–4.9 cm, and every 3 months for AAA >5 cm. β-Blockers are provided to reduce dP/dt, and blood pressure is aggressively reduced (e.g., <130/80 mm Hg). ACE inhibitors may be of particular benefit.[25] Rupture is more likely to occur in active smokers, and smoking cessation is therefore paramount.

References

1. Elefteriades JA, Farkas EA. Thoracic aortic aneurysm. Clinically pertinent controversies and uncertainties. J Am Coll Cardiol 2010; 55: 841–57.
2. Hagan PG, Nienaber CA, Isselbacher EM, et al. The international registry of acute aortic dissection. JAMA 2000; 283: 897–903.
3. Song JK, Kim HS, Kang DH, et al. Different clinical features of aortic intramural hematoma versus dissection involving the ascending aorta. J Am Coll Cardiol 2001; 37: 1604–10.
4. Rogers AM, Hermann LK, Booher AM, et al. Sensitivity of the aortic dissection detection risk score, a novel guideline-based tool for identification of acute aortic dissection at initial presentation. Circulation 2011; 123: 2213–18.
5. Kosuge M, Uchida K, Imoto K, et al. Frequency and implications of ST-T abnormalities on hospital admission electrocardiograms in patients with type A aortic dissection. Am J Cardiol 2013; 112: 424–9.

6. Hiratzka LF, Bakris GL, Beckman JA, et al. ACCF/AHA/AATS/ACR/ASA/SCA/SCAI/SIR/STS/SVM guidelines for the diagnosis and management of patients with thoracic aortic disease. Circulation 2010; 121: e266–369.

7. Dake MD, Kato N, Mitchell RS, et al. Endovascular stent-graft placement for the treatment of acute aortic dissection. N Engl J Med 1999; 340: 1546–52.

8. Della Corte A, Bancone C, Quarto C, et al. Predictors of ascending aortic dilatation with bicuspid aortic valve: a wide spectrum of disease expression. Eur J Cardiothorac Surg 2007; 31: 397–404.

9. Nistri S, Grande-Allen J, Noale M, et al. Aortic elasticity and size in bicuspid aortic valve syndrome. Eur Heart J 2008; 29: 472–9.

10. Davies RR, Goldstein LJ, Coady MA, et al. Yearly rupture or dissection rates for thoracic aortic aneurysms: simple prediction based on size. Ann Thorac Surg 2002; 73: 17–28.

11. Coady MA, Rizzo JA, Hammond GL, et al. What is the appropriate size criterion for resection of thoracic aortic aneurysm? J Thorac Cardiovasc Surg 1997; 113: 476–91. *Ascending aorta >6 cm → risk of rupture/dissection 34%, descending aorta: 6–7 cm: ~15%, > 7 cm: 40%. The hinge point for the sharp rise of rupture/dissection is 6 cm for ascending aorta, 7 cm for descending aorta.*

12. Michelena HI, Khanna AD, Mahoney D, et al. Incidence of aortic complications in patients with bicuspid aortic valves. JAMA 2011; 306: 1104–12.

13. Isselbacher E. Thoracic and abdominal aortic aneurysms. Circulation. 2005; 111: 816–28.

14. Ellozy SH, Carroccio A, Minor M, et al. Challenges of endovascular tube graft repair of thoracic aortic aneurysm: midterm follow-up and lessons learned. J Vasc Surg 2003; 38: 676–83.

15. Flye MW, Choi ET, Sanchez LA, et al. Retrograde visceral vessel revascularization followed by endovascular aneurysm exclusion as an alternative to open surgical repair of thoracoabdominal aortic aneurysm. J Vasc Surg 2004; 39: 454–8.

16. Shores J, Berger KR, Murphy EA, Pyeritz RE. Progression of aortic dilatation and the benefit of long-term β-adrenergic blockade in Marfan's syndrome. N Engl J Med 1994; 330: 1335–41.

17. Groenink M, Alexander W. den Hartog, Franken R, et al. Losartan reduces aortic dilatation rate in adults with Marfan syndrome: a randomized controlled trial. Eur Heart J 2013; 34: 3491–500.

18. Frydman G, Walker PJ, Summers K, et al. The value of screening in siblings of patients with abdominal aortic aneurysm. Eur J Vasc Endovasc Surg 2003; 26: 396–400.

19. Lederle FA, Wilson SE, Johnson GR, et al. Aneurysm Detection And Management Veterans Affairs Cooperative Study Group. Immediate repair compared with surveillance of small abdominal aortic aneurysms. N Engl J Med 2002; 346: 1437–44.

20. UK Small Aneurysm Trial Participants. Mortality results for randomised controlled trial of early elective surgery or ultrasonographic surveillance for small abdominal aortic aneurysms. Lancet 1998; 352: 1649–55.

21. Lederle FA, Johnson JR, Wilson SE, et al. Rupture rate of large abdominal aortic aneurysms in patients refusing or unfit for elective repair. JAMA 2002; 287: 2968–72.

22. United Kingdom EVAR Trial Investigators. Endovascular versus open repair of abdominal aortic aneurysm. N Engl J Med 2010; 362: 1863–71.

23. De Bruin J, Baas A, Buth J. Long-term outcome of open or endovascular repair of abdominal aortic aneurysm. N Engl J Med 2010; 362: 1881–9. *DREAM trial.*

24. United Kingdom EVAR Trial Investigators. Endovascular repair of aortic aneurysm in patients physically ineligible for open repair. N Engl J Med 2010; 362: 1872–80. *In comparison to no repair, EVAR reduces aneurysm-related mortality but has a high early procedural mortality and late need for reintervention. Overall, no effect on late mortality in those high risk patients.*

25. Diehm M, Baumgartner I. ACE inhibitors and abdominal aortic aneurysms. Lancet 2006; 368: 659–65.

Part 9   OTHER CARDIOVASCULAR DISEASE STATES

21   Pulmonary Embolism and Deep Vein Thrombosis

1. PULMONARY EMBOLISM

I. Presentation of pulmonary embolism (PE) and risk factors

A. Signs and symptoms

- Dyspnea and tachypnea are the most common findings; however, they may not be seen at rest and may be purely exertional.
- Tachycardia is common and is occasionally an isolated finding. Frequently, however, tachycardia is either *transient* or *relative* (80–90 bpm).
- Chest pain is usually a pleuritic pain in patients with distal emboli; angina-like pain may be seen in patients with large central emboli and secondary RV ischemia. Hemoptysis is seen with pulmonary infarction, often resulting from small distal emboli.
- Hypotension, syncope, and RV failure with increased JVP/RV heave/right-sided S_3 are seen with large PE and imply reduced hemodynamic reserve.
- Lower extremity edema or tenderness on palpation is seen in 50% of DVTs.

Practical Cardiovascular Medicine, First Edition. Elias B. Hanna.
© 2017 John Wiley & Sons Ltd. Published 2017 by John Wiley & Sons Ltd.

B. Risk factors (see Table 21.1)

Table 21.1 Risk factors for PE/DVT.

- Active cancer within the last 6 months, or active therapy for cancer
- Transient major risk factors within the last 4 weeks: acute medical illness with hospitalization, surgery, trauma
- Transient minor risk factors: pregnancy, oral contraceptive therapy, travel >8 hours
- History of PE/DVT
- Hypercoagulability
  - Genetic: factor V Leiden, prothrombin gene mutation, protein C or S deficiency, antithrombin III deficiency
  - Acquired: antiphospholipid syndrome, active cancer, myeloproliferative disorders, nephrotic syndrome
- Idiopathic: ~10% of patients with idiopathic PE/DVT will end up being diagnosed with cancer within the next year
- Other risk factors: age, smoking, obesity

II. Probability of PE

The clinical probability of PE is assessed using the Wells criteria, which essentially give weight to three features:[1]

- No alternative diagnosis for the patient's presentation, whether it is dyspnea, hypoxia <95%, chest pain, or tachycardia
- Major risk factors for DVT/PE
- Clinical signs of DVT or hemoptysis

The probability is high when two or three features are present, intermediate when only one feature is present, and low when none is present.

III. Initial workup
ECG, chest X-ray, and arterial blood gas (ABG) are initially performed to look for alternative explanations and for suggestive PE signs.

A. ECG
ECG findings in PE:

- Sinus tachycardia or "relative" tachycardia (80–100 bpm) is common.
- Right axis deviation, RVH/RBBB, P pulmonale.
- T-wave inversion in the anterior precordial leads, corresponding to RV strain.[2]
- Deep S in lead I, Q and T-wave inversion in the inferior lead III and sometimes aVF ($S_1Q_3T_3$). The deep S wave in lead I actually represents depolarization of an RV that has expanded down and to the right, and corresponds to right-axis deviation.[3,4]

These findings are not specific for PE and may be seen in any RV volume or pressure overload state, whether acute or chronic. In the right context, however, they are specific for PE. Sinus tachycardia is sensitive (~50–70%); each one of the other criteria is ~10–20% sensitive, and the combination of several of them is ~50% sensitive for the diagnosis of PE. When PE is large enough to produce marked hypoxemia or shock, several of those changes are almost always present, especially T inversion in V_1–V_3, which is present in 85% of massive or submassive PE. A heart rate that is consistently ≤60 bpm in a patient who is not receiving rate-slowing drugs makes PE highly unlikely. *It is important to look at the admission ECG, as tachycardia may be transient.*

B. Arterial blood gas
Arterial blood gas usually shows hypoxia, hypocapnia, and a high A–a gradient (>10 mmHg at ambient air, >50 mmHg on high-dose O_2). O_2 saturation and A–a gradient are, however, normal in up to 20% of the patients.[5] An abnormal A–a gradient is non-specific and is seen in most pulmonary illnesses as a result of ventilation/perfusion mismatch. Hypercapnia is rare and frequently suggests a different diagnosis or an associated illness (e.g., COPD). Only a massive PE with massive increase in dead space can cause hypercapnia, per se.

C. Chest X-ray
Chest X-ray is grossly normal. It often shows some subtle abnormalities (linear atelectasis, pleural effusion, pulmonary artery cutoff sign).

D. D-dimer
D-dimer is a fibrin degradation product that results from the intrinsic, albeit ineffective, lysis of a clot. If the PE pre-test probability is low and D-dimer is negative, PE can be ruled out. A positive D-dimer, on the other hand, is non-specific and may be seen with any inflammation, pregnancy, or active clotting for any reason, e.g., cancer, bleed, trauma, medical procedure, or even venipuncture. D-dimer should not be used in the high pre-test probability population, especially the cancer population (in whom falsely negative and positive results may be seen).

IV. Specific PE workup
A diagnostic strategy is provided in Figure 21.1 (ESC).[1,5] If PE is highly probable and the bleeding risk is low, start IV unfractionated heparin (UFH) therapy, then establish a definitive diagnosis:

- *Spiral CT PE protocol* is very sensitive but may miss subsegmental, small PEs (Figure 21.2). Meta-analyses of long-term follow-ups of CT results have shown that CT is almost as accurate as pulmonary angiogram for ruling out PE. The negative predictive value is 95–99%, and in patients with a negative study the rate of PE diagnosis or mortality on 3-month follow-up is very low (<1%).[6,7] Moreover, spiral CT can establish other diagnoses (pneumonia, pulmonary edema) and establish the severity of PE by looking at RV enlargement and inter-ventricular septal bulge.

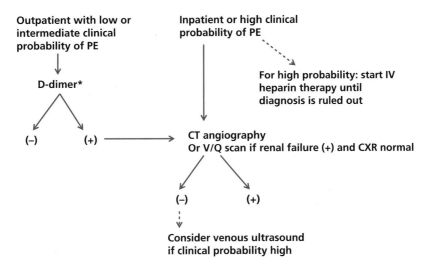

Figure 21.1 Algorithm for the diagnosis of pulmonary embolism.
*Most hospitalized patients have an elevated D-dimer because of comorbidities, inflammation, or blood draws. Hospitalized patients should undergo initial testing with an imaging study.

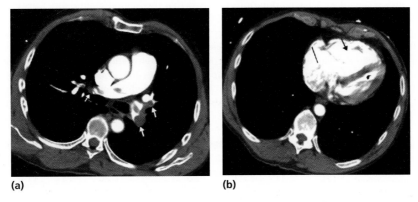

(a)   **(b)**

Figure 21.2 (a) Massive bilateral PEs in the proximal right and left pulmonary arteries, as evidenced by the filling defects (*arrows*). **(b)** RV (*arrow*) and RA (*line*) enlargement. RV and RA are the anterior structures; see how the RV is more than three times the size of the LV (*dot*). RA is also much larger than LA.

Performing a lower extremity venous CT along with the same study increases the sensitivity, especially in high clinical probability cases.[8] The main risk of CT is contrast-induced renal failure.

While the thrombus often lyses within weeks of anticoagulant therapy, defects may persist on CT for over 6 months in up to 50% of patients, albeit becoming eccentric and non-occlusive (recanalized). Thus, on a repeat study, defects in the same territory do not necessarily imply recurrent PE.[9]

- *V/Q scan* is useful when its result is normal or "low probability," which either means there are no perfusion defects or there are perfusion defects that are matched with ventilation defects. V/Q scan is also useful when the result is "high probability," as noted by multiple unmatched perfusion defects. However, ~30–40% of the studies have intermediate probability results. Overall, V/Q scan is valuable if the chest X-ray is normal and the patient does not have any severe cardiopulmonary abnormality that would interfere with the result. It is also valuable in renal failure, when CT may be risky.
- *Pulmonary angiogram* is rarely used and does not have a higher yield than current-generation chest CT. It may be considered if the CT or V/Q scan is indeterminate yet the PE clinical probability is high.
- *Lower extremity venous ultrasound* is positive in ~70% of DVTs. It is useful as an additional test if V/Q scan or CT is indeterminate or negative but the PE clinical probability is high.[8] In addition, it may be performed before CT if renal failure is present and one is trying to avoid the performance of CT. The results are only reliable if positive, ruling in DVT (and PE in the right setting). Negative results do not lessen the PE probability.

Transthoracic echo may show signs of RV strain in ~30–60% of PEs, and in almost all cases of submassive or massive PE.[10] RV strain manifests as: (i) RV dilatation (RV >30 mm on long-axis view, or RV >LV on four-chamber view); (ii) systolic PA pressure >35 mmHg; or (iii) D-shaped septum in systole (pressure overload). Systolic PA pressure >50 mmHg cannot be generated by an acutely failing RV, and thus PA pressure over 50 mmHg suggests some degree of chronicity. Rarely, a thrombus in transit is seen in the right-sided chambers (~4%); this is associated with a high mortality.

In a patient with shock and suspected PE, these echo features can make a presumptive diagnosis of PE and may be enough to justify thrombolytic therapy in this unstable context, even without further definitive diagnostic studies.[11,12] In those unstable patients, emergent TTE may also help rule out other causes of shock, such as MI or tamponade. TEE may show a saddle embolus in the proximal PA branches but is rarely needed.

The **McConnell sign** signifies hypokinesis of the RV free wall with normal RV apical motion. In hospitalized patients with RV dysfunction of any cause, this sign is highly specific for PE (>94%) but not very sensitive (20–77%); i.e., it is frequently absent in PE-induced RV dysfunction.[13,14]

BNP and troponin I as prognostic markers. Troponin increases in 50% of patients with moderate-to-large PE associated with RV strain. Also, BNP often increases in large PE (the degree of increase in PE is less marked than in HF).

V. Submassive PE, pulmonary hypertension, and thrombolysis

Acute pulmonary hypertension occurs when emboli obstruct >30% of the pulmonary vascular bed, or less so in a patient with prior cardiopulmonary disease. The thin RV is poorly tolerant of the acute rise in afterload and, as a result, fails and dilates; the dilatation further increases RV afterload and leads to a vicious circle of RV failure. RV dilatation compresses the LV and further reduces cardiac output. Hypotension may ensue and worsen RV ischemia, as the RV is more dependent on systolic blood pressure than the LV. Peripheral vasoconstriction and tachycardia acutely preserve the systemic pressure.

Thrombolytics achieve quick lysis of the PE (a few hours) and a quick, almost immediate improvement in pulmonary pressure and RV function in 92% of patients.[5,15] However, intrinsic thrombolysis is also potent and often dissolves a large part of the thrombus burden in patients receiving anticoagulation only, in a way that the hemodynamic superiority of thrombolysis over anticoagulation may be limited to a few days only. In addition, while acute pulmonary hypertension mainly results from the embolic obstruction per se, pulmonary vasoconstriction is a secondary contributor that improves over the course of therapy (vasoconstriction results from hypoxemia and from platelet-released serotonin and thromboxane).[16] Several studies suggest that 1 week after therapy, the degree of vascular obstruction on perfusion imaging and the degree of RV dysfunction are similar between thrombolysis-treated and anticoagulation-treated patients. PA pressure dramatically improves within a week of therapy, and heparin-treated patients often catch up with thrombolysis-treated patients.[11,17–20] Thus, thrombolysis is mostly useful in patients who are in shock, since those patients are unlikely to survive the first few days and catch up with thrombolysis-treated patients.

Massive PE is defined as shock, i.e., sustained hypotension (SBP <90 mmHg or 40 mmHg lower than baseline for over 15 minutes). This must be distinguished from the transient hypotension of syncope, which may imply reduced cardiac output reserve (submassive PE), but not massive PE.

Submassive PE is defined as PE without shock but with evidence of any of the following:[11]

- Pulmonary hypertension (systolic PA pressure >40 mmHg, often implying severe pulmonary hypertension since the RV cannot generate pressures >50 mmHg acutely).
- RV dysfunction by imaging, with either hypokinetic or dilated RV (RV/LV diameter >0.9 on echo or CT four-chamber view).
- Biochemical evidence of RV necrosis (elevated troponin beyond the "gray zone," e.g., >0.1–0.4 ng/ml) or RV dysfunction (BNP >90).
- Hypoxemia with O_2 saturation <90% on ambient air, SBP <100 mmHg, pulse >110 bpm, or shock index (pulse/SBP ratio) >1 (the first three clinical features are components of the "PE shock index").

ESC guidelines use the term *intermediate–high-risk PE* to characterize these patients, and mandate the presence of RV involvement both by imaging (RV dilatation or pulmonary hypertension) *and* biomarker assessment (troponin, BNP).[5]

Massive and submassive PE are clinical terms that correlate with the size of PE but also with the patient's underlying cardiopulmonary reserve. Whereas most stable, anticoagulated patients catch up with thrombolysis-treated patients, data suggest that a subgroup of patients with submassive PE are at risk *of persistent pulmonary hypertension, RV failure, and long-term persistence of symptoms* (25–50% of patients).[11,21,22] This subgroup is also at risk of acute clinical deterioration. In two studies, thrombolysis of stable patients with evidence of RV dysfunction or pulmonary hypertension dramatically and more effectively reduced PA pressure than standard anticoagulation, not only acutely but over the long term.[21,22] Thrombolysis also reduces the rate of acute clinical deterioration in submassive PE.[23] In a trial of systematic thrombolysis vs. anticoagulation with selective thrombolysis for submassive PE (defined by a combination of both RV imaging features *and* troponin >0.06 ng/ml), systematic thrombolysis reduced acute deterioration but did not affect the overall acute mortality and was associated with increased bleeding events, including a 2% rate of intracranial bleeding, mostly occurring in patients older than 75.[24] Thus, the widespread use of thrombolysis in submassive PE was not clearly superior to its selective use. As such, standalone anticoagulation is an appropriate initial strategy, as many patients improve their PA and RV parameters quickly; *thrombolysis may be reserved for patients who do not improve their PA pressure within 1–2 days, those who deteriorate clinically, or those with pre-shock findings* (persistent tachycardia, borderline BP, persistent severe hypoxia) (class IIa in ESC guidelines)[5].

While mostly useful in the first few days after the onset of PE symptoms, thrombolysis remains useful in patients who have had symptoms for 6–14 days, with 70% of the latter patients demonstrating improvement with thrombolysis on lung scan.[25] In practice, it is often difficult to define the onset of PE, especially in patients who have subacute symptoms of several weeks and who may have multiple emboli of various ages, some of which are acute;[25] thrombolysis may be attempted in patients with recent symptoms and persistent pulmonary hypertension. The benefit of thrombolysis is less time-dependent in PE than in MI or stroke for the following reasons: (i) thrombolysis is more effective in lysing a PA clot than a coronary or cerebral clot; 100% of the cardiac output goes through the pulmonary circulation, while only 5% and 15% of the cardiac output goes to the coronary and cerebral circulations, respectively; (ii) as opposed to a coronary occlusion, which quickly leads to MI and makes late thrombolysis futile, pulmonary arterial occlusion rarely leads to a large pulmonary infarction, as the pulmonary parenchyma receives most of its supply from the bronchial arterial circulation. Only small infarctions may be seen with distal emboli.

Catheter-directed therapy of the main and lobar PA branches may be performed in patients who have a high bleeding risk with a full thrombolytic dose. Typically, catheter therapy consists of thrombus fragmentation and aspiration, often followed by a low-dose direct catheter infusion of alteplase over 12–24 hours. This relatively low dose of alteplase is assumed to be safer.[5]

Considering the high mortality of patients with submassive PE and free-floating right heart thrombus seen on echo (>20%), those patients are best treated with systemic thrombolysis or surgical thromboembolectomy in an experienced center. Catheter thrombectomy is risky in those patients, as it may dislodge emboli into the right circulation, but also the left circulation if PFO is present.

VI. PE and chronic pulmonary hypertension

A first episode of PE leads to a significant risk of *symptomatic* chronic thromboembolic pulmonary hypertension (CTPH) of about 4% at 2 years, even without recurrence of PE.[26] This risk is higher in patients whose initial presentation is submassive PE, where up to 25–50% of patients have persistent pulmonary hypertension and where acute therapy with thrombolysis reduces this risk.[21,22] Think of CTPH in any case of chronic pulmonary hypertension. CTPH is treatable with surgical pulmonary thromboendarterectomy when the pulmonary obstruction is central (~70% of the cases), but not when it is distal and microvascular.

VII. Acute treatment of PE

A. Initial anticoagulation

One of the following three regimens is recommended:

- IV UFH, 80 units/kg bolus then 18 units/kg IV drip, with PTT monitoring Q6h. The PTT goal is 1.5–2.5 times normal.
- LMWH (enoxaparin), 1 mg/kg SQ Q12h or 1.5 mg/kg SQ Q24h. Reduce the dose to 1 mg/kg Q24h if GFR <30 ml/min, and avoid in ESRD.
- Fondaparinux SQ QD (<50 kg: 5 mg once daily; 50–100 kg: 7.5 mg once daily; >100 kg: 10 mg once daily). Fondaparinux should be avoided if GFR <30 ml/min.

In the absence of renal failure (GFR <30 ml/min) or high bleeding risk, LMWH or fondaparinux is preferred to UFH. They have been shown to be at least as efficacious as UFH in PE, with a trend towards superiority and a similar bleeding risk.[27,28] In patients with a high bleeding risk, UFH is preferred because of its shorter half-life.

Warfarin is started on the first day, usually at a dose of 5 mg per day. A dose of 10 mg for 2 days allows faster achievement of INR goal

Note that the fondaparinux dose used for PE is higher than the dose used for ACS (2.5 mg SQ QD). Also, the starting dose of heparin is higher for PE than ACS. PTT goal is higher for PE (60–85 s) than for ACS (46–70 s). In ACS, aggressive antiplatelet therapy is the mainstay therapy and high-intensity anticoagulation is avoided. Conversely, in PE, anticoagulation is the mainstay therapy and subtherapeutic anticoagulation should be avoided for any duration.

and is recommended in young healthy patients, whereas a 5 mg dose is recommended in elderly patients or those with heart or liver failure (ACCP guidelines).[29,30] Anticoagulation reaches steady state in ~7 days. INR is checked at 3–4 days, when it is expected to be 1.5–1.9, and warfarin is titrated accordingly. UFH or LMWH should be continued until INR is therapeutic for 2 consecutive days.

As an alternative to heparin and warfarin, rivaroxaban (Xarelto) and apixaban (Eliquis) have been approved for the acute and chronic therapy of PE/DVT in patients with GFR >30 ml/min, and may be started acutely instead of UFH or enoxaparin. Alternatively, parenteral anticoagulants may be started then switched to rivaroxaban or apixaban later.

B. Indications for thrombolysis

Thrombolysis results in a quick, almost immediate improvement of PA pressure and RV hemodynamics. However, by 1 week, pulmonary perfusion and RV function improve in most anticoagulated patients almost similarly to thrombolysis-treated patients, albeit more slowly (they often catch up with thrombolysis-treated patients). Thus, thrombolysis is indicated in the following patients (ACCP, AHA guidelines):[11,30]

- Massive PE where immediate improvement of hemodynamics is necessary (SBP <90 mmHg for over 15 minutes) (class I).
- Submassive PE (= intermediate–high-risk PE with both imaging *and* biomarker evidence of RV involvement). In this case, *the main goal of thrombolysis is prevention of chronic pulmonary hypertension and acute clinical deterioration*. Thrombolysis may be indicated if the bleeding risk is low and the patient is younger than 75 (class IIb in AHA guidelines). Alternatively, thrombolysis is better reserved for patients who do not quickly improve their PA pressure within 1–2 days of therapy or show signs of cardiopulmonary deterioration (class IIa in ESC guidelines).

Alteplase is administered as a 100 mg intravenous dose over 2 hours. Heparin is restarted at the end of the alteplase infusion. Alternatively, a weight-based bolus of tenecteplase has been used (30–50 mg, dose similar to STEMI).[23]

In high-bleeding-risk patients, catheter thrombectomy and a low-dose local infusion of alteplase may be considered (~0.5–1 mg/h, for a total of ~10–20 mg).

C. IVC filter

One trial has shown that the addition of an IVC filter to anticoagulant therapy reduces the risk of recurrent PE in the acute (12 days) and long-term (8 years) setting by ~50%. However, it doubles the risk of DVT and leads to a long-term risk of IVC thrombosis (~25%). Overall, it does not reduce the combined rate of thromboembolic events.[31]

An IVC filter is therefore indicated only in the following two scenarios:

- Contraindication to anticoagulation, such as a recent major bleed, trauma, surgery (<3 weeks), or a history of intracranial hemorrhage. If the contraindication is likely to be transient, placement of a retrievable IVC filter is preferred. The retrievable filter has a hook that allows later removal, generally within a few weeks (up to 3–12 months with some devices).
- Patient undergoing pulmonary thromboendarterectomy.

Recurrent PE/DVT despite therapeutic anticoagulation is a relative indication for IVC filter. This situation is usually due to off-and-on periods of subtherapeutic anticoagulation, rather than a truly ineffective anticoagulation. Anticoagulation should be continued along with IVC filter placement, as the IVC filter will only increase the DVT risk. *Massive PE is not, per se, an indication for IVC filter, even massive PE that required thrombolysis.*

VIII. Duration of anticoagulation

In the absence of anticoagulation, the risk of recurrence of PE/DVT is highest in the first 3 months, and may be as high as 20%.[5] Beyond the first 3 months, in the absence of anticoagulation, the yearly risk of recurrence of provoked PE/DVT is ≤3% (major risk factor 1%, transient minor risk factor 3%), while the yearly risk of recurrence of unprovoked PE/DVT is 3–10%.[30] On the other hand, anticoagulation is associated with a 2–3% yearly risk of major bleeding. A similar risk of recurrence is expected after anticoagulation is stopped, whether it is stopped at 3 months or 6–12 months.[5,32] A meta-analysis has shown that 3 months of anticoagulation vs. ≥6 months was associated with a similar risk of DVT/PE during the 2 years following cessation of anticoagulation.[33,34]

In unprovoked PE/DVT, certain risk factors are associated with a doubling of the risk of recurrence, making it close to 10%, whereas the lack of those risk factors reduces the recurrence risk to 3%. The risk factors for recurrence are:

- Recurrent DVT/PE.
- High-risk thrombophilias: antiphospholipid syndrome, protein C or S deficiency, antithrombin III deficiency, homozygote factor V Leiden, or homozygote prothrombin gene mutation.
- An elevated D-dimer 1 month after interruption of anticoagulation, which implies active subclinical clotting and a high risk of thrombotic events.[35]
- Residual thrombus or defect on venous ultrasound, which increases the risk of a new DVT. The residual thrombus, even if old and organized, may serve as a nidus for further thrombus deposition or impair venous flow in a way that favors recurrent DVT.[36]

In the unprovoked PE/DVT patients with a low or moderate bleeding risk, long-term anticoagulation beyond 3 months (possibly lifelong) is warranted (Table 21.2).[30] Cancer patients have the highest risk of recurrence, ~20–30% within a year, and require extended therapy even if the bleeding risk is high (as long as cancer is active). LMWH is twice as effective as warfarin in reducing PE/DVT recurrence in cancer patients, and is the preferred therapy in these patients, as long as cancer is active;[30,37] vomiting, fluctuant nutritional status, or liver dysfunction are common in these patients and alter the efficacy and safety of warfarin. LMWH should be provided for at least 3–6 months, followed by either LMWH or warfarin (ESC guidelines). Studies of novel oral anticoagulants only included a small minority of cancer patients (<5 %), and thus novel oral anticoagulants do not have a clear role in cancer patients.

Bleeding risk is high in the following patients: (i) age >75; (ii) previous GI bleed, especially when the cause is not reversible; (iii) chronic severe HTN; (iv) prior stroke; (v) requirement for dual antiplatelet therapy; (vi) baseline anemia Hb <10 g/dl; (vii) hepatic or renal disease.

While anticoagulation reduces the risk of PE/DVT recurrence by 90%, aspirin has been shown to reduce this risk by ~30%, and may be a reasonable alternative to anticoagulation in patients who have an intermediate, rather than high, risk of recurrence.[38] A target INR 1.5–1.9 is superior to placebo for PE/DVT prevention but inferior to a target INR 2–3, with the same bleeding risk; thus, this low level of anticoagulation is not justified.

Table 21.2 Duration of long-term anticoagulation.

1. Provoked PE or DVT (major or minor transient risk factor)	3 months
2. Unprovoked idiopathic PE or proximal DVT	3 months if the bleeding risk is high >3 months (extended therapy) if the bleeding risk is low/moderate[a] Consider D-dimer testing, venous ultrasound, and testing for thrombophilias to decide about pursuing therapy beyond 3 months (in those with a low/moderate bleeding risk, or possibly, those with a high bleeding risk)
3. Recurrent PE or DVT	>3 months if the bleeding risk is low or moderate[a]
4. High-risk hereditary thrombophilias	>3 months if the bleeding risk is low or moderate[a]
5. Active cancer within the last 6 months	Extended LMWH, or, less favorably, warfarin

[a] Even with recurrent PE or thrombophilias, limiting anticoagulant therapy to 3 months is appropriate in high-bleeding-risk patients. Cancer patients have the highest risk of recurrence (20–30% within a year) and qualify for extended therapy even if bleeding risk is high. Extended therapy implies routine reassessment of bleeding risk and reconsideration of the duration of anticoagulation, and does not necessarily equate with indefinite therapy.

IX. Thrombophilias

Thrombophilias are classified into high-risk and moderate-risk thrombophilias:[39]

- *High-risk thrombophilias:* antiphospholipid syndrome, protein C or S deficiency, antithrombin III deficiency, homozygote factor V Leiden or prothrombin gene mutation. Each one of the high-risk thrombophilias has a 1–3% prevalence among patients with a first PE/DVT, and is associated with a 2.5× increase in the risk of recurrence.
- *Moderate-risk thrombophilias:* Heterozygote factor V Leiden or prothrombin gene mutation. While highly prevalent among patients with PE/DVT (15% and 5%, respectively), they only modestly increase the risk of recurrence by ~30% and do not merit extended anticoagulation per se.[39]

HIT is the highest-risk thrombophilia and should be considered in any hospitalized patient who develops DVT despite receiving heparin, along with a reduction in platelet count.

Thrombophilias do not modify the INR goal (2–3). After a DVT/PE, testing for thrombophilia is indicated in the following cases: (i) idiopathic DVT/PE; (ii) recurrent DVT/PE; (iii) DVT/PE at age <40; (iv) DVT at an unusual site, including upper extremity; (v) family history of DVT/PE. Antithrombin III and, occasionally, proteins C and S may decrease in acute thrombosis. In addition, proteins C and S are reduced with warfarin, and antithrombin III is reduced with heparin. Thus, measurement may be done acutely before intitiation of anticoagulation, but if the levels of antithrombin III or protein C or S are abnormal, they need to be confirmed in a stable phase, after anticoagulation is discontinued (e.g., beyond 3 months). The genetic testing of factor V Leiden and prothrombin mutation may be performed at any time. *Cancer screening should also be performed.*

Antiphospholipid syndrome is tested using two modalities: (i) antibody testing (*anticardiolipin*, β_2-microglobulin); (ii) demonstration of prolongation of a clotting time, not correctable with the addition of normal plasma (= *lupus anticoagulant* = prolongation of PTT or Russell viper venom time). Since the clotting time is also prolonged by heparin therapy, it has no diagnostic value during heparin therapy.

In asymptomatic patients, thrombophilias drastically increase the risk of DVT/PE in relative terms (up to 15 times), but the absolute yearly risk of spontaneous DVT/PE remains low, ≤1%, even in pregnancy.[40] Asymptomatic thrombophilias do not warrant anticoagulation, but warrant the avoidance of additional risk factors (e.g., oral contraception) and appropriate prophylaxis during high-risk situations.

> Thrombophilias are mainly associated with venous thrombosis. For most conditions, the association with arterial thrombosis (MI, stroke) is questionable and weak. Some conditions are associated with combined venous and arterial thromboses: antiphospholipid syndrome, HIT, malignancy (Trousseau syndrome), paradoxical embolism, and hematologic malignancies (myeloproliferative disorders, paraproteinemias, and paroxysmal nocturnal hemoglobinuria).
>
> Also, a patient with HF and AF may be prone to both DVT and arterial embolism.

X. PE prognosis

When appropriately treated with anticoagulation, the mortality of low-risk PE without signs of RV failure is 1–3%. The mortality of submassive PE, including PE in patients with underlying cardiopulmonary disease, is 3–10%, while the mortality of massive PE is >10% and is improved with thrombolysis.[11] While the acute risk is not much increased with submassive PE, the long-term risk of pulmonary hypertension and persistent symptoms is drastically increased.

2. DEEP VEIN THROMBOSIS

I. Types

Proximal DVT involves the popliteal vein or the more proximal veins (i.e., the superficial femoral vein, which is a deep vein, or the iliac vein). It leads to PE in 50% of cases. Upper extremity proximal DVT involves the axillary vein or more proximal veins. Rarely, proximal DVT may result in severe venous congestion, so severe as to impede forward arteriolar flow and induce a pale then cyanotic acute limb ischemia (phlegmasia alba dolens, then phlegmasia cerulea dolens; "alba" means white, "cerulea" means blue). In contrast to acute limb ischemia from arterial occlusion, massive edema is present in phlegmasia and distal arterial pulses remain audible on Doppler exam.

Distal DVT is located below the popliteal vein and usually does not cause PE unless it extends proximally. Upper extremity distal DVT involves the brachial vein or more distal arm veins. Proximal extension occurs in 15% of patients, usually within 2 weeks of presentation.

II. Diagnosis

Clinical probability of DVT is based on three features: local DVT signs, DVT risk factors, and the absence of alternative diagnoses. When clinical probability is low or intermediate, D-dimer may be used to rule out DVT. When D-dimer is positive or the clinical probability is high, venous ultrasound and Doppler of the lower extremities is performed.

Ultrasound is 95% sensitive for proximal DVT, but only 50–70% sensitive for calf DVT. In addition, it cannot always diagnose isolated pelvic vein DVT (indirect signs of pelvic DVT may be seen). A DVT is diagnosed when a thrombus is directly seen, when the vein loses its full compressibility, or when venous flow loses its respiratory variations on spectral Doppler (indirect sign of pelvic DVT). Of note, isolated pelvic DVT is relatively uncommon, as DVT typically starts distally and usually affects the femoral veins when the iliac veins are affected.

If the venous ultrasound does not suggest DVT but the clinical suspicion is high, D-dimer may be performed to definitely rule out DVT. If D-dimer is positive, it is recommended to repeat the ultrasound exam at 7 days (an extension of a calf DVT will be seen by that time). *If isolated pelvic DVT is suspected in a patient with severe thigh edema, venous CT or MRI may be performed.*

III. Treatment

Proximal DVT. Initial and long-term anticoagulation is similar to PE, except that therapy may be started in an outpatient setting, and may be facilitated by the use of rivaroxaban or apixaban, which obviates the need for bridging from a parenteral anticoagulant to warfarin.

Most patients with iliofemoral DVT, especially iliac DVT, do not recanalize, and at least 25% of patients will have venous claudication and post-phlebitic syndrome (50% of patients with iliac DVT).[41] Post-phlebitic syndrome may lead to venous ulcers in a third of patients. Catheter-directed thrombolysis or pharmacomechanical thrombolysis using thrombectomy devices is suggested in patients with a low bleeding risk and a symptomatic iliofemoral DVT that does not quickly improve with anticoagulation (class IIa AHA, not ACCP).[11] It is also indicated in the rare limb-threatening DVT (alba or cerulea). Thrombolysis should not be administered intravenously; rather, it is administered locally through a prolonged catheter infusion (e.g., 12–24 hours of local r-tPA infusion). It is used up to 21 days after onset of symptoms.

Knee-high compression stockings (30–40 mmHg) for 2 years after a proximal DVT have been shown to reduce post-phlebitic syndrome and are recommended, whether post-phlebitic syndrome occurred or not (ACCP, AHA).[11,30]

Distal DVT does not need to be treated with anticoagulation if it is asymptomatic, not extensive, or if the patient has a high bleeding risk. Serial venous ultrasounds for 1–2 weeks are recommended in these patients. If distal DVT is symptomatic or if it extends proximally, anticoagulation is recommended for 3 months (rather than a shorter duration).

Superficial vein thrombosis is not necessarily treated with any anticoagulation, but may be treated with a prophylactic dose of enoxaparin or fondaparinux.

Upper extremity DVT usually occurs in patients with pacemakers or central catheters, mostly central catheters placed in cancer patients. If the catheter is functional and still required, it does not need to be removed. A minimum of 3 months of anticoagulation is recommended for a proximal upper extremity DVT: 3 months if the catheter is removed, or longer than 3 months if the catheter remains in place, for as long as it remains in place (especially in cancer patients) (ACCP).

SVC syndrome usually results from compression of the SVC by a mediastinal tumor, typically lung cancer. Complete SVC obstruction usually occurs when extrinsic compression is accompanied by intravascular thrombosis. If extensive thrombosis is present, catheter-directed thrombolysis followed by SVC stenting with a self-expanding stent is recommended.[42]

Upper extremity DVT may also develop in patients with thoracic outlet obstruction. Those are typically young athletic patients with hypertrophied cervical muscles and a cervical rib or long spinal processes that compress the brachial plexus, subclavian vein or subclavian artery. It may also develop in patients who heavily use their arm for athletic activity (venous microtrauma).[42]

Upper extremity DVT may also be idiopathic; ~25% of idiopathic upper extremity DVTs may be related to an occult cancer.

3. IMMUNE HEPARIN-INDUCED THROMBOCYTOPENIA

Heparin-induced thrombocytopenia (HIT) develops 4–16 days after initiation of heparin but may occur earlier, within minutes to hours, if the patient has been exposed to heparin within the last 3 months. It may develop days to weeks (up to 40 days) after heparin cessation in patients who have already been discharged from the hospital (delayed HIT). It is due to the formation of antibodies against the heparin–platelet PF4 complex.

I. Incidence

Approximately 2.5% of heparin-treated patients develop HIT. HIT is less common with prophylactic SQ heparin and 10 times less common with LMWH.

II. Diagnosis

Decrease in platelet count to <150,000 per microliter or decrease in platelet count >50% (even if the platelet count remains normal).

Also, heparin-induced skin necrosis at heparin injection sites, any thrombosis that occurs during effective therapy with heparin, or bilateral adrenal hemorrhages suggest HIT. Thrombocytopenia is rarely severe and is typically above 20,000 per microliter (median, 60,000 per microliter).

HIT antibodies should be ordered, and have a high diagnostic yield; however, they are not immediately available. The clinical context is used to determine the need for antithrombin therapy while antibodies are obtained for confirmation (particularly when the diagnosis is unsure). HIT antibodies may be negative very early on; thus, a negative test may need to be repeated if the clinical suspicion of HIT is high. On the other hand, using ELISA assay, a slight increase in titers is very sensitive and may not reflect clinical HIT.

HIT is a prothrombotic state rather than a bleeding state. It leads to thrombosis in 50% of patients. This is called *heparin-induced thrombocytopenia and thrombosis syndrome (HITTS).* Thrombosis mainly occurs within the first few days of HIT, when the thrombosis risk is 6% per day. The thrombosis risk persists for up to 6 weeks after the discontinuation of heparin. Venous thrombi are four times more common than arterial thrombi.

III. Treatment

Whenever HIT is suspected, heparin and LMWH are discontinued. Thrombosis is sought on clinical grounds and on a lower extremity venous ultrasound. If there is any evidence of thrombosis, whether thrombosis for which heparin was given or thrombosis induced by HIT:

• Start a direct thrombin inhibitor (DTI): argatroban IV (hepatically cleared; not affected by renal function). Monitor PTT during treatment. Do not start warfarin acutely, as warfarin increases the risk of thrombosis and/or skin necrosis and gangrene in patients with HIT.
• Start warfarin late, after the platelet count has near-normalized (>100,000 per microliter) and after several days of treatment with DTI. Begin with a small dose and overlap with DTI for 5 days. DTI increases INR, and thus the INR goal *during the overlap* is twice the standard INR goal (>4). Give warfarin for at least 3 months (the duration of warfarin therapy depends on the underlying cause of DVT, as detailed above in Section 1, *Pulmonary embolism*).

Even in the absence of thrombosis or HITTS, HIT itself mandates the use of a DTI to prevent the associated high incidence of thrombosis. DTI is initiated as soon as possible, whenever there is a moderate/high suspicion of HIT, without awaiting the result of HIT antibody testing.

DTI is continued until the platelet count returns to baseline, at which time warfarin is initiated and continued for ~30 days.

In HIT, low platelets are not a contraindication to DTI, unless the patient is actively bleeding. Platelet transfusions should be avoided unless there is active bleeding.

Note: Anticoagulant therapies in a patient with a prior history of HIT
- DVT prophylaxis in a patient with a history of HIT: fondaparinux (anti-Xa) 2.5 mg SQ QD.
- Coronary intervention in a patient with a history of HIT: bivalirudin IV or argatroban IV.
- A patient with a history of HIT over 90 days ago can be anticoagulated with heparin for short durations, <3 days, as HIT antibodies have already cleared by that time and it takes 4 days to form new ones.

QUESTIONS AND ANSWERS

Question 1. A 60-year-old man presents with severe dyspnea and one syncopal episode. On admission, O_2 saturation is 87% on ambient air, BP is 125/75, and pulse is 85 bpm. Lungs are clear. Echo shows RV dilatation and hypokinesis with preserved apical contraction; PA pressure is 45 mmHg. CT shows multilobar PE. Troponin I is 0.4 ng/ml. The patient has no prior bleeding history and no prior stroke. What is the next step?
A. IV heparin. No need for thrombolysis, the patient's PA pressure will catch up with thrombolytic-treated patients in a few days.
B. IV heparin + IV thrombolysis (class I indication)
C. IV heparin. Monitor closely for 2-3 days, and consider thrombolysis for clinical deterioration or persistent pulmonary hypertension.
D. IV heparin + IV thrombolysis + IVC filter

Question 2. A 45-year-old woman presents with acute dyspnea and hypoxia. SBP is ~100 mmHg, pulse is 110 bpm, and CT confirms the presence of a saddle pulmonary embolus involving the main PA branches. She is severely hypoxic and requires 5 liters of O_2 per minute to keep O_2 saturation >90%. Troponin I is 1 ng/ml. Echo shows severe RV hypokinesis and a worm-like structure in the RA, intermittently flopping into the RV. What is the next step?
A. IV heparin
B. IV heparin + IV thrombolysis
C. IV heparin + surgical thrombectomy
D. IV heparin + catheter thrombectomy
E. B or C

Question 3. A 60-year-old woman had a PE with no identifiable trigger and no cancer on chest X-ray and mammography. She was given apixaban therapy for 3 months, uneventfully. She is asking about the need to continue therapy beyond 3 months. All the following statements are true, *except which one*?
A. Anticoagulation should be continued for at least 6 months, which is the highest-risk period for recurrence
B. The risk of recurrence after discontinuation of anticoagulation is steady, whether anticoagulation is discontinued at 3 months or 6 months
C. Three months is the mandatory duration of therapy. But anticoagulation is preferably continued >3 months in all patients with low bleeding risk
D. Beyond 3 months, thrombophilia testing, D-dimer testing (3 weeks after stopping anticoagulation), and lower extremity venous study help decide which patients are more likely to benefit from long-term therapy
E. After 3 months, the yearly risk of recurrence is 3% in the absence of any abnormality on thrombophilia or D-dimer testing, vs. 6–10% risk in the presence of any abnormality
F. She has a 10% probability of cancer diagnosis within the next year

Answer 1. C. With heparin therapy, this patient will likely catch up with thrombolytic-treated patients. However, data suggest that thrombolysis may be beneficial in patients with both radiological and biomarker evidence of RV dysfunction (submassive PE), a significant proportion of whom do not catch up with thrombolytic-treated patients. Thrombolysis reduces acute deterioration and the long-term risk of pulmonary hypertension. Yet, considering its risk, thrombolysis is mainly indicated if cardiopulmonary deterioration occurs (class IIa ESC guidelines).

Answer 2. E. While the patients of Questions 1 and 2 both have submassive PE, the current patient is clearly a higher-risk patient within the large spectrum of submassive PE. SBP is lower, tachycardia is persistent with heart rate/SBP ratio >1 (shock index >1), and hypoxemia is more severe, suggesting that she is less stable and less likely to improve with heparin only. Moreover, the thrombus in transit is a very high-risk finding that advocates for more aggressive therapy (sudden death may occur if it moves into the PA). Catheter thrombectomy may dislodge the clot and may lead to right- and left-sided emboli (if PFO is present).

Answer 3. A.

References
1. Piazza G, Goldhaber SZ. Acute pulmonary embolism. Part I: epidemiology and diagnosis. Circulation 2006; 114: 28–32.
2. Ferrari E, Imbert AI, Chevalier T, et al. The ECG in pulmonary embolism, predictive value of negative T waves in precordial leads: 80 case reports. Chest 1997; 111: 537–43.
3. Sreeram N, Cheriex EC, Smeets JL, et al. Value of the 12-lead electrocardiogram at hospital admission in the diagnosis of pulmonary embolism. Am J Cardiol 1994; 73: 298–303.
4. Stein PD, Terrin ML, Hales CA, et al. Clinical, laboratory, and roentgenographic findings in patients with acute pulmonary embolism and no pre-existing cardiac or pulmonary disease. Chest 1991; 100: 598–603.
5. Konstantinides SV, Torbicki A, Agnelli G, et al. 2014 ESC guidelines on the diagnosis and management of acute pulmonary embolism. Eur Heart J 2014; 35: 3033–80.

6. Moores LK, Jackson WL, Shorr AF, Jackson JL. Meta-analysis: outcomes in patients with suspected pulmonary embolism managed with CT pulmonary angiography. Ann Intern Med 2004; 141: 866–74.

7. Quiroz R, Kuchner N, Zou KH, et al. Clinical validity of a negative CT scan in patients with suspected pulmonary embolism: a systematic review. JAMA 2005; 293: 2012–17.

8. Stein PD, Fowler SE, Goodman LR, et al. Multidetector computed tomography for acute pulmonary embolism. N Engl J Med 2006; 354: 2317–27. *PIOPED II: sensitivity 83% (in comparison to a combination of V/Q, Doppler±angiography), specificity 96%, sensitivity increased to 90% with venous CT.*

9. Nijkeuter M, Hovens MMC, Davidson BL, et al. Resolution of thromboemboli in patients with acute pulmonary embolism: a systematic review. Chest 2006; 129: 192–7.

10. Kucher N, Rossi E, De Rosa M, Goldhaber SZ. Prognostic role of echocardiography among patients with acute pulmonary embolism and a systolic arterial pressure of 90 mm Hg or higher. Arch Intern Med 2005; 165: 1777–81.

11. Jaff MR, McMurtry S, Archer SL, et al. Management of massive and submassive pulmonary embolism, iliofemoral deep vein thrombosis, and chronic thromboembolic pulmonary hypertension: a scientific statement from the American Heart Association. Circulation 2011; 123: 1788–830.

12. Rudoni RR, Jackson RE, Godfrey GW, et al. Use of two-dimensional echocardiography for the diagnosis of pulmonary embolus. J Emerg Med 1998; 16: 5–8.

13. McConnell MV, Solomon SD, Rayan ME, et al. Regional right ventricular dysfunction detected by echocardiography in acute pulmonary embolism. Am J Cardiol 1996; 78: 469–73.

14. Kurzyna M, Torbicki A, Pruszczyk P, et al. Disturbed right ventricular ejection pattern as a new Doppler echocardiographic sign of acute pulmonary embolism. Am J Cardiol 2002; 90: 507–51.

15. Goldhaber SZ, Come PC, Lee RT, et al. Alteplase versus heparin in acute pulmonary embolism: randomised trial assessing right-ventricular function and pulmonary perfusion. Lancet 1993; 341: 507–11.

16. Lualdi JC, Goldhaber SZ. Right ventricular dysfunction after acute pulmonary embolism: pathophysiologic factors, detection, and therapeutic implications. Am Heart J 1995; 130: 1276–82.

17. The urokinase pulmonary embolism trial. A national cooperative study. Circulation 1973; 47 (2 Suppl): II1–108.

18. Dalla-Volta S, Palla A, Santolicandro A, et al. PAIMS 2: alteplase combined with heparin versus heparin in the treatment of acute pulmonary embolism. Plasminogen activator Italian multicenter study 2. J Am Coll Cardiol 1992; 20: 520–6.

19. Konstantinides S, Tiede N, Geibel A, et al. Comparison of alteplase versus heparin for resolution of major pulmonary embolism. Am J Cardiol 1998; 82: 966–70.

20. Ribeiro A, Lindmarker P, Johnsson H, et al. Pulmonary embolism: one-year follow-up with echocardiography doppler and five-year survival analysis. Circulation 1999; 99: 1325–30.

21. Kline JA, Steuerwald MT, Marchick MR, et al. Prospective evaluation of right ventricular function and functional status 6 months after acute submassive pulmonary embolism: frequency of persistent or subsequent elevation in estimated pulmonary artery pressure. Chest 2009; 136: 1202–10.

22. Sharifi M, Bay C, Skrocki L, et al. Moderate pulmonary embolism treated with thrombolysis (from the "MOPETT" Trial). Am J Cardiol 2013; 111: 273–7.

23. Konstantinides S, Geibel A, Heusel G, et al. Heparin plus alteplase versus heparin alone in patients with submassive pulmonary embolism. N Engl J Med 2002; 347: 1143–50. *MAPPET 3 trial.*

24. Meyer G, Vicaut E, Danays T, et al. Fibrinolysis for patients with intermediate-risk pulmonary embolism. N Engl J Med 2014; 370: 1402–11. *PEITHO trial.*

25. Daniels LB, Parker JA, Patel SR, Grodstein F, Goldhaber SZ. Relation of duration of symptoms with response to thrombolytic therapy in pulmonary embolism. Am J Cardiol 1997; 80: 184–8.

26. Pengo V, Lensing AWA, Prins MH, et al. Incidence of chronic thromboembolic pulmonary hypertension after pulmonary embolism. N Engl J Med 2004; 350: 2257–64.

27. Matisse investigators. Subcutaneous fondaparinux versus intravenous unfractionated heparin in the initial treatment of pulmonary embolism.N Engl J Med 2003; 349: 1695–702.

28. Low-molecular-weight heparin in the treatment of patients with venous thromboembolism. The Columbus Investigators. N Engl J Med 1997; 337: 657–62.

29. Kovacs MJ, Rodger M, Anderson DR, et al. Comparison of 10-mg and 5-mg warfarin initiation nomograms together with low-molecular-weight heparin for outpatient treatment of acute venous thromboembolism. A randomized, double-blind, controlled trial. Ann Intern Med 2003; 1389: 714–19.

30. Guyalt GH, Akl EA, Crowther M, et al. Executive summary: Antithrombotic therapy and prevention of thrombosis, 9th edition. American College of Chest Physicians Evidence-Based Clinical Practice-Based Guidelines. Chest 2012; 141: 7S–47S.

31. Prepic study group. Eight-year follow-up of patients with permanent vena cava filters in the prevention of pulmonary embolism: the PREPIC randomized study. Circulation 2005; 112: 416–22.

32. Heit JA, Mohr DN, Silverstein MD, et al. Predictors of recurrence after deep vein thrombosis and pulmonary embolism: a population-based cohort study. Arch Intern Med 2000; 160: 761–8.

33. Agnelli G, Prandoni P, Becattini C, et al.; Warfarin Optimal Duration Italian Trial Investigators. Extended oral anticoagulant therapy after a first episode of pulmonary embolism. Ann Intern Med 2003; 139: 19–25.

34. Boutitie F, Pinede L, Schulman S, et al. Influence of preceding duration of anticoagulant treatment and initial presentation of venous thromboembolism on risk of recurrence after stopping therapy: analysis of individual participants' data from seven trials. BMJ 2011; 342: d3036

35. Palareti G, Cosmi B, Legnani C, et al. D-dimer testing to determine the duration of anticoagulation therapy. N Engl J Med 2006; 355: 1780–9.

36. Prandoni P, Lensing AW, Prins MH, et al. Residual venous thrombosis as a predictive factor of recurrent venous thromboembolism. Ann Intern Med 2002; 137: 955–60. *A meta-analysis of 11 RCTs found that the amount of residual thrombus after anticoagulant therapy correlated strongly with the risk of recurrent VTE. It is unknown whether this is a causal relationship, with residual thrombus creating a physical nidus for the development of new thrombus, or whether the presence of residual thrombus is simply a marker for a separate biological process that leads to recurrent VTE.*

37. Lee AY, Levine MN, Baker RI, et al Randomized Comparison of Low-Molecular-Weight Heparin versus Oral Anticoagulant Therapy for the Prevention of Recurrent Venous Thromboembolism in Patients with Cancer (CLOT) Investigators. Low-molecular-weight heparin versus a coumarin for the prevention of recurrent venous thromboembolism in patients with cancer. N Engl J Med 2003; 349: 146–53.

38. Brighton TA, Eikelboom JW, Mann K, et al. Low-dose aspirin for preventing recurrent venous thromboembolism. N Engl J Med 2012; 367: 1979–87.

39. Heit JA. Thrombophilia: common questions in laboratory assessment and management. Hematology Am Soc Hematol Educ 2007: 127–35.

40. Gerhardt A, Scharf RE, Beckmann MW, et al. Prothrombin and factor V mutations in women with a history of thrombosis during pregnancy and the puerperium. N Engl J Med 2000; 342: 374–80.

41. Kahn SR, Ginsberg JS. Relationship between deep venous thrombosis and the post thrombotic syndrome. Arch Intern Med 2004; 164: 17–26.

42. Engelberger RP, Kucher N. Management of deep vein thrombosis of the upper extremity. Circulation 2012; 126: 768–73.

22 Shock and Fluid Responsiveness

1. SHOCK

See Chapter 2 for the specific management of cardiogenic shock. See Chapter 38 for ventricular support devices.

I. Shock definition and mechanisms

Shock is defined as sustained hypotension *along with* evidence of low tissue perfusion (oliguria <30 ml/h for 1 hour, cold or mottled extremities, altered mental status, or elevated serum lactate level). Hypotension is usually defined as a mean systemic pressure <65 mmHg or a systolic pressure <90 mmHg for over 30 minutes, or requirement for catecholamine infusion to maintain systolic pressure ≥90 mmHg.[1,2] Systemic pressure may be higher in shock patients with chronic hypertension; a decline in systolic pressure of >40 mmHg is commonly used to define hypotension in the previously hypertensive patient.

There are *four mechanisms of shock*: (1) hypovolemia; (2) low cardiac output, as in left or right cardiogenic shock; (3) vasodilatory shock, also called distributive shock (septic shock, anaphylactic shock, shock from excessive amount of sedatives and vasodilators); (4) obstructive shock, where LV filling is prevented by a right-sided obstruction, such as pulmonary embolism, tamponade or isolated RV shock.

Right heart catheterization establishes the shock mechanism by assessing the three determinants of shock (Table 22.1):

1. Right- and left-sided filling pressures (CVP, PCWP). The normal CVP is <8–12 mmHg. If CVP <8 mmHg, particularly <5 mmHg, and PCWP <15 mmHg in a patient with shock, there is likely a hypovolemic component of the shock.
2. Cardiac output (CO). The normal cardiac index is 2.2–4.0 liters/min/m². If cardiac index <2.2 → cardiogenic component of the shock
3. Systemic vascular resistance (SVR). Normal SVR is 700–1500 dyn.s.cm⁻⁵. If SVR <700 → vasodilatory component of the shock

Clinically, left-heart cardiogenic shock is defined as a shock with clinical or radiographic evidence of pulmonary congestion.[1,2]

Some shock states may be mixed. In septic shock, one may have a hypovolemic component and a cardiogenic component with reduced myocardial contractility, the so-called septic cardiomyopathy, seen in as many as 30% of cases. Furthermore, in septic shock, cardiac output needs to be high enough to match the increased tissue demands and the vasodilated circulation, and to compensate for the maldistribution of flow (skeletal muscle flow is increased, while splanchnic flow is reduced and heterogeneous because of microvascular congestion). ***A cardiac output that is "normal" in absolute values may be inappropriate in the context of septic shock; this is suggested when the tissue perfusion and SvO₂ are low (SvO₂ <65%) despite normalization of the systemic pressure***. Both an adequate mean arterial pressure *and* an adequate cardiac output are required for end-organ perfusion.

While cardiogenic shock is classically described in patients with acute large MIs, it is also seen in patients with chronic severe cardiomyopathy and decompensating factors, such as acute infection, tachyarrhythmia, excessive vasodilators or sedation, cases where the limited cardiac output reserve cannot match the dilated circulation. In addition, volume overload, by itself, increases ventricular filling pressures and thus reduces myocardial perfusion and cardiac output.

In the SHOCK trial of cardiogenic shock secondary to acute MI, 20% of patients had reduced CO and elevated PCWP but relatively low SVR (<1000). This was related to a concomitant infection or to a systemic inflammatory response associated with nitric oxide release in cardiogenic shock.[3] In cardiogenic shock, SVR increases to maintain systemic pressure; SVR that is "normal" in value in the absence of vasodilator therapy is, in fact, relatively low.

A shock state with a wide pulse pressure is characteristic of septic shock, AI, or any vasodilatory condition (cirrhosis, vasodilatory drug excess).

Always remember adrenal shock (Addisonian shock), in which three mechanisms of shock are present (hypovolemia, low SVR, and myocardial depression). Importantly, functional adrenal failure may result from septic shock. Also, think of adrenal shock in patients who are acutely sick and who have been receiving chronic steroid therapy; their chronically suppressed adrenal glands cannot generate stress doses of steroids.

Practical Cardiovascular Medicine, First Edition. Elias B. Hanna.
© 2017 John Wiley & Sons Ltd. Published 2017 by John Wiley & Sons Ltd.

Table 22.1 Hemodynamic findings in the four different types of shock.

	CVP	PCWP	Cardiac index	SVR
Hypovolemic	↓	↓	↓	↑
Cardiogenic	↑	↑	↓	↑
Low SVR	↓	↓	↓, normal, or ↑	↓
Obstructive[a]	↑	↓	↓	↑

[a] Disproportionately elevated PA pressure and CVP in comparison to PCWP suggest pulmonary embolism or precapillary pulmonary hypertension.
In tamponade or isolated RV shock, equalization of CVP and PCWP is often seen.

II. Goals of shock treatment

Increase mean arterial pressure (MAP) to >65 mmHg *and* provide good tissue perfusion, manifested as:

- Urine output >0.5 ml/kg/h, with a stable creatinine.
- Absence of acidosis. Gastric pH or serum lactate may be monitored as a marker of perfusion.
- Mixed venous O_2 saturation (SvO_2) ≥65–70%.
- Heart rate <120 bpm.
- Warm skin with capillary refill ≤2 seconds.

One study addressed a target MAP of 65–70 mmHg vs. 80–85 mmHg in septic shock and found no difference in mortality and overall adverse events. Only in patients with underlying chronic hypertension did the higher MAP goal reduce the incidence of severe renal failure and the requirement for acute dialysis.[4]

Note on SvO_2

SvO_2 is the mixed venous O_2 saturation, which is the O_2 saturation of the venous return, best sampled from the pulmonary artery (PA being the chamber where the venous blood achieves its best mixing from all sources). It may also be appropriately sampled from an SVC line. It is the result of O_2 delivery to the tissues minus O_2 consumption by the tissues. If O_2 delivery does not match O_2 demands, O_2 extraction will be high, which reduces the venous O_2 content and SvO_2.

SvO_2 is thus a marker of how well O_2 delivery matches O_2 consumption, and a guide to appropriate shock therapy. In the absence of anemia or hypoxemia, a low SvO_2 <60–65% implies that the cardiac output is inappropriate, even if high in absolute value.

Examples of O_2 delivery/consumption mismatch in different contexts:

- Septic shock: O_2 delivery is reduced from flow maldistribution and hypovolemia; O_2 demands are increased with requirements of a higher than normal O_2 delivery
- Reduced cardiac output, anemia, or hypoxemia reduces O_2 delivery

III. Immediate management of any shock

The shock and the volume status are quickly classified by history and physical exam, with a focus on:

- Cardiac history.
- Pulmonary edema, elevated JVP, and peripheral edema, which are signs of volume overload. Unlike pulmonary edema, peripheral edema does not necessarily preclude fluid resuscitation *acutely* in cases of septic or hemorrhagic shock.
- Fever and potential sources of infection.

ECG and chest X-ray are quickly performed.

A. Intravenous fluid boluses

In the absence of pulmonary edema, a normal saline bolus of 0.5–2 liters is quickly administered in less than an hour (<20 minutes for the first liter). Fluid administration is the first therapy of hypovolemic and low-SVR shocks; patients who have peripheral edema or elevated JVP are hypervolemic and are generally not fluid responsive, but may *occasionally* be fluid responsive at the onset of septic or hemorrhagic shock.

Fluids are administered until signs of fluid repletion develop. Alternatively, fluids may be administered until CVP is 8–12 mmHg (or 12–15 mmHg in the case of ventilation with positive end-expiratory pressure) or PCWP is 15–18 mmHg.[5]

B. If the patient remains hypotensive despite quick intravenous fluid resuscitation, especially *if signs of fluid repletion develop* (elevated JVP, pulmonary edema, decreased O_2 saturation)

1. Norepinephrine or dopamine may be started (norepinephrine ≥0.05 mcg/kg/min, dopamine ≥3 mcg/kg/min). These two drugs are effective whether the shock is cardiogenic or distributive, until more is figured out.

2. In a cardiogenic context, inotropes are administered: dobutamine is started at 3 mcg/kg/min if SBP >80 mmHg, whereas dopamine or norepinephrine are started if SBP <70–80 mmHg. Dopamine may be administered at 3–10 mcg/kg/min (at this level, dopamine has mixed α+ and β+ effects, β+>α+).

3. In a septic context, vasopressors are administered: norepinephrine (mixed α+ and β+ effects, that is, vasoconstrictive and inotropic effects), phenylephrine (pure α+ effect, without β+ or inotropic effect), vasopressin

4. At this point, along with these initial measures:
- A central venous line may be placed to monitor CVP and help assess the volume status and SVO$_2$. A pulmonary artery catheter (Swan–Ganz) is not generally needed and has not been shown to improve outcomes in comparison to using a central line to measure CVP and SvO$_2$.
- An intra-arterial line is often necessary for blood pressure monitoring in any shock requiring inotropes and/or vasopressors.
- Echocardiography is performed
- If the diagnosis remains in doubt and the patient does not improve despite the initial measures, a PA catheter may be placed to diagnose the mechanism of shock and pulmonary edema, and to guide therapy.

C. In the context of septic shock, if low perfusion signs persist despite achieving the target systemic pressure and despite a presumably normal volume status

Consider that the cardiac output or the systemic pressure is still inadequate even if normal or high in absolute value. At this point, inotropes may be administered to increase cardiac output and O$_2$ delivery, allowing it to match the O$_2$ demands (Figure 22.1).

D. Provide adequate oxygenation (arterial O$_2$ saturation >90–95%), and adequate hemoglobin level

Intubate and mechanically ventilate in the case of any respiratory distress or obtundation. Respiratory effort can consume up to 30% of the cardiac output. Mechanical ventilation, by relieving the work of breathing, helps improve tissue perfusion.

In the absence of acute hemorrhage, red blood cells should only be transfused when hemoglobin decreases to <7–7.5 g/dl, with a target hemoglobin level of 7–9 g/dl (TRICC and TRISS trials).[6,7] One trial of early goal-directed therapy used a target hemoglobin level of 10 g/dl in the first 6 hours of resuscitation; however, this did not prove necessary in two later trials.[8,9]

> Steps A–D should lead to reversal of hypotension and good tissue perfusion within 6 hours of starting therapy (= early goal-directed therapy of sepsis).[5] CVP and SvO$_2$ may be used as a guide to therapy, as in the first trial of early goal-directed therapy.[5] However, this is not necessary, and reliance on clinical parameters of perfusion is often sufficient, as shown in two other trials (Figure 22.1).[8,9]

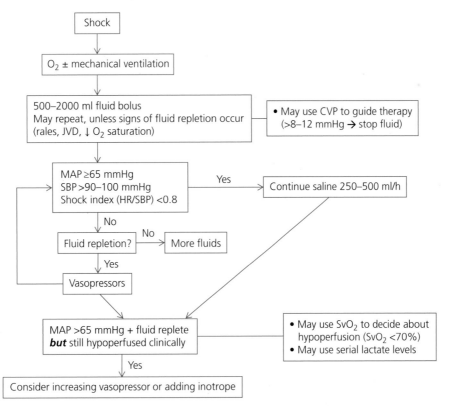

Figure 22.1 Aggressive early therapy of septic shock (the first 6 hours). Early goal-directed therapy implies the use of a central venous line with monitoring of CVP and SvO$_2$, but this is not necessary. Clinical signs of hypoperfusion consist of oliguria, serum lactate >4 mmol/l, mottled skin. Effectiveness of therapy may be assessed by lactate clearance: a reduction of lactate levels ≥10% at 1–2-hour intervals suggests an improvement in tissue perfusion. This algorithm is inspired by references 5–7. MAP, mean arterial pressure.

Table 22.2 Causes of cardiogenic shock.

---

1. Acute MI: shock is related to LV dysfunction (~75%), RV shock, mechanical complication (~12%)

2. Cardiogenic shock without acute coronary event:
- End-stage chronic cardiomyopathy (progressive), especially with decompensating factors (acute infection, arrhythmia, excessive sedation or vasodilator therapy, cases where the limited cardiac output reserve cannot match the dilated circulation). Also, volume overload, by itself, increases ventricular filling pressures and reduces myocardial perfusion and cardiac output.
- Acute cardiomyopathy: fulminant myocarditis or stress cardiomyopathy
- Acute valvular disease, especially valvular insufficiency
- Fast and prolonged tachyarrhythmia, or inappropriate bradycardia
- Prolonged cardiopulmonary bypass (post-pump shock)

E. Perform a quick workup in parallel to the previous steps

ECG, chest X-ray, cardiac enzymes, complete blood count, and blood/urine/sputum cultures are obtained. Line infections are considered, and in case of doubt, lines older than 48 hours are removed and replaced. Infectious foci are sought (e.g., abdomen, joints, skin).

Bedside echocardiography is performed:

- Echocardiography rules out tamponade, cardiogenic shock from LV failure, acute valvular disorders, and massive PE with acute RV failure.
- Echocardiography helps determine:
  - RA, LA, and PA pressures, which help guide fluid therapy.
  - Volume responsiveness. A small LV cavity that is hypercontractile with near cavity obliteration or elevated LV outflow velocity often indicates hypovolemia.

F. Start empiric broad-spectrum antibiotics whenever there is any suspicion of sepsis (start the antibiotics within 1 hour of this suspicion)

Treat the potential source of infection (e.g., drain any abscess, remove central lines).

G. Administer stress doses of steroids for a shock that persists for more than 1 hour despite inotropes/vasopressors or for the patient who uses steroids chronically

H. In cardiogenic shock, look for a cause and treat it (see Table 22.2)

- PCI+IABP±mechanical circulatory support (e.g., Impella) in MI
- Surgical correction of an acute valvular regurgitation or a mechanical complication of MI
- Cardioversion of a fast tachyarrhythmia (>150 bpm)
- Pacing for an inappropriately low heart rate, e.g., shock with a rate <60–70 bpm

A patient with shock is expected to be tachycardic. In fact, tachycardia attempts to compensate for an inappropriately reduced cardiac output. A "normal" heart rate of 50–70 bpm is inappropriate in shock and may dictate temporary pacing.

2. FLUID RESPONSIVENESS

Fluid responsiveness addresses the improvement of cardiac output (>10%) with fluid administration. In chronic systolic HF, PCWP >15 mmHg or CVP >8–12 mmHg predicts the lack of fluid responsiveness; in diastolic HF or acute systolic HF, PCWP >20–22 mmHg predicts the lack of fluid responsiveness (Chapter 5). In fact, diuresis may improve cardiac output in these cases. However, while CVP and PCWP are helpful in establishing the mechanism of a shock, they only weakly predict fluid responsiveness, particularly when they are not severely reduced or severely elevated (e.g., CVP between 5–12 mmHg), or when the patient does not have an underlying systolic HF. In addition, a high CVP does not rule out volume responsiveness in a critically ill patient (e.g., sepsis, trauma) who does not have a history of systolic HF, especially if atrial, venous, or ventricular compliance is impaired, as is sometimes seen with hypoxia (Figure 22.2). Thus, some patients with a normal or high CVP are fluid-responsive, while others are not. **Fluid responsiveness is better assessed using the *dynamic response of stroke volume and systemic arterial waveform to positive pressure ventilation* in mechanically ventilated patients or *to passive leg raising* in both mechanically ventilated and spontaneously breathing patients.**

During mechanical ventilation, the positive intrathoracic pressure reduces cardiac output in patients who are fluid-responsive, and analysis of the respiratory change in stroke volume or analysis of systemic arterial waveform from an arterial line is very helpful in addressing fluid responsiveness.[10] If the ventricles are on the steep portion of the Frank–Starling curve, an increase in venous return increases stroke volume, and thus the respiratory changes in venous return lead to respiratory fluctuations of the stroke volume. If the stroke volume varies by >20% with respiration or if the systolic pressure or the pulse pressure decreases by >13% between an end-expiratory hold and the next ventilatory cycle, the RV and the LV are sensitive to volume changes and are, therefore, volume-responsive. On echocardiography, LVOT or aortic valve VTI velocity may be used as a surrogate of stroke volume;[11,12] in fact, stroke volume=(LVOT VTI × LVOT area) or (aortic VTI × aortic valve area).

While the respiratory fluctuation in stroke volume and systolic arterial and pulse pressure may reflect hypovolemia (pulsus paradoxus), this is not sensitive or specific enough in patients who are **spontaneously breathing**.[13,14] In such patients, rely on the clinical evidence of

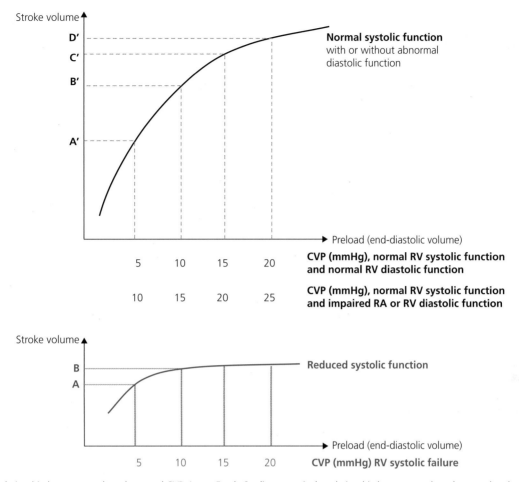

Figure 22.2 Relationship between stroke volume and CVP. A true Frank–Starling curve is the relationship between stroke volume and preload measured as volume rather than pressure. Preload volume and CVP do not linearly correlate, and their relationship depends on ventricular and atrial compliance. In fact, the same preload volume corresponds to a higher CVP value in patients with impaired ventricular or atrial compliance.

In patients with normal systolic function (*upper figure*), stroke volume continues to increase even when CVP rises from 10 to 15 and 20 mmHg, as the ventricle has a steeper Frank–Starling curve (*A′* to *B′* to *C′* to *D′*); this is more marked if ventricular or atrial compliance is impaired. In patients with abnormal systolic function (*lower figure*), stroke volume does not significantly increase with a change in CVP from 5 to 10 or 20 mmHg (*A* to *B*), as the ventricle is already on a flat portion of the Frank–Starling curve.

hypervolemia (peripheral edema), and assess the change in stroke volume or pulse pressure after passive leg raising or after a small volume load (500 ml). Passive leg raising-induced change in stroke volume, cardiac output, or pulse pressure reliably predicts volume responsiveness, whatever the breathing conditions.[15–17] An increase in cardiac output or stroke volume of >12.5% or a change in pulse pressure of ≥9% with passive leg raising suggests volume responsiveness; if a Swan–Ganz catheter is not in place, the change in stroke volume or cardiac output may be assessed using echocardiography. A decrease in CVP during inspiration may also predict fluid responsiveness in patients who are breathing spontaneously but not deeply (in severe RV failure, CVP increases with inspiration or remains unchanged rather than decreases).[18,19]

As described in the prior paragraphs, **echocardiography** may be used to assess volume responsiveness. An increase in stroke volume >12.5% with passive leg raising, but also an IVC diameter <1.2 cm, predicts volume responsiveness in spontaneously breathing or mechanically ventilated patients.[17,20] Furthermore, a change in aortic valve VTI >12% between inspiration and expiration or IVC collapsibility >12% predicts volume responsiveness in mechanically ventilated patients.[9,21,22] Patients who are mechanically ventilated tend to have a larger IVC diameter and reduced IVC collapsibility because of the positive intrathoracic pressure that impedes venous return; that's why 12% collapsibility, as opposed to 50% in spontaneously breathing patients, is considered a sign of volume responsiveness.[21] In any patient, whether spontaneously breathing or mechanically ventilated, a hyperdynamic LV with systolic cavity collapse or a hyperdynamic LV with intracavitary LV pressure gradient and SAM of the mitral valve implies severe hypovolemia, particularly hypovolemia associated with excessive use of inotropes. However, a small LV cavity may also be seen in overloaded patients with restrictive cardiomyopathy.

In mechanically ventilated patients who do not have an arterial line, the pulse oximetry tracing may be used to predict volume responsiveness. The plethysmographic waveform of pulse oximeters is a qualitative indicator of blood volume changes at the fingertip. One study suggested a correlation between pulse waveform variation provided by pulse oximetry and systolic pressure variation; thus, pulse waveform variation predicts volume responsiveness in mechanically ventilated patients.[23] However, the pulse oximetry tracing is not useful in hypotensive patients whose finger perfusion is reduced.

Appendix. Hemodynamic equations, transfusion, and miscellaneous concepts

A. Hemodynamic variables and equations

- O_2 arterial content (ml O_2/dl) = $SaO_2 \times$ Hb $\times$ capacity of 1 g Hb to carry O_2 (=1.36 ml of O_2 per g of Hb)
- O_2 venous content (ml O_2/dl) = $SvO_2 \times$ Hb $\times$ 1.36
- O_2 delivery (ml O_2/min) = O_2 arterial content $\times$ CO $\times$ 10
- O_2 consumption (ml O_2/min) = (O_2 arterial content – O_2 venous content) $\times$ CO $\times$ 10. This is the *Fick equation*.
- CVP = RA pressure: normal <8 mmHg
- RA pressure and RV diastolic pressure are equal (in the absence of tricuspid stenosis)
- Pulmonary capillary wedge pressure (PCWP) = pulmonary artery occlusive pressure: normal <15–18 mmHg
- PA pressure: normal <35/15 mmHg, with a mean pressure <25 mmHg. PA diastolic pressure is normally equal to PCWP, unless precapillary pulmonary hypertension exists (as in lung disease, pulmonary vascular disease, or pulmonary embolism). In these cases, pulmonary arterial disease or vasoconstriction leads to a diastolic PA pressure that exceeds PCWP by >5 mmHg.
- Cardiac index: normal >2.2 l/min/m²
- SVR = (mean BP – CVP) $\times$ 80/cardiac output. Normal SVR: 700–1500 dyn.s.cm^{-5}
- PVR = (mean PA pressure – PCWP)/cardiac output. Normal PVR <2 Wood units

B. Peripheral edema that occurs after resuscitation means hypervolemia and signals the need to back off fluid resuscitation

Contrary to common belief, the concept of "hypervolemia with intravascular volume depletion" is often untrue. Interstitial volume quickly equilibrates with plasma volume; therefore, edematous patients have excess of intravascular volume and are non-responsive to fluid administration. Occasional exceptions are seen, such as at the onset of septic or hemorrhagic shock in a patient who previously had peripheral edema; because of the acute onset, the intravascular volume has not had time to equilibrate with the interstitial volume, and these patients are initially fluid-responsive despite hypervolemia. This may also occur in acute abdominal illnesses, cirrhosis with ascites, or immediately after abdominal surgery (when fluids tend to accumulate in the abdominal cavity).

C. SvO$_2$ vs. ScvO$_2$

Mixed central venous O_2 saturation (ScvO$_2$) represents SVC O_2 saturation and is normally lower than IVC O_2 saturation, which receives the high venous O_2 content of the renal veins (low renal O_2 extraction). SVC O_2 is slightly lower than the overall mixed venous O_2 saturation, i.e., SvO$_2$. However, for patients in shock, a reversal of this relation occurs and ScvO$_2$ becomes greater than SvO$_2$ (by 5–10%). Redistribution of blood away from the splenic, renal, and mesenteric blood (IVC territory) toward the cerebral circulation (SVC territory) leads to this phenomenon (more O_2 extraction in the IVC territory: SVC O_2 >IVC O_2 and PA O_2). In septic shock, the goal SvO$_2$ is >65% while the goal ScvO$_2$ is >70%.

D. Colloid fluids (Dextran, Hetastarch)

In sepsis, colloid fluids have not been shown to be superior to crystalloid fluids (such as normal saline). In fact, colloid fluids may lead to more renal failure, coagulopathy, and mortality than crystalloids.[24]

E. Intensive insulin therapy

Intensive insulin therapy given to achieve a glycemic control of 80–110 mg/dl has been shown to decrease mortality in surgical ICU patients. However, in medical ICU patients and in patients with sepsis, aggressive insulin therapy to achieve a glucose level of <110 mg/dl has not been beneficial and has led to severe episodes of hypoglycemia. A glucose level of <200 mg/dl is, however, desirable.[24]

F. Note about inotropes and vasopressors

The SOAP II trial randomized patients with septic or cardiogenic shock to dopamine vs. norepinephrine. There was no overall difference in mortality, but dopamine was associated with twice the risk of AF (~20% vs. 11%) and VT, and more sinus tachycardia. Also, in the subgroup of patients with cardiogenic shock, norepinephrine was associated with better survival than dopamine.[25]

A meta-analysis of six septic shock trials showed greater mortality with dopamine than with norepinephrine.[26] Thus, norepinephrine is the drug of choice in septic shock, and in cardiogenic shock with severe hypotension.

Vasopressin can reduce the need for a high norepinephrine dose and is suggested in patients requiring a norepinephrine dose >0.15 mcg/kg/min. It is safe and may be associated with a mortality reduction in vasodilatory shock.[27]

G. Indications for transfusion

Three classic randomized trials addressed transfusion in critically ill patients (TRICC trial: all-comers in the intensive care unit; TRISS trial: patients with septic shock; gastrointestinal bleeding trial: patients with acute gastrointestinal bleed but without shock).[6,7,28] All three trials showed that using a Hb transfusion cutoff <7 g/dl, rather than 9 g/dl, is safe, and it was associated with a significant mortality reduction in the gastrointestinal bleeding trial and a strong trend towards mortality reduction in the TRICC trial.

Data on ACS patients are more sparse, but suggest that transfusion should be reserved for Hb <8 g/dl, unless angina is ongoing (ESC guidelines, grade I).[29]

The above thresholds apply to most patients. However, higher cutoffs (~9–9.5 g/dl) should be used in patients with ongoing major bleed (e.g., hemorrhagic shock), and in those with *severely symptomatic anemia*, i.e., angina at rest/ischemia on ECG, angina or dyspnea on mild activity, or severe sinus tachycardia. Conversely, fatigue is a vague symptom and is not, per se, a strong indication for transfusion.

Anemia is associated with worsened outcomes in all settings and may exacerbate myocardial ischemia in patients with CAD or ACS. Yet transfusion, by itself, does not always reverse this ischemia and leads to its own untoward effects. It increases volume overload in HF. The transfused red cells are different from intrinsic red cells without as much capacity for O_2 carrying (the longer they are stored, the worse they get). Plus, transfused red cells have potential prothrombotic (ADP release) and proinflammatory effects. In fact, while normal red blood cells transport and dispense nitric oxide to the microvasculature, this function is disrupted in transfused red blood cells, which leads to impaired regional vasodilatation.

The general approach adopted by the author is presented in Table 22.3.

Table 22.3 General indications for transfusion in critically ill or ACS patients.

1. In any critical illness, septic shock, or hemodynamically stable gastrointestinal bleed, a cutoff of 7–7.5 g/dl is appropriate
2. In patients with active bleed and hemodynamic instability from bleeding, transfusion should be considered at a higher cutoff (9–9.5 g/dl, even more sometimes)
3. In patients with severe tachycardia, especially sinus tachycardia (>110–120 bpm) that can only be attributed to anemia, transfusion may be considered at a higher cutoff (9 g/dl)
4. For ACS patients who are stabilized without angina, a Hb cutoff of 8 g/dl is appropriate. If they continue to exhibit episodes of angina at rest or mild exertion, a higher cutoff may be used (likely 9–9.5 g/dl). Also, in patients about to undergo PCI, a higher cutoff is generally used.
5. In all patients, the cause of a new anemia should be sought and treated (bleeding, hemolysis). In ACS, this cause is sought before performing any PCI and before the administration of antithrombotic therapy. For example, in a patient with Hb 8 g/dl and severe angina: transfuse, perform endoscopy, start proton pump inhibitor, and ensure Hb stability for a few days before PCI.

References

1. Thiele H, Zeymer U, Neumann FJ, et al. Intraaortic balloon support for myocardial infarction with cardiogenic shock. N Engl J Med 2012; 367: 1287–96.
2. Hochman JS, Sleeper LA, Webb JG, et al. Early revascularization in acute myocardial infarction complicated by cardiogenic shock. SHOCK Investigators. Should We Emergently Revascularize Occluded Coronaries for Cardiogenic Shock. N Engl J Med 1999; 341: 625–34. *SHOCK trial.*
3. Kohsaka S, Menon V, Lowe AM, et al.; SHOCK Investigators. Systemic inflammatory response syndrome after acute myocardial infarction complicated by cardiogenic shock. Arch Intern Med 2005; 165: 1643–50.
4. Asfar P, Meziani F, Hamel JF, et al. High versus low blood-pressure target in patients with septic shock. N Engl J Med 2014; 370: 1583–93.
5. Rivers E, Nguyen B, Havstad S, et al. Early goal-directed therapy in the treatment of severe sepsis and septic shock. N Engl J Med 2001; 345: 1368–77.
6. Hebert PC, Wells G, Blajchman MA, et al. A multicenter, randomized, controlled clinical trial of transfusion requirements in critical care. N Engl J Med 1999; 340: 409–17. *TRICC trial.*
7. Holst LB, Haase N, Wetterslev J, et al. TRISS: Transfusion requirements in septic shock. N Engl J Med 2014; 371: 1381–91. *TRISS trial.*
8. ProCESS investigators. A randomized trial of protocol-based care for early septic shock. N Engl J Med 2014; 370: 1683–93.
9. ARISE Investigators, ANZICS Clinical Trials Group. Goal-directed resuscitation for patients with early septic shock. N Engl J Med 2014; 371: 1496–506.
10. Michard F, Teboul J. Predicting fluid responsiveness in ICU patients. Chest 2002; 121: 2000–8.
11. Charron C, Caille V, Jardin F, et al. Echocardiographic measurement of fluid responsiveness. Curr Opin Crit Care 2006; 12: 249–254.
12. Kaplan A, Mayo PH. Echocardiography performed by the pulmonary/critical care medicine physician. Chest 2009; 135: 529–35.
13. Soubrier S, Saulnier F, Hubert H, et al. Can dynamic indicators help the prediction of fluid responsiveness in spontaneously breathing critically ill patients? Intensive Care Med 2007; 33: 1117–24.
14. Rooke GA, Schwid HA, Shapira Y. The effect of graded hemorrhage and intravascular volume replacement on systolic pressure variation in humans during mechanical and spontaneous ventilation. Anesth Analg 1995; 80: 925–32.
15. Monnet X, Rienzo M, Osman D, et al. Passive leg raising predicts fluid responsiveness in the critically ill. Crit Care Med 2006; 34: 1402–7.
16. Preau S, Saulnier F, Dewavrin F, et al. Passive leg raising is predictive of fluid responsiveness in spontaneously breathing patients with severe sepsis or acute pancreatitis. Crit Care Med 2010; 38: 819–25.
17. Lamia B, Ochagavia A, Monnet X, et al. Echocardiographic prediction of volume responsiveness in critically ill patients with spontaneously breathing activity. Intensive Care Med 2007; 33: 1125–32.
18. Magder S, Georgiadis G, Cheong T. Respiratory variations in right atrial pressure predict the response to fluid challenge. J Crit Care 1992; 7: 76–85.
19. Heenen S, De Backer D, Vincent JL. How can the response to volume expansion in patients with spontaneous respiratory movements be predicted? Crit Care 2006; 10: R102.
20. Jue J, Chung W, Schiller NB, et al. Does inferior vena cava size predict right atrial pressure in patients receiving mechanical ventilation? J Am Soc Echocardiogr 1992; 5: 613–18.
21. Barbier C, Loubieres Y, Schmit C, et al. Respiratory changes in inferior vena cava diameter are helpful in predicting fluid responsiveness in ventilated septic patients. Intensive Care Med 2004; 30: 1740–6.
22. Feissel M, Michard F, Mangin I, et al. Respiratory changes in aortic blood velocity as an indicator of fluid responsiveness in ventilated patients with septic shock. Chest 2001; 119: 867–73.
23. Partridge BL. Use of pulse oximetry as a noninvasive indicator of intravascular volume status. J Clin Monit 1987; 3: 263–8.
24. Brunkhorst F, Engel C, Bloos F, et al. Intensive insulin therapy and pentastarch resuscitation in severe sepsis. N Engl J Med 2008; 358: 125–39.
25. De Backer D, Biston P, Devriendt J, et al.; SOAP II Investigators. Comparison of dopamine and norepinephrine in the treatment of shock. N Engl J Med 2010; 362: 779–89.
26. De Backer D, Aldecoa C, Njimi H, Vincent JL. Dopamine versus norepinephrine in the treatment of septic shock: a meta-analysis. Crit Care Med 2012; 40: 725–30.
27. Serpa Neto A, Nassar AP, Cardoso SO, et al. Vasopressin and terlipressin in adult vasodilatory shock: a systematic review and meta-analysis of nine randomized controlled trials. Crit Care 2012; 16: R154.
28. Villanueva C, Colomo A, Bosch A, et al. Transfusion strategies for acute upper gastrointestinal bleeding. N Engl J Med 2013; 368: 11–21.
29. Steg PG, Hubert K, Andreotti F, et al. Bleeding in acute coronary syndromes and percutaneous coronary interventions: position paper by the Working Group on Thrombosis of the European Society of Cardiology. Eur Heart J 2011; 32: 1854–64.

1. HYPERTENSION

Hypertension (HTN) is defined as blood pressure >140/90 mmHg on two or more occasions (each one on a different clinic visit), or on one occasion when there are signs of end-organ damage (LVH, retinopathy, chronic kidney disease). Both the systolic blood pressure (SBP) and diastolic blood pressure (DBP) are associated with increased coronary, HF, and stroke risk. The risk is likely greater with increments in SBP than equivalent increments in DBP. In addition, in older patients (>65) or patients with CAD, a J curve is seen for DBP and SBP: a high DBP (>90 mmHg) increases cardiovascular risk, but a low DBP (<70 mmHg) is also harmful and increases the risk of coronary events.[1–5] A J curve also exists for SBP (probably <110 mmHg). Younger patients have a hockeystick curve, wherein the risk remains flat, unchanged, at low DBP <70 mmHg.

I. Stages of hypertension
The stages of HTN are:

- Pre-hypertension: 120–140/80–90 mmHg. This BP level is a marker of increased cardiovascular risk, but not an indication to treat. While a BP <115/65 mmHg is ideal, actively reducing BP to <120 mmHg with drug therapy does not necessarily improve outcomes.
- Stage 1: 140–160/90–100 mmHg.
- Stage 2 (severe): > 160/100 mmHg.[6]

The systemic arteries stiffen with increasing age, which leads to a sharp increase in pressure during systole and a sharp decline in pressure during diastole. Thus, with age, SBP and pulse pressure increase while DBP decreases; isolated systolic HTN is highly prevalent in older patients. Arterial stiffening is more common in populations with high sodium intake and obesity.

II. Causes of HTN
Hypertension is primary (essential) in 95% and secondary in 5% of patients. Tables 23.1–23.4 list the features that suggest secondary HTN, the causes of secondary hypertension, and the workup of hypertension.

Practical Cardiovascular Medicine, First Edition. Elias B. Hanna.
© 2017 John Wiley & Sons Ltd. Published 2017 by John Wiley & Sons Ltd.

Table 23.1 Situations that warrant workup for secondary HTN.

A. Age <30 with systolic or diastolic HTN; age >60 with diastolic HTN

B. Resistant HTN (= resistant to three drugs at optimal doses, including a diuretic)

C. Acute HTN with DBP >110 mmHg, or malignant HTN

D. Laboratory findings (creatinine, K, urinalysis)
  1. ↓ K or metabolic alkalosis in the absence of diuretic therapy (→ RAS or hyperaldosteronism)
  2. ↑ Creatinine (→ RAS or chronic renal insufficiency)
  3. ↑ Creatinine with ACE-I (→ RAS)
  4. Abnormal urinalysis (glomerular hematuria, proteinuria)
  5. Unilateral small kidney (kidney size difference ≥1.5 cm suggests RAS)

E. History/exam features
  1. Abdominal bruit, peripheral arterial disease → RAS
  2. Paroxysmal headaches, palpitations, sweating, pallor → pheochromocytoma
  3. HTN worsens with β-blockers → pheochromocytoma
  4. Orthostatic hypotension → may be pheochromocytoma, but is usually related to hypovolemia, autonomic dysfunction, stiff non-compliant arteries, or side effect of treatment
  5. Sleep apnea features

RAS, renal artery stenosis.

Table 23.2 Causes of secondary hypertension.

A. Chronic kidney disease (CKD): ~2% of HTN. CKD is the most common cause of secondary HTN (diabetic nephropathy, glomerulonephritis, or polycystic kidney disease). CKD is also a common complication of essential HTN

B. Renal artery stenosis (RAS): 1–2% (uni- or bilateral RAS)

C. Primary hyperaldosteronism (e.g., adrenal hyperplasia, or adrenal adenoma [Conn's syndrome]). This is a common cause of resistant HTN, including severe HTN >180/110 mmHg, and is seen **in up to 20% of patients with resistant HTN**.[7–9] K is often normal, as hypokalemia is only seen late in the disease process. Obesity and sleep apnea trigger an increase in aldosterone synthesis, sometimes mimicking primary hyperaldosteronism

D. Drugs: contraceptive pills, NSAIDs, cocaine, steroid therapy

E. Sleep apnea

F. Cushing's syndrome, including its most common cause, steroid therapy

G. Pheochromocytoma: ~50% of patients present with permanent HTN and paroxysmal spikes, ~45% have permanent HTN only, ~5% have paroxysmal HTN only

H. Hypercalcemia

I. Hyper- and hypothyroidism. Hypothyroidism causes hypervolemia and a predominantly diastolic hypertension, while hyperthyroidism usually causes isolated systolic hypertension

J. Coarctation of the aorta

These causes, especially RAS, generally lead to elevations of both systolic and diastolic BP, as both hypervolemia and vasoconstriction occur. Isolated systolic HTN is unlikely to be secondary to RAS.

Table 23.3 Basic workup for any HTN.

A. Creatinine, potassium, calcium

B. Urinalysis (signs of glomerulopathy [proteinuria, hematuria])

C. Look for end-organ damage
  1. *ECG ± echo* (looking for LVH): LVH voltage on ECG correlates with the left ventricular mass and with the risk of developing HF. Strain ST–T changes correlate with worse LVH and with a higher risk of LV dysfunction. The occurrence of LBBB correlates with a higher likelihood of systolic dysfunction
     - LVH voltage may regress with therapy. This correlates with a reduction of HF risk[10]
     - Echo may show diastolic dysfunction, which precedes LVH and is more prevalent than LVH
  2. *Urinalysis*
     - Proteinuria hints at glomerular damage causing HTN or secondary to HTN
     - Microalbuminuria (ratio of urinary albumin/creatinine on a spot urine): hints at early glomerular damage from diabetes or HTN
     - Decreasing albuminuria is a treatment goal and is associated with renoprotection and improved cardiovascular outcomes
  3. *Funduscopic exam:* Arteriolar narrowing, hemorrhages, excudates, papilledema

Table 23.4 Specific workup when secondary HTN is suspected.

A. Doppler ultrasound of the renal arteries (or MRA or renal perfusion nuclear scan)

B. Aldosterone serum level and plasma renin activity (PRA). If aldosterone/PRA ratio >20 and aldosterone level >10 ng/dl, primary hyperaldosteronism is suggested.[a] ACE inhibitors and β-blockers affect this testing, but not enough to warrant drug interruption (the former ↑ PRA, the latter ↓PRA).[7] Aldosterone antagonists should, however, be stopped

C. Serum-free metanephrines and normetanephrines, and 24-hour urinary metanephrines and normetanephrines (these two tests have the best yield for the diagnosis of pheochromocytoma)

D. TSH

E. Consider sleep study in the appropriate context

---

[a] A primary elevation in aldosterone level leads to a feedback decrease in PRA. Aldosterone is expressed in ng/dl while PRA is expressed in ng/ml/h.

III. Treatment of HTN: goals of therapy
A. Goal ≤140/90 mmHg, including in patients with diabetes, CKD or CAD[11,12]
Possible goal ≤120–130 mmHg in select high-risk patients (e.g., CAD) who can tolerate lower pressure

In the HOT trial, which randomized patients to multiple DBP goals (<90 vs. < 85 vs. < 80), a DBP of 82 mmHg was associated with the lowest risk of cardiovascular events, with a J curve beyond that point. Diabetic patients derived further benefit from DBP <80 mmHg, with no evidence of a J curve. A similar lack of J curve was seen in the UKPDS study. This led to the recommendation of a lower BP goal in diabetic patients.[5,13] However, later on, the ACCORD trial of diabetic patients compared aggressive HTN control, i.e., SBP <120 mmHg (mean 119 mHg), with a more conservative HTN control of 130–140 mmHg (mean 133 mmHg).[14] The aggressive HTN control did not improve mortality or the overall cardiovascular outcomes. It reduced the already low stroke risk in these appropriately treated patients (from 0.5% per year to 0.3% per year), but increased the risk of side effects (dizziness, creatinine rise). Moreover, post-hoc analyses from INVEST trial suggest that SBP <130 mmHg in diabetic patients, or <140 mmHg in patients older than 80 does not improve cardiovascular outcomes.[15,16]

Concerning CKD, three trials addressed BP goals <140/90 mmHg in CKD and did not find any statistically significant benefit on renal outcomes (AASK, MDRD, REIN-2 trials).[12,17–19] In the AASK trial of African-American patients, BP reduction to a mean of 128/78 mmHg did not improve renal outcomes in comparison with BP of 141/85 mmHg; conversely, the specific use of ACE-I improved renal outcomes in comparison with other drugs.

Concerning diastolic HF, the I-PRESERVE trial has shown that ARB does not provide any benefit in patients with controlled HTN (BP 136/76 mmHg), indirectly suggesting that an SBP goal much lower than 140 mmHg may not be warranted in diastolic HF.[20]

In CAD patients with normal EF and SBP 130–140 mmHg who receive aggressive statin and revascularization therapy, the addition of ACE-I did not improve outcomes (55% had prior MI) (PEACE trial).[21]

Yet, recently, the SPRINT trial randomized *non-diabetic* patients with HTN and one additional cardiovascular risk factor to SBP goal <120 mmHg vs. < 140 mmHg (28% of patients had CKD, 20% had coronary or vascular disease, and 28% were older than 75).[22] *In contrast to the above data, intensive SBP control led to a reduction of total mortality, HF, and cardiac mortality.* Note, however, that the mean SBP achieved in the intensive group was 121.4 mmHg, not <120 mmHg. Also note that the absolute mortality reduction was small, 0.37% per year; side effects such as syncope and acute kidney injury were increased, and renal outcomes were not improved.

Optimal BP may differ for various vital organs. Several post-hoc analyses have shown that the risk of stroke continues to decrement with SBP below 120 mmHg, but MI and acute renal events may become more frequent.[4,23] The J curve between BP (SBP, and even more so DBP) and coronary events is particularly evident in patients with underlying CAD or LVH that impairs coronary flow autoregulation. A 2007 AHA statement suggested keeping DBP over 65 mmHg in patients with non-revascularized CAD.[24]

B. The very elderly (≥80 years of age)
In the very elderly, ESC suggests that 150 mmHg is an acceptable target. The only randomized trial addressing HTN in this age group aimed for a target SBP of 150 mmHg (HYVET trial).[25] SBP goal of 150 mmHg also needs to be accepted in elderly frail patients who develop orthostatic symptoms with drug therapy, even if <80 years of age (ESC guidelines).[11] Moreover, JNC 8 considers SBP of 150 mmHg an acceptable target in patients 60–80 years of age who do not have diabetes, CKD, or CAD.[12]

> The improvement in cardiovascular and renal outcomes is related more to the BP achieved and the 24-hour hypertensive control than to a particular drug mechanism.

IV. Treatment of HTN: timing, first-line drugs, compelling indications for specific drugs
A. BP 140–160/90–100 mmHg on two occasions
If BP is in this range, lifestyle modifications are initiated (sodium ≤3 g/d, exercise, and weight loss), and BP is rechecked in 1 month. If BP is still elevated, drug therapy is initiated. Elderly patients with non-compliant arteries, CKD patients, and black patients are particularly susceptible to high sodium intake.

B. BP > 160/100 mmHg on two readings
If BP >160/100 mmHg, drug therapy is initiated immediately.

C. How and what to start
- If BP 140–160/90–100 mmHg, one drug is started.
- If BP >160/100 mmHg, combination therapy may be started (JNC 8), except in the elderly patient, where careful drug initiation is recommended.
- Each drug is expected to reduce BP by ≤20/10 mmHg.

D. First-line drugs
In the absence of any compelling condition, any of the following three classes of agents can be used as a first-line therapy:

a. Thiazide diuretic
b. ACE-I or ARB
c. CCB

In the ALLHAT trial, all three classes achieved similar reduction in mortality and MI. Thiazide diuretic was superior to ACE-I for stroke prevention and slightly superior to ACE-I and CCB for HF prevention.[26]

β-Blockers, especially atenolol given once daily, are less effective for HTN control, patient survival, and stroke/MI risk reduction and should not be used as a first-line therapy unless there is a compelling indication (HF, arrhythmias, angina).[27–31]

E. Follow-up

One or two drugs are started, then BP is rechecked 1 month later (oral agents work slowly and take more than 1 week to achieve the optimal effect).

a. If BP remains uncontrolled, the dosage of the drug(s) is optimized (the target being at least one-half of the maximal dose, which is usually an optimal dose). Subsequently, another first-line drug is added, then a third first-line drug is added if needed. If HTN persists in spite of drug A, doubling the dose of A achieves 5× less BP reduction than adding another drug.[32] In addition, maximizing the dose of one drug increases side effects more than it improves BP control; therefore, in general, once a moderate dose of drug A is achieved, adding a new drug is preferred to maximizing the dose of drug A.

b. If not the first drug used, a thiazide diuretic is typically added as a second agent whenever a combination is needed. This is because hypervolemia is a common mechanism of HTN, *sometimes exacerbated by vasodilator-induced volume retention*. In fact, thiazide diuretics are synergistic with other antihypertensive drugs.

Conversely, the ACCOMPLISH trial suggests that when combination therapy is needed, the combination of ACE-I and amlodipine is superior to the combination of ACE-I and hydrochlorothiazide, with 20% more reduction of death, MI, and stroke.[33] This trial mainly recruited white patients without CKD, with a high prevalence of diabetes and CAD. The results may not apply to other thiazide diuretics (chlorthalidone), or to black patients or patients with obvious hypervolemia or CKD. Diuretic therapy remains an appropriate second agent or, at least, third agent if needed.

> **Note**
>
> Always watch for signs of orthostatic hypotension or fatigue, which may occur with very fast BP reduction and dictate a slower titration as well as general measures to prevent orthostatic hypotension.
>
> Always look at out-of-office home measurements to diagnose the following:[34,35]
>
> - The white-coat effect, in which BP is high in the office and normal at home. This effect is suspected in patients with chronic HTN who do not display any target end-organ damage and repeatedly show signs of overtreatment such as orthostatic hypotension. The white-coat effect has either a small or no long-term adverse effect.
> - Masked HTN, which is the reverse of white-coat HTN. BP is high at home and normal at the office. This occurs in 10–30% of patients with HTN. Masked HTN has a major, long-term adverse cardiovascular effect and needs to be treated.

F. Compelling indications for specific antihypertensive drugs

1. CAD: β-blocker, ACE-I/ARB; aldosterone antagonist for LV dysfunction post-MI.

2. HF: β-blocker (carvedilol, metoprolol XL), ACE-I/ARB, aldosterone antagonist, diuretic. The combination hydralazine–nitrates is a second-line therapy for persistent HF or refractory HTN despite the preceding regimen (especially for black patients).

3. CKD, or microalbuminuria/proteinuria: ACE-I/ARB. Volume overload, sometimes occult, is common in CKD and explains the antihypertensive efficacy of diuretics.

4. Diabetes or metabolic syndrome without nephropathy: the ALLHAT and VALUE trials suggest the lack of difference between ACE-I/ARB, CCB, and thiazide diuretic in terms of cardiovascular outcomes, including in the diabetic subgroup. Thus, any of the three first-line therapies may be initiated in diabetic patients. Yet ACE-I/ARB and CCB may be preferred, as they do not worsen diabetes control (ESC); in fact, ACE-I/ARB therapy potentially improves insulin sensitivity and reduces the risk of diabetes in patients with metabolic syndrome. β-Blockers and thiazide diuretics increase the risk of diabetes and may worsen the lipid profile.[11] ACE-I or ARB therapy is preferred in microalbuminuria.

5. Black patients do not respond well to ACE-I/ARB monotherapy when used for HTN control. Black patients are salt-sensitive, as they have a highly active distal tubular sodium channel (high renal sodium retention) and, consequently, low renin and angiotensin levels. Thiazides and CCBs are the most effective drugs for HTN in this population; aldosterone antagonists are also effective, as they reduce the amount of tubular sodium channels. However, ACE-I therapy is very effective in black patients with CKD or HF and remains first-line therapy in this context. ACE-I therapy is also an effective antihypertensive therapy in black patients already receiving CCB or diuretic therapy, both of which activate the renin–angiotensin system.[24] The AASK trial addressed ACE-Is in black patients with CKD and showed that ACE-Is are as effective as amlodipine in controlling HTN, and more effective in long-term GFR preservation.[17]

6. Supraventricular arrhythmias: β-blockers, non-DHP CCBs.

7. Ventricular arrhythmias: β-blockers.

V. Resistant HTN

Resistant HTN is HTN resistant to three drugs administered at an optimal dosage, including a diuretic

A. Causes[36–38]

- *Non-compliance* with low salt diet or drug therapy. Salt non-compliance may be assessed by measurement of 24-hour urinary sodium, which correlates with dietary sodium intake (a high urinary sodium implies a high sodium intake).
- *Obesity* increases renin–angiotensin activity, aldosterone synthesis, and thus extracellular volume. It also increases sympathetic activity. Every 10 kg of weight loss reduces BP by ~10 mmHg, and thus *weight loss is of critical importance in morbidly obese patients*.
- NSAID, steroid therapy, cocaine, excessive alcohol use (>2 drinks/day for men or >1 drink/day for women).
- *Occult hypervolemia*: patients with resistant hypertension often have subclinical hypervolemia, which may be due to excessive salt intake, inadequate diuretic therapy, or a compensatory response to vasodilator therapy.[39]
- *White-coat HTN* (ambulatory BP measurements or 24-hour Holter BP monitoring are typically indicated in resistant HTN).

- Inappropriately small cuff size leads to BP overestimation in obese patients.
- *Secondary HTN*, particularly renal artery stenosis, hyperaldosteronism, and sleep apnea.
- *Pseudohypertension* of the elderly. In this case, the peripheral arteries are stiff and calcified and can hardly be compressed by the BP cuff, even if the intra-arterial pressure is normal. This results in a falsely elevated BP measurement. Hints to pseudohypertension:
  ○ "Severe HTN" is present without any end-organ damage.
  ○ Small doses of antihypertensive drugs induce dizziness.
  ○ Radial or brachial arteries remain palpable like stiff "pipes" despite cuff inflation beyond the audible systolic BP (i.e., arteries palpable despite being pulseless).
  ○ The definitive diagnosis is established by performing intra-arterial measurements.

B. If HTN is truly resistant, second-line drugs may be added

- β-Blockers, especially nebivolol or the α/β-blocker carvedilol.
- Spironolactone 25 mg daily or amiloride (a potassium-sparing diuretic): the addition of a small dose of spironolactone has been found to be very effective in treating drug-resistant HTN and decreases BP by ~20/10 mmHg in black or white patients (PATHWAY-2 trial).[36,39,40] This may be particularly true in obese patients and in the case of the frequently underdiagnosed primary hyperaldosteronism. The efficacy, however, appears independent of renin level or renin/aldosterone ratio.
- Consider increasing the dose of hydrochlorothiazide (HCTZ) or switching to chlorthalidone or a loop diuretic for better control of hypervolemia, including subclinical hypervolemia. The efficacy of HCTZ, but not chlorthalidone or loop diuretics, is reduced in patients with GFR <30 ml/min. According to the British HTN guidelines, increasing the diuretic dose or adding spironolactone is the immediate next step in resistant HTN management.[27]
- Central sympathomimetics (clonidine: α_2-agonist).
- Direct vasodilators (hydralazine).
- α-Blockers.
- The combination of ACE-I and ARB or renin inhibitor is neither useful nor recommended for patients with refractory HTN.

C. Consider the mechanism of the refractory HTN, and try to treat it accordingly[37] (volume, vascular tone, catecholamine tone)

- If the patient has CKD or volume overload on exam, consider increasing the diuretic therapy or adding spironolactone if creatinine <2 mg/dl.
- If the patient's heart rate is >84 bpm, consider catecholamine excess as a cause of HTN or as a result of diuretic and vasodilator therapy, and add or increase β-blocker therapy.
- In the absence of the above, try to increase vasodilator therapy. Alternatively, or later on, increase diuretic therapy for occult hypervolemia.

VI. Peripheral vs. central aortic pressure: therapeutic implications

The systolic pressure increases in the peripheral arteries as a result of the pressure waves that are reflected from arterial bifurcation points and small peripheral vessels and that add to the systolic wave. After the age of 60, the reflected waves not only amplify the peripheral arterial pressure but also return to the central aorta quickly as a result of heightened arterial stiffness; this is called increased pulse wave velocity. Thus, these waves reach the aortic root in late systole, which leads to augmentation of the central aortic pressure as well as the peripheral pressure.[41–44] In fact, in the elderly, the systolic and pulse aortic pressures are increased because of: (1) ejection of the stroke volume into a stiff aorta; (2) increased pulse wave velocity that allows the reflected waves to return to the aorta in systole. In contrast, in the young patient, the reflected waves return to the central aorta in early diastole, which increases diastolic pressure and potentially coronary filling. The systolic aortic pressure is closer to the peripheral systolic pressure in the elderly than in the young.

β-Blockers, when used for hypertension, reduce the peripheral arterial pressure but less so the central arterial pressure (pseudo-antihypertensive effect).[42–44] This is because β-blockers exert less effect on arterial remodeling and stiffness than calcium channel blockers, ACE inhibitors, or diuretics. Furthermore, a reduction in heart rate prolongs the cardiac ejection phase and may allow the backward wave reflection to reach the central systolic pressure at its peak rather than late. Also, a reduction in heart rate may lead to the ejection of a higher stroke volume into a poorly compliant aorta. Consequently, the central aortic pressure may increase with heart rate reduction.[41–43] Vasodilators (ACE-Is, CCBs), diuretics, and aldosterone antagonists improve arterial compliance, reduce reflected waves, and delay their timing. Thus, these agents reduce peripheral pressure, but even more the central aortic pressure, and supplement diastolic coronary filling.

VII. Antihypertensive drugs

A. ACE-Is and ARBs

1. Mechanism of benefit in CKD

ACE-Is/ARBs are the preferred agents in CKD, including advanced CKD. ACE-I/ARBs vasodilate efferent renal arterioles, without any effect on the afferent arteriole, which reduces GFR and may increase creatinine acutely. However, over the long term, the kidneys are protected from the high glomerular pressure that leads to scarring (Figure 23.1). ACE-Is/ARBs reduce the rate of decline of renal function and the incidence of end-stage renal disease by ~20–50% as compared to other antihypertensive agents, particularly CCBs, despite comparable BP reduction (AASK and IDNT trials, JNC 8).[12,17,45] This benefit is achieved with optimal to high doses and is accentuated in patients with proteinuria >1 g/d; in fact, ACE-Is/ARBs more effectively reduce proteinuria than any other agent.[17,45] The worse the proteinuria, the more striking the benefit. The benefit continues to be seen in advanced renal failure (up to a creatinine of 5 mg/dl).[46] It is also seen in black patients with CKD.[17] ACE-Is may not be more nephroprotective than CCBs or thiazide diuretics in patients with early nephropathy and no proteinuria (ALLHAT study).[26,47]

2. Contraindications and monitoring

ACE-I/ARB initiation is contraindicated in acute kidney injury and in bilateral RAS, in which cases kidney perfusion is dependent on angiotensin II.

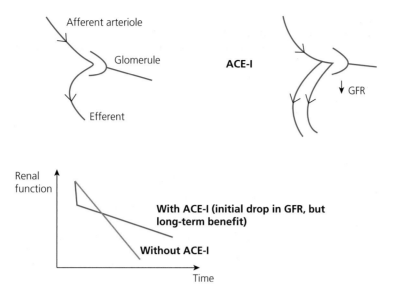

Figure 23.1 Effect of ACE-I on renal function over the short and long term.

Creatinine is checked 7–14 days after starting ACE-I/ARB. An increase in creatinine of up to 30% is tolerated, as these agents are beneficial over the long term. The following three conditions most commonly explain a creatinine rise >30%: hypovolemia (overdiuresis), nephropathy with GFR dependence on the angiotensin system, or severe low-output HF. While less common, bilateral RAS should also be considered. If creatinine rises >30%:

- The patient is assessed for hypovolemia (orthostatic hypotension). A diuretic that was recently initiated may be withheld.
- In the absence of obvious hypovolemia or recent diuretic initiation, ACE-I is discontinued at least temporarily, with an attempt to resume it later, at a lower dose, in patients without RAS.

3. Differences between ACE-I and ARB
- Renin, released by the juxtaglomerular apparatus, converts angiotensinogen to angiotensin I. The angiotensin converting enzyme, secreted by the vascular endothelium, especially in the lungs, converts angiotensin I into active angiotensin II, which stimulates the adrenal secretion of aldosterone and acts as a vasoconstrictor. ACE-Is prevent the conversion of angiotensin I to the active angiotensin II and prevent the degradation of a vasodilator, bradykinin.
- ARBs block angiotensin-II type 1 receptor, which is the receptor involved in salt retention, vasoconstriction, tissue growth, and deleterious vascular and cardiac remodeling.
- The main advantage of ARB over ACE-I is the lower frequency of angioedema and the absence of cough (cough being a side effect of ACE-I-triggered bradykinin release, occurring in 10% of patients). A cross-reactive angioedema rarely occurs with ARB, in <5% of ACE-I reactive patients; ACE-I- related angioedema does not preclude the use of ARB in patients with a strong compelling indication, such as HF or CKD (close monitoring is warranted).

4. The combination of ACE-I and ARB should generally be avoided (JNC 8)
The combination ACE-I/ARB has not been shown to improve cardiovascular outcomes or HTN control, with a worsening of major renal outcomes (ONTARGET trial).[23] In HF, the combination ACE-I–aldosterone antagonist is preferred to ACE-I–ARB, as the former improves survival, whereas the latter improves HF hospitalization without any effect on mortality.

B. CCBs
1. Types of CCBs and mechanisms of action
- Dihydropyridines (DHPs; e.g., nifedipine, amlodipine, felodipine) are vasodilators that have minimal to no negative chronotropic and inotropic effect. Felodipine has the least negative inotropic effect, and both amlodipine and felodipine have been studied in systolic HF and shown to be safe. Amlodipine is a very long-acting DHP, with sustained 24-hour BP reduction, which explains the clinical efficacy of this agent.
- Non-DHPs (diltiazem and verapamil) have negative inotropic and chronotropic effects, particularly prominent with verapamil. They also have a vasodilatory effect, slightly less prominent than that of DHPs.

The combination of a DHP and a non-DHP is not generally used. This combination, however, may be used in patients with refractory HTN who cannot receive β-blockers because of asthma. If a patient can receive a β-blocker, DHP is better combined with a β-blocker than with a non-DHP.

2. Contraindications
- Non-DHPs are contraindicated in systolic HF, significant sinus bradyarrhythmia (rate <55–60 bpm) or second- or third-degree AV block. Non-DHPs are avoided in combination with β-blockers, except for the rate control of AF, where the combination β-blocker–diltiazem may be used.
- Long-acting DHPs are not contraindicated in compensated HF (with the exception of nifedipine) or in bradyarrhythmias. In general, the short-acting nifedipine is avoided in CAD as it leads to reflex tachycardia and subsequent myocardial ischemia, even though its direct effect is slightly rate slowing.

3. Other side effects

Headache, edema (mainly with DHPs), constipation (mainly with verapamil). Edema is not responsive to diuretics but may be reduced with ACE-I/ARB.

C. Diuretics (thiazide diuretics, loop diuretics, aldosterone antagonists)
1. Thiazide diuretics (hydrocholorothiazide, chlorthalidone)

Thiazide diuretics are weak diuretics that block sodium reabsorption in the distal tubule, where ~3–5% of sodium is reabsorbed. Loop diuretics block sodium reabsorption in the ascending loop of Henle, where ~25% of sodium is reabsorbed. Thiazide diuretics are the typical diuretics used in HTN. They are longer-acting than loop diuretics, and they induce less hypovolemia and hypokalemia than loop diuretics, but more hyponatremia. Chronic diuretic administration also produces mild vasodilation and improves arterial compliance by inhibiting sodium entry into smooth muscle cells.

Chlorthalidone is longer acting than hydrocholorothiazide (HCTZ), provides greater 24-hour BP reduction, and is possibly associated with better outcomes.[48] At the recommended dose of 12.5–25 mg, HCTZ reduces 24-hour ambulatory BP less than chlorthalidone 12.5–25 mg and other antihypertensives (ACE-I, CCBs), even though office BP may be similarly reduced.[49] HCTZ 50 mg achieves optimal 24-hour BP reduction and may be reserved for patients with refractory HTN. While more efficacious, chlorthalidone may be associated with a higher early risk of acute kidney injury and hypokalemia warranting close monitoring. Indapamide is a thiazide-like diuretic with a more pronounced vasodilatory effect.

a. Side effects of thiazides:
- Hypovolemia, hypokalemia, hypomagnesemia: mainly with HCTZ doses >25 mg/day or chlorthalidone. Hypokalemia explains why thiazide diuretics were associated with an *increased risk of sudden death* in old studies. Potassium level should be closely monitored after thiazide initiation. *The combination of thiazide with a potassium-sparing diuretic counteracts the increased risk of sudden death.*[50] Creatinine and potassium are checked 7 days after diuretic initiation.
- Hyponatremia may be due to hypovolemia, but may also be due to the fact that the target of thiazide action, the distal tubule, is the diluting segment of the nephron; thus, urine is more concentrated when thiazides are used, which gives a "SIADH-like" picture, especially in the elderly.
- Hypercalcemia (whereas loop diuretics have a direct calcium-reducing effect).
- Other dose-dependent metabolic side effects: hyperuricemia, hyperglycemia (mostly related to hypokalemia and attenuated with K sparing diuretics), increased LDL.

b. Dose of chlorthalidone: 12.5–25.0 mg/day. Dose of HCTZ: 25 mg/day (~2:1 equivalence to chlorthalidone). HCTZ may be increased to 50 mg/day in resistant HTN. The 12.5 mg HCTZ dose has limited efficacy, except when combined with amiloride 5 mg.

> Rather than doubling the dose of a thiazide, combining it with the potassium-sparing diuretic amiloride improves BP control and attenuates metabolic side effects (PATHWAY-3 trial).[51] It also counteracts the increased risk of sudden death. This comes at the price of a small risk of hyperkalemia, especially in patients with CKD, acute prerenal renal failure, or diabetes, which mandates K monitoring early after therapy initiation and with any illness.

2. Loop diuretics (furosemide, bumetanide, torsemide)

Loop diuretics are mainly used in HF, but may also be used for HTN when creatinine is >2.5 mg/dl or GFR is <30 ml/min, because, in that case, the efficacy of thiazides may be reduced. In patients with GFR <30 ml/min, less sodium is filtered overall; in order to maintain appropriate natriuresis, relatively less sodium is reabsorbed from each of the remaining nephrons (compensatory mechanism). In those patients, less absolute and relative sodium can be eliminated by any diuretic, particularly a thiazide diuretic, since even normally, only ~3–5% of sodium is reabsorbed by the distal tubule. Thus, thiazide diuretics are less effective in patients with advanced renal failure, but, contrary to common belief, remain effective after cumulative dosing. All thiazide diuretics are renally eliminated, have a long half-life, especially chlorthalidone, and cumulate in renal failure, which further potentiates their effect after multiple dosing and explains their efficacy in hypertensive patients with advanced CKD;[52,53] in fact, chlorthalidone may be "too" effective and lead to hypovolemia. The following diuretic regimens may be used for BP reduction in advanced CKD: chlorthalidone 12.5–25 mg every other day, furosemide once or twice daily, torsemide once daily.

The main problems with loop diuretics are: (i) short duration of action (4–6 hours), (ii) diuretic effect that is too potent for isolated HTN. Torsemide has a longer duration of action and may be preferred. In the absence of overt hypervolemia, HF, or advanced renal failure, thiazides are better antihypertensive agents than loop diuretics.

In case of sulfa allergy, thiazide diuretics and the typical loop diuretics cannot be used. Ethacrynic acid, a loop diuretic, may be used instead (available in both oral and IV forms).

3. Aldosterone antagonists (spironolactone, eplerenone)

Aldosterone antagonists act on the distal collecting tubule and induce mild diuresis, which may be particularly prominent in patients with hyperactive distal tubular sodium channels or patients resistant to other diuretics. However, in many patients, this mild diuresis cannot account for all of the antihypertensive benefit. Aldosterone has proliferative and fibrotic vascular and cardiac effects, and has vasoconstrictive effects through the vascular sodium ion, all of which are counteracted by spironolactone. In fact, spironolactone improves vascular compliance and tone and increases nitric oxide release.[54] The benefit is seen in patients with or without high levels of aldosterone, with or without adjunctive diuretic therapy, implying that blocking even a slight, unnoticed excess of aldosterone provides clinical benefit.

Regardless of HTN, they are used for systolic HF with functional classes II–IV and for patients with a recent MI, LVEF <40%, and either diabetes or HF.

Aldosterone antagonists and other potassium-sparing diuretics (amiloride, a distal sodium channel antagonist) can also be used with thiazides to improve BP control and to counteract the risk of sudden death associated with hypokalemia.[50] Aldosterone antagonists and amiloride are also excellent agents for refractory HTN in white or black patients, especially obese patients.[36,39,40] The correction of hypokalemia has, by itself, vasodilatory and antihypertensive effects. Because the increased risk of diabetes associated with thiazides is related to hypokalemia, the addition of potassium-sparing diuretics to thiazides attenuates the risk of diabetes.

The main side effect is hyperkalemia. Thus, aldosterone antagonists should be avoided if creatinine >2 mg/dl or GFR <30 ml/min, and potassium should be closely monitored at 3 and 7 days, then every 2–4 weeks for 3 months, then every 3 months.

D. β-Blockers

β-Blockers exert antihypertensive effects through a reduction of cardiac output but also through the blockade of juxtaglomerular β_1-receptors, which reduces renin release. Furthermore, lipophilic β-blockers may inhibit central sympathetic tone. However, β-blockers, particularly the hydrophilic β-blocker atenolol, appear inferior to first-line antihypertensive agents. In one meta-analysis, β-blockers reduced stroke and HF in comparison with placebo but were inferior to diuretics in regards to stroke and mortality.[29] In the LIFE trial, atenolol was inferior to losartan for stroke reduction.[30] In the ASCOT trial, an atenolol-based strategy was associated with more stroke, mortality, total cardiovascular events, and diabetes than an amlodipine-based strategy.[31] This inferiority of β-blockers may be related to atenolol itself, to an inappropriate once-daily use of atenolol, or to the fact that β-blockers are less effective in reducing central BP in poorly compliant arteries.[42]

While heart rate reduction is associated with improved outcomes in HF and in the post-MI setting, heart rate reduction with β-blockers in hypertensive trials is associated with increased event rate, mainly when heart rate is <65 bpm. This probably occurs because a low heart rate may paradoxically increase stroke volume even when a β-blocker is used, with a resultant increase in pulse pressure and central aortic pressure.[55]

On the other hand, data from the UKPDS study of diabetic patients showed that β-blockers were equivalent to ACE-Is in the reduction of cardiovascular events.[56] In younger patients with compliant arteries, β-blockers, in formulations other than atenolol, may remain effective.

1. *β-Blockers are contraindicated in:*
- Decompensated HF (they are indicated for compensated systolic HF, where they should be titrated slowly, every 2 weeks).
- Symptomatic or severe sinus bradycardia or AV nodal block (heart rate <55 bpm, PR interval >0.24 seconds, any second- or third-degree AV block).
- History of severe asthma or decompensated COPD. Patients with mild-to-moderate reactive airway disease or compensated COPD usually tolerate small-to-medium doses of β_1-blockers (e.g., metoprolol up to 100 mg/day).

Other side effects: fatigue, impotence (rarely). Fatigue may be due to a limitation of the cardiac output reserve or to a CNS effect.

Metabolic side effects: β-blockers may worsen hyperglycemia, hypoglycemia, and hypoglycemic unawareness. However, β-blockers are not contraindicated in diabetic patients if there is a compelling indication, and in fact β-blockers have a particular benefit in diabetic patients (UKPDS study). β-blockers can increase triglycerides and reduce HDL.

2. *Cardioselective β_1-blockers* (atenolol, metoprolol, bisoprolol) have fewer metabolic effects, bronchospastic effects, and vasoconstrictive effects (better tolerated in PAD) than non-selective β-blockers, but lose their cardioselectivity at high doses. Atenolol has a shorter duration of action than commonly thought, and, if used, should be given twice daily like metoprolol. Atenolol, unlike metoprolol, is renally cleared, and the dose should be reduced and given once daily in renal failure.

3. *Lipophilic β-blockers* are metabolized by the liver, leading to reduced bioavailability and a short half-life (metoprolol, propranolol: highly lipophilic; carvedilol, labetalol, bisoprolol: moderately lipophilic). Atenolol is a *hydrophilic β-blocker* but has a short half-life as well (6 hours). Lipophilic β-blockers have more CNS effects, such as fatigue, somnolence, and depression, but may also be more beneficial as a result of sympathetic neuromodulation. Beside the inappropriate once-daily dosing, hydrophilicity may explain why atenolol has not been clearly beneficial in the post-MI setting.[57] Yet, consider switching to atenolol if CNS side effects occur.

4. *Mixed α_1- and non-selective β-blockers* (labetalol, carvedilol) are more effective agents for BP reduction. Carvedilol, in comparison with metoprolol, does not worsen glucose or lipid control, improves insulin resistance, provides better renal protection, and does not lead to weight gain;[58] it may also have a beneficial urological effect in patients with benign prostate hyperplasia.[59]

Labetalol and carvedilol lose significant α-blocking effect with long-term administration, while the β-blocking effect remains unchanged; carvedilol preserves some of its α-blocking effect over the long term. Either way, the α-blocking effect is not as pronounced as with prazosin (carvedilol provides enough α-blockade to derive a benefit without the inherent harm).[60,61]

5. *Nebivolol* is the most cardioselective β_1-blocker. It also has direct vasodilatory effects mediated by nitric oxide potentiation. Nebivolol, like carvedilol, seems to have a more pronounced antihypertensive effect, without dyslipidemic and dysglycemic effects.

6. *Sudden β-blocker withdrawal* should be avoided, as it may lead to a withdrawal syndrome of tachycardia, HTN, and myocardial ischemia.

E. α₁-Blockers

α_1-Blockers are used as third-line agents and are mainly indicated in patients who have HTN and benign prostate hyperplasia. α-Blockers reduce BP less effectively than first-line agents and are associated with a higher risk of HF and stroke as compared to first-line agents; this is related to a lesser antihypertensive efficacy but also to the reflex sympathetic stimulation.[62]

Beside the higher risk of HF, α-blockers are associated with the highest risk of orthostatic hypotension (especially with the first dose), which dictates their bedtime use.

Prazosin is used for HTN, doxazosin and terazosin are used for both HTN and prostate hyperplasia, while tamsulosin is a more selective α_{1a}-blocker that is selective for urethral tissue.

F. Clonidine (centrally acting sympathomimetic)

Clonidine leads to vasodilatation and negative ino- and chronotropism. It may worsen bradycardia (especially in combination with β-blockers) and HF.[24] In fact, clonidine is better avoided in HF, as a related central-acting sympathomimetic drug increased mortality in HF.[24]

Clonidine frequently leads to drowsiness. Acute withdrawal syndrome occurs on sudden withdrawal, and therefore clonidine must be tapered off over 1–2 weeks. Clonidine is not an appropriate drug when compliance is uncertain.

G. Hydralazine

Hydralazine is a direct-acting vasodilator that is mainly beneficial in black patients with HF, in combination with nitrates. It is also used as a second-line agent for refractory HTN.

Hydralazine has the following side effects:

- Reflex tachycardia and worsening of myocardial ischemia. Therefore, it must be used cautiously in CAD, along with nitrates and/or β-blockers
- Fluid retention, which means that it *must be used with a diuretic.*
- Reversible drug-induced lupus (especially with high doses or in the case of renal failure).

> Note that ACE-Is and long-acting DHPs are vasodilators that do not lead to reflex tachycardia. This is partly related to a slow-onset, sustained rather than abrupt effect. ACE-Is do not lead to reflex tachycardia because they reset the baroreceptor reactivity to lower levels of blood pressure.

H. Direct renin inhibitor

A direct renin inhibitor (aliskiren) is another blocker of the renin–angiotensin–aldosterone system and has the same antihypertensive effect as an ACE-I. It has renoprotective effects, reduces proteinuria, and is effective in combination with a CCB or a thiazide and seems better tolerated than an ACE-I. In combination with ACE-I or ARB, the additional antihypertensive effect is minimal, but the additional renal protection may be significant.[63] Aliskiren is very long-acting – its effect lasts several days to weeks; this is an advantage of this drug.

No long-term outcome data are available, so an ACE-I or an ARB is preferred. In patients already taking ACE-I or ARB, aliskiren barely provides any additional antihypertensive effect. Thus, the role of aliskiren has yet to be defined.

VIII. Other considerations in therapy

A. Orthostatic hypotension

Before starting therapy and during follow-up, check for orthostatic symptoms (dizziness) and check orthostatic changes in blood pressure. Patients may be hypertensive while recumbent but hypotensive while standing; this may be due to:

- Hypovolemia. Hypovolemia is typically associated with resting or orthostatic tachycardia.
- Autonomic dysfunction related to age or diabetes. The reduced baroreceptor activity prevents the rise in heart rate and vascular tone upon orthostasis.
- Poor arterial compliance associated with age, PAD, or severe, chronic HTN. *Poor arterial compliance leads to a striking rise but also striking fall in BP upon small changes in arterial volume, as may happen during the change from a supine to an upright position. These patients may have severe supine hypertension yet severe orthostatic hypotension.*
- Hypokalemia, psychotropic drugs.

> Antihypertensive therapy tends to worsen orthostatic hypotension, regardless of its cause, as it further impedes the compensatory mechanisms that occur during upright positioning, such as vasoconstriction or cardiac output increase.

Management of orthostatic hypotension:

- Look for treatable causes (hypovolemia, hypokalemia, psychotropic drugs).
- Maintain good hydration and consider stopping the diuretic. In patients with poor arterial compliance or autonomic dysfunction, any increase in salt intake leads to a striking HTN. Conversely, slight hypovolemia, which may occur when moderate activity is performed in a hot environment, leads to a striking hypotension.
- Sleep at 45 degrees, which stimulates the renin–aldosterone system to increase plasma volume. Also, *upright sleep prevents recumbent, nocturnal HTN.*
- Wear waist-high compressive stockings.
- Anticholinesterase therapy (pyridostigmine [Mestinon]).
- Start BP medications at low doses with slow titration (start with one drug at a time rather than a combination). SBP levels of 140–160 mmHg may have to be accepted. In fact, orthostatic hypotension impedes appropriate BP control.
- While all antihypertensive drugs may worsen orthostatic hypotension, diuretics (hypovolemia) and α-blockers should specifically be avoided.

B. Indications for 24-hour ambulatory BP monitoring

- Resistant HTN.
- Labile HTN.

- HTN with symptoms of postural hypotension. Holter may show overtreatment.
- Suspicion of white-coat HTN (clues: normal home BP measurements, no end-organ damage).
- Patients with suspected masked HTN, where BP is normal in the office and elevated in the ambulatory setting. This occurs in up to a third of HTN cases.

Normal mean daytime BP is <135/85 mmHg; normal nighttime BP is <120/75 mmHg; and normally there should be a nocturnal dip of 10–20% between the mean daytime and nighttime BP. Both non-dipping and over-dipping (large pressure surge in the morning) are associated with impaired long-term outcomes. Studies have shown that ambulatory BP was superior to the clinic's BP for the prediction of cardiovascular mortality.[34,64] Moreover, nighttime BP was the most potent predictor of outcomes. Hence, 24-hour BP control should be ensured using long-acting drugs, twice-daily regimens, or scheduling at least one of the antihypertensive drugs at bedtime.

Short of performing 24-hour BP monitoring, BP self-monitoring may be performed by the patient. The target value for self-monitored BP is, in general, < 135/85 mmHg.

2. HYPERTENSIVE URGENCIES AND EMERGENCIES

I. Definitions
A. Malignant HTN = hypertensive emergency
Malignant HTN is severe HTN with acute end-organ damage. Malignant HTN is not defined by the level of BP but by its effect, which is related not only to the severity of HTN but to the acuteness of the rise. In general, diastolic BP is >120 mmHg in HTN emergency. Acute damage to the following organs defines HTN emergency:

1. *Eye* (papilledema or retinal bleed): this is the most useful and specific definition of malignant HTN.
2. *Acute encephalopathy* due to cerebral edema: starts as headache/nausea/vomiting, followed by confusion.
   Hypertensive encephalopathy must be differentiated from stroke. In both cases, severe HTN occurs and is associated with neurological changes. Unlike stroke, hypertensive encephalopathy is a non-focal neurological problem that progresses more insidiously than stroke and reverses when BP is controlled.
3. *Cardiovascular*: acute myocardial ischemia, pulmonary edema, aortic dissection.
4. *Renal*: acute kidney injury, called *malignant nephroangiosclerosis*, is characterized by increased creatinine and hematuria or proteinuria on urinalysis. However, these renal findings are non-specific and may be chronic. Even if acute, it is possible that the renal failure is causing HTN rather than the reverse.

B. Hypertensive urgency
Hypertensive urgency is acute HTN (DBP >120 mmHg) without acute end-organ damage. The patient may have mild symptoms, like headache, epistaxis, or mild dyspnea. The majority of patients with severe HTN are asymptomatic; lowering BP is not an emergency in this case.[65,66]

II. Treatment of hypertensive emergencies
A. Guidelines of treatment
Intravenous drugs, preferably short-acting and titratable drugs, are initially used, the goal being a reduction of mean blood pressure by ~25% within 30–60 minutes with a DBP goal of ~100–105 mmHg.[67–69] The vascular beds are autoregulated and adapted to a high BP, which explains that a sharper BP drop will lead to myocardial, cerebral, and renal ischemia (Figure 23.2). A certain degree of quick BP reduction is necessary in hypertensive emergencies, as active organ damage is ongoing.

In aortic dissection, ongoing myocardial ischemia, and pulmonary edema, BP may have to be reduced further and faster to limit the ongoing damage. In addition, in myocardial ischemia and HF, BP may precipitously fall once ischemia and HF improve, as the catecholaminergic surge drops.

Two or three oral drugs may be introduced within several hours to a day, followed by tapering of the intravenous therapy. A normal BP is achieved over days to weeks. A patient who was supposed to receive multiple antihypertensive drugs chronically may not have been fully compliant with therapy; reintroduce those drugs gradually, e.g., two drugs at a time, rather than altogether.

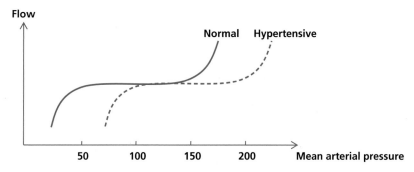

Figure 23.2 Autoregulation curve. Autoregulation of microvascular (mainly arteriolar) resistance allows the preservation of organ perfusion across a wide range of mean systemic pressures, between 50 and 150 mmHg. In severely hypertensive patients, this curve is shifted to the right (*dashed curve*), and systemic perfusion decreases when mean systemic pressure decreases below 100 mmHg (for example, when SBP decreases from 200 mmHg to 140 mmHg).

B. Intravenous drugs

1. *Nitroprusside* drip (0.25–4 mcg/kg/min): nitroprusside is a direct vasodilator.
   - Immediate onset of action, short duration of action (lasts 3–5 minutes on cessation), easy to titrate.
   - Indicated in all hypertensive emergencies (including HF, myocardial ischemia, cerebrovascular events). Tachyphylaxis may occur.
   - Risks: thiocyanate toxicity, especially in renal failure or when high doses are used (>2–3 mcg/kg/min). Thiocyanate levels should be checked after 5 days of therapy, and sooner, after 2 days of therapy, in high-risk patients.

   Rarely, nitroprusside may worsen myocardial ischemia through a diffuse microvascular vasodilatation that further drops the pressure past a coronary stenosis. Therefore, nitroprusside is better used as a second-line agent in ACS; it is better avoided the first 9 hours of an acute MI.[70]

2. *Labetalol* (α-, β-blocker) : labetalol is administered as IV bolus(es) (20–80 mg Q10 min until desired effect is achieved, up to a total of 300 mg), followed by scheduled boluses Q2–6 h or an infusion (0.5–2.0 mg/min).
   - Fast onset (minutes), but effect lasts 2–6 hours, which obviates the need for an infusion. Note that, if an infusion is used, the effect will last several hours after off-titration.
   - May be used in most emergencies, except acute HF.

3. *Nicardipine* is a dihydropyridine CCB administered as a drip (2.5–15 mg/h):
   - Fast onset, but effect lasts 1–4 hours.
   - Caution is suggested in: (i) acute HF, as nicardipine has mild negative inotropic effects; (ii) acute coronary syndrome, as reflex tachycardia may occur (in the latter case, combine nicardipine with a β-blocker).

   Another dihydropyridine, *clevidipine*, has a fast onset and a fast offset and may be used as an IV infusion. It has the same pitfalls as nicardipine, except for the much shorter duration of action and the plasma metabolism (independent of hepatic or renal function).

4. *Nitroglycerin* is indicated in acute HF and acute coronary ischemia. HTN being partly driven by HF and ischemia (catecholamine surge), nitroglycerin relieves HTN through its relief of ischemia and HF. Outside these two conditions, it is not very effective and tolerance to its effect develops rapidly.

5. *Fenoldopam* drip (0.1–0.3 mcg/kg/min, max 1.6 mcg/kg/min): fenoldopam is a short-acting vasodilator that acts as an agonist of dopamine-1 and α_2 receptors. Unlike other intravenous antihypertensive agents, it may preserve or increase renal perfusion while it decreases BP, and is the preferred agent in patients with acute kidney injury.
   - Onset in minutes; effect lasts 30 minutes.
   - Can be used in all emergencies, particularly if renal function is impaired.
   - Caution in glaucoma.

6. *Hydralazine*: in emergencies, hydralazine is administered as intravenous boluses of 10–20 mg Q2–4 h.
   - Onset of action is fast (10–20 minutes), but effect lasts 3–8 hours, more so in renal failure.
   - Less effective and less predictable than other antihypertensive agents, and may occasionally lead to profound and uncontrollable hypotension. It may also lead to reflex tachycardia and myocardial ischemia. Thus, hydralazine is preferably avoided in all hypertensive emergencies, particularly in acute myocardial ischemia.
   - First-line agent in pre-eclampsia/eclampsia.

7. *Enalaprilat* is administered as intravenous boluses of 0.625–1.25 mg Q6h (max 5 mg IV Q6h). A 1.25 mg IV dose is equivalent to a 5 mg oral dose.
   - Onset is fast (15 minutes); effect lasts 6 hours.
   - Unpredictable and uncontrollable BP reduction, sometimes severe (especially in high renin states, such as renovascular HTN or renal failure).
   - Also, avoid it in acute MI because of the risk of precipitous hypotension.

Severe HTN with myocardial ischemia (chest pain, ST changes):
- While acute malignant hypertension may lead to secondary ACS and troponin rise, ACS per se may, on the flip side, lead to hypertension (catecholamine surge). In ACS, hypertension dramatically improves with angina relief and NTG, whereas in malignant hypertension, hypertension is persistent and difficult to control despite multiple antihypertensive therapies, NTG having only a minor effect on it.

Severe HTN with acute HF:
- While HTN may cause acute HF, acute HTN may at least be partially secondary to the acute pulmonary edema and the accompanying sympathetic surge. ***This explains the precipitous BP fall commonly seen during acute diuresis.*** Besides which, the impaired vascular compliance leads not only to sudden BP rise with slight volume change but also to sudden BP fall. While vasodilatation increases cardiac output of the failing heart, excessive vasodilatation, as is seen sometimes in patients who get intubated and sedated, may not be matched by enough rise in the limited cardiac output, which precipitates hypotension. Thus, the aggressive initiation of vasodilators (NTG, nitroprusside, nicardipine), sedative agents, or multiple antihypertensive agents on admission should be avoided until diuresis has been initiated.

III. Treatment of hypertensive urgencies

BP is slowly reduced over 24–48 hours.[67] ***End-organ damage is not imminent, and the main risk of hypertensive urgencies is over-treatment.*** Place the patient in a quiet environment, treat pain/anxiety, recheck BP, and start oral medications. If the patient has withheld antihypertensive medications, restart them; this alone often allows HTN control.

Hospitalization is not necessary. Prescribe two oral medications that will provide a long-term benefit and reduce BP over 24–72 hours, and discharge home with close follow-up.

In hospitalized patients, "as needed" orders for hydralazine or labetalol are often inappropriate. These orders acutely and intermittently reduce severe, asymptomatic HTN, rather than address it in a sustained fashion. This practice was associated with prolonged hospital stays.[71]

IV. Causes and workup

Essential HTN is still the most common cause of malignant HTN. In fact, over 75% of patients with hypertensive urgencies/emergencies are known to have chronic HTN, and non-compliance with medical therapy is a common trigger. However, 20–56% of patients, particularly white patients, have an underlying cause that should be sought:

- Renal artery stenosis
- Renal failure or glomerulopathy
- Pheochromocytoma
- Drugs: cocaine, clonidine or β-blocker withdrawal (rebound HTN)

V. Specific situations (see Table 23.5)

Table 23.5 Treatment in specific settings.

A. Ischemic stroke
- Tolerate BP up to 200/120 mmHg (except if thrombolytics are given, in which case BP should be treated to a level ≤180/105 mmHg)
- Start treating HTN beyond the first 2 days; normalize it in 1–2 weeks

B. Hemorrhagic stroke
- Keep SBP at 140–160 mmHg or lower if the cerebral perfusion tolerates it. As BP is reduced, clinically monitor the mental status or invasively monitor the intracranial pressure and the cerebral perfusion pressure
- Labetalol or nitroprusside is the agent of choice

C. Aortic dissection
- Regimen should always include a β-blocker to reduce the aortic pulse pressure and sharpness of pressure rise (dP/dt). Vasodilators should not be administered alone, as they increase dP/dt
- Consider labetalol or the combination of nitroprusside and a β-blocker (e.g., esmolol)
- Aggressive BP control is indicated even if BP is normal; try to achieve a mean BP of ~70 mmHg (SBP ~90–100 mmHg)

D. Acute HTN with myocardial ischemia (ACS)
Give a combination of:
- NTG IV
- β-blockers orally or IV in the absence of contraindications and risk factors for cardiogenic shock (see Chapter 2)
- Oral ACE-I, preferably oral captopril which is the fastest and shortest-acting oral ACE-I; avoid the intravenous ACE-I enalaprilat
- Add nitroprusside IV or nicardipine IV if the preceding is not enough

E. Scleroderma crisis
- ACE-Is. In scleroderma, HTN results from severe activation of the renin–angiotensin system, and leads to acute, progressive microvascular injury and thrombotic microangiopathy, including renal injury. ACE-Is stabilize or improve renal function in most of those patients

F. Cocaine
First-line therapies:
- Benzodiazepine
- NTG
Second-line therapies for persistent HTN or persistent chest pain:
- Verapamil or diltiazem in the absence of HF; or long-acting dihydropyridine, orally (preferably) or intravenously
- Phentolamine (α-blocker)
Avoid β-blockers acutely, even α- and β-blocker

G. Postoperative HTN
- Analgesics
- β-blockers, especially labetalol
- Post-cardiac surgery: NTG, β-blockers

H. Hypertensive pseudo-emergency
- HTN is related to a massive catecholaminergic surge from pain, anxiety, hypoxia, hypercapnia, postictal state, hypoglycemia. Treat the underlying cause

QUESTIONS AND ANSWERS

Question 1. A 58-year-old obese man (BMI 40), diabetic, has refractory hypertension of 155/70 despite HCTZ, amlodipine 10 mg daily, and lisinopril 20 mg daily. Beside medical therapy, what are the three most important interventions that could improve his HTN?

Question 2. In the above patient, what is the best drug to be added for resistant hypertension?
A. Bisoprolol
B. Carvedilol

C. Clonidine
D. Spironolactone
E. Hydralazine

Question 3. A 55-year-old white man has HTN and is receiving lisinopril 20 mg daily. His BP on follow-up is 150/80 mmHg. He does not have any peripheral edema. What is the best treatment option, beside lifestyle measures?
A. Increase lisinopril to 40 mg then 80 mg daily
B. Add HCTZ 25 mg
C. Add amlodipine 5 mg
D. B or C

Question 4. A 60-year-old man presents with acute pulmonary edema. He has LVH on the ECG, and no ischemic abnormalities. BP is 210/100 mmHg. What is the next step?
A. Intravenous diuresis
B. Diuresis + nitroprusside, aiming for a reduction of mean arterial pressure ~25% at 30 minutes
C. Diuresis + nicardipine, aiming for a reduction of mean arterial pressure ~25% at 30 minutes
D. Diuresis + nitroglycerin

Question 5. Concerning the HTN autoregulation curve:
A. The x-axis is pressure, the y-axis is tissue flow
B. In HTN, the curve is shifted to the right
C. This curve explains why patients with chronic HTN do not tolerate an abrupt pressure drop to the normal level
D. The curve may shift back to the left with time, which explains that the symptoms and the slight creatinine rise sometimes seen upon initiation of antihypertensive drugs improve with time
E. All of the above

Question 6. A 52-year-old African-American man has HTN on several clinic visits, 150/95 mmHg. He is started on hydrocholorothiazide (HCTZ). Which statement is *incorrect*?
A. For better BP control and fewer metabolic effects, it is best to combine thiazide with amiloride or triamterene
B. Potassium and creatinine need to be checked 1 week after therapy initiation
C. A 12.5 mg dose of HCTZ is usually an effective starting dose
D. Thiazide diuretic is initially effective through volume reduction but is later effective through the reduction of vascular resistance

Question 7. In a patient with CKD, which statement is *incorrect*?
A. Aggressive BP control to a mean SBP of 128 mmHg did not clearly improve renal outcomes in comparison with SBP of 140 mmHg in the AASK trial
B. Diuretic therapy should be avoided
C. ACE-I improves renal outcomes in comparison to CCB despite similar BP control, mostly in patients with proteinuria (AASK and IDNT trials)
D. In the ALLHAT trial, analysis of patients with nephropathy showed that ACE-I was not superior to chlorthalidone or amlodipine in respect to renal outcomes (different result from AASK and IDNT)

Question 8. In a patient with diabetes and without CKD, which of the following is *incorrect*?
A. ACE-I or ARB is preferred, as it reduces the incidence of diabetic nephropathy
B. ACE-I is preferred to a thiazide diuretic, as the latter may worsen diabetes control. Yet both reduce cardiovascular and renal events to a similar degree (ALLHAT trial)
C. ACE-I/ARB may reduce the incidence of diabetes in patients with prediabetes according to the NAVIGATOR trial but not the DREAM trial

Question 9. Which statement is *incorrect*? β-Blocker therapy:
A. Has more LVH-reverting effect than losartan
B. Is less effective in reducing central aortic pressure than ACE-I, CCB, or diuretics
C. Is associated with a higher risk of stroke and mortality in comparison to thiazide diuretics or CCB

Question 10. Which of the following statements is *incorrect*?
A. In the ALLHAT trial, chlorthalidone, lisinopril, and amlodipine were associated with similar mortality and MI, but thiazide was superior for HF reduction, and superior to lisinopril for stroke reduction
B. In the VALUE trial, valsartan and amlodipine were associated with similar cardiac mortality and morbidity
C. In the ASCOT trial, atenolol and amlodipine were associated with similar stroke and mortality
D. HCTZ at the doses of 12.5–25 mg achieves less 24-hour BP reduction than chlorthalidone, ACE-I, or CCB
E. In black patients, ACE-I monotherapy has reduced efficacy, except in systolic HF or CKD

Question 11. A 68-year-old man with a history of stable CAD and normal LVEF has BP of 136/80 mmHg. Which statement is *incorrect*?
A. The PEACE trial suggests that the addition of ACE-I at this SBP range does not improve outcomes
B. The SPRINT trial suggests that intensive SBP control <130 mmHg would improve mortality in this patient
C. The HOT trial addressed various DBP goals and showed a J curve for a DBP <82 mmHg
D. The SPRINT trial suggests that SBP <130 mmHg improves renal outcomes, HF, and stroke

Answer 1. (1) Weight loss of 15–20 kg may fully control his HTN and is the most important intervention. (2) Low-salt diet. (3) Check for sleep apnea and treat it.

Answer 2. D. Spironolactone is the most efficacious drug in resistant HTN (PATHWAY-2 trial). Increasing the thiazide diuretic dose and adding carvedilol or nebivolol (especially if pulse >80 bpm) are also alternatives. Clonidine, hydralazine, and pure α-blockers are last resort.

Answer 3. D. Adding a new drug is far more effective than increasing the dose of lisnopril, especially that lisinopril is already at an optimal dose. As shown in ACCOMPLISH trial, the second drug does not have to be a diuretic, and the combination ACE-I–amlodipine was superior to ACE-I–thiazide in white patients without overt hypervolemia.

Answer 4. A. While HTN may cause acute HF, acute HTN may at least be partially secondary to the acute pulmonary edema and the accompanying sympathetic surge. This explains the precipitous BP fall commonly seen during acute diuresis. Thus, the aggressive initiation of vasodilators (NTG, nitroprusside, nicardipine), sedative agents, or multiple antihypertensive agents on admission should be avoided until diuresis has been initiated.

Answer 5. E.

Answer 6. C. A 25 mg dose of HCTZ is usually the effective starting dose.

Answer 7. B. Hypervolemia is frequently at the center of HTN in CKD. Diuretic therapy, usually with a thiazide, is a key antihypertensive therapy in CKD (usually initiated after ACE-I therapy).

Answer 8. A.

Answer 9. A. According to the LIFE trial, losartan has more LVH-reverting effect than atenolol.

Answer 10. C. In the ASCOT trial, atenolol-based therapy was associated with higher stroke and mortality than amlodipine-based therapy.

Answer 11. D. In the SPRINT trial, SBP goal <120 mmHg (SBP achieved = 121.4 mmHg) reduced mortality and HF, but not MI, stroke, or renal events. More acute kidney injury was seen with this intensive BP control.

References

1. Messerli FH, Mancia G, Conti CR. Dogma disputed: can aggressively lowering blood pressure in hypertensive patients with coronary artery disease be dangerous? Ann Intern Med 2006; 144: 884–93. *Data from INVEST trial. Also J curve for SBP <120.*
2. Messerli FH, Panjrath GS. The J-curve between blood pressure and coronary artery disease or essential hypertension. J Am Coll Cardiol 2009; 54: 1827–34.
3. Boutitie F, Gueyffier F, Pocock S, et al. J-shaped relationship between blood pressure and mortality in hypertensive patients: new insights from a meta-analysis of individual-patient data. Ann Intern Med 2002; 136: 438–48. *Also J curve for SBP.*
4. Mancia G. Effects of intensive blood pressure control in the management of patients with type 2 diabetes mellitus in the Action to Control Cardiovascular Risk in Diabetes (ACCORD) trial. Circulation 2010; 122: 847–9.
5. Hansson L, Zanchetti A, Carruthers SG, et al.; HOT Study Group. Effects of intensive blood-pressure lowering and low-dose aspirin in patients with hypertension: principal results of the Hypertension Optimal Treatment (HOT) randomised trial. Lancet 1998; 351: 1755–62. *Patients randomized to DBP <90, < 85, < 80 mmHg. J curve for DBP, with nadir ~82 mmHg, except in diabetics, where risk continues to decrement with DBP <80 mmHg.*
6. Chobanian AV, Bakris GL, Black HR, et al. The seventh report of the joint national committee on prevention, detection, evaluation, and treatment of high blood pressure: the JNC 7 report. JAMA 2003; 289: 2560–71.
7. Calhoun DA, Nishizaka MK, Zaman MA, et al. Hyperaldosteronism among black and white subjects with resistant hypertension. Hypertension 2002; 40: 892– 6.
8. Gallay BJ, Ahmad S, Xu L, et al. Screening for primary aldosteronism without discontinuing hypertensive medications: plasma aldosterone–renin ratio. Am J Kidney Dis 2001; 37: 699–705.
9. Calhoun DA, Jones D, Textor S, et al. Resistant hypertension: diagnosis, evaluation, and treatment. A scientific statement from the American Heart Association Professional Education Committee of the Council for High Blood Pressure Research. Hypertension 2008; 51: 1403–19.
10. Okin PM, Devereux RB, Harris KE, et al. Regression of electrocardiographic left ventricular hypertrophy is associated with less hospitalization for heart failure in hypertensive patients. Ann Intern Med 2007; 147: 311–319.
11. Mancia G, Fagard R, Narkiewicz K, et al. 2013 ESH/ESC Guidelines for the management of arterial hypertension: the Task Force for the management of arterial hypertension of the European Society of Hypertension (ESH) and of the European Society of Cardiology (ESC). J Hypertension 2013: 31: 1281–357.
12. James PA, Oparil S, Carter BL, et al. 2014 evidence-based guideline for the management of high blood pressure in adults: report by the panel appointed to the Eighth Joint National Committee (JNC 8). JAMA 2014; 311: 507–20.
13. UK Prospective Diabetes Study Group. Tight blood pressure control and risk of macrovascular and microvascular complications in type 2 diabetes: UKPDS 38. BMJ 1998; 317: 703–13.
14. Cushman WC, Evans GW, Byington RP, et al. Effects of intensive blood-pressure control in type 2 diabetes mellitus. N Engl J Med 2010; 362: 1575–85. *ACCORD BP.*
15. Cooper-DeHoff RM, Gong Y, Handberg EM, et al. Tight blood pressure control and cardiovascular outcomes among hypertensive patients with diabetes and coronary artery disease. JAMA 2010; 304: 61–8.
16. Denardo SJ, Gong Y, Nichols WW, et al. Blood pressure and outcomes in very old hypertensive coronary artery disease patients: an INternational VErapamil ST-Trandolapril (INVEST) substudy. Am J Med 2010; 123: 719–26.
17. Wright JT, Bakris G, Greene T, et al. Effect of blood pressure lowering and antihypertensive drug class on progression of hypertensive kidney disease: results from the AASK trial. JAMA 2002; 288: 2421–31. *Patients with proteinuria (urinary protein/creatinine ratio >0.22) derived the most benefit from ACE-I in comparison to metoprolol and amlodipine. ACE-I was best for reducing proteinuria.*
18. Klahr S, Levey AS, Beck GJ, et al. The effects of dietary protein restriction and blood-pressure control on the progression of chronic renal disease. Modification of Diet in Renal Disease Study Group. N Engl J Med 1994; 330: 877–84.

19. Ruggenenti P, Perna A, Loriga G, et al. Blood-pressure control for renoprotection in patients with non-diabetic chronic renal disease (REIN-2): multicentre, randomised controlled trial. Lancet 2005; 365: 939–46.

20. Massie BM, Carson PE, McMurray JJ, et al. Irbesartan in patients with heart failure and preserved ejection fraction. N Engl J Med 2008; 359: 2456–67.

21. PEACE Trial Investigators. Angiotensin-converting-enzyme inhibition in stable coronary artery disease. N Engl J Med 2004; 351: 2058–68.

22. SPRINT research group. A randomized trial of intensive versus standard blood pressure control. N Engl J Med 2015; 373: 2103–16.

23. Mann JF, Schmieder RE, McQueen M, et al. Renal outcomes with telmisartan, ramipril, or both, in people at high vascular risk (the ONTARGET study): a multicentre, randomised, double-blind, controlled trial. Lancet 2008; 372: 547–53. *In this trial of patients who were mainly normotensive (BP 141/82 mmHg), the combination of ACE-I and ARB was associated with a higher risk of acute kidney injury and worse major renal outcomes than ACE-I monotherapy.*

24. Rosendorff C, Black HR, Cannon CP, et al. Treatment of hypertension in the prevention and management of ischemic heart disease. Circulation 2007; 115: 2761–88.

25. Beckett NS, Peters R, Fletcher AE. Treatment of hypertension in patients 80 years of age or older. N Engl J Med 2008; 358: 1887–98.

26. Wright JT, Dunn JK, Cutler JA, et al. ALLHAT Collaborative Research Group outcomes in hypertensive black and nonblack patients treated with chlorthalidone, amlodipine, and lisinopril. JAMA 2005; 293: 1595–608.

27. Higgins B, Williams B; Guideline Development Group. Pharmacological management of hypertension. Clin Med (Lond) 2007; 7: 612–16. *British HTN guidelines.*

28. Psaty BM, Smith NL, Siscovick DS, et al. Health outcomes associated with antihypertensive therapies used as first-line agents: a systematic review and meta-analysis. JAMA 1997; 277: 739–45.

29. Messerli FH, Grossman E, Goldbourt U. Are beta-blockers efficacious as first-line therapy for hypertension in the elderly? A systematic review. JAMA 1998; 279: 1903–7.

30. Dahlof B, Devereux RB, Kjeldsen SE, et al.; LIFE study group. Cardiovascular morbidity and mortality in the losartan intervention for endpoint reduction in hypertension study (LIFE): a randomized trial against atenolol. Lancet 2002; 359: 995–1003.

31. Dahlof B, Sever PS, Poulter NR, et al.; ASCOT Investigators. Prevention of cardiovascular events with an antihypertensive regimen of amlodipine adding perindopril as required versus atenolol adding bendroflumethiazide as required, in the Anglo-Scandinavian Cardiac Outcomes Trial–Blood Pressure Lowering Arm (ASCOT-BPLA): a multicentre randomised controlled trial. Lancet 2005; 366: 895–906.

32. Wald DS, Law M, Morris JK, et al. Combination therapy versus monotherapy in reducing blood pressure: meta-analysis on 11,000 participants from 42 trials. Am J Med 2009; 122: 290–300.

33. Jamerson K, Weber MA, Bakris GL, et al. Benazepril plus amlodipine or hydrochlorothiazide for hypertension in high-risk patients. N Engl J Med 2008; 359: 2417–28. *ACCOMPLISH trial.*

34. Dolan E, Stanton A, Thijs L, et al. Superiority of ambulatory over clinic blood pressure measurement in predicting mortality: the Dublin Outcome Study. Hypertension 2005; 46: 156–61.

35. Mancia G, Facchetti R, Bombelli M, et al. Long-term risk of mortality associated with selective and combined elevation in office, home and ambulatory blood pressure. Hypertension 2006; 47: 846–53.

36. Calhoun DA, Jones D, Textor S, et al. Resistant hypertension: diagnosis, evaluation, and treatment. A scientific statement from the American Heart Association professional education committee. Hypertension 2008; 51: 1403–19.

37. Hirsch S. A different approach to resistant hypertension. Cleve Clin J Med 2007; 74: 449–56.

38. Taler SJ, Textor SC, Augustine JE. Resistant hypertension: comparing hemodynamic management to specialist care. Hypertension 2002; 39: 982–8.

39. Williams B, MacDonald TM, Morant S, et al. Spironolactone versus placebo, bisoprolol, and doxazosin to determine the optimal treatment for drug-resistant hypertension (PATHWAY-2): a randomised, double-blind, crossover trial. Lancet 2015; 386: 2059–68.

40. Chapman N, Dobson J, Wilson S, et al, on behalf of the Anglo-Scandinavian Cardiac Outcomes Trial Investigators. Effect of spironolactone on blood pressure in subjects with resistant hypertension. Hypertension 2007; 49: 839–45.

41. Safar ME, Protogerou AD, Blacher J. Statins, central blood pressure, and blood pressure amplification. Circulation 2009; 119: 9–12.

42. Williams B, Lacy PS, Thom SM, et al. Differential impact of blood pressure-lowering drugs on central aortic pressure and clinical outcomes: principal results of the Conduit Artery Function Evaluation (CAFE) study. Circulation 2006; 113: 1213–25.

43. Wilkinson IB, MacCallum H, Flint L, Cockcroft JR, Newby DE, Webb DJ. The influence of heart rate on augmentation index and central arterial pressure in humans. J Physiol 2000; 525: 263–70.

44. Williams B, Lacy PS. Impact of heart rate on central aortic pressures and hemodynamics: analysis from the CAFE (Conduit Artery Function Evaluation) study: CAFE-Heart Rate. J Am Coll Cardiol 2009; 54: 705–13.

45. Lewis EJ, Hunsicker LG, Clarke WR, et al. Renoprotective effect of the angiotensin-receptor antagonist irbesartan in patients with nephropathy due to type 2 diabetes. N Engl J Med 2001; 345: 851–60. *IDNT trial; all participants had proteinuria >900 mg/day.*

46. Hou FF, Zhang X, Zhang GH, et al. Efficacy and safety of benazepril for advanced renal insufficiency. N Engl J Med 2006; 354: 131–40.

47. Rahman M, Pressel S, Davis BR, et al. Renal outcomes in high-risk hypertensive patients treated with an angiotensin-converting enzyme inhibitor or a calcium channel blocker vs a diuretic: a report from the Antihypertensive and Lipid-Lowering Treatment to Prevent Heart Attack Trial (ALLHAT). Arch Intern Med 2005; 165: 936–46.

48. Ernst ME, Carter BL, Zheng S, Grimm RH. Meta-analysis of dose-response characteristics of hydrochlorothiazide and chlorthalidone: effects on systolic blood pressure and potassium. Am J Hypertens 2010; 23: 440–6.

49. Messerli FH, Makani H, Benjo A, et al. Antihypertensive efficacy of hydrochlorothiazide as evaluated by ambulatory blood pressure monitoring. A meta-analysis of randomized trials. J Am Coll Cardiol 2011; 57: 590–600.

50. Siscovick D.S., Raghunathan T.E., Psaty B.M., et al. Diuretic therapy for hypertension and the risk of primary cardiac arrest. N Engl J Med 1994; 330: 1852–7.

51. Brown MJ, Williams B, Morant SV, et al. Effect of amiloride, or amiloride plus hydrochlorothiazide, versus hydrochlorothiazide on glucose intolerance and blood pressure (PATHWAY-3): a parallel-group, double-blind randomised phase 4 trial. Lancet Diabetes Endocrinol 2016; 4: 136–47.

52. Dussol B, Moussi-Frances J, Morange S, et al. A randomized trial of furosemide vs hydrochlorothiazide in patients with chronic renal failure and hypertension. Nephrol Dial Transplant 2005; 20: 349–53.

53. Knauf H, Mutschler E. Diuretic effectiveness of hydrochlorothiazide and furosemide alone and in combination in chronic renal failure. J Cardiovasc Pharmacol 1995; 26: 394–400.

54. Aronow WS, Fleg JL, Pepine CJ, et al. ACCF/AHA 2011 expert consensus document on hypertension in the elderly. J Am Coll Cardiol 2011; 57: 2037–114.

55. Bangalore S, Sawhney S, Messerli FH. Relation of beta-blocker-induced heart rate lowering and cardioprotection in hypertension. J Am Coll Cardiol 2008; 52: 1482–9.

56. Lopez-Sendo J, Swedberg K, McMurray J, et al. Expert consensus document on β-adrenergic receptor blockers. Eur Heart J 2004; 25: 1341–62.

57. UK Prospective Diabetes Study Group. Tight blood pressure control and risk of macrovascular and microvascular complications in type 2 diabetes: UKPDS 38. BMJ 1998; 317: 703–13.

58. Bakris GL, Fonseca V, Katholi RE, et al. Metabolic effects of carvedilol vs metoprolol in patients with type 2 diabetes mellitus and hypertension: a randomized controlled trial. JAMA 2004; 292: 2227–36. Weber K, et al. Comparison of the hemodynamic effects of metoprolol and carvedilol in hypertensive patients. Cardiovasc Drugs Ther 1996; 10: 113–7.

59. Lewandowski J, Sinski M, Symonides M, et al. Beneficial influence of carvedilol on urologic indices in patients with hypertension and benign prostatic hyperplasia: results of a randomized, crossover study. Urology 2013; 82: 660–6.

60. Giannattasio C, Cattaneo BM, Seravalle G, et al. Alpha 1-blocking properties of carvedilol during acute and chronic administration. J Cardiovasc Pharmacol 1992; 19 Suppl 1: S18–22.

61. Kubo T, Azevedo ER, Newton GE, et al. Lack of evidence for peripheral α1-adrenoceptor blockade during long-term treatment of heart failure with carvedilol. J Am Coll Cardiol 2001; 38: 1463–9.

62. ALLHAT Collaborative Research Group. Major cardiovascular events in hypertensive patients randomized to doxazosin vs chlorthalidone: the Antihypertensive and Lipid-Lowering Treatment to prevent Heart Attack Trial (ALLHAT). JAMA 2000; 283: 1967–75.

63. Parving HH, Persso F, Lewis J, et al. Aliskiren combined with losartan in type 2 diabetes and nephropathy. N Engl J Med 2008; 358: 2433–46.

64. Staessen J, Thijs L, Fagard R, et al.; Systolic Hypertension in Europe Trial Investigators. Predicting cardiovascular risk using conventional vs ambulatory blood pressure in older patients with systolic hypertension. JAMA 1999; 282: 539–46.

65. Zampaglione B, Pascale C, Marchisio M, Cavallo-Perin P. Hypertensive urgencies and emergencies. Hypertension 1996; 27: 144–7.

66. Calhoun DA, Oparil S. Treatment of hypertensive crisis. N Engl J Med 1990; 323: 1177–83.

67. Marik PE, Rivera R. Hypertensive emergencies: an update. Current Opinion in Critical Care 2011; 17: 569–80.

68. Devlin JW, Dasta JF, Kleinschmidt K, et al. Patterns of antihypertensive treatment in patients with acute severe hypertension from a nonneurologic cause: Studying the Treatment of Acute Hypertension (STAT) registry. Pharmacotherapy 2010; 30: 1087–96.

69. Peacock WF, Varon J, Baumann BM, et al. CLUE: a randomized comparative effectiveness trial of IV nicardipine versus labetalol use in the emergency department. Crit Care 2011; 15: R157.

70. Cohn JN, Franciosa JA, Francis GS, et al. Effect of short-term infusion of sodium nitroprusside on mortality rate in acute myocardial infarction complicated by left ventricular failure: results of a Veterans Administration cooperative study. N Engl J Med 1982; 306: 1129–35.

71. Weder AB, Erickson S. Treatment of hypertension in the inpatient setting: use of intravenous labetalol and hydralazine. J Clin Hypertens 2010; 12: 29–33.

24 Dyslipidemia

I. Indications for therapy

Evidence supports the following two concepts:

- Statin drugs have pleiotropic effects (improvement of endothelial function, anti-inflammatory effects) and reduce mortality in patients with CAD regardless of the baseline LDL level, even if it is below 70 mg/dl (or even 40 mg/dl).[1–3] *Higher doses of statin provide more benefit than lower doses.*
- The lower the LDL achieved in CAD patients (even levels well below 70 mg/dl), the greater the benefit (PROVE-IT and TNT trials).[4–6] In the TNT trial of stable CAD, patients with the lowest achieved LDL <64 mg/dl had the lowest risk of cardiovascular events and there was no evidence of harm with very low LDL levels.[1,2,7] In the IMPROVE-IT trial, a lower LDL (53 mg/dl) achieved with a statin + ezetimibe combination translated into a lower MI and stroke risk than statin alone (LDL 69 mg/dl).[8]

Conversely, two trials suggest that the addition of niacin or fibrate to statin therapy does not improve outcomes in high-risk patients. In the AIM-HIGH trial, patients with established CAD, controlled LDL levels, and mildly uncontrolled triglyceride or HDL levels did not benefit from the addition of niacin; the same result was seen with the addition of fenofibrate on top of statin therapy in diabetic patients (ACCORD trial).[9,10] In these two trials, LDL was not significantly reduced by the addition of niacin or fibrate.

In light of the importance of both statin therapy and attainment of very low LDL levels, ACC/AHA recommends the use of statin in four high-risk groups regardless of lipid levels.[11] The four major statin benefit groups are:

a. *Patients with established CAD or vascular disease* (→ prescribe high-intensity statin in most patients; moderate-intensity statin in patients >75 years old or those at a high risk of intolerance)

b. *Diabetic patients 40–75 years old* (→ prescribe high-intensity statin)

c. *Patients with LDL ≥190 mg/dl* (→ prescribe high-intensity statin)

d. *Patients without vascular disease or diabetes, whose LDL is 70–189 mg/dl, and whose estimated 10-year risk of cardiovascular events is ≥7.5%, using a clinical risk calculator* (→ prescribe moderate-to-high-intensity statin). The clinical risk calculator accounts for age/sex, diabetes, smoking, HTN and its control, HDL and total cholesterol. Less strongly, a family history of premature CAD in first-degree relatives or hs-CRP ≥2 mg/l may indicate statin therapy.

The combination of statin and non-statin drugs may be considered in patients who cannot tolerate an adequate statin dose (→ add anti-PCSK9 or ezetimibe), patients whose LDL decreases <30–50% with statin therapy or does not decline to <70 mg/dl (→ add anti-PCSK9 or ezetimibe), or, questionably, patients whose triglyceride/HDL levels remain markedly abnormal under statin therapy (→ add niacin or fibrates).

In addition, non-statin drugs are probably useful in patients belonging to the above groups who, nonetheless, cannot tolerate any statin.

II. Notes on LDL, HDL, and triglycerides

A. LDL

The atherogenic risk of a lipoprotein is related to its size. LDL particles, and more particularly the small and dense LDL particles, are more likely to penetrate the endothelium and initiate atherosclerosis than VLDL particles. For a given LDL cholesterol level, small LDL particles or a high number of LDL particles (LDL-p) are more atherogenic than large or less numerous LDL particles, because they lead to more endothelial penetration and injury.[7] In fact, cholesterol is only a portion of any given liproprotein (LDL, HDL, or VLDL), which also contains proteins (Apo B), triglycerides, and phospholipids. *In patients with low LDL who continue to have recurrent events, a high number of small LDL particles is suspected, and is indirectly reflected by a low HDL level and high triglyceride, VLDL, and non-HDL cholesterol levels.* LDL-p has not been studied independently at a large scale, and thus this measurement is not routinely performed, especially in primary prevention. Apo B is the protein found in all atherogenic particles, such as LDL, VLDL, and Lp(a). Apo B levels correlate with the number of LDL particles and may predict cardiovascular outcomes as well as or better than LDL, especially in patients with low LDL levels. Apo A is the central protein of HDL, and low Apo A levels may be associated with impaired outcomes.

B. Non-HDL cholesterol

Non-HDL cholesterol = total cholesterol − HDL = LDL + VLDL + VLDL remnants. It is a strong predictor of adverse outcomes.

C. HDL

HDL scavenges "bad" cholesterol from the endothelium and lipid-laden macrophages (cholesterol efflux), then empties it onto VLDL through the cholesteryl ester transfer protein (CETP). VLDL is then taken up by the liver and eliminated in the bile (reverse transport mechanism). A *spontaneously* high HDL is protective against CAD as it indicates that "bad" cholesterol has been scavenged and will be eliminated through the CETP enzyme. Drugs that increase HDL by inhibiting CETP may saturate HDL and inhibit its capacity to scavenge cholesterol (dysfunctional HDL). This may paradoxically increase cardiovascular events.[12] In fact, the HDL process is complex, and a pharmacological increase in HDL may not improve outcomes. Niacin increases HDL but also the efficacy of the scavenging effect by reducing VLDL, and reduces atherogenic lipoproteins, which explains the possible improvement of outcomes with niacin.

Furthermore, HDL may cease to predict cardiovascular outcomes in patients receiving statin who have an adequately controlled LDL (substudies of JUPITER and CETP inhibitor trials).[12–14]

D. Triglycerides (TGs)

TGs, when >500 mg/dl, warrant therapy because of the marked risk of pancreatitis. TGs, per se, are associated with some increase in the risk of cardiovascular events, though less strikingly than LDL. In fact, a high TG level is associated with high levels of VLDL and VLDL remnants; large VLDLs may not be atherogenic, but the smaller VLDLs and their remnants are small enough to penetrate the endothelium. A high VLDL precludes cholesterol elimination from HDL, which affects the efficacy of HDL scavenging. Thus, a high TG level reflects a high level of atherogenic lipoproteins, and primarily mandates a reduction of non-HDL cholesterol rather than TG.

III. Drugs: LDL-lowering drugs

A. Statins

Statins inhibit HMG-CoA reductase, the enzyme that synthesizes intracellular cholesterol. This leads to an increase in LDL receptors and LDL uptake by cells. Statins lower LDL 30–60%, lower TG 15–25%, and increase HDL 5–10%. Statins are the best agents for lowering non-HDL cholesterol as well.

a. The most potent statins are rosuvastatin (5–40 mg/day) and atorvastatin (10–80 mg) (LDL ↓ 40–60%), followed by simvastatin 10–40 mg (LDL ↓ 35–45%) and pravastatin (LDL ↓ 30%). Rosuvastatin is the most effective statin for raising HDL, while atorvastatin is the most effective statin for reducing TGs.

b. Doubling the statin dose lowers LDL by 6% more, but is associated with a more significant increase in myopathy and hepatitis.

c. Increasing the dose of atorvastatin to 80 mg reduces LDL by 60% vs. 40% reduction with a dose of 10 mg. The same reduction can be obtained by adding ezetimibe to atorvastatin 10 mg, with fewer side effects.

d. Dosing:

   i. In the case of high-risk patients with established vascular disease, high statin doses proven to be the best in clinical trials are used (atorvastatin 40–80 mg; rosuvastatin 20–40 mg). These doses reduce LDL by ≥50% and are particularly important in ACS, where statins may directly stabilize active plaques.

   ii. If the patient is a lower-risk patient, or if there is a concern about side effects (e.g., elderly patients >75, renal failure, or possibility of drug interactions), use a moderate-intensity statin dose, which reduces LDL by 30–50% (pravastatin 40 mg, simvastatin 20 mg, atorvastatin 10 mg). Ezetimibe may be added for further LDL reduction.

   iii. Low-intensity statin is only tried in patients with statin intolerance.

B. Ezetimibe (inhibits cholesterol absorption)

Ezetimibe reduces LDL by ~20% even in patients already receiving a statin. It also reduces non-HDL cholesterol. In the IMPROVE-IT trial, patients with a recent ACS (mainly MI) and a baseline LDL of 95 mg/dl were randomized to simvastatin 40 mg vs. simvastatin 40 mg + ezetimibe. The statin group achieved LDL of 69 mg/dl, while the combined group achieved LDL of 53 mg/dl, which translated into a 10% reduction of MI, and 20% reduction of stroke. Lower LDL was better in this high-risk ACS population, even when a non-statin drug was added.[8]

C. Anti-PCSK9 antibodies (alirocumab, evolocumab)

Anti-PCSK9 antibodies are a new class of drugs. PCSK9 is an enzyme that destroys LDL receptors. Blocking this enzyme increases LDL receptors and dramatically reduces LDL by over 50%, even in patients already receiving a statin. These drugs are administered subcutaneously, once every 2 weeks. They have been associated with a ~50% reduction of cardiovascular events in patients with familial hypercholesterolemia or patients with established cardiovascular disease who do not achieve LDL <70 mg/dl with statin (or do not tolerate statin). They are approved for use in these two groups of patients.

D. Bile acid sequestrants (cholestyramine, colestipol)
These agents reduce bile acid reabsorption, which reduces the cholesterol available to synthesize LDL (LDL ↓ 15–30% but TG may ↑). These agents are avoided if TG >300 mg/dl.

E. Nutrients high in phytosterols (plant sterols)
Phytosterols decrease cholesterol absorption and reduce LDL by ~10%. A high intake of fibers also lowers cholesterol absorption.

> The LDL level in neonates is only ~40 mg/dl, and it appears that human cells only require an LDL plasma level of 25 mg/dl. Wild mammalian species have LDL ~40 mg/dl and rarely develop atherosclerosis. Human hunter–gatherer societies, which carry on the Paleolithic lifestyle, and rural Chinese have LDL cholesterol in that range as well and show no evidence of atherosclerosis, even late in life. The same applies to many patients with genetic loss-of-function of PCSK9. All this led to the suggestion that LDL is at the center of atherosclerosis and a very low LDL may prevent the initiation of atherosclerosis.[15,16] This also suggests that a very low LDL is safe. Data from PCSK9 trials concur that a very low LDL, even <25 mg/dl, is safe (ODYSSEY long-term trial).[17] A very low LDL level, however, may not fully prevent the progression of a pre-existing atherosclerosis.

IV. Drugs: TG/HDL-treating drugs and lifestyle modification
A. Niacin
Niacin reduces fat degradation in the adipose tissue, which reduces the release of free fatty acids in the circulation, reducing VLDL synthesis. The reduction in VLDL indirectly improves the HDL scavenging mechanism, which raises HDL and reduces LDL. Thus, niacin raises HDL 15–25%, lowers TG 20–25% (at high doses, ~2000 mg), and lowers LDL 10–15%. Niacin is the best available agent for raising HDL. It also improves the quality of LDL cholesterol, increasing the size and reducing the number of LDL particles. Niacin doses >2000 mg are better avoided because of the risk of increasing glucose levels.

Niacin was the first lipid-lowering drug to show a reduction in MI and total mortality in the Coronary Drug Project (secondary prevention trial of patients with prior MI).[18] In fact, there is more evidence for improved survival and cardiovascular outcomes with niacin than with fibrates.[7] However, in a contemporary trial of CAD patients already receiving statin with well-controlled LDL levels and mildly reduced HDL levels (~35 mg/dl), niacin did not provide additional benefit (AIM-HIGH trial).[9] It may still have a role in patients unable to take statins, or patients with CAD and markedly abnormal TG or HDL.[19]

B. Fibrates
Fibrates increase liprotein lipase activity, which degrades VLDL into VLDL remnants and buoyant LDLs that are readily taken up by the liver. Fibrates also have other effects, such as reducing VLDL synthesis in the liver and increasing Apo A1 synthesis (HDL protein). Thus, fibrates lower TG 20–50%, increase HDL 10–20%, ± lower LDL 10–15% (especially fenofibrate).

Fibrates are the most effective agents in lowering TGs. However, gemfibrozil may raise LDL in patients with severely increased TGs (by converting some VLDL into LDL). In the Helsinki and VA-HIT studies, patients with low HDL and without CAD (Helsinki study) or with CAD (VA-HIT study) derived a reduction in MI and stroke with gemfibrozil.[20,21] However, these patients were not receiving statin therapy, and no reduction in mortality was seen. Routine fenofibrate therapy failed to show a benefit in diabetic patients receiving statin therapy, most of whom did not have a CAD history (ACCORD); this result may not extend to patients with prior CAD or those with severely abnormal HDL or triglycerides, wherein a trend towards benefit was seen.[9] In general, in all three of these studies, the subgroup of patients with elevated TG derived a large and significant reduction in cardiovascular events with fibrate therapy.

Fibrates, when used in renal failure or in combination with statins, are associated with an increased risk of myositis of 1%. If a decision is made to provide a combination therapy in statin-treated patients who continue to have a markedly reduced HDL or a high TG, niacin is generally the preferred agent. Gemfibrozil is best avoided in combination with a statin;[11] fenofibrate is a safer fibrate in patients who require combined therapy with a statin.[10,22]

C. Omega-3 fatty acids
Omega-3 fatty acids (fish oil, 3–6 g/day) reduce TG by ~30–40%, through reduction of the hepatic synthesis of TG and activation of the lipoprotein lipase. In the GISSI-Prevenzione trial of patients with recent MI (≤3 months), omega-3 fatty acids reduced the risk of cardiovascular events.[23]

D. Tight glycemic control
Tight glycemic control is one of the most effective means of achieving the TG/HDL goal in diabetic patients.

E. Lifestyle modification
Diet and exercise are indicated in all patients. These are mildly effective in reducing LDL (usually a 15–20% reduction, in the range of 30 mg/dl). The most effective diet is the Mediterranean diet (fruits, vegetables, whole grains, fish, nuts, and olive oil) and a diet switch from saturated to monounsaturated fat (olive oil).

Lifestyle modification, particularly the reduction of simple sugars, is quite effective in reducing TG and raising HDL, more so than it is effective in reducing LDL.

Smoking cessation raises HDL. Mild alcohol consumption (1–2 drinks/day) raises HDL and may improve cardiovascular outcomes, but should be avoided if TG >200 mg/dl.

V. Metabolic syndrome

A. Diagnosis
Three of five criteria are needed for the diagnosis (AHA):[24]

1. Obesity (male: waist >40 inches; female: waist >35 inches). Lower cut-points are used in Asian populations.
2. TG level >150 mg/dl
3. HDL <40 mg/dl in men, <50 mg/dl in women
4. HTN >130/85 mmHg
5. Fasting blood glucose >100 mg/dl

B. Treatment
1. Diet, exercise, and weight loss.
2. HTN: ACE-I/ARB may reduce glucose levels and lower the risk of diabetes.[24,25]
3. Glucose intolerance and risk of diabetes: metformin or glitazone therapy is effective in further decreasing the risk of diabetes. However, therapeutic lifestyle changes are the most effective means of reducing this risk. Acarbose has been shown to decrease the risk of cardiovascular events in patients with glucose intolerance.[26]
4. Statin therapy is indicated in most of these patients, based on their 10-year cardiovascular risk.

VI. Diabetes

A. Statin therapy
All diabetic patients older than 40 years of age derive a reduction of cardiovascular events, stroke and mortality with statin therapy, even in the absence of established CAD and regardless of LDL levels (even if <100 mg/dl) (HPS and CARDS trials, the latter mandated the presence of one additional risk factor: HTN, smoking, retinopathy, albuminuria).[27,28] Not infrequently, patients with diabetes have low yet atherogenic levels of LDL.

B. Tight glycemic control improves TG/HDL levels
Tight glycemic control is the first-line therapy for TG/HDL in diabetes.

C. Pioglitazone and metformin
Pioglitazone (unlike rosiglitazone) lowers LDL and TG and increases HDL. Metformin lowers TG.

VII. Elevated hs-CRP (high-sensitivity C-reactive protein test) ≥2 mg/l
The JUPITER trial has shown that in patients with low LDL levels (~100 mg/dl), age >50 (men) or 60 (women), and no CAD equivalent but hs-CRP >2 mg/l, statin therapy reduces cardiovascular events at 5 years by ~47%.[29] The addition of CRP to lipid screening may select seemingly low-risk patients with low LDL and no history of CAD who would benefit from statin therapy.

VIII. Chronic kidney disease (CKD)
In patients aged ≥50 years, CKD (GFR <60 ml/min/1.73 m² or albuminuria) is associated with a 10-year risk of cardiovascular events >20%, and thus CKD should be considered a CAD equivalent and treated with a statin, regardless of LDL level and regardless of the presence of CAD (Kidney society guidelines).[30] Paradoxically, at the extreme of CKD, patients with end-stage renal disease did not derive a benefit from statin therapy in one randomized trial; this does not apply to patients with end-stage renal disease and established CAD.[31]

IX. Causes of dyslipidemia to consider

A. Markedly elevated LDL (>190 mg/dl) suggests familial hypercholesterolemia
In this case, the LDL receptor is underproduced or dysfunctional.

B. Markedly elevated TG level (>500 mg/dl) suggests familial hypertriglyceridemia

C. Remember to rule out secondary causes of dyslipidemia
Hypothyroidism (↑ LDL), nephrotic syndrome (↑ LDL), uremia (↑ TG), alcohol abuse (↑ TG), and medications: β-blockers (↑ TG, ↓ HDL), thiazides (↑ LDL), contraceptive pills (↑ TG).

X. Side effects of specific drugs: muscle and liver intolerance with statins, fibrates, and niacin
With all lipid-lowering drugs, baseline liver profile is obtained and the patient is monitored for muscular symptoms. Follow-up liver profile is not routinely indicated with statin therapy, but is indicated if toxicity is clinically suspected and if niacin is used (6–8 weeks after starting therapy or after changing dose, then every 6 months). Baseline CK may be measured in those at risk of adverse muscle events; CK is obtained during therapy only in those who develop muscular symptoms. Lipid profile is checked 1.5–3.0 months after therapy initiation to ensure compliance and appropriate LDL reduction.

A. Statin (HMG CoA reductase inhibitors)
Adverse effects:

i. *Myopathy.* Muscle symptoms with or without elevated CK are reported in up to 10–20% of real-world, registry patients, and usually occur within weeks or months of statin initiation (median of 1 month).[32] Statin toxicity may manifest as cramping, heaviness, or weakness, particularly with exertion. Some patients may develop dyspnea or fatigue concomitantly with the muscle complaint. Active patients, especially athletes, are more likely to manifest muscular symptoms. Myopathy may be related to pharmacokinetics (high dose or drug interactions) or to an underlying metabolic disorder that is unveiled by statin therapy.[33] The latter patients typically cannot tolerate any statin. While myopathy is symmetric, a focal exacerbation of underlying tendinitis, osteorthritis, or lumbar pain/radiculopathy is possible. In fact, muscle weakness induced by statin may aggravate a pre-existent muskeloskeletal pain. Three degrees of muscular effects occur with statin:[34]

a. Myalgia: muscular symptoms without CK elevation
b. Myositis: muscular symptoms with CK elevation
c. Rhabdomyolysis: muscular symptoms with CK elevation over 10× upper limit of normal. It is often accompanied by acute renal failure. Rhabdomyolysis occurs in <0.1% of patients.

Many patients with mild muscle aches have improvement of symptoms within 2 weeks of continued use, and thus immediate discontinuation may not be warranted. CK elevation 3–10× normal without significant symptoms does not warrant discontinuation either.[32] Statin is discontinued if CK >10× normal or the patient experiences severe muscle aches. Muscle aches usually disappear within a few days to 2 weeks of discontinuation. The persistence of symptoms longer than 2 weeks after discontinuation implies that they are not related to statin; the original statin may be resumed. If the patient has severe muscle aches or myositis without rhabdomyolysis, he may tolerate another statin, which should be started once symptoms resolve. Fluvastatin XL appears to have the least muscle toxicity, and pravastatin is second in safety.[30] Among the potent statins, rosuvastatin may be the safest, especially when administered at a low dose on alternate days.[31]

The risk of myositis is increased with age; renal failure; combined therapy with fibrate (~1%) and, less so, niacin; and combined therapy with CYP450 inhibitors (diltiazem, amiodarone, macrolides, HIV protease inhibitors, azole, grapefruit juice).

> Look for drug interactions (e.g., diltiazem), underlying hypothyroidism, or 25-hydroxy-vitamin D deficiency as common predisposing factors. Supplementation with CoQ 10 may reduce muscle symptoms.

ii. *Hepatitis*. Mildly elevated transaminases, 1–2× normal, do not contraindicate the initiation or continuation of statin therapy. A rise in transaminases to >3× normal usually dictates statin discontinuation (~0.5% risk; ~1% risk in the case of statin+niacin combination). Liver profile should return to normal within 2 weeks of discontinuation. A lower dose of the same statin or another statin may be tried.
iii. Except for pravastatin, all statins are metabolized by the cytochrome P450 system. Pravastatin, rosuvastatin, and fluvastatin are less subject to cytochrome P450 drug interactions than other statins. Pravastatin and rosuvastatin are hydrophilic, which may explain the lower frequency of muscular symptoms with these agents.

B. PCSK9 inhibitors
PCSK9 inhibitors appear to be well tolerated in patients who are intolerant to statins. In such patients, the rate of discontinuation of PCSK9 inhibitors for muscular symptoms is low (<5%), lower than the rate of discontinuation with ezetimibe.[35] In fact, in most studies, muscular symptoms occurred with similar frequency in patients receiving PCSK9 inhibitors and placebo.[36]

C. Niacin (nicotinic acid)
Adverse effects: (a) flushing; (b) increased blood glucose; (c) increased uric acid; (d) peptic ulcer; (e) hepatitis. (b) and (c) mainly occur with
  doses >1500 mg/day or in the case of uncontrolled diabetes (HbA1c >7). Flushing improves with time and is reduced by slow titration, premedication with aspirin, and the use of an extended-release niacin form (Niaspan).
Dosage: Niaspan 500 mg QHS. The dosage is doubled every month up to a maximum of 2000 mg QHS.

D. Fibrates
Adverse effects: gallstones (gemfibrozil), hepatitis, myositis. Gemfibrozil interacts with warfarin (↑ INR). Gemfibrozil is contraindicated in conjunction with statin. Fenofibrate is contraindicated if GFR <30 ml/min/1.73 m², and the dose should not exceed 54 mg/day if GFR is 30–60 ml/min/1.73 m².

E. Cholestyramine
Adverse effects: bloating, constipation.

QUESTIONS AND ANSWERS

Question 1. A 60-year-old diabetic man presents with NSTEMI and undergoes stenting of the mid-LAD. He has a history of stroke 2 years ago. His LDL is 190 mg/dl, HDL 35 mg/dl, and triglycerides 300 mg/dl. He used a statin in the past, but stopped it because of hip pain. What is the best treatment strategy?
A. Ezetimibe and niacin
B. Ezetimibe and PCSK9 inhibitor
C. Niacin and PCSK9 inhibitor
D. Reintroduce statin (atorvastatin or rosuvastatin, starting at low dose, then up-titrated if possible) along with ezetimibe. Recheck lipids 6 weeks later; if LDL still >70, or if the patient cannot tolerate statin, add PCSK9 inhibitor

Question 2. A 45-year-old woman is obese and has prediabetes and controlled HTN. She has premature CAD in first-degree relatives at the age of 50. LDL is 118 mg/dl, HDL is 45 mg/dl. Her 10-year ACC cardiovascular risk score is 2% if she is a non-smoker and 6% if she is a smoker. Which of the following indicates statin therapy in this patient, according to ACC guidelines?

A. The cardiovascular risk of 5–7.5% (in case of smoking)

B. The family history of premature CAD

C. Metabolic syndrome

D. Prediabetes

E. A or B

Question 3. A patient had a recent ACS and AF and was placed on atorvastatin 80 mg. He is also on diltiazem, amiodarone, aspirin, and clopidogrel. On his follow-up clinic visit, he notes significant proximal myalgias. Which of the following is *incorrect*?

A. Diltiazem and amiodarone are inhibitors of cytochrome P450 3A4, and increase the level and toxicity of atorvastatin

B. Simvastatin can be used, as it is not a substrate of cytochrome P450 3A4

C. Pravastatin is not metabolized by any cytochrome, while rosuvastatin and fluvastatin are metabolized by different cytochromes (2C9 rather than 3A4). The latter two can be used with diltiazem or amiodarone

D. PCSK9 inhibitors can be used, and are associated with a low discontinuation rate in patients intolerant to statins

Answer 1. D. Frequently, muscular symptoms are not solely related to statin, and may be related to low vitamin D, thyroid disorder, or drug interaction. The patient may tolerate statin, especially a different statin, upon reinitiation. Two objectives should be achieved: (1) provide statin therapy and (2) reduce LDL <60–70 mg/dl. Hence, the focus should be on LDL-lowering drugs. Answer A would be acceptable if the patient truly cannot tolerate any statin and PCSK9 drugs are not available.

Answer 2. E. A family history of CAD in first-degree relatives (<55 years of age for men, < 65 years of age for women) yields a class IIb recommendation for statin therapy, regardless of the 10-year risk score calculator. Also, a risk score of 5–7.5% is a class IIa recommendation for statin therapy. Prediabetes and metabolic syndrome are markers of high risk that have not been included in the 2013 ACC guidelines for statin therapy.

Answer 3. B. Simvastatin and lovastatin are extensively metabolized by cytochrome P450 3A4, which is inhibited by diltiazem, amiodarone, macrolides, grapefruit juice, and protease inhibitors; atorvastatin is moderately metabolized by this cytochrome. Rosuvastatin is metabolized by another cytochrome and does not have these drug interactions. PCSK9 inhibitors do not have any known drug interaction.

References

1. Leeper NJ, Ardehali R, deGoma EM, Heidenreich PA. Statin use in patients with extremely low low-density lipoprotein levels is associated with improved survival. Circulation 2007; 116: 613–18. *Patients with LDL <40 mg/dl had the lowest mortality.*
2. Lee KH, Jeong MH, Kim HM, et al. Benefit of early statin therapy in patients with acute myocardial infarction who have extremely low low-density lipoprotein cholesterol. J Am Coll Cardiol 2011; 58: 1664–71.
3. Heart Protection Study Collaborative Group. MRC/BHF Heart Protection Study of cholesterol lowering with simvastatin in 20 536 high-risk individuals: a randomised placebo-controlled trial. Lancet 2002; 360: 7–22. *HPS trial.*
4. Cannon CP, Braunwald E, McCabe CH, et al. Intensive versus moderate lipid lowering with statins after acute coronary syndromes. N Engl J Med 2004; 350: 1495–504. *PROVE-IT TIMI trial.*
5. LaRosa JC, Grundy SM, Waters DD, et al. Intensive lipid lowering with atorvastatin in patients with stable coronary disease. N Engl J Med 2005; 352: 1425–35. *TNT trial.*
6. Wiviott SD, Cannon CP, Morrow DA, et al. Can low-density lipoprotein be too low? The safety and efficacy of achieving very low low-density lipoprotein with intensive statin therapy: a PROVE IT-TIMI 22 substudy. J Am Coll Cardiol 2005; 46: 1411–16.
7. LaRosa JC, Grundy SM, Kastelein JJ, et al. Safety and efficacy of atorvastatin-induced very low-density lipoprotein cholesterol levels in patients with coronary heart disease (a post hoc analysis of the Treating to New Targets [TNT] study). Am J Cardiol 2007; 100: 747–52.
8. Cannon CP, Blazing MA, Giugliano RP, et al. Ezetimibe added to statin therapy after acute coronary syndromes. N Engl J Med 2015; 372: 2387–97. *IMPROVE-IT trial.*
9. Ginsberg HN, Elam MB, Lovato LC, et al. Effects of combination lipid therapy in type 2 diabetes mellitus. N Engl J Med 2010; 362: 1563–74. *ACCORD trial.*
10. AIM-HIGH investigators. Niacin in patients with low HDL cholesterol levels receiving intensive statin therapy. N Engl J Med 2011; 365: 2255–67.
11. Stone NJ, Robinson JG, Lichtenstein AH, et al. 2013 ACC/AHA guideline on the treatment of blood cholesterol to reduce atherosclerotic cardiovascular risk in adults: a report of the American College of Cardiology/American Heart Association Task Force on Practice Guidelines. Circulation 2014; 129 (25 Suppl 2): S1–45.
12. Schwartz GG, Olsson AG, Abt M, et al. Effects of Dalcetrapib in Patients with a Recent Acute Coronary Syndrome. N Engl J Med 2012; 367: 2089–99.
13. LaRosa JC. How much statin intervention is enough? J Am Coll Cardiol 2011; 58: 1672–3.
14. Ridker PM, Genest J, Boekholdt SM, et al. HDL cholesterol and residual risk of first cardiovascular events after treatment with potent statin therapy: an analysis from the JUPITER trial. Lancet 2010; 376: 333–9.
15. Forrester JS. Redefining normal low-density lipoprotein cholesterol levels. J Am Coll Cardiol 2010; 56: 630–6.
16. O'Keefe JH, Cordain L, Harris WH. Optimal low-density lipoprotein is 50 to 70 mg/dl: Lower is better and physiologically normal. J Am Coll Cardiol 2004; 43: 2142–6.
17. Robinson JG, Farnier M, Krempf M, et al. Efficacy and safety of alirocumab in reducing lipids and cardiovascular events. N Engl J Med 2015; 372: 1489–99.
18. Canner PL, Berge KG, Wenger NK, et al. Fifteen year mortality in Coronary Drug Project patients: long-term benefit with niacin. J Am Coll Cardiol 1986; 8: 1245–55.

19. Brown BG, Zhao XQ, Chait A, et al. Simvastatin and niacin, antioxidant vitamins, or the combination for the prevention of coronary disease. N Engl J Med 2001; 345: 1583–92.

20. Rubins HB, Robins SJ, Collins D, et al. Gemfibrozil for the secondary prevention of coronary heart disease in men with low levels of high-density lipoprotein cholesterol. N Engl J Med 1999; 341: 410–18.

21. Frick MH, Elo O, Haapa K, et al. Helsinki Heart Study: primary-prevention trial with gemfibrozil in middle-aged men with dyslipidemia. Safety of treatment, changes in risk factors, and incidence of coronary heart disease. N Engl J Med 1987; 317: 1237–45.

22. Jones PH, Davidson MH. Reporting rate of rhabdomyolysis with fenofibrate+statin versus gemfibrozil+any statin. Am J Cardiol 2005; 95: 120–2.

23. GISSI-Prevenzione Investigators. Dietary supplementation with n-3 polyunsaturated fatty acids and vitamin E after myocardial infarction: results of the GISSI-Prevenzione trial. Lancet 1999; 354: 447–55.

24. Grundy SM, Cleeman JI, Daniels SR, et al. Diagnosis and management of the metabolic syndrome: an American Heart Association/National Heart, Lung, and Blood Institute Scientific Statement. Circulation 2005; 112: 2735–52.

25. NAVIGATOR Study Group. Effect of valsartan on the incidence of diabetes and cardiovascular events. N Engl J Med 2010; 362: 1477–90.

26. Chiasson J, Josse RG, Gomis R, et al. Acarbose treatment and the risk of cardiovascular disease and hypertension in patients with impaired glucose tolerance: the STOP-NIDDM trial. JAMA 2003; 290: 486–94.

27. Heart Protection Study Collaborative Group. MRC/BHF Heart Protection Study of cholesterol-lowering with simvastatin in 5963 people with diabetes: a randomised placebo-controlled trial. Lancet 2003; 361: 2005–16.

28. Colhoun HM, Betteridge DJ, Durrington PN, et al. Primary prevention of cardiovascular disease with atorvastatin in type 2 diabetes in the Collaborative Atorvastatin Diabetes Study (CARDS): multicentre randomised placebo-controlled trial. Lancet 2004; 364: 685–96.

29. Ridker PM, Danielson E, Fonseca FA, et al.; JUPITER Study Group. Rosuvastatin to prevent vascular events in men and women with elevated C-reactive protein. N Engl J Med 2008; 359: 2195–207.

30. Kidney Disease: Improving Global Outcomes (KDIGO) Lipid Work Group. KDIGO Clinical Practice Guideline for Lipid Management in Chronic Kidney Disease. Kidney Int, Suppl. 2013; 3: 259–305.

31. Fellstrom BC, Jardine AG, Schmieder RE. Rosuvastatin and cardiovascular events in patients undergoing hemodialysis. N Engl J Med 2009; 360: 1395–407.

32. Bruckert E, Hayem G, Dejager S, Yau C, Bégaud B. Mild to moderate muscular symptoms with high-dosage statin therapy in hyperlipidemic patients: the PRIMO study. Cardiovasc Drugs Ther 2005; 19: 403–14.

33. Fernandez G, Spatz ES, Jablecki C, Phillips PS. Statin myopathy: a common dilemma not reflected in clinical trials. Clev Clin J Med 2011; 76: 393–403.

34. Pasternak RC, Smith SC, Bairey-Merz CN, et al. ACC/AHA/NHLBI clinical advisory on the use and safety of statins. J Am Coll Cardiol 2002; 40: 567–72.

35. Nissen SE, Stroes E, Dent-Acosta RE, et al. Efficacy and tolerability of evolocumab vs ezetimibe in patients with muscle-related statin intolerance. JAMA 2016; 315: 1580–90.

36. Sabatine MS, Giugliano RP, Wiviott SD, et al. Efficacy and safety of evolocumab in reducing lipids and cardiovascular events. N Engl J Med 2015; 372: 1500–9. *Osler trial.*

25 Pulmonary Hypertension

I. Definition

Pulmonary hypertension (PH) is defined as a mean PA pressure ≥25 mmHg at rest.[1,2] An increase in mean PA pressure to >30 mmHg with exercise used to be considered a diagnostic feature of PH but is less specific, particularly in patients >50 years of age who may normally have an increase in mean PA pressure to 40 mmHg with exercise. The classification of PH severity is shown in Table 25.1.

II. Categories of PH

There are two major categories of pulmonary hypertension.

A. PH secondary to left heart disease (also called pulmonary venous hypertension or postcapillary PH)

Left-sided ventricular or valvular diseases may produce an increase in LA pressure with passive backward transmission of pressure to the pulmonary circulation. As a result, PA pressure rises. In this case:[3]

- PCWP is elevated (>15 mmHg).
- Diastolic PA pressure is passively increased and is equal to PCWP or is up to 7 mmHg higher than PCWP.
- Pulmonary vascular resistance (PVR) is <3 Wood units. The transpulmonary gradient, i.e., mean PA pressure minus PCWP, is <12 mmHg (some investigators use a cutoff of 20 mmHg).[1] Note that the transpulmonary gradient is the numerator in PVR calculation: PVR = transpulmonary gradient/cardiac output.

Left heart failure is the most common cause of PH. HF may be obvious in some patients, but may be occult in others, especially when isolated LV diastolic dysfunction is present.[4] Furthermore, with chronic venous PH, pulmonary arteries may undergo reactive changes and PH may become a mixed venous and arterial PH, in which case PCWP is elevated but diastolic PA pressure is >7 mmHg higher than PCWP and PVR is >3 Wood units.[5,6] In fact, a precapillary component accompanies PH in 20–35% of patients with advanced left HF,[6–8] and may accompany PH of mitral stenosis and diastolic HF. In addition, this situation may be seen in patients with mixed disorders, such as left HF and COPD. The active, precapillary PH component resolves after treatment of HF, but may take weeks or months to fully resolve.[3]

Resting PCWP may be normal despite LV failure, especially in patients appropriately treated with diuretics. The improvement of pulmonary pressure lags behind the improvement of PCWP, and these patients may have a normal PCWP with elevated PA pressure, simulating precapillary PH, except for a PVR that is only mildly increased. Exercise testing, volume loading, or pulmonary vasodilator challenge are appropriate strategies that increase PCWP in occult LV dysfunction and thus unveil the diagnosis of postcapillary PH. Patients who are suspected of having left heart disease-associated PH or mixed postcapillary PH and precapillary PH are approached as in Figure 25.1.

Up to 70% of patients with systolic LV dysfunction or isolated LV diastolic dysfunction may develop PH, and the presence of PH is associated with a poor prognosis in these patient populations.[2,9,10] One study documented a high prevalence of PH in patients with heart failure and preserved EF; 83% of patients in this study had PH, the median PA systolic pressure being 48 mmHg.[10] Interestingly, PA pressure was out of proportion to what would be expected from the rise in PCWP. For the same PCWP, patients with heart failure had a much higher PA pressure than patients with hypertension and no heart failure. Thus, in addition to the postcapillary PH, a precapillary pulmonary hypertension frequently coexists or develops during the course of heart failure with preserved EF.

Practical Cardiovascular Medicine, First Edition. Elias B. Hanna.
© 2017 John Wiley & Sons Ltd. Published 2017 by John Wiley & Sons Ltd.

Table 25.1 Classification of severity of pulmonary hypertension.

	Systolic PA pressure	Mean PA pressure
Mild PH	35–50 mmHg	25–35 mmHg
Moderate PH	50–70 mmHg	35–45 mmHg
Severe PH	>70 mmHg	>45 mmHg or PVR >6–7 Wood units

WHO classification- WHO group 1 is PAH; WHO group 2 is left heart disease-related PH; WHO group 3 is PH secondary to lung disease or hypoxemia; WHO group 4 is chronic thromboembolic PH.

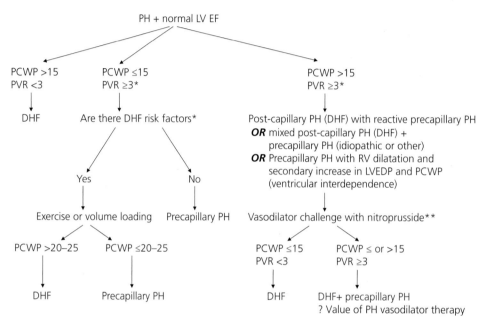

Figure 25.1 Diagnostic approach to distinguish between precapillary PH (pulmonary arterial hypertension) and PH related to diastolic heart failure (DHF). PVR <3 correlates with a transpulmonary gradient (mean PA pressure minus PCWP) <20 mmHg and diastolic PA pressure within 5–7 mmHg of PCWP. Wood unit is the PVR unit used in this figure.

*HTN, age >65, diabetes, LVH, left atrial enlargement, atrial fibrillation, low E', E/E' >15. With exercise, PCWP may normally rise up to 20–25 mmHg. Exertional PCWP is abnormal if it exceeds 20–25 mmHg.

**Adenosine or epoprostenol may further increase LV preload and PCWP in left heart failure, and may be used to show that DHF is the primary driver of PH. Otherwise, when addressing vasoreactivity in patients with an established HF diagnosis, nitroprusside as a pulmonary vasodilator is preferred as it reduces afterload and may actually reduce PCWP. Modified with permission of Elsevier from Hoeper et al. (2009).[3]

B. Precapillary PH

Precapillary PH is characterized by PCWP and LVEDP ≤15 mmHg, PVR ≥3 Wood units, and a transpulmonary gradient >12 mmHg.[1,2,11] In cases of precapillary PH associated with severe RV failure, pericardial distension and functional pericardial constriction may occur, leading to ventricular interdependence and equalization of RV and LV end-diastolic pressures, with a subsequent rise in LV end-diastolic pressure and PCWP to 15–20 mmHg.[12] As opposed to left heart disease, the increase in PCWP is, in this case, the result of PH rather than the cause of PH. Yet, in such an instance, PH may be erroneously labeled as left heart disease-associated PH. The presence of signs of LV diastolic dysfunction on echocardiography supports the diagnosis of left heart disease-associated PH, while severe RV dilatation and severe elevation of PVR >7 Wood units support the diagnosis of precapillary PH.

There are three major categories of precapillary PH:

1. Pulmonary arterial hypertension (PAH), which is related to a pulmonary vascular disease affecting the pulmonary arterioles. PAH may be idiopathic, familial, or related to connective tissue disease, toxins (amphetamines, anorexigen), cirrhosis (portopulmonary hypertension), HIV, or Eisenmenger syndrome. Idiopathic PAH may be seen at any age or sex but is more common in female patients (female/male ratio 3:1; age 36 ± 15 years).

In congenital heart disease with a large left-to-right shunt (e.g., VSD, PDA, or less often ASD), PA pressure initially increases as a result of the increase in right-sided flow, PVR remaining initially low (pressure = flow × resistance; an increase in flow leads to an increase in pressure). This "dynamic" PH resolves with shunt closure. Over time, the increased pulmonary flow induces progressive pulmonary vascular disease and severe increase in PVR to a point that PVR approaches SVR, PA pressure approaches systemic pressure, and the shunt reverses and becomes directed right-to-left or bidirectional. This is Eisenmenger syndrome and, except in ASD, is usually established in infancy or childhood. It is unusual for VSD or PDA to be diagnosed as a cause of PH in an adult.

Pulmonary veno-occlusive disease is characterized by primary venular abnormalities similar to the arteriolar abnormalities seen in idiopathic PAH and may be idiopathic or associated with scleroderma. Similar to PAH, true pulmonary arterial wedging is difficult during catheterization, but, if successful, it still creates a column of stagnant blood between the catheter and the LA; thus, the truly wedged PCWP approximates the LA pressure, albeit damped through the venular obstruction, and is normal in value. The wedged PA pressure, i.e., LA pressure, is normal, but the pulmonary capillary pressure is increased and pulmonary edema may be seen.

2. *PH secondary to thromboembolic disease*. Approximately 4% of patients who develop acute PE do not fully resolve their thrombus burden and go on to develop chronic PH. This often occurs after single PE episodes. Most often, the thrombus involves the main lobar pulmonary artery or the proximal arteries (80%), with small-vessel arteriopathy and thrombosis that subsequently occur and contribute to disease progression. In a smaller category of cases, the thromboembolic process is purely distal, involving the small distal pulmonary arteries (the distal type is less likely to benefit from surgical thromboendarterectomy).

3. *PH secondary to hypoxic lung disease*. Mild PH is common in patients with COPD, but severe PH is very unusual. In fact, moderate and severe PH are only seen in 5–10% and 2% of severe COPD cases, respectively.[13,14] Also, sleep apnea does not usually lead to more than mild PH. Conversely, severe PH may be seen with advanced-stage fibrotic lung disease that obliterates the pulmonary capillaries, sarcoidosis, or obesity–hypoventilation syndrome.

III. Two tips in the evaluation of PH

The following two ideas are essential to the evaluation of PH:

1. In chronic severe PH, the PA pressure number may start declining into the mild range as the RV develops severe failure and becomes unable to generate high PA pressure. PVR, on the other hand, remains severely elevated.

2. In acute PH (e.g., pulmonary embolism), the RV is not able to generate a systolic PA pressure higher than 45–50 mmHg. Therefore, in a case of acute pulmonary embolism, a systolic PA pressure higher than 40 mmHg implies severe pulmonary hypertension.[11] A systolic PA pressure higher than 50 mmHg suggests a subacute or chronic process.

In both cases, the PA pressure number underestimates the true severity of the pulmonary vascular abnormality. The presence of severe RV dysfunction, a severely elevated RA pressure, or a severely elevated PVR >6–7 Wood units is diagnostic of severe PH. In fact, in patients with severe PH that is evidenced by elevated PVR and RV failure, a high systolic PA pressure predicts recovery of RV function with therapy and better outcomes than a low systolic PA pressure. A higher systolic PA pressure corresponds to a better RV function.[15,16]

IV. Hypoxemia in patients with PH

Hypoxemia may be related to the cause of PH, such as pulmonary edema (left heart disease), lung disease, hypoventilation syndrome, or Eisenmenger syndrome and right-to-left shunting. On the other hand, PAH may, by itself, lead to hypoxemia, mainly in patients with patent foramen ovale. In those patients, the increased RA pressure "opens" the PFO, leading to a secondary right-to-left shunt (this shunt is the result rather than the cause of PAH). Also, *a degree of arteriovenous shunting may occur at the pulmonary level, as a diversion from the "plugged" pulmonary microvascular flow.*

While hypoxemia may be seen in any PH, cyanosis at rest or with exercise characterizes Eisenmenger syndrome more than other causes of PH. Exercise-induced cyanosis or marked drop in O_2 desaturation is characteristic of an intracardiac shunt, wherein further right-to-left shunting occurs during exercise, as venous return increases.

V. Diagnosis: echocardiography; right and left heart catheterization

A. Echocardiography

PH is often initially suggested by echocardiography. Echocardiography estimates PA pressure, and:

1. Suggests a left-sided etiology. In addition to valvular function and LV systolic function, echocardiography assesses LA pressure, LV diastolic function, and left atrial size.

2. Looks for signs of severity of PH: RV and RA dilatation, severe TR, RV systolic dysfunction, and abnormal interventricular septal motion (the high, right-sided pressure or volume makes the septum bow to the left). Frequently, PA pressure cannot be directly measured by echo; those signs indirectly suggest PH.

B. Catheterization

Catheterization is needed to confirm the diagnosis and the etiology of PH, particularly in cases of moderate-to-severe PH without a clear cause. Patients with a clear clinical and echo diagnosis of left HF do not require cardiac catheterization for PH assessment. Also, patients with an acute PE diagnosis do not require cardiac catheterization (this may, however, be required for chronic thromboembolic PH). The goals of catheterization are:

1. Confirm the diagnosis of PH by measuring PA pressure and calculating PVR (PVR = [mean PA – PCWP]/cardiac output). The spectral Doppler profile of TR is too weak or insufficient to measure the PA pressure in approximately 25–55% of patients referred for PA pressure evaluation; TR may not be present even when PH is severe.[17] The echocardiographic diagnosis of PH is falsely positive in up to 50% of patients, and, overall, the PA pressure value differs from the catheterization value by >10 mmHg in 50% of patients. Echocardiography may under- or overestimate PA pressure in various PH etiologies.[17,18]

2. Assess PCWP to determine if PH is secondary to left HF. The assessment of PCWP may be difficult in patients with severe PH:[19–21] (i) segmental PA branches are dilated, which makes them difficult to wedge; thus, a hybrid PCWP–PA pressure tracing may be obtained and lead to overestimation of the true PCWP; (ii) on the other hand, the true PCWP waveform may be flattened without distinct waves, as the retrograde transmission of LA pressure through the constricted pulmonary vasculature is damped. Moreover, wedging a PA catheter in a patient with PH is associated with an increased risk of PA rupture.

In the absence of an appropriate PCWP tracing, LVEDP needs to be measured. A case can be made to perform left heart catheterization and measure LVEDP in all patients with PH. ***Not only can PCWP overestimate LVEDP***, but according to a large analysis of 4000 heart catheterizations in patients with PH, ***PCWP underestimates LVEDP in over 50% of patients*** and misclassifies postcapillary PH as pre-capillary PH. This is related to wedging issues, damping of the pressure transmission from LA to the wedged PA, but also to the fact that LVEDP is larger than PCWP in patients with compensated LV dysfunction.[22]

Patients with normal LVEDP and PCWP may still have occult HF. ***If suspected clinically, give a volume load or perform exercise testing or vasodilator challenge and see if PCWP or LVEDP increases, unveiling left HF as the cause of PH.***

3. Assess for a left-to-right shunt (oximetry screen of SVC, IVC, and PA). Right-to-left shunt, on the other hand, is suspected when hypoxemia is present at rest and does not quickly improve with deep breathing or O_2 therapy.

4. Perform acute vasoreactivity testing if PAH is suspected. Vasodilator challenge should not be performed in overt left HF with marked PCWP elevation, as it may increase pulmonary blood flow and thus PCWP, which leads to pulmonary edema. It should not be performed in case of PH secondary to severe lung disease, as vasodilators worsen V/Q mismatch and hypoxemia. It may, however, be performed when *severe* PH is concomitant with lung disease, as severe PH often implies a primary pulmonary vascular disease independent of lung disease.

Only 10% of patients with PAH have a positive response to vasodilator challenge. ***Since non-responders still respond well to the chronic administration of potent pulmonary vasodilators (prostacyclin, bosentan, sildenafil), one may wonder what the rationale for vasodilator challenge is. The rationale for vasodilator challenge is threefold:*** (1) positive responders to vasodilator challenge may respond to chronic calcium channel blocker therapy; (2) positive responders have a better long-term prognosis; (3) the hemodynamic tolerance to vasodilator therapy is assessed. One should ensure that PCWP does not increase and cardiac output and systemic pressure do not decrease with vasodilators. **In fact, a vasodilator challenge may be used as a form of left heart stress testing, unveiling occult left HF.**

An acute response to vasodilator testing is defined by the ACC and pulmonary societies as a drop of mean PA pressure by >10 mmHg to <40 mmHg without a decrease in cardiac output. Other investigators have defined a positive response as a decrease in PA pressure and PVR by ≥20%.[19] Some patients have a decrease in PVR and an increase in cardiac output with vasodilators, such that PA pressure (cardiac output × PVR) remains unchanged. Thus, the sole reliance on PA pressure to assess vasoreactivity has its limitation, yet it more specifically predicts a response to oral vasodilators. Beside the assessment of PA pressure and PVR during testing, it is also important to assess:

    a. *Cardiac output* generally increases with vasodilator therapy, except in severe RV failure with lack of contractile reserve.

    b. *PCWP*: an increase in PCWP unveils an overlooked left heart failure and predicts intolerance to vasodilator therapy.

    c. O_2 *saturation* may drop in patients with lung disease.

    d. *RA pressure*: vasodilators increase venous return which may not be tolerated in a patient with severe RV failure.

    e. *Systemic blood pressure*.

Acute vasodilator testing is performed using one of the three following agents: IV epoprostenol, IV adenosine (starting at 50 mcg/kg/min, and titrated by 50–100 mcg/kg/min every 2 minutes, to a maximum of 250 mcg/kg/min), and inhaled nitric oxide. These agents are titrated up until the maximal dose is reached, systemic intolerance occurs (dyspnea, nausea), or one of the five negative endpoints occurs (hypotension, ↓ CO, ↑ PCWP, ↑ RA pressure, ↓ O_2 saturation)

Additional note: Vasoreactivity testing is useful in two more situations. Patients with left-to-right shunt (ASD, VSD, PDA) who have PH with a PVR >2/3 SVR or >6 Wood units need to have vasoreactivity testing before shunt correction to ensure that PH is reversible; otherwise shunt closure may precipitate right heart failure. Patients with advanced left HF who are considered for cardiac transplantation and who have PH with high PVR require vasoreactivity testing to assess the reversibility of PH and their operability. In this case, however, the use of prostanoids may increase PCWP and is poorly tolerated. Nitroprusside and milrinone are the vasodilators of choice, as they reduce PVR in reactive PH but also reduce LV afterload, which prevents the increase in PCWP.

C. Other tests
Depending on the context, these tests are performed before or after confirmation of PH:

1. Chest CTA or V/Q scan for the diagnosis of thromboembolic PH. These studies do not usually miss the proximal form of thromboembolic PH, which is the most common form and the treatable form of thromboembolic PH. To definitely rule out PE and diagnose multiple distal PEs missed by the above, a pulmonary angiogram may need to be performed if the clinical suspicion is high.

2. Chest X-ray, arterial blood gases, pulmonary function testing with diffusion capacity, ± high-resolution CT scan of the chest for the diagnosis of lung diseases. Remember, however, that lung diseases do not usually lead to severe PH.

On chest X-ray, look for pulmonary edema or parenchymal lung disease. Pulmonary hypertension, per se, leads to enlarged central pulmonary arteries, i.e., enlarged hila, with marked tapering of the peripheral arteries and oligemia of the lung fields. This is opposed to the diffuse vascular engorgement seen with pulmonary edema.

3. Sleep study in most patients.

4. HIV, liver function testing, antinuclear antibodies, TSH, BNP.

VI. Treatment
A. PH secondary to left heart failure, pulmonary thromboembolic disease, or lung disease: treat the underlying cause
1. Treat LV failure, aggressively treat hypertension, and perform valvular surgery in case of severe valvular disease. PH is expected to be reversible, but the process may be slow, and temporary support with vasodilators may be needed perioperatively.

2. Pulmonary thromboendarterectomy in thromboembolic PH with proximal thromboembolic disease.

3. Bronchodilators and O_2 in the case of lung disease.

4. Pulmonary vasodilators are not recommended and may be harmful. They may worsen V/Q mismatch by vasodilating the hypoventilated areas of the lungs, which worsens hypoxemia. They may increase pulmonary blood flow and lead to pulmonary edema in the case of LV dysfunction.

B. Pulmonary arterial hypertension

Without specific therapy, idiopathic PAH has a poor prognosis with a median survival of 2.8 years. PAH related to Eisenmenger syndrome has a better prognosis, as the right-to-left shunt relieves the RV overload. Conversely, PAH associated with connective tissue disease (scleroderma) or HIV has a worse prognosis.[23] Several high-risk features imply a poor prognosis:

- NYHA class IV; syncope (implies a severe reduction of the cardiac output reserve)
- 6-minute walking distance <300 m
- Clinical signs of RV failure or severe RV or RA dilatation on echo
- Elevated RA pressure >14 mmHg, low cardiac index <2 l/min/m²
- Pericardial effusion
- BNP >180 pg/ml
- The severity of PA pressure rise, per se, is not an indicator of poor prognosis. In fact, a declining PA pressure in the face of a severely increased PVR is a marker of reduced cardiac output and RV failure (poor prognosis).

Pulmonary vasodilator therapy improves symptoms and survival very significantly (meta-analysis).[24] It is targeted to patients with pulmonary arterial hypertension and NYHA classes II–IV (Figure 25.2). Calcium channel blockers (CCBs) are associated with a dramatic improvement in survival of the few patients who acutely respond to vasodilator testing and achieve a sustained clinical response; thus, those select patients (5%) are initially treated with CCBs.[21,25]

Non-responders to vasodilator testing are treated with one of the four categories of selective pulmonary vasodilators:[26] (i) prostacyclin (IV, SQ, inhaled, and more recently oral), (ii) endothelin-receptor antagonists (ERA) (bosentan, ambrisentan, macitentan), (iii) phosphodiesterase-5 inhibitors (sildenafil and tadalafil), which reduce the degradation of the vasodilator cGMP, (iv) stimulator of guanylate cyclase (riociguat), which enhances cGMP production.

The latter two categories of drugs are related, as they both act on the cGMP system, i.e., the downstream nitric oxide system. In fact, nitric oxide binds to the intracellular guanylate cyclase and activates it, generating cGMP. Riociguat should not be combined with phosphodiesterase inhibitors, as they both act on the cGMP system (risk of hypotension without much benefit). Nitrates increase cGMP in the systemic but not pulmonary arteries and are not effective in PAH.

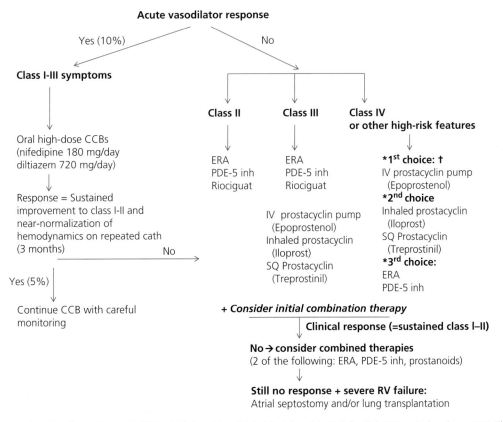

Figure 25.2 Treatment algorithm for patients with PAH, which is mainly validated for idiopathic PAH, familial PAH, and scleroderma PAH. This algorithm is cautiously extrapolated to other forms of PAH, Eisenmenger syndrome, and thromboembolic PAH that cannot be treated surgically or that persists after surgical therapy. This algorithm is adapted from recommendations from references 1 and 25.

†In class IV, intravenous epoprostenol is preferred because it is the therapy that has shown a mortality reduction in a randomized fashion, and is the therapy most widely studied in class IV.[28]

CCB, calcium channel blocker; ERA, endothelin-receptor antagonist; PDE-5 inh, phosphodiesterase-5 inhibitors.

Even in the absence of a positive vasodilator response upon testing, these potent pulmonary vasodilators reduce PVR over the long term, and, more importantly, prevent arterial remodeling, scarring, and the further increase in PA pressure. Therapy needs to be started as soon as possible, as it dramatically reduces mortality over the short-term follow-up (14 weeks in a meta-analysis).[24] Clinical non-responders to pulmonary-specific vasodilators, i.e., those who do not improve to a functional class I or II, may be treated with combined therapies. A recent study has suggested that initial combination therapy with tadalafil and ambrisentan, vs. initial therapy with either one of them, is associated with a 50% reduction in clinical events and twice the increase in walking distance.

Note that, except for the rare dramatic responder to CCB, PAH therapies only mildly reduce PA pressure (by ~10%), and thus PA pressure is not used as a therapeutic endpoint. PAH therapies improve PVR, RV function and size on echo, RA pressure, and cardiac output without much of an effect on PA pressure.[1,27,28] Along with the reduction in PVR, cardiac output increases, which may mask any PA pressure improvement (PA pressure ~ PVR × cardiac output). Thus, therapy targets clinical improvement (sustained class I–II, improved 6-minute walking distance), and improvement of echo parameters and BNP. Invasive reassessment, after several months of therapy, is done in high-risk patients or those who do not improve clinically.

Chronic anticoagulation (warfarin) is associated with improved survival. This is based on retrospective analyses that included patients with idiopathic or familial PAH.[24,26] This therapy has been extrapolated to other patients with PAH.[1] Anticoagulation prevents the progressive, thrombotic pulmonary arteriopathy that occurs with PAH.

Supportive measures are frequently used: O_2 for severe hypoxemia and diuretics for RV volume overload. Diuretics are useful for symptom relief and are usually well tolerated, as the dilated RV is not preload-dependent. In case of florid edema, gently diurese by 1000 ml/day.

QUESTIONS AND ANSWERS

Question 1. Among elderly patients referred for the evaluation of pulmonary hypertension, what is the most commonly missed diagnosis?
A. Sleep apnea
B. Chronic lung disease
C. HFpEF
D. PE

Question 2. A 57-year-old obese woman has dyspnea on exertion, NYHA III. She has a history of hypertension. Her BP is currently 136/85 mmHg. No clinical signs of HF are present. Her echo shows a systolic PA pressure of 75 mmHg with RV pressure overload pattern, mild concentric LV remodeling, and mild LA enlargement with normal LA pressure. What is the next step?
A. Prescribe a diuretic and reassess PA pressure
B. Sleep study
C. Right and left heart catheterization with vasoreactivity and exercise testing
D. Prescribe sildenafil

Question 3. The patient in Question 2 underwent cardiac catheterization that confirmed severe PAH: PA pressure 75/35, mean 45 mmHg; PCWP and LVEDP 13 mmHg at rest and 19 mmHg with exercise; no significant drop of PA pressure with adenosine testing. A chest X-ray and a lung perfusion scan are normal. She is placed on bosentan therapy. Three months later, her functional capacity and dyspnea have improved significantly (NYHA II). No signs of right HF are present on exam. An echo is performed and still shows severe PH, PA pressure 75 mmHg. What is the next step?
A. Switch to sildenafil
B. Switch to prostacyclin products
C. Add sildenafil
D. Continue the same therapy

Question 4. Vasodilator therapy is initiated in a patient with severe PAH, elevated RA pressure, and severe RV dilatation on echo. All of the following parameters are endpoints of therapy, *except for which one?*
A. Improving functional class to NYHA I–II
B. Reducing RA pressure to <8 mmHg
C. Increasing 6-minute walking distance to >380–440 m (or more in young patients)
D. Reducing PA pressure by 20%
E. Reducing RV dilation to normal or near-normal
F. Increasing cardiac index to >2.5–3 l/min/m²
G. Normal BNP

Question 5. A 55-year-old woman presents with class III dyspnea. She is diagnosed with PAH. Based on recent data, which therapy is the best first-line therapy?
A. Sildenafil
B. Ambrisentan
C. IV epoprostenol
D. Combination tadalafil–ambrisentan

Question 6. A 49-year-old man has a history of thromboembolic PH with RV failure. A year ago, his cardiac catheterization demonstrated RA pressure 25 mmHg, PA pressure 95/55 mmHg, PCWP 20–22 mmHg, and PVR 11 Wood units. He is placed on bosentan and sildenafil. More recently, due to progressive symptoms, subcutaneous treprostinil is added. However, his symptoms continue to worsen. A right heart

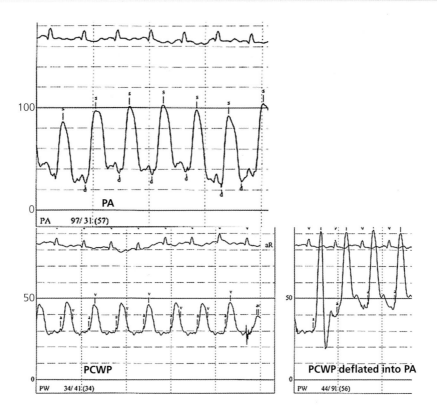

Figure 25.3

catheterization is repeated, revealing the PA and PCWP shown in Figure 25.3. His RA pressure is 14 mmHg and his cardiac output is 8 l/min by thermodilution. What is the next step?

A. The patient's PH is refractory. Up-titrate the dose of treprostinil

B. Continue the current regimen. RA pressure, CO, and PVR have improved

C. Reduce the dose of vasodilator therapy and consider adding furosemide

Question 7. A 35-year-old woman presents with class III dyspnea. She is found to have severe PAH with PA pressure 100 mmHg and PVR 9 Wood units. Echo shows ASD of 1 cm with right-to-left shunt across it. The RV is mildly dilated, and it mostly displays signs of pressure overload. What is the diagnosis and next management?

A. Eisenmenger syndrome. ASD closure is contraindicated at this point

B. Idiopathic PAH. ASD is an incidental finding and should not be closed

C. PAH secondary to ASD, but not a definite Eisenmenger. Attempt vasodilator testing: if PVR declines and the shunt converts from right-to-left to left-to-right with testing, ASD may be closed.

Question 8. Of the following PAH medications, select the one which has the most liver toxicity (10%), the one which has most been associated with peripheral edema, the one which has most interactions with cytochrome P450 3A4 and 2C9, and the one which reduces the blood levels of oral contraceptives:

A. Sildenafil

B. Bosentan

C. Ambrisentan

D. Macitentan

Answer 1. C.

Answer 2. C. The patient's PH may be precapillary (PAH) or may be related to left heart diastolic dysfunction. In the absence of overt hypervolemia or HTN, and without proof that PCWP is elevated, adding a diuretic is not appropriate. A diuretic would be an appropriate first step in a patient with florid left HF/pulmonary edema. Sildenafil is not prescribed before a right heart catheterization confirms the diagnosis of PH and the precapillary origin of PH. Right and left heart catheterization is the next step: resting pressures are obtained, then, if PCWP and LVEDP are normal or borderline at rest, exercise testing is performed to unveil LV diastolic dysfunction, especially in a patient with LA enlargement and concentric LV remodeling. Vasoreactivity testing is also a left heart stressor that may increase PCWP/LVEDP and unveil LV diastolic dysfunction. A sleep study needs to be performed and sleep apnea treated; however, this is not the most important next step, especially because sleep apnea does not usually explain severe PH. In fact, sleep apnea may aggravate LV diastolic failure.

Answer 3. D. Except for a rare dramatic response seen in patients who have a positive response to vasoreactivity testing, PAH therapies only mildly reduce PA pressure (by ~10%), if at all, and thus PA pressure is not used as a therapeutic endpoint. The improvement in functional class to I–II and the improvement of RV failure and RA pressure are endpoints of therapy. Vasodilators reduce PVR and increase cardiac output, both of which are desirable effects that correlate with clinical improvement. However, PA pressure, which is ~ PVR × cardiac output, remains unchanged. The 75 mmHg value that follows therapy is different from the initial 75 mmHg value, as the underlying components (CO × PVR) have favorably changed. Combination therapy may be considered simply because it is a superior *initial* strategy, not because of the persistent PA pressure elevation.

Answer 4. D.

Answer 5. D. Initial combination therapy was superior to initial monotherapy in the AMBITION trial. Prostanoids are first-line therapy in patients with NYHA class IV or other high-risk, RV failure features (Section VI.B), not this patient.

Answer 6. C. Initially (a year ago), the patient had severe pulmonary arterial (precapillary) hypertension, with RV failure and severely elevated RA pressure. PCWP was mildly elevated as a result of RV failure and the inherent equalization of left and right diastolic pressures (with RA pressure remaining slightly higher than PCWP). The elevation of PCWP did not match the severity of PVR elevation.

On the current study, note the very wide PA pulse pressure and the near-ventricularization of the PA pressure waveform. This may imply either (i) severe pulmonic valve insufficiency or (ii) high-cardiac-output state. The high cardiac output obtained by thermodilution suggests the latter. In pulmonary insufficiency, the thermodilution injectate keeps recirculating away from the PA sensor and a low cardiac output is obtained, or sometimes no CO can be obtained.

PCWP is very elevated (mean ~35 mmHg) with a very large V wave that approximates 50 mmHg. This implies severe LV failure. In fact, PCWP > >RA pressure, definitely implying that LV failure is the primary process at this point. Moreover, PVR is calculated at ~2.5 Wood units (PVR = [mean PA – PCWP]/CO). Thus, at this point, the severe pulmonary hypertension is secondary to both LV failure and the high-output state, rather than elevated PVR (PA pressure being proportional to CO × PVR, a high cardiac output may lead to a high PA pressure, even if PVR is reduced). LV failure, by itself, is secondary to the excessive vasodilator therapy that floods the left heart with a high pulmonary and systemic flow.

Answer 7. B. When a small defect is found in an adult with severe PH and severe PVR elevation (usually VSD <1 cm or ASD <2 cm), the defect is likely an incidental finding rather than a cause of PAH (ESC guidelines 2015); the defect allows decompression of the right chambers and should not be closed. In the current case, the severity of PVR elevation is disproportionate to the size of the ASD. ASD rarely causes Eisenmenger, and when it does, the defect is usually large (>2 cm) and has already caused RV failure for some time before Eisenmenger develops. Answer C would be an appropriate management strategy if the defect was large.

Answer 8. The drug with most liver toxicity is bosentan; the one with most peripheral edema is ambrisentan; the one with most cytochrome drug interactions is bosentan (sildenafil also has cytochrome drug interactions); and the one which reduces the effect of oral contraception is bosentan.

References

1. McLaughlin VV, Archer SL, Badesch DB, et al. ACCF/AHA 2009 consensus document on pulmonary hypertension. J Am Coll Cardiol 2009; 53: 1573–619.
2. Badesch DB, Champion HC, Sanchez MAG, et al. Diagnosis and assessment of pulmonary arterial hypertension. J Am Coll Cardiol 2009; 54: S55–66.
3. Hoeper MM, Barbera JA, Channick RN, et al. Diagnosis, assessment, and treatment of non-pulmonary arterial hypertension pulmonary hypertension. J Am Coll Cardiol 2009; 54: S85–96.
4. Boilson BA, Schirger JA, Borlaug BA. Caveat medicus! Pulmonary hypertension in the elderly: a word of caution. Eur J Heart Fail 2010; 12: 89–93.
5. Delgado JF, Conde E, Sanchez V, et al. Pulmonary vascular remodeling in pulmonary hypertension due to chronic heart failure. Eur J Heart Fail 2005; 7: 1011–16.
6. Simonneau G, Robbins IM, Beghetti M, et al. Updated clinical classification of pulmonary hypertension. J Am Coll Cardiol 2009; 54: S43–54.
7. Oudiz RJ. Pulmonary hypertension associated with left-sided heart disease. Clin Chest Med 2007; 28: 233–41.
8. Costard-Jackle A, Fowler MB. Influence of preoperative pulmonary artery pressure on mortality after heart transplantation: testing of potential reversibility of pulmonary hypertension with nitroprusside is useful in defining a high risk group. J Am Coll Cardiol 1992; 19: 48–54.
9. Moraes DL, Colucci WS, Givertz MM. Secondary pulmonary hypertension in chronic heart failure: the role of the endothelium in pathophysiology and management. Circulation 2000; 102: 1718–23.
10. Lam CS, Roger VL, Rodeheffer RJ, et al. Pulmonary hypertension in heart failure with preserved ejection fraction: a community-based study. J Am Coll Cardiol 2009; 53: 1119–26.
11. McLaughlin VV, Archer SL, Badesch DB, et al. ACCF/AHA 2009 consensus document on pulmonary hypertension. J Am Coll Cardiol 2009; 53: 1573–619.
12. Jaff MR, McMurtry S, Archer SL, et al. Management of massive and submassive pulmonary embolism, iliofemoral deep vein thrombosis, and chronic thromboembolic pulmonary hypertension. Circulation 2011; 123: 1788–830.
13. Scharf SM, Iqbal M, Keller C, et al. Hemodynamic characterization of patients with severe emphysema. Am J Respir Crit Care Med 2002; 166: 314–22.
14. Chaouat A, Bugnet AS, Kadaoui N, et al. Severe pulmonary hypertension and chronic obstructive pulmonary disease. Am J Respir Crit Care Med 2005; 172: 189–94.
15. Shiran A, Sagie A. Tricuspid regurgitation in mitral valve disease. J Am Coll Cardiol 2009; 53: 401–8.
16. Kaul TK, Ramsdale DR, Mercer JL. Functional tricuspid regurgitation following replacement of the mitral valve. Int J Cardiol 1991; 33: 305–13.
17. Arcasoy SM, Christie JD, Ferrari VA, et al. Echocardiographic assessment of pulmonary hypertension in patients with advanced lung disease. Am J Respir Crit Care Med 2003; 167; 735–40.
18. Rich JD, Shah SJ, Swarny RS, et al. Inaccuracy of Doppler echocardiographic estimates of pulmonary arterial pressure in patients with pulmonary hypertension. Implications for clinical practice. Chest 2011; 5: 988–93.

19. Kafi SA, Melot C, Vachiery J, et al. Partitioning of pulmonary vascular resistance in primary pulmonary hypertension. J Am Coll Cardiol 1998; 31: 1372–6.
20. Grimbert FA. Effective pulmonary capillary pressure. Eur Respir J 1988; 1: 297–301.
21. Sitbon O, Humbert M, Jais X, et al. Long-term response to calcium channel blockers in idiopathic pulmonary arterial hypertension. Circulation 2005; 111: 3105–11.
22. Halpern SD, Taichman DB. Misclassification of pulmonary hypertension due to reliance on pulmonary capillary wedge pressure rather than left-ventricular end diastolic pressure. Chest 2009; 136: 37–43.
23. McLaughlin VV, Presberg KW, Doyle RL. Prognosis of pulmonary arterial hypertension: ACCP evidence-based clinical practice guidelines. Chest 2004; 126: 78S–92S.
24. Galiè N, Manes A, Negro L. A meta-analysis of randomized controlled trials in pulmonary arterial hypertension. Eur Heart J 2009; 30: 394–403.
25. Rich S, Kaufmann E, Levy PS. The effect of high doses of calcium-channel blockers on survival in primary pulmonary hypertension. N Engl J Med 1992; 327: 76–81.
26. Barst RJ, Gibbs SR, Ghofrani HA, et al. Updated evidence-based treatment algorithm in pulmonary arterial hypertension. J Am Coll Cardiol 2009; 54: S78–84.
27. Galiè N, Hinderliter AL, Torbicki A, et al. Effects of the oral endothelin-receptor antagonist bosentan on echocardiographic and Doppler measures in patients with pulmonary arterial hypertension. J Am Coll Cardiol 2003; 41: 1380–6.
28. Barst RJ, Rubin LJ, Long WA, et al. Primary Pulmonary Hypertension Study Group A comparison of continuous intravenous epoprostenol (prostacyclin) with conventional therapy for primary pulmonary hypertension. N Engl J Med 1996; 334: 296–301.

26 Syncope

Syncope is a transient loss of consciousness *and* postural tone with spontaneous, complete recovery. *Lightheadedness* and *dizziness*, on the other hand, are terms that may imply any one of the following four conditions: (i) near-syncope, i.e., the feeling of impending faint; (ii) vertigo, i.e., an illusion of motion, usually from an inner ear disorder; (iii) disequilibrium (ataxia) from peripheral neuropathy or cerebellar disorder; (iv) non-specific lightheadedness from anxiety.

There are three major types of syncope: neurally mediated syncope, orthostatic hypotension, and cardiac syncope.

I. Neurally mediated syncope (reflex syncope)

Neurally mediated syncope is the most common type of syncope, accounting for two-thirds of the cases.[1-3] It results from an inappropriate response of autonomic reflexes, leading to vasodilatation and bradycardia. It is usually preceded by premonitory symptoms (lightheadedness, diaphoresis, nausea, malaise, abdominal discomfort, tunnel vision). However, this may not be the case in a third of patients, more so elderly patients who may not recognize or remember the warning. Palpitations are frequently reported with reflex syncope and do not necessarily imply an arrhythmic syncope.[4,5] This syncope does not usually occur in a supine position,[4,5] but may occur in a seated position.[6] Subtypes of neurally mediated syncope are as follows:

A. Vasovagal syncope (neurocardiogenic syncope)

This syncope is usually triggered by sudden emotional stress, prolonged sitting or standing, dehydration, or a warm environment, but may also occur without any trigger. It is the most common syncope in young patients (female > male) and, contrary to a common misconception, may occur in the elderly as well.[7] Usually, it is not only preceded but followed by nausea, malaise, fatigue, or diaphoresis;[4,5,8] the patient's full revival may be slow. When the syncope is prolonged >30–60 seconds, clonic movements and loss of bladder control are common.[9]

Mechanism. Vasovagal syncope is initiated by anything that leads to strong myocardial contractions on an "empty" heart. Emotional stress, reduced venous return (from dehydration or prolonged standing), or vasodilatation (hot environment) stimulates the sympathetic system and reduces the LV cavity size, which leads to strong hyperdynamic contractions in a relatively empty heart. This hyperdynamic cavity obliteration activates the myocardial mechanoreceptors, initiating a paradoxical *vagal reflex with vasodilatation and relative bradycardia*.[10] Vasodilatation is usually the predominant mechanism (*vasodepressor response*), particularly in older patients, but severe bradycardia is also possible (*cardioinhibitory response*), particularly in younger patients.[7] **Diuretic and vasodilator therapies increase the predisposition to vasovagal syncope, particularly in the elderly**.

On tilt table testing, vasovagal syncope is characterized by hypotension and a relative bradycardia, sometimes severe.[10]

B. Situational syncope

This syncope is caused by a reflex triggered in specific circumstances such as micturition, defecation, coughing, weightlifting, laughing, or deglutition. The reflex may be initiated by a receptor on the visceral wall (e.g., bladder wall) or by the strain that reduces venous return.

Practical Cardiovascular Medicine, First Edition. Elias B. Hanna.
© 2017 John Wiley & Sons Ltd. Published 2017 by John Wiley & Sons Ltd.

C. Carotid sinus hypersensitivity

Carotid sinus hypersensitivity (CSH) is an abnormal response to carotid massage that is predominantly found in patients over 50 years of age. *Spontaneous carotid sinus syndrome* is a form of CSH where syncope clearly occurs in a situation that stimulates the carotid sinus (head rotation, head extension, shaving, tight collar); this is a rare cause of syncope (~1% of syncope cases). Conversely, *induced carotid sinus syndrome* is much more common and represents CSH in a patient with unexplained syncope and without obvious triggers; the abnormal response is *induced* during carotid massage rather than spontaneously. In induced carotid sinus syndrome, carotid sinus hypersensitivity is a marker of a diseased sinus node or AV node that cannot withstand any inhibition; this diseased node is the true cause of syncope rather than CSH per se, and carotid massage is a "stress test" that unveils conduction disease.

Thus, carotid sinus massage is indicated in unexplained syncope regardless of circumstantial triggers. It consists of applying firm pressure over each carotid bifurcation (just below the angle of the jaw) consecutively for 10 seconds. It is performed at the bedside, and may be performed in both supine and erect positions during tilt table testing; erect positioning increases the sensitivity of carotid massage. An abnormal response to carotid sinus massage is defined as any of the following: [11–13]

i. Vasodepressor response: systolic blood pressure (SBP) decreases by ≥50 mmHg
ii. Cardioinhibitory response: pause ≥3 seconds (sinus pause or AV block)
iii. Mixed vasodepressor and cardioinhibitory response

Overall, a cardioinhibitory component is present in ~2/3 of CSH cases. CSH is found in 25–50% of patients over 50 years of age with unexplained syncope or fall, and is almost equally seen in men and women.[11] One study correlated CSH with the later occurrence of asystolic syncope during prolonged internal loop monitoring; subsequent pacemaker therapy reduced the burden of syncope.[12] Another study, in patients >50 years old with unexplained falls, found that 16% of them had cardioinhibitory CSH; pacemaker placement reduced falls and syncope by 70% compared with no pacemaker therapy in these patients.[13] On the other hand, CSH is seen in 39% of elderly patients who do not have a history of syncope or fall, and thus it is important to rule out other causes of syncope before attributing it to CSH.

D. Post-exertional syncope

While exertional syncope is alarming for a malignant cardiac or arrhythmic cause, post-exertional syncope is usually a form of vasovagal syncope. Upon exercise cessation, venous blood stops getting pumped back to the heart through the peripheral muscular contraction, yet the heart is still exposed to the catecholamine surge and hypercontracts on an empty cavity. This triggers a vagal reflex.

Post-exertional syncope may also be seen in hypertrophic obstructive cardiomyopathy (HOCM) and aortic stenosis (AS), where the small left ventricular cavity is less likely to tolerate the reduced preload after exercise and is more likely to obliterate.

II. Orthostatic hypotension

Orthostatic hypotension accounts for ~10% of cases of syncope.[1–3] Normally, after the *first few minutes* of standing, ~25–30% of blood pools in the veins of the pelvis and the lower extremities, strikingly reducing venous return and stroke volume. Upon prolonged standing, additional blood volume extravasates in the extravascular space, further reducing venous return. This normally leads to a reflex increase of sympathetic tone, peripheral and splanchnic vasoconstriction, *and* an increase in heart rate of 10–15 bpm. Overall, cardiac output (CO) is reduced while blood pressure (BP) is maintained (BP = CO × vascular resistance: vascular resistance ↑, CO ↓).

Orthostatic hypotension is characterized by *autonomic failure*, with a lack of compensatory increase in vascular resistance or heart rate upon orthostasis; or by significant *hypovolemia* that cannot be overcome by sympathetic mechanisms. It is defined as a drop of SBP ≥20 mmHg or DBP ≥10 mmHg after 30 seconds to 5 minutes of orthostasis. BP is checked immediately upon standing and at 3 and 5 minutes of orthostasis; this may be done at the bedside or during tilt table testing.[2,4] Some patients may have an immediate BP drop of >40 mmHg upon standing, with a quick return to normal within 30 seconds. This "initial orthostatic hypotension" may be common in elderly patients receiving antihypertensive drugs and may elude detection upon standard BP measurement.[2] Other patients with milder orthostatic hypotension may develop a more delayed hypotension 10–15 minutes later, as more blood pools in the periphery.[14]

Along with the BP drop, a failure to increase heart rate identifies autonomic dysfunction. On the other hand, an excessive increase in heart rate >20–30 bpm may signify a hypovolemic state even if BP is maintained, the lack of BP drop being related to the excessive heart rate increase.

Orthostatic hypotension is the most common cause of syncope in the elderly and may be due to: (i) autonomic dysfunction (age, diabetes, uremia, Parkinson's disease), (ii) volume depletion, (iii) drugs that block autonomic effects or cause hypovolemia (vasodilators, β-blockers, diuretics, neuropsychiatric medications, alcohol).

Since digestion leads to peripheral vasodilatation and splanchnic blood pooling, syncope that occurs within 1 hour postprandially has a similar mechanism to orthostatic syncope.

Supine HTN with orthostatic hypotension. Some patients with severe autonomic dysfunction or **severely non-compliant arteries** are unable to regulate vascular tone. They display severe HTN when supine and significant hypotension when upright.

Postural orthostatic tachycardia syndrome (POTS) is another form of orthostatic failure that occurs most frequently in young women (<50 years old). In POTS, autonomic dysfunction affects the peripheral vascular resistance, which fails to increase in response to orthostatic stress. This autonomic dysfunction does not affect the heart, which manifests a striking compensatory increase in rate of >30 bpm within the first 10 minutes of orthostasis, or an absolute heart rate >120 bpm. Unlike in orthostatic hypotension, BP and cardiac output are maintained through this increase in heart rate, yet the patient still develops symptoms of severe fatigue or near-syncope, possibly because of flow maldistribution and reduced cerebral flow.[2] While POTS, per se, does not induce syncope,[2] it may be associated with a vasovagal form of syncope that occurs beyond the first 10 minutes of orthostasis in up to 38% of these patients.[15] In a less common, hyperadrenergic form of POTS, there is no autonomic failure but the sympathetic system gets overly activated, with orthostasis leading to this excessive tachycardia.[10,16]

III. Cardiac syncope

Accounting for ~10-20% of cases of syncope, a cardiac etiology is the main concern in patients presenting with syncope, and **the main predictor of mortality and sudden death**.[1,2,8,17,18] Syncope often occurs suddenly without any warning signs (sudden syncope is also called *malignant syncope*). As opposed to neurally mediated syncope, the post-recovery period is not usually marked by lingering malaise.

There are three forms of cardiac syncope:

1. Structural heart disease with cardiac obstruction: AS, HOCM, severe pulmonary arterial hypertension. Peripheral vasodilatation occurs *during* exercise, but CO cannot increase because of the fixed or dynamic obstruction to the ventricular outflow. Since BP = CO × peripheral vascular resistance, BP drops with the reduction in vascular resistance. Exertional ventricular arrhythmias may also occur in these patients. Syncope may also occur *after* exercise.

2. Ventricular tachycardia (VT) secondary to:

i. Underlying structural heart disease, with or without reduced LVEF, such as coronary arterial disease, hypertrophic cardiomyopathy, hypertensive cardiomyopathy, or valvular disease.

ii. Primary electrical disease (long QT syndrome, Wolff–Parkinson–White syndrome, Brugada syndrome, arrhythmogenic right ventricular dysplasia, sarcoidosis).

Occasionally, *fast supraventricular tachycardia* causes syncope at its onset, before vascular compensation develops. This occurs in patients with underlying heart disease.[2,10,11]

3. Bradyarrhythmias, with or without underlying structural heart disease. Bradyarrhythmias are most often related to degeneration of the conduction system or to medications, rather than cardiomyopathies.

MI/ischemia causes syncope only when complicated by arrhythmias or by a shock.

> When a patient with a history of heart failure presents with syncope, VT and bradyarrhythmias are top considerations. Nevertheless, about half of cases of syncope in patients with cardiac disease have a non-cardiac cause,[17] including the hypotensive or bradycardic side effect of drugs.

IV. Other causes of syncope

Acute medical or cardiovascular illnesses may cause syncope and are sought in the appropriate clinical context: (1) severe hypovolemia or gastrointestinal bleed; (2) large pulmonary embolus with hemodynamic compromise; (3) tamponade; (4) aortic dissection; (5) hypoglycemia.

Bilateral critical carotid disease or severe vertebrobasilar disease very rarely causes syncope, and, when it does, it is associated with focal neurologic deficits.[2] Vertebrobasilar disease may cause "drop attacks," i.e., a loss of muscular tone with fall but without loss of consciousness.[19]

Severe proximal subclavian disease leads to reversal of the flow in the ipsilateral vertebral artery as blood is shunted toward the upper extremity. It manifests as dizziness and syncope during the ipsilateral upper extremity activity, usually with focal neurological signs (subclavian steal syndrome).[2]

Psychogenic pseudosyncope is characterized by a high frequency of attacks that typically last longer than a true syncope and occur multiple times per day or week, sometimes with a loss of motor tone.[2] It occurs in patients with anxiety or somatization disorders.

Note

Reflex syncope is the most frequent *etiology* of syncope. However, long asystolic pauses due to sinus or AV nodal block are the most frequent *mechanism* of unexplained syncope and are seen in >50% of syncope cases on prolonged rhythm monitoring.[1,20] These pauses may be related to intrinsic sinus or AV nodal disease or, more commonly, to extrinsic effects, such as the vasovagal mechanism. Some experts favor classifying and treating syncope based on the mechanism rather than the etiology, but this is not universally accepted.[1,21]

V. Syncope mimic: seizure (see Table 26.1)

Table 26.1 Features that suggest seizure rather than syncope.

- Unconsciousness often lasts longer than 5 minutes
- Postictal confusion or paralysis
- Prolonged tonic–clonic movements. Clonic movements may be seen with any prolonged syncope (>30 sec), in a more limited and brief form (<15 seconds), without the tonic arching of the back
- Tongue biting strongly suggests seizure

Urinary incontinence is not helpful, as it frequently occurs with syncope as well as seizure

VI. Clinical clues (see Table 26.2)

Table 26.2 Clinical clues to the diagnosis of syncope.[2–5,8]

Position during syncope
- Supine → reflex syncope is unlikely
- Sitting or standing position → any cause is possible
- Within a few minutes of sitting or standing → orthostatic hypotension
- Prolonged sitting or standing → vasovagal

Situation during syncope
- Exertion (strenuous activity, not just walking) → cardiac syncope (cardiac obstacle, ventricular arrhythmias)
- Post-exertion → vasovagal
- Postprandial → orthostatic hypotension
- Sudden fear, pain, unpleasant sight, hot environment → vasovagal
- Strain situation (micturition) → reflex syncope
- Head turning, shaving, tight collar → carotid sinus syndrome

Prodromes (abdominal discomfort, malaise, palpitations, nausea, blurry vision)
- Yes and >5 seconds → reflex syncope
- No or <5 seconds → cardiac syncope. *However, reflex or orthostatic syncope may be associated with prodromes <5 seconds or no prodrome in 33–50% of patients, more so in the elderly*

How consciousness is regained after syncope
- Promptly → cardiac syncope
- Prolonged fatigue or nausea after syncope → reflex syncope
- Confusion → seizure

Color during syncope
- Pale, diaphoresis → reflex syncope, orthostatic syncope
- Blue → arrhythmia, seizure

Duration
- >5 minutes → seizure, hypoglycemia; not syncope (except occasionally aortic stenosis)

Underlying heart disease, chest pain → cardiac syncope

Multiple neuropsychiatric or blood pressure medications → orthostatic syncope (cardiac syncope possible)

The presence or the lack of injury does not help differentiate cardiac from reflex syncope

Multiple syncopal recurrences (≥3) suggest a reflex or orthostatic syncope (one is less likely to survive three spells of cardiac syncope). This is particularly true if the interval between spells is >4 years[8]

VII. Diagnostic evaluation of syncope (Figure 26.1)

Underlying structural heart disease is the most important predictor of ventricular arrhythmias and death.[18,22–24] Thus, the primary goal of syncope evaluation is to rule out structural heart disease by history, examination, ECG, and echocardiography.

A. Basic initial strategy

The etiology of syncope is determined by history and physical examination alone in up to 50% of cases, mainly vasovagal syncope, orthostatic syncope, or seizure.[2,3,17] Always check blood pressure both lying and standing and in both arms, and obtain an ECG. Perform carotid massage in all patients older than 50 years if syncope is not clearly vasovagal or orthostatic and if cardiac syncope is not likely. Carotid massage is contraindicated if the patient has a carotid bruit or any history of stroke.

ECG establishes or suggests a diagnosis in 10% of patients (Table 26.3).[2,8,17,25] A normal ECG, or mild non-specific ST–T abnormality, suggests a low likelihood of cardiac syncope and is associated with an excellent prognosis. Abnormal ECG findings are seen in 90% of cases of cardiac syncope and only 6% of cases of neurally mediated syncope.[26] In one study of syncope patients with a normal ECG and a negative cardiac history, none had an abnormal echocardiogram.[27]

B. If the heart is normal clinically and by ECG

If the history suggests neurally mediated syncope or orthostatic hypotension, and the history, examination, and ECG are not suggestive of CAD or any other cardiac disease, the workup is stopped.

C. If the patient has signs or symptoms of heart disease

If the patient has signs or symptoms of heart disease (angina, dyspnea, clinical signs of HF, murmur), a history of heart disease, or exertional, supine, or malignant features, *heart disease should be sought* and the following performed:

- *Echocardiography* to assess LV function, severe valvular disease, and LV hypertrophy.
- *Stress test* (possibly) in case of exertional syncope or associated angina. However, the overall yield of stress testing in syncope is low (<5%).[28]

D. If no heart disease is suggested by ECG and echocardiography

Often, the workup may be stopped and syncope considered neurally mediated. ***The likelihood of cardiac syncope is very low in patients with normal ECG and echocardiography, and several studies have shown that patients with syncope who have no structural heart disease have a normal long-term survival.***[18,24,29] The following workup may, however, be ordered if the presentation is atypical and syncope is (i) malignant, (ii) recurrent, (iii) associated with physical injury, or (iv) occuring in a supine position:[17]

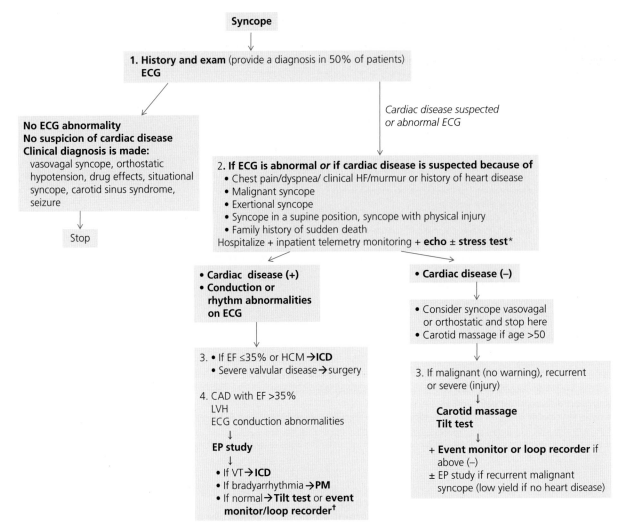

Figure 26.1 Management of syncope.

*Also, consider severe hypovolemia, bleeding, pulmonary embolism, and tamponade and rule them out clinically. Carotid Doppler and head CT scan are not indicated, especially given that carotid stenoses, per se, very rarely lead to syncope.

†EP study may have missed bradyarrhythmias and some forms of VT.

CAD, coronary arterial disease; EF, ejection fraction; EP, electrophysiological; LVH, left ventricular hypertrophy; HCM, hypertrophic cardiomyopathy; ICD, implantable cardioverter defibrillator; PM, pacemaker.

Table 26.3 ECG or Holter findings suggestive of cardiac syncope.

1. **Bradyarrhythmia-related syncope is *established* with any of the following:**
   - Sinus bradycardia <40 bpm or sinus pauses >3 s while awake
   - Mobitz II, high-grade, or complete AV block
   - Alternating LBBB or RBBB (on the same ECG or on ECGs obtained on separate occasions)
2. **Bradyarrythmia-related syncope is *suggested* with:**
   - Isolated RBBB or LBBB (VT also possible, depending on the underlying cardiac disease)
   - Mobitz I AV block
3. **Tachyarrhthmia-related syncope is *established* with:**
   - Sustained VT or fast SVT (>160 bpm)
4. **Underlying heart disease and VT is *suggested* with:**
   - Q waves
   - AF
   - LBBB, RBBB, QRS >0.11 s
   - LVH, RVH, large R wave in V1
5. **Primary electrical disorders are *suggested* with:**
   - Long QTc, pre-excitation, RBBB with Brugada pattern, or T-wave inversion in V_1–V_3 or epsilon waves (ARVD)
6. **Acute ST–T abnormalities**

- *Carotid sinus massage* in patients >50 years old, if not already performed. Up to 50% of these patients with unexplained syncope have CSH.[11]
- *24-hour Holter monitoring.* A significant arrhythmia is rarely detected; on the other hand, syncope or dizziness may occur without any arrhythmia, ruling out arrhythmia as a cause of the symptoms.[30] The diagnostic yield of Holter monitoring is low (1–2%) in patients with infrequent symptoms,[1,2] and is not improved with 72-hour monitoring.[30] The yield is higher in patients with very frequent, daily symptoms, many of whom have psychogenic pseudosyncope.[2]
- *Tilt table testing* to diagnose vasovagal syncope. It is positive for a vasovagal response in up to 66% of patients with unexplained syncope.[1,17] Patients with heart disease taking vasodilators or β-blockers may have abnormal baroreflexes; therefore, a positive tilt test is not necessarily indicative of vasovagal syncope in patients with heart disease (tilt testing is less specific in these patients).
- If the etiology remains unclear or there are some concerns about arrhythmia, an *event monitor* (4 weeks of external rhythm monitoring) or an *implantable loop recorder* (implanted subcutaneously in the prepectoral area for 1–2 years) is placed. Those monitors record the rhythm when the rate is lower or higher than predefined cutoffs or when the rhythm is irregular, regardless of symptoms. The patient or an observer may also activate the event monitor during or after an event, which freezes the recording of the 2–5 minutes preceding the activation and the 1 minute following it.

  In a patient who has had syncope, a pacemaker is indicated for episodes of high-grade AV block, pauses >3 seconds, or bradycardia <40 bpm while awake, and an ICD is indicated for sustained VT, even if syncope does not occur concomitantly with these findings. The finding of non-sustained VT on monitoring increases the suspicion of VT as a cause of syncope, but does not prove it or dictate an ICD, per se.
- Electrophysiologic (EP) study has a low yield in patients with normal ECG and echocardiography (bradycardia indices are detected in 10%).[30]

Carotid Doppler and head CT are not indicated, especially because carotid stenoses, per se, almost never lead to syncope. Head CT is performed whenever a seizure is suggested clinically.

E. If heart disease is diagnosed by echocardiography or if significant ECG abnormalities are found
Perform the following:

1. *Pacemaker placement for these ECG abnormalities*:[1,2,17]
   - Second-degree Mobitz II or third-degree AV block
   - Sinus pause >3 seconds or bradycardia <40 bpm while awake
   - Alternating left bundle branch block (LBBB) and right bundle branch block (RBBB) on the same ECG or separate ECGs
2. *Inpatient telemetry monitoring*
3. *Electrophysiologic (EP) study* is mainly valuable for patients with structural heart disease, including EF 36–49%, CAD, AF, or LV hypertrophy with normal EF.[25] Overall, in patients with structural heart disease and unexplained syncope, the yield is 55% (inducible VT in 21%, abnormal indices of bradycardia in 34%).[30]
   Limitations. The yield of EP study is low in bradyarrhythmias and in patients with EF ≤35%.[31] In the latter case, the syncope is often arrhythmia-related and the patient often has an indication for an ICD regardless of EP study results, especially if the low EF has been persistent despite medical therapy.[25]
4. If the above tests are negative, the differential diagnosis still includes arrhythmia, as the yield of EP study is low for bradyarrhythmias and some VTs, but also, at this point, neurally mediated syncope. The next step may be *prolonged rhythm monitoring or tilt table testing*. An *event monitor* or an *implantable loop recorder* may be placed for prolonged monitoring. The yield of the 30-day event monitor is highest in patients with frequently recurring syncope, where it reaches a yield of up to 40% (10–20% will have a positive diagnosis of arrhythmia, while 15–20% will have symptoms with a normal rhythm).[30,32] The implantable recorder has a high diagnostic yield overall, and is used in patients with infrequent syncopal episodes (yield up to 50%).[1,33,34]

In brief, there are *two diagnostic approaches to unexplained syncope:* the monitoring approach (loop recorder) and the testing approach (tilt table testing). A combination of both strategies is frequently required in patients with unexplained syncope, and, according to some investigators, a loop recorder may be implanted early on.[20]

F. In patients with LV dysfunction and EF ≤ 35%, an ICD may be placed without the need for an EP study
ICD is needed anyway in these patients for the prevention of sudden death even if the cause of syncope is not an arrhythmia. Patients with a low EF and a history of syncope are at a high risk of sudden cardiac death.[25] Yet, in some patients with newly diagnosed cardiomyopathy, LV function may improve with medical therapy (myocarditis, hypertensive cardiomyopathy); the arrhythmic risk being essentially high during the period of ventricular dysfunction, a wearable external defibrillator may be placed while the decision about ICD is finalized within the ensuing months.

In patients with hypertrophic cardiomyopathy, place ICD after any unexplained syncopal episode.

Valvular heart disease needs surgical correction.

If ischemic heart disease is suspected, coronary angiography is performed, with revascularization if appropriate. An ICD should be placed anyway if EF is ≤35%. Except in a large acute myocardial infarction, the substrate for VT is not ameliorated with revascularization.[25,35] Consider EP study when syncope occurs with CAD and a higher EF.

G. Note on LBBB and RBBB

Patients with RBBB or LBBB and unexplained syncope (not clearly vasovagal or orthostatic) likely have syncope related to intermittent high-grade AV block.[36] One study monitored these patients with an implanted loop recorder and showed that ~40% of them had recurrence of syncope within 48 days, often concordantly to complete AV block; ~55% of these patients had major events (syncope or high-grade AV block).[37] Many of the patients had a positive tilt test; thus, tilt testing is not specific for vasovagal syncope in these patients and should not be used to exclude a bradyarrhythmic syncope. Also, patients selected for this study had undergone carotid sinus massage and EP study with a negative result. In another analysis, EP study detected a proportion of the bradyarrhythmias, but more importantly, induced VT in 14% of patients with RBBB or LBBB; while not sensitive enough for bradyarrhythmia, EP study was highly specific and fairly sensitive for the emergence of VT upon follow-up.[36] Thus, unexplained syncope in a patient with RBBB or LBBB may warrant carotid sinus massage, then EP study to rule out VT, followed by placement of a dual-chamber pacemaker if the EP study is negative for VT, or at least placement of a loop recorder.

VIII. Tilt table testing (see Table 26.4)[10,38]

Tilt testing consists of strapping the patient to a table that is subsequently inclined to 60–80° for 30–45 minutes. It is a form of orthostatic stress that simulates prolonged standing and is actually more stressful than standing, as the patient is deprived of the skeletal muscle pumping that normally occurs with standing. The patient may be further stressed by infusing isoproterenol or administering sublingual nitroglycerin, which increases the likelihood of syncope during testing.

The specificity of tilt table testing for vasovagal syncope is up to 90% and the false positive rate is ~10% (the specificity is reduced with pharmacological facilitation). The sensitivity is ~80%, and it is positive in up to 66% of patients with unexplained syncope.[10,39] The false-positive rate is higher in patients with structural heart disease, LBBB, or RBBB; in fact, tilt table testing of patients with arrhythmic syncope and abnormal EP study elicits syncope in up to 25% of these patients. The yield of tilt testing is highest in patients with an intermediate pre-test probability of vasovagal syncope, such as *patients without structural heart disease who have an unexplained malignant or recurrent syncope, elderly patients with unexplained syncope or fall, or patients with structural heart disease (e.g., treated CAD, LV hypertrophy) but normal or only mildly reduced EF, no significant valvular disease, and normal EP study*. Patients with a high or low pre-test probability of vasovagal syncope have the lowest yield from tilt testing.

IX. Indications for hospitalization

Patients should be hospitalized if they have severe hypovolemia or bleeding, or if there is any suspicion of heart disease by history, examination, or electrocardiography, including:

- History of HF, low EF, or CAD
- ECG suggestive of arrhythmias (Table 26.3)
- Family history of sudden death
- Lack of prodromes, physical injury, exertional syncope, syncope in a supine position, or syncope associated with dyspnea or chest pain.[2,40]

In these situations, there is concern about arrhythmia, structural heart disease, or acute myocardial ischemia. The patient is admitted for *immediate telemetry monitoring*; *echocardiography* and sometimes stress testing are performed. Then the patient is discharged if this initial workup does not suggest underlying heart disease. Alternatively, EP study is performed or a device is placed in patients found to have structural heart disease. Prolonged rhythm monitoring or tilt table testing may be performed when syncope with underlying heart disease or worrisome features remains unexplained.

Several web-based interactive algorithms have been used to determine the indication for hospitalization. They incorporate the above clinical and ECG features and, sometimes, echocardiographic features.[2,22,23,40–42]

> Among high-risk patients, the risk of sudden death, a major cardiovascular event, or significant arrhythmia is high in the first few days after the index syncopal episode, justifying the hospitalization and inpatient rhythm monitoring and workup in the presence of the above criteria.[22,40,42]

Table 26.4 Types of response to tilt table testing.

1. **Vasodepressor syncope:** abrupt, rapid hypotension without a significant drop in heart rate (<10%)
2. **Cardioinhibitory syncope:** hypotension with a drop in heart rate to <40 bpm or a pause >3 seconds. A mixed response is characterized by a significant drop in heart rate that remains, however, >40 bpm without a prolonged pause. In all forms of vasovagal syncope, except some cardioinhibitory forms, BP falls before the rate falls. BP falls suddenly
3. **Orthostatic hypotension:** hypotension within 10 minutes of tilt, without bradycardia (usually a slight increase in heart rate is seen). The drop in blood pressure is more gradual in orthostatic hypotension than in vasovagal syncope
4. **POTS:** significant increase in heart rate during the first 10 minutes of tilt (an increase of >30 bpm or an absolute rate >120 bpm). Significant hypotension does not occur (blood pressure is normal or low normal)
5. **Cerebral syncope:** no significant hemodynamic change, but intense cerebral vasoconstriction on transcranial Doppler
6. **Psychogenic syncope:** syncope without hemodynamic or transcranial Doppler change

To be considered positive for vasovagal syncope, hypotension (with or without bradycardia) needs to occur *along with reproduction of syncope or near-syncope*. A hemodynamic effect without symptoms is not considered an abnormal tilt test result.

X. Treatment of neurally mediated syncope

A. Treatment of vasovagal syncope
Vasovagal therapy consists of the following:

- Maintain euvolemia and good fluid intake at all times. Patients with premonitory symptoms should sit or lie down at the onset of symptoms. Crossing the legs or isometric handgrip at the onset of symptoms often abort the episode.
- Compression stockings (30 mmHg). Since venous blood pools in the pelvic veins, these stockings should be waist-high.
- Tilt training. Tilt training consists of two 30-minute sessions of upright standing against a vertical wall every day. Also, head-up, semi-recumbent tilt sleeping may help.
- Non-pharmacological measures are the key therapy. If syncope recurs despite these interventions, consider:
  - Midodrine (α-agonist) or fludrocortisone (mineralocorticoid).
  - While β-blockers have been used, one randomized trial has shown that β-blocker therapy is not more effective than placebo.[43]
  - Intracerebral serotonin appears to facilitate the sympathetic withdrawal that eventually leads to vasovagal syncope. Selective serotonin reuptake inhibitors have reduced the occurrence of vasovagal syncope in several studies (one randomized trial with paroxetine).[44]
- Role of pacing. In the ISSUE-3 trial, patients with vasovagal syncope and ≥3 recurrences underwent loop recorder implantation. About one-third of these patients had a recurrence of syncope during recording, with asystole (≥3 seconds) in half of them. In this subgroup with cardioinhibitory recurrence, pacemaker therapy reduced the 2-year recurrence from 57% to 25%.[21] This study supports the paradigm of treating syncope based on the mechanism rather than the etiology (according to these investigators, asystole secondary to a vasovagal mechanism is treated similarly to asystole secondary to sinus node disease). Other studies have shown that pacemaker therapy is highly effective when asystole is documented at the time of syncope, regardless of the etiology.[20] Thus, pacing *may be* considered in recurrent vasovagal syncope with asystolic mechanism.

B. Carotid sinus hypersensitivity
Carotid sinus syndrome, which is a syncope clearly occurring in a circumstance wherein the carotid sinus is manipulated, along with a cardioinhibitory response to carotid sinus massage, is an indication for dual-chamber pacing.

Unexplained syncope with a cardioinhibitory carotid sinus hypersensitivity is a class IIa indication for dual-chamber pacing.

C. Orthostatic hypotension and POTS
Therapy consists of the following:

- Treat hypovolemia and maintain good fluid and salt intake. Treat hypokalemia. Rule out adrenal insufficiency.
- Arise slowly in stages, avoid activities after eating.
- May need to withhold diuretics and other antihypertensives. In elderly patients with orthostatic hypotension and supine HTN, antihypertensive drugs are initiated slowly, diuretics are avoided, and some degree of supine HTN may be accepted (e.g., 150 mmHg). Sleeping in an upright position may attenuate nocturnal HTN (as BP drops in the upright position) and decrease renal perfusion, thereby activating the renin–angiotensin system and increasing the extracellular volume.
- Waist-high compression stockings may help.
- If the above fails, fludrocortisone is the medication of first choice, but it may worsen supine HTN or promote HF and edema. Other options: midodrine (may worsen supine HTN), cholinesterase inhibitor (pyridostigmine).

D. Syncope and driving
In survivors of VT/VF, the highest risk of arrhythmic events and syncope recurrence is in the first 6–12 months.[45] Thus, patients with cardiac syncope or possible cardiac syncope should refrain from driving for at least 6 months, even if ICD is implanted.

In general, the risk of recurrence after a vasovagal syncope is ~10–30%, being highest in patients with multiple prior recurrences.[6] A study showed that the most common cause of syncope while driving is vasovagal syncope. In all patients, the risk of another syncope was relatively higher in the first 6 months after the event, with a 12% recurrence rate during this period. However, ~50% of all recurrences occurred >6 months later, with a 12% recurrence rate between 6 months and 4–5 years.[6] Despite this recurrence risk that persists for several years, the recurrence during driving was unusual in appropriately diagnosed and treated patients (up to 7% per 8 years), and, importantly, patients who had syncope while driving and no underlying structural heart disease had the same long-term survival as the general population. Long drives increase the risk of recurrence by increasing the peripheral venous pooling; also, recurrence of syncope is more likely and more dangerous for commercial drivers who spend a significant proportion of their time driving.

In general, patients with syncope should be prohibited from driving for at least a period of time (e.g., 6 months), during which the risk of recurrence is highest and serious cardiac disease or arrhythmia, if present, would emerge. The above study shows that it is relatively safe to resume driving beyond 6 months, particularly short drives with proper hydration, after appropriate evaluation for cardiac disease. Commercial driving may need to be permanently prohibited.

QUESTIONS AND ANSWERS

Question 1. A 62-year-old man presents with syncope while working in his yard (standing position). He did not have any prodrome and sustained a head bruise. He does not report any recent chest discomfort or dyspnea. He has a history of myocardial infarction 5 years previously, and he takes aspirin, metoprolol, lisinopril, thiazide diuretic, and atorvastatin. His electrocardiogram shows inferior Q waves, but no ischemic ST–T abnormalities and no conduction abnormality. His echocardiogram shows inferior hypokinesis with an overall LVEF of 45%. His troponin I level is normal. What is the next best step?
A. Coronary angiography
B. Admit for telemetry monitoring then discharge home next day if no arrhythmia is seen, with a diagnosis of vasovagal syncope

C. Place a 30-day event monitor
D. Place an implantable loop recorder
E. Tilt table testing
F. Admit for telemetry monitoring and perform an electrophysiologic (EP) study

Question 2. A 66-year-old man presents with syncope. It occurred while he was walking his dog. He has a facial laceration and does not recall any premonitory symptom. A similar episode occurred 8 months previously. He has no known cardiac history and takes a thiazide diuretic for hypertension. His exam is overall unremarkable and shows a blood pressure of 135/80 without any orthostatic hypotension. An ECG shows non-specific low T-wave voltage and an echocardiogram is normal. Telemetry monitoring for 24 hours did not reveal any significant arrhythmia. What is the next management step?
A. Reassurance, no further workup
B. Tilt table testing
C. Carotid sinus massage followed, if negative, by tilt table testing
D. 30-day event monitor
E. Stress testing
F. Electrophysiologic study

Question 3. A 30-year-old man who grew up in Mexico, and who has no prior medical problems, presents with syncope while playing basketball. He had very brief premonitory dizziness. He is admitted to the hospital. Telemetry monitoring does not show any arrhythmia. ECG and echo are normal. What is the next step?
A. Reassurance
B. Exercise stress test
C. Event monitoring
D. Tilt table testing

Question 4. The patient in Question 3 undergoes stress testing, which shows monomorphic VT at peak exercise, along with dyspnea and no syncope. This VT appears to be originating from the LV inferolateral wall. Coronary angiography shows normal coronary arteries. What is the next step?
A. Ablation for idiopathic LV VT
B. Cardiac MRI

Question 5. A 66-year-old woman has a history of permanent AF that is rate-controlled without any AV nodal blocking agent. She has a history of obesity and mild LVH. Her medications consist of warfarin and amlodipine. She had syncope upon standing up after eating a large meal. Another episode of near-syncope occurred while driving for 10 minutes, 3 months later. ECG shows AF, rate 55 bpm, LAFB, and incomplete RBBB. Telemetry monitoring shows AF pauses of up to 2.6 seconds during sleep. Echo shows normal LVEF with LVH. What is the next step?
A. Reassurance (vasovagal syncope)
B. Tilt table testing
C. Pacemaker placement
D. Carotid sinus massage, followed by EP study, followed by tilt table testing then implantable loop recording

Answer 1. F. An acute coronary event is not likely in the absence of cardiac complaints surrounding the syncope and in the absence of acute electrocardiographic or troponin abnormalities. Coronary angiography has a low yield in this context. While vasovagal syncope is possible (syncope in a hot environment, vasodilatory and diuretic medications), the first diagnosis to eliminate is cardiac syncope secondary to ventricular tachycardia from a myocardial scar, especially when the syncope is sudden and has an exertional trigger. An EP study is the next step in a patient with structural heart disease and EF >35%. If EP study does not induce a tachyarrhythmia or does not detect a conduction abnormality, it is reasonable to proceed with either tilt table testing (vasovagal syncope) or implantable loop recorder (arrhythmia undetected by EP study).

Answer 2. C. In light of the benign ECG and echocardiogram, it is unlikely that this patient has a cardiac or arrhythmic syncope. However, in light of the syncope recurrence, the abruptness (no premonitory symptom), and the physical injury, further workup is necessary to establish a definite cause and treat it. Carotid sinus massage is necessary in any unexplained syncope over the age of 50. If carotid massage is negative, and in the absence of structural heart disease, tilt table testing is an appropriate next step. Vasovagal syncope of the elderly is a likely diagnosis. An alternative strategy would be implanting a loop recorder for long-term rhythm monitoring. The yield of EP study is low when the ECG and echocardiogram are normal. The yield of a 30-day event monitor is low in patients with infrequent syncope recurrences. In the absence of angina, the yield of stress testing is low.

Answer 3. B. The syncope occurrence during exercise is suggestive of arrhythmia or heart disease. Even if ECG and echo are normal, stress testing is warranted.

Answer 4. B. The normal ECG and echo suggest that VT may be idiopathic, but the occurrence of syncope and the inferolateral origin make idiopathic VT less likely. In this case, cardiac MRI is performed. It shows a large inferolateral scar. In addition, the patient develops a complete RBBB on his ECG few months later. Cardiac sarcoidosis or Chagas disease is most likely in this patient.

Answer 5. D. The patient's syncope, especially the first episode, may be suggestive of vasovagal syncope. However, the conduction abnormality present on the ECG (AF with slow conduction), is suggestive of AV nodal disease. Also, LAFB and incomplete RBBB suggest the possibility of AV block. In this context, syncope is likely due to AV block, manifesting as a long AF pause. However, a pacemaker is not indicated as none of the findings, per se, is diagnostic of AV block and syncope could still be vasovagal. EP study should be performed, seeking a long HV interval or an infra-His block, or VT in a patient with underlying cardiac abnormality. This is followed by implanting a loop recorder, then a pacemaker if a long pause (>3 seconds) is documented during wakefulness. Tilt table testing may also be performed, even in a patient with structural heart disease, as long as EF is >35% and EP study has not suggested any arrhythmia (case where the likelihood of vasovagal syncope is not low).

References

1. Brignole M, Hamdan MH. New concepts in the assessment of syncope. J Am Coll Cardiol 2012; 50: 1583–91.
2. Moya A, Sutton R, Ammirati F, et al. Guidelines for the diagnosis and management of syncope (version 2009): the Task Force for the Diagnosis and Management of Syncope of the European Society of Cardiology (ESC). Eur Heart J 2009; 30: 2631–71.
3. Kapoor W. Syncope. N Engl J Med 2000; 343: 1856–62.
4. Graham LA, Kenny RA. Clinical characteristics of patients with vasovagal syncope presenting as unexplained syncope. Europace 2001; 3: 141–6.
5. Calkins H, Shyr Y, Frumin H, et al. The value of clinical history in the differentiation of syncope due to ventricular tachycardia, atrioventricular block and neurocardiogenic syncope. Am J Med 1995; 38: 365–73.
6. Sorajja D, Nesbitt GC, Hodge DO, et al. Syncope while driving: clinical characteristics, causes, and prognosis. Circulation 2009; 120: 928–34.
7. Kochiadakis GE, Papadimitriou EA, Marketou ME, et al. Autonomous nervous system changes in vasovagal syncope. Is there a difference between young and older patients Pacing Clin Electrophysiol 2004; 10: 1371–7.
8. Alboni P, Brignole M, Menozzi C, et al. Diagnostic value of history in patients with syncope with and without heart disease. J Am Coll Cardiol 2001; 37: 1921–8.
9. Brignole M, Alboni D, Benditt D, et al. Task force on syncope, European Society of Cardiology. Part 1. The initial evaluation of patients with syncope. Europace 2001; 3: 253–60.
10. Grubb BP. Neurocardiogenic syncope and related disorders of orthostatic intolerance. Circulation 2005; 111: 2997–3006.
11. Brignole M, Menozzi C, Gianfranchi L, et al. Carotid sinus massage, eyeball compression, and head-up tilt test in patients with syncope of uncertain origin and in healthy control subjects. Am Heart J 1991; 122: 1644–51.
12. Maggi R, Menozzi C, Brignole M, et al. Cardioinhibitory carotid sinus hypersensitivity predicts an asystolic mechanism of spontaneous neurally mediated syncope. Europace 2007; 9: 563–7.
13. Kenny RM, Richardson DA, Steen N, et al. Carotid sinus syndrome: a modifiable risk factor for nonaccidental falls in older adults (SAFE PACE). J Am Coll Cardiol 2001; 38: 1491–5.
14. Gibbons CH, Freeman R. Delayed orthostatic hypotension: a frequent cause of orthostatic intolerance. Neurology 2006; 67: 28–32.
15. Ojha A, McNeeley K, Heller E, et al. Orthostatic syndromes differ in syncope frequency. Am J Med 2010; 123: 245–9.
16. Kanjwal Y, Kosinski D, Grubb BP. The postural tachycardia syndrome: definitions, diagnosis and management. Pacing Clin Electrophysiol 2003; 26: 1747–57.
17. Brignole M, Alboni P, Benditt DG, et al.; European Society of Cardiology. Guidelines on management (diagnosis and treatment) of syncope. Eur Heart J 2001; 22: 1256–306.
18. Soteriades ES, Evans JC, Larson MG, et al. Incidence and prognosis of syncope. N Engl J Med 2002; 347: 878–85.
19. Kubak MJ, Millikan CH. Diagnosis, pathogenesis, and treatment of "drop attacks". Arch Neurol 1964; 11: 107–13.
20. Brignole M, Menozzi C, Bartoletti A, et al. Early application of an implantable loop recorder allows effective specific therapy in patients with recurrent suspected neurally mediated syncope. Eur Heart J 2006; 27: 1085–92.
21. Brignole M, Menozzi C, Moya A, et al. Pacemaker therapy in patients with neurally mediated syncope and documented asystole: Third International Study on Syncope of Uncertain Etiology (ISSUE-3): a randomized trial. Circulation 2012; 125: 2566–71.
22. Quinn J, McDermott D, Stiell I, Kohn M, Wells G. Prospective validation of the San Francisco Syncope Rule to predict patients with serious outcomes. Ann Emerg Med 2006; 47: 448–54.
23. Colivicchi F, Ammirati F, Melina D, et al.; OESIL (Osservatorio Epidemiologico sulla Sincope nel Lazio) Study Investigators. Development and prospective validation of a risk stratification system for patients with syncope in the emergency department: the OESIL risk score. Eur Heart J 2003; 24: 811–19.
24. Kapoor WN, Hanusa BH. Is syncope a risk factor for poor outcomes? Comparison of patients with and without syncope. Am J Med 1996; 100: 646–55.
25. Strickberger SA, Benson DW, Biaggioni I, et al. AHA/ACCF scientific statement on the evaluation of syncope. J Am Coll Cardiol 2006; 47: 473–84.
26. Sarasin FP, Louis-Simonet M, Carballo D, et al. Prospective evaluation of patients with syncope. Am J Med 2001; 111: 177–84
27. Sarasin FP, Junod AF, Carballo D, et al. Role of echocardiography in the evaluation of syncope: a prospective study. Heart 2002; 88: 363–7.
28. AlJaroudi WA, Alraies MC, Wazni O, Cerqueira MD, Jaber WA. Yield and diagnostic value of stress myocardial perfusion imaging in patients without known coronary artery disease presenting with syncope. Circ Cardiovasc Imaging 2013; 6: 384–91.
29. Ungar A, Del Rosso A, Giada F, et al. Early and late outcome of treated patients referred for syncope to emergency department. The EGSYS 2 follow-up study. Eur Heart J 31 2010: 2021–6.
30. Linzer M, Yang EH, Estes NA III, et al. Diagnosing syncope. 2. Unexplained syncope: Clinical Efficacy Assessment Project of the American College of Physicians. Ann Intern Med 1997; 127: 76–86.
31. Fujimara O, Yee R, Klein GJ, et al. The diagnostic sensitivity of electrophysiologic testing in patients with syncope caused by transient bradycardia. N Engl J Med 1989; 62: 1703–7.
32. Linzer M, Pritchett EL, Pontinen M, et al. Incremental diagnostic yield of loop electrocardiographic recorders in unexplained syncope. Am J Cardiol 1990; 66: 214–19.
33. Edvardsson N, Frykman V, van Mechelen R. Use of an implantable loop recorder to increase the diagnostic yield in unexplained syncope: results from the PICTURE registry. Europace 2011; 13: 262–9.
34. Brignole M, Sutton R, Menozzi C, et al. Early application of an implantable loop recorder allows a mechanism-based effective therapy in patients with recurrent suspected neurally mediated syncope. Eur Heart J 2006; 27: 1085–92.
35. Brugada J, Aguinaga L, Mont L, et al. Coronary artery revascularization in patients with sustained ventricular arrhythmias in the chronic phase of a myocardial infarction: effects on the electrophysiologic substrate and outcome. J Am Coll Cardiol 2001; 37: 529–33.

36. Moya A, Garcia-Civera R, Croci F, et al. Diagnosis, management, and outcomes of patients with syncope and bundle branch block. Eur Heart J 2011; 32: 1535–41.

37. Brignole M, Menozzi C, Moya A, et al. Mechanism of syncope in patients with bundle branch block and negative electrophysiological test. Circulation 2001; 104: 2045–53.

38. Brignole M, Menozzi C, Del Rosso A, et al. New classification of haemodynamics of vasovagal syncope: beyond the VASIS classification. Analysis of the presyncopal phase of the tilt test without and with nitroglycerin challenge. Europace 2000; 2: 66–76.

39. Grubb BP, Kosinski D. Tilt table testing: concepts and limitations. Pacing Clin Electrophysiol 1997; 20: 781–7.

40. Brignole M, Chen WK. Syncope management from emergency department to hospital. J Am Coll Cardiol 2008; 51: 284–7.

41. Daccarett M, Jetter TL, Wasmund SL, Brignole M, Hamdan MH. Syncope in emergency department: comparison of standardized admission criteria with clinical practice. Europace 2011; 13: 1632–8.

42. Costantino G, Perego F, Dipaola F, et al.; STePS Investigators. Short- and long-term prognosis of syncope, risk factors, and role of hospital admission results from the STePS (Short-Term Prognosis of Syncope) study. J Am Coll Cardiol 2008; 51: 276–83.

43. Sheldon R, Connolly S, Rose S, et al. Prevention of Syncope Trial (POST). A randomized, placebo-controlled study of metoprolol in the prevention of vasovagal syncope. Circulation 2006; 116: 1164–70.

44. Di Gerolamo E, Di Iorio C, Sabatini O, et al. Effects of paroxetine hydrochloride, a selective serotonin reuptake inhibitor, on refractory vasovagal syncope: a randomized, double-blind, placebo-controlled study. J Am Coll Cardiol 1999; 33: 1227–30.

45. Larsen GC, Stupey MR, Walance CG, et al. Recurrent cardiac events in survivors of ventricular fibrillation or tachycardia: implications for driving restrictions. JAMA 1994; 271: 1335–9.

27   Chest Pain, Dyspnea, Palpitations

1. CHEST PAIN

I. Causes (see Table 27.1)

Table 27.1 Causes of chest pain.

A. Cardiac
1. CAD: stable angina, ACS
2. Aortic dissection
3. Acute pericarditis
4. Secondary ischemia from cardiac causes: acute HF,[a] acute HTN, AS, HOCM
5. Secondary ischemia from non-cardiac causes: tachyarrhythmia, anemia

B. Pulmonary
1. Pneumothorax
2. Pneumonia
3. Exudative pleural effusion
4. Pulmonary embolism
5. Pulmonary hypertension (→ chest pain + dyspnea + syncope on exertion)

C. Gastrointestinal
1. Esophageal spasm or reflux
2. Esophageal ulceration after vomiting (Mallory–Weiss syndrome)
3. Peptic ulcer disease
4. Acute pancreatitis, cholecystitis, biliary colic

D. Chest wall
1. Strain of muscles or ligaments
2. Costochondritis ("Tietze's syndrome" is a costochondritis with swollen red costochondral joints)
3. Shoulder or cervical joint problem (pain is exacerbated by a particular movement of neck/shoulder rather than exertion)

E. Psychogenic

[a] The increase in LVEDP reduces the pressure gradient between aortic diastolic pressure and LVEDP, and thus reduces coronary flow even in the absence of CAD. Also, elevated LVEDP increases microvascular resistance.

Practical Cardiovascular Medicine, First Edition. Elias B. Hanna.
© 2017 John Wiley & Sons Ltd. Published 2017 by John Wiley & Sons Ltd.

Only 25% of patients presenting to the ED with chest pain have true unstable angina/ACS. However, ACS should be the first consideration and should always be ruled out. Approximately 5% of patients discharged home with a presumed non-cardiac chest pain are eventually diagnosed with MI or unstable angina.[1] Also, consider other emergencies like aortic dissection, PE, pericarditis, and gastrointestinal urgencies (pancreatitis, complicated peptic ulcer), and rule them out at least clinically and by chest X-ray and ECG.

II. Features

A. Angina and acute coronary syndrome

- Typical angina occurs with exertion and is relieved with rest. It is precipitated by walking uphill, in the cold, or after a meal. *Chest pain that occurs at rest* and is not reproduced with exertion is unlikely to be angina, the exception being vasospastic angina. *Postprandial angina* is often a marker of severe, sometimes multivessel CAD; as opposed to biliary colic or peptic ulcer disease, angina occurs immediately after the meal and is exacerbated by postprandial physical activity. *Nocturnal angina* may imply severe CAD or vasospasm on top of fixed CAD; the increased venous return in the recumbent position increases O_2 demands and triggers ischemia in patients with critical, sometimes multivessel, CAD.
- The duration of angina is typically a few minutes. If chest pain lasts over 20–30 minutes, the cardiac markers should be positive; otherwise, angina is an unlikely diagnosis. If chest pain lasts < 15 seconds, the pain is atypical (likely musculoskeletal).
- Severe distress or profuse diaphoresis could mean ACS or another serious illness (aortic dissection). Nausea and vomiting usually imply severe angina. Eructation could mean angina or gastroesophageal disease.
- *Dyspnea* may be an angina equivalent and may indicate extensive CAD with a secondary increase in ventricular stiffness and LVEDP. Always consider angina in the differential diagnosis of dyspnea. Indigestion, deep fatigue, or pain in the arms, neck, or jaw are other atypical presentations for which ACS should be considered.

- Atypical presentations are more common in the elderly, female, and diabetic patients.
- A positive response to nitroglycerin is defined as chest pain relief within less than 5 minutes of sublingual nitroglycerin. The relief of chest pain with sublingual nitroglycerin does not reliably predict ACS; similarly, the relief of chest pain with a GI cocktail does not predict the absence of ACS.
- S_4 is commonly heard during active angina. In a patient with angina, S_3 or MR murmur implies a high-risk ACS with LV dysfunction.
- ECG may be normal or non-diagnostic in 50% of ACS cases, and cardiac biomarkers may be negative in up to 30% of high-risk ACS cases. Ischemia related to circumflex distribution is notoriously silent, since the posterolateral wall is underrepresented on the 12-lead ECG. Also, some patients have baseline ECG abnormalities, such as LBBB, LVH, or a paced rhythm that affects ECG interpretation.

True angina and PE pain may seem reproducible with palpation, as the chest wall is frequently hypersensitive in these conditions. *A combination of multiple low-likelihood features* (**P**ositional pain, **P**leuritic stabbing pain, or **P**alpable localized pain), rather than reliance solely on pain reproducibility, better defines the low-likelihood group.[2]

B. Aortic dissection

Three clinical features point to the possibility of aortic dissection:[3]

- Predisposing condition: aortic valve disease, known aortic aneurysm, Marfan, or family history of aortic dissection.
- Suggestive symptoms: chest, back, or abdominal pain that is either very abrupt (within seconds), severe, or tearing. Note, however, that the pain of aortic dissection is commonly sharp rather than tearing.
- Suggestive exam findings: AI murmur (in 25–45%), pulse deficit or blood pressure differential between arms (~20%), neurologic deficit concomitant with chest pain (5%).

The presence of two or three features makes aortic dissection highly probable. The probability is intermediate when one feature is present; aortic imaging is warranted in the latter case if symptoms are not clearly explained by chest X-ray (CXR) or ECG. Up to 5% of aortic dissections have none of the features, but may be suspected by a widened mediastinum on CXR.

Aortic dissection should be suspected in any patient with chest pain and concomitant stroke, mental status changes, or peripheral ischemia.

In addition to the classic hypertension, hypotension may be seen with complicated aortic dissection (AI, tamponade). Hypotension may also be a pseudohypotension resulting from the obstruction of flow to one limb. Measuring blood pressure in all limbs may unveil this phenomenon.

C. Pulmonary embolism (PE)

1. Clinical features

- Dyspnea and tachypnea are the most common findings; however, they may not be seen at rest and may be purely exertional.
- Tachycardia is common and is occasionally an isolated finding. Frequently, however, tachycardia is either *transient* or *relative* (80–90 bpm).
- Chest pain is usually a pleuritic pain in patients with distal emboli; angina-like pain may be seen in patients with large central emboli and secondary RV ischemia. Hemoptysis is seen with pulmonary infarction, often resulting from small distal emboli.
- Hypotension, syncope, and RV failure with increased JVP/RV heave/right-sided S_3 are seen with a large PE and imply reduced hemodynamic reserve.
- Lower extremity edema or tenderness on palpation is seen in 50% of DVTs.

2. The clinical probability of PE is assessed using the Wells criteria, which essentially give weight to three features

- No alternative diagnosis for the patient's presentation, whether it is dyspnea, hypoxemia < 95%, chest pain, or tachycardia
- Clinical signs of DVT or hemoptysis
- Major risk factors for DVT/PE

The probability is high when two or three features are present, intermediate when only one feature is present, and low when none is present.

3. Initial workup

- Arterial blood gas: usually shows hypoxia, hypocapnia, and a high A–a gradient (>10 mmHg on ambient air, > 50 mmHg on high-dose O_2). O_2 saturation and A–a gradient are, however, normal in up to 20% of patients. A–a gradient increases in most pulmonary pathologies as a result of V/Q mismatch, and thus is not specific for PE. Hypercapnia is rare, and only a massive PE with a massive increase in dead space can cause hypercapnia, per se.
- Chest X-ray is grossly normal.
- ECG shows sinus tachycardia or relative tachycardia (80–100 bpm). In large PE, it shows more pronounced tachycardia and signs of RV strain in up to 85% of patients: T inversion in the anterior leads V_1–V_3, RVH/right axis deviation/RBBB, $S_1Q_3T_3$, and P pulmonale. Atrial arrhythmias may also be seen. *Look at the admission ECG, as tachycardia may be transient.*

D. Acute pericarditis

Pericarditis is characterized by pleuritic chest pain that increases with recumbency and movements, and improves with leaning forward. It typically radiates to the trapezius. It has a rapid onset.

- On exam, a pericardial friction rub with a systolic and a diastolic component is heard.
- ECG shows diffuse ST elevation and/or PR depression in 90% of patients. These changes may resolve after one to several days.
- CRP is highly sensitive for the diagnosis of acute pericarditis.
- **The diagnosis of pericarditis requires two of the following four features**:

    (1) chest pain; (2) rub; (3) typical ECG findings (widespread ST-segment elevation and/or PR depression); (4) pericardial effusion (which is only present in 40% of pericarditis cases and usually small). CRP is a confirmatory finding.

E. Pneumonia, pleural effusion, pneumothorax

Pleural and pulmonary illnesses are characterized by dyspnea, cough, and pleuritic chest pain, i.e., sharp pain that increases with deep inspiration, cough, or movement.

III. Management of chronic chest pain

See Chapter 3, Section II and Figures 3.1 and 3.2.

IV. Management of acute chest pain

A. ECG

If the ECG shows ST elevation consistent with STEMI, perform emergent reperfusion with primary PCI or fibrinolysis.

If the ECG shows ST depression or deep T inversion consistent with ischemia, especially if dynamic, consider the diagnosis of non-ST elevation ACS, but keep in mind the possibility of aortic dissection, PE, or pericarditis if clinically plausible.

B. CXR, cardiac biomarkers, ± bedside echo during active pain

In ACS, a bedside echo performed during active chest pain should reveal a wall motion abnormality. In fact, a normal echo *during active chest pain* strikingly reduces the likelihood of ACS. Echo is not sensitive if performed after pain resolution. Conversely, echo is not very specific for ongoing ischemia, as a wall motion abnormality may correspond to an old infarct.

C. If any clinical, X-ray, or ECG feature suggests aortic dissection, PE, pericarditis, or a pulmonary cause of chest pain, proceed to the appropriate workup and therapy. Avoid anticoagulation if the clinical or radiographic likelihood of aortic dissection is more than low. Before starting anticoagulation, verify the lack of mediastinal enlargement on CXR.

If aortic dissection is suggested, perform aortic CT or emergent TEE and start aggressive BP control and intravenous β-blockers.

If PE is suggested, perform chest CT angiography, PE protocol. The same CT and contrast injection are usually appropriate for the diagnosis of aortic dissection as well (but not vice versa). V/Q scan may be performed instead of CT in renal failure and in the absence of severe CXR abnormalities; CXR abnormalities decrease the specificity and the diagnostic yield of the V/Q scan. Anticoagulation is started early on, before the workup, if PE is probable and the bleeding risk is low.

If pericarditis is suggested, the diagnosis will be established by clinical, ECG, and CRP features.

If a pulmonary cause is suggested, the diagnosis will be established by CXR and chest CT if needed.

If cholecystitis or acute pancreatitis is suggested, the diagnosis will be established by a liver function panel, amylase/lipase, and abdominal ultrasound.

D. In the absence of aortic dissection, PE, pericarditis, or pulmonary features, consider the diagnosis of ACS regardless of the initial ECG and cardiac biomarkers, and obtain serial ECGs and cardiac biomarkers. Repeat the ECG during each recurrence of pain. Proceed to full ACS therapy and early coronary angiography within 24–72 hours of presentation, with revascularization if appropriate (CABG or PCI), in high-risk ACS, i.e., ACS with any of following features:

- Ischemic ST depression, transient ST elevation (< 20 minutes), or deeply inverted or biphasic T waves.
- Elevated troponin. Any troponin elevation (e.g., 0.05 ng/ml) in a patient with chest pain and no other obvious cardiac or systemic insult (HF, critical illness) implies a high-risk ACS.
- Recurrent true rest angina.
- Prior PCI in the last 6–12 months, or CABG.
- Hemodynamic or electrical instability.
- LV dysfunction, LV wall motion abnormalities.

PCI becomes emergent in the following cases: refractory true angina, ST elevation, hemodynamic instability or electrical instability (recurrent VT).

In the absence of high-risk features, perform stress testing or coronary CT angiography at 6–12 hours after a brief clinical, ECG, and troponin monitoring in a chest pain unit (troponin must be negative 3–6 hours after chest pain onset). Alternatively, low-risk or low-probability patients may be discharged home with plans for outpatient stress testing within 72 hours, as they have a low risk of coronary events in the short term.[4]

2. ACUTE DYSPNEA

I. Causes (see Table 27.2)

Table 27.2 Causes of acute dyspnea.

A. Cardiac
1. Acute pulmonary edema due to acutely decompensated HF, or to acute new-onset HF (acute MI, acute hypertension, acute valvular insufficiency, arrhythmia)
Diagnosis: history (orthopnea, paroxysmal nocturnal dyspnea, recent quick weight gain, and past cardiac history), exam ($\uparrow$ JVP, S_3, $\pm$ S_4, crackles, peripheral edema), elevated BNP, chest X-ray
2. Tamponade ($\uparrow$ JVP, pulsus paradoxus)
3. Always remember that dyspnea could be an angina equivalent
B. Pulmonary embolism
Diagnosed by the following three features: (i) PE/DVT risk factors; (ii) DVT signs; and (iii) absence of other causes of dyspnea (no gross abnormalities on chest X-ray)
C. Pulmonary
1. Pneumonia
2. Asthma attack or COPD exacerbation: asthma may occasionally lead to cough and/or dyspnea in the absence of wheezes on examination (variant or atypical asthma). Wheezing may be uncovered with maximal forced expiration. Also, severe asthma exacerbation may not produce wheezes (airways are so narrow that there is total interruption of airflow and decrease in breath sounds)
3. Pneumothorax or large pleural effusion
4. ARDS in the context of pneumonia, aspiration, septic shock, or trauma
D. Laryngeal causes (laryngospasm, laryngeal edema [anaphylaxis]) lead to an inspiratory stridor $\pm$ urticaria
E. Metabolic causes
Metabolic acidosis (such as diabetic ketoacidosis), hypocalcemia, dyskalemia, severe acute anemia, hyperthyroid storm.
+ Shock of any cause leads to hyperventilation and tachypnea

Beside HF, there are two additional causes of *nocturnal dyspnea*:[5]

- Patients with COPD may have mucus hypersecretion, so that, after a few hours of sleep, secretions accumulate and produce dyspnea and wheezing, which are relieved by cough and sputum expectoration.
- Patients with asthma may have their most severe bronchospasm between 2 a.m. and 4 a.m. and wake up with severe dyspnea and wheezing. Inhaled bronchodilators usually improve symptoms quickly.

In HF, paroxysmal nocturnal dyspnea (PND) usually develops 2–4 hours after sleep and improves after 15–30 minutes of sitting upright or walking. Dyspnea is often accompanied by cough (dry or productive of frothy sputum), wheezing, and diaphoresis.

Orthopnea is mainly seen in HF but may also be seen with pericardial diseases, advanced asthma/COPD with diaphragmatic flattening and weakness, bilateral diaphragmatic paralysis, severe obesity and severe ascites, all cases where the diaphragm tends be pushed up in a supine position.

Platypnea is dyspnea that worsens in the upright position. Platypnea is seen with pulmonary right-to-left shunts such as pulmonary AV fistulas (including hepatopulmonary syndrome), or the rare case of PFO that allows right-to-left shunting in the upright position.

Trepopnea is orthopnea that mainly occurs in one lateral decubitus position. Patients with HF are typically more comfortable in the right lateral decubitus position, as this position raises the level of the heart (especially the left ventricle), which slows venous return. This position may partly explain the predominance of right pleural effusion in HF.[6]

Note that nocturnal or exertional cough, rather than dyspnea, may be the primary complaint of patients with HF.

II. Notes

A. Differential diagnosis of shock + respiratory distress
- Cardiogenic shock with pulmonary edema
- Septic shock due to pneumonia or septic shock with ARDS
- Tamponade
- Massive PE
- Anaphylactic shock with bronchospasm, laryngeal edema
  + Any shock leads to tachypnea (the patient hyperventilates in order to improve O_2 supply)

B. Wheezing
Wheezing may indicate COPD/asthma but may also indicate pulmonary edema ("cardiac asthma"), PE, or pneumonia. In cardiac asthma, cyanosis and diaphoresis occur more often than in bronchial asthma, and adventitious breath sounds are more common (crackles, rhonchi). True asthma has more musical, pure wheezes.[5]

C. Pulmonary shunt and pulmonary shunt effect
Most of the disorders listed in Table 27.2, A–C, lead to a *pulmonary shunt effect* in which pulmonary blood is not oxygenated because of obstruction of the airways, or to a *true pulmonary shunt* in which the alveoli, per se, are obstructed and filled with fluid. A pulmonary shunt or shunt effect initially leads to hypocapnia, hypoxemia, or normoxemia (pO2 may be normal early on), and elevated A–a gradient. A–a gradient increases in most pulmonary pathologies; it implies V/Q mismatch but does not identify it (could be PE, pulmonary edema, COPD exacerbation, pneumonia, ARDS). The more severe the process, the higher the A–a gradient rises.

$$\text{A–a gradient} = \text{alveolar } PO_2 - \text{arterial } PO_2$$
$$= (FiO_2 \times [\text{atmospheric pressure} - 47] - PaCO_2/0.8) - PaO_2$$
$$= (\sim150 \text{ mmHg on ambient air, sea level} - PaCO_2/0.8) - PaO_2$$

Normal < 10–15 mmHg on ambient air, < 50–75 mmHg on high-flow O_2. A–a gradient normally increases by 5–7 mmHg with each 10% increase in FiO_2.

As the illness progresses, the patient gets tired and starts hypoventilating, which leads to a worsening of the hypoxemia and development of hypercapnia. Hypercapnia occurs sooner in pulmonary edema and COPD than in asthma and pneumonia, and is rare in PE. A patient with COPD may have chronic hypercapnia that worsens during exacerbations.

D. Cyanosis
Cyanosis corresponds to a deoxygenated Hb concentration of > 5 g/dl. There are two forms of cyanosis: (i) central cyanosis related to severe hypoxemia (respiratory issue or cardiac right-to-left shunt); (ii) peripheral cyanosis related to a shock state where arterial O_2 saturation is normal but peripheral tissue hypoxia occurs. There is tongue cyanosis in the former, not the latter.

Cyanosis manifests less easily in anemic patients.

Respiratory distress without gross abnormalities on CXR:
- PE
- Bronchospasm, COPD exacerbation
- Severe sepsis, shock states, or metabolic acidosis
- Acutely decompensated chronic HF, where CXR findings are frequently subtle (exam and BNP findings help with the diagnosis)
- Also, myocardial ischemia or systolic or diastolic LV dysfunction can increase the pulmonary capillary pressure and the pulmonary engorgement on exertion without leading to frank pulmonary edema.

III. Management
The hemodynamics and the volume status are quickly assessed clinically. The following is obtained: ECG (seeking ischemia and arrhythmias), CXR, arterial blood gas, basic lab tests including cardiac markers and BNP. BNP helps differentiate a cardiac from a pulmonary origin of dyspnea in the acute setting (BNP < 100 pg/ml makes left HF a very unlikely cause of acute dyspnea, while BNP over 500 pg/ml makes left HF a likely cause of dyspnea).

A. Quick and specific therapies are instituted
When pulmonary edema is suspected, furosemide (40–80 mg IV) and/or vasodilator therapy (e.g., IV nitroglycerin) is administered. The administration of furosemide may await CXR if the diagnosis is uncertain and the patient is stable. ACS should be considered and treated if the ECG or the clinical symptoms support it (ischemic ST abnormality, hyperacute new HF). Echocardiography is performed.

If pneumonia is suspected, broad-spectrum antibiotics are administered and blood and sputum cultures are obtained.

A hypoxia that is severe and out of proportion to lung findings on exam and CXR is suggestive of PE. When the probability of PE is intermediate or high, anticoagulation is initiated, then a CT PE protocol or a V/Q scan is performed.

Wheezes secondary to a true asthma are treated with continuous albuterol nebulization for 1 hour or more. Conversely, wheezes secondary to HF should not be aggressively treated with albuterol, as it worsens myocardial ischemia and tachyarrhythmias with no clear benefit.

B. Intubation and non-invasive ventilation

Consider intubation in the following cases:

1. Respiratory distress with a respiratory rate > 35/min, not improving quickly with furosemide, O_2, and nebulizer therapy regardless of O_2 saturation (the patient is getting more tired, breathing is getting more shallow with accessory muscle use and paradoxical respiration).
2. Hypoxemia not responding to maximal O_2 therapy (O_2 saturation < 88% despite the administration of 100% O_2 via a face mask).
3. Acute hypercapnia or worsening of chronic hypercapnia with pH < 7.25.
4. Any shock associated with respiratory distress.
5. Alteration of mental status.

In COPD and in acute pulmonary edema, while waiting for the initial measures to take effect, non-invasive ventilation may be tried (CPAP, BiPAP). Non-invasive ventilation is particularly helpful for:

- Decompensated COPD with ventilatory failure and hypercapnia, where non-invasive ventilation may reduce the need for intubation.[7]
- HF, where the positive thoracic pressure reduces the preload and the afterload. In HF, non-invasive ventilation with either CPAP or BiPAP improves dyspnea and oxygenation more quickly than standard therapy, without an effect on survival or a reduction in the need for intubation.[8]

Non-invasive ventilation is not useful in patients with ARDS, where severe hypoxemia rather than hypoventilation is the main issue.[9] Regardless of the underlying illness, if no improvement is seen within the first 30 minutes of non-invasive ventilation and initial measures, or if there are mental status changes, severe acidosis (pH < 7.2), or hemodynamic compromise, proceed with immediate intubation.

A prolonged ineffective use of CPAP or BiPAP may paradoxically increase *expiratory work,* gastric distension and aspiration, and may prolong hypoxemia and delay a salutary intubation. *All this leads to increased mortality in patients who are intubated after a prolonged and ineffective non-invasive ventilation.*[10,11]

3. PALPITATIONS

I. Causes
A. Benign premature beats: 20–30% of palpitations are secondary to PACs or PVCs.

B. Sustained cardiac arrhythmia, consisting of one of the following (10–20% of palpitations):[12–14]

1. *Benign arrhythmia* that is sustained and sometimes poorly tolerated: AVNRT/AVRT, atrial tachycardia, inappropriate sinus tachycardia.
2. *Serious but non-malignant arrhythmia*: AF, atrial flutter, pacemaker syndrome in patients with a single-lead VVI pacemaker.
3. *Malignant arrhythmia*: VT.

The serious and malignant arrhythmias typically occur in patients with underlying structural heart disease: LV systolic dysfunction, CAD, hypertensive cardiomyopathy, valvular disease, or hypertrophic cardiomyopathy.

Also, HF can lead to sinus tachycardia and palpitations on mild exertion, i.e., palpitations disproportionate to the degree of exertion. In severe aortic insufficiency, the augmented stroke volume may be felt as palpitation.

C. Psychiatric (anxiety, somatization): 30–40% of palpitations are attributed to psychosomatic disease. Note, however, that anxiety may be triggered by the arrhythmia. In fact, one study has shown that two-thirds of patients who were eventually diagnosed with SVT were falsely diagnosed with panic disorder early on.[15]

D. Metabolic/drugs (10% of palpitations): hyperthyroidism, anemia, obesity and deconditioning (may lead to disproportionate sinus tachycardia with mild activity), pheochromocytoma, and medications (decongestants, anticholinergic drugs, albuterol, acute vasodilator such as hydralazine, withdrawal of β-blockers or clonidine, drugs [caffeine, cocaine, alcohol withdrawal]).

II. Diagnosis
A. The diagnosis mainly relies on the history and examination (see Table 27.3)

B. Workup of palpitations (see Table 27.4)
In most patients with palpitations, the cause is benign and the history, physical exam, and basic workup suggest a cause and rule out malignant arrhythmias. **A normal or non-specific ECG and a normal echo almost exclude a malignant arrhythmia (VT secondary to myocardial disease) and make serious arrhythmias unlikely**. Brief or occasional palpitations with normal ECG, echo, and basic blood work are likely secondary to premature beats or anxiety and do not warrant any further workup.

When palpitations are **sustained or poorly tolerated**, a Holter or an event monitor may be used to diagnose paroxysmal AF or SVT. An event monitor provides a high yield for the diagnosis of palpitations when a sustained arrhythmia is suspected (up to 80% yield), much higher than the diagnostic yield of a Holter monitor (~30% yield).[13,16] This is true when the palpitations are frequent, more than once

Table 27.3 Diagnostic features of palpitations (duration, onset/offset, regularity, relation to exertion).

a. Palpitations lasting a second; "flip-flopping" in the chest or skipped beats lasting an instant → premature beats (PACs/PVCs)
b. Sustained, fast palpitations → sustained arrhythmia (SVT, AF, VT), hyperthyroidism, anemia. Ask if regular or irregular
c. Abrupt onset/offset → sustained arrhythmia
d. *Poorly tolerated palpitations* → sustained arrhythmia (SVT, AF, VT)
   Syncope → VT
e. Pounding in the neck means that the atria and ventricles contract at the same time → VT or SVT with short RP interval (AVNRT)
f. Palpitations initiated by exertion with persistence after exercise cessation → CAD, any arrhythmia (benign or serious)
g. Palpitations on mild exertion disproportionate to the degree of exertion → HF, anemia, hyperthyroidism, AF, obesity or severe deconditioning
h. Palpitations on standing → postural hypotension
i. Palpitations accompanied by a regular and normal heart rate → anxiety

Context
History of CAD or severe heart disease; murmur or gallop on exam → arrhythmia

Table 27.4 Workup of palpitations.

Basic workup
1. ECG: look for signs of underlying heart disease, suggesting the possibility of arrhythmias:
   - Q wave, ischemic ST–T abnormalities
   - LVH, bundle branch blocks
   - ↑ QT, WPW
2. TSH, blood count
3. Echo: look for structural heart disease (large LA, low EF, valvular disease, severe LVH)

Selective workup
1. Stress test is indicated for chest pain, exertional palpitations, or poorly tolerated palpitations (rule out an angina equivalent)
2. 24-hour Holter or 30-day event monitor is indicated if:
   - Underlying heart disease is evident on ECG or echo
   - No heart disease is evident, but the patient develops *sustained and poorly tolerated* palpitations suggestive of sustained arrhythmia (SVT, AF, or idiopathic VT occurring without any structural heart disease).
3. Electrophysiologic study may be performed in patients with *sustained and poorly tolerated palpitations* and a non-diagnostic Holter/event monitor
   - This is particularly indicated if, in addition, the poorly tolerated palpitations are associated with syncope, underlying heart disease, or a documented rapid pulse
   - May be used for ablation of the diagnosed arrhythmia (AVNRT, AVRT, atrial tachycardia, atrial flutter, idiopathic VT)

a month. An event monitor is also more cost-effective than a Holter monitor. In the assessment of palpitations, almost all events are detected in the first 2 weeks (mainly 1 week), making 4 weeks of monitoring unnecessary.[16] Syncope, on the other hand, may require more prolonged monitoring, including an implantable loop recorder for recurrent unexplained syncope.

References

1. Pope JH, Aufderheide TP, Ruthazer R, et al. Missed diagnosis of acute cardiac ischemia in the emergency department. N Engl J Med 2000; 342: 1163–70.
2. Lee TH, Cook F, Weisberg M, et al. Acute chest pain in the emergency room. Identification and examination of low-risk patients. Arch Intern Med 1985; 145: 65–9.
3. Rogers AM, Hermann LK, Booher AM, et al. Sensitivity of the aortic dissection detection risk score, a novel guideline-based tool for identification of acute aortic dissection at initial presentation. Circulation 2011; 123: 2213–18.
4. Koukkunen H, Pyorala K, Halinen MO. Low-risk patients with chest pain and without evidence of myocardial infarction may be safely discharged from emergency department. Eur Heart J 2004; 25: 329–35.
5. Ingram R, Braunwald E. Dyspnea and pulmonary edema. In: Harrison's Principles of Internal Medicine, 16th edn. Philadelphia, PA: McGraw-Hill, 2001, p. 203.
6. De Araujo BS, Reichert R, Eifer DA, et al. Trepopnea may explain right-sided pleural effusion in patients with decompensated heart failure. Am J Emerg Med 2012; 30: 925–31.
7. Brochard L, Mancebo J, Wysocki M. et al. Noninvasive ventilation for acute exacerbations of chronic obstructive pulmonary disease. N Engl J Med 1995; 333: 817–22.
8. Gray A, Goodacre S, Newby DE, et al. Noninvasive ventilation in acute cardiogenic pulmonary edema. N Engl J Med 2008; 359: 142–51.
9. Delclaux C, L'Her E, Alberti C, et al. Treatment of acute hypoxemic nonhypercapnic respiratory insufficiency with continuous positive airway pressure delivered by a face mask: a randomized controlled trial. JAMA 2000; 284: 2352–60.
10. Esteban A, Anzueto A, Frutos F, et al. Characteristics and outcomes in adult patients receiving mechanical ventilation: a 28-day international study. JAMA 2002; 287: 345–55.
11. Esteban A, Frutos-Vivar F, Ferguson ND, et al. Noninvasive positive-pressure ventilation for respiratory failure after extubation. N Engl J Med 2004; 350: 2452–60.

12. Zimetbaum P, Josephson ME. Evaluation of patients with palpitations. N Engl J Med 1998; 338: 1369–73.

13. Kinlay S, Leitch JW, Neil A, et al. Cardiac event recorders yield more diagnoses and are more cost-effective than 48-hour Holter monitoring in patients with palpitations: a controlled clinical trial. Ann Intern Med 1996; 124: 16–20.

14. Josephson ME, Goldberger AL. Utility of patient-activated cardiac event recorders in general clinical practice. Am J Cardiol 1997; 79: 371–2.

15. Lessmeier TJ, Gamperling D, Johnson-Liddon V, et al. Unrecognized paroxysmal supraventricular tachycardia. Potential for misdiagnosis as panic disorder. Arch Intern Med 1997; 157: 537–43.

16. Zimetbaum PJ, Kim KY, Josephson ME, et al. Diagnostic yield and optimal duration of continuous-loop event monitoring for the diagnosis of palpitations. Ann Intern Med 1998; 128: 890–5.

28 Infective Endocarditis and Cardiac Rhythm Device Infections

1. INFECTIVE ENDOCARDITIS

I. Clinical diagnosis

The diagnosis of infective endocarditis (IE) is based on the Duke criteria, which consist of two major and five minor criteria.[1]

In brief, the two major criteria are: (i) two positive blood cultures for a typical IE organism; (ii) echo finding of a vegetation or a new valvular regurgitation (worsening of a prior regurgitation or murmur is not enough).

The five minor criteria are: (i) fever; (ii) predisposing valvular condition or intravenous drug use; (iii) immunologic phenomenon, such as Osler nodes or glomerulopnephritis; (iv) vascular embolism, major (e.g., stroke, pulmonary embolism) or minor (e.g., Janeway lesions, conjunctival hemorrhage); (v) only one positive blood culture, or positive blood culture for an organism that is not a usual IE organism, or positive *Coxiella* titers. The diagnosis is made in the presence of two major criteria, or one major and three minor criteria, or all five minor criteria.

II. Echocardiography: timing and indications

When IE is suspected, TTE and TEE are often both required. TTE is the recommended initial imaging modality and may be sufficient in patients with a low clinical suspicion, good quality images, and negative valvular findings.[2]

TEE is recommended in patients with a high clinical suspicion of IE and normal TTE. In fact, the sensitivity of TTE for the diagnosis of TEE-confirmed endocarditis is ~55–60%, both for aortic and for mitral endocarditis.[3,4] TEE should also be performed in the majority of patients with positive TTE, in order to diagnose local abscess complications that will dictate urgent surgery. On both TTE and TEE, vegetations but also destructive valvular lesions and local infectious complications should be sought.

TEE may miss vegetations in 5–10% of patients, particularly in the following cases:[2,3] (1) very early stage; (2) very small vegetation <3 mm; (3) pre-existing, severe valvular lesion (myxomatous mitral valve, calcified AS, prosthetic valve). If the clinical suspicion remains high, TEE should be repeated 3–5 days after the initial examination (e.g., *S. aureus* bacteremia in a patient with prosthetic valve and negative initial TEE).[2,5] The diagnostic yield of a third examination is low.

Several abnormalities may mimic a vegetation:

a. Mitral valve abnormalities, such as myxomatous mitral leaflet thickening, prolapsed mitral cusp, or flail mitral chordae. In addition, a tumor may mimic a vegetation (e.g., papillary fibroelastoma which originates from the valve, or myxoma which originates from interatrial septum and extends towards the valve).

b. Aortic valve abnormalities, such as Lambl excrescence or prolapsed aortic cusp.

Also, a healed endocarditis may be hard to differentiate from active endocarditis. As compared to a recent vegetation, an old vegetation tends to be more echogenic or even calcified, but this cannot be reliably used to exclude acute IE.

Practical Cardiovascular Medicine, First Edition. Elias B. Hanna.
© 2017 John Wiley & Sons Ltd. Published 2017 by John Wiley & Sons Ltd.

For right-sided endocarditis, TTE and TEE may have a similar diagnostic yield.[6] However, TEE is superior for the assessment of vegetations on pacemaker leads or indwelling catheters, and thus is required in those cases. It is also required when concomitant left-sided involvement or abscess complications need to be addressed.

A particular diagnostic case is *Staphylococcus aureus* bacteremia. Regardless of whether the source of bacteremia is known (osteomyelitis, cellulitis, central catheter infection, pneumonia), ~25% of all patients with *S. aureus* bacteremia and 23% of those with central catheter infection as the primary focus have evidence of endocarditis by TEE, without clinical or transthoracic echocardiographic findings.[7] Contrary to a common misconception, IE most commonly involves the *left-sided valves*, in 65% of these patients. Thus, it seems warranted and cost-effective for all patients with *S. aureus* bacteremia to undergo TEE.[7,8] *S. aureus* is virulent and can even cause endocarditis of a normal native valve.

III. Organisms

The most common organisms responsible for IE are: streptococci (viridians streptococci and *Streptococcus bovis*: 40–60%), enterococci (5–15%), *S. aureus* (30–40%), HACEK organisms (5–10%), and coagulase-negative staphylococci (5%).[2] Streptococci and enterococci involve left-sided, abnormal valves and lead to subacute IE that progresses over weeks to months. *S. aureus* involves the right- or left-sided valves, and has a predilection to seed normal as well as abnormal valves; *S. aureus* IE is rapidly invasive and destructive and leads to acute IE that progresses over days to weeks. Coagulase-negative *Staphylococcus* infection of native valves may be seen in patients with a central line or intracardiac device and is often aggressive and complicated. Occasionally, *Coxiella* endocarditis may be seen in farmers.

Intravenous drug users are prone to *S. aureus* IE (~70%), which in this case more commonly involves the tricuspid valve (~60%) rather than the left-sided valves (~40%), many of which are previously normal valves. This is in contradistinction to patients with focal *S. aureus* infections, such as osteomyelitis or catheter infections, who tend to be older with intrinsic left valvular disease, in whom *S. aureus* more frequently seeds the abnormal, left-sided valves. IV drug users with abnormal left-sided valves may have streptococcal and enteroccoccal infection of these left-sided valves. *Pseudomonas aeruginosa* and fungi may also be seen in intravenous drug users.

Prosthetic valves may be infected early postoperatively (<60 days to 1 year) or late (>1 year). Early infections are usually surgical infections, predominantly caused by *Staphylococcus* coagulase-negative (~35%) and positive (~20%); enterococci and Gram-negative bacilli are second in frequency. Late infections are caused by the same organisms as native valve endocarditis: streptococci (viridians, *S. bovis*) are the most common, followed by staphylococci and enteroccoci. Coagulase-negative staphylococci may still be seen, especially with central line or device placement.

IV. Morphology

Vegetations are typically located on the upstream side of the valve, in the path of a regurgitant jet, but may be located anywhere on the components of the valvular or subvalvular apparatus, as well as the mural endocardium of the cardiac chambers (LA, LV) or ascending aorta. Large vegetations are almost always associated with significant valvular regurgitation or, less often, valvular stenosis. Regurgitation results from the bulk of the vegetation impeding valvular closure, from valvular perforation/tear, or from rupture of an infected chorda. In fact, a large mass without valvular regurgitation argues against vegetation (in this case, other cardiac masses should be considered). Smaller vegetations, on the other hand, may not be associated with any significant regurgitation in up to 25% of cases.[3]

V. Anatomical complications

Periannular extension is common, occurring in 10–40% of all native valve endocarditis, more commonly aortic endocarditis than mitral or tricuspid endocarditis. Periannular infection is even more common with prosthetic valve endocarditis, occurring in 56–100% of cases, and leading to prosthetic dehiscence and paraprosthetic regurgitation.[2] Perivalvular abscesses are common with prosthetic valves because the annulus, rather than the leaflet, is usually the primary site of infection.[2]

Aortic valve vegetation can extend to the aortic annulus and lead to aortic abscess. The infection tends to spread through the weakest annular structure, the membranous interatrial septum, which contains the AV node.[9] This explains why AV block is common with perivalvular abscess. This abscess may communicate with the aortic lumen and lead to pseudo-aneurysm formation. An abscess or pseudoaneurysm may rupture and communicate with the pericardium surrounding the base of the aorta (full-blown rupture or microperforation), leading to a hemorrhagic pericardial effusion. It may communicate with a cardiac chamber such as LV, leading to paravalvular AI; LA, leading to severe pulmonary edema; or RA or RV, leading to a massive left-to-right shunt and severe left ± right failure (Figures 28.1, 28.2). The annular abscess may lead to dehiscence of a prosthetic valve with perivalvular regurgitation. Therefore, worsening HF, persistent infection, new murmur, pericardial effusion, or new AV block in a patient with IE is a hint to abscess formation and warrants repeating TEE. AV block (including a new first-degree AV block or bundle branch block) has a high positive predictive value for abscess formation (88%) but low sensitivity (45%).[2,9]

A narrow fibrous space, called the mitral–aortic intervalvular fibrosa (or interannular fibrosa), separates the aortic root and mitral annulus. Aortic root abscess or mitral annular abscess may extend into this space and lead to pseudoaneurysm of this space, with subsequent seeding of the mitral valve from the aortic valve (or vice versa) and extension throughout the cardiac cytoskeleton (Figure 28.1).

Aortic root abscess manifests initially as aortic root wall thickening. If only slight thickening is visualized, TEE may need to be repeated a few days later, at which time a clear aortic free space, with or without fistulization on color Doppler, confirms the diagnosis.

VI. Indications for valvular surgery and special situations
A. Indications for valvular surgery in left-sided endocarditis

Valvular surgery is definitely indicated in the following cases (class I indications):[2,10]

1. Severe valvular regurgitation or obstruction with cardiogenic shock or refractory pulmonary edema (emergent), or with any degree of heart failure (urgent). Delaying surgery to allow extended antibiotic therapy carries the risk of permanent ventricular dysfunction and progressive cardiac deterioration and should be discouraged. In fact, even mild congestive heart failure at initial presentation may progress insidiously despite appropriate antibiotic therapy. Early mitral closure in acute AI, rapidly decelerating MR signal on spectral Doppler of MR

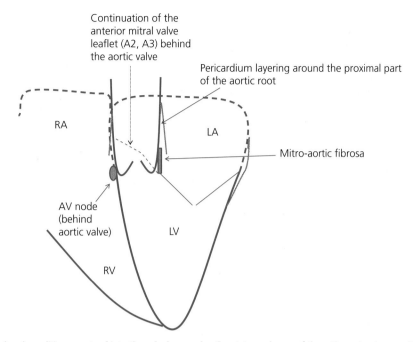

Figure 28.1 Aortic or mitral endocarditis can extend into the valvular annulus then into each one of these three structures: mitral–aortic interannular fibrosa, AV node, or pericardial space. Fistulization into a cardiac cavity (LA, LV, RA, RV) may also occur.

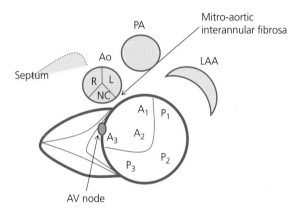

Figure 28.2 The AV node, and particularly the His bundle coming off the AV node, are anterior structures, located anterior to the ostium of the coronary sinus at the distal interatrial septum (triangle of Koch). Two-thirds of the circumference of the aortic valve is connected to the muscular ventricular septum, while the remaining one-third is in fibrous continuity with the anterior mitral leaflet (interannular fibrosa, close to the non-coronary cusp). At one point posteriorly, the aortic valve is in continuity with the His bundle and the interatrial septum.

(V-wave cutoff), or pulmonary hypertension are signs of poor hemodynamic tolerance of the valvular insufficiency that indicate the need for surgery. HF is the most frequent and serious complication of IE.

2. Local infectious complications (abscess, pseudoaneurysm, fistula) indicate urgent surgery. Delaying surgery carries the risk of abscess extension.

3. Refractory or relapsing bacteremia (>7 days) despite appropriate antibiotic therapy, often indicative of a local complication. This situation is more common with aggressive organisms, including *S. aureus*, and when vegetations are bulky and resistant to antibiotic penetration. It is also important to rule out local or distant abscesses.

4. Certain organisms:
- Left-sided *S. aureus* endocarditis is difficult to control, highly destructive, and is likely to require urgent surgery. It is, per se, an absolute indication for early surgery in prosthetic valve endocarditis and a relative indication for early surgery in native valve endocarditis, unless an immediate response is obtained with antibiotic therapy.
- Fungal endocarditis.

B. Case of a large vegetation >1 cm or prior embolization

Systemic embolization occurs in 20–40% of patients with IE and most frequently involves the brain (65% of the cases), then the spleen and kidneys; some emboli are asymptomatic and diagnosed by CT. The risk of embolization is dramatically reduced after 2–3 weeks of antibiotic therapy. Beside the timing, vegetation >10 mm in size, hypermobile vegetation, *S. aureus* or fungal infection, or IE of the anterior mitral leaflet are risk factors for embolization.[11] In fact, the risk of embolization of aortic IE (10%) is lower than that of mitral IE (25%) or anterior leaflet mitral IE (37%). Also, one study has shown that vegetation length >10 mm or >15 mm is associated with a 60% or 83% risk of embolization, respectively.[11] Therefore:

- Surgery seems reasonable (class IIa) in patients who already had an embolization, have a persistently large vegetation >1 cm, and are in the early phase of IE treatment (first 2 weeks).
- Surgery may be performed in patients with vegetation >10 or 15 mm without prior embolization, particularly when the regurgitation is severe (class IIa). If surgery is considered for this indication, it should be done urgently, at the time the risk of embolization is highest. This indication is supported by one randomized trial.[12]
- Since most patients with severe valvular regurgitation eventually need surgery sooner or later, the *early performance of surgery appears to be the preferred strategy if a large vegetation is associated with severe valvular regurgitation*.[12] Seventy-six patients with a vegetation >1 cm in diameter and severe valvular disease were randomized to early surgery (within 48 hours of randomization) or conventional treatment with surgery as needed, later on (77% eventually underwent surgery, mostly during hospitalization). Patients with classic indications for early surgery (HF, abscess) and patients without severe valvular disease were excluded. Patients with major stroke were also excluded. Patients with smaller strokes, TIA, or renal/splenic embolism were included, and ~45% of randomized patients had a prior embolism (~28% cerebral). Early surgery dramatically reduced the risk of symptomatic recurrent events (eight cases [21% vs. 0%], seven of which occurred between 2 and 9 days, especially at 2–5 days, after randomization, and included five major strokes, one anterior MI, one limb ischemia).

Surgery in patients with a large vegetation and without severe valvular disease is more controversial. *The clearest indication is the patient with a large vegetation, severe valvular disease, and peripheral embolism or cerebral embolism not associated with a major stroke.*

The problem is, however, that when patients have already had a cerebral embolization, early surgery within the first 2 weeks after a stroke is associated with a high risk of neurologic deterioration. Neurologic deterioration may result from hemorrhagic transformation during cardiopulmonary bypass/anticoagulation, or exacerbation or expansion of ischemia from perioperative hypotension. These factors make a recent embolic stroke a relative contraindication to valvular surgery in infective endocarditis (STS guidelines).[13] In fact, after an ischemic stroke, the risk of deterioration with surgery is 20% in the first 3 days, 20–50% between 4 and 14 days, 6–10% between 15 and 28 days, and <1% after 28 days. Two other series suggest, however, that surgery performed at a median of 4 days after a stroke did not compromise neurological recovery.[14,15] Thus, surgery is probably safe within the first 4 days after an ischemic event (especially a small or silent infarct or a transient ischemic attack) but not after a hemorrhagic event.[16] Cardiac surgery may need to be delayed 2 weeks after a large cerebral infarction, but may be performed earlier, especially in the first 4 days, in case of recurrent embolization, increased vegetation size despite appropriate antibiotic therapy, refractory infection, or HF.[14,15] Surgery needs to be delayed at least 4 weeks after a hemorrhagic stroke.

Hemorrhagic transformation is common following cerebral embolization, with rates as high as 50% in some studies. Less common is the formation of an abscess within the infarct cavity over the days or weeks following the infarct. Because of this risk of hemorrhagic transformation, anticoagulation of patients with mechanical prostheses is discontinued for 2 weeks after a cerebral embolism.[2]

C. Types of valvular surgery

Valvular surgery often consists of valve replacement, but valvular repair with vegetectomy and patch repair may be performed, particularly for the mitral valve (class I recommendation for mitral valve repair when technically feasible, STS guidelines).[13] Repair rates range from 33% to 94% in published series (STS guidelines). In the previously described study, ~50% of mitral surgeries consisted of valvular repair.[12] In the case of aortic endocarditis with periannular extension, drainage of abscess cavities, excision of necrotic tissue, and closure of fistulous tracts often accompany valve replacement surgery. Aortic valve homograft and root homograft, when available, may be preferred because they are associated with a low incidence of sewing-ring infection and mural endocarditis, possibly related to the improved antibiotic penetration.

D. Indications for tricuspid valve surgery

Isolated right-sided endocarditis has a relatively benign course with a low in-hospital mortality. Therefore, a conservative approach is appropriate for the large majority of patients with tricuspid and pulmonic valve endocarditis.[17] When PA pressure is normal, TR and RV volume overload are usually well tolerated without an imminent risk of RV failure.

Surgical indications:[18]

- Refractory infection despite 2–3 weeks of antibiotic therapy, in the absence of a pulmonary abscess (otherwise, pulmonary abscess may explain the persistence of infection).[10] This is the main indication for tricuspid endocarditis surgery.
- Massive TR with deteriorating RV dilatation.[18]
- Recurrent pulmonary emboli are a surgical indication according to one source,[18] but not according to another source.[10]

Surgical options include:[17,18] (i) debridement and vegetation excision with valve repair if the vegetation/destruction does not involve more than half of the tricuspid apparatus, or (ii) total valvectomy with prosthetic valve replacement. Vegetectomy with valve repair is preferred whenever possible. Total excision of the tricuspid valve without immediate replacement may be tolerated by some patients.[18,19] RV dysfunction does not usually occur for several months after valvular excision, unless the patient has pulmonary hypertension secondary to multiple pulmonary emboli; a bioprosthetic valve may be inserted 6–9 months later, after infection control.

2. CARDIAC RHYTHM DEVICE INFECTIONS

I. Organisms and mechanisms of infection

Cardiac device infection is often caused by *Staphylococcus* species, most commonly coagulase- negative staphylococci (45%) or *S. aureus* (29%). The pocket may become infected at the time of implantation, either endogenously from the skin of the patient or exogenously.[20] It may also get infected if the generator or leads erode through the skin; note that device erosion, per se, may result from an underlying infection.

On the other hand, the generator or leads may become infected as a result of hematogenous seeding during bacteremia or fungemia secondary to a distantly infected focus. This characteristically occurs with *S. aureus* bacteremia and is unlikely with Gram-negative bacteremia. The prevalence of device infection secondary to *S. aureus* bacteremia is difficult to determine, as it is not easy to differentiate this mechanism of device infection from intraoperative contamination at the time of device placement.

Device infection may track along the intravascular portion of the lead and result in lead or valvular vegetation in up to one-fourth of cases.

II. Diagnosis

A. Clinical

Most often (~70%), local inflammatory changes of the generator/pocket site are present, or cutaneous erosion with percutaneous exposure of the generator and/or leads is seen.

Fever or increased white count may not be seen. Infrequently, device infection manifests as fever of undefined origin without local inflammatory changes at the generator/pocket site.

Among all-comers with *S. aureus* bacteremia and an implanted cardiac rhythm device, ~45% had confirmed device infection by echocardiography (vegetations) or upon explantation. Only 40% of confirmed device infections had local signs of infection. Also, only 40% of device infections had the device as a source of infection, the remaining patients having a central catheter or a soft tissue infection as a distant source of bacteremia.[21] The device was more likely the source of infection in case of early *S. aureus* bacteremia (<1 year post-implantation).

B. Echocardiography

In the above study, one-third of patients with confirmed device infection did not have any vegetation on TEE.[21] Thus, in case of *S. aureus* bacteremia, the clinician should have a high index of suspicion that the implant is infected, even if local signs of generator pocket infection are absent and no generator, wire, or valvular vegetations are detected by TEE.

While TEE may not be superior to TTE in demonstrating tricuspid valve endocarditis, it is superior in demonstrating lead endocarditis (RA, SVC vegetations) and is a valuable diagnostic tool when a device infection is suspected, particularly in case of bacteremia, more so *S. aureus* bacteremia.

On the other hand, lead masses are frequently seen on TEE in patients without any infectious concern. In one study, masses were seen on the leads of 5% of pacemakers and were considered thrombus rather than vegetation.[22] In another report, lead masses were seen in 13/132 patients (10%) in whom TEE was performed for an indication other than ruling out endocarditis, and only one of those patients was clinically adjudicated to have an infected device.[23] Thus, it is important to take the clinical context into account, and an unsuspected lead mass on TTE or TEE is often a thrombus.

III. Diagnosis in patients with bacteremia but no local or TEE signs of infection

Although bloodstream infection can be a manifestation of device infection, it can occur without device infection in ~55% of the cases. The device is more likely to be infected if the patient has *S. aureus* bacteremia with any one of the following: (1) no clear source of *S. aureus* bacteremia can be identified; (2) persistent bacteremia despite antibiotic therapy and removal of a culprit central catheter; (3) the patient develops recurrent bacteremia; (4) bacteremia within the first 3 months of device placement. Cardiac devices may sometimes be retained in patients with an identifiable source of *S. aureus* infection (e.g., infected intravascular catheter) and no clear involvement of the leads or device by TEE or physical examination. Such patients, however, require careful follow-up to detect relapsing infection, which would generally occur within 12 weeks after discontinuation of antibiotic therapy if the prosthetic device was seeded at the time of the initial *S. aureus* bacteremia. Patients found to have relapsing infection should undergo complete device extraction.[20,21]

Device infection is unlikely in patients with Gram-negative bacteremia and no other signs of infection; thus, device removal is not recommended in this setting. However, a relapsing or refractory Gram-negative bacteremia despite appropriate antibiotic therapy and despite the absence of a defined source of infection should trigger device removal. The same probably applies to patients with coagulase-negative staphylococcal bacteremia, enteroccocemia or fungemia.[20]

IV. Management

The whole system (generator and leads) should be removed in all patients with device infection, including patients with only localized pocket infection and no sign of systemic infection.[24] The only exception is superficial infection of the wound or incision site (e.g., stitch abscess, superficial cellulitis) early after implantation which can be managed by conservative antibiotic therapy without removing the device.

Complete removal of hardware is needed because the relapse rate from retained hardware is high. Device infections are associated with a high mortality, particularly in patients with a confirmed device-related endocarditis and in those treated without device removal. The in-hospital mortality varies between 7% and 14%. Leads may be extracted percutaneously with <1% procedure-related mortality.[24]

After extraction, two decisions have to be made: duration of antibiotic therapy and timing of reimplantation (Figure 28.3). Antibiotic therapy is generally continued for 2 weeks after device explantation, longer if there is evidence of endocarditis. Also, before reimplanting a device, one should assess *whether* the patient still needs one. Studies indicate that up to 30% of patients may no longer require a cardiac device.[24]

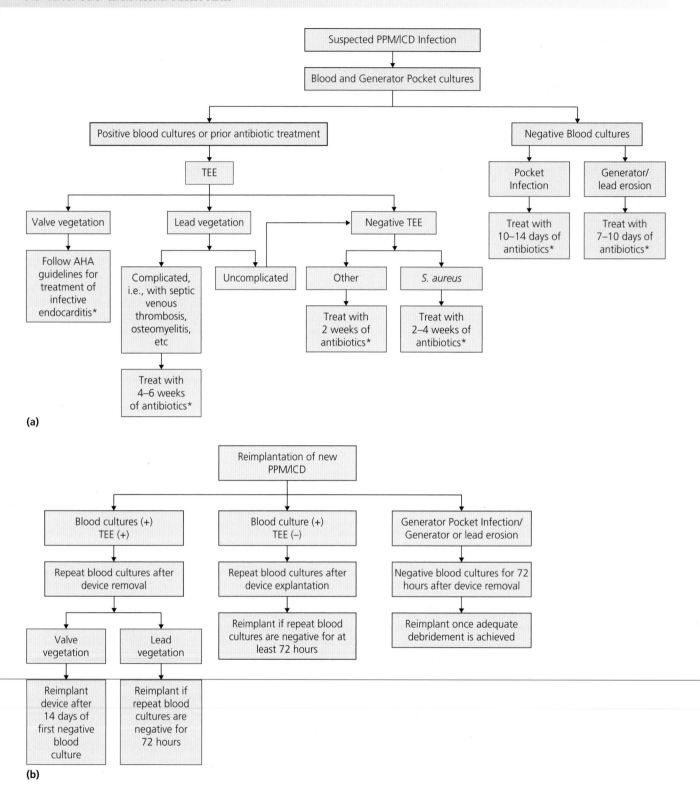

Figure 28.3 (a) Duration of antibiotic therapy in patients with device infection. This algorithm applies only to the patients with complete device explantation. *Duration of antibiotics should be counted from the day of device explantation. **(b)** Timing of reimplantation in patients with device infection. PPM, permanent pacemaker.

Reproduced with permission of Elsevier from Sohail et al. (2007).[24]

References

Infective endocarditis

1. Durack DT, Lukes AS, Bright DK. New criteria for diagnosis of infective endocarditis: utilization of specific echocardiographic findings. Duke Endocarditis Service. Am J Med 1994; 96: 200–9.
2. Baddour LM, Wilson WR, Bayer AS, et al. AHA scientific statement. Infective endocarditis in adults: diagnosis, antimicrobial therapy, and management of complications. Circulation 2015; 132:1435–86.
3. Erbel R, Rohmann S, Drexler M, et al. Improved diagnostic value of echocardiography in patients with infective endocarditis by transoesophageal approach: a prospective study. Eur Heart J 1988; 9: 43–53.
4. Reynolds HR, Jagen MA, Tunick PA, Kronzon I. Sensitivity of transthoracic versus transesophageal echocardiography for the detection of native valve vegetations in the modern era. J Am Soc Echocardiogr 2003; 16: 67–70.
5. Habib G, Badano L, Tribouilloy C, et al. Recommendations for the practice of echocardiography in infective endocarditis. Eur J Echocardiogr 2010; 11: 202–19.
6. San Roman JA, Vilacosta I, Zamorano JL, Almeria C, Sanchez-Harguindey L. Transesophageal echocardiography in right-sided endocarditis. J Am Coll Cardiol 1993; 21: 1226–30.
7. Fowler VG, Li J, Corey GR, et al. Role of echocardiography in evaluation of patients with Staphylococcus aureus bacteremia: experience in 103 patients. J Am Coll Cardiol 1997; 30: 1072–8.
8. Rosen AB, Fowler VG, Corey GR, et al. Cost-effectiveness of transesophageal echocardiography to determine the duration of therapy for intravascular catheter-associated Staphylococcus aureus bacteremia. Ann Intern Med 1999; 130: 810–20.
9. Blumberg EA, Karalis DA, Chandrasekaran K, et al. Endocarditis-associated paravalvular abscesses: do clinical parameters predict the presence of abscess? Chest 1995; 107: 898–903.
10. Prendergast BD, Tornos P. Surgery for infective endocarditis: who and when? Circulation 2010; 121: 1141–52.
11. Di Salvo G, Habib G, Pergola V, et al. Echocardiography predicts embolic events in infective endocarditis. J Am Coll Cardiol 2001; 37: 1069–76.
12. Kang DH, Kim YJ, Kim SH, et al. Early surgery versus conventional treatment for infective endocarditis. N Engl J Med 2012; 366: 2466–73.
13. Byrne, JG, Rezai K, Sanchez JA, et al. Surgical management of endocarditis: the Society of thoracic surgeons clinical practice guidelines. Ann Thorac Surg 2011; 91: 2012–19.
14. Gammie JS, O'Brien SM, Griffith BP, Peterson ED. Surgical treatment of mitral valve endocarditis in North America. Ann Thorac Surg 2005; 80: 2199–204. *In this series, early surgery at a median of 4 days did not compromise neurologic recovery.*
15. Ruttmann E, Willeit J, Ulmer H, et al. Neurological outcome of septic cardioembolic stroke after infective endocarditis. Stroke 2006; 37: 2094–9. *Surgery at a median 4 days (0–38 d) did not compromise neurological recovery; neurological recovery did not vary with the timing of surgery. No significant incidence of intracranial hemorrhage postoperatively.*
16. Angstwurm K, Borges A, Halle E, et al. Timing the valve replacement in infective endocarditis involving the brain. J Neurol 2004; 251: 1220–6.
17. Musci M, Siniawski H, Pasic M, et al. Surgical treatment of right-sided active infective endocarditis with or without involvement of the left heart: 20 year single center experience. Eur J Cardiothorac Surg 2007; 32: 118–25.
18. Akinosoglou K, Apostolakis E, Koutsogiannis N, et al. Right-sided infective endocarditis: surgical management. Eur J Cardiothorac Surg 2012; 42: 470–9.
19. Arbulu A, Holmes RJ, Asfaw I. Surgical treatment of intractable right-sided infective endocarditis in drug addicts: 25 years' experience. J Heart Valve Dis 1993; 2: 129–37.

Cardiac rhythm device infections

20. Baddour LM, Epstein AE, Erickson CC, et al. Update on cardiovascular implantable electronic device infections and their management: a scientific statement from the American Heart Association. Circulation 2010; 121: 458–77.
21. Chamis AL, Peterson GE, Cabell CH, et al. Staphylococcus aureus bacteremia in patients with permanent pacemakers or implantable cardioverter-defibrillators. Circulation 2001; 104: 1029–33.
22. Lo R, D'Anca M, Cohen T, Kerwin T. Incidence and prognosis of pacemaker lead-associated masses: a study of 1,569 transesophageal echocardiograms. J Invasive Cardiol 2006; 18: 599–601.
23. Downey BC, Juselius WE, Pandian NG, et al. Incidence and significance of pacemaker and implantable cardioverter-defibrillator lead masses discovered during transesophageal echocardiography. Pacing Clin Electrophysiol 2011; 34: 679–83.
24. Sohail MR, Uslan DZ, Khan AH, et al. Management and outcome of permanent and implantable cardioverter-defibrillator infections. J Am Coll Cardiol 2007; 49: 1851–9.

29 Preoperative Cardiac Evaluation

In patients undergoing vascular surgery, ~60% have significant CAD. Two major mechanisms underlie perioperative myocardial infarction:

1. Catecholamine surge, tachycardia, and hypertension increase coronary shear stress, which triggers plaque rupture. This is more likely to happen in plaques with a large atherosclerotic burden or plaques associated with severe stenosis, but may happen on non-obstructive plaques.[1,2]

Surgery-induced procoagulant state may lead to coronary thrombosis over a ruptured or even a non-ruptured lesion, particularly if the stenosis is tight with a low flow state.

2. Prolonged periods of demand/supply mismatch in patients with severe but previously stable CAD, without any plaque rupture.

Overall, each one of the two mechanisms is primarily responsible for ~50% of postoperative MIs.[1] A combination is likely responsible for MI in a substantial proportion of patients. Most events occur in the first 24–48 hours postoperatively, the period of highest sympathetic tone. The infarct is most commonly NSTEMI/non-Q-wave MI. In a series of 21 patients who underwent preoperative coronary angiography and developed postoperative MI after vascular surgery, slightly over half of the infarcts corresponded to the territory of a totally occluded coronary artery, in which collaterals could not provide enough supply during a period of high stress; additionally, those patients had severe multivessel disease, potentially impairing collateral flow.[3] The remaining infarcts occurred in the territory of a non-significant lesion, in patients who nonetheless had extensive atherosclerosis. This highlights not only the frequency of demand/supply mismatch, but also the fact that plaque rupture may very well occur at non-obstructive sites. Plaque rupture usually occurs in a patient with significantly obstructive CAD, and the overall extent of CAD correlates with the risk of events and plaque rupture; however, the infarct does not necessarily occur at the actual site of severe stenosis. In fact, a non-obstructive lesion may be vulnerable (high plaque burden, thin cap). This explains why revascularization may not fully prevent postoperative MI.

According to the ACC/AHA 2014 preoperative guidelines,[4] the cardiac evaluation for noncardiac surgery is based on the assessment of (1) active cardiac conditions, (2) known cardiovascular disease and cardiac risk factors, and (3) functional capacity in metabolic equivalents (METs).

Practical Cardiovascular Medicine, First Edition. Elias B. Hanna.
© 2017 John Wiley & Sons Ltd. Published 2017 by John Wiley & Sons Ltd.

I. Steps in preoperative evaluation

A. First step: if the surgery is emergent, no cardiac workup is performed preoperatively

B. Second step: if the surgery is not emergent, evaluate for active cardiac conditions

Active cardiac conditions:

- Active, unstable coronary syndrome, or recent MI (<1 month) with persistent ischemic symptoms or ischemia on non-invasive stress testing
- Severe unstable arrhythmia
- Decompensated HF
- Severely symptomatic valvular heart disease

These patients need to have their cardiac condition treated before surgery, depending on the urgency of the surgery (PCI for ACS, medical therapy for HF, surgical therapy for symptomatic, severe valvular disease).

In case of an emergent surgery, proceed to the high-risk surgery with maximal medical therapy.

C. Third step: in the absence of active cardiac conditions, look for clinical risk factors, and use the revised cardiac risk index or Lee index

The Lee index includes six factors:[5]

- History of CAD
- Compensated or prior HF
- Diabetes
- Renal insufficiency
- Cerebrovascular disease
- Intermediate- or high-risk surgery

1. **In the case of a Lee risk score of 0 or 1, *or* in the case of a low-risk surgery** regardless of risk factors, surgery is performed without any further cardiac workup. The surgery is a low-cardiac-risk surgery.
2. **In the case of a Lee risk score ≥2 *and* poor functional capacity <4 METs (or unknown) *and* intermediate- or high-risk surgery,** non-invasive preoperative cardiac testing may be performed for further cardiac risk assessment (class IIa recommendation). If the functional capacity is ≥4 METs, especially ≥7 METs, stress testing is not needed even if the Lee risk score is high. Preoperative testing determines the functional capacity when it is unclear (exercise testing), and allows risk stratification of patients with a clearly reduced functional capacity <4 METs (pharmacologic testing). Four METs corresponds to climbing one flight of stairs, walking up a hill, walking fast at ground level, dancing, or performing heavy housework or yardwork (pushing a power mower, scrubbing floors, carrying heavy groceries). Sexual intercourse corresponds to 3–5 METs.

Note that preoperative testing is mainly useful to assess how risky the surgery will be and to see whether it should be avoided or altered, if possible. ***Testing is only performed if it will change management, i.e., if surgery can be deferred. Preoperative testing is, therefore, much less useful in patients who require a necessary, vital surgery (e.g., cancer surgery)***.

A high-risk finding on preoperative testing indicates preoperative coronary angiography only if preoperative revascularization is feasible. If extensive CAD is present (left main or multivessel CAD), revascularization, typically CABG, should generally be performed before a non-vital elective surgery (class I recommendation). This revascularization is mainly meant to improve the long-term cardiac risk of the patient. Outside ACS or left main disease, preoperative revascularization does not clearly change the operative cardiac risk (CARP trial), even in high-risk ischemic patients with at least five abnormal segments on stress imaging (LV being divided into 17 segments).[5,6] There is no evidence that PCI of a single- or two-vessel disease (non-proximal LAD) improves perioperative outcomes, outside ACS.

II. Surgical risk: surgery's risk and patient's risk

A. Classification of the surgery's risk

The surgery is classified into one of three risk categories:

- High risk: aortic or major peripheral vascular surgery
- Intermediate risk: intraperitoneal, intrathoracic, carotid endarterectomy, common femoral endarterectomy, head and neck surgery, orthopedic surgery, prostate surgery
- Low risk: endoscopic procedures, breast surgery, cataract surgery, ambulatory surgery

The risk of perioperative major cardiac events (death or MI) is generally ≤1% with low-risk surgery, regardless of the underlying patient's risk; and is generally 1–5% with intermediate-risk surgery and 5% with high-risk surgery, although the actual risk of intermediate- and high-risk surgeries also depends on the patient's intrinsic risk (Lee risk score). For example, a low-risk patient undergoing major vascular surgery has <2–5% risk of major cardiac events.

B. Classification of the patient's overall risk (integrates the surgery's risk with the patient's risk factors)

In the presence of an active cardiac condition (Section I.B, above), the patient is a high-risk patient.

In the absence of an active condition, a Lee risk score ≥3 identifies high-risk stable patients, a score of 2 identifies intermediate-risk patients, while a score of 0 or 1 identifies low-risk patients. The risk of postoperative major adverse cardiac events (MACE) (death, MI, or definite pulmonary edema) in high-, intermediate-, and low-risk patients is ≥9%, 4–5%, and 0.5–1.3%, respectively.[7]

C. Risk of MACE according to stress testing results

A high-risk stress test result (stress echo or nuclear stress test) is associated with a 10–25% risk of perioperative death or MI, while a normal stress test result is associated with a 0–4% (~2%) risk of death or MI.[4] Therefore, a low-risk stress test steps down the risk in a patient with a high Lee index, but the absolute risk may remain significant.

III. CARP and DECREASE V trials

The CARP and DECREASE V trials have shown that patients with established but stable CAD, including multivessel/triple-vessel CAD, who are undergoing high-risk vascular surgery, do not benefit from revascularization preoperatively.

In the CARP trial, 509 intermediate-to-high-risk patients (by Lee risk score or stress testing) undergoing vascular surgery (33% AAA) and found to have CAD on coronary angiography were randomized to medical therapy or coronary revascularization (59% CABG, 41% PCI). Surgery was delayed a median of 6 weeks after revascularization. The postoperative risk of death was ~3% in both groups, and MI rate was ~8% (high MACE risk not modified by revascularization).[6]

In DECREASE V, the MACE risk was even higher and unchanged with revascularization. This is related to the fact that postoperative MI in a CAD patient may result from a plaque rupture occurring at the site of an obstructive lesion but also frequently a non-obstructive one. Moreover, preoperative revascularization is associated with its own set of complications, such as stent thrombosis. Therefore, the usefulness of preoperative coronary revascularization in patients not having active ACS is not established, even in high-risk subgroups with strongly positive stress tests.[7]

Caveats

1. Only 35% of CARP patients had three-vessel CAD and only 44% had moderate/large ischemia on stress testing. At least 25% had low-risk Lee score and nuclear imaging.[6] In a post-hoc analysis of CARP, patients who underwent CABG had fewer MIs after vascular surgery than those who underwent PCI and probably those treated medically, despite the more extensive CAD in CABG patients.[8] In another CARP analysis, patients with large anterior ischemia seemed to benefit from preoperative revascularization.[9] This underlines a potential role of preoperative CABG in patients with extensive CAD undergoing elective vascular surgery.

2. Left main disease was excluded from the CARP trial, and, in an analysis of the CARP registry, left main disease benefited from preoperative revascularization.[10]

Preoperative coronary testing may be useful to show the general prognosis of the patient. A high surgical risk based on preoperative stress testing may lead to a change in management but not necessarily revascularization. It should lead to a risk/benefit discussion with the patient, with a potential cancellation of non-vital surgery and consideration of percutaneous angioplasty for PAD or endovascular repair of abdominal aortic aneurysm, even if the result is expected to be inferior to surgery. Preoperative coronary testing is much less useful in patients who require a vital surgery, such as cancer surgery.

> Patients with high-risk stable CAD (left main or triple-vessel CAD) are expected to have long-term improvement with revascularization and have an indication for revascularization to improve their long-term outcome rather than their immediate postoperative outcome.
>
> These patients require revascularization regardless of surgery, and if possible this should be performed before surgery. Conversely, finding one- or two-vessel disease does not dictate preoperative revascularization per se, since, again, this revascularization does not clearly improve perioperative outcomes.

IV. Only the highest-risk coronary patients require revascularization preoperatively

The highest-risk patients are those with recent acute coronary syndrome, or MI in the last month with persistent ischemia clinically or on stress testing. Stenting, however, is associated with several pitfalls:

1. Dual antiplatelet therapy after stenting increases the surgical bleeding risk.
2. The prothrombotic milieu created by surgery increases the risk of stent thrombosis.

Surgery soon after stenting (2 weeks) may lead to catastrophic results, with a high risk of death and MI. In one analysis, death (mostly secondary to stent thrombosis, and partly secondary to bleeding) occurred in 32% of patients who underwent surgery <2 weeks after stenting, and in four out of five patients who underwent surgery 1 day after stenting.[11] One or both antiplatelet agents were only briefly interrupted before surgery (~1 day), and interruption of antiplatelet therapy may therefore not have been solely responsible for this high rate of stent thrombosis. Bleeding was also very common, and early post-PCI bleeding is known to be associated with MI and stent thrombosis.

V. Preoperative percutaneous revascularization

If percutaneous revascularization needs to be performed preoperatively, dual antiplatelet therapy is given and **surgery is postponed for at least 1 month after bare-metal stent (BMS) and 3 months, preferably 6 months, after drug-eluting stent (DES)** (class I for antiplatelet interruption at 6 months, IIb at 3 months). This delay gives time for the stent struts to endothelialize and allows an effective duration of dual antiplatelet therapy.

If surgery is needed more urgently (<4 weeks), balloon angioplasty is performed without any stenting if possible, and BMS is placed only as a bailout for complicated angioplasty. Surgery can be performed 2–4 weeks after balloon angioplasty; there is a risk of acute vessel thrombosis with earlier surgery.

VI. Surgery that needs to be performed soon after stent placement

- If surgery needs to be performed earlier than 4 weeks after BMS placement or earlier than 3 months after DES placement, try to perform the surgery while the patient is still on dual antiplatelet therapy.
- Dual antiplatelet therapy does not usually need to be held before dental procedures.
- Except for aortobifemoral bypass surgery, peripheral vascular surgery (femoropopliteal bypass, CEA) may be performed under a dual antiplatelet regime.
- Gastrointestinal endoscopic procedures:
  - Gastroscopy, colonoscopy with biopsies, and ERCP with endoprosthesis placement may be performed under dual antiplatelet regime.
  - Polypectomy or ERCP with sphincterotomy may be done under aspirin monotherapy.
  - Endoscopic gastrostomy tube may require holding both antiplatelet agents.
- Aspirin monotherapy does not increase major surgical bleeding, except during intracranial surgery, posterior chamber ophthalmic surgery, and transurethral prostatectomy (but may be continued in the latter case).

In a patient with a prior history of PCI with BMS or DES, the risk of MACE is highest in the first 30–45 days (10–20%), then is reduced to ≤5% (~3%) beyond 45 days for BMS and beyond 6 months for DES, with ~1.5% risk of stent thrombosis (low in absolute numbers, but much higher than the natural incidence of stent thrombosis during this post-PCI period).[12–15] With second-generation DES (Xience V, Resolute), data suggest that the risk of stent thrombosis with clopidogrel discontinuation 6 months after PCI is very low, possibly even 1 month, especially if DES was implanted for stable CAD rather than ACS (stenting of STEMI carries the highest risk of stent thrombosis).[16] Surgery 1–6 months after DES placement carries an increased but not dramatic risk of MACE (~4–5% MACE, with 2% stent thrombosis, despite the interruption of clopidogrel in the majority of patients reported);[12,13] this is lower with a second-generation DES, especially if DES was implanted for stable CAD.

If clopidogrel is discontinued perioperatively within 1–6 months after DES placement, resume it as soon as possible after surgery, using a 300 mg load. In fact, when clopidogrel is interrupted beyond the first month after PCI, stent thrombosis typically occurs >7 days after interruption, if at all.[16–18] Therefore, brief interruption of clopidogrel beyond the first month after DES placement, when inevitable, is usually safe.

Always ensure that at least one antiplatelet agent is continued throughout surgery, regardless of the type of stent used and even if surgery is performed >6 months after PCI. There is a lifetime risk of stent thrombosis upon discontinuation of both antiplatelet agents.

Bridging with a glycoprotein IIb/IIIa inhibitor (GPI) has been suggested, starting 2 days after clopidogrel discontinuation until 12 hours before surgery. However, no evidence supports this strategy. Since GPI is not used postoperatively, i.e., during the highest-risk period, the risk of stent thrombosis may not be reduced. Moreover, the bleeding risk makes it unfavorable in most situations. GPI may be reserved for individual high-risk situations.

VII. Preoperative β-blocker therapy

The administration of β-blockers perioperatively, starting >1 day preoperatively and for 7 days postoperatively, is indicated in high-risk patients (Lee index ≥3) undergoing intermediate- or high-risk surgery; β-blockers appear to improve postoperative outcomes in these patients.[19] They are also indicated in patients with highly positive stress tests, and should be continued in patients already taking them chronically.

They are not useful, and are in fact harmful, in the low-risk category. β-Blockers should be started a few days preoperatively and progressively titrated to achieve a heart rate of 60–70 bpm.[20] The initiation of a high β-blocker dose in the immediate preoperative period (<24 hours) without proper titration increases the risk of hypotension, stroke, and mortality, even in high-cardiac-risk patients (POISE trial).[21]

VIII. Other interventions that improve outcomes

A. Statin therapy

In addition to improving long-term outcomes, the perioperative use of statins decreases the immediate postoperative cardiovascular events. High-risk patients who initiated statin therapy at a median of 37 days before vascular surgery had >50% reduction of their postoperative cardiovascular events, including death and MI.[22]

B. Optimize the volume status of patients with HF

Always look for S_3, high JVP, and pulmonary edema, and treat any volume overload preoperatively.

HF patients are at a particularly high risk of developing pulmonary edema during the *stress of extubation*. Positive-pressure ventilation reduces both preload and afterload, providing optimal loading conditions. Conversely, extubation is a major stressor associated with a sudden rise of both preload and afterload, and a risk of myocardial ischemia or HF decompensation.

IX. Severe valvular disease

Patients with severe, symptomatic valvular disease should generally undergo valvular surgery before elective non-cardiac surgery. The perioperative risk is highest with symptomatic AS.

In asymptomatic severe MR, AI, or MS, elective surgery may be performed with attention to volume and rate control (avoid tachycardia with MS and bradycardia with AI) (class IIa recommendation).

In asymptomatic severe AS, elective surgery may be performed without a significant increase in the risk of death or MI (class IIa). In one series, the perioperative rates of death and MI were 0% and 3%, respectively. These patients frequently developed intraoperative hypotension and required vasopressors.[23]

Patients with severe symptomatic AS who cannot undergo valvular surgery – because of comorbidities or patient refusal – can undergo non-cardiac surgery with an acceptable risk. In the combined results of two series, 2 of 36 patients with severe and mostly symptomatic AS died late postoperatively (aortic valve area ~0.6 cm², EF mostly normal). No death occurred intraoperatively. Careful volume control, aggressive BP monitoring, often with an intra-arterial line, and prompt therapy of hypotension with vasopressors are required.[24,25] Reduction of preload and systemic vascular resistance should be avoided. The severe fixed obstruction prevents an increase in cardiac output should systemic vasodilatation occur, which precipitates severe hypotension.

On a similar note, patients with symptomatic HOCM do well with non-cardiac surgery, with a very low mortality risk, but have an increased risk of postoperative HF.[26] BP should be carefully monitored and preload and afterload reduction avoided. This implies appropriate volume control and the use of phenyleprine as needed.

X. Perioperative hypertension

Appropriate HTN control is necessary to prevent perioperative myocardial ischemia. Patients with severe HTN are more prone to intraoperative hypotension than normotensive patients; this may be related to the heightened vascular resistance that suddenly drops with anesthesia, or to the impaired vascular compliance, which makes the systemic pressure quickly rise up but also quickly fall with volume fluctuations. Perioperative ACE-I/ARB may exaggerate this intraoperative hypotension; therefore, ACE-I/ARB may be withheld the morning of surgery then resumed once the patient is hemodynamically stable.[4]

XI. Preoperative management of patients with pacemakers or ICDs

See Chapter 14, Section VII.

QUESTIONS AND ANSWERS

Question 1. A 65-year-old diabetic patient is planning to undergo elective cholecystectomy for recurrent postprandial pain. He has mild dyspnea on exertion (>4 METs) but no chest pain. He undergoes preoperative testing with a nuclear SPECT, which shows severe inferior ischemia and preserved LVEF. Coronary angiography shows 80% mid-RCA stenosis. What is the next step?
A. Aggressive medical regimen. Revascularization is not indicated. His surgical risk is intermediate but revascularization will not improve his surgical risk
B. Aggressive medical regimen. Revascularization is not indicated. His surgical risk is low
C. Aggressive medical regimen and PCI of the RCA with BMS
D. Aggressive medical regimen and PCI of the RCA with DES

Question 2. A 70-year-old diabetic man is found to have a colon cancer and will need to undergo colon resection. He has been weak and minimally active for the last few months (<4 METs). He does not have angina or prior HF; he has HTN and CKD. What is the next step?
A. Considering his low METs and his Lee risk score, he needs preoperative stress testing
B. Proceed with surgery with optimal statin and β-blocker therapy

Question 3. The patient of Question 3 underwent stress testing, which showed moderate anterior ischemia. Coronary angiography is performed and shows 70% mid-LAD stenosis. What is the next step?
A. PCI of LAD with BMS and colon surgery in 6 weeks
B. Proceed with surgery with optimal statin and β-blocker therapy, and careful perioperative monitoring

Question 4. A 70-year-old patient has a history of mid-LAD DES (everolimus stent) placed 6 weeks previously for stable angina. His angina has resolved. He now develops abdominal pain and is found to have cholecystitis with abscess formation. The surgeon wants to perform cholecystectomy during this hospital stay and wants to discontinue clopidogrel. What is your recommendation?
A. Try to postpone surgery until 3 months after the PCI date
B. Perform surgery under dual antiplatelet therapy
C. May interrupt clopidogrel for 5–7 days, then resume it the second day postoperatively

Question 5. A patient had a TIA, manifesting as aphasia, yesterday. His carotid ultrasound and CT show 80% left internal carotid stenosis. CEA is planned. He has a history of exertional chest pain for the last 6 months. His troponin I is negative. What is the best strategy?
A. Proceed with CEA as soon as possible, without any cardiac workup
B. Perform preoperative stress testing
C. Perform preoperative coronary angiography

Question 6. A patient had a TIA, manifesting as aphasia, yesterday. His carotid ultrasound and CT show 80% left internal carotid stenosis. He also experienced resting chest pain and had a mild troponin rise. Coronary angiography is performed and shows 80% proximal LAD and 80% mid-RCA stenoses. What is the best strategy?
A. Proceed with CEA without coronary revascularization
B. Simultaneous CEA–CABG
C. Coronary stenting followed by CEA within the same hospital stay
D. Coronary stenting followed by CEA in 1 month
E. Coronary stenting and carotid stenting within the same hospital stay

Question 7. A 65-year-old patient, smoker, has severe bilateral claudication with non-healing ulcer and rest pain of the left foot. He does not report any angina, but his activity is limited. Angiography shows occlusion of both common and external iliacs (TASC D lesions). He is referred for aortobifemoral bypass grafting. A preoperative nuclear stress test shows anterior ischemia, and a subsequent coronary angiography shows 80% mid-LAD stenosis. Rank these three management strategies in order of preference:
A. Stent the LAD with BMS, then perform aortofemoral bypass surgery in 4 weeks
B. Proceed with aortofemoral bypass surgery without any LAD stenting
C. Reconsider the percutaneous treatment option for iliac disease, even it was deemed anatomically unfavorable.

Answer 1. A. The patient does not have a clear angina. The inferior ischemia implies that the patient has an increased surgical risk, including a risk of functional ischemia/infarction of the RCA territory during surgery. However, except for left main disease or extensive three-vessel CAD, preoperative revascularization does not change postoperative cardiac complications. Medical therapy with a statin and a β-blocker, initiated more than a week before surgery, and careful perioperative monitoring are the strategies that improve outcomes. PCI of the RCA may be appropriate from an angina standpoint in this patient with severe ischemia and dyspnea (presumably angina equivalent), but it is not appropriate for preoperative optimization. If PCI is performed, surgery will have to be postponed >1 month.

Answer 2. B. the patient has a Lee risk score of 3 and a functional status <4 METs, which may seem to qualify him for preoperative stress testing (class IIa). But testing is only performed if it will change management, i.e., if surgery can be deferred and if preoperative revascularization is feasible. Preoperative testing is much less useful in a patient who requires a necessary, vital surgery, where delays are unacceptable and where the potential peri-PCI antithrombotic therapy will make the active cancer bleed.

Answer 3. B.

Answer 4. C. The patient has an active condition that may not allow a 3-month surgical delay. Since the bleeding risk is increased with dual antiplatelet therapy and may not be accepted by the surgeon, and since PCI is over 1 month old, clopidogrel may be interrupted and resumed soon after surgery. With second-generation DES, the risk of stent thrombosis with brief clopidogrel interruption (<10 days) beyond 1 month of PCI is low.

Answer 5. A. Stress testing soon after a stroke or TIA may not be safe, particularly in light of the BP swings that accompany stress testing. The stroke risk is high in the early period after TIA, implying a prompt need for surgery. Coronary revascularization at this time is not indicated. More specifically, coronary stenting followed by surgery within the ensuing 2–4 weeks may lead to catastrophic outcomes. It is best to proceed with CEA without the delays of cardiac workup or revascularization.

Answer 6. E. The patient has two active conditions: ACS and cerebrovascular event. Surgery for one may worsen the other. Stenting for both conditions, if anatomically feasible, likely presents less risk than surgery. Simultaneous CEA–CABG is associated with a high risk of stroke and mortality, in comparison with sequential CEA–CABG, and should be avoided if possible.

Answer 7. C > B > A. While TASC D iliac lesions are preferably treated surgically, they often can be treated percutaneously by experienced operators, in a high-surgical-risk patient. In this patient, percutaneous therapy is the safest strategy from a cardiac standpoint. If percutaneous therapy fails or is deemed impossible, bypass surgery should be performed as soon as possible in this patient with critical limb ischemia. As per CARP trial, stenting does not improve perioperative outcomes and only delays surgery. As per CARP trial and registry analyses, the highest-risk patients, probably left main or three-vessel disease patients, may benefit from preoperative revascularization. If the patient only had claudication and surgery could be delayed, stenting the LAD with BMS or DES and waiting 1 or 3 months, respectively, might be acceptable, especially considering the limitations of the CARP trial (Section III).

References

1. Landesberg G, Beattie WS, Mosseri M, et al. Perioperative myocardial infarction. Circulation 2009; 119: 2936–44.
2. Fukumoto Y, Hiro T, Fujii T, Hashimoto G, Fujimura T, Yamada J, Okamura T, Matsuzaki M. Localized elevation of shear stress is related to coronary plaque rupture. J Am Coll Cardiol 2008; 51: 645–50.
3. Ellis SG, Hertzer NR, Young JR, Brener S. Angiographic correlates of cardiac death and myocardial infarction complicating major nonthoracic vascular surgery. Am J Cardiol 1996; 77: 1126–8.
4. Fleisher LA, Fleischmann KE, Auerbach AD, et al. 2014 ACC/AHA guideline on perioperative cardiovascular evaluation and management of patients undergoing noncardiac surgery: a report of the American College of Cardiology/American Heart Association Task Force on practice guidelines. J Am Coll Cardiol 2014; 64: e77–137.
5. Lee TH, Marcantonio ER, Mangione CM, et al. Derivation and prospective validation of a simple index for prediction of cardiac risk of major noncardiac surgery. Circulation 1999; 100: 1043–9.
6. McFalls EO, Ward HB, Moritz TE, et al. Coronary-artery revascularization before elective major vascular surgery. N Engl J Med 2004; 351: 2795–804. CARP trial.
7. Poldermans D, Schouten O, Vidakovic R, et al. A clinical randomized trial to evaluate the safety of a noninvasive approach in high-risk patients undergoing major vascular surgery: the DECREASE-V Pilot Study. J Am Coll Cardiol 2007; 49: 1763–9.
8. Ward HB, Kelly RF, Thottapurathu L, et al. Coronary artery bypass grafting is superior to percutaneous coronary intervention in prevention of perioperative myocardial infarctions during subsequent vascular surgery. Ann Thorac Surg 2006; 82: 795–801.
9. Garcia S, Rider JE, Moritz TE, et al. Preoperative coronary artery revascularization and long-term outcomes following abdominal aortic vascular surgery in patients with abnormal myocardial perfusion scans: a sub-group analysis of the CARP trial. Catheter Cardiovasc Interv 2011; 77: 134–41.
10. Garcia S, Moritz TE, Ward HB, et al. Usefulness of revascularization of patients with multivessel coronary artery disease before elective vascular surgery for abdominal aortic and peripheral occlusive disease. Am J Cardiol 2008; 102: 809–13.
11. Kaluza GL, Joseph J, Lee JR, et al. Catastrophic outcomes of noncardiac surgery soon after coronary stenting. J Am Coll Cardiol 2000; 35: 1288–94.

12. Singla S, Sachdeva R, Uretsky BF. The risk of adverse cardiac and bleeding events following noncardiac surgery relative to antiplatelet therapy in patients with prior percutaneous coronary intervention. J Am Coll Cardiol 2012; 60: 2005–16.

13. Wijeysundera DN, Wijeysundera HC, Yun L, et al. Risk of elective major noncardiac surgery after coronary stent insertion: a population-based study. Circulation 2012; 126: 1355–62.

14. Wilson SH, Fasseas P, Orford JL, et al. Clinical outcome of patients undergoing non-cardiac surgery in the two months following coronary stenting, J Am Coll Cardiol 2003; 42: 234–40.

15. Sharma AK, Ajani AE, Hamwi SM, et al. Major noncardiac surgery following coronary stenting: when is it safe to operate? Catheter Cardiovasc Interv 2004; 63: 141–5.

16. Ferreira-Gonzales, Marsal JR, Ribera A, et al. Dual antiplatelet therapy after drug-eluting stent implantation. Risk associated with discontinuation within the first year. J Am Coll Cardiol 2012; 60: 1333–9.

17. Kimura T, Morimoto T, Nakagawa Y, et al. Antiplatelet therapy and stent thrombosis after sirolimus-eluting stent implantation. Circulation 2009; 119: 987–95.

18. Airoldi F, Colombo A, Morici N, et al. Incidence and predictors of drug-eluting stent thrombosis during and after discontinuation of thienopyridine treatment. Circulation 2007; 116: 745–54.

19. Lindenauer PK, Pekow P, Wang K, et al. Perioperative beta-blocker therapy and mortality after major noncardiac surgery. N Engl J Med 2005; 353: 349–61.

20. Beattie WS, Wijeysundera DN, Karkouti K, et al. Does tight heart rate control improve beta-blocker efficacy? An updated analysis of the noncardiac surgical randomized trials. Anesth Analg 2008; 106: 1039–48.

21. POISE Study Group. Effects of extended-release metoprolol succinate in patients undergoing non-cardiac surgery (POISE trial): a randomized controlled trial. Lancet 2008; 371: 1839–47.

22. Schouten O, Boersma E, Hoeks SE, et al. Fluvastatin and perioperative events in patients undergoing vascular surgery. N Engl J Med 2009; 361: 980–9.

23. Calleja AM, Dommaraju S, Gaddam R, et al. Cardiac risk in patients aged >75 years with asymptomatic, severe aortic stenosis undergoing noncardiac surgery. Am J Cardiol 2010; 105: 1159–63.

24. O'Keefe JH, Shub C, Rettke SR. Risk of noncardiac surgical procedures in patients with aortic stenosis. Mayo Clin Proc 1989; 64: 400–5.

25. Torsher LC, Shub C, Rettke SR, Brown DL. Risk of patients with severe aortic stenosis undergoing noncardiac surgery. Am J Cardiol 1998; 81: 448–52.

26. Dhillon A, Khanna A, Randhawa MS, et al. Perioperative outcomes of patients with hypertrophic cardiomyopathy undergoing noncardiac surgery. Heart 2016, epub ahead of print June 2016.

30 Miscellaneous Cardiac Topics: Cardiac Masses and Tumors, Pregnancy, HIV and Heart Disease, Cocaine and the Heart, Chemotherapy and Heart Disease, Chest X-Ray

Practical Cardiovascular Medicine, First Edition. Elias B. Hanna.
© 2017 John Wiley & Sons Ltd. Published 2017 by John Wiley & Sons Ltd.

1. CARDIAC MASSES

I. Differential diagnosis of a cardiac mass

The differential diagnosis of a cardiac mass includes four entities: (1) echo artifact or normal variant; (2) thrombus; (3) vegetation; (4) cardiac tumor (Table 30.1).

A *thrombus* usually occurs at specific cardiac locations in association with specific cardiac conditions (LV apex in patients with apical akinesis, right-sided chambers in patients with pacemaker leads). A *vegetation* arises from the free edge of a valve, on the side of the upstream chamber, and may occasionally involve the subvalvular apparatus; when large and visible, it is usually associated with a significant valvular regurgitation. A *myxoma* usually originates from the interatrial septum through a stalk, while a *fibroelastoma* often originates from the free edge of a valve, on the side of the downstream chamber.

II. Cardiac tumors; focus on atrial myxoma

A. General features

About 85% of primary cardiac tumors are benign, and of those, myxoma is the most common subtype. The relative frequency of *myxoma* in pathological and surgical series is 50% of all primary tumors (~50–75 % of benign tumors).[1,2] The second most common cardiac tumor is *papillary fibroelastoma* (involves the mitral or aortic valve). Other benign cardiac tumors include lipomas, rhabdomyoma, and hemangiomas. Most valvular tumors are papillary fibroelastomas. Primary malignant cardiac tumors are very rare and include angiosarcoma, the most common type, and rhabdomyosarcoma.

Secondary metastatic malignancies are 20 times more common than primary cardiac tumors. However, these malignancies often involve the pericardium leading to effusions, less commonly involve the myocardium, and least commonly involve the endocardium.[3] In fact, a cavitary or endocardial mass is usually a primary cardiac tumor rather than a metastatic malignancy.

Cardiac myxomas, more specifically, are characterized by polygonal cells in an extracellular matrix of acid-mucopolysaccharides. They are thought to arise from remnants of subendocardial primitive mesenchymal cells in the fossa ovalis and endocardium.[4] Anatomically, myxomas typically originate from the interatrial septum (fossa ovalis) and extend into the LA (75%) or RA (15%) (Figure 30.1).[5,6] About 3–4% of myxomas arise from the LV or RV wall. Rarely, atrial myxomas may arise from the mitral valve or the atrial wall. Myxomas are present at multiple locations in 5% of patients, more so in familial cases.

Table 30.1 Echocardiographic features allowing the differential diagnosis of a cardiac mass.

---

1. **Variants or artifacts**
   - RA: Eustachian valve, Chiari network, crista terminalis
   - LA: calcified aortic valve projecting inside the LA (beam width artifact)
   - Aortic valve: nodules of Arantius, Lambl excrescences[a]
   - Mitral valve: thick myxomatous valve, elongated chordae, flail chordae
   - RV: moderator band (between apex and septum)
   - Interatrial septum: lipomatous hypertrophy of the septum secundum sparing the fossa ovalis (dumbbell-shaped)
2. **Features favoring cardiac thrombus**
   Thrombus occurs in association with specific cardiac conditions at the following locations:
   - LA appendage in atrial fibrillation
   - LA appendage ± main LA in mitral stenosis
   - LV in case of apical akinesis
   - Prosthetic valve
   - Right-sided pacemaker leads or indwelling catheters
   - Right heart in case of venous thrombus in transition
3. **Features favoring a vegetation**
   - Originates from a valve, usually the free edge of a valve, on the upstream side (LA in mitral endocarditis, LV in aortic endocarditis). May rarely come off the chordae, or the LA wall if underlying MR is present
   - Significant valvular regurgitation is usually present with a large vegetation
   - Abnormal valvular structure (abnormal baseline structure ± valvular perforation or distortion related to the infectious process)
   - Morphology: irregularly shaped, highly mobile. Motion chaotic, does not track the leaflet motion (sometimes opposite)
4. **Features favoring a cardiac tumor**
   - ***Myxoma*** originates from the interatrial septum through a narrow stalk and extends into LA (75%) or RA (15%). Myxoma may also originate from RV or LV
     Morphology: myxoma is mobile, irregularly shaped ("grape cluster" appearance) with lucencies ± calcifications. This morphology may simulate vegetation. Unlike vegetation, myxoma may also be round and smooth-surfaced
   - ***Fibroelastoma*** originates from the aortic or mitral valve, mitral chordae, or papillary muscles. It is most often on the downstream side of the valve without significant regurgitation (≠ vegetation). At the aortic level, it may simulate Lambl excrescence but is larger (0.5–2 cm)

---

[a] Nodules of Arantius are small fibrous thickenings of the aortic valvular body, at the points where the leaflets abut. Lambl excrescences are small fibrous fibers arising from the edges of the aortic valve leaflets, mostly seen in patients older than 40 years.

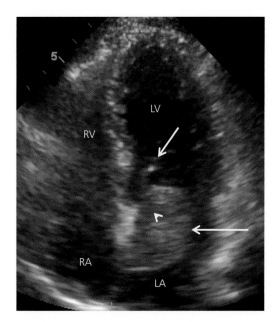

Figure 30.1 Apical four-chamber view showing a large left atrial mass (*horizontal arrow*). The mass does not seem to originate from the mitral valve (*oblique arrow*). It is round, smooth-surfaced with areas of lucencies (*arrowhead*). This is consistent with left atrial myxoma rather than vegetation.

B. Clinical presentation and diagnosis of myxoma

The median age at the time of diagnosis is 50–60 years, with an age range of 15–80 years and a slight female predominance.[5] Most patients are symptomatic at the time of diagnosis (85%). Three types of symptoms are encountered:

I. Obstructive signs and symptoms that result from the tumor obstructing the mitral inflow (70% of patients). This leads to paroxysmal dyspnea or syncope that may occur with specific body positions. A diastolic tumor plop may be heard, simulating S_3.

II. Peripheral embolization of the friable myxoma (in 30% of patients, cerebral in two-thirds of them). This is more common with lobulated than round tumors. One study found more emboli with smaller tumors.[5]

III. Constitutional symptoms, such as fever, rash, or weight loss (in 30% of patients, related to interleukin-6 release by the myxoma).

On echo, myxoma is characterized by an irregular shape with a "grape cluster" appearance, but it may also be round, smooth-surfaced. It is non-homogeneous, with areas of lucency (corresponding to hemorrhage) and sometimes calcifications.

The diagnosis is usually established by the typical location and echocardiographic features (Figure 30.1). TEE helps confirm the diagnosis, as it shows the narrow stalk originating from the fossa ovalis, defines whether there is valvular invasion, and excludes multiple masses, which is important for surgical planning. MRI may also be used for that purpose; in light of its high extracellular water content, myxoma has a high intensity on T2 images.

C. Treatment

Treatment of cardiac *myxomas* is surgical. Despite being a benign tumor, a myxoma is potentially lethal because of intracavitary or valvular obstruction, embolization, and induction of conduction and rhythm disturbances, all of which may occur while awaiting surgical correction. Therefore, surgery is usually performed promptly, or urgently in some series, after the diagnosis is made. Recurrence may occur in case of incomplete resection, intraoperative dissemination, or growth from a new focus, and is seen in 1–3 % of sporadic cases (~20% of familial cases), mostly in the first 4 years after resection.[7]

Valvular *fibroelastomas* also appear to have a significant embolization risk, and warrant removal in case of a prior embolic event, large size ≥ 1 cm, or mobility.

Rhabdomyoma is the most common pediatric cardiac tumor. It may occur sporadically or in conjunction with tuberous sclerosis. It generally arises from the ventricular myocardium and regresses spontaneously (very good prognosis).

2. PREGNANCY AND HEART DISEASE

Pregnancy is associated with a 50% increase in blood volume and with reduced systemic and pulmonary vascular resistances. Preload is increased while afterload is reduced, which leads to increased stroke volume. In addition, heart rate increases by 20%. All this increases cardiac output by 40–50%. The increase in blood volume and cardiac output peaks in the second trimester (24 weeks) then plateaus.[8] Cardiac output decreases with supine position (caval compression) and increases with lateral position. Both SBP and DBP decline, reaching a nadir in mid-pregnancy, with a more marked drop of DBP (from the reduced vascular resistance). Systemic vascular resistance starts to rise in the third trimester, at which time BP slightly rises, although it remains lower than pre-conception, and cardiac output stops increasing.

Cardiac output further increases during labor and delivery (60–80%), partly because of the high adrenergic tone, and partly because each uterine contraction pumps blood into the intravascular space. Epidural analgesia may reduce preload and limit the rise in cardiac output.

After delivery, preload abruptly increases as IVC compression is relieved and as blood leaves the congested uterus over the next 1–3 days ("autotransfusion"). Thus, cardiac output continues to rise after delivery. Preload may also transiently decrease with bleeding, and this is more likely to occur with cesarean delivery as it incurs more blood loss (1000 ml vs. 500 ml). The eventual increase in preload explains how pulmonary edema may occur in the first few days after delivery. Afterload increases with uterine contractions, then abruptly drops as the uterus relaxes post-delivery.

A loud S_1, an S_3, and a mild midsystolic murmur (2 or 3/6) may be normally heard. A mild RV heave and a displaced apical impulse may be felt.

A split S_2, an S_4, a loud systolic murmur, or any diastolic murmur are abnormal.

I. High-risk cardiac conditions during which pregnancy is better avoided[9]

A. Eisenmenger syndrome, or primary or secondary severe pulmonary hypertension
Severe pulmonary hypertension is associated with a 30–50% maternal mortality and is an absolute contraindication to pregnancy.[9,10]

B. Severe AS, mainly if symptomatic
The increased preload may lead to pulmonary edema, while the striking afterload reduction in a patient with fixed obstruction and fixed cardiac output may lead to hypotension and collapse.[11] This may even be more prominent around delivery, when a sudden increase in preload and a drop in afterload may occur. Pregnancy should be delayed until AS is corrected; patients with non-calcified AS may be treated with percutaneous valvuloplasty to avoid the hazard of prosthetic valves. If AS is discovered during pregnancy, percutaneous valvuloplasty may need to be performed in patients who develop severe symptoms.

Pregnancy is risky even in asymptomatic patients. Yet, a subset of asymptomatic severe AS patients may have a low mortality during pregnancy; this subset consists of patients who are asymptomatic on stress testing with good functional capacity and BP response. There is no need to discourage pregnancy in these patients.[9]

C. Severe MS, even if asymptomatic
The increased preload and tachycardia associated with pregnancy exaggerate the transmitral gradient, particularly in the third trimester and during delivery.[11] MS should be corrected before pregnancy. Otherwise, if pregnancy occurs before correction, β-blockers and judicious doses of diuretics are used during pregnancy. PMBV may need to be performed in pregnant patients with uncontrolled symptoms.

D. Any cardiomyopathy or valvular disease with EF < 30%
In one study, patients with dilated cardiomyopathy and moderate or severe LV dysfunction or NYHA class III/IV (mostly idiopathic) had a 70–80% risk of cardiac events during pregnancy or postpartum. These consisted mainly of HF decompensations, arrhythmias (AF, atrial flutter), and one transient ischemic attack (among 18 patients). These complications were managed medically and no maternal death occurred; one fetal death occurred during maternal pulmonary edema.[12,13] Pregnancy is preferably avoided in these patients, but some patients may want to proceed in light of the limited mortality risk. Those who proceed with pregnancy may continue β-blocker therapy, hydralazine, digoxin, and low-dose diuretic; ACE-I and aldosterone antagonists are stopped.

E. Aortic root dilatation ≥ 45 mm

F. Complex cyanotic congenital heart disease (tetralogy of Fallot, Ebstein, Fontan circulation)
Cyanosis, by itself, reduces fetal growth, particularly when arterial O_2 saturation is <85% at rest or stress. In the absence of HF or ventricular dysfunction, the maternal risk may be low, but the fetal risk is always high when O_2 saturation <85%. In fact, fetal survival is only 12% in the latter case. In corrected tetralogy of Fallot, carefully assess for any residual defect before giving advice about the safety of pregnancy. In the absence of significant VSD, pulmonic stenosis, or pulmonic regurgitation, and in the case of a normal PA pressure and RV function, pregnancy is well tolerated. In a Fontan patient with normal ventricular function, no cyanosis, and no significant valvular regurgitation, pregnancy may be possible.

> *Patients with any of the above conditions (A–F) should be counseled against pregnancy, unless the condition is a valvular condition (MS or AS) that is corrected before conception. On the other hand, if an unplanned pregnancy occurs, early termination is considered in some, but not all of these conditions.* Early termination is most definitely considered in patients with severe pulmonary hypertension, severe LV dysfunction that is also severely symptomatic, cyanosis with hypoxemia <85%, or prior peripartum cardiomyopathy with persistent LV dysfunction. Conversely, severe AS, severe MS, or compensated LV dysfunction may be managed at a tertiary center without termination, with close follow-ups and medical therapy (+ procedural therapy, if needed for AS and MS); termination may be considered if severe symptoms develop early on, in the first trimester.

II. Cardiac conditions that are usually well tolerated during pregnancy, but in which careful cardiac evaluation and clinical and echo follow-up are warranted[9]

A. ASD, even if a large left-to-right shunt is present with RA and RV enlargement.[14] In pregnancy, the systemic resistance decreases more than the pulmonary resistance, which may reduce the left-to-right shunt. Closure before pregnancy is preferred, but pregnancy should be allowed to continue if a large ASD is diagnosed during pregnancy, as complications are uncommon.[14,15]

B. Small VSD; small PDA.

C. Severe asymptomatic TR, even if RV and RA are dilated.

D. Severe MR and AI are usually well tolerated when LV function is normal and the patient is asymptomatic. This is because pregnancy is associated with reduced afterload and increased heart rate (reduces AI symptoms). The increased preload may, however, accelerate LV dilatation and warrants careful monitoring. Exercise testing is recommended before pregnancy to confirm the asymptomatic state.[9]

E. Mild or moderate asymptomatic AS.

F. Severe pulmonic stenosis. In the absence of RV dysfunction, pulmonic stenosis is usually well tolerated during pregnancy.

G. Hypertrophic obstructive cardiomyopathy. While afterload reduction may increase the LVOT gradient, the increase in preload counteracts it, and pregnancy is usually well tolerated in HOCM. Symptoms, if present, are controlled with β-blockers.

H. Marfan syndrome with aortic root <4 cm. Two studies showed no fatality during these patients' pregnancy and no significant acceleration of aortic dilatation.[16,17] β-blockers are administered during pregnancy to reduce aortic growth, and frequent ultrasound surveillance is performed (Q 1–2 months). Patients with aortic size of 4–4.4 cm have a significant aortic growth during pregnancy, occasionally a striking growth with a risk of dissection.

Note: Antibiotic prophylaxis is not recommended in women with native valvular disease undergoing vaginal delivery, except for a prior history of endocarditis.

III. Cardiac indications for cesarean section

Cesarean delivery attenuates the rise in cardiac output at the price of more blood loss and more abrupt hemodynamic fluctuations than vaginal delivery, especially because spinal anesthesia is usually needed with cesarean delivery. Also, cesarean delivery increases the risk of venous thrombosis. Thus, vaginal delivery with assisted second stage is preferred in the majority of patients; epidural anesthesia is advised to limit the increase in cardiac output (unless the patient is anticoagulated). Cesarean delivery is indicated for obstetric reasons and in the following three cardiac conditions:[15]

- Unstable aorta
- Warfarin anticoagulation around delivery time (vaginal delivery is associated with a high risk of neonatal intracranial hemorrhage)
- Severe HF or severe AS with active HF and life-threatening symptoms, wherein the limited cardiac output reserve cannot provide the high output required for vaginal delivery

IV. Mechanical prosthetic valves in pregnancy: anticoagulation management

Patients with mechanical prosthetic valves have a strikingly increased risk of valve thrombosis and thromboembolism during pregnancy. One large meta-analysis has shown that even when adequately anticoagulated with warfarin throughout pregnancy, the thromboembolic risk is ~4%. *The risk drastically increases when heparin is substituted for warfarin between weeks 6 and 12 (the risk increases from 4% to 9%, even if heparin is only used for 6 weeks), with a doubling of the maternal mortality risk (from 2% to 4%).*[18] The thromboembolic risk is much higher if adjusted-dose unfractionated heparin is used throughout pregnancy (25%). Those historical risks were mainly seen with cage–ball and single-leaflet disk prostheses, and the dosing of heparin was unclear. The risk may currently be lower with St. Jude bileaflet valves, especially in the aortic position, and with appropriate heparin dosing during the 6-week substitution.

Conversely, while warfarin is a much more effective anticoagulant in pregnancy than heparin, it traverses the placental barrier and is associated with a fetopathy risk of ~6% (mainly bone and facial hypoplasia, sometimes mental retardation), and a risk of spontaneous abortion. This risk mostly results from warfarin administration between 6 and 12 weeks, especially if the required dose is >5 mg/day. The same meta-analysis has shown that when unfractionated heparin is substituted at or before 6 weeks of gestation, the risk of fetopathy is totally eliminated, at the price of a drastic increase in maternal thromboembolism. A study of LMWH has shown a similarly high risk of maternal thromboembolism with weight-based dosing, but less so with monitoring of Xa activity.[19] Heparin is a large molecule that does not traverse the placental barrier, and it is safe from the fetal standpoint.

Thus, continuous intravenous UFH (rather than subcutaneous heparin) or subcutaneous LMWH may be substituted for warfarin as soon as pregnancy is recognized, ideally before 6 weeks, and administered until 12 weeks (both agents receive a class IIa recommendation if the required warfarin dose is >5 mg/d, class IIb if the required warfarin dose is ≤5 mg/d). Warfarin is resumed after 12 weeks, until 36 weeks. Alternatively, when the risk of valve thrombosis is high and the warfarin dose is ≤5 mg, continuous warfarin therapy throughout 36 weeks may be considered and discussed with the patient (class IIa recommendation).

Intravenous heparin is started at 36 weeks, 2–3 weeks before the anticipated delivery, to prevent the fetal intracranial hemorrhage associated with warfarin (the latter has a longer half-life in the fetus).

When UFH is used in the substitution period, PTT should be monitored and kept over twice the control. When LMWH is used, anti-Xa activity should be measured 4–6 hours post-injection and kept at 0.8–1.2 units/ml. With warfarin, the INR goal is 2.5–3.5. Aspirin should be continued along with anticoagulation.

Both warfarin and heparin are compatible with ***breastfeeding***, as none of them is secreted in breast milk.[20]

V. Peripartum cardiomyopathy (PPCM)

PPCM is LV systolic dysfunction that develops in the last month of pregnancy or within 5 months postpartum, without any prior heart disease. Hypertension frequently coexists with PPCM and is a risk factor for PPCM. Older age, African-American race, multiparity, and multifetal pregnancies are other risk factors. Depending on its severity, hypertension does not necessarily imply a diagnosis of hypertensive cardiomyopathy and is consistent with PPCM.[20,21] In fact, severe acute HTN usually causes pulmonary edema through acute diastolic rather than systolic dysfunction.[22] The mechanism of PPCM is likely immunological.

A. Prognosis, LV recovery

LV function fully recovers in ~55–60% of PPCM cases within 6 months of the diagnosis. Before recovery, however, PPCM is associated with a significant risk of complications, including a mortality of 3–10% (sudden death or HF death, mainly within 6 months of the diagnosis), severe progressive HF requiring heart transplantation in 6%, and thromboembolic complications.[20,21] PPCM may be associated with a higher risk of LV thrombus than other forms of dilated cardiomyopathy, and potentially a higher risk of embolization. This higher thromboembolic risk may be due to the hypercoagulable state of pregnancy and the first 2 postpartum months.

B. Treatment

Similarly to any systolic HF, standard HF therapy is used, even if it is unclear whether this therapy specifically increases the recovery of PPCM. ACE inhibitors are contraindicated during pregnancy and are of unclear safety during lactation. PPCM is thus treated with β-blockers, hydralazine, digoxin, and loop diuretics, during pregnancy or lactation. Spironolactone may be used in the postpartum, including in breastfeeding women. Since PPCM is associated with a high thromboembolic risk, an expert review suggests anticoagulation therapy until EF improves to over 35%.[20] If PPCM recovers, the tapering and discontinuation of these drugs may be safe, but close monitoring is required, as late deterioration of LV function has been described.[23]

PPCM is associated with a high early risk of sudden death before LV function eventually recovers. Since this risk of sudden death is only transient in patients who eventually recover, a wearable defibrillator vest rather than an ICD may be justified. ICD is indicated in patients who do not recover their LV function within 6 months of medical therapy.

Breastfeeding is safe, and has even been associated with a higher rate of LV recovery.

Subsequent pregnancies should be avoided in patients with PPCM, even in those who recover their LV function. In one report, pregnancy was associated with a 20% mortality and 50% risk of worsening of LV function in patients with persistent LV dysfunction; in those who recovered LV function, pregnancy was safer, with no fatality, but a 20% risk of relapse.[24]

VI. Cardiovascular drugs during pregnancy (see Table 30.2)

Table 30.2 Cardiovascular drugs and pregnancy.

- ACE-I, ARB, aldosterone antagonists: contraindicated during pregnancy[a]
- Adenosine: safe
- Aspirin 81 mg is safe (higher doses should be avoided)
- β-Blockers (labetolol, metoprolol) have been extensively and safely used in pregnancy, but may rarely cause intrauterine growth retardation or neonatal hypoglycemia. Atenolol may be teratogenic and should be avoided. Limited data available for carvedilol
- Calcium channel blockers: less studied than β-blockers, but appear safe. β-blockers are preferred for arrhythmias. Most experience exists with verapamil and nifedipine
- Digoxin: safe
- Diuretics: may be used to treat HF. Avoid the aggressive use of diuretics, as they may reduce placental flow
- Amiodarone: crosses the placenta and may cause neonatal goiter. May be used if necessary
- Sotalol, flecainide: relatively safe
- Hydralazine, methyldopa: safe
- Nitrates: may be used in HF, but preferably avoided
- Clopidogrel: probably safe, but limited data
- Statins, ezetimibe: contraindicated

[a] ACE-I is secreted in breast milk and is also better avoided during lactation. β-Blockers, digoxin, and hydralazine are only secreted in a small amount in milk, and may be used during lactation (except for atenolol and sotalol)

VII. Arrhythmias during pregnancy

Pregnancy is associated with an increased risk of arrhythmias, whether structural heart disease is present or not. There is a significant increase in the risk of SVT, especially in the third trimester (AVNRT, AVRT, incessant atrial tachycardia). AF and atrial flutter are rare during pregnancy and are usually associated with cardiomyopathies, valvular or congenital heart disease, or hyperthyroidism. AF may rarely be seen in healthy pregnancies (lone AF).

Carotid sinus massage is safe in pregnancy. Adenosine, β-blockers, or calcium channel blockers may be used for SVT. DC cardioversion is also safe and may be used, if needed, for hemodynamic instability.

VIII. MI and pregnancy

The risk of MI increases three- to fourfold during pregnancy, especially during the third trimester and the first 6 weeks postpartum. The MI is most commonly a STEMI (75%), and usually occurs in patients older than 30. It is associated with a high mortality of 11–20%. In case series where angiography or autopsy was performed, the following processes were found:[25,26]

i. Coronary atherosclerosis with or without thrombosis in 40% of the cases
ii. Coronary artery dissection in 27% of the cases, frequently involving multiple coronary arteries (~50%), and most commonly involving the left main or LAD
iii. Coronary thrombosis without underlying atherosclerosis in ~15%
iv. Normal coronary arteries in 13% (likely coronary spasm)

In a more recent series, coronary artery dissection was the most common cause of pregnancy-related MI (43%).[26] Coronary dissection is relatively more frequent in the postpartum than the antepartum period. Patients with coronary artery dissection have an increased risk of iatrogenic coronary dissection during the contrast injections of diagnostic angiography and a risk of further propagating the dissection during PCI; thus, PCI may be reserved for severe obstruction/occlusion of proximal segments with impaired flow and active ischemia.[26] Also, fibrinolytic therapy is contraindicated in coronary dissection.

IX. Hypertension and pregnancy

A. Types
- Chronic HTN, present before pregnancy
- Gestational HTN: new HTN arising beyond 20 weeks of pregnancy, without proteinuria
- Pre-eclampsia: new HTN or worsening of a chronic HTN, associated with proteinuria >0.3 g/24 hours

B. Treatment
Methyldopa, hydralazine, β-blockers (especially labetalol), nifedipine

3. HIV AND HEART DISEASE

I. Pericardial disease
Pericardial effusion is the most common cardiac manifestation of HIV infection, with an incidence of 11% per year in patients with CD4 count <200 not receiving antiretroviral therapy. It is usually asymptomatic and small but is seen with lower CD4 counts, which implies a more advanced disease and a 2.2× increase in adjusted mortality despite the usually small size.[27] Patients with a moderate or large effusion may have a high risk of progression to tamponade. Also, a large or symptomatic effusion frequently, in over 50% of the cases, has a specific diagnosis: infectious (tuberculosis, purulent, opportunistic infection), or malignant (especially lymphoma or Kaposi sarcoma).[28]

II. HIV cardiomyopathy
See Chapter 5.

III. Pulmonary hypertension (PH)
The prevalence of pulmonary arterial hypertension (PAH) in HIV is ~0.5%. PH may also be due to lung disease or left HF, which increases the overall prevalence of any PH in HIV, particularly mild PH, up to 30%.[29] As opposed to myocardial and pericardial processes, PAH does not appear to correlate with CD4 count, and was described in patients with CD4 count over 900.[30] Pathologically, lesions are similar to idiopathic PAH (plexiform arteriopathy). PAH results from circulating cytokines or circulating HIV antigens activating endothelial cells. Antiretroviral therapy improves PAH and survival in these patients. Epoprostenol and bosentan were also effective in small studies.[31]

IV. CAD
Patients with HIV have accelerated atherosclerosis and an almost doubled risk of MI, particularly HIV patients older than 50.[32] The risk of MI is further increased by protease inhibitors, which increase triglycerides and the number of small LDL particles, and reduce HDL. Truncal fat redistribution (lipodystrophy) may occur with HIV regardless of the type of therapy and may lead to metabolic syndrome.

4. COCAINE AND THE HEART

I. Myocardial ischemia

A. Causes
Cocaine induces myocardial ischemia through several mechanisms:

1. α+ effect leads to coronary vasoconstriction.
2. Severe HTN and tachycardia increase myocardial O2 demands.
3. Cocaine promotes platelet aggregation and thrombus formation through increased plasminogen activator inhibitor (PAI).
4. Chronic cocaine use promotes atherosclerosis.

All of these effects are strongly promoted by concomitant cigarette or alcohol use (alcohol is synergistic with cocaine). Fifty percent of patients with cocaine-related MI have normal coronaries.

B. Presentation
Chest pain mainly occurs within 1 hour of cocaine use, but can occur up to several hours later (up to 36–96 hours later), because the concentration of active metabolites increases hours later and may lead to delayed vasoconstriction. Between 7% and 20% of patients presenting with chest pain to urban emergency units have a positive cocaine screen.[33]

C. Diagnosis
Approximately 6% of patients with cocaine-associated chest pain have MI (as manifested by elevated CK or troponin), half of whom have normal coronary arteries.[33] The remaining patients have ischemia that is not sustained enough to lead to MI, or non-cardiac pleuritic pain.

MI is difficult to diagnose by ECG, because many cocaine users have an abnormal baseline ECG with ST elevation (early repolarization, LVH). On the other hand, ST elevation can be related to spasm rather than thrombotic occlusion. Thus, ST elevation is sensitive but not very specific in cocaine users.

Cocaine use is diagnosed by a urinary screen of both cocaine and its metabolites. Cocaine half-life is 60–90 minutes, but its metabolites persist 24–72 hours. In chronic high-dose users, cocaine metabolites may be found for up to 2 weeks.

Always think of aortic dissection and rule it out at least clinically and by chest X-ray.

D. Treatment of cocaine-related MI or ischemia
1. Medical therapy
The following three treatments are first-line, class I therapies that should be administered to most patients with cocaine-induced chest pain:[34]

1. Aspirin.
2. Nitroglycerin, which reduces vasospasm and hypertension.
3. Benzodiazepines, which reduce the central sympathetic stimulatory effects of cocaine, and thus reduce tachycardia and hypertension.

The following therapies are class IIb therapies that may be used selectively in patients with persistent hypertension or chest pain despite the first-line therapies:

4. Verapamil or diltiazem in the absence of HF, or long-acting dihydropyridine, orally (preferably) or intravenously.
5. Phentolamine (α-blocker) may also be used as a second-line agent for persistent ischemia or hypertension.

Avoid β-blockers acutely. β-Blockers increase vasospasm, as they lead to unopposed α activation. While combined α- and β-blockers may seem safe, labetalol was associated with an increased risk of seizure and death in animal studies, probably because it is much more a β-blocker than an α-blocker; thus, even α/β-blockers should be avoided acutely. Most cocaine users continue to use cocaine after discharge, and chronic β-blocker therapy should therefore be avoided in most patients, except in case of a strong compelling reason, such as LV systolic dysfunction.

2. Role of invasive management and thrombolysis
If chest pain persists despite the first four treatments listed above, and ECG shows persistent ST elevation, emergent coronary angiography ± PCI should be performed. Thrombolytics are preferably avoided in cocaine users because of the concomitant hypertension that contraindicates their use, and because ST elevation may be a persistent spasm rather than a thrombus. Yet, as per AHA guidelines, thombolytics may be used in persistent ischemia with a clear-cut ischemic ST elevation despite nitroglycerin, benzodiazepines, and calcium channel blockers, if a coronary angiogram is not available.

3. Role of stress testing
If chest pain resolves with the initial measures and cardiac enzymes are negative, the patient may be discharged at 12–24 hours (a stress test is optional rather than mandatory).

II. Other cardiac complications of cocaine
A. LV dysfunction is seen in 7% of chronic cocaine users. LV dysfunction results from ischemia and/or catecholamine toxicity (contraction band necrosis, tachycardia-mediated cardiomyopathy).
B. Supraventricular or ventricular arrhythmias. Arrhythmias mainly occur in patients with cocaine-induced myocardial ischemia or LV dysfunction.
C. Aortic dissection.
D. Hypertensive crisis. Hypertension may be treated with nitroglycerin, nitroprusside, nicardipine, or phentolamine.
E. Brugada pattern on ECG (RBBB with ST elevation in V_1–V_2).
F. Endocarditis with intravenous cocaine use. The intravenous use of cocaine is associated with a higher risk of endocarditis than the intravenous use of other drugs. Unlike the endocarditis associated with other drugs, the endocarditis of cocaine users more often involves the left-sided cardiac valves than the right-sided valves.

5. CHEMOTHERAPY AND HEART DISEASE

I. Cardiomyopathy
A. Anthracyclines
Anthracyclines cause myocardial free radical formation with subsequent myocardial necrosis and irreversible, progressive myocardial injury. The progression may, however, be stopped with early detection and interruption of therapy, and with the use of ACE inhibitors and carvedilol.

Cardiomyopathy may occur *early on*, i.e., during therapy or within a year of completion of therapy, in 2% of the patients, or may develop *late*, i.e., over a year after therapy, sometimes even decades later. In fact, the prevalence of anthracycline toxicity increases with time, especially in children.[35,36] The risk is dose-dependent and increases after a cumulative doxorubicine dose of 300 mg/m², and particularly a dose of 550 mg/m² (26% frequency at this dose). ACE-I and carvedilol have been positively studied as a preventive therapy for anthracycline toxicity in patients receiving high doses of an anthracycline or those with a rise in troponin after chemotherapy.[36,37] An intracellular chelator, dexrazoxane, may be used in patients receiving cumulative doses over 300 mg/m².

Rarely, acute immediate cardiotoxicity occurs during infusion; this is usually transient.

LVEF should be measured before therapy initiation. Therapy should be avoided in patients with EF <30%, and preferably avoided in patients with EF 30–50%. In patients with EF >50%, EF measurement is repeated after a cumulative dose of 250–300 mg/m², and therapy stopped if EF decreases by ≥10% or to <50%.[38] The occurrence of new diastolic dysfunction may precede systolic dysfunction and indicates early cardiotoxicity.

B. Cyclophosphamide
Cyclophosphamide, when used in high individual doses, may induce acute cardiac toxicity consisting of myopericarditis and pericardial effusion within 10 days of therapy. This acute toxicity lasts less than a week, without long-term sequelae or cumulative effect in patients who survive the acute cardiomyopathy.[38] Unfortunately, the acute cardiomyopathy has a significant mortality of up to 12% when very high doses are used.

C. Trastuzumab (Her-2 receptor antagonist used in breast cancer)

Trastuzumab inhibits epidermal growth factor (EGF), and thus reduces normal myocardial growth, repair, and survival. The incidence of trastuzumab-induced cardiotoxicity is 2–7%, and this increases up to 27% when it is combined with other cardiotoxic agents. The cardiotoxicity is usually reversible after cessation of therapy, after a mean of 1.5 months. Some institutions allow the reuse of trastuzumab along with HF therapies after EF improves.

II. Myocardial ischemia

A. 5-Fluorouracil (5-FU) and capecitabine. These antimetabolites may cause coronary thrombosis or coronary macro- or microvascular spasm, within 2–5 days of therapy and lasting up to 48 hours.[36] High doses and continuous 5-FU infusions have higher cardiotoxicity than bolus administration. The risk is higher in patients with underlying CAD.

B. Bevacizumab (Avastin) can cause arterial thrombosis through endothelial injury. It is associated with up to 1.5% risk of acute MI.[36]

C. Paclitaxel and docetaxel may cause myocardial ischemia and infarction during and up to 14 days after therapy.[39] Paclitaxel may also cause bradycardia and ventricular arrhythmias and may increase the risk of anthracycline-induced cardiomyopathy.

D. Cisplatin and carboplatin may cause vasospasm or vascular injury leading to myocardial ischemia. Hypertension is also a common side effect.

6. CHEST X-RAY

I. Chest X-ray in heart failure (see Figures 30.2, 30.3)

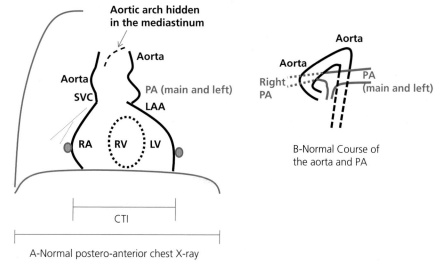

Figure 30.2 (a) Normal posteroanterior chest X-ray. Note that the RV does not have a shadow, and LA does not have a shadow (except for LA appendage [LAA]). The lung vessels are seen in the lower lung fields and do not extend to the outer third of the lungs. The cardiothoracic index (CTI) measures the width of the cardiac silhouette from the outermost right point to the outermost left point (*dots*), and divides it by the widest thoracic cage diameter (usually at the costophrenic angles). **(b) Normal course of the PA and aorta**, explaining how they project on chest X-ray posteroanterior view. The right hilum is slightly lower than the left.

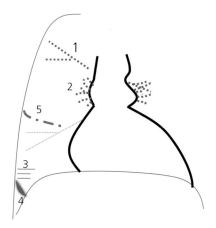

Figure 30.3 Chest X-ray in HF. (1) Cephalization and vessel extension to the outer third of the lung fields; (2) perihilar haziness and peribronchial cuffing; (3) Kerley B lines; (4) right pleural effusion; (5) minor fissure effusion.

A. Early signs of LV failure

a. *Cardiomegaly* (cardiothoracic index >0.5)

b. *Cephalization of pulmonary vessels.* Normally, the pulmonary capillary pressure is low at the upper lobe (~0 mmHg), allowing the alveolar pressure to collapse those capillaries and prevent flow (zone 1); thus, the lower lobe vessels are wider than the upper lobe vessels. In addition, pulmonary vessels do not normally extend to the outer third of the lungs. When the LA pressure increases, the high pulmonary capillary pressure prevents capillary collapse at the upper lobes while creating a leak into the interstitium of the lower lobes. This leak compresses the lower lobe vessels and diverts blood to the upper lobes, which explains why the upper lobe vessels become at least as wide as the lower lobe vessels.

c. *Vessels extend towards the outer third of the lung fields and are hazy.* Beware that an underpenetrated CXR may exaggerate pulmonary vascular findings.

B. At a later stage, interstitial pulmonary edema occurs and manifests as:

a. *Perihilar haziness, perivascular haziness, and peribronchial cuffing:* the bronchi, as well as both the hilar and peripheral pulmonary arteries, lose their sharpness and become hazy and "fluffy" from the interstitial edema. The thick bronchial walls may lead to "doughnut-like" densities throughout the lung fields.

b. *Kerley B lines:* represent edema in the interlobular septa and manifest as 1–2 cm horizontal, pleural-based lines, at the lower lungs ("stepladder").

c. *Pleural effusions,* right greater than left. Isolated left pleural effusion is possible but rare (<10%).

Normally, the minor fissure, a right-sided fissure, may be seen on the frontal chest X-ray (CXR) view. The oblique fissures are not seen on the frontal view, as the frontal view is parallel to the oblique fissures rather than orthogonal to them. Both fissures may be seen on the lateral view. During HF, edema may be seen in the minor fissure and may collect as a round opacity that simulates a tumor ("pseudotumor") but resolves with diuresis.

C. At the latest stage, alveolar pulmonary edema is seen and manifests as "white" patches, predominantly over the perihilar area ("batwing" appearance).

Note that all of these signs may be absent in patients with chronically elevated PCWP, in whom the lymphatic drainage prevents the occurrence of any edema. Even the heart size may be normal in patients with diastolic HF (LV hypertrophy, restrictive cardiomyopathy). On the other hand, in patients with acute HF, many or all of these signs are present.

The absence of cardiomegaly in patients with radiographic HF implies three possibilities: (i) de novo acute HF (acute MI, myocarditis, acute MR/AI); (ii) diastolic HF (no LV dilatation); (iii) non- cardiogenic pulmonary edema.

The presence of interstitial and/or alveolar edema with sharp costophrenic angles, i.e., without any pleural effusion, argues against HF and favors the diagnosis of non-cardiogenic pulmonary edema or severe bilateral pneumonia.

A radiographic delay of 1–2 days may be seen between normalization of pulmonary capillary pressure and resolution of pulmonary edema. Pleural effusions may take a long time to resolve.

In pulmonary arterial hypertension, the hila are enlarged as in HF, but as opposed to HF, there is constriction and pruning of the peripheral vessels.

II. Various forms of cardiomegaly (see Figure 30.4)

A. False impression of cardiomegaly

CXR is normally taken in full inspiration, in which case the right hemidiaphragm normally projects over the ninth posterior rib or sixth anterior rib. Expiration or supine position makes the heart more horizontal and exaggerates the cardiac silhouette. Also, the cardiac silhouette is exaggerated in anteroposterior imaging (portable CXR), as the source is closer to the heart than in posteroanterior imaging. Supine positioning, anteroposterior imaging, and expiration exaggerate the cardiac silhouette and the vascular markings, including cephalization.

B. Enlarged RV

An enlarged RV expands to the left heart contour and makes the apex look up ("boot-shape"); however, the majority of adults have biventricular enlargement rather than isolated RV enlargement, and in that case this shape is uncommon.

C. Enlarged LV

In LV enlargement, the LV contour is displaced downward, sometimes even without an increase in cardiothoracic index. Conversely, anteroapical akinesis or aneurysm is characterized by a horizontal LV contour.

Generalized cardiac enlargement with a globular or water-bottle shape may indicate pericardial effusion but also cardiomyopathy.

In the absence of LV dilatation, LV hypertrophy may be associated with a normal cardiac silhouette or a slightly prominent apex, depending on whether the hypertrophy extends inward or outward.

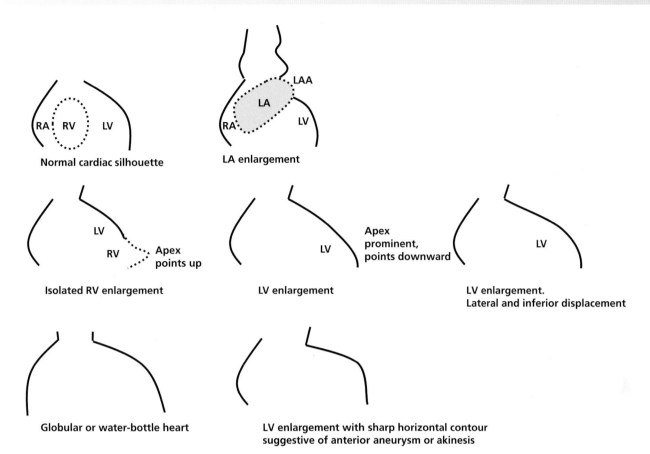

Figure 30.4 Various morphologies of cardiomegaly. LA enlargement is characterized by convex bulging of the LAA, and double density over the RA contour.

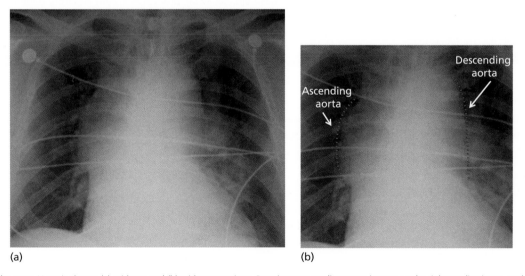

Figure 30.5 The same X-ray is shown (a) without and (b) with annotations. Prominent ascending aorta is seen on the right mediastinum, and descending aorta on the left mediastinum, as indicated by the interrupted lines. This indicates ascending and descending aortic dilatation, dissection, or simply elongation (uncoiling). This patient had ascending and descending aortic dissection.

III. Left atrial enlargement; aortic dilatation

Left atrial enlargement is recognized on the posteroanterior view as: (i) convex bulging of the shadow of the LA appendage (rather than straight line); (ii) widening of the carinal angle (>100°); (iii) double density over the RA shadow, implying that the LA is extending towards the RA (Figure 30.4). It is also recognized on the lateral view by a local posterior bulge of the upper cardiac silhouette (towards the spine).

Aortic dilatation is characterized by widening of the ascending aorta (on the right) or the descending aorta (left aortic knob fills the space between the aorta and the PA) (Figure 30.5). The widening of the ascending aortic shadow may also indicate elongated rather than dilated aorta.

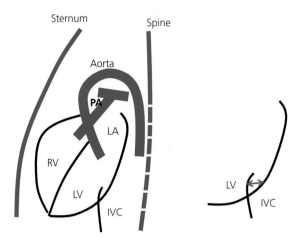

Figure 30.6 Lateral chest X-ray. Note that the LA shadow is surrounded by the aortic and PA shadows.
- When RV is enlarged, it expands superiorly and fills the retrosternal space for over a third of the sternal length, i.e., the distance from the top of the sternal notch to the xyphoid.
- When LV is enlarged, it bulges posteriorly towards the spine but also inferiorly below the shadow of the diaphragm. LV enlargement is suggested when the distance between the LV border and the IVC border becomes >17 mm (double arrow, right image).
- When LA enlarges, it causes a focal, round bulge of the upper cardiac silhouette towards the spine.
- Dilatation or elongation of the ascending or descending aorta may be seen. A dilated ascending aorta fills the anterior mediastinal space.

IV. Lateral chest X-ray
Note the features of LV, RV, and LA dilatation on the lateral CXR (Figure 30.6).

V. Chest X-ray in congenital heart disease
See Chapter 18, Figure 18.10.

QUESTIONS AND ANSWERS

Question 1. A 29-year-old woman of Columbian origin is at 30 weeks of gestation. She presents with cough productive of blood-tinged sputum, severe dyspnea, and hypoxia (O_2 saturation 80% on ambient air). On exam, BP = 150/90, pulse = 125 bpm, JVP is elevated, P_2 is loud, and diffuse crackles are heard. The differential diagnosis includes all of the following, *except* (multiple answers possible):
A. Peripartum cardiomyopathy
B. Pre-existing dilated cardiomyopathy
C. Chagas disease
D. Myocardial infarction from coronary dissection
E. Mitral stenosis from rheumatic heart disease
F. Severe HTN/pre-eclampsia with pulmonary edema

Question 2. The ECG of the patient in Question 1 shows sinus tachycardia at 125 bpm and P mitrale. She remains hypoxic despite high-flow O_2 therapy. Echo confirms severe mitral stenosis with a valvular gradient of 20 mmHg (heart rate 125 bpm), a valve area of 1.2 cm², and systolic PA pressure of 80 mmHg. What is the next step?
A. Intravenous metoprolol
B. Intravenous furosemide
C. Immediate sedation and intubation
D. All of the above

Question 3. The patient's pulmonary edema improved with furosemide and heart rate reduction to 75 bpm (maximally tolerated dose of metoprolol [50 mg bid]). She is extubated and ambulates with mild dyspnea. What is the next step?
A. Continue conservative management
B. Mitral valvuloplasty

Question 4. All the following antihypertensive drug(s) are used in pregnancy, *except*?
A. Methyldopa
B. Hydralazine
C. Labetalol
D. Nifedipine
E. Atenolol

Question 5. In which of the following conditions is pregnancy contraindicated? (multiple answers)
A. Severe pulmonary hypertension of any origin
B. Severe asymptomatic AS with normal EF

C. Severe symptomatic AS

D. Severe asymptomatic MS

E. Severe asymptomatic MR with normal EF

F. HOCM

G. Large ASD with large left-to-right shunt

H. Cyanotic congenital heart disease with O_2 saturation <85% (rest or stress)

I. Dilated cardiomyopathy with LVEF 25% and persistent NYHA class III–IV

Question 6. Should pregnancy occur anyway, in which of the conditions of Question 5 should termination of pregnancy be considered?

Question 7. Concerning HIV and heart disease, all of the following is true *except*:

A. Pericardial effusion is the most common cardiac manifestation of HIV

B. Pericardial effusion is usually small but associated with increased mortality

C. A large HIV-related effusion has a low risk of progression to tamponade and is rarely due to coinfections

D. HIV cardiomyopathy is often seen in patients with CD4 counts <400 and is associated with a high mortality risk (may approximate 50% at 2 years)

E. Endomyocardial biopsy may be needed in a HIV patient with progressive HF (to rule out opportunistic myocardial infections)

Question 8. A 33-year-old woman, 36 weeks pregnant, presents with severe dyspnea and hypoxemia. She has pulmonary edema by exam and X-ray. BP is 170/105, pulse is 110 bpm. ECG shows diffuse ST depression. Echo shows a non-dilated LV with global hypokinesis and EF of 25%, with no MS. What is the *least likely* diagnosis out of the following four?

A. Peripartum cardiomyopathy

B. Acute MI of pregnancy (NSTEMI)

C. Acute myocarditis

D. Pre-eclampsia

Question 9. A 29-year-old woman has severe MR from an anterior mitral leaflet prolapse. She is asymptomatic with normal LV dimension and EF of 65%. She is able to perform 11 minutes on treadmill Bruce protocol with exertional PA pressure <50 mmHg. She wants to conceive. What is the best advice?

A. She has a relatively low cardiac risk during pregnancy, overall favoring pregnancy now rather than pregnancy following mitral valve replacement. She should conceive now with close monitoring

B. Perform bioprosthetic mitral replacement, followed by pregnancy

C. Perform mechanical mitral replacement, followed by pregnancy

Question 10. A 26-year-old woman is pregnant at 12 weeks. She is asymptomatic. A murmur is heard during routine exam with split S_2. Echo shows a large ASD with L–R shunt, RV enlargement, and normal PA pressure. What is the next step?

A. Recommend pregnancy termination, considering the high maternal cardiac risk

B. Pursue the pregnancy with clinical cardiac follow-up

C. Close the ASD during pregnancy

Question 11. A 26-year-old woman is pregnant at 12 weeks. She is asymptomatic. A continuous murmur is heard at the left upper sternal border. Echo shows a PDA with L–R shunt, Qp/Qs of 1.3, mild LV enlargement, and normal PA pressure. What is the next step?

A. Recommend pregnancy termination, considering the high maternal cardiac risk

B. Pursue the pregnancy with clinical cardiac follow-up

C. Close the PDA during pregnancy

Question 12. A 34-year-old pregnant woman (33 weeks) develops severe chest pain that has been ongoing for the last 2 hours. ECG shows anterior ST elevation. She receives aspirin, clopidogrel, heparin, NTG, and metoprolol. Chest pain resolves and ST elevation dramatically improves. Coronary angiography is performed and shows a 35 mm long smooth 70% stenosis in the mid-LAD without impaired distal flow. What is the next step?

A. Low-pressure balloon dilatation

B. Low-pressure stenting

C. Conservative management with no intervention

Answer 1. A and F. The presentation is too early for peripartum cardiomyopathy. HTN is relatively mild and rather secondary to the patient's distress and pulmonary edema.

Answer 2. D. MS is one of two conditions that respond to immediate β-blocker therapy during active pulmonary edema (the other condition being HOCM). In a non-pregnant, mildly hypoxic patient, one may administer medical therapy and await 15 minutes before proceeding with intubation. In a pregnant woman, hypoxemia or acidemia of any degree or duration should not be tolerated. Fetal oxygenation requires a maternal PaO_2 >70 mmHg (O_2 saturation >95%) and a pH >7.3.

Answer 3. A. In most pregnant women with severe MS, stability can be achieved with medical therapy. Only if the patient had recurrent or refractory pulmonary edema or hypoxia would mitral valvuloplasty be performed during pregnancy.

Answer 4. E.

Answer 5. A, C, D, H, I.

Answer 6. A, H, I.

Answer 7. C. A large HIV-related effusion has a high risk of progression to tamponade, which warrants pericardiocentesis. Also, frequently (>50%), this effusion is due to associated infections or cancers.

Answer 8. D. A non-dilated LV with severe dysfunction is consistent with acute-onset cardiomyopathy. In the absence of pre-existing cardiomyopathy, severe acute HTN is unlikely to cause acute systolic LV dysfunction. In the absence of quick stabilization with diuretic therapy ± NTG and intubation, coronary angiography is warranted.

Answer 9. A.

Answer 10. B. Pregnancy is usually well tolerated in patients with ASD and no clinical HF, especially given that right–left shunting may decrease during pregnancy.

Answer 11. B. A small PDA without significant LV failure or pulmonary hypertension is usually well tolerated during pregnancy. The LV enlargement is likely secondary to the pregnancy itself, rather than the PDA.

Answer 12. C. The smooth, long morphology suggests dissection of the media (intramural hematoma). Commonly, an intimal flap is not seen in spontaneous coronary dissection. Considering the high risk of propagating the dissection during PCI, conservative management is appropriate in a patient with non-critical disease and no ongoing ischemia. As opposed to plaque rupture or erosion, the majority of spontaneous coronary dissections spontaneously heal on follow-up angiography (≥1 month).

References

1. Odim J, Reehal V, Laks H, et al. Surgical pathology of cardiac tumors: two decades at an urban institution. Cardiovasc Pathol 2003; 12: 267–70.
2. Molina JE, Edwards JE, Ward HB. Primary cardiac tumors: experience at the University of Minnesota. Thorac Cardiovasc Surg 1990; 38 Suppl 2: 183–91.
3. Otto C. Cardiac masses and potential cardiac source of embolus. In: Otto C. Practice of Clinical Echocardiography, 3rd edn. Philadelphia, PA: Saunders, 2007.
4. Amano J, Kono T, Wada Y, et al. Cardiac myxoma: its origin and tumor characteristics. Ann Thorac Cardiovasc Surg 2003; 9: 215–21.
5. Oliveira R, Branco L, Galrinho A, et al. Cardiac myxoma: a 13-year experience in echocardiographic diagnosis. Rev Port Cardiol 2010; 29: 1087–100.
6. Grebenc ML, Rosado-de-Christenson ML, Green CE, et al. Cardiac myxoma: imaging features in 83 patients. RadioGraphics 2002; 22: 673–89.
7. Elbardisi AW, Dearani JA, Daly RC, et al. Survival after resection of primary cardiac tumors: a 48-year experience. Circulation 2008; 118: S7–15.
8. Robson SC, Hunter S, Dunlop W, et al. Serial study of factors influencing changes in cardiac output during human pregnancy. Am J Physiol 1989; 256: H1060–5.
9. Zagrosek V, Blomstrom Lundqvist C, Borghi C, et al. ESC Guidelines on the management of cardiovascular diseases during pregnancy: the Task Force on the Management of Cardiovascular Diseases during Pregnancy of the European Society of Cardiology (ESC). Eur Heart J 2011; 32: 3147–97.
10. Warnes CA. Pregnancy and pulmonary hypertension. Int J Cardiol 2004; 97 (Suppl 1): 11–13.
11. Reimold SC, Rutherford JD. Valvular heart disease in pregnancy. N Engl J Med 2003; 349: 52–9.
12. Grewal J, Siu SC, Ross HJ, et al. Pregnancy outcomes in women with dilated cardiomyopathy. J Am Coll Cardiol 2009; 55: 45–52.
13. Avila WS, Rossi EG, Ramires JA. Pregnancy in patients with heart disease: experience with 1000 cases. Clin Cardiol 2003; 26: 135–42.
14. Webb G, Gatzoulis MA. Atrial septal defects in the adult. Circulation 2006; 114: 1645–53.
15. Uebing A, Steer PJ, Yentis SM, Gatzoulis MA. Pregnancy and congenital heart disease. BMJ 2006; 332: 401–6.
16. Meijboom LJ, Vos FE, Timmermans J, et al. Pregnancy and aortic root growth in the Marfan syndrome: a prospective study. Eur Heart J 2005; 26: 914–20.
17. Rossiter JP, Repke JT, Morales AJ, Murphy EA, Pyeritz RE. A prospective longitudinal evaluation of pregnancy in the Marfan syndrome. Am J Obstet Gynecol 1995; 173; 1599–606.
18. Chan WS, Anand S, Ginsberg JS. Anticoagulation of pregnant women with mechanical heart valves: a systematic review of the literature. Arch Intern Med 2000; 160: 191–6.
19. Oran B, Lee-Parritz A, Ansell J. Low-molecular weight heparin for the prophylaxis of thromboembolism in women with prosthetic mechanical heart valves during pregnancy. Thromb Hoemost 2004; 92; 747–51.
20. Elkayam U. Clinical characteristics of peripartum cardiomyopathy in the United States. J Am Coll Cardiol 2011; 58: 659–70.
21. Goland S, Modi K, Bitar F. Clinical profile and predictors of complications in peripartum cardiomyopathy. J Card Fail 15 2009: 645–50.
22. Gandhi SK, Powers JC, Nomeir AM, et al. The pathogenesis of acute pulmonary edema associated with hypertension. N Engl J Med 2001; 344: 17–22.
23. Amos A, Jaber WA, Russell SD, et al. Improved outcomes in peripartum cardiomyopathy with contemporary. Am Heart J 2006; 152: 509–13.
24. Elkayam U, Tummala PP, Rao K, et al. Maternal and fetal outcomes of subsequent pregnancies in women with peripartum cardiomyopathy. N Engl J Med 2001; 334: 1567–71.
25. Roth A, Elkayam U. Acute myocardial infarction associated with pregnancy. J Am Coll Cardiol 2008; 52: 171–80.
26. Elkayam U, Jalnapurkar S, Barakkat MN, et al. Pregnancy-associated acute myocardial infarction. A review of contemporary experience in 150 cases between 2006 and 2011. Circulation 2014; 129: 1695–702.
27. Heidenreich PA, Eisenberg MJ, Kee LL, et al. Pericardial effusion in AIDS. Incidence and survival. Circulation 1995; 92: 3229–34.
28. Chen Y, Brennessel D, Walters J, et al. Human immunodeficiency virus-associated pericardial effusion: report of 40 cases and review of the literature. Am Heart J 1999; 137: 516–21.
29. Hsue PY, Deeks SG, Farah HH, et al. Role of HIV and human herpesvirus-8 infection in pulmonary arterial hypertension. AIDS 2008; 22: 825–33.
30. Mehta NJ, Ijaz KA, Rajal N, et al. HIV-related pulmonary hypertension analytic review of 131 cases. Chest 2000; 118: 1133–41.
31. Nunes H, Humbert M, Sitbon O, et al. Prognostic factors for survival in human immunodeficiency virus-associated pulmonary arterial hypertension. Am J Respir Crit Care Med 2003; 167: 1433–9.
32. Freiberg MS, Chang CC, Kuller LH, et al. HIV infection and the risk of acute myocardial infarction. JAMA Intern Med. 2013; 173(8): 614.

33. Lange RA, Hillis LD. Cardiovascular complications of cocaine use. N Engl J Med 2001; 345: 351–8.

34. McCord J, Jneid H, Hollander JE, et al. Management of cocaine-associated chest pain and myocardial infarction. Circulation 2008; 117: 1897–2007.

35. Wouters K.A., Kremer L.C., Miller T.L., et al. Protecting against anthracycline-induced myocardial damage: a review of the most promising strategies. Br J Haematol 2005; 131: 561–78.

36. Yeh ETH, Bickford CL. Cardiovascular complications of cancer therapy: incidence, pathogenesis, diagnosis, and management. J Am Coll Cardiol 2009; 53: 2231–47.

37. Cardinale D, Colombo A, Sandri MT. Prevention of high-dose chemotherapy-induced cardiotoxicity in high-risk patients by angiotensin-converting enzyme inhibition. Circulation 2006; 114: 2474–81.

38. Gharib MI, Burnett AK. Chemotherapy-induced cardiotoxicity: current practice and prospects of prophylaxis. Eur J Heart Fail 2002; 4: 235–42.

39. Rowinsky EK, McGuire WP, Guarnieri T, et al. Cardiac disturbances during the administration of taxol. J Clin Oncol 1991; 9: 1704–12.

Part 10   CARDIAC TESTS: ELECTROCARDIOGRAPHY, ECHOCARDIOGRAPHY, AND STRESS TESTING

31   Electrocardiography

I. Overview of ECG leads and QRS morphology

An ECG lead consists of two poles (a positive pole and a negative pole). It captures the cardiac electrical potential spreading between these two poles (Figures 31.1, 31.2). If a wave spreads towards the negative pole then turns towards the positive pole, a negative deflection is initially seen, followed by a positive deflection. If the vector of the propagating wave is parallel to the line formed by the two poles, the amplitude of the deflection will be largest; if it is orthogonal, the deflection will be small and almost isoelectric. The electrodes that are positioned on the limbs and the precordium are the poles, whereas the axis formed between two poles is called a lead. Leads I, II, and III are bipolar leads that register the electrical spread between two limb poles. Limb leads aVR, aVL, and aVF register the electrical spread between a central pole and one limb pole; the central pole is the center of the two other limb poles (Figures 31.3, 31.4).

Precordial leads V_1–V_6 register the electrical spread between a central pole and one chest pole; the central pole is the center of all limb poles, located in the center of the chest (Figures 31.5, 31.6). The limb leads aVR, aVL, and aVF, and the precordial leads, are called unipolar leads because they mainly depend on the position of one pole.

Precordial leads V_5–V_6 and limb leads I and aVL point to the left and are left lateral leads, leads I and aVL being high lateral leads. Precordial leads V_1–V_2 are right-sided leads but also septal leads; they overlie the right heart but also the interventricular septum. V_1–V_3 are anteroseptal leads. Limb leads II, III, and aVF point inferiorly, and are thus inferior leads.

Practical Cardiovascular Medicine, First Edition. Elias B. Hanna.
© 2017 John Wiley & Sons Ltd. Published 2017 by John Wiley & Sons Ltd.

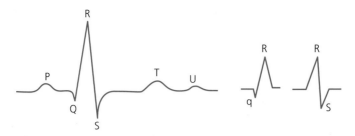

Figure 31.1 P–QRS–T complex. P wave represents the atrial depolarization and includes a part of the AV nodal conduction. PR interval consists of P wave and AV conduction. AV conduction consists of AV nodal conduction, His conduction, and infra-Hisian conduction (bundle branches before the myocardium); most of the AV conduction time is consumed by conduction through the AV node. The PR segment also includes the atrial repolarization; in normal states, the PR segment is isoelectric or slightly depressed <0.8 mm (as a result of atrial repolarization).

QRS complex represents ventricular depolarization. ST–T segments represent ventricular repolarization. ST segment = phase 2 of the action potential or plateau phase of repolarization. T wave = phase 3 of the action potential. TP segment = phase 4 of the action potential. The normal U wave is a diastolic wave related to the mechanical stretch of the myocardium in phase 4 (diastole).

Normal calibration:
- Height of one small box = 1 mm = 0.1 mV. One big box = 5 small boxes = 0.5 mV.
- Width of one small box = 1 mm = 0.04 seconds. One big box = 5 small boxes = 0.2 seconds (sweep speed: 25 mm/s).

Watch for half-standardization, especially when comparing ECGs.

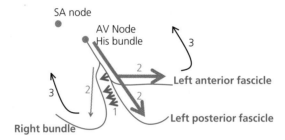

Figure 31.2 Arrows show the spread of the electrical depolarization. Ventricular depolarization starts at the left-sided septum, then spreads to the whole septum from left to right (through the left bundle, *blue arrows 1*). It then spreads to each ventricle through the left and right bundles (*gray arrows 2*). The apex of each ventricle is depolarized first, followed by the lateral wall and the posterior basal region (apical-to-basal spread of depolarization bilaterally, *black arrows 3*). Note that *septal depolarization occurs from left to right.*

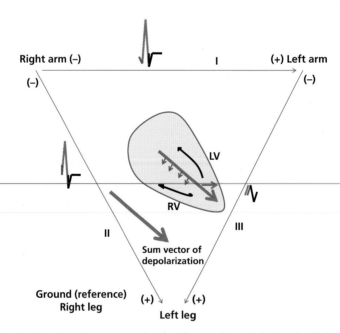

Figure 31.3 Illustration of how the electrical depolarization spreads in the heart (frontal plane, bipolar limb leads). The *blue arrows* represent the left-to-right septal depolarization. The *gray arrow* is the main axis of depolarization along the septum towards the LV and apex. The *black arrows* represent the late depolarization spreading towards the base. The QRS deflections that correspond to each one of these depolarizations are colored likewise.

The QRS complex in each lead represents how the electrical activity is spreading in relation to the lead. The **septal depolarization** (*blue*) **explains the normal small q wave** seen in normal individuals in lead I, other limb leads (sometimes), and left precordial leads. The basal depolarization explains the late "s" wave in those leads. The main deflection (big R or big S) is explained by the main depolarization spread. One can imagine how the amplitude of a deflection changes with a slight change in the way depolarization spreads.

To grossly conceive how QRS appears in a lead (amplitude, positive vs. negative direction), contrast the sum vector of depolarization with the axis of the lead.

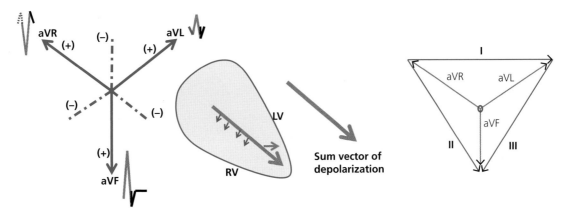

Figure 31.4 Illustration of how electrical depolarization spreads in the heart (frontal plane, unipolar limb leads).

The limb leads' poles are placed on the shoulders and thighs but may be placed more distally across the limbs. Compared to the shoulders/thighs, placing the limb poles on the torso falsely magnifies QRS, but placing them further away on the limbs (wrists and feet) does not significantly reduce QRS amplitude. This is similar to projecting a photograph on a wall; if the wall is close to the photograph, a small change in the wall-to-photograph distance translates into a large change in the size of the projected image, but this is not the case if the wall is far away from the photograph.

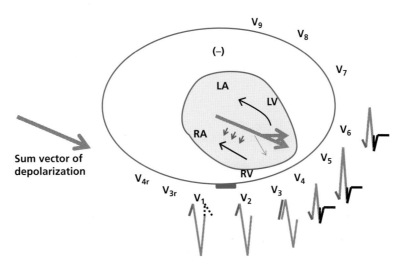

Figure 31.5 Illustration of how electrical depolarization spreads in the heart (horizontal plane, unipolar precordial leads). **V₁ and V₂** overlie the **right** heart and the septum, whereas **V₄ through V₆** overlie the **apex and the LV**. The QRS complex starts as rS in leads V_1–V_3 and progresses to qRs in the left leads. The small r in V_1–V_2 and the small q past the transition zone (V_4–V_6) represent septal depolarization. At the transition zone (e.g., V_3 in this picture), the R wave represents septal depolarization and part of the main axis of depolarization. The amplitude of R or S in each lead depends on how parallel the sum vector of depolarization is to the axis of the lead.

Since leads V₁ and V₂ overlie the right heart, any abnormality that makes electrical forces go towards the right heart makes QRS positive in V₁ or V₂; this is the case in RBBB and RVH. Conversely, any abnormality that makes electrical forces go towards the left makes QRS positive in V₅ or V₆; this is the case in LBBB and LVH.

$V_1 \rightarrow$ 4th intercostal space, right sternal border. $V_2 \rightarrow$ 4th intercostal space, left sternal border. $V_4 \rightarrow$ 5th intercostal space, midclavicular level. $V_3 \rightarrow$ between V_2 and V_4. $V_5 \rightarrow$ 5th space, anterior axillary line. $V_6 \rightarrow$ 5th space, midaxillary line. $V_7 \rightarrow$ posterior axillary line, $V_9 \rightarrow$ paraspinal line; $V_8 \rightarrow$ between V_7 and V_9 (~ below the scapula)

Appendix 2 provides an illustration of cardiac depolarization and the QRS morphology in the limb and precordial leads in various disease states.

The electrical spread of ventricular depolarization (QRS) and ventricular repolarization (ST–T) is captured by the ECG leads. Ventricular repolarization (phases 2 and 3 of the action potential) has an opposite polarity to ventricular depolarization (phase 0 of the action potential), yet the T wave has the same polarity as QRS. In fact, ventricular depolarization spreads from the endocardium to the epicardium; however, the epicardium has a shorter action potential than the endocardium, and although it is activated later, repolarization starts earlier in the epicardium and spreads to the endocardium. Therefore, in normal individuals, the electrical vectors of repolarization and depolarization have the same direction. QRS and ST–T are concordant, with the ST segment being isoelectric as all myocardial cells reach the same phase 2 plateau level without any intramyocardial gradient.

In disease states where some myocardial areas are activated very late, such as bundle branch block or ventricular dilatation or hypertrophy, the late areas are repolarized very late as well, so that the difference in action potential duration between epicardium and endocardium

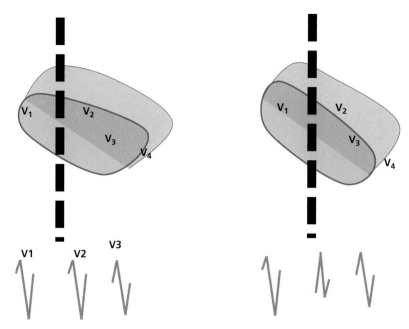

Figure 31.6 Frontal view of the precordial leads. Normally, R wave progressively increases in height between V_1 and V_3, V_1 and V_2 overlying the right heart. Occasionally, depending on the heart orientation, the electrode V_2 may be on the left of the septum, while V_3 may be on the right of the septum. R wave may be large in V_2 but becomes small again in V_3. This is more likely to happen if V_3 is placed at the same vertical level as V_2.

is unable to restore the polarity of repolarization. For example, in LBBB, both the endocardium and epicardium that depolarize late repolarize late as well; in severe concentric LVH, the epicardium depolarizes so late that it repolarizes late as well. In these patients, the electrical vectors of depolarization and repolarization have opposite polarity and directions (QRS and ST–T are discordant), and different parts of the myocardium reach phase 2 (ST segment) at different times, which creates an oblique deviation of the ST segment. This is particularly true in patients with the most delayed depolarization (severe ventricular hypertrophy or enlargement, LBBB).

On the other hand, the length of the QT corresponds to how dispersed the repolarization is across various myocardial areas, regardless of which areas are repolarized first and last.

II. Stepwise approach to ECG interpretation

The following steps are followed in ECG interpretation:[1]

1. Rhythm: look at QRS regularity and rate.
   - Then look for P waves, and assess the P–QRS relationship.
   - Determine if the rhythm is sinus (P [+] in I and II and [–] in aVR).
2. Determine QRS axis in the frontal plane (leads I, II, and aVF). Also assess R-wave progression in V_1–V_6 (normal vs. poor progression vs. early transition).

   Then start analyzing each ECG segment:
3. Analyze P wave in leads II and V_1–V_2 (left or right atrial enlargement).
4. Analyze PR interval.
5. Analyze *QRS width*: if ≥ 120 ms, look at the QRS morphology in the right leads V_1–V_2 and the left leads V_5–V_6, and characterize it as RBBB (wide upright QRS on the right, V_1–V_2), LBBB (wide upright QRS on the left, V_5–V_6), non-specific conduction delay, or pre-excitation (WPW).

   Look for LAFB features.

   Analyze *QRS amplitude*: look for big R wave on the right (RVH) or big R wave on the left (LVH), and use the hypertrophy criteria.
6. Look for abnormal Q waves.
7. Analyze ST–T segments. Are they depressed or elevated? In which leads and which family?
   - In case of ST depression, does the abnormality appear secondary to LVH/LBBB/RVH/RBBB and is it opposite to the QRS direction? Or does it appear ischemic?
   - In case of ST elevation, does the abnormality appear secondary to LVH/LBBB and is it opposite to QRS direction? Is it concave upward without reciprocal changes or Q waves (this may suggest pericarditis or secondary ST elevation)? Is PR segment depressed?
8. Assess QT segment. Look for patterns of electrolyte abnormalities.

III. Rhythm and rate

A. Look at the rhythm strip and survey for the following:

1. Assess the regularity of QRS complexes. Then look for P waves and assess the P and QRS relationship, i.e., look for an association between P and QRS, and look for hidden P waves manifesting as notches over the QRS or the ST–T segment. P wave is often best seen in lead II, which is often parallel to the P-wave axis.

Examples of cardiac rhythms:

  a. **Sinus rhythm or tachycardia**: one sinus-looking P wave before each QRS (Figure 31.7).
  b. **Atrial tachycardia, atrial flutter**: one or more P waves are seen before each QRS with consistent P–QRS association. R–R intervals are equal or, if not equal, there is a consistent repetition of the same pattern of R–R intervals.
   • Example: 2:1 conduction, meaning that every second P wave gets conducted, so there is one QRS for every two P waves with regular P–P intervals and R–R intervals.
   • Or 4:1 or 1:1 conduction.
   • Or variable conduction (2:1, mixed with 3:1, 4:1). In this case, R–R intervals are irregular, but there is repetition of the same R–R intervals.
  c. **Atrial fibrillation**: irregularly irregular rhythm or tachycardia (total chaos; no repetition of the same R–R intervals; Figure 31.8). Another irregularly irregular rhythm is MAT. Unlike AF, in MAT, polymorphic P waves are seen and conduct in a 1:1 fashion.
  d. **AVNRT/AVRT**: regular, narrow complex tachycardia. P waves are not seen or are seen just after or within ST–T, with a 1:1 QRS–P association (Figure 31.9).
  e. **Ventricular tachycardia**: wide complex tachycardia with no relation between P waves and QRS complexes (AV dissociation) *and/or* more QRS complexes than P waves (Figure 31.10).
  f. **Bradycardia with regular P waves and regular QRS complexes, unrelated to each other**: complete AV block (Figures 31.11, 31.12).
  g. **Bradycardia without any P wave**: sinus arrest with junctional escape rhythm, AF with complete AV block and junctional escape rhythm, or hyperkalemia.

2. Premature ventricular or atrial complexes (PVCs or PACs). *PVC* is wide with ST–T directed opposite to QRS. *PAC* is narrow, but may be wide in case of aberrancy (Figure 31.13).

3. Irregular rhythm with some pattern or regularity, meaning that R–R intervals are not all equal, but some of them are:
 • Atrial tachycardia or atrial flutter with variable AV conduction (e.g., conduction changes from 2:1 to 3:1, then 2:1 again). The rhythm is irregular, but there is a pattern to it (Figure 31.14).
 • PVCs or PACs (PVCs and PACs are usually followed by a pause).
 • Sinus arrhythmia (P–P interval varies cyclically, PR distance remains constant).

4. Groups of beats separated by pauses:
 • Second-degree AV block (Figure 31.15)
 • Frequent PACs, PVCs, or non-conducted premature Ps, each followed by a pause (Figure 31.13)

5. Look for **pacemaker spikes** (small vertical lines before P or QRS or both P and QRS).

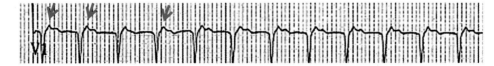

Figure 31.7 Regular QRS rhythm with a P wave before each QRS complex: sinus tachycardia or atrial tachycardia. Analyze P morphology in leads I, aVR, and II to determine if the rhythm is sinus or ectopic atrial.

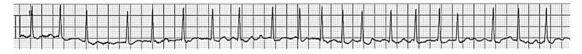

Figure 31.8 Irregular tachycardia with no repetition of any R–R pattern. No clear P wave is seen; rather, waves that vary greatly in shape are seen. This is AF with fibrillatory atrial waves.

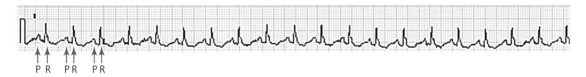

Figure 31.9 Narrow complex tachycardia with a pseudo-r′ in lead V₁ that represents a retrograde P wave (*arrows*). This is a narrow complex tachycardia with a very short interval between QRS and the retrograde P wave → AVNRT.

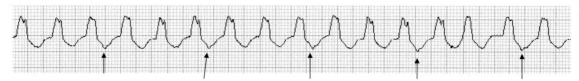

Figure 31.10 Wide complex tachycardia: VT vs. SVT with bundle branch block. Look for P waves on top of the ST–T segments: one can identify deflections that have a consistent *morphology* and *timing* and that can be marched out. They occur after every third QRS. Since the number of QRS complexes > number of P waves, this is VT. The P waves are retrograde P waves.

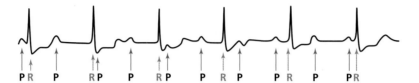

Figure 31.11 Bradycardia with regular P waves and regular QRS complexes, unrelated to each other. Some P waves fall on top of the ST–T segments and manifest as notches. This is a third-degree AV block. If P wave occasionally conducts, the QRS rhythm would have some irregularity.

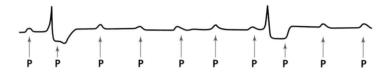

Figure 31.12 Severe bradycardia with regular P waves and regular QRS complexes, unrelated to each other: third-degree AV block.

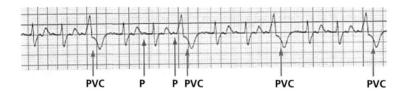

Figure 31.13 Irregularity with a pattern. Wide premature complexes with ST–T changes opposite to QRS are seen; these occur in a trigeminal pattern. A wide premature beat is typically a PVC, but could be a PAC with bundle branch block (aberrancy). In this case, the premature beat falls after a normally occurring, non-premature P wave (*blue arrows*) with a shorter PR interval than the sinus beat: this is typical of a PVC. **A PVC does not affect the sinus P wave, which keeps marching through it, sometimes falling before it at a short PR interval.** A PAC, on the other hand, should be preceded by a non-sinus premature P wave that does not march out with the preceding sinus P waves; the premature P may fall prematurely into the preceding T wave and deform it. *A deformed T wave is a clue to a PAC.*

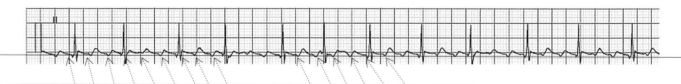

Figure 31.14 Atrial flutter with variable conduction (3:1, 4:1). The sawtooth flutter waves are marked by the *arrows*. R–R intervals are not equal, but there is some repetition of the same R–R intervals.

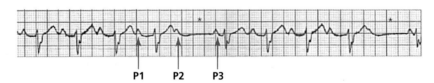

Figure 31.15 There are two groups of beats followed by pauses (*asterisks*), which raises the suspicion of second-degree AV block (e.g., Wenckebach). P2 is not conducted: this could be AV block or a very premature PAC that gets blocked. The fact that P2 is not premature rules out a blocked PAC. The clue to AV Wenckebach is the progressive PR prolongation, especially manifest when comparing P3R to P1R (P3R < P1R); also, the progressive R–R shortening before the block is a feature of Wenckebach.

B. Calculate the ventricular rate

The ventricular rate is equal to 300 divided by the number of big boxes between two QRS complexes. If the rhythm is irregular (e.g., AF), count the number of QRS complexes in 3 seconds (15 large boxes), then multiply this number by 20; or count the number of QRS complexes on the standard 12-lead ECG run (10 seconds) and multiply it by 6.

C. The rhythm is sinus if P wave is upright in leads I, II, and aVF and inverted in lead aVR, corresponding to a P-wave axis of 0–75°.

Also, a sinus P wave is typically biphasic (positive then negative) in V_1 and V_2, but sometimes entirely positive in V_1–V_2 or entirely negative in V_1. A sinus P wave is always upright in V_3–V_6.

A different P-wave morphology means ectopic atrial rhythm/tachycardia, accelerated junctional rhythm with retrograde P wave, or AVNRT/AVRT with retrograde P wave. **A retrograde P wave** is negative in the inferior leads II, III, and aVF and is usually seen shortly after the QRS. If P waves have three different morphologies, the rhythm is a wandering atrial pacemaker (rate < 100 bpm) or a wandering atrial tachycardia (rate > 100 bpm, also called *MAT*) and is irregular.

IV. QRS axis in the limb leads and normal QRS progression in the precordial leads

A. Determine the frontal QRS axis by looking at the net QRS voltage (upward minus downward deflection) in leads I, II, and aVF (see Figure 31.16)

The normal QRS axis is between –30° and +90°. To determine QRS axis, start by looking at leads I and aVF. If the net QRS is negative in lead aVF, the axis is < 0°; one must look at lead II to determine if the axis is < –30°, which defines left-axis deviation.

1. *If the net QRS is negative in lead I and upright in lead aVF,* **right-axis deviation** *is present.* Six causes (the first four are abnormal):
   - RVH (including pulmonary embolism)
   - Lung disease even without RVH
   - Left posterior fascicular block (LPFB) (usually associated with right bundle-branch block [RBBB])
   - Lateral MI: Q wave is seen in lead I. Instead of a Q wave, a diminutive small r wave (rS pattern) sometimes appears in leads I–aVL. In this case, the Q waves in leads V_5–V_6 and the frequently seen T-wave inversion in I–aVL allow the diagnosis (≠ RVH)
   - Normal variant: vertical heart with a 90–100° axis in young individuals
   - Arm electrodes misplacement: P wave will also be negative in lead I, and upright in lead aVR

   If right-axis deviation is present, evaluate for RVH by looking for a tall R wave in V_1 ± V_2 (R wave > 7 mm or R wave > S wave) or a deep S wave in V_6.

> Note that isolated RBBB does not lead to right-axis deviation (think of an associated RVH or LPFB when right axis accompanies RBBB).

2. *If the net QRS is upright in lead I but negative in leads II and aVF,* **left-axis deviation** *is present.* Four causes:
   - LVH
   - Left anterior fascicular block (LAFB)
   - Left bundle branch block (LBBB)
   - Inferior MI

   The QRS axis progressively shifts more leftward with obesity, which pushes the diaphragm up, and with age, but does not normally exceed –30°. Conversely, thin individuals tend to have a more vertical heart. **Inspiration and upright position make the heart more vertical and may explain a change in axis without intervening disease.**

3. *If the net QRS is negative in leads I and aVF, the* **axis is in the northwest quadrant** *(extreme right or left deviation).* The northwest axis may occur in various right or left pathologies.

   If QRS is equiphasic in all limb leads, the axis is perpendicular to the frontal plane and is called *indeterminate*. This may be a normal variant or may occur with right ventricular pathology. One variant, $S_1S_2S_3$, signifies that S ≥ R in leads I, II, and III, and implies an indeterminate axis (S = R) or northwest axis (S > R). It may be a normal variant when the axis is indeterminate.

> To fine-tune the axis, look at the lead where QRS is closest to equiphasic, i.e., the lead where R = S with a neutral net force. The axis is close to + or –90° from this lead (Figure 31.16). If QRS is closest to equiphasic in two leads, the axis is in between the perpendicular lines to these two leads, in the appropriate quadrant.

B. Look at the normal QRS progression across V_1–V_6

Normally, QRS is negative in V_1–V_2 (rS) and becomes progressively positive in V_5–V_6 (Rs). Note: rS denotes small R, big S. Rs denotes big R, small S.

1. *If QRS starts positive in V_1–V_2 (***early transition***), consider six causes, the first two being "Right problems":*
   - RVH (which also leads to right-axis deviation).
   - RBBB.
   - Posterior wall infarction: large, and more importantly, wide R wave in V_1, reciprocal of a posterior Q wave. Often, Q waves are present in V_7–V_9 and in the inferior leads.
   - WPW: short PR and delta wave are present.

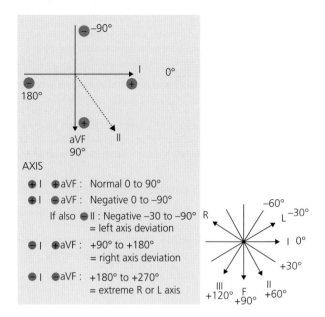

Figure 31.16 Start by looking at leads I and aVF. If QRS is negative in lead aVF, the axis is < 0°; one must look at lead II to determine if the axis is < −30°, which defines left-axis deviation. In all other cases, looking at leads I and aVF is enough to grossly define the type of axis deviation. Reproduced with permission of Scrub Hill Press from Hanna et al. (2009).[1]

- Septal hypertrophic cardiomyopathy (thick septum, thicker than the lateral wall, projects as big R in V_1–V_2 and big Q in the lateral leads); or Duchenne muscular dystrophy (posterior wall fibrosis).
- However, the most common cause of early transition is a normal variant. It is more common in young individuals, where the heart is swung more anteriorly than older individuals. A low malposition of electrodes V_1–V_2 is also a common cause of early transition.

2. Poor precordial R-wave progression *means that the R-wave height remains < 3 mm (= 0.3 mV, three small boxes) in lead V_3, and more specifically ≤ 1.5 mm, with failure of the R/S height ratio to increase.*

It may be an equivalent of Q wave and may signify an anterior MI, particularly if one of the following two features coexists: (i) T inversion in V_1–V_3; (ii) R wave in lead I < 4 mm. The small R wave in lead I suggests diminution from a lateral MI, although it may also be secondary to COPD. Conversely, the following two features argue against MI: (i) improvement of R-wave progression with lower placement of the chest electrodes; (ii) sudden R-wave transition in V_4 or V_5, which suggests a high misplacement of electrodes V_1–V_2 and a normal placement of electrodes V_3–V_6, as in patients with large breasts. In MI, R wave remains small in V_4–V_5 and transitions slowly, yet a slow transition does not necessarily imply MI. Reverse R progression, which means that R wave not only progresses poorly but gets smaller between V_1 and V_2 or V_2 and V_3, slightly increases the likelihood of MI.

However, poor R progression is most often related to the following causes, the first three being "left problems" (Figure 31.17):
- LAFB.
- LVH.
- LBBB.
- High misplacement of electrodes V_1–V_2 or low heart/low diaphragm position (thin and tall individuals); or heart swung posteriorly, away from V_1–V_2 (older subjects). Normal R-wave progression may be seen when the chest leads are placed one interspace lower.
- COPD, in which case the heart is pushed down and posteriorly, away from the precordium: COPD leads to poor R-wave progression with right-axis deviation. Poor R-wave progression with right-axis deviation may also be seen when anterior MI is associated with a high lateral MI. The overall size of the QRS allows the distinction between COPD and anterior MI (QRS voltage is often reduced in COPD). Also, in COPD, recording the chest leads one interspace lower often corrects R-wave progression, at least partially.

V. P wave: analyze P wave in leads II and V_1 for atrial enlargement, and analyze PR interval (see Figures 31.18, 31.19)

A. Lead V_1 (and/or V_2)
- Left atrial enlargement = terminal negative P-wave deflection > 1 box wide (40 ms) and 1 box deep (0.1 mV).
- Right atrial enlargement = initial positive P-wave deflection ≥ 1.5 small boxes high.

B. Lead II (and I, III)
P waves should be < 2.5 small boxes high (0.25 mV high) and < 3 small boxes wide (120 ms wide).

- Left atrial enlargement = P wave ≥ 120 ms and notched
  P may have a negative terminal deflection in leads III and aVF, i.e., left P-axis deviation. While an abnormal P-wave axis suggests ectopic atrial origin, in context, it may rather imply atrial enlargement.

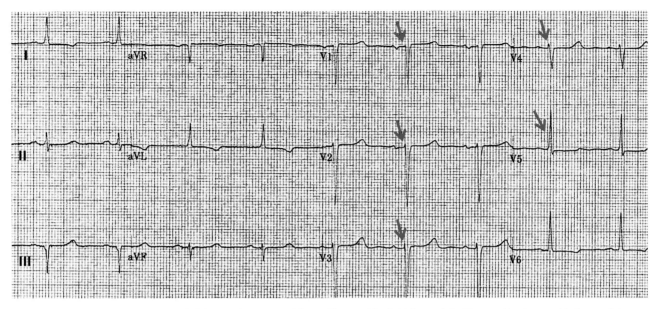

Figure 31.17 Poor R-wave progression probably secondary to LVH with a sudden transition in V₅ (*arrows*). Sudden transition is a good indicator of the absence of anterior MI. The lack of T-wave inversion in the anterior leads and the normal-size R wave in lead I also make MI unlikely.

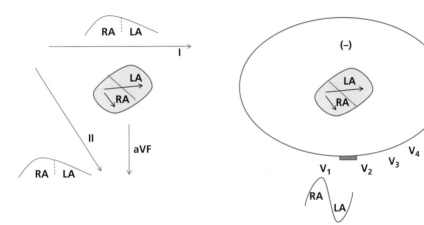

Frontal plane:
Both RA and LA depolarizations are oriented to the left. RA depolarization occurs first and determines the height of the P depolarization. LA depolarization occurs second and determines the duration of the depolarization.

Horizontal plane:
RA depolarization occurs first; it is directed anteriorly, thus RA deflection is positive in V₁ and V₂. LA deflection occurs next; it is directed posteriorly, thus, LA deflection is the 2nd deflection and is negative in V₁–V₂

Figure 31.18 Normal and abnormal RA and LA deflections. Atrial depolarization starts from the sinus node, at the junction of SVC–RA, and spreads in a radial fashion to depolarize the RA, interatrial septum, and LA.

RA enlargement (RAE) is characterized by increased voltage of the first atrial deflection in lead II and in leads V₁–V₂. LA enlargement (LAE) is characterized by prolongation of P duration in lead II with a double hump, the second hump corresponding to LA depolarization. Depending on the severity of LAE and on the heart orientation, the P wave may peak high and relatively early in lead II, simulating RAE (e.g., vertical heart). Also, it may have a positive component in lead V₁. Thus, anatomical LAE may mimic RAE electrocardiographically; up to 30% of cases of electrocardiographic RAE are actually LAE.

Moreover, depending on the severity of RAE, the duration of P wave may be increased and a negative component may be seen in lead V₁. Thus, anatomical RAE may simulate LAE electrocardiographically.

P-wave amplitude normally increases during sinus tachycardia or exercise, while the P-wave duration decreases; this is due to a more synchronized RA and LA depolarization. Thus, RAE criteria are less valid in sinus tachycardia, but LAE criteria remain valid. In fact, an increase in P duration with exercise suggests left HF with LA volume overload unveiled by exercise.

RAE and LAE may be seen on ECG as a result of increased atrial pressure or atrial ischemia, even in the absence of true enlargement. RAE may be seen in patients with lung disease (vertical heart) even in the absence of true enlargement. Thus, the ECG terms RAE and LAE are better replaced with RA abnormality and LA abnormality, respectively.

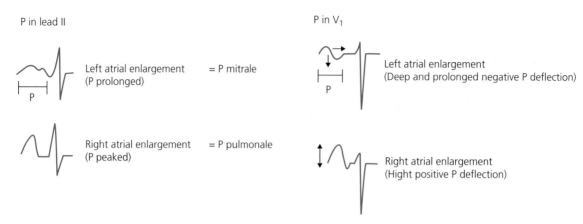

Figure 31.19 Right atrial enlargement and left atrial enlargement. Reproduced with permission of Scrub Hill Press from Hanna et al. (2009).[1]

- Right atrial enlargement = P wave is peaked ≥ 0.25 mV
  P axis may be rightward > +75°, and P may become flat in lead I and inverted in aVL. This could suggest a non-sinus P wave. However, in the presence of other signs of right heart pathology (i.e., right-axis deviation of QRS), the P wave is rather a sinus P wave with a right P-axis deviation.

C. Normal PR interval

Normal PR interval is 120–200 ms (3–5 small boxes; assess it in multiple leads and take the longest).

- PR < 3 small boxes: pre-excitation (WPW pattern), but may just be a fast-conducting AV node. Look for delta waves.
- PR > 5 small boxes: first-degree AV block.
- PR interval includes AV conduction but also atrial repolarization. Atrial enlargement, atrial infarction, or sinus tachycardia with increased P-wave amplitude may depress the PR interval; also, atrial repolarization may prolong and extend over the ST segment, causing ST depression.

VI. Height of QRS: LVH, RVH

Grossly, look at the height and the width of QRS in leads V_1, V_6 and I–aVL.

A. Look for LVH (see Figure 31.20)

LVH can be identified using any of the following criteria (assuming standard calibration):

- In lead I, R wave > 14 mm, or R wave in lead I + S wave in lead III > 25 mm.
- In lead aVL, R wave > 11 mm or > 13 mm in case of LAFB (very specific criterion).
- S wave in V_3 + R wave in aVL ≥ 28 mm in men or ≥ 20 mm in women. This is Cornell criterion, the most sensitive and specific LVH criterion. Specificity is reduced if LAFB is additionally present.
- In the precordial leads: **big R on the left** (V_5–V_6) and big S on the right (V_1–V_2) translate into:
  - S wave in V_1 + R wave in V_5 or V_6 ≥ 35 mm
  - Any S wave (V_1–V_3) + any R wave (V_4–V_6) ≥ 45 mm
  - R wave in V_6 > R wave in V_5.
  - R wave in V_5 or V_6 > 26 mm
- Notes:
  - LVH may be associated with delayed precordial QRS transition, as the vector of depolarization is turned leftward.
  - LAFB shifts the electrical depolarization superiorly and posteriorly; thus, R wave is increased in the limb leads I and aVL, and S wave is deepened across the precordial leads. This reduces the specificity of Cornell and aVL criteria.

- LVH should not be formally diagnosed in the presence of complete LBBB. For practical purposes, however, 80% of patients with LBBB have LVH.
- A strain repolarization pattern may be present. Strain means the ST segment and T wave are directed opposite to QRS. A strain pattern correlates with a more severe LVH.
- Electrocardiographic LVH correlates with LV mass but also LV volume, and may imply LV dilatation rather than thickening

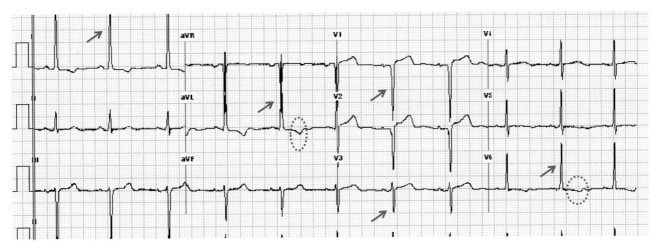

Figure 31.20 LVH with secondary ST–T depression in the left lateral leads, directed opposite to the QRS complex, called *strain pattern* (marked by the *circles*). The following LVH criteria are met (as indicated by the arrows):

- R aVL + S $V_3 \geq 28$ mm (5.5 big boxes)
- R aVL > 11 mm (>2.2 big boxes)
- R in I ≥ 15 mm (3 boxes); R in I + S in III > 25 mm
- S in V_1 + R in V_5 or $V_6 \geq 35$ mm; R in V_5 > 26 mm

B. Look for RVH (Figure 31.21)
RVH is characterized by:

1. Right-axis deviation (net QRS [–] in lead I, [+] in lead aVF)
   and
2. **Big R** wave in the **right** lead V_1 (≥7 mm), or big S wave in the left leads V_5–V_6 (≥7 mm)
   Or big R > S in V_1, big S > R in V_6, or small S in V_1 ≤2 mm
   Or R in V_1 + S in V_6 > 10.5 mm

   In the absence of RBBB, a monophasic R wave in V_1 or a qR pattern in V_1 signifies severely increased RV pressure (higher than systemic pressure in the case of qR pattern).

RVH differential diagnosis and coexisting patterns

- *Posterior MI* may lead to a prominent R wave in V_1. In posterior MI, R wave is not only high but is also wide > 1 mm (≠ RVH), T wave is positive in V_1–V_2 (vs. inverted in RVH), the axis is not right, and there are often Q waves in V_7–V_9 and in the inferior or lateral leads.
- *An incomplete RBBB pattern* with RSR' may be seen along with RVH. This pattern is often secondary to the slow conduction across the enlarged RV rather than a diseased right bundle. In fact, incomplete RBBB with right axis is frequently secondary to RVH, more specifically a volume overload pattern of RVH. RVH is definitely diagnosed if the *axis is right and R' > 10 mm*. As RVH progresses, R' becomes taller and a monophasic R may develop, particularly with pressure overload patterns.
- *Lung disease, such as COPD*, is characterized by: (1) right-axis deviation in the frontal plane as the heart is pushed down and made more vertical; (2) deep S wave in all precordial leads, V_1 through V_6, as the heart rotates posteriorly; (3) reduced overall QRS voltage in all leads, especially limb leads, because of increased chest air; while dominant, S wave is not particularly deep in the precordial leads. This chronic lung disease pattern simulates an old anterolateral MI, wherein R is diminished across all precordial leads and in the lateral leads I and a VL (rS pattern throughout all those leads).

  The presence of true RVH in conjunction with lung disease is characterized by one of the following: large R or small S in V_1 (≤2 mm), RSR' pattern, or T-wave inversion in V_1–V_2. P pulmonale may be seen with lung disease even without RVH.

Additional notes

- Right-axis deviation may be less evident in patients with an associated LVH or LAFB.
- Higher voltage and more strain pattern is seen with pressure overload (pulmonary hypertension) than with volume overload (ASD). ASD is often only characterized by rSR' pattern, and rarely leads to tall monophasic R waves.
- Left atrial enlargement supports the diagnosis of LVH, and right atrial enlargement supports the diagnosis of RVH in cases of borderline voltage criteria. LVH with right atrial enlargement or RVH with left atrial enlargement suggests biventricular hypertrophy, unless MS is present (MS may lead to left atrial enlargement + RVH).

C. Biventricular enlargement

Biventricular enlargement is characterized by any one of the following:

1. Voltage criteria for both LVH and RVH. This usually implies tall R waves in V_5–V_6 (LVH) with a small S wave in V_1, or R>S in V_1 (R is not usually large in V_1, but is larger than S).
2. LVH with right-axis deviation.
3. LVH with right atrial or biatrial enlargement.
4. LVH with T inversion in V_1–V_2 (T going in the same direction as QRS). This T inversion can be secondary to RV strain or anterior ischemia.
5. Tall R wave and tall S wave in the mid-precordial leads V_3–V_4 (Katz–Wachtel sign).

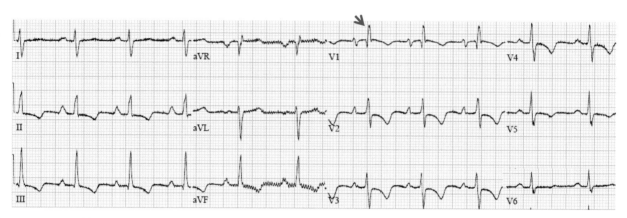

Figure 31.21 QRS is (–) in lead I and (+) in lead aVF, implying a right-axis deviation. The smallest net QRS is in leads I and aVR. QRS axis is thus between perpendicular to I (+90°) and aVR (+120°). Axis is ~+105°. RVH is diagnosed by the fact that axis is right and R>S in V_1. In fact, there is a qR pattern in V_1 (S=0) (*arrow*), signifying severely increased RV pressure. P pulmonale and secondary T inversion are also seen.

VII. Width of QRS. Conduction abnormalities: bundle brunch blocks

The normal QRS duration is <110 ms. In complete bundle branch block, the QRS is wide (≥120 ms or 3 small boxes). In incomplete bundle branch block, the QRS is 110–119 ms.

Look at the QRS complex in lead V_1. **Is the net QRS complex upright (i.e., positive)?**
- If yes, consider RBBB.
- If no (negative QRS in lead V_1), consider LBBB. *A conduction block makes the QRS vector look towards it: RBBB makes the QRS vector look towards the right, leading to an upright wide QRS in the right leads* (Figures 31.22–31.26).

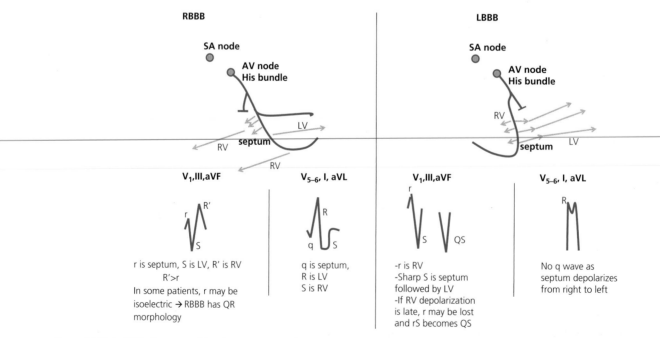

Figure 31.22 In RBBB, the vector of depolarization spreads from the left septum to the right and left ventricles. RSR' is seen in V_1, R being septal depolarization, S being LV depolarization, and R' being the late RV depolarization. RS is seen in V_6, R being LV depolarization, and the wide S being the slow RV depolarization.

In LBBB, the vector of depolarization spreads from the right septum to the left septum and the left ventricle. The vector looks toward V_6 and away from V_1. Thus, in LBBB, QRS is positive in V_5–V_6 and widely negative in V_1. The septal q wave that is normally seen in the left lateral leads is lost, as the septum depolarizes from the right to the left. The presence of any q wave in leads V_5–V_6 or lead I is not typical of LBBB and suggests an old MI. Only rarely, a q wave may be seen in lead aVL.

A. RBBB

In **RBBB**, QRS has a slurred positivity in the **right** leads. Beside QRS $\geq$ 120 ms, *both* the following two criteria are required to make the diagnosis of RBBB:

- rSR', rsR', or rsr' pattern in the **right** leads V_1 and/or V_2. R' is usually wider and taller than the initial R wave. A qR pattern may replace rSR' in lead V_1 when the initial r wave is isoelectric. A single wide R wave, often notched, may be seen instead of rSR'.
- A *wide* S wave in the left leads I and V_6. *S wave must be wider than R wave or wider than 40 ms.*

In addition, T-wave inversion in V_1–V_2 is common but not mandatory (T directed in an opposite direction to QRS).

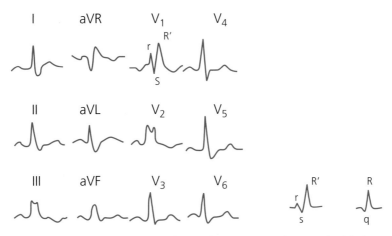

Figure 31.23 RBBB. rSR' is seen in V_1, notched R wave is seen in V_2, and rsR' and qR patterns are shown on the right (rsR' means small R, small S, big R'). Any of those patterns is consistent with RBBB in V_1–V_2. S wave is wide and slurred in leads I, aVL, and V_5–V_6.

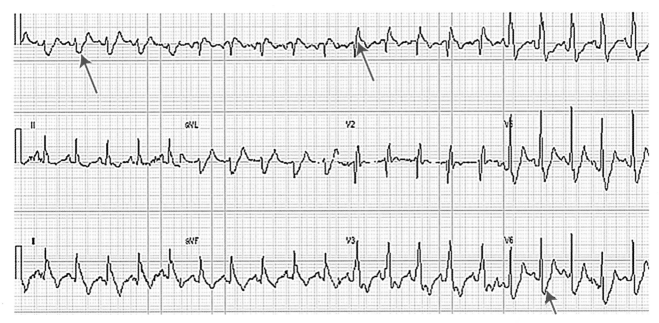

Figure 31.24 Sinus tachycardia with RBBB (rSR' in V_1–V_2, wide and slurred S in V_5–V_6 and I–aVL, *arrows*). Right-axis deviation (QRS [–] in lead I, [+] in lead aVF) signifies an associated RVH (most commonly) or LPFB. T-wave inversion in V_1–V_3 and II/III/aVF is secondary to RBBB and RVH. The patient is diagnosed with PE. Reproduced with permission of Scrub Hill Press from Hanna et al. (2009).[1]

B. LBBB

In **LBBB**, QRS has a slurred positivity in the **left** leads. The first four criteria are required to make the diagnosis of LBBB:

1. Wide notched R wave in leads I, aVL, and V_5–V_6 (M-shaped or slurred, plateaued R wave).
2. QRS is negative in leads V_1, V_2, V_3 with an rS or QS pattern.
   QS pattern may also occur in leads III and aVF, simulating an inferior MI, but not in lead II.
   QR pattern does not occur with LBBB and always implies an associated MI.

3. The septal q wave should be absent in the left leads I and V₅–V₆. A narrow q wave may be seen in aVL.

4. The ST segment and T wave should be directed opposite to QRS. Unlike LVH, RBBB, and RVH, secondary ST–T changes are mandatory in LBBB.

5. Two less usual features may be seen in LBBB and do not preclude the diagnosis of LBBB:

- q wave in aVL.
- RS pattern (rather than a plateaued R pattern) in leads V₅–V₆. This occurs in patients with delayed QRS transition, such as patients with enlarged LV or LV depolarization that spreads from apex to base; the frontal QRS axis is leftward in both of these cases.

An incomplete RBBB or LBBB, also called bundle branch delay, is characterized by a QRS of 110–119 ms with QRS features of the respective bundle branch block in V₁, V₆, and I. Similarly to a complete block, an incomplete block is accompanied by the secondary repolarization abnormalities.

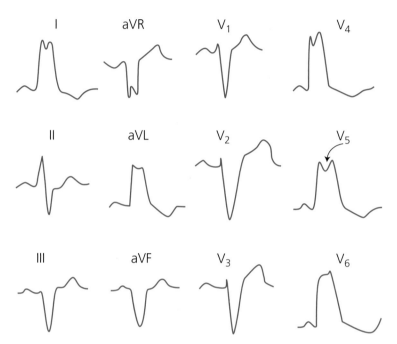

Figure 31.25 LBBB. In the lateral leads, there may be an "M-shaped" R wave (as seen here in I and V₅) or a broad slurred R wave (as seen in V₆). When the LV is enlarged or the depolarization is turned further leftward, the transition zone and the wide R wave may not be reached in lead V₆, and an RS pattern is seen in leads V₅–V₆. The wide, M-shaped R wave will still be seen in leads I-aVL and will also be seen more laterally in leads V₇–V₉. Reproduced with permission of Scrub Hill Press from Hanna et al. (2009).[1]

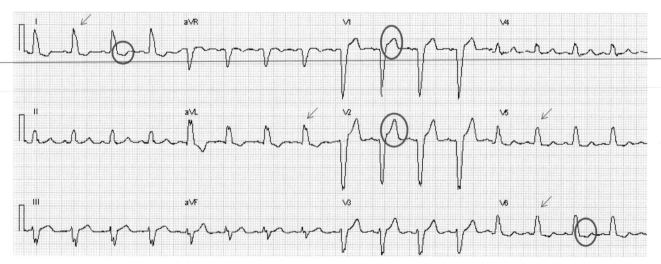

Figure 31.26 LBBB (slurred R wave in the left leads: V₅–V₆ and I–aVL) (*arrows*). ST depression in V₅–V₆, I, and aVL, and ST elevation in V₁–V₃, directed opposite to QRS, are secondary to LBBB (*circles*).

- rSR′ or rSr′ patterns in V₁–V₂ may be normal variants if QRS is < 110 ms and r and r′ are small (r′ < 5 mm) and smaller than S wave, without right-axis deviation, right atrial enlargement, or T-wave inversion.
- Posterior MI may simulate rSR′ in V₁. As opposed to RBBB, r is usually wide.
- RVH may lead to rSR′ pattern in V₁ with incomplete or complete RBBB. In those cases, RVH is diagnosed if the axis is right, as determined by the net voltage of the initial, unblocked 80 ms of QRS in the limb leads, *along with* a suggestive clinical context or R′ > 10 mm in V₁. In fact, right axis in a RBBB is most commonly due to RVH, more so when RBBB is *incomplete*. Incomplete RBBB may reflect a prolonged depolarization of a large RV rather than a histological abnormality of the right bundle.

LVH cannot be formally diagnosed in the presence of complete LBBB, but can be diagnosed in the presence of incomplete LBBB. In fact, *LVH with QRS 110–119 ms and with loss of septal q waves in leads I and V₅–V₆ is a combined LVH + incomplete LBBB.* Outside LBBB, septal q waves are prominent in patients with LVH and may be of pathological dimension. In some patients, LBBB is due to a block across the left bundle, but in many other patients, LBBB is due to diffuse slowing across a diseased, enlarged LV. In the latter patients, *there is a progression from LVH to incomplete LBBB then complete LBBB over months to years, as cardiomyopathy progresses, and LBBB tends to have more left-axis deviation.*

A wide QRS ("complete block" ≥ 120 ms) typically has either RBBB or LBBB pattern. A mildly widened QRS (110–119 ms) may be an incomplete block (RBBB or LBBB pattern), or a widened QRS accompanying LVH, RVH, or fascicular block.

However, a mildly or a definitely **widened QRS may also signify**:

- Pre-excitation (WPW). In that case, the wide QRS starts with a "slur" (= delta wave = slow QRS upslope). This slur is riding the P wave (= short PR). *Unlike bundle branch block, where QRS has a steep initial portion and a slow terminal portion, the QRS complex of WPW is widened at its initial uptake* (Figure 31.27).
- Hyperkalemia.
- Drugs (class Ic antiarrhythmic drugs, tricyclics, phenothiazines).
- Non-specific intraventricular conduction delay.

In contrast to bundle branch block and WPW, the wide QRS of hyperkalemia is characterized by being wide both in its initial portion (≠ bundle branch block) and in its terminal portion (≠ WPW). A very wide QRS (> 180–200 ms) should always suggest hyperkalemia or WPW pattern.

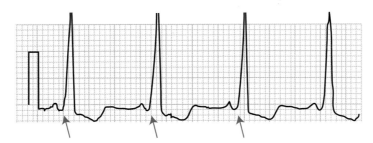

Figure 31.27 WPW with short PR segment and slurred R wave. The upslope of R wave is slow (≠ LBBB).

VIII. Conduction abnormalities: fascicular blocks

The left bundle divides into the left anterior and the left posterior fascicles. In fascicular blocks, unlike bundle branch blocks, QRS must not be very wide and must be < 120 ms; usually, QRS is 80–100 ms wide (Figures 31.28, 31.29, 31.30).

A. Left anterior fascicular block (LAFB)

- LAFB is defined as "*an unexplained left-axis deviation*" with QRS axis between –45° and –90°. In other words, LAFB manifests as left-axis deviation beyond –45° without LBBB or inferior MI.
- A qR pattern is seen in lead I and particularly lead aVL, while rS pattern is typically seen in the inferior leads II, III, and aVF (net QRS is negative in the latter leads). Beside being positive in I and negative in aVF, the net QRS is larger in aVF than in I, which defines axis ≤ –45°.
- Additional notes:
  ○ LVH does not preclude LAFB diagnosis. In fact, LVH with left-axis deviation over –45° usually implies LVH + LAFB.
  ○ Inferior MI makes LAFB diagnosis more difficult. Inferior MI may lead to a QS pattern in leads II, III, and aVF and a left axis over –45°, whether LAFB coexists or not. If LAFB coexists, R wave will peak in aVL earlier than in aVR.
  ○ LAFB does not, by itself, produce QS waves in leads III and aVF and should not mimic inferior MI.
  ○ While the ACC guidelines mandate the presence of a small septal q wave in lead aVL for the definition of LAFB, a study has suggested that up to 27% of patients with LAFB do not have a q wave in leads I and/or aVL. These may be patients who have a horizontal heart, in whom the septal depolarization is orthogonal to lead I ± aVL, or patients who have a degree of septal conduction block.
  ○ LAFB is common with and without underlying heart disease and does not portend an independent prognostic significance. LAFB does not lead to secondary ST–T abnormalities.

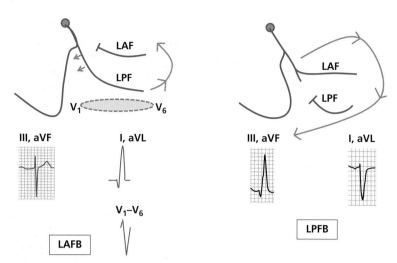

Figure 31.28 In LAFB, the vector of depolarization spreads from the posterior fascicle *superiorly* and *to the left* in a counterclockwise fashion. The superior spread in the *frontal plane* explains the left-axis deviation and the fact that R wave peaks earlier in lead aVL (left) than aVR (right). Also, the R wave amplitude is increased in leads I and aVL. Unlike LBBB, septal depolarization is still left-to-right, hence the septal q wave in leads I and aVL is not usually lost. The q wave may be lost in lead I if the septal depolarization is orthogonal to lead I, but not usually in lead aVL.

The superior spread away from the *precordial plane* explains the deep S waves across all of the precordial leads V_1–V_6 and the delayed R-wave progression. The small "r" corresponds to the initial, inferiorly directed septal depolarization. Occasionally, if the leads are moved up, away from this initial depolarization, the initial "r" is lost, which produces a QS pattern in V_1–V_2 mimicking anterior MI. Moreover, a tiny initial q wave may appear before "r" in V_1–V_3 (qrS pattern), further mimicking MI. The resolution of Q wave by moving the leads one intercostal space down argues against MI.

In LPFB, the depolarization spreads left/up through the anterior fascicle then down and to the right. This initial upward spread explains the q waves in leads III and aVF, while the inferior spread explains the prominent R wave in those leads, the right-axis deviation, and the deep S wave in leads I and aVL. LAF, left anterior fascicle; LPF, left posterior fascicle.

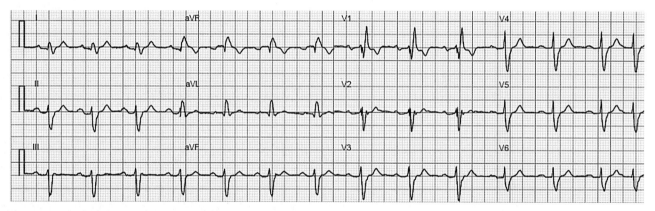

Figure 31.29 LAFB + RBBB.

- QRS is wide > 120 ms with rSR' in V_1 and a wide S in V_5–V_6 = RBBB.
- The net QRS is (–) in lead aVF and equiphasic in lead I, implying a left axis of ~ –90°. In the absence of LBBB, this is diagnostic of LAFB. Also, a q wave is seen in lead aVL, which is often necessary to define LAFB.

Reproduced with permission of Scrub Hill Press from Hanna et al. (2009).[1]

A combination of RBBB and left-axis deviation suggests the presence of LAFB in addition to the RBBB (= bifascicular block). This is a common conduction abnormality.

B. LPFB

- LPFB is uncommon and typically occurs in conjunction with RBBB.
- LPFB is defined as "*an unexplained right-axis deviation*" (more than +90°) = right-axis deviation without RVH, COPD, or lateral MI (R wave in V_1 and S wave in V_6 are not large). A qR pattern is seen in the inferior leads III/aVF. LPFB does not lead to ST–T abnormalities.

C. Bifascicular and trifascicular blocks

A bifascicular block is a block in two of the three conduction fascicles (right bundle, left anterior fascicle, and left posterior fascicle). It can take one of the following forms: (i) LBBB; (ii) RBBB + LAFB = RBBB with left-axis deviation; (iii) RBBB + LPFB = RBBB with right-axis deviation (which could also be RBBB + RVH).

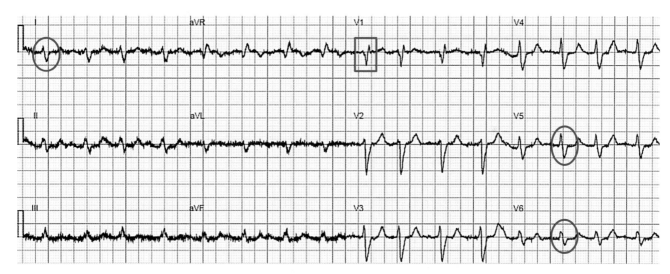

Figure 31.30 RBBB + LPFB. Since QRS is wide > 120 ms, look in V$_1$ and in V$_6$ to determine if the morphology fits more with LBBB or RBBB. In this case, QR morphology is seen in V$_1$ (*box*), with a wide slurred S wave in V$_5$–V$_6$ and I, aVL (*circles*): this is RBBB. The axis is right (net QRS is negative in I and positive in aVF). Exact axis: QRS is closest to equiphasic in lead II → axis perpendicular to +60° → +150°. The cause of right axis could be RVH or LPFB. Because there are no RVH criteria (R′ < S in V$_1$, S not larger than R in V$_6$), LPFB is the probable diagnosis. Reproduced with permission of Scrub Hill Press from Hanna et al. (2009).[1]

A trifascicular block implies that all three fascicles have a conduction block. The block is incomplete in at least one fascicle, otherwise complete AV block would be present. Trifascicular block may manifest as:

- Bifascicular block + increased PR interval: this is often a trifascicular block (may also be bifascicular block with first-degree AV block)
- Alternating RBBB + LBBB, i.e., RBBB and LBBB alternate on the same ECG or on different ECGs obtained up to several years apart
- RBBB with alternating LAFB and LPFB

D. Wide QRS 110–119 ms or ≥ 120 ms that does not fulfill the typical LBBB or RBBB morphology
For example, one bundle branch block morphology is seen in the precordial leads and the contralateral bundle branch block morphology is seen in the limb leads. This wide QRS may be:

- A form of RBBB + LAFB
- Non-specific intraventricular conduction delay, especially in a patient with cardiomyopathy
- Pre-excitation, hyperkalemia, or drugs (class I antiarrhythmics, tricyclics)

Note that QRS notching with a normal QRS duration < 110 ms does not imply a conduction delay and is often normal. It is related to the way the vector of depolarization spreads around the lead.

> Always think of hyperkalemia in any patient with atypical bundle branch block.

IX. Low QRS voltage and electrical alternans
Low QRS voltage is defined as an **absolute sum of R and S waves < 5 mm in every limb lead and < 10 mm in every precordial lead.** Also, a decrease in voltage in the limbs and/or precordial leads in comparison to an old ECG may be indicative of disease, even if it does not fulfill the listed criteria. A patient with baseline LVH may have a relatively reduced QRS voltage without fulfilling the low-voltage definition.

A. Differential diagnosis of small QRS voltage
- Pericardial effusion. Electrical alternans may also be seen.
- Any "shield" around the heart: COPD, obesity, large pleural effusion, and notably hypothyroidism ("low" and "slow").
- Constrictive pericarditis; some restrictive infiltrative cardiomyopathies (such as amyloidosis and hemochromatosis, but not Fabry disease).

B. High QRS voltage in the precordial leads with low QRS voltage in the limb leads is relatively specific for a dilated LV with low EF

C. Electrical alternans is an every-other-beat alternation of two different but *equally wide* and *equidistant* QRS complexes
Electrical alternans may also involve the P and T waves, in which case it is called total alternans and is very specific for pericardial effusion (Figure 31.31).

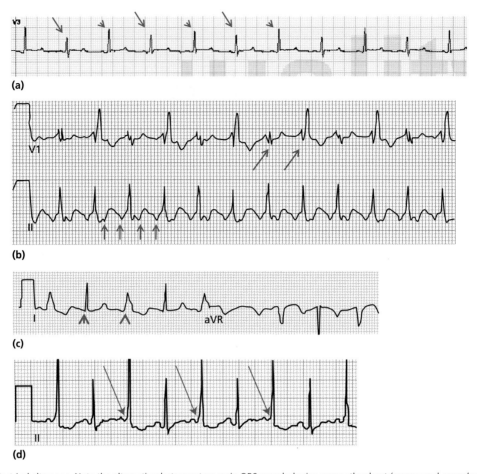

Figure 31.31 (a) Electrical alternans. Note the alternation between two main QRS morphologies every other beat (*arrows* and *arrowheads*). This is different from the cyclical QRS changes seen in patients breathing deeply and rapidly. The two QRS complexes have approximately the same width.

(b) Atrial flutter. Negative flutter waves are seen in lead II (*vertical arrows*). Note the alternation of two QRS morphologies, both equally wide and equidistant (*oblique arrows*). The larger QRS in V$_1$ is a typical RBBB, the smaller QRS is an atypical RBBB with RSR'S' pattern. This is electrical alternans secondary to tachyarrhythmia, wherein the ventricular conduction alternately follows a slightly different path.

(c) Alternation between a narrow QRS and an equidistant wide QRS with LBBB morphology (*arrowheads*). Ventricular bigeminy is unlikely, as the wide QRS is equidistant from the narrow one. This is not electrical alternans either, as QRS width is changing significantly. This is an intermittent, alternating LBBB.

(d) Alternation of a narrow and an equidistant wide QRS. PR interval shortens and a delta wave is seen on the wider QRS complexes (*arrows*). This is intermittent pre-excitation. One QRS is antegradely conducted over an accessory pathway with a short PR and a delta wave (WPW). The next beat proceeds down the AV node rather than the accessory pathway, the accessory pathway being in a refractory period.

QRS amplitude may vary with respiration, particularly in patients who are breathing heavily. In this case, the heart position, and more particularly the septal position, varies with respiration; this may be seen in tamponade, but also in severe COPD or any respiratory distress. This cyclic change of QRS morphology and axis is not electrical alternans and correlates more with pulsus paradoxus ("electrical paradoxus"). Conversely, electrical alternans implies every-other-beat alternation of two distinct QRS morphologies and corresponds to a swinging heart in a patient with pericardial efffusion. Electrical alternans may also be seen with:

- Severe HF, where it is mechanically induced by an alternate change in cardiac contraction (like pulsus alternans).
- SVT, especially AVRT or any fast SVT, wherein a slight variation in ventricular conduction occurs alternately.
- Acute myocardial ischemia or PE, where again there is a conduction alternans.
- Intermittent pre-excitation or intermittent conduction block, such as LAFB or bundle branch block, occurring in an alternating fashion. This is rather a mimic than a true electrical alternans.

A slight change in QRS morphology may normally be seen between the beats of an irregular rhythm, making the diagnosis of true electrical alternans more difficult (e.g., AF).

X. Assessment of ischemia and infarction: Q waves

Normally, a small Q wave (q) may be seen in all leads except the right precordial leads before the R/S transition zone, which usually corresponds to leads V$_1$, V$_2$, and V$_3$. An abnormal Q wave signifies an old MI, a recent MI, or an acute evolving STEMI (in the latter, concomitant ST elevation would be present in the same leads) (Figures 31.32–31.35).

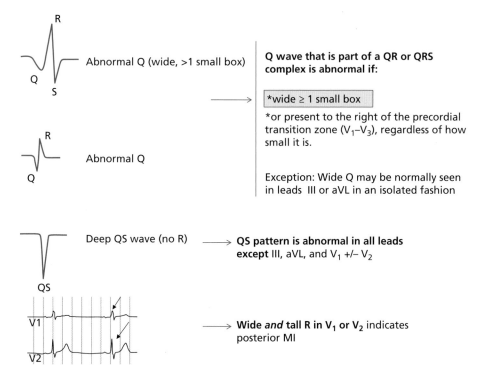

Figure 31.32 Wide Q wave (QS or QR) may be normally seen in lead III of a horizontal heart looking away from lead III. QS or QR pattern may normally be seen in lead aVL in a patient with a vertical heart that looks away from lead aVL.

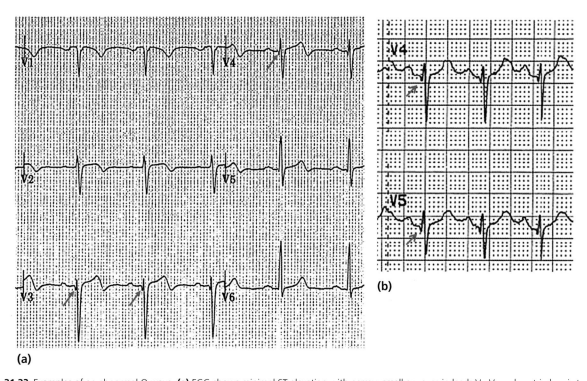

Figure 31.33 Examples of an abnormal Q wave. **(a)** ECG shows minimal ST elevation with narrow small q waves in leads V_3–V_4 and post-ischemic terminal T-wave inversion (not a Wellens syndrome since Q waves are present). **Q of any size, when seen in the precordial leads before the transition zone as part of a qrS complex, is abnormal and is almost 100% indicative of MI** (the rare exception being the tiny q wave sometimes seen with LAFB). This ECG is a late STEMI, at a time when Q waves/T inversion have appeared and ST elevation is resolving. **(b)** Small q waves in leads V_4–V_5 where QRS is still overall negative. Thus, these q waves occur before the transition zone and imply MI, even if very small.

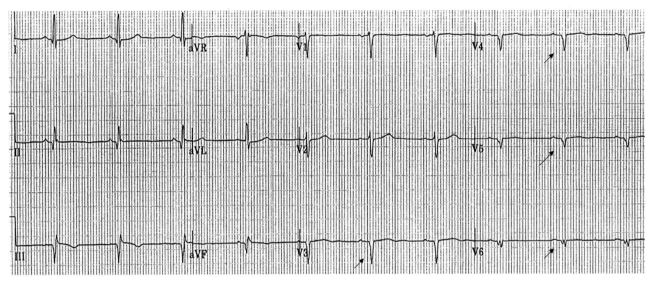

Figure 31.34 Inferior Q waves and anterolateral QS waves (QS waves are wide monophasic Q waves, *arrows*). QS waves may be normal in leads V$_1$–V$_2$, but not in leads V$_3$–V$_6$.

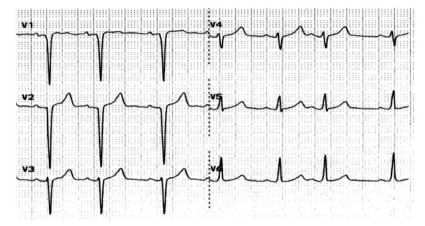

Figure 31.35 QS pattern is seen in leads V$_1$–V$_2$, small R wave is seen in leads V$_3$–V$_4$. As opposed to QS pattern extending to V$_3$ or beyond, QS pattern limited to V$_1$ or V$_2$ is not definitely an anterior MI. Only 20% of patients with a QS pattern in leads V$_1$–V$_2$, without other abnormalities on the ECG, have an anterior MI. The differential diagnosis of a QS pattern in leads V$_1$–V$_2$ is similar to the differential diagnosis of delayed R-wave progression.

Q wave is abnormal when it is:

- ≥0.03 seconds wide (~1 small box) and ≥0.1 mV deep (1 mm)
  or
- whenever any q wave is seen before the precordial transition zone, no matter how small it is (= any q wave in leads V$_1$–V$_3$ is abnormal when QRS is still overall negative in V$_1$–V$_3$).

The criterion Q wave > ¼ of the R-wave height is not, per se, specific for the diagnosis of MI.

A wide *and* tall R wave in leads V$_1$ or V$_2$ is a mirror image of a posterior Q wave and implies posterior MI (R ≥ 0.04 seconds in width and R > S in height). As opposed to RVH, R wave is not just tall but wide, T wave is upright rather than inverted, and Q waves are often present in the inferior or lateral leads, and in leads V$_7$–V$_9$.

Differential diagnosis of pathologic Q waves

- A QRS that consists of only one deep negative deflection is, in fact, a monophasic deep Q wave. Since there is no intervening R wave, this negative wave is a Q wave rather than an S wave, but is sometimes called a QS wave.
- QS in V$_1$–V$_2$ may represent an anterior MI in 20% of the cases, but often does not. Similarly to poor R-wave progression, it often results from LBBB, LAFB, LVH shifting the heart leftward and posteriorly, COPD pushing the heart down and posteriorly, or, frequently, low heart/low diaphragm with high lead placement away from the heart. Moving the precordial leads below the standard position may correct Q waves in many of the latter cases (COPD, low heart, LAFB). QS that extends to V$_3$ is often an anterior MI, while QS extending to V$_4$ is definitely an anterior MI. **Importantly, as opposed to QS, qrS in V$_1$–V$_3$ always signifies anterior MI, regardless how small the q wave is** (rarely, anterior qrS may be seen with LAFB). While infrequently suggestive of anterior MI, poor R-wave progression may be the only sequela of ~25% of anterior MIs.

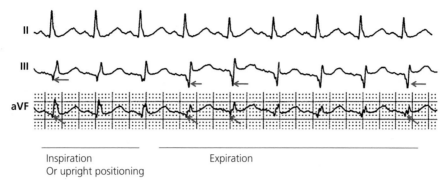

Inspiration
Or upright positioning

Expiration

Figure 31.36 In expiration, Q wave is wide and deep in leads III and aVF (*arrows*); no Q wave is seen in lead II at any time (Q wave in lead II makes inferior MI definite). During inspiration or upright position, the Q wave becomes smaller and narrower in both leads III and aVF, implying that this Q wave is most likely related to a horizontal heart position during expiration. This lessens the probability of inferior MI but does not rule it out.

- Whereas QS or QR in the inferior leads III and aVF often signifies an MI, it may be a normal variant in obese/stocky individuals with horizontal hearts directed away from the inferior leads. A deep breath or standing up verticalizes the heart and minimizes these Q waves (Figure 31.36).

  QS in leads III and aVF, but not in lead II and not QR, may also occur with LBBB and LVH, cases where the depolarization vector looks away from the inferior leads.

  QR in leads III and aVF may be seen with RVH or PE, wherein the LV is pushed up and the RV expands down. The up-looking LV depolarization explains the inferior Q waves.

  Note, however, that a wide Q in the inferior lead II almost always implies MI, and a QrS pattern, even when limited to leads III and aVF, usually implies MI and is not seen with obesity or conduction abnormalities. Also, the presence of a wide R wave in lead aVR increases the likelihood of a true inferior MI.
- QS or QR may normally occur in lead aVL in patients with vertical hearts, or in cases of chest deformity or left pneumothorax. Severe septal hypertrophy (HCM) may produce deep/wide Q waves in the lateral leads (QR pattern in leads I, aVL, V_5–V_6), and sometimes the inferior leads, ± prominent R waves in the right precordial leads V_1–V_2 (all correspond to the septal forces).
- The negative delta wave of pre-excitation may simulate a wide and pathologic Q wave. It may be seen in the inferior, lateral, or anterior leads.
- Any cardiomyopathy, especially infiltrative cardiomyopathy (e.g., amyloidosis), may lead to Q waves as a result of fibrosis or myocardial replacement with the infiltrative process. Myocarditis occasionally leads to Q waves.
- Takotsubo cardiomyopathy, which leads to anterior ST-segment elevation and T-wave inversion, may also lead to transient anterior Q waves.

XI. Assessment of ischemia: ST-segment depression and T-wave inversion

Abnormalities of the ST segment and T wave represent abnormalities of ventricular repolarization. The ST segment corresponds to the plateau phase of ventricular repolarization (phase 2), while the T wave corresponds to the phase of rapid ventricular repolarization (phase 3). ST-segment or T-wave changes may be secondary to abnormalities of depolarization, i.e., pre-excitation or abnormalities of QRS voltage or duration. On the other hand, ST-segment and T-wave abnormalities may be unrelated to any QRS abnormality, in which case they are called primary repolarization abnormalities. They are caused by ischemia, pericarditis, myocarditis, drugs (digoxin, antiarrhythmic drugs), and electrolyte abnormalities, particularly potassium abnormalities.[2]

ST-segment deviation is usually measured at its junction with the end of the QRS complex, i.e., the J point, and is referenced against the TP or PR segment.[3] Some authors, however, prefer measuring the magnitude of the ST segment deviation 40–80 ms after the J point, when all myocardial fibers are expected to have reached the same level of membrane potential and to form an isoelectric ST segment; at the very onset of repolarization, small differences in membrane potential may normally be seen and may cause deviation of the J point and of the early portion of the ST segment.[4] A diagnosis of ST-segment elevation myocardial infarction (STEMI) that mandates emergent reperfusion therapy requires ST-segment elevation equaling or exceeding the following cut-points, in at least two contiguous leads (using the standard of 1.0 mV = 10 mm):[5]

- 1 mm in all standard leads other than leads V_2–V_3.
- 2.5 mm in leads V_2 and V_3 in men younger than age 40, 2 mm in leads V_2 and V_3 in men older than age 40, and 1.5 mm in these leads in women.
- 0.5 mm in the posterior chest leads V_7–V_9. ST-segment elevation is attenuated in the posterior leads because of their greater distance from the heart, explaining the lower cut-point.

Concerning ST-segment depression, a depression of up to 0.5 mm in leads V_2 and V_3 and 1 mm in the other leads may be normal.[3]

While ST-segment deviation that falls below these cut-points may be a normal variant, any ST-segment elevation or depression (≥0.5 mm) may be abnormal, particularly when the clinical setting or the ST-segment morphology suggests ischemia, or when other ischemic signs such as T-wave abnormalities, Q waves, or reciprocal ST-segment changes are concomitantly present. Conversely, ST-segment elevation that exceeds these cut-points may not represent STEMI. In an analysis of chest pain patients manifesting ST-segment elevation, only 15% were eventually diagnosed with STEMI. Beside size, careful attention to the morphology of the ST segment and the associated features is critical.

In adults, the T wave is normally inverted in lead aVR; is upright or inverted in leads aVL, III, and V_1; and is upright in the remaining leads. The T wave is considered inverted when it is deeper than 1 mm and is considered flat when its peak amplitude is between 1 mm and −1 mm.[3]

A. Secondary ST-segment and/or T-wave abnormalities

In secondary ST-segment or T-wave abnormalities, QRS criteria for ventricular hypertrophy (LVH or RVH), bundle branch block (LBBB or RBBB), or pre-excitation are usually present, and the ST segment and T wave have *all of* the following morphologic features (Figure 31.37A):

i. The ST segment and T wave are directed opposite to the QRS: this is called discordance between the QRS complex and the ST–T abnormalities. In the case of RBBB, the ST and T are directed opposite to the terminal portion of the QRS, i.e., the part of the QRS deformed by the conduction abnormality.
ii. The ST segment and T wave are both abnormal and deviate in the same direction, i.e., the ST segment is downsloping and the T wave is inverted in leads with an upright QRS complex, which gives the ST–T complex a "reverse checkmark" asymmetric morphology.
iii. The ST and T abnormalities are not dynamic, i.e., they do not change in the course of several hours to several days.

Thus, in LVH or LBBB, since the QRS complex is upright in the left lateral leads I, aVL, V_5, and V_6, the ST segment is characteristically depressed and T wave inverted in these leads (Figure 31.38). In RVH or RBBB, T waves are characteristically inverted in the right precordial leads V_1–V_3. LBBB is always associated with secondary ST–T abnormalities, the absence of which suggests associated ischemia. LVH and RVH, on the other hand, are not always associated with ST–T abnormalities, but when present, they correlate with more severe hypertrophy or ventricular systolic dysfunction,[6] and have been called *strain pattern*. In addition, while these morphologic features are consistent with secondary abnormalities, they do not rule out ischemia in a patient with angina.

There are **some exceptions** to these typical morphologic features:

- In LVH/LBBB, the transition of QRS from negative to positive may occur in a different lead than the transition of T wave from positive to negative. Thus, in one lead, the QRS and T wave may both be upright, or the QRS and T wave may both be negative. This, however, is usually limited to one lead.
- RVH and RBBB may be associated with isolated T-wave inversion without ST-segment depression in the precordial leads V_1–V_3. In fact, RBBB and RVH are usually associated with only mild degrees of ST-segment depression in comparison to their left counterparts (the R wave and myocardial mass are smaller with RVH/RBBB than LVH/LBBB).
- LVH may be associated with symmetric T-wave inversion without ST-segment depression or with a horizontally depressed ST segment. This may be the case in up to one-third of ST–T abnormalities secondary to LVH and is seen in hypertrophic cardiomyopathy in leads V_3–V_6 (this pattern is classically seen with the apical variant but is common with any variant).[7]

B. Ischemic ST-segment depression and/or T-wave inversion

ST-segment depression or T-wave inversion that adopts *any* of the features shown in Figure 31.37B–E is consistent with ischemia:

i. The ST-segment depression *or* T-wave inversion is directed in the same direction as the QRS complex: this is called concordance between the QRS complex and the ST or T abnormality (Figure 31.37B).
ii. The ST segment is depressed but the T wave is upright (Figure 31.37C).
iii. The T wave has a positive–negative biphasic pattern (Figure 31.37D).
iv. The T wave is symmetrically inverted and has a pointed configuration, while the ST segment is not deviated or is upwardly bowed (coved) or horizontally depressed (Figure 31.37E).
v. The magnitude of ST-segment depression progresses or regresses on serial tracings, or ST-segment depression progresses to T-wave abnormality during ischemia-free intervals (dynamic ST-segment depression).

Unlike ST-segment elevation, ST-segment depression does not localize ischemia.[8] However, the extent and the magnitude of ST-segment depression correlate with the extent and the severity of ischemia. In fact, ST-segment depression in eight or more leads, combined with ST-segment elevation in leads aVR and V_1 and occurring during ischemic pain, is associated with a 75% predictive accuracy of left main or three-vessel disease (Figure 31.39).[9,10] This finding may also be seen in cases of tight proximal left anterior descending stenosis.[11] It implies diffuse subendocardial ischemia, with reciprocal ST-segment elevation in the two leads that look away from the normal myocardial repolarization. ST-segment elevation that is more prominent in aVR than V_1 often implies critical left main coronary disease and often mandates urgent angiography.[11]

> When ST-segment elevation occurs in two contiguous leads while ST-segment depression occurs in other leads, and when the ST–T abnormalities are ischemic rather than secondary to LVH or LBBB, ST-segment elevation is considered the primary ischemic abnormality whereas ST-segment depression is often considered a reciprocal "mirror image" change in opposite leads. ST-segment elevation is reciprocal to ST-segment depression only when ST depression is diffuse and ST elevation is limited to the two non-contiguous leads, V_1 and aVR, implying an extensive subendocardial ischemia.

Note: T-wave inversion and Wellens syndrome

Either the positive–negative biphasic T waves of the type shown in Figure 31.37D or the deeply inverted (≥5 mm) T waves that often follow them, when occurring in the precordial leads V_2 and V_3, with or without similar changes in V_1, V_4, V_5, are virtually pathognomonic for very recent severe ischemia or injury in the distribution of the left anterior descending artery (LAD) and characterize what is known as Wellens syndrome (Figure 31.40).[12–15] Wellens et al. showed that 75% of patients who developed these T-wave abnormalities and who were treated

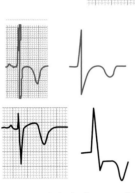

(a) ST-segment depression and asymmetric T-wave inversion secondary to left ventricular hypertrophy (left) and left bundle branch block (right).

(b) ST-segment depression and T-wave inversion concordant to QRS, suggestive of ischemia.

(c) ST-segment depression with an upright or biphasic negative-positive T wave, suggestive of ischemia.

(d) Positive-negative biphasic T wave with a minimally elevated J point and an angle of 60 to 90 degrees between the initial ascending portion and the descending portion of the T wave (Wellens-type T-wave abnormality, usually seen in precordial leads V_1–V_4). This finding is very specific for ischemia.

(e) Symmetric and pointed deep T-wave inversion with an isoelectric or a slightly up-sloping or horizontally depressed ST segment (isoelectric: top two panels; slightly up-sloping: third panel; horizontally depressed: fourth panel); often follows the biphasic T waves seen in D by hours to days. As the T-wave changes subsequently regress, the positive-negative biphasic T-waves are again seen before repolarization returns to normal.

Figure 31.37 ST-segment and T-wave morphologies in cases of **(a)** secondary abnormalities and **(b–e)** ischemic abnormalities. Modified with permission of Scrub Hill Press from Hanna et al. (2009).

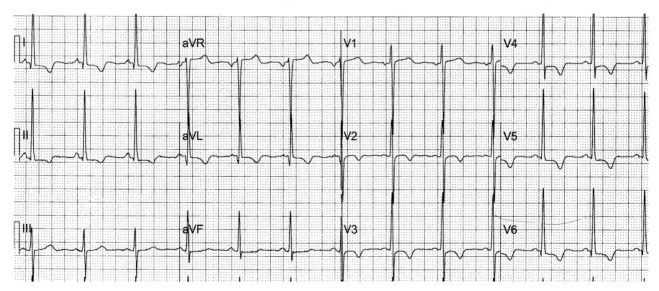

Figure 31.38 Example of left ventricular hypertrophy with typical secondary ST–T abnormalities in leads I, II, aVL, V_4–V_6. The QRS complex is upright in these leads while the ST segment and T wave are directed in the opposite direction, i.e., the QRS and the ST–T complexes are discordant. Reproduced with permission of the Cleveland Clinic Foundation from Hanna and Glancy (2011).[2]

medically without angiographic investigation went on to develop extensive anterior wall myocardial infarction within a mean of 8.5 days.[12] In a later investigation of 1260 patients presenting with unstable angina, 180 patients (14%) had this characteristic T-wave pattern.[13] All of the latter patients had stenosis of 50% or more in the LAD (proximal to the 2nd septal branch), and 18% had total LAD occlusion. Thus, although medical management may provide symptomatic improvement at first, early coronary angiography and revascularization should be strongly considered in anyone with Wellens syndrome because it usually predicts impending anterior myocardial infarction.

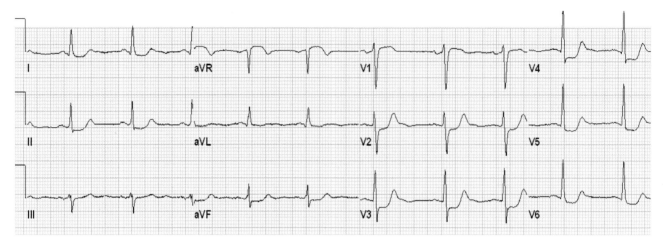

Figure 31.39 Electrocardiogram of a patient with angina at rest and elevated cardiac biomarkers. ST-segment depression in nine leads with elevation in leads aVR and V_1 suggested subendocardial ischemia related to three-vessel or left main coronary artery disease. He had severe left main and three-vessel disease on coronary arteriography. Reproduced with permission of the Cleveland Clinic Foundation from Hanna and Glancy (2011).[2]

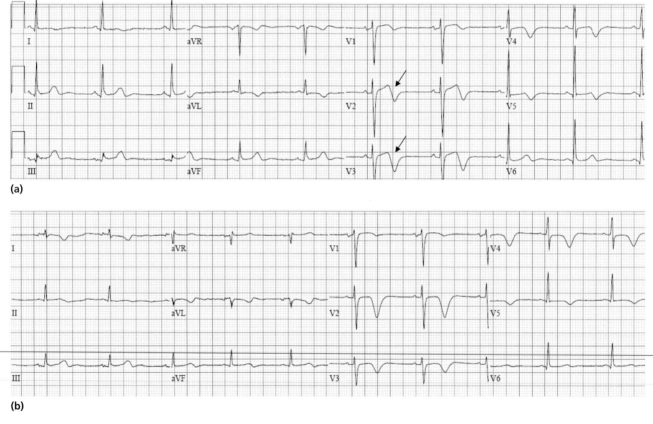

Figure 31.40 Examples of Wellens-type T-wave abnormalities. **(a)** Wellens-type biphasic T wave in leads V_2 and V_3 *(arrows)* and deep T-wave inversion in lead V_4, with a straight or convex ST segment. **(b)** Wellens-type deep T-wave inversion in leads V_2–V_4. Each patient had a 90% proximal left anterior descending stenosis at coronary arteriography. Reproduced with permission of the Cleveland Clinic Foundation from Hanna and Glancy (2011).[2]

Wellens syndrome is characterized by two patterns of T-wave changes. In 75% of the cases, T waves are deeply (≥ 5 mm) and symmetrically inverted in leads V_2 through V_4. In 25% of the cases, the T wave has a characteristic positive–negative biphasic morphology in leads V_2 through V_4 (Figure 31.37D).[12] In both patterns, the ST segment is upsloping with a straight or convex morphology, but is not significantly elevated (<1 mm); the downslope of the T wave is sharp (60–90°); and the QT interval is often prolonged. Even in the first pattern, a biphasic T wave is usually seen in at least one lead. This abnormality is characteristically seen hours to days after the ischemic chest pain resolves. In fact, the ischemic episode is usually associated with transient ST-segment elevation or depression that progresses to the T-wave abnormality after the pain subsides.[13] In Wellens' original description, only 12% of patients had small increases in the creatine kinase level. Therefore, the ECG may be the only indication of an impending large anterior infarction in a chest-pain-free patient.[14]

No Q wave is seen and the ST segment is not significantly elevated. The same T-wave morphology may be seen with Q-wave MI or STEMI, but is not called Wellens syndrome in those instances. Rather, it is part of the ECG progression of Q-wave MI (Figure 31.33).

T waves that are symmetrically but less deeply inverted than Wellens-type T waves may still represent ischemia. However, this finding is less specific for ischemia and is associated with better outcomes than Wellens syndrome or ST-segment deviation, particularly when the T wave is less than 3 mm deep.[16] In fact, one prospective cohort study found that isolated mild T-wave inversion in patients presenting with ACS is associated with a favorable long-term outcome, similar to patients with no ECG changes.[17] Similarly to Wellens syndrome, U-wave inversion in leads V_1–V_3, a subtle finding, often implies anterior ischemia.

Biphasic T waves may rarely be seen in the precordial leads outside Wellens syndrome (Figure 31.41).

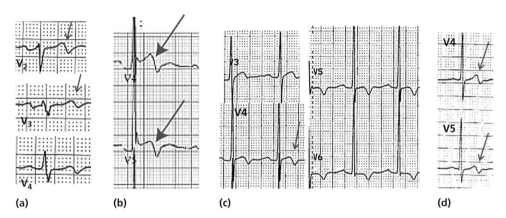

(a)   (b)   (c)   (d)

Figure 31.41 Non-Wellens biphasic T waves. **(a)** Biphasic T wave in leads V_2–V_3, not absolutely typical of Wellens syndrome as the ST segment is concave and T-wave downslope is not very steep. However, this patient had 95% proximal LAD stenosis. **(b)** Normal variant T-wave inversion in an asymptomatic young black male, with prominent, early repolarization-type ST elevation (seen here in leads V_4–V_5, but may be seen in V_2–V_3). **(c)** Biphasic T wave in lead V_4 in a patient with LVH; T wave is transitioning to an inverted pattern in lead V_4, while ST segment is still elevated in this lead and transitions to depression in lead V_6. This early T-wave transition gives a biphasic shape in lead V_4. **(d)** Normal variant biphasic T wave in leads V_4–V_5 in a 50-year-old white man with negative cardiac markers and normal coronary arteries on angiography. This pattern was transient; three ECGs performed the same day, before and after this ECG, were normal. As opposed to Wellens syndrome, the biphasic T waves are not seen in leads V_2–V_3, and the downslope of the T wave is not very steep. A pattern of biphasic T waves may also be seen in pericarditis before T waves fully invert.

C. Frequently missed diagnoses manifesting as ST-segment depression or T-wave inversion

1. True posterior ST-segment elevation myocardial infarction (STEMI)

When accompanied by inferior STEMI, posterior infarction is easily recognized, but it can be difficult to diagnose when it occurs alone, the so-called true posterior STEMI. ST-segment depression that is most prominent in leads V_1 through V_3 often indicates posterior STEMI rather than non-ST-segment elevation ischemia and indicates the need for emergent revascularization. *In fact, in the setting of posterior infarction, leads V_1–V_3 predominate as the areas of maximum depression, whereas greater ST-segment depression in the lateral precordial leads (V_4 through V_6) or inferior leads (II, III, aVF) is more indicative of non-occlusive and non-regional subendocardial ischemia* (Figure 31.42A–B).[10,18–20] In most or all of the cases of posterior infarction, the posterior chest leads V_7–V_9 reveal ST-segment elevation.[21] One study has found that ST-segment depression in the anterior precordial leads is as sensitive as ST-segment elevation in leads V_7 through V_9 in identifying posterior myocardial infarction (sensitivity 80%),[22] while other studies revealed that ST-segment deviation on the standard 12-lead ECG has a lower sensitivity (~60%) in identifying posterior infarction.[20,23] The posterior leads are far from the myocardium, which explains how ST elevation may be minimized and missed in these leads; to improve the sensitivity, 0.5 mm of ST elevation is considered significant in those leads (ACC guidelines).[3]

Tall *and* wide (≥0.04 s) R waves in leads V_1 or V_2, particularly when associated with upright T waves, suggest posterior infarction and may further corroborate this diagnosis, but this finding may take up to 24 hours to manifest and is only seen in about 50% of patients with posterior infarction.[23]

Studies have shown that ST-segment elevation on the standard 12-lead ECG is found in fewer than 50% of patients with acute left circumflex occlusion and inferoposterior infarction,[20] yet these are cases of "missed" STEMI that indeed benefit from emergent angiography and reperfusion. In addition, studies of non-ST-segment elevation ACS consistently identify patients who have acute vessel occlusion (~15–20% of cases),[20] yet their initial angiography is usually delayed for hours or days after the initial presentation.[24] Recognizing that ST-segment depression that is greatest in leads V_1, V_2, or V_3 represents posterior infarction helps identify a portion of the missed STEMIs in a timely fashion. In addition, in cases of anterior ST-segment depression and in cases of chest pain with non-diagnostic ECG, the recording of ST elevation in leads V_7–V_9 is highly sensitive for detecting a true posterior injury.

2. Acute pulmonary embolism

An anterior ischemic pattern of symmetric T-wave inversion in the precordial leads V_1 through V_4 may also be a sign of acute or chronic right ventricular strain, particularly acute PE. Sinus tachycardia is usually present, but other ECG signs of pulmonary embolism, such as RVH and RBBB, may be absent. In fact, T-wave inversion in leads V_1–V_4 is noted in 19% of patients with non-massive PE and in 85% of patients

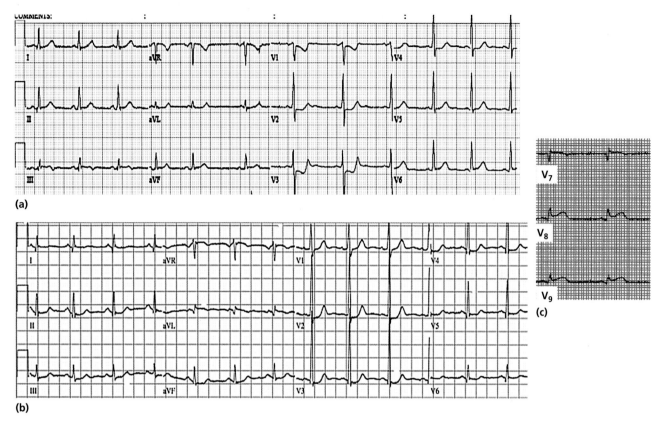

Figure 31.42 Examples of posterior infarction. **(a)** ST-segment depression in the precordial leads V_1–V_4, with a maximal depression in lead V_3, in a patient with severe ongoing chest pain for the preceding 3 hours. This suggests a true posterior ST-segment elevation myocardial infarction. There is also a subtle ST-segment elevation in lead III, which further points to the diagnosis of inferoposterior infarction. Emergency coronary arteriography shows a totally occluded mid-left circumflex coronary artery.

(b) The ST segment is depressed in leads V_1–V_6 and leads II, III, aVF, with a maximal depression in leads V_2 and V_3. In addition, tall R waves are seen in leads V_1 and V_2 and Q waves are seen in the lateral leads I and aVL. In a patient with severe persistent chest pain, this suggests a posterolateral infarct. Coronary arteriography shows a totally occluded second obtuse marginal branch.

(c) In both A and B, ST elevation and wide Q waves are seen in the posterior leads V_7–V_9. ST elevation is barely 1 mm, as the posterior leads are further away from the heart than the anterior leads, which makes posterior ST changes subtle (0.5 mm of ST elevation in those leads is significant). ST elevation appears pronounced when compared to the size of the QRS.

Reproduced with permission of the Cleveland Clinic Foundation from Hanna and Glancy (2011).[2]

with massive PE, and is the most sensitive and specific ECG finding in massive PE.[25] In addition, acute PE may be associated with T-wave inversion in leads III and aVF,[26] and changes of concomitant anterior and inferior ischemia should always raise the suspicion of this diagnosis.[27] Rapid regression of these changes on serial tracings favors PE rather than MI.

> ***Top two differential diagnoses for anterior ST-segment depression (V_1–V_3):***
> - Posterior STEMI if ST depression predominates in the anterior leads.
> - Anterior ischemia if ST depression is diffuse rather than predominant in the anterior leads
>
> ***Top two differential diagnoses for anterior T-wave inversion (V_1–V_3):***
> - Anterior ischemia (may be Wellens syndrome)
> - PE

3. ST-segment depression reciprocal to a subtle ST-segment elevation

Reciprocal ST-segment depression is present in all patients with inferior MI and in 70% of patients with anterior MI.[28] This "reciprocal" change might also represent remote ischemia in a distant territory in patients with multivessel coronary disease.[29,30] However, it is important to recognize that the magnitude of ST-segment elevation and reciprocal ST-segment depression is affected by the distance of the leads recording these changes from the ischemic region and their angle of deviation from the ischemic region.[31] This explains why occasionally – and particularly when the overall amplitude of the QRS complex is low – the magnitude of ST-segment elevation is small whereas the reciprocal ST-segment depression is more prominent. In fact, in the absence of LVH or LBBB, the reciprocal ST-segment depression should always be sought. It is of great utility in patients with acute cardiac symptoms and mild elevation of ST segments of 1–1.5 mm in two contiguous leads, as it strongly suggests the diagnosis of STEMI rather than other causes of mild ST-segment elevation (1–1.5 mm)

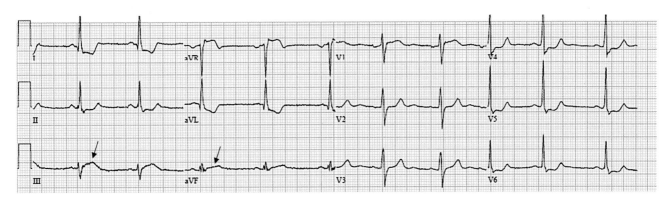

Figure 31.43 Example of subtle ST-segment elevation in two contiguous leads with a prominent ST-segment depression in other leads. The ST segment is depressed in leads I and aVL and V₄–V₆. There is a subtle ST-segment elevation with a broad dome-shaped T wave in leads III and aVF *(arrows)*, suggesting that the primary abnormality is actually an acute inferior injury. Coronary arteriography shows a totally occluded right coronary artery in its mid-segment and severe left circumflex disease. The ST-segment depression is partly reciprocal to the inferior injury and partly a reflection of left circumflex-related ischemia. Reproduced with permission of the Cleveland Clinic Foundation from Hanna and Glancy (2011).[2]

(Figure 31.43).[32] The less-pronounced ST-segment elevation is often overlooked, and the patient is erroneously diagnosed with non-ST-segment elevation ACS rather than STEMI. This has a marked impact on the patient's management, as STEMI requires emergent revascularization, while non-ST-segment elevation ischemia requires early (but not emergency) coronary angiography.

4. Hypokalemia and digitalis effect

ST-segment depression, T-wave flattening, and prominent U waves are the hallmarks of hypokalemia and can be mistaken for ischemic changes, including ischemic lengthening of the QT interval (Figure 31.44).[33–36] Digitalis also produces ST-segment depression, low or inverted T waves, and prominent U waves, but the U waves rarely are of the giant variety seen with severe hypokalemia, and the ST-segment depression has a sagging shape. In addition, digitalis shortens the QT interval.

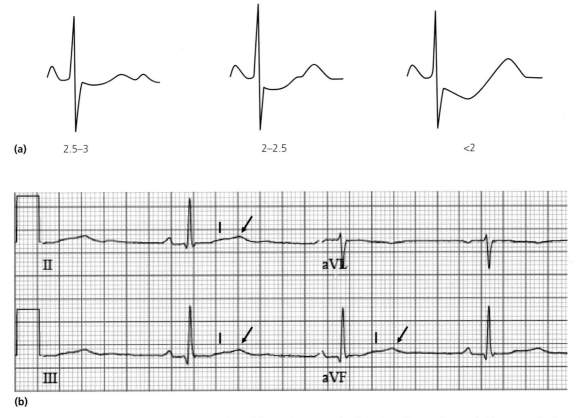

(a)   2.5–3   2–2.5   <2

(b)

Figure 31.44 Hypokalemia and electrocardiographic abnormalities. **(a)** Note the progressive flattening of T wave, increase in U wave amplitude, and depression of ST segment with progressive levels of hypokalemia (potassium levels are expressed in mEq/liter). **(b)** Electrocardiogram of a patient with potassium level of 2.8 mEq/l. Note the flattened T waves *(bars)* and the prominent U waves *(arrows)*. Reproduced with permission of the Cleveland Clinic Foundation from Hanna and Glancy (2011).[2]

5. Memory T waves

RV pacing, LBBB, frequent PVCs, VT, or even SVT are associated with secondary ST-segment and T-wave abnormalities. When these events are intermittent, T waves may remain inverted for hours to weeks after resolution of the event, and these are called memory T waves.[37,38] The ST segment may also get depressed. "Memory T wave" is a misnomer in that the repolarization abnormality does not necessarily have the same morphology as the provoking event and does not necessarily occur in the leads where the T wave was inverted during the provoking event; in fact ST–T may have been normal during tachycardia.

D. Diffuse (global) T-wave inversion

This term is applied when the T wave is inverted in most of the standard ECG leads except aVR, which shows a reciprocal upright T wave. The QT interval is often prolonged, and T-wave inversion is often symmetric and "giant" (>10 mm) (Figure 31.45).[3,39] Walder and Spodick have found this pattern to be caused most often by either *myocardial ischemia* or *neurological events*, particularly intracranial hemorrhage, and it seems more prevalent in women.[40] Two other mechanisms can cause this pattern: *hypertrophic cardiomyopathy* and *high catecholamine state* (takotsubo cardiomyopathy, cocaine abuse). Less commonly, global T inversion may be due to pericarditis, PE, and advanced or complete AV block.[40,41] The prognosis in patients with global T-wave inversion is determined by the underlying disease, and the striking T-wave changes per se do not imply a poor prognosis.[42] This pattern may suggest ischemia, yet, unlike Wellens sign, and in spite of the more extensive T inversion, it is not pathognomonic for ischemia.

On a particular note, takotsubo cardiomyopathy is characterized by ECG changes that mimic ischemia, especially anterior STEMI, and is often impossible to differentiate from myocardial ischemia related to a coronary event without performing coronary arteriography. The most common abnormality on the admission ECG is ST-segment elevation (~80% of patients), typically seen in the precordial leads. Within 24–48 hours of presentation, almost all patients also develop post-ischemic diffuse T-wave inversion and prolongation of the QT interval. New Q waves may be seen in 6–31% of the patients and are usually transient.[43,44] Inferior ST-segment elevation may be seen but is unusual. ST elevation is usually less marked than STEMI.

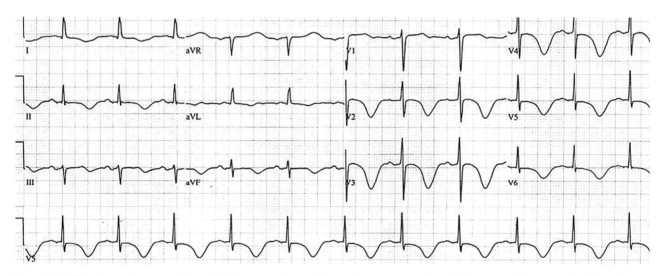

Figure 31.45 Global T-wave inversion with marked QT prolongation in a 77-year-old woman presenting with dyspnea and elevated cardiac biomarkers. **In contrast to Wellens T wave, T wave is not biphasic in any lead, T inversion extends beyond the precordial leads, and the ST segment does not have an upwardly coved shape with a sharp T descent.** Her coronary arteriography showed a 90% distal left main stenosis. Reproduced with permission of Baylor University Medical Center from Glancy et al. (2009).[39]

E. Other causes of T-wave inversion or ST-segment depression

Various other entities may cause T-wave inversion, notably acute pericarditis or myocarditis,[45,46] and normal variants of repolarization (Table 31.1, Figure 31.46).[47] Additionally, a non-pathological junctional ST-segment depression may be seen in tachycardia (Figure 31.47). When baseline ST-segment depression is present, the occurrence of any tachycardia will accentuate ST-segment depression regardless of ischemia.

The term non-specific ST–T changes applies to mild changes, especially ST-segment depression < 1 mm and T-wave inversion < 3 mm. A non-specific T-wave inversion and sometimes a mild ST-segment depression may occur with upright posture, high catecholamine tone, fear, tachycardia, or after a meal, and are partly explained by a *direct effect of catecholamines or tachycardia on myocardial repolarization*. Hyperventilation may produce T-wave inversion but also ST-segment depression; this may create false-positive stress test results. Conversely, a baseline T-wave inversion may normalize with those same processes or with exercise. This normalization is commonly a true normalization of a benign abnormality; however, in a patient with ischemic symptoms, the upright change may represent an ischemic response ("pseudo-normalization" of T-wave inversion).

Table 31.1 Differential diagnosis of ST-segment depression and/or T-wave inversion.

Condition	Features
Secondary repolarization abnormalities	• ST segment and T wave move in the same direction, discordant with QRS
Ischemic ST-segment or T-wave abnormalities[a]	• ST segment or T wave may be concordant with QRS • ST segment and T wave may go in opposite directions • Symmetric and pointed T-wave inversion • Positive–negative biphasic T wave

Wellens syndrome	• Symmetric and deeply inverted T waves
	  OR
	  Positive–negative biphasic T wave in leads V_2 and V_3, occasionally V_1, V_4, V_5, and V_6
	  PLUS
	• Isoelectric or minimally elevated (<1 mm) ST segment
	• No precordial Q waves
	• Prolonged QT interval
	• History of recent chest pain in the last hours to days
	• Pattern present in pain-free state
	• Normal or slightly elevated cardiac serum markers

True posterior STEMI	• Maximal ST-segment depression in V_1–V_3 • ST-segment elevation in V_7–V_9
ST-segment elevation reciprocal to a subtle ST-segment depression	• Subtle ST-segment elevation concomitant to a more marked ST-segment depression in the reciprocal leads
Pulmonary embolism	• T-wave inversion in the anterior and/or inferior leads • Sinus tachycardia, rSR' in V_1–V_2, right ventricular hypertrophy, "P pulmonale" • Rapid regression of abnormalities on serial tracings favors PE rather than MI
Hypokalemia	• ST-segment depression • T-wave flattening • Prominent U wave (with the flattened T wave, may mimic a wide and notched upright T wave) • Prolonged QTU interval
Digitalis effect	• Similar to hypokalemia, except that ST-segment depression is typically sagging, T–U wave separation is more distinct, and QT interval is shortened
Takotsubo cardiomyopathy	• ST-segment elevation in the precordial leads or more diffusely • Diffuse T-wave inversion • Prolonged QT
Acute pericarditis	• Diffusely inverted or biphasic T waves • ST-segment elevation has often resolved at this stage
Memory inverted T waves	• Appear after pacing, transient LBBB, or transient tachycardia (VT or SVT)
Mild rapidly reversible T-wave abnormalities	• T-wave inversion occurs with standing, hyperventilation, exercise or after a meal. May improve with exercise. ST depression may also be seen, especially with hyperventilation
Persistent juvenile T-wave pattern	• T-wave inversion in V_1–V_3 • Decrements between V_1 and V_3 • Young female (<40 years old) • No other ECG or clinical abnormality
Global T-wave inversion	• T-wave inversion in most leads except aVR. • T wave sometimes giant (>10 mm) • May be seen with ischemia, intracranial processes, hypertrophic cardiomyopathy, cocaine use, Takotsubo cardiomyopathy. • Less often: pericarditis/myocarditis, PE, advanced AV block

[a] Any one of these features suggests ischemia.

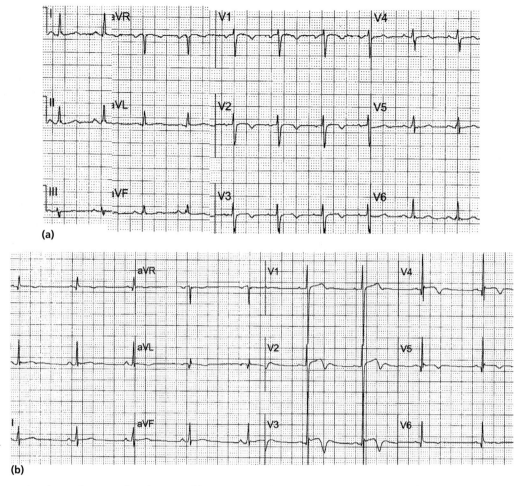

Figure 31.46 Examples of normal variants of repolarization. **(a)** Persistent juvenile T-wave pattern in a 40-year-old female with T-wave inversion extending from lead V_1 to lead V_4. The depth of the inverted T waves decrements between V_1 and V_4. Also, T wave progressively becomes less deeply inverted as the patient ages. **(b)** Normal variant terminal T-wave inversion with ST-segment elevation in leads V_2 through V_5 in a 21-year-old black man. This pattern is most often seen in young black men, a few of whom at other times manifest the typical early repolarization pattern. The age and clinical presentation distinguish this pattern from Wellens-type T waves. Reproduced with permission of the Cleveland Clinic Foundation from Hanna and Glancy (2011).[2]

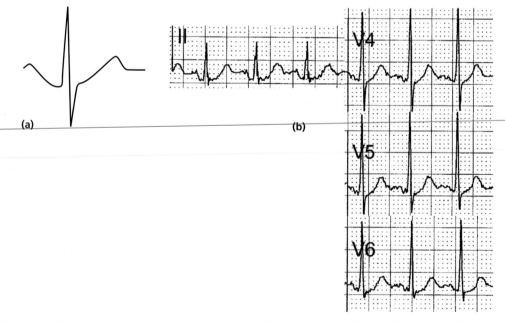

Figure 31.47 **(a)** Upsloping ST-segment depression in sinus tachycardia. During tachycardia, the amplitudes of the P wave and the negative atrial repolarization wave increase. This exaggerated atrial repolarization extends over the PR and ST segments and depresses the PR segment and the initial portion of the ST segment. Here, the ST segment is better referenced to the PR segment than the TP segment, as the PR segment is depressed to the same extent by atrial repolarization. **(b)** ECG of a patient with sinus tachycardia and junctional ST-segment depression in leads II and V_4 through V_6. It has no pathological significance. Reproduced with permission of the Cleveland Clinic Foundation from Hanna and Glancy (2011).[2]

XII. Assessment of ischemia: differential diagnosis of ST-segment elevation

The differential diagnosis of ST-segment elevation on the ECG includes **four major processes**: ST-segment elevation myocardial infarction (STEMI), early repolarization, pericarditis, and ST-segment elevation secondary to a QRS abnormality (left bundle branch block, left ventricular hypertrophy, or pre-excitation). Additional processes, such as hyperkalemia, pulmonary embolism, and Brugada syndrome, may be associated with ST-segment elevation. The clinical setting, as well as careful attention to the ST–T configuration, often allow an etiologic diagnosis (Table 31.2, Figure 31.48).[48]

A. STEMI (acute subepicardial injury pattern)

In STEMI, the ST-segment elevation is typically a convex or a straight oblique line, blending with a wide T wave to form a dome.[49] ST-segment elevation may, however, be concave, in up to 40% of anterior STEMIs, particularly in the early stage.[49–51] The non-concave morphology is highly specific but not sensitive for the diagnosis of anterior STEMI.[49–52]

Four other features characteristic of STEMI may be present (Figures 31.49, 31.50):

- Concomitant T-wave abnormalities (wide, ample, or inverted T wave).
- Q waves.
- ST depression in the reciprocal leads. Reciprocal ST depression is seen in all inferior STEMIs and in 70% of anterior STEMIs.[53,54] *Diffuse ST elevation mimicking pericarditis may be seen with mid-vessel occlusion of a LAD that wraps around the apex* and supplies part of the inferior wall.
- ST- or T-wave amplitude may approximate or exceed the QRS amplitude in at least one lead.[49,55,56] This finding is characteristic of STEMI, wherein the QRS complex "shrinks" as the infarcted area becomes electrically neutral, whereas the ST–T segments become ample.[49,55] In fact, early STEMI may be characterized by a small R wave that seems to be pulled up by the elevated ST segment. A small or absent R wave, along with an ample, convex ST segment that fuses with the T wave and exceeds the height of the remaining R wave is called "tombstoning."

Note that ST elevation may not be acute STEMI but an old STEMI with a chronically dysfunctional myocardium (dyskinetic or aneurysmal myocardium). In fact, an old STEMI may manifest as a chronic, persistent ST elevation along with Q waves; T waves may be inverted or upright, but not ample.[56] A history of an old myocardial infarction, old ECGs, if available, and a quick bedside echo may allow the diagnosis. In the case of an old dyskinetic infarct, echocardiography shows a thin, bright (scarred) and possibly aneurysmal myocardium, whereas in acute STEMI the myocardium is neither thin nor scarred yet. If the patient does not report a history of myocardial infarction, if the T wave is ample (>75% the size of QRS), or if the patient presents with a typical ongoing angina, presume it is acute STEMI.

B. Early repolarization

Early repolarization is a normal variant of ST-segment elevation ≥ 1 mm (measured at the J point). It is highly prevalent in individuals under age 40 and remains prevalent in a middle-aged population. Two distinct and sometimes coexistent forms of early repolarization have been described: (i) ST elevation in the anterior leads V_1–V_3;[57–60] (ii) ST elevation in the lateral leads (V_4–V_6, I, aVL) or inferior leads.[59–63] The prevalence of the first form, i.e., ST elevation ≥ 1 mm in any of the leads V_1 through V_3, is 60–90% in men < 45 years of age, 20–40% in men > 45 years of age, and ~10% in women of any age.[57] Thus, this form of early repolarization is called "normal male pattern."

Even early repolarization that involves the lateral or inferior leads is common, with a prevalence of ~15% in individuals 30–40 years of age and ~5–10% in those 40–65 years of age.[61–64] It is 2–4 times more prevalent in men and 3 times more prevalent in African-Americans. It is also highly prevalent in athletes younger than 25 (~30–40%).[63]

Either way, early repolarization closely resembles the ST-segment elevation of pericarditis and has the following features (Figure 31.51):

- The ST segment is concave upward. The J point is well demarcated and may be *notched* or *slurred* (Figure 31.48).
- The ST elevation is usually ≤ 3 mm.
- The ST elevation may be limited to the anterior leads or, in many instances, may extend to the inferior leads, lateral leads, or both. *Early repolarization is very rarely limited to the limb leads, and involvement of some precordial leads is the rule.*[59,60] The ST segment is depressed in lead aVR in 50% of patients.
- The T wave is usually ample and may exceed 10 mm in the precordial leads in one-third of patients.[58] As opposed to the ample T wave of STEMI, the T wave is not broad and remains smaller than the QRS complex. The ample T wave distinguishes early repolarization from pericarditis, and explains the low ST–T ratio in lead V_6. In up to 10% of young black men, T wave has a terminal inversion in leads V_3 to V_5, and occasionally leads V_1 and V_2, mimicking infarction or Wellens pattern (Figures 31.46, 31.52).
- The QRS complex tends to have a prominent precordial voltage, in sharp contrast with STEMI where QRS "shrinks."[49,58,63]

The early repolarization pattern may be intermittent and may vary between serial ECGs. It typically decreases with a rise in sympathetic tone, as observed during exercise, and increases with a rise in vagal tone.[59,60,65,66] While it is usually a benign finding, the early repolarization pattern in leads other than V_1–V_3 has been associated with an increased risk of sudden death, particularly when the ST-segment elevation is horizontal/descending rather than upsloping, and possibly, when early repolarization involves the inferior leads with a J point that is notched and wide (≥1 mm) or elevated ≥ 2 mm.[61,63] The absolute increase in the risk of sudden death, however, is very small (0.07% per year).[67]

Table 31.2 Differential diagnosis of ST-segment elevation.

STEMI[a]	Early repolarization	Pericarditis	LVH, LBBB, pre-excitation	Hyperkalemia
1. ST elevation straight or convex upward, blends with T to form a dome 2. Wide upright T *or* inverted T 3. Q waves 4. ST elevation or T wave may approximate or exceed QRS height 5. Reciprocal ST depression	• Notched J point • ST elevation ≤ 3 mm	• PR depression > 1mm[b] • ST elevation < 5 mm	• Both ST and T are directed opposite to QRS • ST elevation < 25% of QRS height (and ST elevation < 2.5 mm in LVH) • Delta wave, short PR, and pseudo-Q waves are seen in pre-excitation	• Narrow-based, peaked T wave pulling the ST segment

[a] **The presence of just one of the first four STEMI features makes the diagnosis of STEMI. Conversely, the lack of all STEMI features does not necessarily rule out STEMI.** The fifth STEMI feature, reciprocal ST depression, may be seen with LBBB and LVH, where ST depression in the lateral leads usually accompanies the anterior ST elevation. Typical reciprocal ST depression is not seen in pericarditis and early repolarization (except for the ST depression in leads aVR and V_1 in pericarditis, and in lead aVR in early repolarization). **While the QTc may be prolonged in STEMI, it is normal in pericarditis and early repolarization.**
[b] PR depression < 1 mm may be seen in early repolarization, and PR depression of any degree may be seen with the atrial injury coinciding with STEMI.

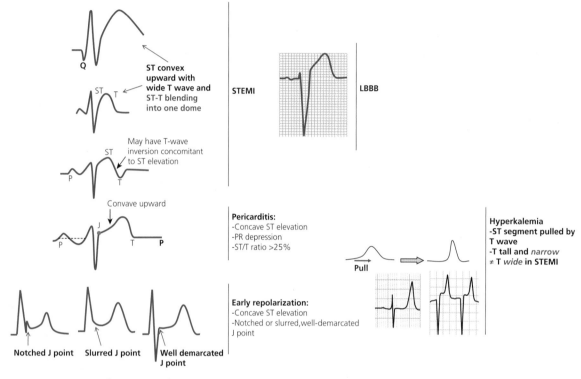

Figure 31.48 Various patterns of ST-segment elevation. Reproduced with permission of the Cleveland Clinic Foundation from Hanna and Glancy (2011).[2]

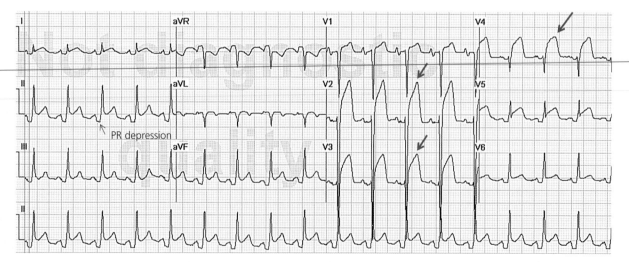

Figure 31.49 Diffuse ST elevation in ~ all leads and ST depression in lead aVR. This initially suggests pericarditis. PR depression in leads II, aVF, V_5, and V_6 further suggests pericarditis. However, having pericarditis features does not necessarily rule out STEMI. One should search for the five STEMI features and make sure none of them is present. In this case, the ST-segment morphology and the abnormally wide T wave are STEMI features. The ST elevation has an upwardly convex shape with a wide and high T wave fused with the ST segment, very typical of STEMI (leads V_2–V_4, *arrows*). Also, the size of the ST elevation (i.e., > 5 mm in V_2–V_4, and larger than the QRS complex in V_4, a feature called "tombstoning") is more consistent with STEMI than with pericarditis. PR depression may be seen in STEMI as a result of atrial infarction (atrial injury leads to atrial repolarization abnormality). The LAD is found to be occluded on coronary arteriography. Reproduced with permission of the Cleveland Clinic Foundation from Hanna and Glancy (2015).[48]

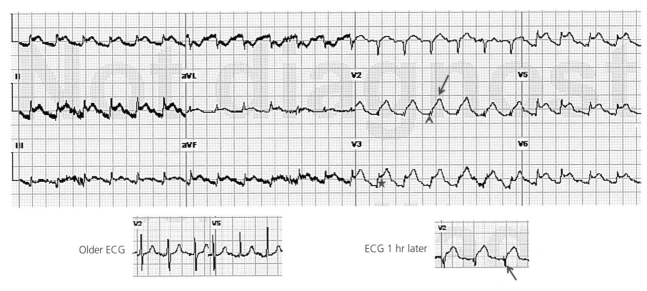

Older ECG

ECG 1 hr later

Figure 31.50 ECG of a patient who has lung cancer. Sinus tachycardia with diffuse ST elevation is seen, along with ST depression in aVR. The QRS voltage is low, particularly when compared to the ECG performed a few days earlier (left lower panel). PR depression is seen in lead II. This could be pericarditis with pericardial effusion. However, go through the STEMI checklist before calling this pericarditis. The ST–T morphology in lead V_2, where the ST and T are blended to form one dome, is characteristic of STEMI (*top arrow*). Moreover, the ST elevation and T wave in leads V_2–V_4 are larger than the QRS, the QRS voltage is "shrinking" (*arrowhead*), and the R wave is pulled up by the ST segment (*star*); this is called "tombstoning." All these features are characteristic of STEMI, wherein the R wave and the QRS complex shrink before forming a deep Q wave. In fact, an ECG recorded 1 hour later shows a fully developed Q wave in lead V_2 (right lower panel, *arrow*). Reproduced with permission of the Cleveland Clinic Foundation from Hanna and Glancy (2015).[48]

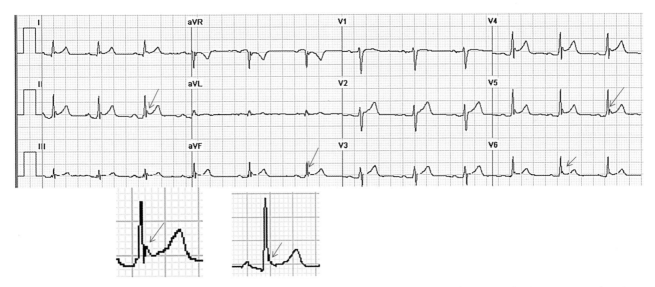

Figure 31.51 Early repolarization with ST-segment elevation in the inferior leads and in the anterolateral leads V_2–V_6. ST elevation is most prominent in leads V_4 and II, with a concavely upward ST morphology and a notch at the J point (*arrows* and *left magnified image*). In half of early repolarization cases, the J point is well demarcated but smooth (*right magnified image*). Note the 1 mm PR depression in leads II and V_5. Slight PR depression may be seen in normal individuals and corresponds to the normal atrial repolarization. Reproduced with permission of the Cleveland Clinic Foundation from Hanna and Glancy (2015).[48]

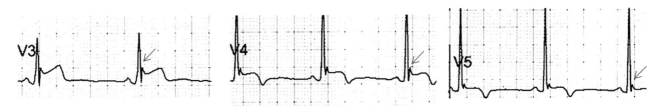

Figure 31.52 Early repolarization with a normal variant T-wave inversion in a 33-year-old black man. The ST segment is elevated with a prominent J-point notch in leads V_3–V_5 (*arrows*). T wave is inverted in leads V_4–V_5. Depending on the autonomic tone, the T waves may at times become upright. Reproduced with permission of the Cleveland Clinic Foundation from Hanna and Glancy (2015).[48]

C. Pericarditis (Figure 31.53)

In pericarditis, ST elevation is concave upward and is widespread to more than one region without reciprocal ST depression, except for the frequent ST depression in leads aVR and V_1 (64%);[68] ST elevation is seldom greater than 4–5 mm.[68,69] The subepicardial injury being diffuse in pericarditis, the axis of the ST segment follows the anatomic axis of the heart and is generally +45° in the frontal plane. Thus, ST depression is seen in leads aVR and V_1, ST elevation is highest in leads II, V_5 and V_6, and is less in leads III and aVL, where the ST segment may occasionally be depressed.[70] The ST segment is elevated at some stage in >90% of patients, and normalizes within 1–7 days.

Transient PR depression >1 mm is often seen and may be the earliest change. It is most frequent in leads II, aVF, and V_4–V_6, and represents atrial subepicardial injury. PR depression in those leads is always associated with PR elevation in lead aVR and sometimes V_1. PR changes often coexist with ST changes, but may be isolated and may precede ST changes.[71] PR depression is characteristic of pericarditis but may be seen in early repolarization, where it is less marked than in pericarditis (<0.8 mm) and implies early repolarization of the atrial tissue;[72] and in MI, where it implies atrial infarction with atrial injury pattern.

Classically, it is said that in pericarditis, unlike in STEMI, the T wave does not invert until the ST elevation subsides. In reality, up to 40% of patients develop a notched or biphasic positive–negative T wave before full return of the ST segment to the baseline, mimicking ischemia.[68,73] Also, if T-wave inversion antedates pericarditis, concomitant ST elevation and T inversion may be seen once pericarditis develops. However, the T wave inverts less deeply and less completely than in STEMI, and the QTc interval remains normal even when the T wave inverts.

Three criteria distinguish pericarditis from early repolarization (*but not from STEMI*):

a. PR depression >1 mm.
b. ST-segment depression in lead V_1.
c. Ratio of ST-segment height to T-wave height ≥25% in lead V_6, V_5, or V_4. This feature allows the distinction between pericarditis and early repolarization with a very high sensitivity and specificity. In pericarditis, the T waves have normal or reduced amplitude, and the ST/T ratio is therefore high.[74] In early repolarization, T waves are tall, and thus the ST/T ratio is <25%.

Widespread ST elevation may be seen with both pericarditis and early repolarization. ST elevation limited to the anterior leads is more likely to be early repolarization than pericarditis.

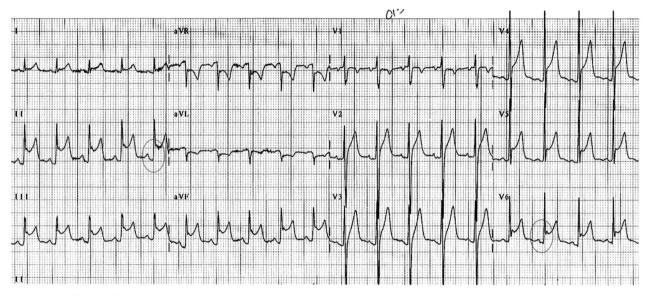

Figure 31.53 Diffuse ST elevation in most leads, with ST depression in lead aVR and an isoelectric ST segment in V_1. None of the STEMI features is present: ST elevation is concave upward, no reciprocal ST depression is seen except in lead aVR, T wave is not wide, inverted, or ample (in relation to QRS), and no Q wave is seen. Furthermore, ST elevation does not exceed 5 mm, ST and T heights are smaller than QRS height, and PR depression is present (*circled areas*). This is consistent with pericarditis, and the hospital course of this patient confirmed this diagnosis.

Early repolarization may lead to a similarly concave ST elevation. However, in early repolarization: (i) ST elevation is ≤3mm; (ii) ST elevation is often limited to the anterior and lateral or inferior leads, but rarely extends to all of them; (iii) there is no deep PR depression; and (iv) the T wave in lead V_6 is high with an ST–T ratio <25%, which is not the case here.

D. Left ventricular hypertrophy (LVH) and left bundle branch block (LBBB) (see Figures 31.54, 31.55, 31.56)

A deep S wave is seen in leads V_1–V_3 and sometimes in the inferior leads, with ST elevation and T waves that are discordant with the QRS complex, i.e., directed opposite to the QRS. The ST elevation is typically concave upward.[52,75] Occasionally, in LBBB or, less so, LVH, ST elevation may be straight or convex, mimicking the dome of STEMI. In the lateral leads, the discordant ST segment is depressed, mimicking a reciprocal ST change.

The following findings imply myocardial infarction:

a. *ST elevation or depression that is concordant with the QRS complex.* Moreover, since ST deviation is mandatory with LBBB, a *"normal-looking" ST segment* implies ischemia.

b. *Inverted T waves* concordant with the QRS in more than one lead, *or biphasic T waves* in more than one lead (e.g., V_1–V_3). Across the precordial leads, T wave may transition from positive to negative one lead earlier or later than the QRS and ST transition. Therefore, even in the absence of ischemia, the T wave may be inverted in lead V_3, wherein the QRS is still deeply negative and the ST is elevated (negative T-wave concordance in one lead). Also, the T wave may be upright in leads V_5, V_6, and I where QRS is upright and the ST segment is depressed (positive T-wave concordance does not imply ischemia).

c. In addition to concordance, a *discordant ST segment or T wave that is very large* may imply ischemia. Whether in LBBB or LVH, *discordant ST elevation ≥ 25% of the QRS height or T wave ≥ 50% of the QRS height often implies ischemia.*

In the particular case of LVH, ST elevation is usually < 2.5 mm in leads V_1–V_3 and is rarely seen in the lateral or inferior leads, where it would be < 1 mm.[75]

Unlike LVH, ST elevation that accompanies LBBB can be ample; thus, absolute ST elevation cutoffs are less helpful in LBBB. For the diagnosis of STEMI in LBBB, a discordant ST elevation ≥ 5 mm has been suggested by Sgarbossa et al.; however, this feature is seen in 10% of control patients with LBBB and no STEMI, and is therefore poorly specific but also poorly sensitive, frequently missing STEMI.[76,77] A discordant ST elevation ≥ 25% of the QRS height has been suggested as a far more sensitive and accurate feature.[78,79]

On another note, **RVH and RBBB may lead to ST depression and T inversion, but not ST elevation. Thus, ST elevation occurring with RBBB or RVH implies STEMI**. While only LBBB poses a diagnostic challenge, both types of bundle branch blocks, if secondary to STEMI, represent equally high-risk categories.[80]

RV pacing leads to discordant ST elevation, similar to LBBB; the same criteria may be used to diagnose MI in the setting of RV pacing.

Note concerning Q waves

RBBB does not affect septal depolarization and only affects the late part of the QRS complex; therefore, it does not create Q waves. LBBB, on the other hand, changes the septal depolarization and may create QS waves in leads V_1–V_3 and III–aVF, mimicking MI. However, LBBB does not typically create any q in the lateral leads or lead II, nor QR anywhere (the latter findings suggest MI). Also, a notch on the *upslope of S* wave in leads V_3–V_5, or the *upslope of R* wave in leads I and aVL, may signify MI (Cabrera's sign).

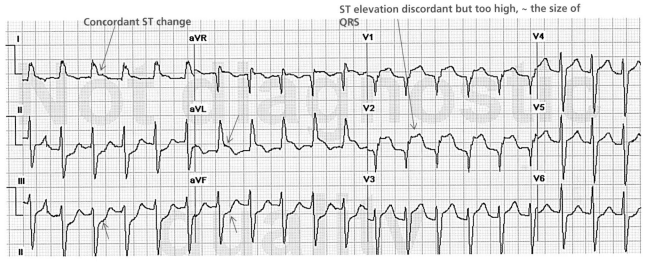

Figure 31.54 SVT with a typical LBBB in leads I and aVL. Concordant ST elevation is seen in leads I and aVL, while concordant ST depression is seen in the inferior leads (*arrows*). The ST elevation in lead V_2 is discordant but is disproportionately high in relation to the QRS (well above 25% of the QRS height). All these features are diagnostic of STEMI. Reproduced with permission of the Cleveland Clinic Foundation from Hanna and Glancy (2015).[48]

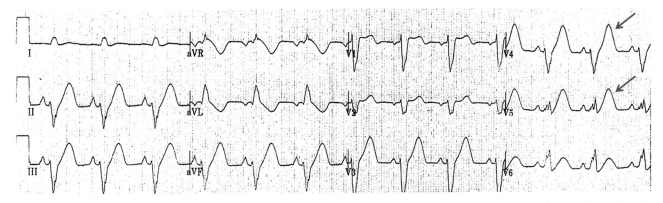

Figure 31.55 LBBB with discordant ST-segment changes. However, the T wave is wide and fused with the ST segment in a domed morphology, and the T wave is larger than the QRS in leads V_4, V_5, and II (*arrows*). This implies a diagnosis of STEMI with hyperacute T waves. This patient had an occluded left anterior descending coronary artery. Reproduced with permission of the Cleveland Clinic Foundation from Hanna and Glancy (2015).[48]

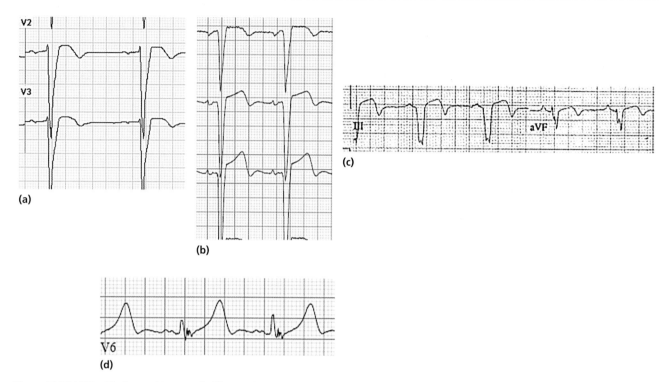

Figure 31.56 LBBB with abnormal T waves. **(a, b)** Discordant ST elevation in V_1–V_3 but concordant T-wave inversion **(a)** or biphasic T wave **(b)**. This is consistent with an anterior injury pattern. **(c)** Concordant T-wave inversion in the inferior leads, consistent with inferior injury. **(d)** A large concordant T wave in lead V_6, larger than the QRS, consistent with injury. Reproduced with permission of the Cleveland Clinic Foundation from Hanna and Glancy (2015).[48]

E. Pre-excitation (Figure 31.57)

Pre-excitation may be associated with negative delta waves that mimic Q waves, and with ST elevation in the leads where the negative delta waves are seen, i.e., ST elevation discordant with the delta wave. The QRS morphology and the delta wave allow the distinction from STEMI.

F. Hyperkalemia (Figure 31.58)

The most common finding in hyperkalemia is a peaked, narrow-based T wave that is usually, albeit not necessarily, tall. ST elevation may be evident in leads V_1–V_3. In contrast to hyperkalemia, the T wave of STEMI is typically wide.

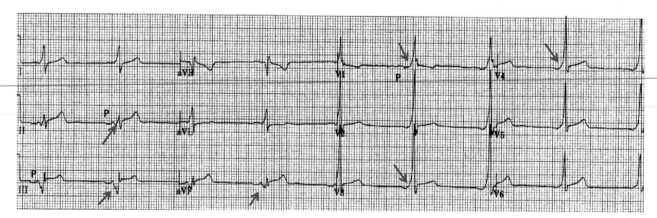

Figure 31.57 At first glance, it seems there is ST elevation in the inferior leads II, III, and aVF, with a wide Q wave. Moreover, there is a wide and tall R wave in lead V_1 with ST-segment depression, suggesting an associated posterior infarct. An ECG performed a few days previously did not show any Q wave or ST-segment elevation. All of this is consistent with an acute inferoposterior STEMI. On further analysis, however, a slur is seen on the upslope of QRS in leads V_1–V_6 (*arrows*), and P wave is "riding" this slur. In the inferior leads, P wave is "riding" the Q wave, which is in fact a negative delta wave. Thus, this ECG represents pre-excitation. The ST deviations are secondary to the pre-excitation and have an orientation opposite to the delta wave. The degree of pre-excitation depends on how fast the AV node is conducting, and thus often varies between ECGs. Reproduced with permission of the Cleveland Clinic Foundation from Hanna and Glancy (2015).[48]

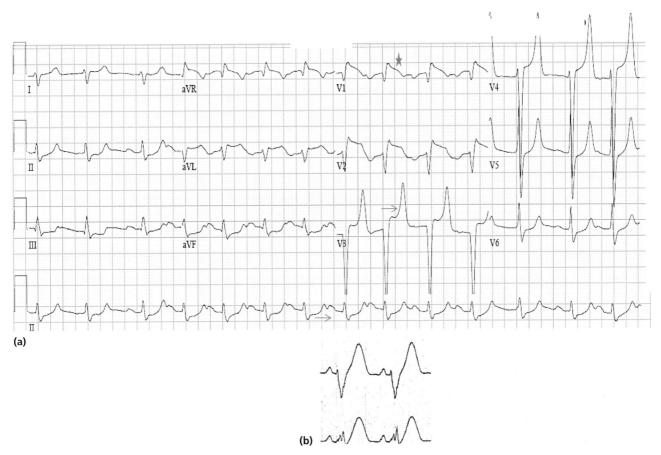

(a)

(b)

Figure 31.58 **(a)** There are ST elevations in leads V_1–V_4, ST depressions in the inferior leads, and peaked T waves in leads V_3–V_5. These T waves have a narrow base and seem to "pull" the ST segment, creating ST elevation in the anterior leads and ST depression in the inferior leads (*arrows*); this shape is consistent with hyperkalemia. In addition, the dowsloping ST elevation seen in V_1–V_2 is consistent with hyperkalemia (*star*). Occasionally, STEMI may have a similar ST–T shape. An RBBB pattern is seen in V_1–V_2 (rSR'); this is consistent with STEMI but also with hyperkalemia, where conduction blocks are common. The serum K level was 7.4 mmol/l and coronary angiography revealed normal coronary arteries.

(b) Hyperacute T wave of STEMI. Note that it is wide and it blends with the ST segment to form one wave. The QRS is shrinking and T wave may become larger than the QRS, a finding characteristic of STEMI.

Reproduced with permission of the Cleveland Clinic Foundation from Hanna and Glancy (2015).[48]

G. Other causes of ST-segment elevation

- ***Takotsubo cardiomyopathy*** mimics all ECG features of anteroapical STEMI. ST elevation may extend to the inferior leads but cannot be isolated in the inferior leads.[81] As in apical STEMI, reciprocal ST depression is uncommon. Within 24–48 hours, ST elevation evolves into deep anterior T-wave inversion and prolonged QT interval. Transient Q waves may be seen.
- ***Myocarditis*** may have one of the following two ECG patterns: (i) pericarditis pattern, or (ii) typical STEMI pattern with Q waves, sometimes localized to one area.
- ***Atrial flutter waves***, particularly of 2:1 atrial flutter, may deform the ST segment in such a manner as to mimic an injury pattern on the ECG. Flutter waves may mimic ST elevation or ST depression (Figures 31.59, 31.60).
- ***A large pulmonary embolism*** may be associated with T-wave inversion in the anterior leads and/or the inferior leads, reflective of cor pulmonale. Less commonly, ST elevation in the anterior or inferior leads is seen, and is most typically isolated to the "right" leads V_1–V_2.[26,82]
- ***Brugada syndrome*** is characterized by ST elevation *and* an RBBB or a pseudo-RBBB pattern in at least two of the leads V_1–V_3. In pseudo-RBBB, the QRS adopts an rSR' morphology in the anterior leads but is normal in the lateral leads. Type 1 Brugada pattern, the pattern that is most specifically associated with sudden death, is characterized by a coved, downsloping ST elevation ≥ 2 mm with T-wave inversion (Figure 31.61).[83] The Brugada pattern can be transient, triggered by fever, cocaine, or class I antiarrhythmic drugs.

Hyperkalemia, Brugada syndrome, and sometimes pulmonary embolism are characterized by an ST elevation that slopes down (Figures 31.58, 31.61), which contrasts with the upsloping, convex ST elevation of STEMI.

XIII. Assessment of ischemia: large or tall T wave
A. Differential diagnosis of a tall upright T wave
Grossly, a T wave is considered tall upright if it is >10 mm in a precordial lead or >6 mm in a limb leads. Yet a T wave may be larger than 10 mm in leads V_2–V_3 in normal young men. It is therefore important to also consider the height of the T wave in relation to the QRS. A T

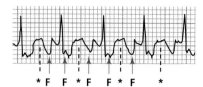

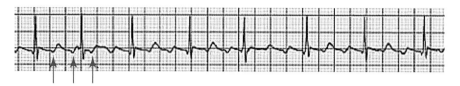

Figure 31.59 Atrial flutter that simulates ST-segment elevation. "F" indicates the negative flutter wave; asterisk (*) indicates the upslope of the flutter wave that gets superimposed on the ST segment, mimicking ST elevation. Reproduced with permission of the Cleveland Clinic Foundation from Hanna and Glancy (2015).[48]

Figure 31.60 Atrial flutter that simulates ST-segment depression. The undulations of the baseline are flutter waves (*arrows*).

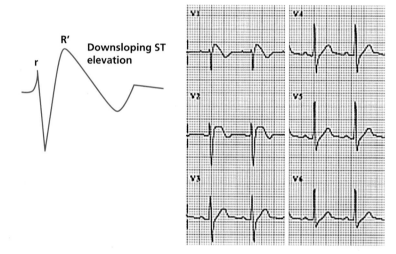

Figure 31.61 Type 1 Brugada pattern in V_1 and V_2, with a downsloping ST elevation that creates a pseudo-R' wave (pseudo-RBBB). The QRS does not have RBBB morphology in leads V_5 and V_6. Reproduced with permission of the Cleveland Clinic Foundation from Hanna and Glancy (2015).[48]

wave that is taller than the dominant QRS waveform (R or S) is abnormal, except in a lead where the QRS is nearly isoelectric. A T wave that is >75% of this waveform is often abnormal.

1. Hyperacute T wave in acute STEMI: T wave is ample and, more importantly, *wide*. It frequently exceeds QRS height in at least one lead. It precedes and/or coincides with ST-segment elevation.

2. Hyperkalemia: T wave is peaked and narrow.

3. Ample T wave in leads V_1–V_3 secondary to LVH/LBBB: the ample T wave is directed opposite to the ample, negative QRS complex.

4. Normal variant: a normal-variant ample T wave is particularly seen in association with early repolarization and high QRS voltage. The normal-variant ample T wave is mostly seen in young men in leads V_2–V_4, where it may exceed 10 mm.

B. deWinter complex

This complex is characterized by an upsloping ST depression in leads V_1 through V_6 followed by a tall upright T wave, which may be narrow or wide (Figure 31.62).[84] It is similar to the hyperacute T-wave pattern; however, while hyperacute T waves quickly progress to a typical ST elevation pattern within a few minutes, deWinter complex does not progress to ST elevation and remains static. The morphology mimics hyperkalemia. deWinter complex is associated with an acute LAD occlusion, and is thus equivalent to an acute anterior STEMI and should warrant emergent catheterization. For unclear reasons (mutation of I_{K-ATP}?), these patients are unable to generate ST-segment elevation.

XIV. QT analysis and U wave

A. QT interval measurement

QT interval is best measured in the lead that shows a distinct T-wave termination, with the best separation of T and U waves. The QT interval may be artificially shortened in some leads, because the beginning of the QRS complex or the end of the T wave may be isoelectric in those leads. On the other hand, QT is often longest in leads V_2–V_3, but those leads have the largest U waves, show the least T–U separation, and may, therefore, overestimate the length of the QT interval. Leads I, aVR, and aVL do not have the diastolic U wave but do not always show a distinct T wave. Thus, QT interval is often best measured in leads II and V_5 or V_6 (Figure 31.63).

QT interval shortens with increasing heart rate. The corrected QT (QTc) at a particular heart rate corresponds to the patient's predicted QT interval had the heart rate been 60 bpm. If the patient's rate is 60 bpm, QTc equals absolute QT. The normal QTc is > 350 ms, and < 460 ms in women and < 450 ms in men.

QTc may be calculated using Bazett's formula:

$$QTc = QT/\sqrt{R–R \text{ interval in seconds}}$$

Bazett is acceptable for rates 50–100 bpm. It falsely prolongs the QTc when the rate is > 100 bpm and falsely reduces it when the rate is < 50 bpm. Hodges' formula is a linear equation that is simpler and more accurate than Bazett's formula at both high and low rates:

$$QTc = QT + 1.75 \, (\text{rate} - 60)$$

This means that normally, QT decreases by 17.5 ms for every 10-beat increase in heart rate, and increases 17.5 ms for every 10-beat decrease in heart rate. If a patient has a QT of 400 ms at a rate of 100 bpm, the QT at a rate of 60 bpm would be $(400 + 17.5 \times 4) = 470$ ms. Bazett would yield a QTc of 515 ms ($400/\sqrt{0.6}$ s). Another quick rule is that for heart rates < 100 bpm, QT interval should be shorter than 1/2 the R–R interval. However, for rates > 100 bpm, the QT interval is normally > 1/2 R–R interval; for rates < 60 bpm, a QT interval < 1/2 R–R interval does not guarantee a normal QTc.

In case of a prolonged QRS, as in bundle branch block, use a higher upper limit of normal for QTc (500 ms), or use the JT interval instead of QT to assess repolarization (normal JTc < 360 ms). In AF, QT interval varies from beat to beat due to R–R interval changes. One may measure the QT intervals that follow the longest and shortest R–R intervals, then divide each by the square root of the preceding R–R interval (QTc1 and QTc2). The average of these two values is QTc.

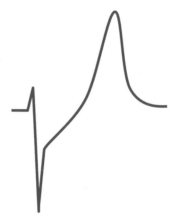

Figure 31.62 deWinter complex in V_1–V_6.

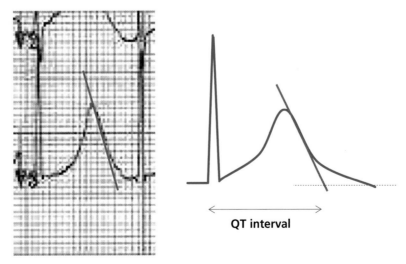

Figure 31.63 QT is not measured using the end of the T wave. Instead, a line is drawn across the maximal T-wave downslope, using the last T-wave peak. The intersection of this line with the baseline is used to calculate QT interval; otherwise, the QT interval may be overestimated.

B. U wave

The normal U wave is a diastolic wave related to the mechanical stretch of the myocardium in phase 4 (diastole). The abnormal U wave could be part of phase 4 (delayed afterdepolarization [DAD]), or part of phase 3 in patients with prolonged repolarization (early afterdepolarization [EAD] seen in patients with prolonged QT).

The U wave of phase 3 is a repolarization wave and is actually a part of the T wave, called T2 wave, that gives the T wave a notched or biphasic shape; it may be seen in leads I/aVL/aVR and should be measured as part of the QT interval. This T2 wave is seen with hypokalemia and QT-prolonging drugs. *In practice, a U wave that is prominent* and *that merges with the T wave or gives a "bifid" T-wave appearance should be included in the measurement of the QT interval.* Conversely, a normal U wave (<25% of T wave), or a prominent U wave that is distant from the T wave (>150 ms peak-to-peak distance), is a phase 4 U wave and should not be counted as part of the QT interval. Thus, leads V_2–V_3 are best avoided for QT measurement.

The normal U wave is particularly visible in leads V_2–V_3 at heart rates < 65 bpm, and is not usually seen at rates > 100 bpm; bradycardia makes U waves more visible but also more ample. The U wave is normally a positive wave, with an amplitude < 25% the T-wave amplitude and < 1.5 mm. An abnormal U wave is a negative U wave of any depth, or an upright U wave that is ≥ 25% of the T wave or ≥ 1.5 mm.

C. Differential diagnosis of a prolonged QTc (Figures 31.64, 31.65)

There are five major causes of a prolonged QTc:

1. Ischemia or post-ischemic evolution
2. Hypokalemia (also gives a prominent U wave), hypocalcemia
3. QT-prolonging drugs (also give a prominent U wave)
4. Congenital long QT syndrome (LQT)
5. Miscellaneous causes: hypothyroidism, hypothermia, cerebrovascular event with large upright or deeply inverted T waves, and any cardiomyopathy (hypertrophic, dilated)

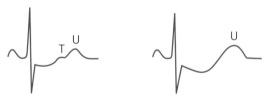

Hypokalemia: ST depressed, U prominent

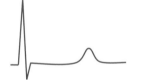

Hypocalcemia: ST prolonged, T narrow
LQT3
Some LQT1

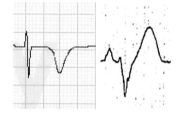

Ischemic long QT: usually along with deep T inversion or hyperacute wide T wave.
Similar shape seen with **cerebrovascular events**

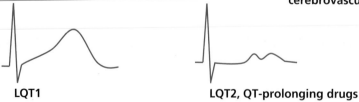

LQT1   **LQT2, QT-prolonging drugs**

Figure 31.64 Typical ST–T morphologies in hypokalemia, hypocalcemia, congenital long QT syndromes, and ischemic QT prolongation.

- In hypokalemia, the ST segment is depressed and U wave is large while T wave is flattened.
- In hypocalcemia and LQT3, QT interval is prolonged as a result of the ST-segment prolongation. As opposed to other congenital long QT syndromes or QT prolongation secondary to drugs, T wave is not significantly widened.
- In LQT1, T wave is wide and ample without ST-segment depression, but may also take the shape of LQT3. In LQT2 and in many drug-induced long QT cases, T wave is wide and notched (double hump) and may simulate hypokalemia.

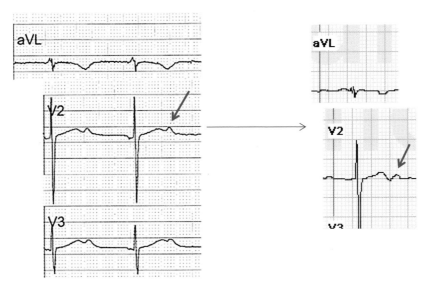

Figure 31.65 On the left, markedly prolonged QT with a notched T wave is seen (QTc ~600 ms). Note that the second T peak is part of the T wave rather than a U wave (*arrow*), as QT is as prolonged in lead aVL, which does not usually show U wave. This patient was receiving amiodarone. On the right, after amiodarone cessation, QT is reduced to normal (QTc 440 ms). Note that lead V_2 now shows a U wave rather than a T wave (*arrow*), as evidenced by the fact that the dip between the two peaks reaches the baseline, and that this wave is not seen in lead aVL.

Note the morphology of a prolonged QT induced by hypokalemia (Figure 31.64). A prolonged QT with a wide ample T wave and no ST depression is not hypokalemia; a deep negative T wave is not hypokalemia either. Consider other causes of long QT in this case, such as congenital long QT syndrome, drugs, or ischemia.

> Most of the causes of prolonged QT are related to a prolonged T-wave duration. Three causes are characterized by a prolonged ST segment with a normal T-wave duration: hypocalcemia, hypothermia, LQT3 and sometimes LQT1.

D. Differential diagnosis of an abnormal U wave
1. *Negative U wave*
  - Ischemia
  - LVH
  - Regurgitant valvular disease with volume overload

2. *Prominent upright U wave*
  - Digoxin (DAD), catecholamines (DAD)
  - Antiarrhythmic drugs (actually T2 wave rather than U wave)
  - Hypokalemia (actually T2 wave rather than U wave)
  - Bradycardia
  - LVH
  - Other: hypercalcemia (DAD), cerebrovascular event

Ischemia does not typically cause a tall upright U wave. Digoxin and hypercalcemia are causes of U wave that are associated with a shortened QT interval.

XV. Electrolyte abnormalities, digitalis effect and digitalis toxicity, hypothermia, PE, poor precordial R-wave progression
A. Electrolyte abnormalities
Hypokalemia initially produces diffusely flattened T wave. With severe hypokalemia<3 mEq/l, the ST–T pattern may mimic an ischemic pattern of ST-segment depression with a wide upright T wave and a prolonged QT interval (Figures 31.66, 31.67). Hypokalemia may lead to PACs/PVCs, polymorphic VT, or, similarly to digoxin, AT with block. Hypokalemia increases vagal sensitivity, and thus may be associated with bradyarrhythmias.

> In patients hospitalized for any surgical or medical illness, a hypokalemia pattern is very common on ECG and is commonly mistaken for ischemia.

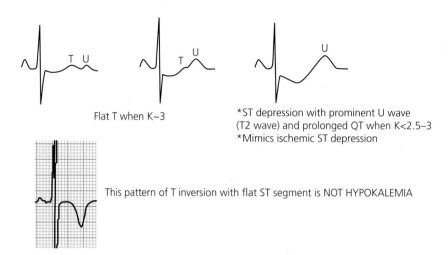

Flat T when K~3

*ST depression with prominent U wave
(T2 wave) and prolonged QT when K<2.5–3
*Mimics ischemic ST depression

This pattern of T inversion with flat ST segment is NOT HYPOKALEMIA

Figure 31.66 Hypokalemia and a pattern that should not be confused with hypokalemia are shown.

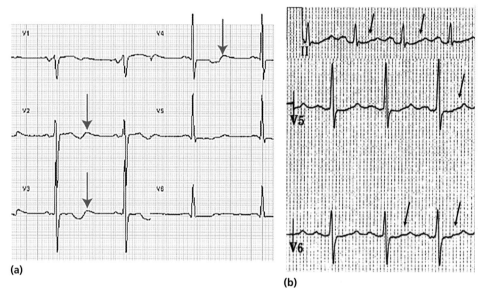

(a)

(b)

Figure 31.67 Two ECG examples of hypokalemia. **(a)** Prolonged QT (QT ~600 ms, QTc 550 ms) with diffuse ST depression and prominent, positive U waves (well seen in V$_2$–V$_5$; *arrows*) (K=2.5 mEq/l). The abnormal U wave merging with T wave is included in QT measurement. **(b)** ST depression with upright "T" wave. On further examination, a notch on the upslope of the ST segment is seen in multiple leads, suggesting that the "T" wave is actually a prominent U wave and the notch is a flattened true T wave (*arrows*).

Hyperkalemia is characterized by the following (Figures 31.58, 31.68, 31.69):

- Potassium 5.5–6 mEq/l: narrow, peaked T waves that are usually, but not necessarily, tall. T wave pulls and tents the ST segment.
- Potassium >6 or 6.5 mEq/l:
  - Conduction abnormalities and wide QRS complex: RBBB, LBBB, LAFB. The wide QRS of hyperkalemia is not usually a typical RBBB or LBBB. With hyperkalemia, the whole QRS is wide, including the initial portion, whereas with a typical bundle branch block, the initial portion is narrow.
  - PR segment prolongs and P wave progressively flattens then becomes absent. The rhythm becomes an accelerated junctional (narrow QRS) or idioventricular (wide QRS) rhythm, sometimes due to a sinoventricular conduction with a total lack of atrial activity.
  - ST-segment elevation that slopes down and/or ST-segment depression.
  - The QRS becomes progressively wider, evolving into a sine wave pattern, then VT/VF. *A very wide QRS >200 ms is always suggestive of hyperkalemia.*

Hypocalcemia and **hypercalcemia** only affect the length of the ST segment (Figure 31.70).

B. Digitalis effect and digitalis toxicity (Figure 31.71)

Digitalis effect pertains to the ECG changes associated with therapeutic digoxin dosing. Digitalis effect is similar to hypokalemia, i.e., ST-segment depression, T-wave flattening, and prominent U wave. Unlike hypokalemia, the ST segment has a "scooping" shape (like a spoon) and QT is shortened. Atypical changes may be seen, such as inverted T wave or reverse-checkmark shape of ST–T, particularly when LVH is also present.

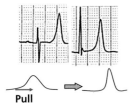

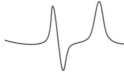

Pull

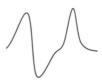

Absent P wave + wide QRS (typical or atypical bundle branch block). Both the initial and late QRS portions are wide

Progressively more QRS widening leading to a sine wave shape

Figure 31.68 Stages of hyperkalemia.

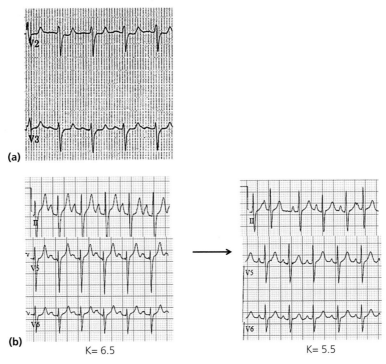

(a)

(b)

K= 6.5   K= 5.5

Figure 31.69 (a) Hyperkalemia of 6.1 mEq/l. Note that T waves are not tall, but are narrow and peaked with ST-segment tenting. **(b)** Hyperkalemia with peaked T waves that are not tall but narrow. Note the improvement after appropriate therapy.

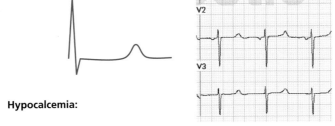

Hypocalcemia:

Long QT that is due to a long ST segment, which is different from long QT secondary to drugs or hypokalemia. T wave is not wide, there is no T wave abnormality.

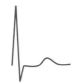

Hypercalcemia: short QTc <390 ms. No significant ST or T wave abnormality

Figure 31.70 Hypocalcemia and hypercalcemia.

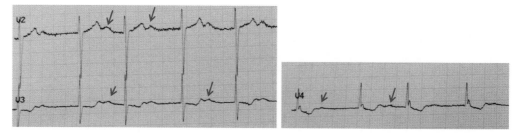

Figure 31.71 Digitalis effect in a patient with AF. Note the prominent U wave (*arrows*), well separated from T wave. ST is depressed and the overall ST–U shape mimics hypokalemia, except for the relatively short QT and the better T–U separation (QT ~380–400 ms, at an overall heart rate of 65 bpm).

Digitalis toxicity pertains to the occurrence of arrhythmias with digoxin therapy. *The three most characteristic arrhythmias are*: (i) AT with block, (ii) accelerated junctional rhythm, (iii) slow or regular ventricular response in AF (implying complete AV block with a junctional escape or accelerated junctional rhythm). Other arrhythmias include frequent PVCs (*the most common and earliest arrhythmia*), VT, bidirectional VT or bidirectional wide SVT, AIVR, and AV block. Digitalis toxicity is exacerbated by hypokalemia, hypomagnesemia, and hypercalcemia.

C. Hypothermia (see Figure 31.72)

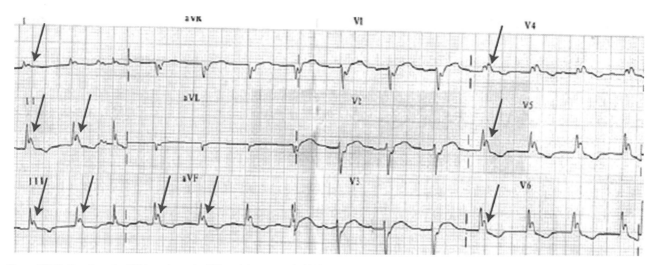

Figure 31.72 Hypothermia. QRS is prolonged > 120 ms. It is not a typical LBBB, as QRS is negative in aVL, and it is not a typical RBBB. Characteristic "dome" waves are seen at the end of QRS in multiple leads (*arrows*): these are Osborne or J waves in a patient with hypothermia. Hypothermia slows impulse conduction throughout all the cardiac tissue, resulting in prolongation of PR, QRS, and QT. It also causes AV block, AF with slow ventricular response, and accelerated junctional rhythm. The height of the Osborne wave is proportional to the degree of hypothermia.

D. Pulmonary embolism (see Figure 31.73, Table 31.1)

E. Poor precordial R-wave progression in COPD and anterior MI (see Figures 31.74, 31.75)

F. ASD and Ebstein anomaly

Secundum ASD is characterized by RV volume overload pattern:
- Incomplete RBBB. RBBB may occasionally be complete (in 5–20% of the cases).
- Right-axis deviation. A severe RVH picture with tall R' or monophasic R wave is not usually seen in volume overload patterns.
- P pulmonale in one-third of the cases.
- R-wave notching near its peak is frequently seen in the inferior leads (~73%) and is called "crochetage." Notching of a normal QRS may, however, be seen in 7% of normal individuals. Also, notching may be seen with other congenital or acquired heart disease. It is mostly specific for ASD when seen in multiple inferior leads and when accompanied by incomplete RBBB.

Primum ASD is characterized by:
- Incomplete RBBB
- Left-axis deviation, as opposed to the right-axis deviation seen with secundum ASD. This is secondary to a distortion of the left bundle with early excitation of the posterior wall. The effect on the conduction system also explains a higher prevalence of prolonged PR interval.

Sinus venosus ASD has ECG findings similar to secundum ASD. Additionally, an ectopic atrial rhythm frequently replaces the sinus rhythm.

Ebstein anomaly is characterized by:
- Right atrial enlargement with very tall P waves ("Himalayan" P waves)
- RBBB that is frequently atypical with a RSR'S' pattern. The latter may occasionally be seen with ASD.
- Prominent Q waves in the inferior leads, which may also be seen with any RVH or PE.

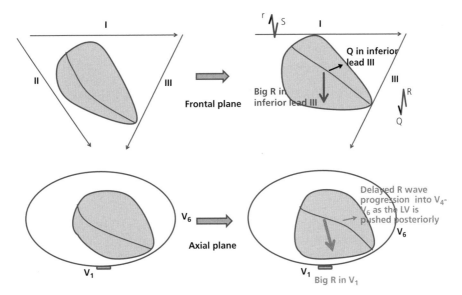

Figure 31.73 Change of vector of depolarization between a normal heart and pulmonary embolism. ***In the frontal plane*** (*top figures*), the LV is pushed up while the RV expands down and to the right, explaining the right axis (S in I, QR in III and aVF); inferior Q wave is explained by the LV being pushed up away from those leads. ***In the axial plane*** (*bottom figures*), the LV is pushed posteriorly while the RV expands to the right. The size of the R wave in V$_1$ may not be large if the RV is strained without being enlarged, and delayed R-wave progression may be the only finding. T inversion in the anterior and inferior leads reflects RV strain and is the most common finding in massive PE.

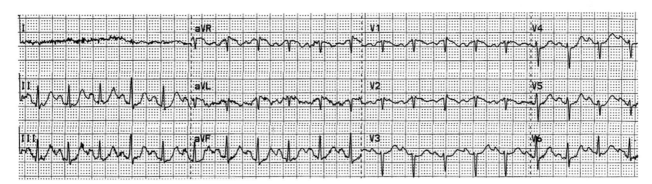

Figure 31.74 Poor precordial R-wave progression with a very small R wave < 1.5 mm in leads V$_1$–V$_4$. The axis is rightward with Q wave in lead aVL. This could be: (1) anterior MI with lateral MI explaining the right-axis deviation; or (2) severe lung disease pattern with prominent posterior forces across the precordial leads. The small QRS voltage in all leads, including the precordial leads, where S is dominant but not particularly deep, suggests lung disease pattern but may be seen with extensive infarction. This patient has severe lung disease with significant hypoxemia at rest and normal LV function.

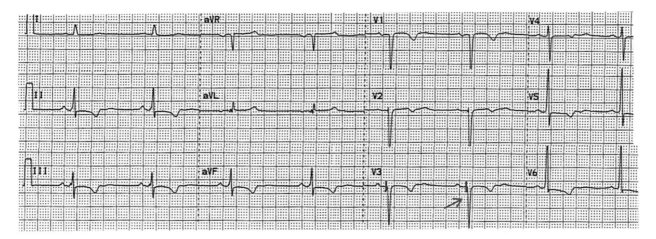

Figure 31.75 Poor precordial R-wave progression with a monophasic Q (QS) in V$_1$ and a small R wave in V$_2$ and V$_3$ (~1 mm). The T-wave inversion in V$_1$–V$_3$ and the small QRS in lead I (~4 mm) are supportive of an anterior MI. As opposed to the ECG shown in Figure 31.74, note that the QRS voltage is not reduced and a deep S wave is seen in V$_2$–V$_3$ (*arrow*). A large voltage is against COPD, while a small voltage may be seen in both COPD or MI.

XVI. Approach to tachyarrhythmias
(See also Chapter 8)

When analyzing a tachycardia, start by looking at three features:

1. Narrow QRS vs. wide QRS (≥120 ms) (choose the lead where QRS is widest).

2. Regular vs. irregular ventricular rate.

3. Look for P waves and their relationship with QRS complexes. P waves are usually seen as notches or deflections that fall over the ST–T segments and have a *consistent morphology* and *timing,* i.e., those deflections are regularly placed and can be marched out. Try to confirm that these deflections are P waves, rather than artifacts or parts of T wave, by analyzing multiple leads. Once P waves are found, their relationship with QRS complexes is analyzed. In wide QRS tachycardia, analyze: (i) AV dissociation, and (ii) the number of P waves compared to the number of QRS complexes. In narrow QRS tachycardia, assess the length of the RP interval.

A. Approach to narrow QRS-complex tachycardias (Figures 31.76–31.79)
Note the Ashman phenomenon (Figure 31.79).

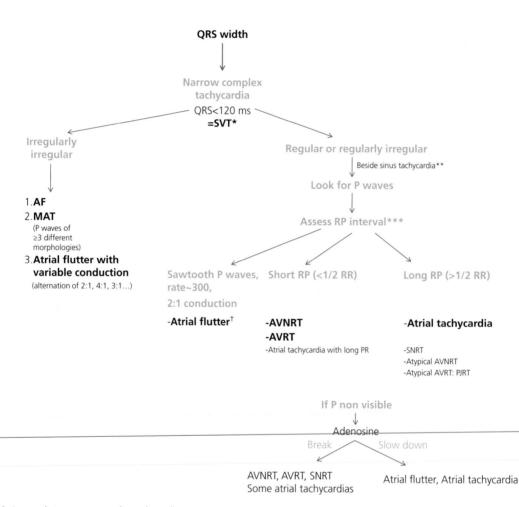

Figure 31.76 Approach to narrow complex tachycardias.

*A narrow QRS tachycardia may occasionally be VT. If QRS is relatively narrow (~110–120 ms) but different in morphology from the baseline QRS, consider it VT or SVT with aberrancy.

As opposed to other tachycardias, sinus tachycardia has a gradual onset and termination and does not have a fixed rate. **Tachyarrhythmias typically have a sudden onset and offset and a very fixed rate, although they may have a quick warm-up at the beginning. For example, a tachycardia with a fixed rate of 122 bpm on a telemetry monitor suggests arrhythmia. In particular, the P wave of atrial tachycardia or SNRT may have a sinus P morphology, but the abrupt onset and the steady rate help differentiate the arrhythmia from sinus tachycardia.

***RP interval is the interval between onset of QRS and onset of the following P wave (retrograde P wave in AVNRT or AVRT). If this interval is < 1/2 of the R–R interval, the tachycardia is a short RP tachycardia.

†**Atrial flutter** may mimic short RP tachycardia if only the flutter wave following the QRS is seen, or may mimic long RP tachycardia/atrial tachycardia if only the flutter wave preceding the QRS is seen. *Atrial tachycardia with negative P waves preceding the QRS complexes in the inferior leads may, in fact, be atrial flutter.* Look carefully for flutter waves to make the diagnosis.

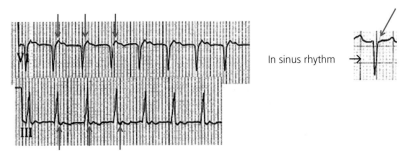

In sinus rhythm →

Figure 31.77 Narrow complex tachycardia. A deflection is seen at the end of QRS in leads V$_1$ and III; this deflection is seen in multiple leads and likely represents P wave. RP interval is very short (~1.5 small boxes, < 90 ms), thus implying AVNRT. Also, the P wave falls so close within the QRS, giving a pseudo-r' shape in V$_1$ and a pseudo-S shape in lead III, typical of AVNRT (*arrows*). The QRS morphology in sinus rhythm does not show r' (*arrow, right panel*) and thus confirms that the r' seen during tachycardia is a P wave rather than a true r' wave.

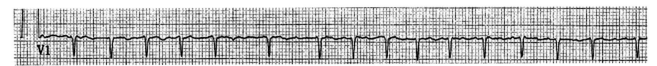

Figure 31.78 Narrow complex tachycardia, irregular. Differential diagnosis:
1. AF.
2. MAT: in MAT, a well-formed P wave is seen before every QRS complex, yet P waves have various morphologies (≥3) and various PR intervals. The rate is usually 100–150 bpm.
3. Atrial flutter with variable conduction (alternation of 2:1, 4:1, 3:1, …).
4. Sinus tachycardia with frequent PACs, including several PACs in a row.

AF is the diagnosis in this case. The small "blips" seen over the baseline are atrial fibrillatory waves rather than real P waves. They do not have a consistent *morphology* or *timing*.

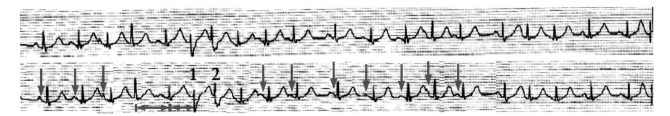

Figure 31.79 The rhythm is irregular. Look for P waves: P waves are present, have more than three different morphologies (*arrows*), with varying PR intervals; this is diagnostic of MAT. Some of the P waves of MAT are of sinus origin, the rest originate from multiple atrial foci.

How about the two wide complexes (*1* and *2*)? Are these PVCs or aberrant complexes, i.e., complexes with functional bundle branch block? In the context of an irregular rhythm (e.g., AF, sinus rhythm with PACs), complexes occurring at a short R–R interval may be aberrant, especially if the short R–R is preceded by a long R–R interval (**long–short sequence**): this is the **Ashman phenomenon**. This is related to the fact that one of the bundles, often the right bundle, is still in a refractory period when the supraventricular stimulus hits early. A long R–R interval further prolongs the bundles' refractory period and makes a QRS that falls shortly after it aberrant (*long–short sequence*). The right bundle normally has a longer refractory period than the left bundle and is more likely to become aberrant. The R–R interval preceding complex 1 (*short caliper*) is short, shorter than any non-aberrant R–R interval, and is preceded by a relatively long R–R interval (*longer caliper*). This is typical of aberrancy. Finding shorter R–R interval(s) not followed by aberrancy argues against aberrancy but may be seen, because aberrancy also depends on the length of the "long" part of the long–short sequence. Complex 2 is preceded by a shorter R–R interval than complex 1, leading to a wider aberrancy. Both complexes 1 and 2 have RBBB morphology, which is the most common pattern in functional aberrancy.

B. Approach to wide QRS-complex tachycardias

A wide QRS-complex tachycardia could be:

1. VT.
2. SVT (including AF) with aberrancy. Aberrancy signifies the occurrence of a functional RBBB, LBBB, or RBBB + LAFB during supraventricular tachycardia, leading to a wide complex morphology simulating VT. Aberrancy occurs when the refractory period of one of the bundles or fascicles is surpassed during the tachycardia. In addition, the bundle branch block may be a pre-existing bundle branch block, in which case the QRS morphology during the tachycardia is similar to the QRS morphology during the sinus rhythm, sometimes slightly wider.
3. SVT (especially AF) with pre-excitation. This means that the SVT is conducted antegradely over an accessory pathway that connects one atrium to one ventricle, short-circuiting the AV node.
4. Other diagnoses: hyperkalemia; drug toxicity (class I antiarrhythmic agents, tricyclic drugs); ventricular pacemaker tracking an atrial arrhythmia (lack of mode switch), or pacemaker- mediated tachycardia.

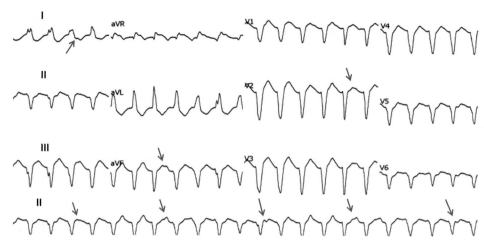

Figure 31.80 Regular wide complex tachycardia. SVT vs.VT?

1. Look for P waves, i.e., look for "blips" or notches that: (a) have a consistent morphology and timing, and (b) can be marched out. P waves are usually best seen in lead II and in the lead with the smallest T and QRS. On this ECG, blips are seen in lead II (*arrows*). These blips can be marched out and have a consistent morphology; they are not part of the T wave, as they are not seen after every QRS and they disfigure T wave variably, depending on where they fall. They are also seen in other leads (leads V_2, I, and aVF: *arrows*), further adding to the evidence that these are P waves, not artifacts or parts of T wave. They do not have a consistent relationship with QRS complexes, and some of them fall inside QRS complexes and are not seen; in fact, an additional P wave is probably hidden between every two evident P waves. Thus, P waves are dissociated from QRS and are less numerous than QRS complexes → VT.

   The variable T-wave morphology is usually a hint to the presence of P waves that are dissociated from QRS/T and falling variably over some T waves.

2. QRS morphology. QRS has a monophasic, negative QS morphology in V_1–V_6. A monophosic negative or positive QRS in all precordial leads is not consistent with RBBB or LBBB and implies VT. This is called QRS concordance (e.g., QS pattern or monophasic R-wave pattern throughout V_1–V_6). QRS being negative in all precordial leads, this VT looks away from the precordium and thus originates from the apex.

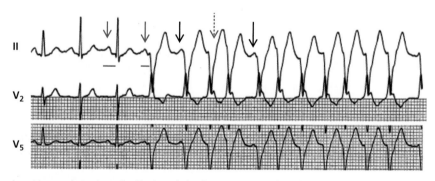

Figure 31.81 Run of irregular wide complex tachycardia. The irregularity does not necessarily imply AF. During a short run of VT or at the initiation of VT, the rhythm may be irregular. Analyze the following:

1. How the tachycardia starts. The tachycardia starts after a regularly occurring sinus P wave (*blue arrows*), **at a shorter PR interval** (compare *bars*). This implies that it starts with a PVC, without interrupting the regularly occurring sinus P waves. The tachycardia has the same morphology as this PVC, thus, this is VT.
2. Look for P waves. Two P waves are seen within the tachycardia (*black arrows*). The first P wave has a morphology similar to the sinus P wave and comes at an interval that is equal to the sinus P–P interval. The second P wave falls at an interval that is a multiple of the sinus P–P interval; there is another P wave preceding it and hidden in the QRS complex (*dashed arrow*). Those P waves fall around the QRS and ST–T segments at their own rate and are dissociated from QRS.
3. QRS morphology. The QRS has a **QS morphology in V_5**, which is not seen with LBBB or RBBB, and is pathognomonic of VT. Final diagnosis: VT.

   A wide complex tachycardia that is very grossly irregular is AF: AF with aberrancy, AF with pre-excitation, or AF with class I antiarrhythmic drug therapy. Polymorphic VT is a distant second possibility. On the other hand, a slightly irregular tachycardia, with only slight variations of R–R interval, may be seen with VT or any SVT at its onset (the first 20 beats).

Summarized approach to wide QRS-complex tachycardias (Figures 31.80, 31.81):

1. ~80% of wide complex tachycardias are VT (95% if CAD or HF). Thus, if one is unsure of the diagnosis, it is safer to consider the arrhythmia VT than SVT and treat it as such. However, it is best to look for features characteristic of VT and establish a definitive diagnosis.
Features that further support VT:
   • P waves are seen scattered between QRS complexes and unrelated to QRS complexes (**AV dissociation**), and/or number of P waves < number of QRS complexes.
   • Morphology of QRS is not consistent with a typical LBBB or a typical RBBB. In patients with a wide baseline QRS, a wide QRS tachycardia that is narrower than baseline is VT.

- Tachycardia starts with a PVC rather than a PAC, and has a morphology similar to the PVC. *How to distinguish a PVC from an aberrant PAC?* A PVC falls on the top of a normally occurring sinus P wave (the regularly occurring sinus P wave appears as a "blip" within the PVC or just before it, at a short PR interval). On the other hand, an aberrantly conducted PAC starts after a premature, non-sinus P wave that may fall within the preceding T wave and deform it. *A deformation of the T wave preceding the premature complex is a hint to a PAC.*

2. SVT with aberrancy: this diagnosis is most confidently made if a baseline bundle branch block is present and the tachycardia has the same morphology as the baseline bundle branch block. Otherwise, the lack of any VT feature supports the diagnosis of SVT.

3. AF with pre-excitation: tachycardia is irregular, polymorphic, bizarre-looking, with a morphology that is wide but not consistent with aberrancy (not a typical RBBB or LBBB).

XVII. Approach to bradyarrhythmias: AV block

(See also Chapter 13)

Identify the **type** but also the **location** of the block (nodal vs. infranodal block) (Figures 31.82–31.87):

1. *First-degree AV block* = PR interval > 200 ms (may be as long as 1000 ms).

2. *Second-degree AV block*

i. Mobitz type I (Wenckebach type): PR progressively prolongs until QRS drops, i.e., a P wave occurring at the intrinsic atrial rate is not followed by a QRS complex. To make the diagnosis, compare PR that follows the blocked P (the shortest PR) with the one that immediately precedes the blocked P (the longest PR). While PR lengthens, R–R progressively shortens before the pause.

ii. Mobitz type II: QRS suddenly drops without a preceding PR change. *The baseline QRS is usually wide.* It may present as intermittently non-conducted P waves or as one non-conducted P wave that is not preceded by progressive PR prolongation and not followed by PR shortening. It is more ominous than Mobitz I and is almost always a distal infranodal AV block. It progresses to a complete infranodal AV block commonly and suddenly.

iii. 2:1 AV block (alternative drop of one QRS complex) could be equivalent to Mobitz I or Mobitz II AV block. If QRS is wide, the block is likely infranodal and is thus a Mobitz II equivalent. If QRS is narrow, the block is likely a Mobitz I equivalent. More specifically, a PR interval > 250 ms with a narrow QRS complex implies a nodal AV block, while a PR interval < 200–250 ms implies that the block is unlikely to be at the nodal level. Also, look for periods of 3:2 conduction on a long rhythm strip; the PR-segment pattern on the long strip helps elucidate the diagnosis.

3. *Third-degree or complete AV block*

No P wave is conducted and a junctional or ventricular escape rhythm takes over. The ventricular rate is regular and unrelated to P waves (AV dissociation). **The PR distance is variable yet the R–R interval is regular**, providing evidence that none of the P waves is conducted. If the AV block is infranodal, the escape is ventricular, wide, at a rate of 20–40 bpm usually. If the AV block is nodal, the escape is junctional, narrow, at a rate of 40–60 bpm (Figures 31.84, 31.85). A wide-complex escape may be considered junctional if a similar bundle branch block is present on the baseline ECG; otherwise, the wide escape is considered ventricular. Both cases, when symptomatic, are urgently treated with a temporary pacemaker followed by permanent pacemaker placement, but infranodal AV block is a real emergency with an imminent risk of cardiac arrest regardless of symptoms.

High-grade AV block means that most P waves are not conducted and an escape rhythm is seen, but some P waves are conducted. The regular escape rhythm is interrupted by some irregularities (Figure 31.86).

Notes

3:2 AV block means that two consecutive P waves conduct while the third P wave gets blocked (i.e., three P waves with two QRS complexes). 4:3 block means three consecutive P waves conduct while the fourth P wave gets blocked. This could be Mobitz I or II depending on the occurrence of progressive PR prolongation. 3:1 block means that only one of three P waves is conducted (three P waves with one QRS). This is also called high-grade AV block or advanced second-degree AV block and has the same negative implication as complete AV block.

Second-degree AV block is characterized by group beating, in which a group of QRS complexes is followed by a pause, then the cycle repeats. The cycle length may be variable (2:1 AV block alternating with 3:2, 4:3, 8:7, etc.). Think of second-degree AV block whenever there is a repetition of groups of beats. Clue to Wenckebach: compare the PR immediately after the pause (the shortest) to the one immediately before it (the longest). Also, R–R progressively shortens before the pause and the duration of the pause is less than twice the R–R interval preceding the pause.

A pause on a rhythm strip may be: (1) a sinus pause; (2) a blocked P wave secondary to AV block; (3) a blocked P wave of a very premature PAC that falls in the ventricular refractory period and does not get conducted. As opposed to AV block, the blocked P wave of a PAC does not march out with the sinus P waves.

Group beating on ECG may be a second-degree AV or SA block, or frequent PVCs or PACs, blocked or conducted, followed by pauses.

One particular type of group beating, *bigeminal rhythm*, is characterized by a repetition of two beats followed by a pause. It is caused by: 3:2 AV or SA block, PACs/PVCs occurring in a bigeminal pattern, or atrial flutter with alternation of 4:1 and 2:1 AV conduction.

Look carefully for 2:1 AV block in any case of sinus bradycardia. 2:1 AV block may mimic sinus bradycardia when the blocked P waves fall on the preceding T waves and go unnoticed or are mistaken for U waves. Conversely, in sinus bradycardia, U waves may be misinterpreted as blocked P waves, causing a false diagnosis of 2:1 AV block. Blocked P waves are distinguished from U waves by the fact that they march out almost equidistantly with the P waves that precede the QRS complexes and have the same shape/amplitude as those P waves, whereas U waves have a different shape and are often less peaked than P waves (Figure 31.87).

AV dissociation is present in all cases of AV block, but AV dissociation does not imply AV block. A competing accelerated junctional or ventricular rhythm that is equal in rate to the sinus rhythm, or faster than it, leads to AV dissociation. It is a competing form of AV dissociation, rather than an AV-block form of AV dissociation. One form of competing AV dissociation is isorhythmic AV dissociation, in which the junctional or ventricular rhythm almost has the same rate as the sinus rhythm, allowing intermittent conduction of sinus P waves that are falling far enough from the QRS complexes (e.g., AIVR, accelerated junctional rhythm). One beat may be a sinus beat preceded by a P wave, the other may be a junctional beat dissociated from the P wave and showing up at any deceleration of the sinus rate (Figure 31.88). *A P wave that falls far enough from the QRS complex yet does not get conducted implies AV block.* In some cases, the junctional rhythm may lead to retrograde P waves that reset the sinus node and inhibit sinus P-wave formation.

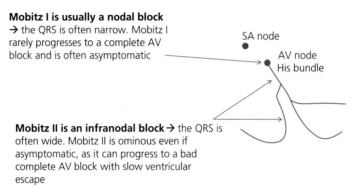

Mobitz I is usually a nodal block
→ the QRS is often narrow. Mobitz I rarely progresses to a complete AV block and is often asymptomatic

SA node

AV node
His bundle

Mobitz II is an infranodal block → the QRS is often wide. Mobitz II is ominous even if asymptomatic, as it can progress to a bad complete AV block with slow ventricular escape

Figure 31.82 Location of the AV block.

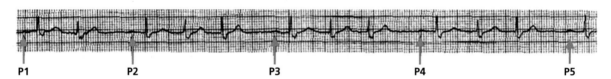

P1   P2   P3   P4   P5

Figure 31.83 Repetition of groups of beats separated by a pause. Think of second-degree AV block. P waves are not seen between P1–P2–P3–P4–P5. However, a slight R–R shortening is progressively seen before each pause, and the pause is shorter than twice the smallest R–R interval: this is typical of Wenckebach type of AV block. Outside the marked P waves, additional P waves are concealed with a very prolonged PR; P waves are falling onto the preceding T waves and deforming them, explaining why T waves appear to have different morphologies. PR is, therefore, progressively lengthening.

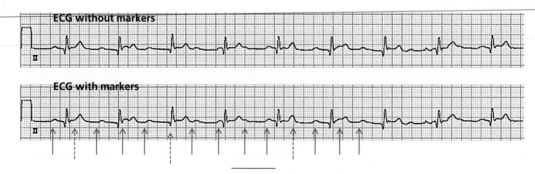

Figure 31.84 Regular, narrow complex rhythm, rate ~55 bpm. P waves are seen around the QRS complexes, falling onto the T waves or the QRS complexes (*arrows*). Some are not seen but expected to be present based on a consistent P–P interval (*dashed arrows*). None of them is conducted; this is evidenced by the fact that the **PR distance is variable yet the ventricular rate is regular**. The P waves are identified by their consistent shape as well as the consistent timing. Look for an R–R space where two P waves are clearly seen, such as the interval *underlined*, then start marching out P waves using this P–P interval. Final diagnosis: sinus tachycardia ~125 bpm with complete AV block and junctional escape rhythm.

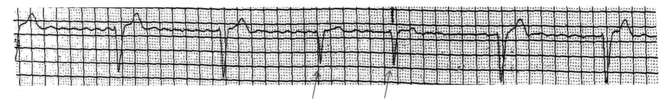

Figure 31.85 AF with a ventricular rate that is slow and mostly regular. This is AF with an almost complete AV block and a wide, regular escape rhythm, likely ventricular. Two QRS complexes occur at a shorter R–R distance and signify occasional AV conduction (*arrows*). Those supraventricular complexes are narrower than the escape rhythm. This is a high-grade rather than a complete AV block.

ECG without markers

ECG with markers

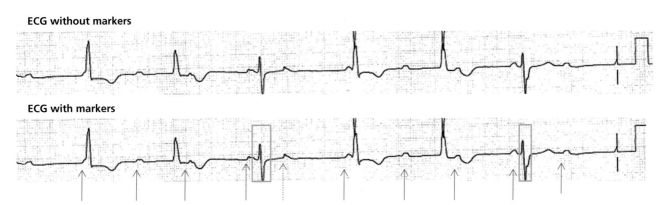

Figure 31.86 Regular wide complex rhythm interrupted by narrower complexes that occur at shorter R–R intervals (*rectangles*). P waves are seen and are grossly regular (*blue and gray arrows*). They are mostly non-conducted, with the exception of the P waves that lead to the shorter R–R intervals and the narrower QRS complexes (*gray arrows*). Beside the wide escape, the short PR interval of the conducted P waves implies an infranodal AV block.

Note a slight irregularity of the P waves. In fact, the P–P interval containing a QRS is shorter than the P–P interval not containing a QRS (ventriculophasic sinus arrhythmia). There is also one PAC (*dashed arrow*). Final diagnosis: high-grade infranodal AV block with ventricular escape rhythm and incomplete AV dissociation (two P waves are conducted).

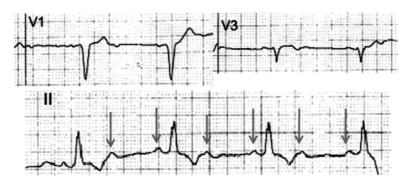

Figure 31.87 2:1 AV block that can be easily mistaken for sinus bradycardia, especially because the non-conducted P waves are well seen in lead II only. The non-conducted P waves are recognized by the fact that they have the same shape and peak as the conducted P waves, implying that they are P waves rather than U waves. The P waves do not perfectly march out, as the P–P interval containing a QRS complex is slightly shorter than the one not containing a QRS complex (*ventriculophasic sinus arrhythmia*). P waves are marked by *arrows*.

XVIII. Abnormal automatic rhythms that are not tachycardic

Three types of abnormal, non-tachycardic rhythms may be seen (Figures 31.89, 31.90, 31.91):

1. Ventricular escape rhythm (<60 bpm, usually <40 bpm) or accelerated idioventricular rhythm (60–120 bpm)
2. Junctional escape rhythm (<60 bpm) or accelerated junctional rhythm (60–130 bpm)
3. Atrial escape rhythm (<60 bpm) or ectopic atrial rhythm (60–100 bpm)

The escape rhythms may be seen in patients with sinus bradyarrhythmia (all three types of escape) or AV block (first two types of escape). **Isorhythmic AV dissociation** may be seen when a junctional or a ventricular rhythm competes with the sinus rhythm at approximately the same rate (see Figure 31.88).

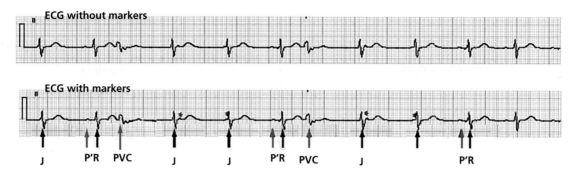

Figure 31.88 Outside the PVCs, the rhythm seems grossly regular. Analyze the P–QRS relationship: some QRS complexes seem to be preceded by P waves with a consistent PR relationship (conducted P, noted as *P'*). On the other hand, some QRS complexes are not preceded by any P wave (junctional QRS, noted as *J*). This suggests that a sinus rhythm and a junctional rhythm are competing at the same rate. After a post-PVC pause, or when the sinus rhythm slightly slows down, the junctional rhythm takes over (= isorhythmic AV dissociation, no AV block). Note that during the junctional rhythm, sinus P waves keep occurring regularly, dissociated from QRS and falling around it, marked by asterisks (*).

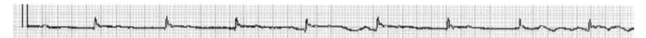

Figure 31.89 Regular narrow complex rhythm without any P wave. This is a junctional rhythm (rate of ~60 bpm), likely a junctional escape rhythm. The cause is either: (i) complete sinus arrest with escape through the AV junction, or (ii) AF with complete AV nodal block and with small fibrillatory waves that are not well seen.

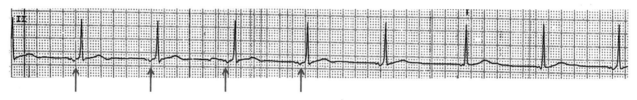

Figure 31.90 Regular narrow complex rhythm (~50 bpm). Negative P waves are seen in lead II, with a short PR interval of ~100 ms. This is either a low atrial rhythm or a junctional rhythm with retrograde P waves. Sinus arrest is not necessarily present; the sinus node may be suppressed by a faster atrial rhythm or by the retrograde P waves of the junctional rhythm.

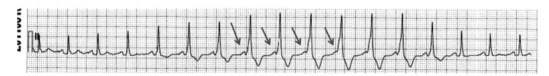

Figure 31.91 Sinus rhythm is interrupted by a wide complex rhythm. The wide complex rhythm has a rate that approximates the sinus rate. P waves (*arrows*) keep occuring through the wide complex rhythm at a very short PR interval. Possible diagnoses:

a. Accelerated idioventricular rhythm (AIVR) that appears once the sinus rate slightly slows down. In fact P waves are falling too close to the QRS complexes and are not getting the opportunity to conduct (isorhythmic AV dissociation). Once the sinus rate increases again, the sinus P waves get conducted and suppress AIVR. Some fusion QRS complexes are seen (5th to 7th QRS, and last QRS of the wide complex run).

b. A less likely diagnosis is intermittent pre-excitation; the latter usually appears when the AV conduction decreases (e.g., more vagal tone), which is typically accompanied by slowing of the P rate.

XIX. Electrode misplacement

A switch of the right and left arm electrodes induces P, QRS, and T changes that follow the change in the axis of the leads. Lead I reverses 180°, and thus P and QRS invert in lead I. Leads II and III switch positions and thus switch their ECG complexes. Leads aVR and aVL switch position, and lead aVF remains the same. While an inverted QRS complex in lead I may suggest right-axis deviation, inverted P, QRS, and T waves often point to switched arm electrodes (Figure 31.92).

When the right arm electrode is switched with the *right leg* electrode (which is the neutral, ground electrode), the ground becomes at arm level, and lead II becomes a lead that runs between two legs, far away from the cardiac depolarization. The ECG of lead II becomes flat, i.e., P, QRS, and T are almost isoelectric. A similar phenomenon happens when the left arm electrode is switched with the right leg electrode, in which case lead III becomes flat. Any time the whole P–QRS–T is almost isoelectric in lead II or III, arm-to-right-leg electrode misplacement is suggested (Figures 31.93, 31.94).

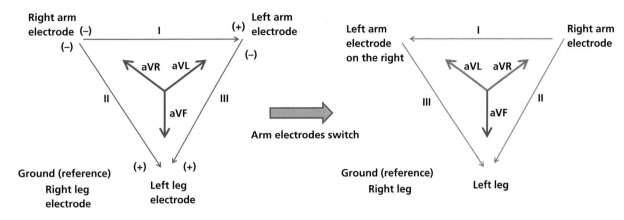

Figure 31.92 Right and left arm electrodes switched. The leads' axis changes are shown. The leads that have changed axis are colored in gray.

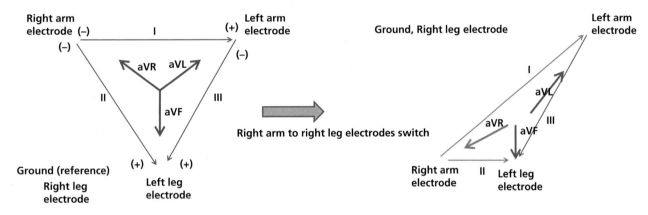

Figure 31.93 Right arm and right leg electrodes switched. The leads' axis changes are shown. The leads that have changed axis are colored in gray.

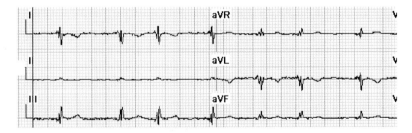

Figure 31.94 Right arm and right leg electrodes switched. Note how lead II is fully isoelectric. Leads aVL, aVF, and III continue to accurately display their respective QRS.

Appendix 1. Supplement on STEMI and Q-wave MI: phases and localization

A. Electrophysiology of the ST-segment changes

Through the opening of K_{ATP} channels, ischemia lowers the amplitude of the action potential, more specifically the plateau phase 2, in the ischemic area, which creates a systolic voltage gradient and a current during phase 2 (injury current) from the normal to the ischemic area (ST deviation); the resting potential of the injured area is less negative, which creates a diastolic injury current from the ischemic area to its surroundings (TP depression). In transmural ischemia, the gradient is between the surrounding areas and the ischemic area, with a resultant current directed towards the leads overlying the ischemic area, creating ST-segment elevation in those leads. In subendocardial ischemia, this current is directed from the subepicardium towards the subendocardium, away from the leads, creating ST-segment depression. This ST-segment depression is, however, non-localizing; the subepicardium wherein the current originates does not necessarily overlie the ischemic subendocardium. The LV and apex having the largest myocardial mass and repolarizing earlier than the rest of the LV (base), the current often originates from this area, leading to ST depression in V_4–V_6 even in inferior ischemia (Figure 31.95). A large area of ischemia creates a larger current and more diffuse and deep ST depression. Those injury currents can lead to triggered activity and can initiate multiple reentry wavelets and polymorphic arrhythmias.

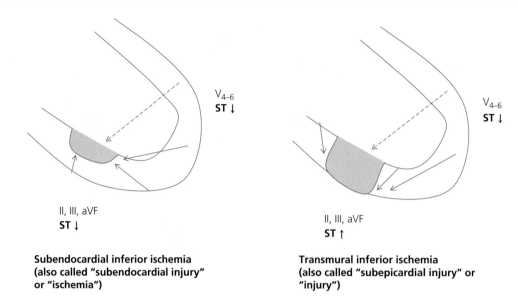

Subendocardial inferior ischemia (also called "subendocardial injury" or "ischemia")

Transmural inferior ischemia (also called "subepicardial injury" or "injury")

Figure 31.95 Subendocardial ischemia (diffuse ST depression, not localized to the ischemic area) vs. transmural ischemia (ST elevation localized to the ischemic area).

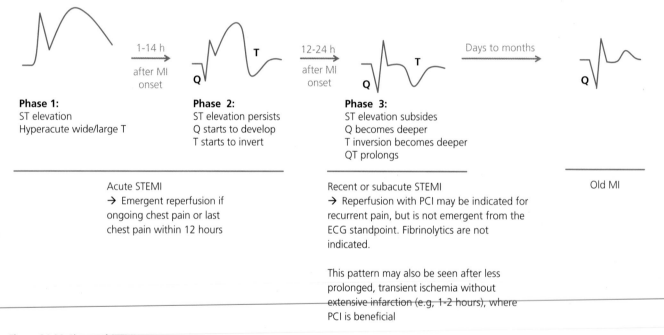

Figure 31.96 Phases of STEMI.

Q waves develop when a transmural area becomes electrically neutral, but not necessarily necrotic. The ventricular depolarization looks away from this neutral area, hence the negative Q deflection. Q waves are seen with transmural infarction, but also stunning or hibernation. They may also be seen with a large area of subendocardial infarction. Conversely, they may not be seen with a small or reperfused area of transmural infarction. Thus, Q-wave MI implies a *large* infarction that is often, but not always, *transmural*.

Q-wave MI is usually the result of a STEMI and is usually a transmural or large MI; non-Q-wave MI is usually NSTEMI and is typically a subendocardial smaller MI. However, some overlap exists. STEMI may lead to non-Q-wave MI, particularly when reperfused with recovery of most of the myocardium. NSTEMI may evolve into Q-wave MI if the non-transmural infarction is large.

B. Phases of STEMI (see Figures 31.96, 31.97)
Note 1. T-wave inversion
T inversion usually starts while the ST segment is still elevated but is starting to subside. T-wave inversion progressively deepens and prolongs QT.

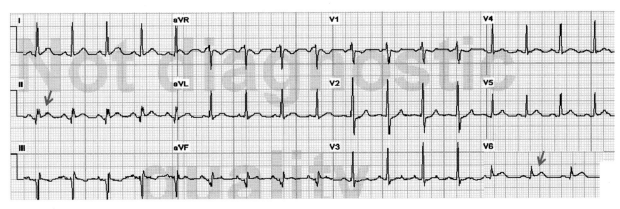

Figure 31.97 The patient presents with chest discomfort that has started 4 hours previously. Subtle ST elevation is seen in leads II, aVF, V$_5$ and V$_6$, with subtle ST depression in V$_1$–V$_2$. Three features suggest that this mild ST elevation is actually STEMI: (i) Q waves in leads II, III, aVF, and posteriorly (R wave in V$_2$); (ii) ST depression in reciprocal leads (V$_1$–V$_2$); (iii) wide T-wave morphology and fused ST–T segments in leads II, V$_5$ and V$_6$ (*arrows*), along with a "shrinking" R wave (R and T waves have ~equal height). He is found to have an acutely occluded large OM branch.

a. T wave that inverts within 4 hours of reperfusion therapy is a sign of reperfusion.

b. T wave that spontaneously inverts within a few hours of symptom onset may imply spontaneous reperfusion.

c. T wave that inverts late, or >4 hours after therapy, is part of the normal post-infarction evolution.

d. T-wave inversion should persist for at least a few days. *If it subsides quickly, in less than a few days, pericarditis or recurrent ischemia with T-wave pseudo-normalization should be suspected.*

e. T-wave inversion that persists >3 weeks is an adverse prognostic sign, suggesting the absence of any functional recovery. T-wave inversion may persist for days, weeks, months, or even years.

Note 2. Hyperacute R waves

Hyperacute R waves, i.e., R waves of shrinking amplitude pulled up by the elevated ST segment, may be seen acutely.

Note 3. Q waves

Q waves develop at 1–14 hours (mean, 9 hours) after the onset of an acute MI, usually STEMI. Most often, they develop acutely while the ST is still elevated and persist indefinitely in 60–90% of patients. Q waves do not necessarily mean subacute or old MI; Q waves concomitant with ST elevation usually signify an acute MI a few hours old (old MI with LV aneurysm is a distant possibility). The appearance of Q waves early in the course of MI does not lessen the benefit of reperfusion and the reduction of the infarct size. Q waves are not synonymous with irreversible myocardial damage and may be seen with a severely ischemic or stunned, non-infarcted myocardium. Q waves may appear after an hour of transient ischemia or a prolonged coronary spasm. Outside STEMI, they may be seen with a viable but hibernating, chronically ischemic myocardium. Q waves may be absent if a reciprocal territory has an old infarction, leading to cancellation of electrical forces (e.g., anterior MI associated with an old posterior MI), or if the myocardium surrounding the scar is hypertrophied.

While the acute appearance of Q waves does not imply irreversible damage, their late persistence for several months implies some irreversible damage with worse LV dysfunction and more HF. In patients with similar baseline Q waves and similar extent of infarction, those who experience Q-wave regression at 1, 6, or 24 months have greater myocardial recovery and more striking EF improvement than those without Q-wave regression (9±11% vs. 2±8%), greater improvement in regional wall thickening, and significant regression of infarct size. Q waves are more likely to regress if the stunned myocardium is larger than the infarcted myocardium.

Q-wave regression is seen in ~40% of patients with anterior or inferior infarct and is generally defined as Q-wave disappearance with reappearance of R wave ≥1 mm in height in at least one lead; the regression is frequently partial, with persistent Q waves in some leads.[85,86] Other studies defined Q-wave regression as reclassification of the ECG from Q-wave MI to no MI.[87,88] Q-wave regression in leads I or aVL may manifest as rS pattern with persistent right-axis deviation and sometimes persistent Q waves in V$_5$–V$_6$. Q-wave regression in the inferior leads may manifest as a "shrinking" of Q wave to a non-significant width in ≥one lead, or may manifest as rS complex with persistent left-axis deviation. Q-wave regression in leads V$_1$–V$_3$ may manifest as poor R-wave progression. In fact, while poor R-wave progression does not usually represent an old anterior MI, up to one-third of old anterior MIs have poor R-wave progression as their only sequela (better prognosis than persistent Q waves). Note that the regeneration of a very small and narrow R wave <0.01 seconds, called embryonic R wave, does not imply Q-wave regression and is, for practical purposes, a form of persistent Q wave.

To summarize: although the depth and the extent of Q waves have a prognostic value in STEMI, and although a Q-wave MI is larger than a non-Q-wave MI and more likely transmural, with a worse short-term prognosis, the dynamics of the appearance, disappearance, or deepening of the Q waves early on are not as useful as the dynamics of ST-segment elevation and T-wave changes for the evaluation of MI reperfusion or viability. The late persistence of Q waves has a more definite prognostic value.

C. Localization of STEMI

1. MI territories

a. V_1–V_3 or V_2–V_4: anterior or anteroseptal MI, also involving the apex (LAD). ***Anterior or anteroseptal STEMI always has ST elevation in V_3. ST elevation in V_1–V_2 without V_3 is not usually an anterior STEMI.***

b. V_4–V_6: anterolateral or lateral MI. If ST elevation is present in $V_3 \rightarrow$ LAD. If ST elevation is isolated to V_4–$V_6 \rightarrow$ LAD or LCx.

c. I–aVL: lateral or high lateral MI → high OM branch, high diagonal branch, or ramus intermedius.

d. II, III, aVF: inferior MI → RCA in 75% of the cases; or LCx, often a dominant LCx, in 25% of the cases. The LCx may be a non-dominant LCx with an OM branch that extends to the inferior wall distally.

e. V_7–V_9: posterior MI, with reciprocal ST depression in V_1–V_3 and wide *and* tall R waves in V_1 or V_2. Think of true posterior STEMI when ST depression is isolated or most prominent in V_1–V_3. ST elevation is usually seen in V_7–V_9, but not always; leads V_7–V_9 are distant from the heart, which sometimes minimizes the ST elevation. Posterior STEMI is often accompanied by some degree of ST elevation in the inferior or lateral leads. An isolated posterior STEMI is more likely due to LCx than RCA occlusion.

f. V_1, ±V_2, right-sided V_4 (V_{4R}), ± right-sided V_3 (V_{3R}): RV infarct associated with an inferior infarct. Note that, beside being a septal lead, V_1 (±V_2) is a right-sided lead that shows ST elevation in RV infarct.

2. Reciprocal changes

a. Anterior ST elevation from a proximal LAD occlusion that involves the high basal septal wall is associated with *inferior ST depression*. Anterior ST elevation from a mid-to-distal LAD occlusion is associated with *lateral ST depression (no inferior ST depression usually)*.

b. Posterior injury and posterior Q waves lead to reciprocal ST-segment depression in V_1–V_3 and wide (≥1 mm), tall R waves in V_1 or V_2.

c. Inferior ST elevation may lead to a high lateral ST depression.

3. Exact location and extent (see Tables 31.3, 31.4; Figures 31.98, 31.99)

Table 31.3 Localization of anterior MI.

Anterior MI proximal to first septal	• ST depression in the inferior leads and in V_5
	• ST elevation in $V_1 > 2.5$ mm
	• RBBB
	• ST elevation in aVR (similar to left main ischemia), and in I and aVL[a]
	• Inability to form Q waves in lateral leads, as these Q waves depend on septal depolarization
Anterior MI distal to first septal and proximal to first diagonal	• No ST depression in the inferior leads ± ST elevation if LAD wraps around the apex
	• ST elevation in the lateral leads I and aVL
	• **May have a pattern of diffuse ST elevation without any reciprocal change**
Anterior MI distal to both first septal and diagonal	• No ST depression in the inferior leads ± ST elevation if LAD wraps around the apex
	• ST depression in the lateral leads

[a] ST elevation in aVR indicates injury of the very proximal high septum, which looks towards the right shoulder. It may represent septal injury from *proximal LAD* occlusion or *left main subtotal occlusion*, or may be reciprocal to diffuse subendocardial ischemia in *left main disease*. Either way, it is a negative prognostic marker.

Table 31.4 Differentiate RCA from LCx in inferior MI.

The inferior RCA injury is looking rightward, while the inferior LCx injury is looking leftward. Features supportive of RCA:

i. Lateral ST depression in lead I (vs. lack of ST depression or ST elevation with LCx)

ii. ST elevation ≥ 0.5 mm in lead V_1 or V_{4R} (implies RV infarct, and thus, RCA). This is a very specific finding

iii. ST elevation in lead III > II (lead III is more parallel to the slightly rightward RCA current of injury, whereas lead II is parallel to the leftward LCx current of injury)

iv. No or minimal (<1 mm) ST depression in aVR implies RCA. The LCx current of injury is directly opposite to the right arm, thus LCx injury leads to ≥ 1 mm ST depression in aVR

LAD occlusion distal to the first septal branch and proximal to the first diagonal branch leads to anteroseptal ST elevation along with lateral and inferior ST elevation. Consequently, diffuse ST elevation without any reciprocal change is seen and may simulate pericarditis. This is alternatively explained by the fact that an apical infarction that does not involve the basal anterior wall is "seen" by all leads without any reciprocal change.

4. Conduction blocks and diagnostic dilemmas in LBBB and RBBB

See Section XII.D in this chapter, and Chapter 2, Sections 1.V and 2.V.

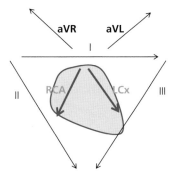

Figure 31.98 In inferior MI, the LCx current of injury looks to the left and has an axis of ~ +45°, while the RCA current of injury looks to the right. RCA injury is parallel to lead III, while LCx injury is parallel to lead II. Thus,

1. ST elevation is more prominent in lead III with RCA injury and in lead II with LCx injury.
2. ST depression in lead I implies RCA injury (cannot be seen with LCx). ST elevation in lead aVL implies LCx injury (cannot be seen with RCA).
3. ST depression is seen in lead aVR with LCx injury, while ST elevation or more subtle ST depression is seen with RCA injury.

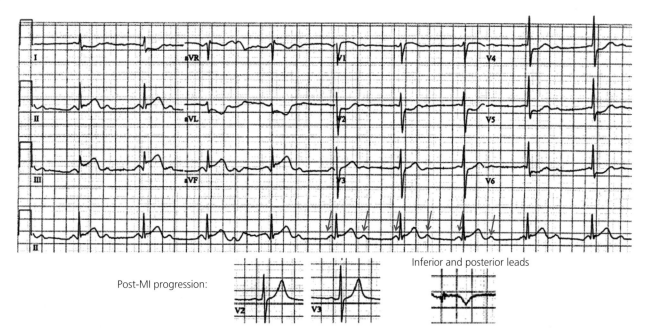

Post-MI progression:

Inferior and posterior leads

Figure 31.99 The rhythm initially appears to be sinus bradycardia (~55 bpm). On closer inspection, there is another P wave between QRS complexes; it is a P wave, rather than a U wave, by the fact that it marches out equidistantly with the P wave that precedes QRS and is as peaky as the P wave (*arrows*). Thus, the rhythm is sinus tachycardia with 2:1 AV block. QRS is narrow, so this 2:1 AV block is likely a Mobitz I equivalent. Sinus tachycardia implies that this AV block is not due to a high vagal tone, but rather to AV nodal ischemia/edema.

Inferior ST elevation with lateral ST depression is seen. ST depression is seen in V_2, which, in the setting of inferior STEMI, implies a posterior extension. 0.5 mm ST elevation is seen in V_1, which, in the setting of inferior STEMI, implies RV infarction. In fact, in a patient with posterior injury, the ST segment is expected to be depressed in V_1; an isoelectric ST segment in V_1 suggests RV infarction. Posterior MI leads to ST depression in V_1 while RV MI leads to ST elevation in V_1; the posterior LV is thicker than the RV but the RV is much closer to lead V_1, explaining how the RV injury overwhelms the posterior injury in lead V_1.

Is the culprit RCA or LCx? The following four findings suggest RCA: (1) reciprocal ST depression in lead I; (2) ST elevation in III > II; (3) RV infarction; and (4) the lack of ST depression in aVR.

During the post-MI evolution, T wave becomes inverted in the inferior leads. ***In the anterior leads, T wave becomes large and wide; this large T wave is, in fact, reciprocal to the deep posterior T wave.***

Appendix 2. Spread of electrical depolarization in various disease states using vector illustration (Figures 31.100–31.103)

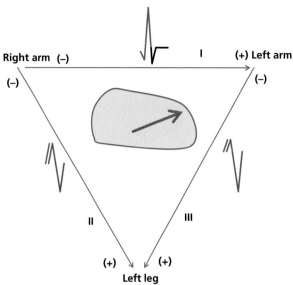

Figure 31.100 Frontal plane of left-axis deviation. This may be secondary to an anatomical shift of the heart, such as LV hypertrophy or enlargement, or to an electrical shift of the electrical depolarization, as in left anterior fascicular block, where the electrical depolarization spreads from down to up. A lesser shift is seen in patients with a horizontal heart, such as older or obese stocky patients.

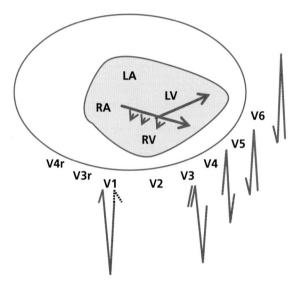

Figure 31.101 Horizontal plane of LV hypertrophy. The vector of depolarization is directed more leftward than normal; thus, R increases in height in V_5–V_6 and S deepens in V_1–V_2, with a later transition (V_4 or V_5 rather than V_3). The septum being thick, the blue septal depolarization is large, and thus the q wave in the lateral leads is deeper than normal; a lack of q wave in the lateral leads in patients with LVH implies incomplete LBBB.

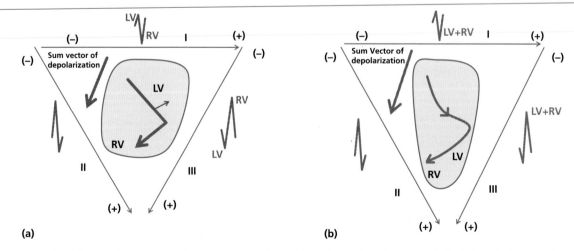

Figure 31.102 (a) Frontal plane of RV hypertrophy or RV strain such as PE. The RV extends to the right, while the LV is pushed up. The big RV explains the big S wave in lead I and the big R wave in the inferior leads, while the upwardly pushed LV depolarization explains the Q wave in leads III and aVF, but not usually in lead II ($S_I Q_{III} Q_{aVF}$ pattern in PE). **(b) Frontal plane of right-axis deviation from upright posture, COPD, or left posterior fascicular block.**

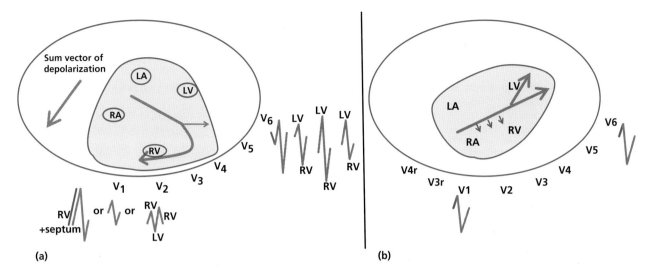

Figure 31.103 (a) Horizontal plane of RV hypertrophy. The sum vector of depolarization is rightward, and therefore R wave is large in V₁ and S wave is large in V₅–V₆, which is opposite to the normal QRS progression across the precordial leads. If the LV and RV depolarize simultaneously and the RV is not severely hypertrophied, the sum simultaneous electrical depolarization will be neutral, and thus R in V₁ will be small; the clue to RVH is that S is small as well. In dilated RV (volume overload), QRS may be wide because RV activity spread in time rather than height, explaining the incomplete RBBB pattern. In severe RV hypertrophy (pressure overload), a monophasic R pattern or a qR pattern may be seen in V₁ (the "q" in the qR pattern may be due to a loss of the normal left-to-right septal depolarization). **(b) Horizontal plane of COPD.** The heart is pushed posteriorly, which explains the deep S wave in both V₁ and V₆. While S wave is larger than R wave, the overall QRS voltage is reduced in all leads as a result of increased chest air.

QUESTIONS AND ANSWERS

Question 1. Analyze Figure 31.80. Is this VT or SVT?

Question 2. Analyze Figure 31.81. Is this VT or SVT?

Question 3. Analyze Figure 31.84. Is the rhythm 2:1 AV block, complete AV block, or Mobitz 1 AV block?

Question 4. Analyze Figure 31.86. Is the rhythm Mobitz 1 AV block, high-grade AV block, or complete AV block?

Question 5. A patient has occasional dizziness. ECG is performed (Figure 31.88):
A. ECG shows AV dissociation and AV block
B. ECG shows a competing form of AV dissociation without AV block

Question 6. Analyze Figure 31.91. What is the rhythm?

Question 7. Analyze Figure 13.15 (Chapter 13). Is there AV block or isorhythmic AV dissociation?

Question 8. Analyze Figure 8.9 (Chapter 8). Is this VT or SVT?

Question 9. An ECG shows a prominent R wave in lead V₁. What features differentiate RVH from posterior MI?

Question 10. An ECG shows right-axis deviation. What features differentiate isolated lung disease pattern from lung disease + RVH?

Question 11. A patient has RBBB. How to make a diagnosis of superimposed RVH?

Question 12. Is a QRS > 120 ms with rsR′ pattern in V₁ enough to make a diagnosis of RBBB?

Question 13. An ECG has a QRS > 120 ms with a wide slurred R wave in leads I and V₅–V₆. A q wave is present in lead I. Is this LBBB?

Question 14. An ECG has a QRS > 120 ms with a wide slurred R wave in leads I and V₅–V₆. A q wave is present in lead aVL. Is this LBBB?

Question 15. Which of the following is consistent with LAFB?
A. QRS 100 ms, left axis –45°, with qR pattern in lead aVL and rS pattern in the inferior leads. LVH may be present
B. QRS 100 ms, left axis –45°, R pattern in aVL and I (no q)
C. QRS 100 ms, left axis –45°, qR pattern in aVL, and QS pattern in leads III and aVF

Question 16. Analyze Figure 31.33. Is Wellens syndrome present?

Question 17. Draw the morphology of ST depression secondary to LVH. Draw the four ST-depression morphologies suggestive of ischemic ST depression.

Question 18. A patient has ST depression concordant with QRS with upright T wave. Does this suggest ischemia?

Question 19. A patient has a flat ST segment with symmetrically inverted T wave. Does this suggest ischemia?

Question 20. Analyze Figures 31.40a, 31.45, and 31.46b. All show prominent biphasic or inverted T waves in the precordial leads. Which statement is *incorrect*?
A. Figure 31.40A is Wellens sign. Figure 31.45 is global T inversion. As opposed to Wellens sign, global T inversion is more widespread, the ST segment is not upwardly convex and T descent is not sharp.
B. Figure 31.46B is a form of early repolarization with precordial biphasic/inverted T wave. As opposed to Wellens sign, the patient is asymptomatic and young. The ST elevation is prominent (more than Wellens), with a notched J point consistent with early repolarization.
C. Global T inversion (Figure 31.45), with its deeper and more prominent T inversion, is more worrisome for ischemia than Wellens (Figure 31.40a).

Question 21. When ST elevation is present on ECG, any of the following characteristics implies STEMI, *except*:
A. ST elevation straight or convex upward, blends with T to form a dome
B. Wide upright T or inverted T
C. Q waves
D. ST elevation or T wave may approximate or exceed QRS height
E. Reciprocal ST depression
F. PR depression

Question 22. A patient presents with chest pain and is found to have the ECG shown in Figure 31.53. Is this STEMI, pericarditis, or early repolarization?

Question 23. A patient presents with chest pain and is found to have the ECG shown in Figure 31.57. An ECG performed few weeks previously is grossly normal. What is the diagnosis?

Question 24. In a patient with LVH and discordant ST elevation, what absolute and relative ST elevation values suggest STEMI?
A. Discordant ST elevation ≥ 2.5 mm in V_1–V_3 in absolute terms, ST elevation ≥ 1 mm in the limb leads; Relative ST discordance $> 25\%$ of the QRS complex and relative T-wave discordance $> 50\%$
B. Absolute ST discordance > 5 mm and relative ST discordance $> 25\%$

Question 25. In a patient with LBBB and discordant ST elevation, what ST elevation values suggest STEMI?
A. Discordant ST elevation > 5 mm in V_1–V_3 in absolute terms
B. Relative ST discordance $> 25\%$ of the QRS complex and relative T-wave discordance $> 50\%$

Question 26. Concerning the long QT morphology in various disease states, which of the following is *incorrect*?
A. Notched T wave in LQT2, hypokalemia, and drug-induced QT prolongation
B. ST depression with upright T-U wave in hypokalemia
C. Long ST segment with a narrow T wave in LQT3
D. Broad, prolonged T wave in LQT1
E. Broad, prolonged T wave in hypocalcemia

Question 27. Draw the ECG patterns of progressive hypokalemia.

Question 28. QT interval is longest in leads V_2–V_3. Yet QT is best measured in other leads. Which leads are best for measurement of QT and why?

Question 29. Define QTc and calculate QTc in a patient whose QT is 400 ms at a heart rate of 100 bpm.

Question 30. A patient has a long QT. Next to the T wave, there is another wave, fused with the T wave and measuring ~50% of the T height. Should QT calculation include this wave?

Question 31. A 55-year-old woman presents with off-and-on chest pain for the last 3 hours. Her ECG is shown in Figure 31.42B. What is the diagnosis?
A. Non-ST-segment elevation acute coronary syndrome. An invasive strategy is performed, but is not urgent
B. Pulmonary embolism
C. Hypokalemia
D. LVH with secondary repolarization abnormality
E. Posterior ST-segment elevation myocardial infarction. Record leads V_7–V_9 and perform emergent coronary angiography and percutaneous coronary intervention

Question 32. A 62-year-old woman with lung cancer presents with chest pain and near-sycope. She is hypotensive. The presenting ECG is shown in Figure 31.50. Which of the following is *incorrect*?
A. The PR depression in lead II, the diffuse ST elevation, and the ST depression in lead aVR are diagnostic of pericarditis. The low QRS voltage suggests an associated pericardial effusion.

B. The domed ST elevation that is fused with the T wave in lead V$_2$ is suggestive of STEMI

C. The ST elevation and the T wave approximate the QRS height in leads V$_2$ to V$_4$, which suggests STEMI

D. The shrinking QRS voltage with a "pulled-up" R wave suggests STEMI

E. Diffuse ST elevation may be seen with occlusion of the midportion of a wrap-around left anterior descending artery

Question 33. A 76-year-old woman presents with acute dyspnea and is found to have pulmonary edema. The presenting ECG is shown in Figure 31.54. A new LBBB is seen. In the context of the new LBBB, which of the following features is (or are) least specific for the diagnosis of STEMI on this ECG (multiple answers possible)?

A. ST elevation concordant with the QRS complex in leads I and aVL

B. ST depression concordant with the QRS complex in the inferior leads

C. Discordant ST elevation of 5 mm in lead V$_2$

D. Discordant ST elevation that exceeds 25% of the QRS height in lead V$_2$, especially one that approximates the whole QRS height

E. Discordant ST elevation that is convex in lead V$_1$

Question 34. A 46-year-old woman presents with dysphagia, vomiting, and atypical chest pain. ECG is performed (Figure 31.67A). Cardiac biomarkers remain negative. What is the most likely cause of the ECG abnormality?

A. Non-ST-segment elevation acute coronary syndrome

B. Pulmonary embolism

C. Takotsubo cardiomyopathy

D. Hypokalemia

E. Pericarditis

Question 35. Analyze Figure 31.71. What is the differential diagnosis?

A. Hypokalemia

B. LQT2

C. Digitalis effect

For questions referring to specific figures, detailed explanations are provided in the figure legends.

Answer 1. VT.

Answer 2. VT.

Answer 3. Complete AV block.

Answer 4. High-grade infranodal AV block with ventricular escape rhythm.

Answer 5. B. ECG shows a sinus rhythm and a junctional rhythm occurring at a close rate, with isorhythmic AV dissociation. There is no AV block.

Answer 6. Sinus rhythm and AIVR with isorhythmic AV dissociation.

Answer 7. High-grade AV block with a fast ventricular escape rhythm.

Answer 8. VT.

Answer 9. In posterior MI, R wave is not only high in V$_1$ but is also wide > 1 mm (≠ RVH), T wave is positive in V$_1$–V$_2$ (vs. inverted in RVH), the axis is not right, and there are often Q waves in V$_7$–V$_9$ and in the inferior or lateral leads (Section VI.B).

Answer 10. In isolated lung disease pattern, the QRS axis is deviated to the right, S is deep throughout all of the precordial leads, and QRS voltage is reduced, especially in the limb leads. Superimposed RVH is suggested by large R or small S in V$_1$ (≤2 mm), RSR' pattern, or T-wave inversion in V$_1$–V$_2$ (Sections VI.B, XV.E).

Answer 11. RVH is diagnosed if the axis is right, as determined by the net voltage of the initial, unblocked 80 ms of QRS in the limb leads, along with R' > S or R' > 10 mm in V$_1$, or S > R in V$_6$. R' > S or R' > 10 mm more strongly suggests RVH in incomplete RBBB than in complete RBBB.

Answer 12. No. A wide S wave, wider than R wave or wider than 40 ms, is also needed in the lateral leads to define RBBB.

Answer 13. No. A septal q wave should not be seen in the lateral leads in LBBB (except, occasionally, in lead aVL).

Answer 14. Yes (Section VII.B).

Answer 15. A. LAFB should have QRS < 120 ms, left axis –45° to –90°, and a small septal q wave in lead aVL. It does not lead to QS pattern in the inferior leads; the latter implies inferior MI rather than LAFB. LVH may coexist with LAFB and does not preclude LAFB diagnosis.

Answer 16. No, because Q waves are also present. In Wellens syndrome, neither Q waves nor prominent ST elevation is present (Wellens is a form of non-ST elevation/non-Q wave ischemia).

Answer 17. Figure 31.37.

Answer 18. Yes.

Answer 19. Yes.

Answer 20. C. Global T inversion is less specific for ischemia than Wellens.

Answer 21. F (see Table 31.2 and Figure 31.48). PR depression may be seen with STEMI (atrial injury), but is more characteristic of pericarditis. Reciprocal ST depression may be seen with LVH and LBBB, but outside the latter two settings, suggests STEMI. The remaining chracteristics suggest STEMI as well.

Answer 22. Pericarditis.

Answer 23. Pre-excitation, with negative delta waves mimicking Q waves, and secondary ST deviations mimicking STEMI.

Answer 24. A (Section XII.D).

Answer 25. B. For LBBB, absolute ST discordance > 5 mm is not very sensitive or specific for the diagnosis of STEMI. Relative discordance is more helpful.

Answer 26. E (Figures 31.64, 31.65).

Answer 27. See Figures 31.66 and 31.67. Hypokalemia leads to T flattening, then ST depression with prominent T-U wave.

Answer 28. Leads II, V_5–V_6 are the best leads for measurement of QT. Leads V_2–V_3 have the most prominent phase 4 U waves and may not show a good separation of T and U waves, leading to overestimation of QT interval. Leads II, V_5–V_6 show distinct T waves with good separation from U waves.

Answer 29. QTc corresponds to the patient's QT interval had the heart rate been 60 bpm. QT decreases by 17.5 ms for every 10-beat increase in heart rate, and increases 17.5 ms for every 10-beat decrease in heart rate. If a patient has a QT of 400 ms at a rate of 100 bpm, QTc would be $(400 + 17.5 \times 4) = 470$ ms.

Answer 30. Yes. This is a T2 wave, which some may call a repolarization U wave (not phase 4 U wave). This may be seen with hypokalemia or QT-prolonging drugs. This type of **U wave, when prominent in size *and* fused with T, should be included in the QT measurement** as it is a part of repolarization.

Answer 31. E. The ECG shows diffuse ST-segment depression that is most prominent in leads V_2–V_3. This should point towards true posterior STEMI rather than non-ST-elevation ischemia and lead to recording of the leads V_7–V_9 and emergent cardiac catheterization. T-wave inversion in the anterior and/or inferior leads, rather than ST-segment depression, may suggest pulmonary embolism in the right clinical context. Hypokalemia is unlikely as T wave is not flattened, no prominent U wave is seen and QT interval is not prolonged.

Answer 32. A. This ECG has a few features suggestive of pericarditis (PR depression and diffuse ST elevation). However, the ECG also shows features suggestive of STEMI. The presence of even one STEMI feature, any of the top four features described in Table 31.2, usually implies STEMI and outweighs other diagnoses. In addition, PR depression may be seen in STEMI (ischemic atrial injury). Diffuse ST elevation without reciprocal ST depression (except possibly in lead aVR) may be seen with occlusion of the mid-portion of the left anterior descending artery.

Answer 33. C and E. In LBBB, discordant ST elevation ≥ 25% of the QRS height (relative discordance) has good sensitivity and specificity for the diagnosis of STEMI, particularly when the size of ST elevation approximates the size of the QRS complex. Convex discordance or absolute discordance > 5 mm is less specific for STEMI.

Answer 34. D. There is diffuse ST depression with upright "T" wave. QT is prolonged, and on further inspection a notch on the upslope of the ST segment is seen in V_5, suggesting that the prominent wave is actually a U wave and the notch is a flattened T wave.

Answer 35. C. Prominent U wave is seen along with ST depression. The ECG may mimic hypokalemia, except that QT is not prolonged and the TU separation is more clear than in hypokalemia.

References

1. Hanna EB. Electrocardiography. In: Hanna EB, Quintal R, Jain N. Cardiology: Handbook for Clinicians. Arlington, VA: Scrub Hill Press, 2009, pp. 328–54.

ST-segment depression and T-wave inversion

2. Hanna EB, Glancy DL. ST-segment depression and T-wave inversion: classification, differential diagnosis, and caveats. Clev Clin J Med 2011; 78: 404–14.
3. Rautaharju PM, Surawicz B, Gettes LS, et al. AHA/ACCF/HRS recommendations for the standardization and interpretation of the electrocardiogram: part IV: the ST segment, T and U waves, and the QT interval. J Am Coll Cardiol 2009; 53: 982–91.
4. Surawicz B, Knilans TK. Non-Q wave myocardial infarction, unstable angina pectoris, myocardial ischemia. In: Chou's Electrocardiography in Clinical Practice: Adult and Pediatric, 5th edn. Philadelphia, PA: WB Saunders, 2001, pp. 194–207.
5. O'Gara PT, Kushner FG, Ascheim DD, et al. 2013 ACCF/AHA guideline for the management of ST-elevation myocardial infarction: a report of the American College of Cardiology Foundation/American Heart Association Task Force on Practice Guidelines. J Am Coll Cardiol 2013; 61: e78–140.
6. Okin PM, Devereux RB, Nieminen MS, et al. Electrocardiographic strain pattern and prediction of new-onset congestive heart failure in hypertensive patients: the Losartan Intervention for Endpoint Reduction in Hypertension (LIFE) study. Circulation 2006; 113: 67–73.
7. Huwez FU, Pringle SD, Macfarlane PW. Variable patterns of ST–T abnormalities in patients with left ventricular hypertrophy and normal coronary arteries. Br Heart J 1992; 67: 304–7.

8. Li D, Li CY, Yong AC, et al. Source of electrocardiographic ST changes in subendocardial ischemia. Circ Res 1998; 82: 957–70.

9. Gorgels AP, Vos MA, Mulleneers R, et al. Value of the electrocardiogram in diagnosing the number of severely narrowed coronary arteries in rest angina pectoris. Am J Cardiol 1993; 72: 999–1003.

10. Glancy DL. Electrocardiographic diagnosis of acute myocardial infarction. J La State Med Soc 2002; 154: 66–75.

11. Yamagi H, Iwasaki K, Kusachi S, et al. Prediction of acute left main coronary artery obstruction by 12-lead electrocardiography: ST-segment elevation in lead aVR with less ST-segment elevation in lead V1. J Am Coll Cardiol 2001; 38: 1348–54.

12. de Zwann C, Bar FW, Wellens HJ. Characteristic electrocardiographic pattern indicating a critical stenosis high in left anterior descending coronary artery in patients admitted because of impending myocardial infarction. Am Heart J 1982; 103: 730–6.

13. de Zwaan C, Bar FW, Janssen JH, et al. Angiographic and clinical characteristics of patients with unstable angina showing an ECG pattern indicating critical narrowing of the proximal LAD coronary artery. Am Heart J 1989; 117: 657–65.

14. Lilaonitkul M, Robinson K, Roberts M. Wellens' syndrome: significance of ECG pattern recognition in the emergency department. Emerg Med J 2009; 26: 750–1.

15. Glancy DL, Khuri B, Cospolich B. Heed the warning: Wellens' type T-wave inversion is caused by proximal left anterior descending artery lesion. Proc (Bayl Univ Med Cent) 2000; 13: 416–18.

16. Savonitto S, Ardissino D, Granger CB, et al. Prognostic value of the admission electrocardiogram in acute coronary syndromes. JAMA 1999; 281: 707–13.

17. Mueller C, Neumann F, Perach W, et al. Prognostic value of the admission electrocardiogram in patients with unstable angina/non–ST segment elevation myocardial infarction treated with very early revascularization. Am J Med 2004; 117: 145–50.

18. Boden WE, Spodick DH. Diagnostic significance of precordial ST-segment depression. Am J Cardiol 1989; 63: 358–61.

19. Shah A, Wagner GS, Green CL, et al. Electrocardiographic differentiation of the ST-segment depression of acute myocardial injury due to the left circumflex artery occlusion from that of myocardial ischemia of nonocclusive etiologies. Am J Cardiol 1997; 80: 512–13.

20. Krishnaswamy A, Lincoff AM, Menon V. Magnitude and consequences of missing the acute infarct-related circumflex artery. Am Heart J 2009; 158: 706–12.

21. Matetzky S, Freimark D, Feinberg MS, et al. Acute myocardial infarction with isolated ST-segment elevation in posterior chest leads V7–9: "hidden" ST-segment elevations revealing acute posterior infarction. J Am Coll Cardiol 1999; 34: 748–53.

22. Matetzky S, Freimark D, Chouraqui P, et al. Significance of ST segment elevations in posterior chest leads (V7 to V9) in patients with acute inferior myocardial infarction: application for thrombolytic therapy. J Am Coll Cardiol 1998; 31: 506–11.

23. Huey BL, Beller GA, Kaiser DL, et al. A comprehensive analysis of myocardial infarction due to left circumflex artery occlusion: comparison with infarction due to right coronary artery and left anterior descending artery occlusion. J Am Coll Cardiol 1988; 12: 1156–66.

24. Gibson C, Pride YB, Mohanavelu S, et al. Angiographic and clinical outcomes among patients with acute coronary syndrome presenting with isolated anterior ST-segment depressions. Circulation 2008; 118: S-654. Abstract 1999.

25. Ferrari E, Imbert AI, Chevalier T, et al. The ECG in pulmonary embolism, predictive value of negative T waves in precordial leads 80 case reports. Chest 1997; 111: 537–43.

26. Sreeram N, Cheriex EC, Smeets JL, et al. Value of the 12-lead electrocardiogram at hospital admission in the diagnosis of pulmonary embolism. Am J Cardiol 1994; 73: 298–303.

27. Stein PD, Terrin ML, Hales CA, et al. Clinical, laboratory, and roentgenographic findings in patients with acute pulmonary embolism and no pre-existing cardiac or pulmonary disease. Chest 1991; 100: 598–603.

28. Surawicz B, Knilans TK. Chou's Electrocardiography in Clinical Practice: Adult and Pediatric, 5th edn. Philadelphia, PA: WB Saunders, 2001, pp. 122–53.

29. Norell MS, Lyons JP, Gardener JE, et al. Significance of « reciprocal » ST-segment depression: left ventriculographic observations during left anterior descending coronary angioplasty. J Am Coll Cardiol 1989; 13: 1270–4.

30. Haraphongse M, Tanomsup S, Jugdutt BI. Inferior ST-segment depression during acute anterior myocardial infarction: clinical and angiographic correlations. J Am Coll Cardiol 1984; 4: 467–76.

31. Wagner GS, Macfarlane P, Wellens H, et al. AHA/ACCF/HRS recommendations for the standardization and interpretation of the electrocardiogram: part VI: acute ischemia/infarction. J Am Coll Cardiol 2009; 53: 1003–11.

32. Brady WJ, Perron AD, Syverud SA, et al. Reciprocal ST-segment depression: impact on the electrocardiographic diagnosis of ST segment elevation acute myocardial infarction. Am J Emerg Med 2002; 20: 35–8.

33. Surawicz B. Electrolytes and the electrocardiogram. Postgrad Med 1974; 55: 123–9.

34. Dierks DB, Shumaik GM, Harrigan RA, et al. Electrocardiographic manifestations: electrolyte abnormalities. J Emerg Med 2004; 27: 153–60.

35. Glancy DL, Wang WL. Abnormal electrocardiogram in a woman with urinary tract infection. J La State Med Soc 2007; 159: 5–6.

36. Surawicz B, Braun H, Crum B, et al. Quantitative analysis of the electrocardiographic pattern of hypopotassemia. Circulation 1957; 16: 750–63.

37. Rosenbaum MB, Blanco HH, Elizari V, et al. Electronic modulation of the T wave and cardiac memory. Am J Cardiol 1982; 50: 213–22.

38. Paparella N, Ouyang F, Fuca G, et al. Significance of newly acquired negative T waves after interruption of paroxysmal reentrant tachycardia with narrow QRS complex. Am J Cardiol 2000; 85: 261–3.

39. Glancy DL, Rochon BJ, Ilie CC, et al. Global T-wave inversion in a 77-year-old woman. Proc (Baylor Univ Med Cent) 2009; 22: 81–2.

40. Walder LA, Spodick DH. Global T wave inversion. J Am Coll Cardiol 1991; 17: 1479–85.

41. Lui CY. Acute pulmonary ambolism as the cause of global T wave inversion and QT prolongation. J Electrocardiol 1993; 26: 91–5.

42. Walder LA, Spodick DH. Global T wave inversion: long-term follow-up. J Am Coll Cardiol 1993; 21: 1652–6.

43. Bybee KA, Kara T, Prasad A, et al. Systematic review: transient left ventricular apical ballooning: a syndrome that mimics ST segment elevation myocardial infarction. Ann Intern Med 2004; 141: 858–65.

44. Wittstein IS, Thiemann DR, Lima JAC, et al. Neurohumoral features of myocardial stunning due to sudden emotional stress. N Engl J Med 2005; 352: 539–48.

45. Spodick DH. The electrocardiogram in acute pericarditis: distributions of morphologic and axial changes in stages. Am J Cardiol 1974; 33: 470–5.

46. Magnani JW, Dec GW. Myocarditis: current trends in diagnosis and treatment. Circulation 2006; 113: 876–90.

47. Kaid KA, Maqsood A, Cohen M, Rothfeld E. Further characterization of the "persistent juvenile T-wave pattern in adults." J Electrocardiol 2008; 41: 644–5.

ST-segment elevation

48. Hanna EB, Glancy DL. ST-segment elevation: differential diagnosis, caveats. Clev Clin J Med 2015; 82: 373–84.
49. Smith SW, Khalil A, Henry TD, et al. Electrocardiographic differentiation of early repolarization from subtle anterior ST-segment elevation myocardial infarction. Ann Emerg Med 2012; 60: 45–56.
50. Smith SW. Upwardly concave ST segment morphology is common in acute left anterior descending coronary occlusion. J Emerg Med 2006; 31: 69–77.
51. Kosuge M, Kimura K, Ishikawa T, et al. Value of ST-segment elevation pattern in predicting infarct size and left ventricular function at discharge in patients with reperfused acute anterior myocardial infarction.Am Heart J 1999; 137: 522–7.
52. Brady WJ, Syverud SA, Beagle C, et al. Electrocardiographic ST-segment elevation: the diagnosis of acute myocardial infarction by morphologic analysis of the ST segment. Acad Emerg Med 2001; 8: 961–7.
53. Birnbaum Y, Sclarovsky S, Mager A, et al. ST segment depression in a VL: a sensitive marker for acute inferior myocardial infarction. Eur Heart J 1993; 14: 4–7.
54. Engelen DJ, Gorgels AP, Cheriex EC, et al. Value of the electrocardiogram in localizing the occlusion site in the left anterior descending coronary artery in acute anterior myocardial infarction. J Am Coll Cardiol 1999; 34: 389–95.
55. Collins MS, Carter JE, Dougherty JM, et al. Hyperacute T wave criteria using computer ECG analysis.Ann Emerg Med 1990; 19: 114–20.
56. Smith SW. T/QRS ratio best distinguishes ventricular aneurysm from anterior myocardial infarction. Am J Emerg Med 2005; 23: 279–87.
57. Surawicz B, Parikh SR. Prevalence of male and female patterns of early ventricular repolarization in the normal ECG of males and females from childhood to old age. J Am Coll Cardiol 2002; 40: 1870–6.
58. Klatsky AL, Oehm R, Cooper RA, et al. The early repolarization normal variant electrocardiogram: correlates and consequences. Am J Med 2003; 115: 171–7.
59. Mehta M, Jain AC, Mehta A. Early repolarization. Clin Cardiol 1999; 22: 59–65.
60. Mehta MC, Jain AC. Early repolarization on scalar electrocardiogram. Am J Med Sci 1995; 309: 305–11.
61. Rollin A, Maury P, Bongard V, et al. Prevalence, prognosis, and identification of the malignant form of early repolarization pattern in a population-based study. Am J Cardiol 2012; 110: 1302–8.
62. Tikkanen JT, Anttonnen O, Junttila MJ, et al. Long-term outcome associated with early repolarization on electrocardiography. N Engl J Med 2009; 361: 2529–37.
63. Tikkanen JT, Junttila MJ, Anttonen O, et al. Early repolarization: electrocardiographic phenotypes associated with favorable long-term outcome. Circulation 2011; 123: 2666–73.
64. Noseworthy PA, Tikkanen JT, Porthan K, et al. The early repolarization pattern in the general population: clinical correlates and heritability. J Am Coll Cardiol 2011; 57: 2284–9.
65. Kralios FA, Martin L, Burgess MJ, Millar K. Local ventricular repolarization changes due to sympathetic nerve-branch stimulation. Am J Physiol 1975; 228: 1621–6.
66. Spratt KA, Borans SM, Michelson EL. Early repolarization: normalization of the electrocardiogram with exercise as a clinically useful diagnostic feature. J Invasive Cardiol 1995; 7: 238–42.
67. Wu SA, Lin XX, Cheng YJ, et al. Early repolarization pattern and risk of arrhythmia death: a meta-analysis. J Am Col Cardiol 2013; 61: 645–50.
68. Surawicz B, Lassiter KC. Electrocardiogram in pericarditis. Am J Cardiol 1970; 26: 471–4.
69. Hull E. The electrocardiogram in pericarditis. Am J Cardiol 1961; 7: 21–6.
70. Spodick DH. Diagnostic electrocardiographic sequences in acute pericarditis. Significance of PR segment and PR vector changes. Circulation 1973; 48: 575–80.
71. Spodick DH. Acute pericarditis: current concepts and practice. JAMA 2003; 289: 1150–3.
72. Charles MA, Besinger TA, Glasser SP. Atrial injury current in pericarditis. Arch Intern Med 1973; 131; 657–62.
73. Noth PH, Barnes HR: Electrocardiographic changes associated with pericarditis. Arch Intern Med 1940; 65: 291–320.
74. Ginzton LE, Laks MM. The differential diagnosis of acute pericarditis from the normal variant: new electrocardiographic criteria. Circulation 1982; 65: 1004–9.
75. Armstrong EJ, Kulkarni AR, Bhave PD, et al. Electrocardiographic criteria for ST- elevation myocardial infarction in patients with left ventricular hypertrophy. Am J Cardiol 2012; 110: 977–83.
76. Sgarbossa EB, Pinski SL, Barbagelata A, et al. Electrocardiographic diagnosis of evolving acute myocardial infarction in the presence of left bundle-branch block. N Engl J Med 1996; 334: 481–7.
77. Madias JE, Sinha A, Agarwal H, Ashtiani R. ST-segment elevation in leads V_1–V_3 in patients with LBBB. J Electrocardiol 2001; 34: 87–8. *5 mm ST elevation not useful in LBBB.*
78. Smith SW, Dodd KW, Henry TD, et al. Diagnosis of ST-elevation myocardial infarction in the presence of left bundle branch block with the ST-elevation to S-wave ratio in a modified Sgarbossa rule. Ann Emerg Med 2012; 60: 766–76.
79. Hanna EB, Lathia V, Ali M, Deschamps EH. New or presumably new left bundle branch block in patients with suspected acute coronary syndrome. J Electrocardiol 2015; 48: 505–11.
80. Sgarbossa EB, Pinski SL, Topol EJ, et al. Acute myocardial infarction and complete bundle branch block at hospital admission: clinical characteristics and outcome in the thrombolytic era. J Am Coll Cardiol 1998; 105–10.
81. Bybee KA, Kara T, Prasad A, et al. Systematic review: transient left ventricular apical ballooning: a syndrome that mimics ST segment elevation myocardial infarction. Ann Intern Med 2004; 141: 858–65.
82. Glancy DL, Mikdadi GM. Syncope in a 67-year-old man. Proc (Bayl Univ Med Cent). 2005; 18: 74–5.
83. Wilde AA, Antzelevitch C, Borggrefe M, et al. Proposed diagnostic criteria for the Brugada syndrome: consensus report. Circulation 2002; 106: 2514–19.

Large or tall T wave

84. de Winter RJ, Verouden NJ, Wellens HJ, Wilde AA. A new ECG sign of proximal LAD occlusion. N Engl J Med 2008; 359: 2071–3.

Q waves and their regression

85. Nagase K, Tamura A, Mikuriya Y, et al. Significance of Q-wave regression after anterior wall acute myocardial infarction. Eur Heart J 1998: 19: 742–6.
86. Voon WC, Chen YW, Hsu CC, et al. Q-wave regression after acute myocardial infarction assessed by Tl-201 myocardial perfusion SPECT. J Nucl Cardiol 2004; 11: 165–70.

87. Coll S, Betriu A, De Flores T, et al. Significance of Q-wave regression after transmural acute myocardial infarction. Am J Cardiol 1988: 61: 739–42.
88. Delewi R, Ijff G, van de Hoef TP, et al. Pathological Q waves in myocardial infarction in patients treated by primary PCI. JACC Cardiovasc Imaging 2013; 6: 324–31.

Further reading

Surawicz B, Childers R, Deal BJ, Gettes LS. AHA/ACCF/HRS recommendations for the standardization and interpretation of the electrocardiogram: part III: intraventricular conduction disturbances. Circulation 2009; 119: e235–40.

Rautaharju PM, Surawicz B, Gettes LS. AHA/ACCF/HRS Recommendations for the Standardization and Interpretation of the Electrocardiogram: Part IV: The ST Segment, T and U Waves, and the QT. J Am Coll Cardiol 2009; 53: 982–91.

Hancock EW, Deal BJ, Mirvis DM, et al. AHA/ACCF/HRS recommendations for the standardization and interpretation of the electrocardiogram: part V: electrocardiogram changes associated with cardiac chamber hypertrophy. Circulation 2009; 119: e251–61.

Poor precordial R-wave progression

Zema MJ, Collins M, Alonso DR, Kligfield P. Electrocardiographic poor R-wave progression: correlation with postmortem findings. Chest 1981; 79: 195–200.

Anatomical LA enlargement mimicking RA enlargement

Chou TC, Helm RA. The pseudo P pulmonale. Circulation 1965; 32: 96–105.

LAFB

Jacobson LB, LaFollette L, Cohn K. An appraisal of initial QRS forces in left anterior fascicular block. Am Heart J 1977; 94: 407–13. *Q wave may be absent in I and/or aVL.*

Elizari MV, Acunzo RS, Ferreiro M. Hemiblocks revisited. Circulation 2007; 115: 1154–63.

Long QT Hodges formula

Chiladakis J, Kalogeropoulos A, Arvanitis P, et al. Preferred QT correction formula for the assessment of drug-induced QT interval prolongation. J Cardiovasc Electrophysiol 2010; 21(8): 905–13.

U wave is T2 wave in hypokalemia and LQT

Yan GX, Antzelevitch C. Cellular basis for the normal T wave and the electrocardiographic manifestations of the long-QT syndrome. Circulation 1998; 98: 1928–36.

Localization of anterior MI

Engelen DJ, Gorgels AP, Cheriex EC, et al. Value of the electrocardiogram in localizing the occlusion site in the left anterior descending coronary artery in acute anterior myocardial infarction. J Am Coll Cardiol 1999; 34: 389–95.

Inferior STEMI RCA vs. LCx

Nair R, Glancy DL. ECG discrimination between right and left circumflex coronary arterial occlusion in patients with acute myocardial infarction. Chest 2002; 122: 134–9.

32 Echocardiography

1. GENERAL ECHOCARDIOGRAPHY

I. The five major echocardiographic views and the myocardial wall segments

A. Parasternal short-axis view (Figures 32.1–32.5)

B. Parasternal long-axis view (Figures 32.6, 32.7, 32.8)

C. Apical four-chamber view (Figure 32.9). Beware of an apical view that does not cut through the true apex, and thus may miss apical akinesis. A true apex is usually thinner than the septal and lateral walls, and, as opposed to the other walls, moves horizontally rather than longitudinally.

D. Apical two-chamber view (Figure 32.10).

E. Subcostal four-chamber view. This view is particularly useful in COPD patients and patients receiving ventilator support, in whom the previous views have a poor quality (Figures 32.11, 32.12).

Arterial distribution (Figures 32.2, 32.13). Note that LAD supplies the anterior two-thirds of the septum, while RCA supplies the inferior one-third of the septum.

II. Global echo assessment of cardiac function and structure

A. Global assessment of myocardial function

A normal wall motion is characterized by an appropriate inward endocardial movement but also appropriate myocardial thickening. A segment can be hypokinetic, akinetic, or dyskinetic. Dyskinesis is outward movement of a myocardial wall during systole, when the remaining walls have an inward movement. Dyskinesis is therefore myocardial outpouching in systole, whereas aneurysm is myocardial outpouching in *both* systole and diastole (see Chapter 2).

Views that are orthogonal to a structure allow better endocardial definition of that structure.

1. Overall assessment of LV function

- EF:
  - Normal: > 50%
  - Mildly decreased: 40–50%
  - Moderately decreased: 30–40%
  - Severely decreased: < 30%
- The loss of the inferior and posterior walls typically leads to an EF of 35–50%, while the loss of the anteroseptal and apical walls typically leads to an EF < 35–40%.

Practical Cardiovascular Medicine, First Edition. Elias B. Hanna.

© 2017 John Wiley & Sons Ltd. Published 2017 by John Wiley & Sons Ltd.

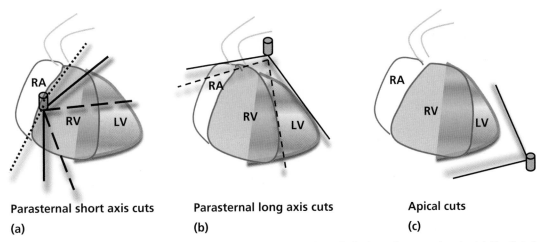

Parasternal short axis cuts

(a)

Parasternal long axis cuts

(b)

Apical cuts

(c)

Figure 32.1 (a) Frontal view showing how the parasternal short-axis views cut through the heart (cross-sectional cuts). The first structure encountered is the right ventricle, which is actually the anterior ventricle; the base of the LV and the mitral valve are encountered more posteriorly. Angling the probe more superiorly allows visualization of the aortic valve, the RA and LA, as well as the RV inflow and outflow (aortic short-axis view, *dotted lines*). Angling the probe more inferiorly allows visualization of the LV body and apex (*dashed lines*).

(b) Parasternal long-axis cuts. The first structure encountered is the RV (more specifically, RVOT), which is actually the anterior ventricle. The LV, LA, and aortic base are encountered more posteriorly, and the interventricular septum is seen in between. Angling the probe more inferiorly (*dashed lines*) allows visualization of the inferior RV wall and the tricuspid valve, as well as the RA (RV inflow view). Angling the probe more superiorly allows visualization of the RVOT and pulmonic valve (RV outflow view).

(c) Apical four-chamber cut. The first structures encountered are the apices of the LV and RV, while the atria are seen in the back. Superior angulation allows visualization of the aortic valve (five-chamber). A 90° rotation would focus on the LV–LA (two-chamber view). Further rotation opens the aortic valve (three-chamber view).

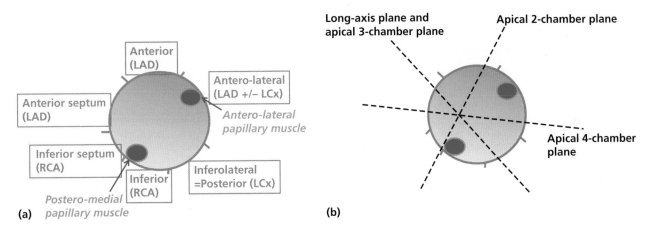

Figure 32.2 (a) Diagram of the **parasternal short-axis view** and various LV segments, with their corresponding arterial supply. **(b)** Orientation of various echo cuts.

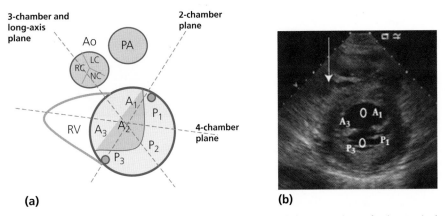

Figure 32.3 (a) Parasternal short-axis view at the level of the mitral valve. Each leaflet has three cusps (A_1–A_3 for the anterior leaflet, and P_1–P_3 for the posterior leaflet). A_3 and P_3 are medial, towards the RV; A_1 and P_1 are lateral The orientations of various echo cuts through the mitral plane are shown. **(b)** Echocardiogram showing the parasternal short-axis view (anterior and posterior leaflets, *circles*). The triangular-shaped RV is partially seen (*arrow*).

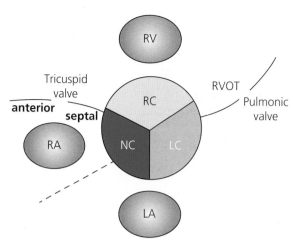

Figure 32.4 Diagram of the **parasternal short-axis view** at the level of the aortic valve (cut closer to the base than Figure 32.3, across the aortic valve, the LA/ RA, and RVOT). The non-coronary or posterior cusp is always the cusp looking towards the interatrial septum. LC, left coronary cusp; NC, non-coronary cusp; RC, right coronary cusp. Reproduced with permission from Hanna EB, Quintal R, Jain N. Cardiology: Handbook for Clinicians. Arlington, VA: Scrub Hill Press, 2009.

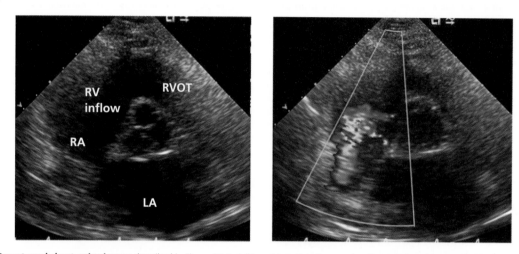

Figure 32.5 Parasternal short-axis view as described in Figure 32.4. A bicuspid aortic valve may be diagnosed on this view, by assessing how the valve opens in systole: a bicuspid valve opens in an oval rather than a "Y" fashion. In diastole, a bicuspid valve may look tricuspid because a fused raphe may be seen between the fused leaflets.

In severe AS, the aortic valve barely opens in this view; planimetry of the aortic valve area may be performed (especially by TEE). Rarely, however, the aortic valve may falsely look open if the cut is a bit below or above the valve level, masking severe AS.

The left image shows backward (= *blue*) blood flow across the tricuspid valve (= TR). Reproduced with permission from Hanna EB, Quintal R, Jain N. Cardiology: Handbook for Clinicians. Arlington, VA: Scrub Hill Press, 2009.

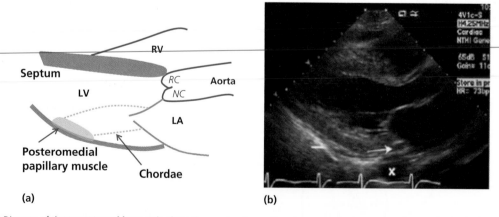

Figure 32.6 (a) Diagram of the **parasternal long-axis view**. Concerning the aortic valve cusps: the lower one, close to the LA, is the non-coronary cusp (NC); the upper one, close to RVOT, is the right coronary cusp (RC). The mitral leaflet close to the aorta is the anterior mitral leaflet (A₂ cusp); the mitral leaflet close to the posterior wall is the posterior leaflet (P₂ cusp).

(b) Echocardiogram showing the parasternal long-axis view. Note the coronary sinus in the AV groove (*arrow*), and note the descending aorta behind it (*x*). The coronary sinus is anterior to the bright pericardium (*line*), whereas the descending aorta is posterior to it and is more rigid. ***From top to bottom, the following structures are seen around the pericardium: coronary sinus → pericardium/pericardial effusion → aorta → pleural effusion.*** The aorta separates pericardial from pleural effusion.

The coronary sinus goes on to drain in the RA. Coronary sinus may enlarge in case of RA dilatation/pulmonary hypertension or persistent left SVC; in the latter case, coronary sinus is severely enlarged > 1 cm.

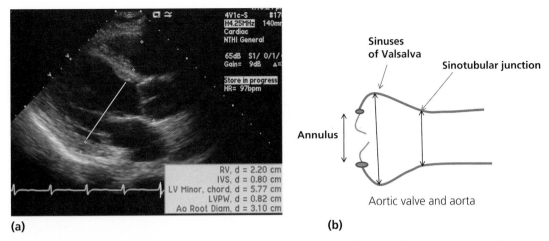

(a)   **(b)**

Figure 32.7 (a) Parasternal long-axis view. Measurements are obtained from top to bottom, between delineated points, at an oblique line crossing the mitral leaflet tips and orthogonal to the axis of the LV (*line*).

(b) Aortic measurements. The annulus is a stable structure that is part of the ventricle/outflow tract and does not usually dilate. The aortic diameter at the level of the sinuses of Valsalva (i.e., the aortic dilatations that suspend the aortic cusps) is normally up to 3.7 cm, while the diameter of the proximal ascending aorta and the sinotubular junction (junction of the ascending aorta with the sinuses of Valsalva) is normally up to 3.2 cm. Aortic dilatation may occur at the level of the ascending aorta and sinotubular junction (e.g., HTN), or may involve the sinuses of Valsalva in addition to the ascending aorta (bicuspid aortic valve, Marfan disease).

The normal diameter at the sinuses is affected by age and body surface area and should generally be < 1.9 cm/m^2 (lower cutoff in younger patients). Reproduced with permission from Hanna EB, Quintal R, Jain N. Cardiology: Handbook for Clinicians. Arlington, VA: Scrub Hill Press, 2009.

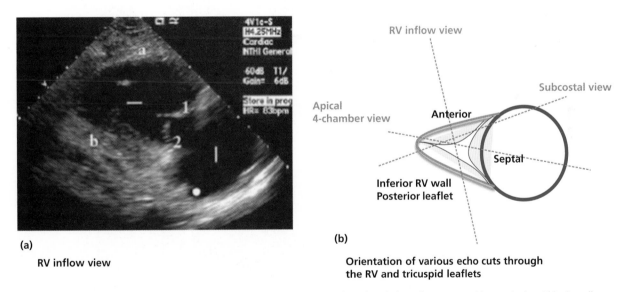

(a)   **(b)**

RV inflow view   **Orientation of various echo cuts through the RV and tricuspid leaflets**

Figure 32.8 (a) Parasternal RV inflow view, which is obtained by angling the probe inferiorly from the parasternal long-axis view. This view allows visualization of the RV (*horizontal bar*) and RA (*vertical bar*). The *dot* indicates the area of IVC entrance into the RA; a rigid Eustachian valve or a filamentous Chiari network may be present at this level. Eustachian valve is seen here, to the left of the dot. The RV walls are the anterior (*a*) and inferior (*b*) walls, and the two tricuspid leaflets are the anterior (*1*) and posterior leaflets (*2*).

(b) Only the RV inflow view shows the posterior leaflet. All other tricuspid valve views show the anterior and septal leaflets (four-chamber, subcostal, and aortic level short-axis views).

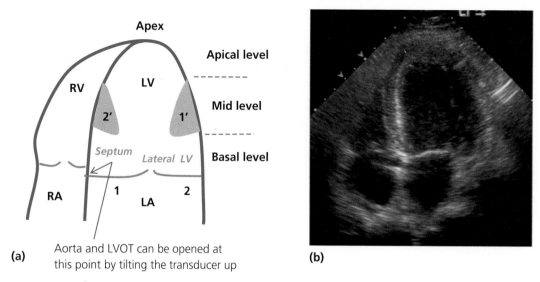

(a) Aorta and LVOT can be opened at this point by tilting the transducer up

(b)

Figure 32.9 (a) Diagram and **(b)** echocardiogram of the **apical four-chamber view**. Aorta and LVOT can be opened up by tilting the transducer up. The anterior leaflet is seen medially (*1*), the posterior leaflet is seen laterally (*2*), the anterior papillary muscle is lateral (*1'*), the posterior papillary muscle is medial (*2'*). ***Note that the valvular leaflets and their respective papillary muscles crisscross in this view.***

The tips of the papillary muscles define the separation between basal LV and mid-LV; the distal part of the papillary muscles separates mid-LV from apex.

Sometimes, *LV false tendon*, a fibrous/fibromuscular band, is seen extending distally from the septum to the lateral LV wall. RV has coarse apical trabeculations (more coarse than LV); it has >3 small papillary muscles. A muscular band where the right bundle is embedded, the *moderator band*, may sometimes be seen at the RV apex (spanning from the septal to the lateral RV wall, similar to the false tendon on the left).

The tricuspid valve is more apical than the mitral valve. When both valves are at the same level, endocardial cushion defect is suspected.

Advanced note: The anterior cusp (*1*) is $A_2 \pm A_3$, the posterior cusp (*2*) is P_1, the most lateral one; see Figure 32.3 to understand how the cusps are cut and the relation between leaflets and papillary muscles.

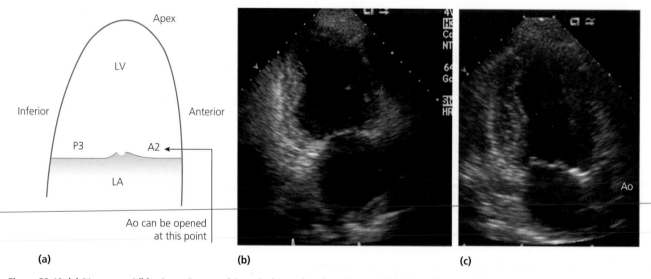

(a)

Ao can be opened at this point

(b)

(c)

Figure 32.10 (a) Diagram and **(b)** echocardiogram of the **apical two-chamber view**; and **(c)** echocardiogram of the **apical three-chamber view**. By opening the aorta with a counterclockwise rotation, the apical two-chamber view becomes the apical three-chamber view, where the anterior and inferior walls are replaced by the septal and posterior walls, respectively. *The apical three-chamber view, also called apical long-axis view, is similar to the parasternal long-axis view, except for a different heart orientation* (the beam is parallel to the aortic flow and the true apex is intercepted). Depending on the cut, three mitral cusps with two orifices may be seen on the two-chamber view (P_3 next to the inferior wall, A_2 in the middle, and P_1 or A_1 next to the anterolateral wall). Use Figure 32.3 for guidance. Reproduced with permission from Hanna EB, Quintal R, Jain N. Cardiology: Handbook for Clinicians. Arlington, VA: Scrub Hill Press, 2009.

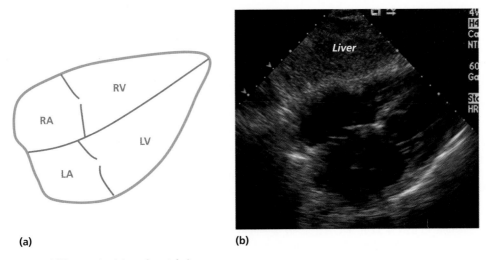

(a)   **(b)**

Figure 32.11 **(a)** Diagram and **(b)** example of the **subcostal view**.

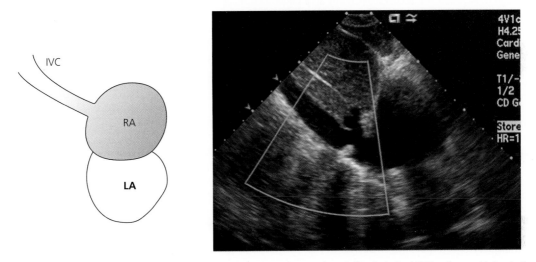

Figure 32.12 **Subcostal view** with a medial tilt to visualize the IVC. A large IVC (>2.1 cm), as well as its lack of 50% collapse with inspiration or sniff, signals high RA pressure. Reproduced with permission from Hanna EB, Quintal R, Jain N. Cardiology: Handbook for Clinicians. Arlington, VA: Scrub Hill Press, 2009.

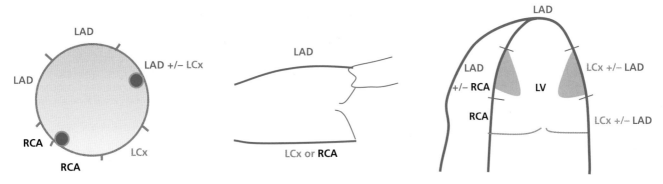

Figure 32.13 **Arterial distribution of various echo segments** on the short-axis view, long-axis view, and apical four-chamber view. Note that the inferior septum (on the short-axis view) and the basal septum (on the four-chamber view) are supplied by the RCA. If the four-chamber cut is angled a bit posteriorly, some of the visualized mid-septum may be supplied by the RCA as well.

2. Assess for LV dilatation and RV dilatation, which are associated with LV and RV systolic dysfunction, respectively.

a. *LV dilatation* is characterized by LV diameter (obtained from the short- or long-axis view)>4 cm in systole or>5.3 cm (women) or >5.8 cm (men) in diastole. Measurements are obtained at the level of the mitral leaflet tips, at the base of the LV.
b. *RV dilatation* (Figure 32.14) is characterized by:
* RV size larger than LV size on the apical four-chamber view
* RV rounded rather than wedge-shaped on the parasternal long-axis view.
* RVOT diameter ≥ 3.0 cm on the long-axis view or the aortic short-axis view; RV maximal diameter on the four-chamber view, around the tricuspid annulus, ≥ 2.9 cm (mild dilatation) or ≥ 3.9 cm (severe). However, these measurements vary according to the way the RV is cut, particularly because the RV has a complex pyramidal shape, which limits their accuracy.
* *RV pressure overload pattern* associated with severe pulmonary hypertension: the RV compresses the LV in *systole* and leads to a compressed D-shaped septum in systole.
* *RV volume overload pattern*: the RV compresses the LV in *diastole* and leads to a paradoxical septal motion towards the RV in systole. In mixed RV volume and pressure overload pattern, the septum remains compressed towards the LV in both diastole and systole.
* RA is enlarged if it is larger than LA on the four-chamber view, or if the interatrial septum bows to the left, or if the septal-lateral diameter is>2.2 cm/m² of BSA (4.5 cm). IVC is typically dilated in RA enlargement.
c. A left ventricular segment that is *bright and thin* (<6 mm) often implies necrotic, non-viable myocardium (due to an infarct or to irreversible non-ischemic cardiomyopathy).

3. Left ventricular hypertrophy (LVH) is characterized by an increased LV mass>115 g/m² in men, or>95 g/m² in women. *Increased wall thickness*, which often underlies LVH, is characterized by an interventricular septal thickness or a posterior wall thickness ≥ 1.1 cm in men, or ≥ 1 cm in women. The wall thickness is severely increased if it is ≥ 1.7 cm in men, or ≥ 1.6 cm in women.

LVH is *concentric* when the walls are thick but the LV is not dilated. LVH is *eccentric* when the walls are thick and the LV is dilated. *Concentric LV remodeling* is characterized by thick walls without overall LVH; i.e., the LV mass is normal

LV mass is calculated using the LV wall thickness and the LV diameter on the parasternal long-axis view.

4. Left atrial size is the "hemoglobin A1c" of the left heart; if LA size is normal, it is unlikely that there are any major systolic, diastolic, or left valvular issues.

A quick way of assessing LA size is by comparing it to the aorta on the long-axis view. LA is enlarged if it is > 1.1× the aortic size. Normal LA end-systolic diameter is<3.8 cm on the parasternal long-axis view (anteroposterior diameter) and on the apical four-chamber view (septal-lateral diameter); LA enlargement is severe if LA diameter>5 cm. LA volume should be assessed using the planimetered LA areas on both the four- and two-chamber views (disk summation technique). This is the preferred method for LA size assessment: LA volume is normally<34 ml/m² of BSA; LA is severely enlarged if LA volume is >48 ml/m².

B. Paradoxical septal motion

Normally, the septum moves in towards the LV in systole, and relaxes towards the RV in diastole. Abnormal septal motion is characterized by a septum that moves out towards the RV in systole, or at least at one point of systole, leading to ineffective septal contraction; and moves in towards the LV in diastole, compressing the LV.

Five differential diagnoses (Figures 32.15–32.18):

1. LBBB and RV pacing. The abnormal septal motion of RV pacing is similar to LBBB, except that it involves the distal/apical septum (rather than the entirety of the septum).
2. RV dilatation with RV volume overload.
3. Pericardial processes (constrictive pericarditis, tamponade). Large respiratory swings (e.g., COPD) may simulate the abnormal septal motion of pericardial processes.
4. Abnormal septal motion post-cardiac surgery.
5. Septal akinesis in a patient with septal MI. Unlike all the other causes of septal motion abnormality, anterior and apical akinesis is also seen in this case.

As opposed to other diagnoses, *pericardial processes*, whether constriction or tamponade, *are characterized by an abnormal septal motion that increases with inspiration and thus varies between beats*, i.e., the septal collapse towards the LV in diastole varies with respiration. In other processes, the abnormal septal motion does not vary as much across beats. In addition, characteristic of constrictive pericarditis, a *septal bounce* may be seen during each diastole, representing an instantaneous change in the RV-to-LV push with instantaneous pressure changes.

A septal motion abnormality may also be seen in patients breathing deeply, wherein the RV pushes the septum towards the LV in deep inspiration. Like pericardial processes, this septal position varies with respiration, but septal bounce is not seen.

In a tachycardic patient, sorting out the respiratory effect may prove difficult. *M-mode imaging is particularly helpful because of its high frame rate.*

The abnormal postoperative septal motion is related to the fact that, after cardiac surgery, the heart is fixed anteriorly to the thorax (meaning, the RV is fixated). During systole, the whole heart moves toward that fixation site, leading to what looks like septal motion abnormality. In fact, it is an abnormal anterior motion of the whole heart, including the posterolateral wall.

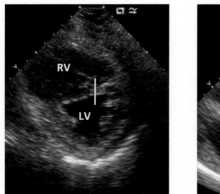
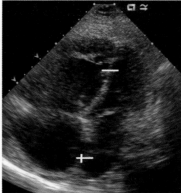

Figure 32.14 Example of **RV enlargement and RV volume overload** on the parasternal short-axis view and apical four-chamber view. The interventricular septum is flattened and pushed toward the LV in diastole (*lines*). The interatrial septum is also bowing towards the LA (*cross*).

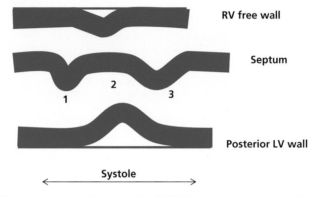

Figure 32.15 During systole, in **LBBB**: (*1*) the septum moves in towards the LV; (*2*) then the septum relaxes while the posterior wall moves in; (*3*) the septum moves in again at the end, not because it is contracting but because the RV is relaxing and pushing it. Thus, the septum moves in twice (*1* and *3*), while the posterior wall moves in between (*2*), when the septum is relaxed. The distance between the peak of (*1*) and the peak of (*2*) is the septal-to-lateral M-mode delay, an index of dyssynchrony (>130 ms → significant).

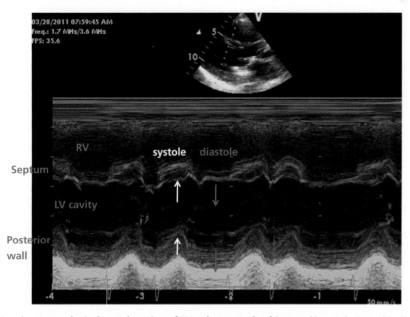

Figure 32.16 M-mode imaging shows **paradoxical septal motion of RV volume overload** (outward in systole, inward in diastole). This paradoxical motion is seen in both inspiration and expiration; it may be a bit more prominent in inspiration, but unlike constrictive pericarditis or tamponade, it is not much more prominent. M-mode allows a fine analysis of how various structures move during the cardiac cycle. QRS is used to time events.

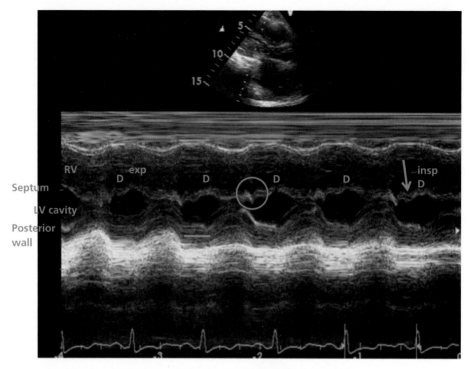

Figure 32.17 Constrictive pericarditis. Three septal abnormalities and one posterior wall abnormality are seen on M-mode (*D* corresponds to the septal position in diastole):

- Septum collapses towards the LV in diastole rather than expands towards the RV (*arrow*).
- This septal collapse is particularly evident in inspiration (insp) and the septal position varies between inspiration and expiration.
- The RV-to-LV diastolic push varies with instantaneous pressures (= septal bounce, *circle*).
- The posterior wall is stiff/horizontal in diastole after the initial brisk expansion (= plateau, *line*).

In RV volume overload, the RV pushes the septum towards the LV in all diastolic cycles, only slightly more so in inspiration. Moreover, only one sharp septal motion towards the LV is seen in diastole.

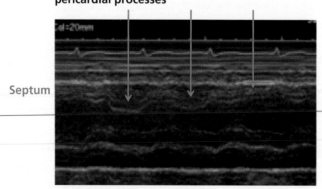

Figure 32.18 Pericardial processes are characterized by septal compression towards the LV in diastole, similar to RV volume overload. However, this RV septal compression varies with respiration, and consequently septal position varies across different cycles.

C. Valvular structure assessment

1. Mitral valve (Figures 32.19–32.21)

- *Degenerative valve*: leaflet(s) are thick, elongated, ± prolapsed into the LA. If, in addition to the prolapse of the leaflet body, the free edge is overriding the other leaflet and turned towards the LA rather than the LV, the leaflet is called *flail leaflet*; this is usually secondary to chordal rupture (a piece of chorda is usually seen flopping in the LA).
- *Rheumatic valve*: thick, calcified valve with a stiff posterior leaflet and a stiff anterior leaflet tip. The anterior leaflet body is, however, mobile. The combination of a stiff anterior leaflet tip and a flexible body gives the anterior leaflet a hockeystick shape on the

parasternal long-axis view. On the short-axis view, the commissures are fused and the valve only opens in its center ("fish mouth" mitral valve).

- *Mitral annular calcifications* involve the mitral annulus rather than the leaflets (in contrast to a rheumatic process). The annulus is calcified, but the leaflets' tips are free. Calcifications are mainly seen at the posterior aspect of the annulus and increase in incidence with age, high LV pressure (HTN, AS), and renal disease. *Only the posterior annulus, which is a muscular structure, calcifies; the anterior annulus is a fibrous structure that only calcifies in radiation heart disease.* Calcifications may, however, extend to the base of both the posterior and anterior leaflets on the four-chamber view (not the leaflet tips, and not the anterior annulus on the long-axis view).

2. Aortic valve

- Aortic valve thickening (sclerosis) and calcification are precursors of AS. Also, aortic sclerosis and calcification are associated with coronary atherosclerosis
- A bicuspid aortic valve is characterized by fusion of two cusps, most commonly the right and left cusps (85%); a raphe is frequently seen between the two fused cusps, and this may create the false impression of a tricuspid valve. Therefore, on the aortic short-axis view, instead of analyzing how many cusps are seen when the valve is closed, it is best to analyze how the aortic valve opens. An elliptical rather than a triangular opening is a hint to a bicuspid valve (Figure 32.22).

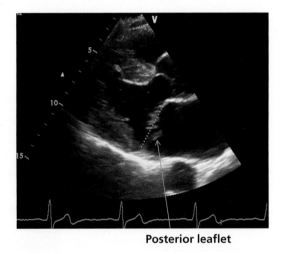

Posterior leaflet

Figure 32.19 Posterior mitral leaflet prolapse. In systole, the leaflet prolapses posteriorly to the mitral annular plane (*blue line*).

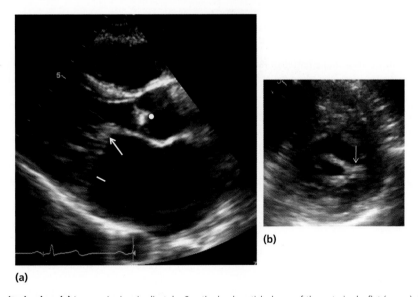

(b)

(a)

Figure 32.20 Rheumatic mitral valve. (a) Long-axis view in diastole. See the hockeystick shape of the anterior leaflet (*arrow*), the tip of which looks attached to the stiff posterior leaflet (*line*), with no diastolic opening. In fact, **both leaflets are tied together by the commissural fusion.** Note the severe LA enlargement, due to MS in this case. Also, note the aortic valve calcification (white aortic valve leaflet tips [*dot*]). Make sure the aortic calcification is not a false impression related to a high echo gain; the fact that the aortic walls appear bright may be a hint to the increased echo gain. **(b)** Short-axis view. Commissural fusion (*arrow*) explains the "fish mouth" opening.

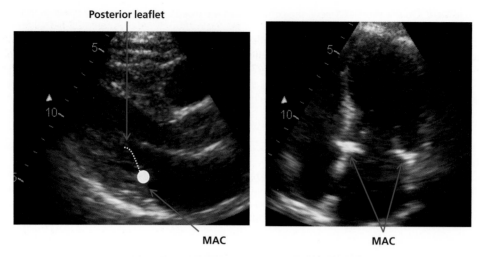

Figure 32.21 Posterior mitral annular calcifications (MAC) in the long-axis and four-chamber views. These posterior calcifications project at the base of the posterior leaflet on the long-axis view and the base of both the posterior and anterior leaflets on the four-chamber view.

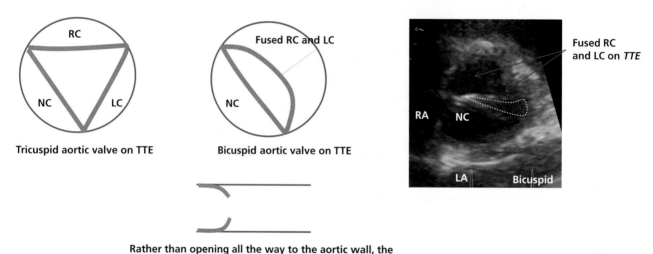

Figure 32.22 Difference in aortic orifice shape between the tricuspid and bicuspid aortic valves (short-axis view). Note that one cusp is larger than the other in bicuspid aortic valve, and hence the aortic opening/closure becomes eccentric; this is evident on the M-mode analysis of the aortic valve.

The leaflets open in a domed fashion on a longitudinal view (long-axis view), as they are restricted by the lack of a third commissure.

A severely stenotic bicuspid valve may appear to open well on the long-axis view. The stenosis being eccentric, it is three-dimensionally more severe than it may appear on a two-dimensional view. LC, left coronary cusp; NC, non-coronary cusp; RC, right coronary cusp.

III. Doppler: mainly assesses blood flow direction (→ regurgitation), timing, and velocity

A. Types

1. *Color Doppler:* color Doppler assigns color to blood flow velocity and direction. The maximal Doppler velocity that can be sampled unambiguously and attributed a blue or red color is called the Nyquist or aliasing limit. Beyond this limit, the color becomes mosaic.

2. *Continuous-wave (CW) spectral Doppler:* CW Doppler traces the highest flow velocity *along one line* swept by the Doppler probe. Therefore, it captures the velocity across the narrowest point or obstruction. It continuously captures waves and is not dependent on the Nyquist limit.

3. *Pulsed-wave (PW) spectral Doppler:* PW Doppler traces the velocity *at one point along the line* swept by the cursor, rather than the whole line swept. It samples waves intermittently, at a specified sampling rate. Therefore, the maximal velocity that can be detected across this one point cannot exceed a certain limit, called the Nyquist limit.

B. Routine Doppler interrogations
1. Color Doppler is performed at the level of each valve to assess regurgitation (see Figures 32.23–32.33)
By "eyeballing" the view, regurgitation appears as a color going backward between chambers, opposite to the normal flow (e.g., any flow from LV to LA, RV to RA, or aorta to LV). It is *blue* (*backward*) for the mitral and tricuspid valves on TTE. It usually has a higher velocity than the Nyquist limit, which leads to *color aliasing* (= mixed, mosaic color). Also, when severe, it is usually turbulent, with high *variance of velocities* (*turbulent flow*, coded as *green color*).

> Reducing the Nyquist limit from 60 cm/s to 30 cm/s increases the area of regurgitant flow by Doppler. Increasing the color gain also increases the area of regurgitant flow. Therefore, an inappropriately low Nyquist limit or a high Doppler gain overestimates the regurgitation severity, while the opposite underestimates the regurgitation severity. Inappropriately low color gain is particularly common in patients with poor windows, wherein the color definition is reduced, similarly to the reduction in echo resolution. Increase the color gain until noise is seen and until color pixels appear within the cardiac tissue, then slightly reduce the gain just until the noise disappears; the latter gain corresponds to the appropriate color gain. For evaluation of regurgitation, the best Nyquist limit is 50–60 cm/s. Also, narrow the Doppler sector to focus on the valve of interest; a large sector reduces the color resolution across the valve of interest.

2. CW Doppler is performed at the level of each valve to assess forward-flow velocity, and, consequently, valvular stenosis (see Figures 32.34, 32.35, 32.36)
Normally, the forward peak velocity across each valve is 1 m/s. An increase in flow velocity corresponds to valvular stenosis.

The peak pressure gradient across a valve can be estimated using this equation (modified ***Bernoulli equation***):

$$\text{Peak gradient} = 4 \times V_{valve}^2$$

This is how gradient is estimated across the aortic valve and the severity of a stenosis is assessed. For spectral Doppler assessment, it is important to obtain a view parallel to the flow.

3. PW Doppler is used to see the velocity at one particular point, such as the mitral inflow (E/A), tricuspid inflow, pulmonary vein inflow (systolic, diastolic, atrial waves), and LVOT flow (Figures 32.37, 32.38)
PW has a limited capacity to measure high velocities that exceed twice the Nyquist limit (>2 m/s), particularly at greater depths.

Two types of velocities are analyzed on CW or PW Doppler: peak velocity and velocity–time integral (VTI). VTI corresponds to the area enclosed by the CW or PW Doppler velocity profile. It is measured in cm (velocity × time) and corresponds to the distance traveled by blood across the interrogated point during one cardiac cycle.

> All Doppler modalities are ***angle-dependent*** and best measure the flow that is aligned with the ultrasound beam. For best assessment of stenosis or regurgitation and for velocity measurement, the ultrasound beam should be parallel to the flow (or within a 20° angle).

4. Tissue Doppler assesses the movement of cardiac structures rather than blood flow (Figures 32.39, 32.40)
Tissue Doppler is useful to assess:

a. Mitral annular velocities during diastole (E' and A'). E' is the annular recoil toward the base during early diastolic filling; A' is the annular recoil during atrial systole. Lateral E' is normally ≥ 10 cm/s, medial E' is ≥ 7 cm/s. The reduction of E' indicates diastolic dysfunction or high left-sided filling pressures.

b. Dyssynchrony of various myocardial segments, manifested as different times from QRS onset to peak systolic velocity (or peak strain) between different walls. The assessment of mechanical dyssynchrony is particularly useful in patients with low EF and QRS 130–150 ms, as it may help identify the responders to biventricular pacing. In patients with HF and QRS < 130 ms, the use of echocardiographic dyssynchrony for identifying potential responders to biventricular pacing has not shown any value.

c. Occult or manifest myocardial dysfunction. The *radial* myocardial *displacement*, *velocity*, and *strain* can be determined on the short-axis view; the *longitudinal* displacement, velocity and strain can be determined on the apical views. A dysfunctional segment may get pulled and displaced by a normal adjacent segment; therefore, a normal displacement or velocity of one myocardial segment does not necessarily imply normal function. Myocardial strain, on the other hand, assesses the percent change in distance between 2 points, and the strain rate assesses the change in velocity between 2 points, i.e., myocardial deformation. Myocardial strain allows an accurate determination of segmental function and may be determined using tissue Doppler or automated ultrasound tissue imaging.

The global ventricular function may also be simply and routinely assessed using annular tissue Doppler. On the annular Doppler, S' is the forward systolic movement of the annulus in systole (longitudinal fibers). S' ≤ 7 cm/s correlates with LV systolic dysfunction. At the tricuspid annulus, S' < 10 cm/s correlates with RV systolic dysfunction.

C. Routine Doppler calculations

1. Volume and flow calculations

Volume and flow can be derived from velocity using the ***continuity equation***, which states that blood volume that crosses a cardiac area during one cardiac cycle = area × VTI. Thus:

$$\text{Blood volume} = \pi r^2 \times \text{VTI} = 0.785 \times d^2 \times \text{VTI} \,(r \text{ is radius, } d \text{ is diameter})$$

$$\text{Per minute flow across a point} = \text{blood volume} \times \text{heart rate}$$

Stroke volume is, thus, equal to: $0.785 \times \text{LVOT d}^2 \times \text{LVOT VTI}$

Cardiac output is equal to: stroke volume × heart rate

2. Aortic valve area (AVA) calculation using the continuity equation

$$\text{AVA} \times \text{aortic velocity} \,(\text{aortic peak velocity or aortic VTI on CW Doppler})$$
$$= \text{LVOT area} \times \text{LVOT velocity} \,(\text{LVOT peak velocity or LVOT VTI on PW Doppler})$$

LVOT diameter should be measured at the insertion of the aortic valve leaflets (i.e., at the annulus, not below it), parallel to the leaflets' plane, in early systole (largest diameter). A falsely low or high LVOT measurement is a common cause of a falsely low or high AVA.

3. Calculation of the systolic PA pressure using the TR jet

Capture of TR jet by CW Doppler is necessary for the calculation of PA pressure. While many normal individuals have mild TR that allows this calculation, over 50% of patients, including some patients with severe pulmonary hypertension, do not have an adequate TR jet envelope.

According to the Bernoulli equation, the pressure difference between RV and RA in systole equals $4 \times V_{TR}^2$.

Thus, RV systolic pressure $= 4 \times V_{TR}^2 + \text{RA pressure}$. In the absence of pulmonic stenosis, RV systolic pressure is equal to PA systolic pressure.

4. Assessment of RA pressure

RA pressure is assessed on the basis of IVC diameter and inspiratory collapse:

i. IVC ≤ 2.1 cm with > 50% inspiratory collapse → RA pressure = 0–5 mmHg

ii. IVC ≤ 2.1 cm but < 50% inspiratory collapse,
or IVC > 2.1 cm with > 50% inspiratory collapse → RA pressure = 5–10 mmHg

iii. IVC > 2.1 cm with < 50% collapse → RA pressure ≥ 15 mmHg, or ≥ 20 mmHg if 0% collapse. Also, even in the intermediate category (ii), if the collapse is ~0% or if the systolic flow of the hepatic veins is blunted, RA pressure is severely elevated.

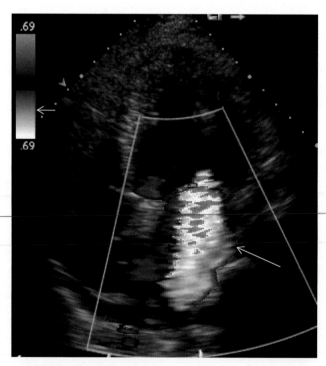

Figure 32.23 MR, four-chamber view. The blue, backward flow between the LV and the LA is MR. The regurgitation can be graded by measuring the regurgitant (blue) area (*arrow*) and comparing it to the LA area. If the regurgitant area is > 40% LA area → severe MR (this also applies for TR: jet area > 30% of RA area → severe TR). This provides a quick idea of the severity of MR, but is not very reliable. Increasing the color gain or lowering the Nyquist limit of the backward flow on the color scale (*horizontal arrow*) increases the regurgitant/turbulent area and makes the MR look more severe. The best Nyquist limit for regurgitation assessment is 50–60 cm/s. To obtain the best color gain, increase the gain until noise is seen in cardiac tissues, then slightly reduce it just until the noise disappears. Reproduced with permission from Hanna EB, Quintal R, Jain N. Cardiology: Handbook for Clinicians. Arlington, VA: Scrub Hill Press, 2009.

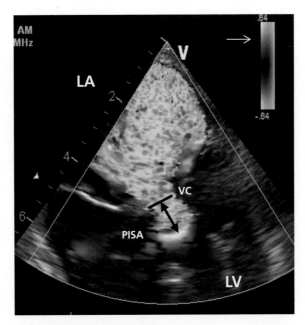

Figure 32.24 Severe MR on four-chamber TEE view. **Severity criteria of MR:**

1. Look at the small spherical portion of the regurgitant jet that is on the side of the ventricle rather than the atrium. As the blood is flowing back from the LV to the LA, it goes through a narrow neck that corresponds to the vena contracta (VC) of the mitral orifice. The flow converging towards the mitral orifice forms hemispheres of increasing velocities, the areas of which are called *proximal isovelocity surface areas (PISA)*. The hemisphere of interest is the one where aliasing occurs (*double arrow*). Thus, the radius of the PISA corresponds to the distance between the narrowest neck of flow and the outer aliasing line (*double arrow*). The larger this hemisphere (>0.9–1.0 cm), the more severe the MR. PISA allows calculation of the effective regurgitant orifice (ERO). If the backward aliasing limit is set at 40 cm/s on the regurgitant color bar (*arrow*), ERO is estimated as:

    $(PISA\ radius)^2/2$

    If PISA radius is 0.9 cm, ERO is ~0.4 cm^2. MR is severe if ERO ≥ 0.4 cm^2. ERO can be used to calculate the regurgitant volume (= ERO × VTI of the regurgitant flow) and the regurgitant fraction. Regurgitant volume > 60 ml or regurgitant fraction > 50% signifies severe MR. PISA is affected by eccentricity of the jet, but less than MR jet area; another limitation is that the PISA should be a 180° hemisphere, not less and not a cylinder.

2. The diameter of the MR flow at its *vena contracta* neck, i.e., the narrowest part (mitral valve level), can be estimated. The larger the diameter, the more severe the MR (≥7 mm → *severe MR*).

3. A severe regurgitation should lead to enlargement of the backward chamber (LA in MR, RA in TR, LV in AI). In addition, the forward chamber often enlarges because of the volume overload. Except in acute cases, a normal-size backward chamber rules out severe regurgitation.

4. Other severity criteria of MR:
    - Increased forward flow and velocity across the mitral valve in diastole: **E velocity > 1.2 m/s**
    - Reversal of the systolic S flow of one or more pulmonary vein(s): specific for severe MR, but not sensitive, as LA compliance may prevent this flow reversal (compensated chronic MR). Moreover, if the jet is eccentric, reversal of flow may be seen in some but not all of the veins. Blunting of S flow, rather than reversal, is also consistent with severe MR but is not specific.

When MR seems severe but LA is not enlarged, make sure that MR is present throughout systole. What seems like severe MR by color or PISA is moderate if it only encompasses 50% of systole or end-systole (this may occur with mitral valve prolapse and with functional MR). The duration of MR is evaluated by CW Doppler or by color M-mode across the mitral valve.

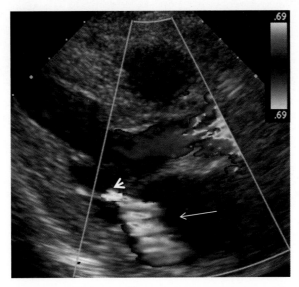

Figure 32.25 MR, long-axis view. The blue flow between LV and LA is MR (*arrow*). *It is eccentric, posteriorly directed, and at least moderate in severity.* When MR is eccentric, consider it more severe than it appears (MR that appears mild is likely moderate). An eccentric jet that turns around the left atrial wall in a circular way is severe MR (Coanda effect). A well-visualized PISA hemisphere (*arrowhead*) despite a Nyquist limit of 69 cm/s is concerning for severe MR. A posteriorly directed MR usually implies either anterior leaflet prolapse or posterior leaflet tethering from inferior akinesis.

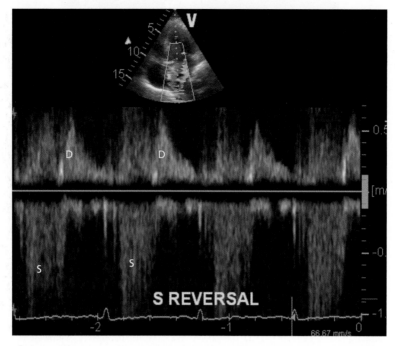

Figure 32.26 Systolic flow reversal of pulmonary venous flow in a patient with severe **MR**. Normally, S flow has the same direction as D flow.

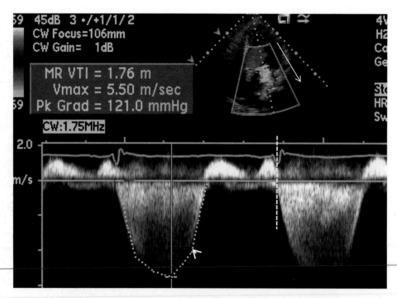

Figure 32.27 CW Doppler across the mitral valve on an apical four-chamber view. The flow is directed backward (*arrow*) from the LV to the LA, and projects below the baseline on CW Doppler. It is dense (white) but not as white as the forward flow, and thus is probably moderate MR. Acute or decompensated severe MR may lead to a late indentation of the CW signal (would be at the location of the arrowhead), related to a large V wave and decreased LV–LA pressure gradient at end-systole. This is called the *V-wave cutoff sign*, and leads to an early-peaking, triangular MR shape.

On the apical views, because of similarities in direction of AS and MR jets and because of beam width artifact, **AS Doppler interrogation may capture MR jet, creating the false impression of severe AS velocity.** Unlike AS, MR jet starts immediately at MV closure, immediately after the mitral inflow A wave, at the peak of R wave on the ECG (*dashed line*). The timing of the two jets and a back-and-forth sweeping of the transducer help differentiate the two.

Reproduced with permission from Hanna EB, Quintal R, Jain N. Cardiology: Handbook for Clinicians. Arlington, VA: Scrub Hill Press, 2009.

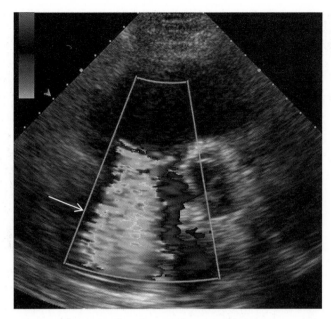

Figure 32.28 Severe TR seen from the short-axis view (aortic valve level) (*arrow*). The same criteria described under Figure 32.24 can be used for TR to assess severity. To estimate ERO, set the backward flow aliasing limit at 28 cm/s (instead of 40). Also, annular dilatation ≥ 3.5 cm correlates with severe functional TR. Use the same vena contracta and ERO values as in MR, use jet area > 30% RA area, and look for hepatic vein flow reversal and RA enlargement. Reproduced with permission from Hanna EB, Quintal R, Jain N. Cardiology: Handbook for Clinicians. Arlington, VA: Scrub Hill Press, 2009.

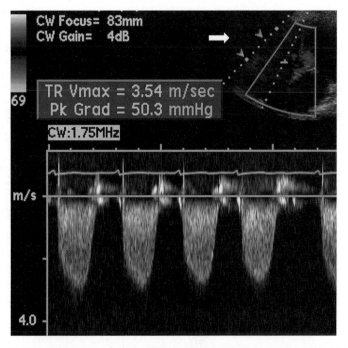

Figure 32.29 TR. CW Doppler across the tricuspid valve on a four-chamber view (see that the line swept is on the right side, *arrow*). TR looks very dense (white) on CW Doppler, which often means large-volume moderate or severe regurgitation. Unlike the *density* of the regurgitation, the *peak velocity* does not correlate with the severity of the regurgitation. This peak velocity correlates with the pressure gradient between the two chambers (here: RV to RA), and hence PA pressure. Severe pulmonary hypertension may occur with mild, non-dense TR, yet the velocity would be high (>4 m/s); conversely, severe, dense TR may be seen with a low TR velocity when PA pressure is not elevated (e.g., primary TR).

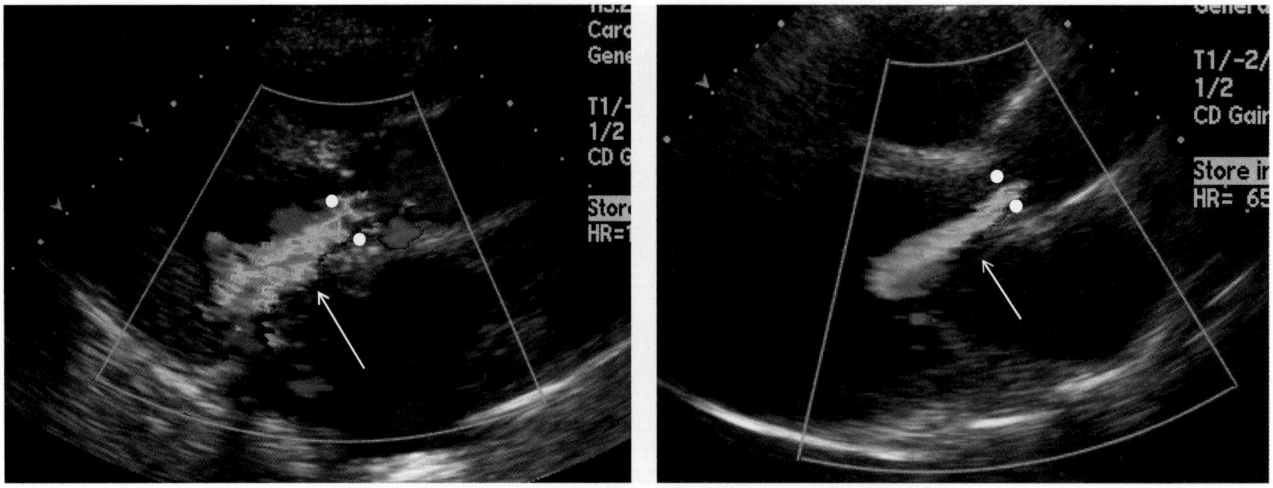

(a)   **(b)**

Figure 32.30 Aortic insufficiency (AI). Long-axis views (a and b) show blue–backward flow from the aorta to the LV (*arrows*), i.e., AI. Assess AI severity by looking at:

1. *The width of the AI jet* just below the aortic valve, on the long-axis view (between the two dots). If AI jet>60% of the LVOT diameter (which is the diameter between the two walls at the aortic valve insertion)→severe AI. AI jet is better evaluated on the parasternal views than the apical views, which tend to falsely "widen" the AI jet.
2. *Pressure half-time* (on CW Doppler, Figure 32.33)
3. *Diastolic reversal of flow* in the thoracic aorta (suprasternal view) or abdominal aorta (subcostal view). A holodiastolic flow reversal signals severe AI. **This is the most important parameter in AI assessment.**

In **(a)**, AI is moderate; in **(b)**, AI is mild.

Reproduced with permission from Hanna EB, Quintal R, Jain N. Cardiology: Handbook for Clinicians. Arlington, VA: Scrub Hill Press, 2009.

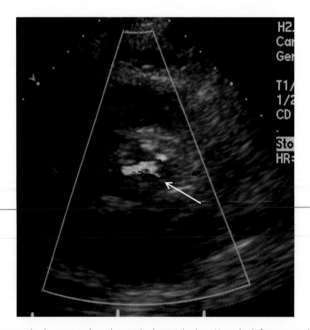

Figure 32.31 AI. The width of the AI jet may also be assessed on the aortic short-axis view. Here, look for a central blue or mixed-color "flame" in diastole (*arrow*), which corresponds to AI jet. AI jet area that is>60% of the whole aortic circle area implies severe AI. AI jet may look falsely enlarged if the cut is well below the regurgitant orifice, or falsely reduced if AI is eccentric. In order to obtain the accurate AI width, the transducer may be angled up until the AI flow is lost; the AI that is seen just before the flow is lost corresponds to the jet width. The latter maneuver is best performed on the TEE' aortic short-axis view. Reproduced with permission from Hanna EB, Quintal R, Jain N. Cardiology: Handbook for Clinicians. Arlington, VA: Scrub Hill Press, 2009.

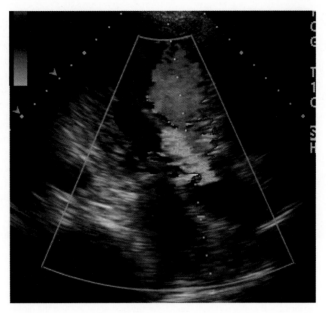

Figure 32.32 AI on three-chamber apical view. This view is not accurate for measurement of the jet width area and vena contracta. Being parallel to the flow, it is excellent for recording of Doppler flow and measurement of AS gradient or AI pressure half-time, but it is not accurate for width measurement. When assessing thickness of a structure or flow, it is best to be orthogonal to the structure or flow.

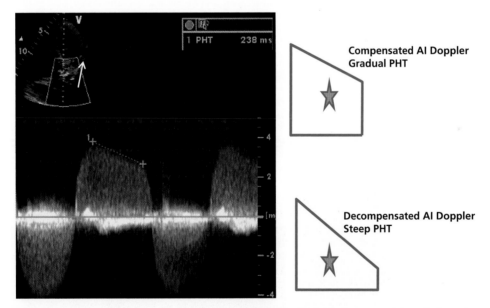

Figure 32.33 AI spectral Doppler assessment on an apical five-chamber view. The flow between the aorta and the LV is directed upward (along the direction of the *arrow*). The slope of this regurgitant flow depends on how closely the LV and aortic pressures approximate during diastole, and thus how severe and acute AI is. The steeper the slope, the more severe and quick is the rise of LV diastolic pressure.

This is called *pressure half-time (PHT)*, which is the time needed for the pressure gradient to decrease in half. If PHT < 250 ms → steep slope → severe AI. Note, however, that a chronic severe but compensated AI with compensated LV may have PHT > 250 ms. PHT correlates more with acuity and decompensation of AI than its severity.

PHT of AI is different from PHT of MS, where a steeper slope implies less severe MS.

Also, the density of this regurgitant flow correlates with severity (the whiter it is in comparison to the forward flow, the larger the AI volume and the more severe the regurgitation).

In this case, note that the patient has AI with PHT < 250 ms but also significant AS, with a peak forward velocity of 4 m/s. AI exaggerates the AS velocity (increased stroke volume), while AS may exaggerate AI severity by the PHT method, as it impairs LV compliance.

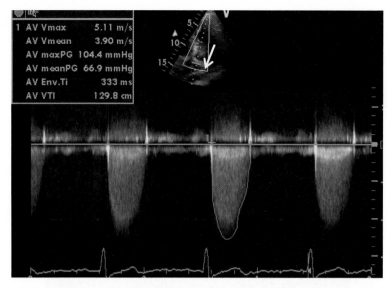

Figure 32.34 AS. CW Doppler across the aortic valve on the apical five-chamber view. The flow directed down is the aortic flow in systole (along the direction of the *arrow*). The normal peak velocity is 1 m/s. Velocity > 2 m/s signals AS; velocity ≥ 4 m/s implies severe AS, which is the case here.

The *peak pressure gradient* may be calculated from peak velocity using the modified Bernoulli equation (= 4 V²). The *mean pressure gradient* integrates all the gradients underneath the velocity envelope. Echo may underestimate the pressure gradient if the interrogation angle is not parallel to the flow, or if the jet envelope is incomplete (may need to increase the gain settings). Search for the best envelope and the highest gradient in multiple views (apical five-chamber, apical three-chamber, right parasternal, and suprasternal views).

Caution: increased CW velocity is not necessarily AS, because CW samples the highest velocity along the whole line swept and not only the aortic valve. It may be LVOT obstruction, where the velocity is increased across the LVOT rather than the aortic valve. In this case, the PW velocity is increased across the LVOT, whereas the localized aortic PW velocity is not increased (PW localizes the site of obstruction, even though it may not be able to record the exact velocity). Also, **in LVOT obstruction, the gradient peaks late and the CW velocity has a late-peaking dagger shape.**

High velocity across the aortic valve may occur in high-output states (sepsis, fever, anemia) and in severe AI (increased stroke volume). In these cases, the velocity is increased across the LVOT and the aorta. The way to figure out the presence of AS is to use the dimensionless index (LVOT PW velocity divided by aortic valve CW velocity). Either VTI or peak velocity may be used. The index is normally ~1, and an index < 0.25 implies severe AS. Also, it is possible to use the true Bernoulli equation, where:

Peak aortic gradient
= 4 × (peak velocity at the obstruction level² – proximal peak velocity²)
= 4 × (aortic velocity² – LVOT velocity²).

The converse occurs in low-output states, where the gradient may be low despite severe AS. Dimensionless index and valve area calculation help make the diagnosis.

In AF, the velocity and the gradient decrease after the short R–R cycles (as opposed to MS). For AVA calculation, use LVOT VTI and aortic valve VTI obtained after the same R–R cycle lengths. For peak/mean gradient estimation, control the rate and average the gradients from several beats.

Another mistake that may lead to overestimation of AS is the confusion of the AS and MR jets on the apical five-chamber or three-chamber view. MR jet starts exactly at the peak of R wave, whereas AS jet starts a bit later.

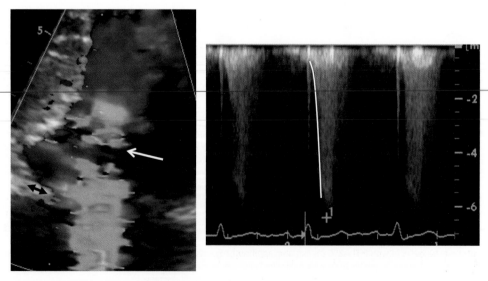

Figure 32.35 Severely increased velocity on aortic Doppler. Several features suggest LVOT obstruction rather than AS: (1) the velocity has a late-peaking dagger shape (*tilted line*), and is "skinnier" than the aortic velocity seen in Figure 32.34; (2) on color Doppler, the aliasing (*arrow*) occurs below the aortic valve level (*double arrow*). **To confirm LVOT obstruction, PW Doppler may be swept throughout the LVOT and the aortic valve. PW Doppler cannot record velocities over 1.5–2 m/s, but will indicate that the velocity is increased across the LVOT rather than the aortic valve. Exact assessment of the velocity with CW ensues.**

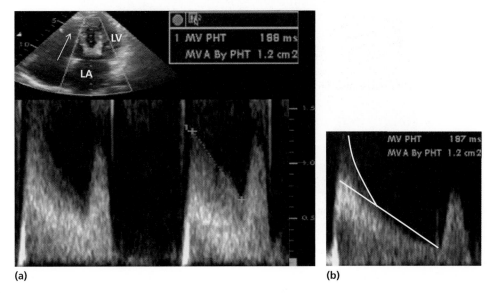

(a) **(b)**

Figure 32.36 MS assessment.

(a) CW Doppler across the mitral valve (MV) on the apical four-chamber view. The flow is directed from the LA (which is down on this view) to the LV (up) along the direction of the *arrow*. A mean gradient > 5 mmHg at rest, or 10–15 mmHg with exercise, corresponds to severe MS. ***Passive leg raising should be performed to assess stress gradient.*** *CW, not PW, should be used to capture the gradient.*

Also, the downslope of the rapid diastolic filling (E wave, first wave) may be used to estimate MV area: a slow downslope means that LA pressure does not equalize with LV pressure even in late diastole (no diastasis), which corresponds to severe MS. The ***pressure half-time*** is the time it takes the pressure gradient to decrease in half [i.e., time it takes E velocity to decrease by 30%], and ***is long in severe MS***. MV area = 220 divided by pressure half-time. However, for the same valve area, LA and LV pressures more readily equalize in case of increased LV diastolic pressure (AI, severe LVH), which makes the downslope look steeper → MV area will be seemingly larger and MS will be seemingly less severe.

(b) If E wave has a "ski slope" shape, (i.e., initially steep then slow downslope), use the slow downslope portion to calculate the pressure half-time. An associated MR or high output state increases the early E-wave velocity and the overall gradient, but the later E slope remains unchanged.

In AF, the pressure gradient varies between different beats (↑ with short R–R cycles, as LA emptying decreases), but the shape and slope of the CW envelope remain unchanged. Mean gradient increases as in any tachycardia (or exercise), but pressure half-time and MV area remain unchanged. PHT = pressure half-time.

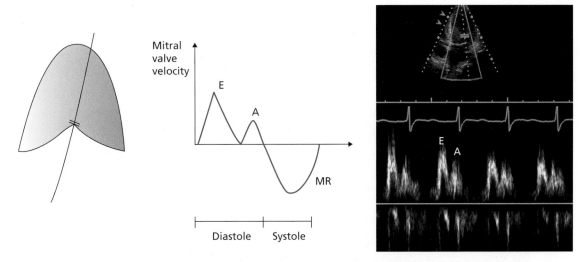

Figure 32.37 PW Doppler at the level of the mitral valve. During diastole, forward flow is recorded across the MV: E is the rapid diastolic filling, A is the filling related to atrial contraction. E occurs after T wave, while A occurs after P wave and almost coincides with QRS. Reproduced with permission from Hanna EB, Quintal R, Jain N. Cardiology: Handbook for Clinicians. Arlington, VA: Scrub Hill Press, 2009.

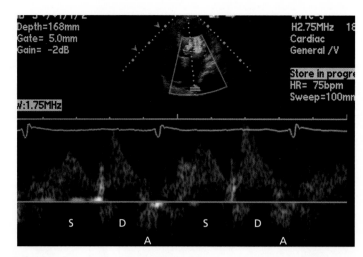

Figure 32.38 PW Doppler across the pulmonary veins on a four-chamber view, pulmonary veins being behind the LA (*cursor*). S and D represent, as it is seen, forward systolic and diastolic flow toward the LA. A wave corresponds to atrial systole, when LA pressure increases and prevents forward blood flow: A is a reversed flow wave. Normally, S is slightly>D or slightly<D. A severely reduced S wave implies elevated LA pressure.

The hepatic venous flow on the subcostal view looks similar to the pulmonary venous flow (S, D, A), except that S and D waves are below the baseline, whereas A wave is above the baseline.

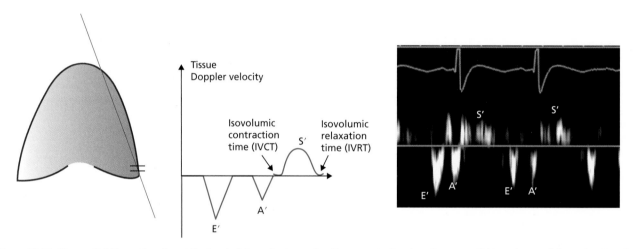

Figure 32.39 Myocardial tissue Doppler at the level of the mitral annulus. The cursor is placed on the myocardial lateral or medial annulus. E' and A' waves occur in diastole, on the downward negative side (diastolic recoil). In systole, a forward positive motion S' occurs. Lateral E' annular velocity is usually higher than medial E'. Measure both lateral and medial E', and calculate E/E' for each E', and for the average E'.

The cursor should be positioned within 0.5 cm of the leaflet insertion site and should be parallel to the plane of cardiac motion.

In myocardial dysfunction (systolic or diastolic), IVCT and IVRT increase, leading to an increase of the following ratio: (IVCT+IVRT)/ejection time (ejection time corresponds to S' time). This ratio, called myocardial performance index or Tei index, may be calculated using myocardial annular Doppler and is normally<0.4.

Reproduced with permission from Hanna EB, Quintal R, Jain N. Cardiology: Handbook for Clinicians. Arlington, VA: Scrub Hill Press, 2009.

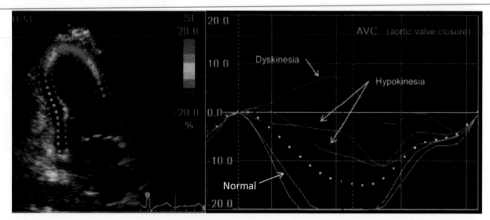

Figure 32.40 2D tissue strain imaging of the LV on a two-chamber view. Strain between two myocardial points=% change in distance between the two points=(distance$_{between these points in systole}$ − distance$_{in diastole}$)/distance$_{in diastole}$. Normal strain values are −20 to −12; abnormal values are −8 to +20. The red color corresponds to normal strain, while the blue/purple corresponds to abnormal strain. In this figure, the antero-apex is blue and therefore dysfunctional.

The time display (*right image*) shows the peak systolic strain of each segment and the strain curve throughout systole then diastole; the segment moving in the opposite direction to the baseline is a dyskinetic segment (apex). Courtesy of Carmen Ilie and Fred Helmcke, who provided this image.

IV. Summary of features characterizing severe valvular regurgitation and stenosis (see Tables 32.1, 32.2)

Table 32.1 Severe valvular regurgitation.

Mitral regurgitation

1. **Jet area >40% of LA area *or* eccentric jet swirling around the LA wall (Coanda effect),** at a Nyquist limit of 50–60 cm/s and a proper color gain.
   Pros: area <20% makes severe MR very unlikely
   Cons: eccentricity reduces jet area; low color gain and high Nyquist falsely reduce the jet area. Conversely, inappropriately high color gain and low Nyquist limit falsely increase the jet area.
2. **Vena contracta ≥7 mm** at a Nyquist limit of 50–60 cm/s. Vena contracta is the narrowest part of the regurgitant flow, i.e., the neck at the origin of MR.
   Pros: accurate, even in eccentric MR. Vena contracta < 3 mm makes severe MR unlikely.
   Cons: does not reliably distinguish moderate from severe MR. Also, should be measured in a view orthogonal to the regurgitation (parasternal long-axis), not an apical view, which tends to falsely widen the vena contracta. It is not accurate if multiple jets are present.
3. **Flow convergence**
   • **PISA radius ≥ 0.9 cm** (regurgitant Nyquist limit set at 40 cm/s)
   • **ERO ≥ 0.4 cm²**
   • **Regurgitant volume ≥ 60 ml/beat** (regurgitant volume = ERO × MR VTI)
   • **Regurgitant fraction = regurgitant volume/(regurgitant volume + stroke volume at the LVOT) > 50%**
   Cons: may underestimate MR if jet is eccentric (but better than jet area in this case), may overestimate MR if jet is not a full hemisphere. Not valid if multiple jets are present.
4. **Mitral E-wave velocity > 1.2 m/s**
   Pros: very sensitive, regardless of eccentricity. A lower E velocity or E/A reversal ~ excludes severe MR.
   Cons: not specific. E velocity increases with high LA pressure and AF.
5. **Pulmonary venous flow:** Blunted S is consistent with severe MR, reversed S is specific for severe MR
   Cons:
   • Blunted or reversed S may not be seen in compensated severe MR, where LA compliance absorbs the regurgitant flow and prevents pulmonary venous abnormalities
   • Blunted S may be seen with high LA pressure or AF, and is not specific for severe MR
   • All four pulmonary veins must be sampled on TEE (eccentric MR flow may enter and reverse the flow of one pulmonary vein only)
6. **CW MR Doppler as dense as the forward mitral flow; *or* dense and triangular with early peaking (V wave cutoff),** indicative of decompensation
   This supports severe MR, but dense flow may also be seen with moderate MR

Important supportive features
• LA enlargement is universal in all severe MR, except, occasionally, acute MR. A normal LA size ~ excludes severe MR except in the acute setting
• LV enlargement, particularly with normal EF, strongly supports severe MR (not as sensitive as LA enlargement, which occurs earlier)
• If MR appears severe yet LA is not enlarged, it is possible that MR is not holosystolic. A large MR jet with a large PISA is not severe if it is brief, as seen sometimes with mitral valve prolapse (end-systolic)

Aortic insufficiency

1. **Vena contracta width (narrowest neck at the origin of AI on the long-axis view) ≥ 7 mm**
   AI jet width ≥ 60% of LVOT diameter (long-axis view)
   AI jet cross-sectional area ≥ 60% of LVOT area (short-axis view) at a Nyquist limit of 50–60 cm/s
   Note: AI jet size is different from vena contracta. AI jet size is the AI size just below the vena contracta, as the jet starts to expand (within 1 cm of the aortic valve)
   Cons: eccentric AI, such as bicuspid AI, may be underestimated, particularly when assessed in a 2D plane where it is narrowest (in the long-axis view). AI may be overestimated when the measurement is performed too low below the vena contracta, or in the apical views
2. **Flow convergence (PISA): ERO ≥ 0.3 cm²**
   Cons: the rounded flow convergence is more difficult to measure in AI than in MR
3. **CW Doppler pressure half-time (PHT) < 250 ms**
   Cons: depends on LV compliance and LVEDP. PHT may be > 250 ms in chronic, compensated severe AI. PHT may be < 250 ms in moderate AI with decompensated LV dysfunction and high LVEDP (e.g., severe HTN). Also, vasodilators may reduce diastolic aortic pressure and thus, PHT
   PHT > 500 ms ~ excludes severe AI
4. ***Holo*diastolic flow reversal in the descending aorta (suprasternal view) or, worse, in the abdominal aorta (subcostal view).** This is assessed by PW Doppler and is the **most sensitive and specific feature** for severe AI. Early to mid-diastolic reversal suggests moderate AI.
5. **Other features**
   • **CW Doppler signal as dense as the forward flow.** Cons: significant overlap between moderate and severe AI
   • **M-mode of the mitral valve shows leaflet fluttering or early closure.** This not only indicates severe AI but decompensated AI

Important supportive feature
   • LV enlargement is universal in chronic severe AI. A normal LV size ~ excludes severe AI, except in the acute setting. LA enlargement is very common in severe AI

Tricuspid regurgitation (same type of features and limitations as MR)

1. Large jet area (Nyquist limit of 50–60 cm/s)
2. Vena contracta > 7 mm (Nyquist limit 50–60 cm/s)
3. PISA radius > 0.9 cm (at a Nyquist limit of 28 cm/s ≠ MR)
4. TR jet dense ± triangular with early peaking (V-wave cutoff)
5. Hepatic venous S blunting, or, worse, reversal (reversal is specific for severe TR)
RA/IVC size is always increased in severe chronic TR

Pulmonic regurgitation

• As opposed to AI, where the *jet width* below the neck determines severity, in PR, the *jet length* and the total jet area in the RV correlate with severity. In severe PR, the color jet goes deep into the RV, beyond the RVOT (use a large Doppler sector to visualize). In mild PR, the jet length is < 1 cm
• CW Doppler: *dense* PR signal with *steep* deceleration and termination of PR flow in mid-diastole (severe PR leads to equalization of PA and RV diastolic pressures in mid-diastole). This early termination of PR flow may, however, be seen when milder PR is associated with severe RV failure and elevated RVEDP
RV is always enlarged in chronic severe PR. In a patient with significant PR, RV enlargement without any other cause suggests severe PR

Table 32.2 Severe valvular stenosis: severe AS, including low-gradient AS, and severe MS.

Aortic stenosis

Peak velocity ≥ 4 m/s, mean gradient ≥ 40 mmHg, and AVA ≤ 1 cm² by continuity equation[a]

Typically, in severe AS:

- Peak LVOT velocity is < 1 m/s
- LVOT velocity/aortic valve velocity ≤ 0.25 (dimensionless index [DI]). DI is, in fact, a component of AVA calculation (AVA = LVOT area × DI). As opposed to AVA calculation, the dimensionless index is not subject to the bias of LVOT diameter measurement

LVOT velocity may be > 1 m/s when severe AS is associated with moderate AI or high-output states (anemia, fever), cases in which DI remains < 0.25; or when severe AS is associated with significant septal bulge and subaortic obstruction. It may be falsely elevated if the LVOT cursor is placed too close to the aortic valve, in the aliasing

Differential of paradoxical low-gradient AS with normal EF (AVA ≤ 1 cm² with low gradient < 40 mmHg):

- Truly severe AS with hypertension and concentric LV hypertrophy explaining the low output
- To make this diagnosis: (1) Ensure proper echo measurements of LVOT and aortic velocity, (2) measure the stroke volume (↓) and valvuloarterial impedance (↑). To be consistent with this diagnosis, LVOT velocity must be < 1 m/s with low DI

Mitral stenosis (see Section VIII.C)

- Mild and moderate MS: MVA > 1.5 cm², gradient usually < 5 mmHg at a normal heart rate (60–85 bpm)
- Severe MS: MVA 1.0–1.5 cm², gradient usually ≥ 5 mmHg at a normal heart rate
- Very severe MS: MVA < 1.0 cm², gradient usually > 10 mmHg

Doppler assesses the transmitral gradient very accurately, as it is easy to align the cursor with the transmitral flow. However, a high gradient does not necessarily imply severe MS; **mild anatomic MS (MVA > 1.5 cm²) may have a severe gradient in the presence of** *tachycardia or high-output state.* Thus, MVA characterizes the anatomic severity of MS better than the gradient

The estimation of MVA using one of 4 methods (mitral inflow pressure half-time, continuity equation, PISA method, and planimetry) is subject to measurement errors. Pressure half-time may falsely ↓ and MVA may falsely ↑ in patients with LV dysfunction (HTN, elderly)

---

[a] AVA = (0.785 × LVOT diameter²) × LVOT velocity/aortic valve velocity.

LVOT diameter should be measured at the insertion of the aortic valve leaflets (= annulus), parallel to the leaflets and within 5–10 mm of the aortic orifice. LVOT is measured in the long-axis view, in early systole (largest diameter, inner edge to inner edge).

LVOT velocity is obtained by positioning the pulsed Doppler ~5 mm proximal to the stenotic valve (not too close to the valve). Avoid catching the high-velocity convergence. Either VTI or peak velocity may be used.

V. M-mode echocardiography is derived from 2D echo (see Figures 32.41, 32.42, 32.43; also Figures 32.15–32.18).

M-mode graphically displays the movement of cardiac structures along one line swept by the probe. It can assess valvular opening, chamber size, and subtle abnormalities of cardiac motion (such as RV compression by pericardial effusion). It has a very high temporal resolution and rapid sampling rate that allows recording of **subtle motion** *and* **timing of cardiac events.**

VI. Pericardial effusion

A. Size (see Figures 32.44, 32.45)

A pericardial effusion is small if < 1 cm, moderate if 1–2 cm, and large if > 2 cm. The effusion is measured as the summation of the anterior and posterior dimensions at end-diastole, i.e., when it appears *smallest*. A small effusion is usually localized posteriorly, while a large effusion is usually circumferential. A swinging heart, i.e., a heart that changes position in a phasic manner, may be seen with large effusions. An echo-free space that is present only anteriorly suggests an epicardial fat pad rather than a pericardial effusion; unless loculated, a pericardial effusion usually gravitates and predominates posteriorly in the supine position, or is circumferential.

B. IVC plethora

IVC plethora has a sensitivity of 97% for tamponade, but a specificity of only 40%, as it may occur with any right heart failure. On hepatic vein Doppler, *a flat D wave* (Y descent) corresponds to impeded right-sided diastolic filling and thus tamponade.

C. Pre-tamponade echocardiographic signs (see Figure 32.46)

- RV compression in early diastole. On M-mode, the RV continues to collapse after systole (inward indentation), while the LV is expanding. This is the most specific and latest tamponade sign. RVOT gets compressed earlier than the remaining RV walls.
- RA compression during ventricular systole, when RA is supposed to expand. RA collapse occurs immediately after atrial systole, and manifests as an RA wall that stays inward after atrial systole. RA collapse that persists for > 1/3 of systole is specific for tamponade.
- > 25% inspiratory decrease of mitral inflow E velocity and aortic velocity. This is due to the LV compression by the RV. This Doppler finding is the corollary of pulsus paradoxus.
- > 25% inspiratory increase of tricuspid inflow E velocity.

The last two findings are the earliest pre-tamponade findings.

Tamponade is a clinical diagnosis. The echocardiographic signs suggest hemodynamic abnormalities that are the substrate for tamponade, but on their own they do not establish the diagnosis of tamponade.

Tamponade may occur as a result of a localized effusion compressing one particular chamber, such as RV, LV, LA, RA, or pulmonary veins, as after cardiac surgery. This is more difficult to diagnose, and only some of the tamponade echocardiographic signs are seen. TEE may be more helpful in showing the localized effusion and cardiac chamber compression (e.g., isolated pulmonary venous compression).

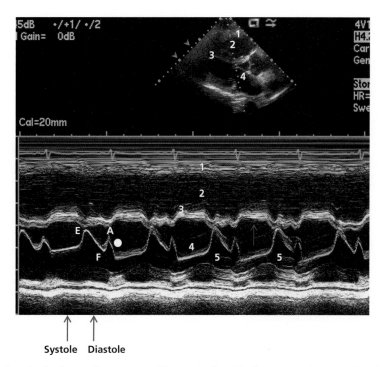

Figure 32.41 M-mode across the mitral valve on the parasternal long-axis view. The first structure intercepted, at the top, is the RVOT wall (white line); the second structure is the RV cavity (dark); the third structure is the septum; the fourth structure is the anterior leaflet of the MV (closes in systole and opens in diastole), and the fifth structure is the posterior mitral leaflet.

The anterior mitral leaflet has two waves in diastole: E (rapid filling) and A, similar to the mitral inflow Doppler. Examples of disease states:
- In MS, the E-wave downslope becomes flat horizontal (flat EF slope), and the posterior leaflet is drawn to the anterior leaflet.
- In high LVEDP, there will be a small extra wave (B bump) at the end of A wave (at the location of the *dot*).
- In SAM, the anterior leaflet will be drawn to the septum in end-systole or, worse, all systole (in the direction of the *arrow*).
- In severe AI, one may have early closure of the mitral valve or diastolic mitral fluttering.
- In tamponade, early diastolic inward indentation of the RVOT is seen.

By moving the interrogation line towards the mid LV, the systolic movement of the septum and the LV posterior wall can be assessed (see Figures 32.15–32.18).

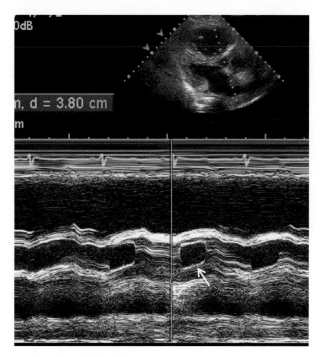

Figure 32.42 M-mode across the aortic valve on the long-axis view. The first structures encountered are the RVOT wall and cavity. Then the aortic walls (rather than LV walls) are encountered and, inside them, the aortic valve. The aortic valve opens well here (open box in systole [*arrow*]). Disease states:
- In severe AS, the box becomes flat. In bicuspid aortic valve, the line of closure in diastole is eccentric
- In HOCM, there is mid-systolic notching (partial closure) of the box.
- In low cardiac output, there is early gradual closure of the aortic valve (the box becomes a triangle: >).

Reproduced with permission from Hanna EB, Quintal R, Jain N. Cardiology: Handbook for Clinicians. Arlington, VA: Scrub Hill Press, 2009.

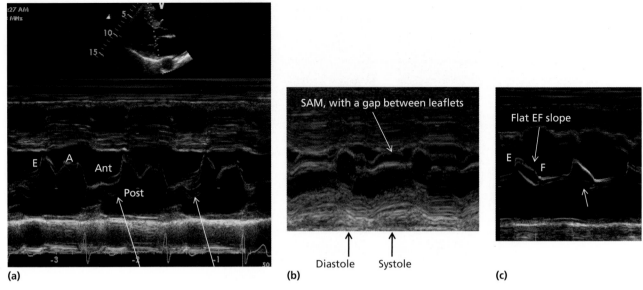

(a)   **(b)**   **(c)**

Figure 32.43 Examples of M-mode across the mitral valve. (a) Posterior mitral leaflet prolapse. See how the posterior leaflet moves posteriorly in mid-to-late systole, creating a "gap" in the mitral closure, and thus MR (*arrows*). **(b)** SAM of the anterior leaflet in HOCM, with the anterior leaflet touching the septum in systole, creating a gap away from the posterior leaflet. **(c)** Flat EF slope in diastole suggests MS (mitral valve is open throughout diastole, with no diastasis). Also, the posterior leaflet is pulled towards the anterior leaflet (commissural fusion) (*arrow*). Ant, anterior mitral leaflet; Post, posterior mitral leaflet.

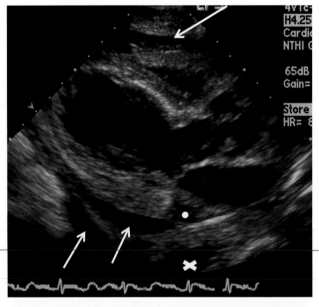

Figure 32.44 Diffuse pericardial effusion on long-axis view, identified as a black band above the RV (*upper arrow*) and a black band posterior to the LV. In this case, posterior to the LV, there are two black bands separated by the pericardium: pericardial effusion and pleural effusion (*lower arrows*). Differentiate pleural from pericardial effusion: the pericardial effusion is anterior to the descending aorta (*X*), whereas the pleural effusion extends behind the aorta. The coronary sinus is in the AV groove, anterior to the pericardium (*dot*). Reproduced with permission from Hanna EB, Quintal R, Jain N. Cardiology: Handbook for Clinicians. Arlington, VA: Scrub Hill Press, 2009.

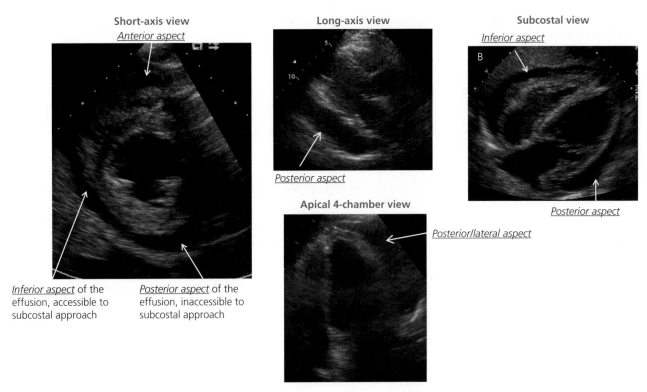

Figure 32.45 Pericardial effusion on multiple views. In a supine position, a free-flowing effusion gravitates and predominates over the posterior aspect of the LV. The posterior aspect is the one seen on the long-axis view (posterolateral aspect) and the four-chamber view. This has to be distinguished from the effusion at the inferior/diaphragmatic aspect of the LV, which is more anterior and is the one seen on the subcostal view (used for subcostal pericardiocentesis).

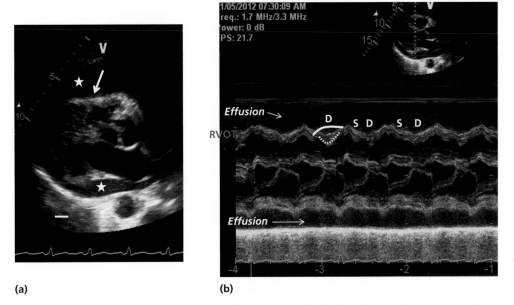

Figure 32.46 (a) Pericardial effusion (*stars*) and pleural effusion (*bar*). The latter is behind the level of the descending aorta. RVOT is compressed in diastole, at a time when the mitral valve is open (RVOT diastolic indentation is marked by *arrow*).

(b) RVOT collapse in early diastole on M-mode. Always time events to the ECG; systole starts at the peak of R wave and occupies the ST–T segment, whereas diastole starts beyond the T wave. Events may also be timed to the mitral opening on M-mode. After the systolic dip, the RVOT should be expanding outward in diastole (as in the *solid line*), rather than pushed inward (*dashed line*). The presence of two dips, a systolic dip and a diastolic dip soon after the RV starts to expand out, is characteristic of tamponade. *For the diastolic dip to be diagnostic, the M-mode has to cut the RVOT in an orthogonal fashion.* D, diastole; S, systole.

VII. Echocardiographic determination of LV filling pressure and diastolic function

A. Main parameters
(see Chapter 5, Figure 5.1)

Diastolic E flow and E/A ratio-Diastolic E flow is affected by: (1) LA pressure, (2) LV relaxation, which is impaired in both diastolic dysfunction and systolic dysfunction, and (3) heart rate and PR interval. Impaired LV relaxation reduces E velocity; however, severe hypovolemia with low left-sided filling pressure may reduce E and E/A ratio even in the absence of a relaxation problem. Prolonged PR interval and sinus tachycardia reduce E and E/A ratio and may be associated with E–A fusion without any relaxation problem. On the other hand, high left-sided filling pressures but also high elastic recoil in normal young patients may elevate E velocity.

Two echocardiographic parameters correlate solely with relaxation and are thus reduced in any LV dysfunction, systolic or diastolic, regardless of filling pressure: mitral annular recoil velocity (E′) and the velocity of Doppler propagation from the mitral valve to the apex on four-chamber color M-mode (Vp). Therefore:

$$E / E' = (LA\ filling\ pressure \times LV\ relaxation) / LV\ relaxation = LA\ filling\ pressure$$

The same applies for E/Vp. E/E′ ratio strongly correlates with LA pressure in both systolic and diastolic dysfunction. E/E′ ratio > 14 establishes the diagnosis of LV failure and high LA pressure. When E/E′ is between 9 and 14, other echocardiographic or BNP features are required to assess left-sided filling pressures. E/E′, E deceleration time, Vp, and E/Vp are still reliable in case of atrial fibrillation, where measurements should be averaged from three non-consecutive beats with cycle lengths within 20% of the average heart rate. E/E′ has pitfalls in some contexts (Table 32.3). E′ value may be obtained from the septal or lateral side of the mitral annulus on the four-chamber view; septal E′ is normally lower than lateral E′. Both values should be used and averaged and usually trend in the same direction.

Note that all these parameters correlate with LA pressure. Only one parameter correlates with LVEDP: (pulmonary vein A duration) minus (mitral valve A duration). If prolonged > 30 ms, it corresponds to a prolonged retrograde atrial flow, which correlates with elevated LVEDP even at a stage of normal mean LA pressure (compensated LV dysfunction). This parameter remains useful regardless of EF, mitral valve disease, or HCM.

LA enlargement is a landmark of diastolic dysfunction and/or increased LA pressure. However, LA size may be normal in mild or moderate, compensated diastolic dysfunction. Conversely, LA may remain enlarged for some time after normalization of a previously elevated LA pressure, or in case of atrial arrhythmia or mitral disease.

B. Other parameters that correlate with left-sided filling pressure

- *S and D on pulmonary venous flow.* The more depressed the systolic S wave, the higher the LA pressure. Patients with elevated LA pressure have a large V wave and a deep Y descent; X descent, on the other hand, is flattened and pulled up by the large V. This explains the large D wave (D = Y) and the flat S (S = X).
- *Isovolumic relaxation time (IVRT).* IVRT is prolonged (>110 ms) with stage 1 diastolic dysfunction, and reduced (<70 ms) with more advanced diastolic dysfunction and high LA pressure (in which case the intersection of LA and LV pressures occurs earlier).
- *E deceleration time (DT) (time it takes the E velocity to fall to zero).* A reduced DT < 160 ms implies a high LA pressure that quickly equalizes with LV pressure.
- *B bump on M-mode.* B bump is a small mitral opening occurring at the end of A opening and corresponds to a high LVEDP.
- *M-mode swept across the mitral valve in apical four-chamber view, with color Doppler recording (color M-mode).* Normally, the colored diastolic inflow looks, roughly, like a steep vertical line ("a flame"). A reduction of the steepness of this line with a velocity of propagation (Vp) < 45 cm/s signifies diastolic dysfunction (any grade). E/Vp > 2.5 correlates with increased LA pressure.
- In severe MR, E increases and E′ recoil increases. E/E′ still correlates with LA pressure if EF is reduced. Otherwise, IVRT and (pulmonary vein A duration) minus (mitral valve A duration) correlate with increased left pressures, regardless of EF.

Table 32.3 Pitfalls of E/E′ in the evaluation of LA pressure.

1. Cases where E′ is inherently reduced and E/E′ does not correlate with LA pressure
- Mitral stenosis
- Prosthetic mitral valve
- Mitral ring
- Severe mitral annular calcification

2. Case where E′ is inherently increased and E/E′ does not correlate with LA pressure
- Severe primary mitral regurgitation with normal LV function

3. Cases of discrepancy between medial and lateral E′
- Error in acquisition[a]
- Constrictive pericarditis: increased septal E′, reduced lateral E′[b]
- Severe pulmonary hypertension[c]

[a] Cursor should be positioned within 0.5 cm of the septal or lateral mitral leaflet insertion site and should be parallel to the plane of cardiac motion.

[b] In constrictive pericarditis, the LV lateral and anteroposterior expansion is constricted with a compensatory increase in septal expansion.

[c] Septal E′ is reduced regardless of LV failure because of reduced RV contribution to septal velocity. Lateral E′ and lateral E/E′ correlate with LV failure and should be used instead.

C. Putting it all together (Figures 32.47, 32.48)

When assessing LV function, a clinician is often faced with two problems: (1) In patients with normal EF, is there any LV diastolic dysfunction, whether compensated or not? (2) In patients with normal or abnormal EF, is LA pressure elevated, and does the patient have a diagnosis of heart failure as opposed to just LV dysfunction? Note that a high LA pressure establishes the diagnosis of diastolic dysfunction in patients with normal EF. Conversely, diastolic dysfunction, when compensated, is not associated with increased LA pressure at rest.

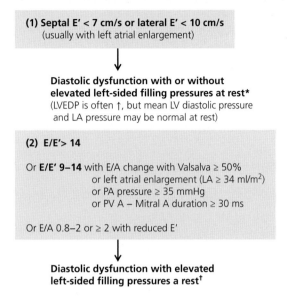

Figure 32.47 Assessment of diastolic dysfunction in a patient with normal LVEF.
*E/A<0.8 assists in establishing the diagnosis of diastolic dysfunction in patients with borderline findings and often correlates with normal left-sided filling pressures (grade 1 diastolic dysfunction). E/A reversal with normal E' may be seen in cases of hypovolemia or older age and should not be universally used to infer the presence of diastolic dysfunction. Also, LA enlargement assists in the diagnosis of diastolic dysfunction in all cases, compensated or not.
†**The measurement of E/E' and PA pressure during *exercise testing or passive leg raising* may establish the diagnosis of diastolic dysfunction in symptomatic patients with otherwise borderline findings**, or establish diastolic dysfunction as a cause of dyspnea in a patient with diastolic dysfunction but normal filling pressures at rest. PV, pulmonary vein.

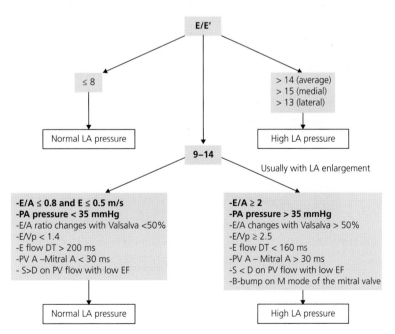

Figure 32.48 Assessment of left-sided filling pressures in patients with normal or abnormal systolic function.
*E/A≤0.8 correlates with normal filling pressures in patients with low LVEF and in most patients with normal LV EF; a patient with severely impaired LV relaxation may have a low LA–LV gradient in early diastole, i.e., low E velocity and E/A ratio, despite a high LA pressure. A depressed S wave (= X descent) on pulmonary venous recording corresponds to a high LA pressure, mainly in the case of a depressed EF. LA enlargement correlates with high LA pressure but LA may remain enlarged even after normalization of LA pressure. E/A and pulmonary venous patterns are not helpful in atrial fibrillation or sinus tachycardia > 100 bpm. DT, mitral inflow deceleration time; PV, pulmonary vein.

D. Assess the volume status and cardiac output of critically ill patients

- The following findings suggest high left-sided filling pressures: high E/A, high E/E′ with a small E′, low/flat systolic wave on the pulmonary vein flow, high PA pressure.
- LV cavity collapse, with or without high LVOT velocity, suggests hypovolemia. However, this may be seen in patients with a stiff, restricted myocardium and volume overload.
- IVC plethora or poor inspiratory collapse implies high RA pressure and probable RV volume overload. Note, however, that IVC dilates with positive-pressure ventilation. Thus, for patients who are mechanically ventilated, IVC dilatation and IVC respiratory variations correlate poorly with RA pressure, yet a small IVC < 1.2 cm at end-expiration still correlates with low RA pressure; even slight IVC collapsibility (>12%) correlates with volume responsiveness.
- Cardiac output can be estimated from the LVOT pulsed-wave Doppler. Aortic or LVOT flow variation > 12% with respiration (mechanical ventilation), or stroke volume increase > 12% with passive leg raising predicts volume responsiveness.

VIII. Additional echocardiographic hemodynamics

Doppler hemodynamics mostly rely on the Bernoulli equation:

$$\text{Peak instantaneous pressure gradient} = 4\left(\text{peak velocity}^2_{\text{across the obstruction}} - \text{peak velocity}^2_{\text{proximal to this obstruction}}\right)$$

The velocity proximal to the obstruction being usually ~1 m/s, the square of this velocity is negligible in patients with a high velocity across the obstruction. Therefore, the simplified Bernoulli equation is:

$$\text{Peak instantaneous pressure gradient} = 4\,\text{peak velocity}^2_{\text{across the obstruction}}$$

A. Proximal isovelocity surface area (PISA) of MR (Figure 32.49)

As blood flows back from the LV to the LA, it converges into multiple sequential hemispheres before reaching the narrow neck of the mitral orifice. This is the convergence flow seen on the LV side, and it is equal to the regurgitant flow seen in the LA. The closer this flow is to the mitral orifice, the higher its velocity, at one point equaling then superseding the aliasing velocity, with all points across one hemispheric line having the same velocity.

  If the line where aliasing occurs is chosen, the velocity of this line would be equal to the Nyquist limit. The inner boundary of the flow convergence is the vena contracta, and the outer boundary is the aliasing color. The area of this flow, PISA, being a hemisphere rather than a 2D circle, is equal to $2\pi r^2$ rather than πr^2, and its velocity is equal to the aliasing limit. The aliasing velocity of the regurgitant color (usually blue on TTE, red on TEE) is the one used for calculation.

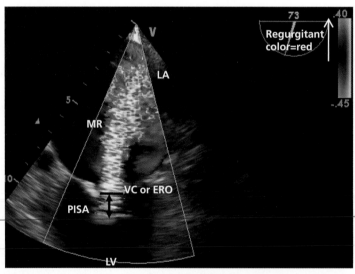

MR flow at the LA side   **= MR flow coming from the LV**
ERO x Peak MR velocity on CW Doppler = PISA area x aliasing velocity of the red color
                                        = 2π (PISA radius)² x aliasing velocity

→ERO = 2π (PISA radius)² x aliasing velocity/ peak MR velocity
       ~ (PISA radius)² /2   if aliasing 40 cm/s

Regurgitant volume = ERO x MR VTI
Regurgitant fraction = Regurgitant volume/ total forward mitral flow
                       = Regurgitant volume/ (Regurgitant volume + Stroke volume)

Figure 32.49 Aliasing velocity of the regurgitant color, which is red in this case and equal to 40 cm/s, is used for PISA calculation. It is the one that should be set at 40 cm/s for the simplified equation. The PISA calculation may also be performed for AI: the peak velocity of the AI spectral envelope is used to calculate ERO, and the VTI of the AI envelope is used to calculate the regurgitant volume. ERO, effective regurgitant orifice area; VC, vena contracta.

The effective regurgitant orifice area (ERO), which corresponds to the narrow regurgitant orifice (or vena contracta), can be calculated using the continuity equation. An ERO ≥ 0.4 cm^2 indicates severe MR. In order to accurately visualize a rounded PISA and measure its radius, the Nyquist limit should be reduced to 40 cm/s; moreover, at this Nyquist limit, the simplified ERO equation applies (ERO ~ PISA radius^2/2).

The PISA principle may also be used to calculate the aortic ERO in AI in an apical view, but it is more technically challenging to delineate the hemisphere of PISA AI than MR; ERO ≥ 0.3 cm^2 indicates severe AI. PISA may also be used to calculate MVA in MS.

Peak velocity of MR is used to calculate ERO by the PISA method. Subsequently, VTI velocity of MR is used to calculate the regurgitant volume (Figure 32.49).

B. Other modality of regurgitant volume calculation

As an alternative to PISA, the regurgitant volume of MR or AI may be calculated using the continuity equation at the level of the LVOT and the mitral valve (**volumetric method**):

Stroke volume at the LVOT = LVOT VTI $\times$ 0.785 $\times$ LVOT diameter^2

Stroke volume at the mitral valve = transmitral VTI $\times$ 0.785 $\times$ mitral annular diameter^2

Transmitral VTI is obtained by tracing the diastolic PW mitral inflow, E–A, in an apical view; mitral annular diameter is also measured in diastole, in an apical view.

The difference between these two stroke volumes is the regurgitant volume of MR or AI. LVOT stroke volume is the larger stroke volume in AI, while mitral stroke volume is the larger stroke volume in MR. This calculation has pitfalls, particularly the measurement of the mitral annular diameter. Moreover, it cannot be used in patients with combined MR and AI, or in patients with MS whose diastolic mitral area is different from the annular area.

C. Pitfalls in MS assessment, pitfalls in mitral valve area calculation using pressure half-time, and various methods of mitral valve area calculation (Figures 32.50, 32.51)

Since it is easy to align the Doppler beam with the mitral inflow on the apical views, the echocardiographic determination of transmitral gradient is usually highly accurate.

On continuous-wave Doppler, the downslope of the mitral inflow E wave can be used to estimate the mitral valve area. The time it takes the pressure gradient to decrease in half, i.e. the time it takes the velocity to decrease by 30%, is the pressure half-time (PHT); mitral valve area (MVA) is equal to 220/PHT. A slow decay corresponds to severe MS, wherein the LA pressure remains higher than LV pressure throughout diastole (no diastasis). However, for the same valve area, LA and LV pressures more readily equalize in case of poor LV compliance or severe AI that briskly increases LV diastolic pressure, which makes the decay look steeper and leads to overestimation of the mitral valve area (i.e., less severe). *This is more commonly the case in elderly or severely hypertensive patients with MS.*

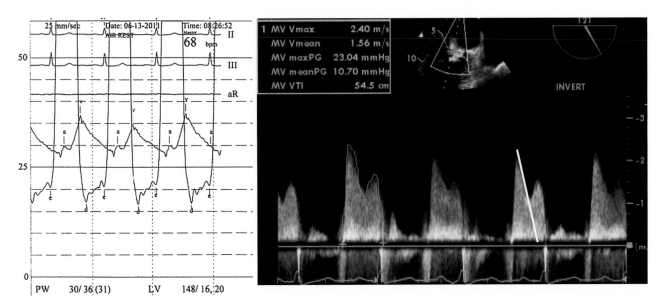

Figure 32.50 Simultaneous LV pressure and PCWP recording is shown on the left, with a mean transmitral pressure gradient of 10 mmHg. The transmitral Doppler flow velocity is shown on the right. The peak velocity is > 2 m/s, which suggests MS (may also signify MR or severely restricted LV filling with hypervolemia). The mean pressure gradient obtained by tracing the Doppler envelope is ~11 mmHg at a rate of 70 bpm, suggesting severe MS.

The valve area calculation using the pressure half-time method, i.e., the steepness of deceleration of E velocity (*gray line*), yields a valve area of 2.6 cm^2. In fact, E velocity falls steeply with a pressure half- time of 80 ms. However, the valve area is calculated invasively at 1.3 cm^2. This discrepancy is expected in light of the patient's severe systemic hypertension (180/100 mmHg) and increased LVEDP. When LV compliance is impaired, LV diastolic pressure increases steeply and therefore, for the same orifice area, LA–LV diastolic pressure gradient decrements faster. This leads to a faster pressure half-time for the same orifice area and creates the false impression of a larger orifice area. The pressure half-time method of orifice area calculation is inaccurate in cases of impaired LV compliance and high LVEDP. A similar limitation of the pressure half-time is seen when MS is associated with AI.

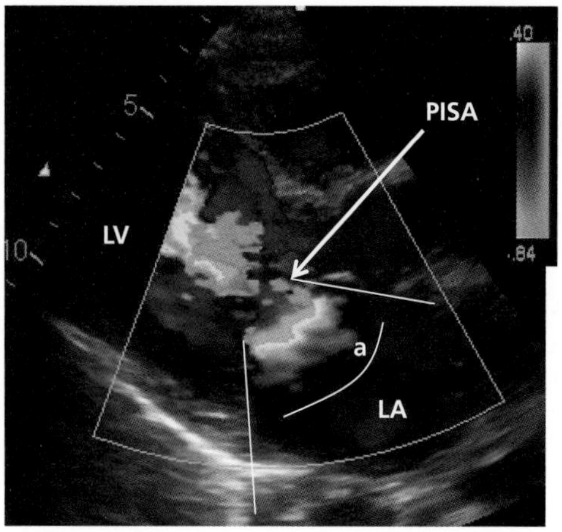

Figure 32.51 PISA of MS on a long-axis view. PISA of MS consists of flow acceleration on the LA side of the mitral valve (≠ PISA of MR, which is on the LV side). On the LA side, the mitral leaflets form an acute angle (≠ obtuse angle on the LV side for MR); thus, PISA of MS is not usually a hemisphere but a cone with an angle (a) that corresponds to the angle formed by the mitral leaflets, and angle adjustment is applied during PISA calculation:

$$\text{MVA} \times \text{peak diastolic velocity across the mitral valve} = 2\,\pi\,(\text{PISA radius})^2 \times \text{red aliasing velocity} \times \textbf{a/180°}$$

In the case of MS associated with concomitant MR or high-output state, the early LA–LV gradient is increased, creating a steep early E flow decay; however, because of MS, the slope of the E flow decay in mid/late diastole is slow. MVA calculation by the pressure half-time method remains accurate using this later slope. In atrial fibrillation, the pressure gradient varies between beats but the shape and the slope of the mitral Doppler envelope remain unchanged, and thus MVA calculation remains accurate.

There are three other modalities for the calculation of MVA:

a. *Continuity equation.* The stroke volume across the LVOT is: (LVOT area × LVOT VTI). The stroke volume across the mitral valve is: (MVA × MV VTI). Therefore:

$$\text{MVA} = \left(0.785 \times \text{LVOT diameter}^2 \times \text{LVOT VTI}\right) / \text{MV VTI}$$

This equation cannot be used in case of concomitant MR, where the flow across the LVOT is lower than the flow across the mitral valve, or AI, where the flow across the LVOT is higher than the flow across the mitral valve.

b. *PISA of the mitral valve.* As opposed to PISA of MR, which is seen on the LV side, a hemisphere of flow acceleration is seen on the LA side in MS. An adjusted PISA equation may be used (Figure 32.51).

c. *Planimetry.* Planimetry consists of tracing the restrictive orifice on the mitral valve short-axis view ("fish mouth"). However, the image should be frozen at the actual leaflet tips, not more proximally where the valvular area would be overestimated. On the other hand, calcium or a high gain may blur the orifice boundaries and underestimate the valvular area.

In summary, echocardiography assesses the transmitral gradient very accurately. However, the estimation of the valvular area using one of the four methods (mitral inflow pressure half-time, continuity equation, PISA method, and planimetry) may be subject to measurement errors. A high gradient does not necessarily imply severe MS; mild MS with MVA > 1.5 cm² may have a severe gradient in the presence of tachycardia or high-output state. Invasive hemodynamics are, thus, valuable for the assessment of MS whenever there is discrepancy between echocardiographic MVA and transmitral gradient; and whenever it is not clear whether the patient's symptoms or pulmonary hypertension are purely secondary to MS, or rather secondary to mild MS + high output state, MS + LV diastolic dysfunction, or intrinsic pulmonary arterial hypertension

D. Pitfalls in PHT use for AI assessment (Figure 32.52)

A compensated or mildly decompensated chronic AI is characterized by a gradual LV diastolic pressure slope and an increase in LVEDP that remains much lower than the aortic pressure, e.g., LVEDP of 20 mmHg with a diastolic aortic pressure of 70 mmHg. On Doppler, this corresponds to a gradual drop of the regurgitant flow velocity with a PHT that is > 250 ms, even if AI is severe. Acute AI or decompensated chronic AI with LV failure is characterized by a steeply rising LV diastolic pressure and equilibration of LVEDP and aortic end-diastolic pressure. On Doppler, this corresponds to a steep drop of regurgitant flow velocity with a short pressure half-time < 250 ms. Thus, a reduced PHT not only correlates with the severity of AI but with its acuity and the LV state (compensated vs. decompensated). Occasionally, AI with severe underlying LV dysfunction may have PHT < 250 ms even if AI is only moderate.

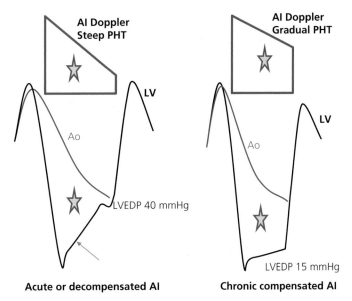

Figure 32.52 LV–aortic pressure tracings in acute AI and chronic AI. In acute AI, the steep diastolic approximation of LV and aortic pressures (triangle, *star*) translates into a similarly steep AI Doppler. PHT: pressure half-time.

E. Correlation between hepatic venous Doppler and RA pressure. Correlation between pulmonary venous Doppler and LA pressure (see Figure 32.53)

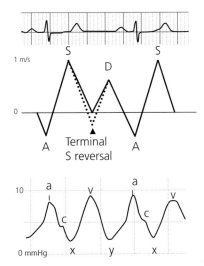

Figure 32.53 Correlations between A, X, V, and Y waves on the LA pressure tracing and S, D, and A flow velocities on the pulmonary venous Doppler. S flow corresponds to the X descent, D flow corresponds to the Y descent, and the A wave corresponds to A-flow reversal (S = X, D = Y). S and D flows are antegrade, while A flow is retrograde. The S wave may be notched and divided into S_1 and S_2 as a result of the C wave. Disease states:
- In the case of *LV failure* with elevated atrial pressure, the V wave is large, the Y descent is deep, and the X descent is usually blunted because it is carried up by the large V wave. The blunted X descent leads to **S-flow blunting** with terminal S reversal, and the deep Y descent leads to a large D flow.
- S flow is blunted or fully reversed in the case of MR.
- *Tamponade*, on the other hand, is characterized by a **blunted Y descent/D flow** because of impeded diastolic filling.
  Similar correlations apply to RA pressure and IVC/hepatic venous Doppler flow.

F. Systolic PA pressure

$$\text{Systolic PA pressure} = 4\,TR_{velocity}{}^{2} + RA\text{ pressure.}$$

G. Diastolic PA pressure

Measure the end-diastolic velocity of the pulmonary regurgitant flow. The end-diastolic gradient between PA and RV is $4\times$(end-diastolic velocity of PR)^2. Thus:

$$\text{Diastolic PA pressure} = 4\times\left(\text{end-diastolic velocity of PR}\right)^2 + \text{RV end-diastolic pressure}$$

RV end-diastolic pressure being equal to RA pressure:

$$\text{Diastolic PA pressure} = 4\times\left(\text{end-diastolic velocity of PR}\right)^2 + \text{RA pressure}$$

PR velocity being a small number, smaller than TR velocity, the calculation of PA diastolic pressure is more subject to error than the calculation of PA systolic pressure.

H. Calculation of LVEDP from AI Doppler flow

The end-diastolic AI velocity corresponds to the gradient between the diastolic aortic pressure and the LVEDP. Using the non-invasive blood pressure:

$$\text{LVEDP} = \text{diastolic BP} - 4\times\left(\text{end-diastolic AI velocity}\right)^2$$

I. Calculation of LA pressure from MR Doppler flow in patients with any degree of MR

The peak MR velocity corresponds to the gradient between LV systolic pressure and LA pressure. LV systolic pressure being equal to the aortic systolic pressure in the absence of AS (~ non-invasive systolic BP), LA pressure is equal to:

$$\text{Systolic BP} - 4\times\left(\text{MR velocity}\right)^2$$

J. Calculation of the peak LV systolic pressure in patients with AS

The peak-to-peak gradient in AS corresponds to ~70% of the peak instantaneous gradient. Therefore:

$$\left(\text{systolic LV pressure} - \text{systolic BP}\right) = 0.7\times\left(4\times\text{peak velocity}^2\right)$$

If the systolic BP is 140 mmHg, and the peak velocity is 5 m/s, the systolic LV pressure is:

$$0.7\times\left(4\times5^2\right) + 140 = 210\,\text{mmHg}$$

K. Calculation of Qp/Qs ratio in the case of a shunt

Normally, the pulmonary flow (Qp) is equal to the systemic flow (Qs). In left-to-right shunt, Qp is larger than Qs, while in isolated right-to-left shunt Qs is larger than Qp. Qp/Qs is the pulmonary-to-systemic flow ratio. Qp/Qs is equal to:

$$\left(\text{VTI}\times\text{diameter at the RVOT}\right) / \left(\text{VTI}\times\text{diameter at the LVOT}\right)$$

PW Doppler is used. RVOT measurements are done on the aortic short-axis view, tilted to the RVOT. The reverse ratio is used for Qp/Qs calculation in PDA. In PDA, the flow across the RVOT is proximal to the shunt and corresponds to Qs, whereas the flow across the LVOT corresponds to Qp.

IX. Prosthetic valves

A. Differentiate a biprosthetic valve from a mechanical valve (see Figures 32.54, 32.55, 32.56)

A bioprosthetic valve is characterized by an echodense sewing ring and *three large struts/vertical columns* in the center of the valvular orifice. The prosthetic leaflets are attached to those struts. Two leaflets may be seen in a single view. The sewing ring and the struts are usually mounted over a metallic frame (stented bioprosthesis). Occasionally, an aortic prosthesis may be stentless.

A mechanical valve has an echodense ring but *does not have struts*. It has one or two metallic hinges that are seen as points or lines in the center of the orifice when the valve opens. The leaflets shadow and reverberate around those hinges during motion. There are two hinges and three orifices – one central and two lateral – in a St. Jude metallic valve, and one hinge in a single-leaflet tilting disk. In addition, with mechanical valves, prosthetic valve clicks are seen on spectral Doppler (dark narrow band on spectral display); these are not seen with normally functioning bioprostheses.

A mitral valve annuloplasty ring is seen as a dense echogenic annulus. A partial posterior ring often mimics posterior mitral annular calcifications, while a full ring may mimic the ring of a bioprosthetic valve (on the parasternal long-axis view, an echodense dot is seen both posteriorly and anteriorly at the annular level).

Prosthetic leaflets are difficult to see because of the sewing ring at the level of the annulus. This may shadow the valvular structure and the Doppler flow. Also, there is shadowing and/or reverberation from the valve itself in case of a mechanical valve or a heavily calcified bioprosthetic valve, which limits visualization. Shadowing means that metal or calcium creates a black shadow that hides all structures behind it, including the Doppler flow. Reverberation means that the ultrasound signal "ping-pongs" back and forth between metallic or calcified structures, creating multiple duplicates of these structures.

B. Prosthetic valve gradients

Inherently, prosthetic valves are mildly obstructive. In fact, a peak velocity of up to 3 m/s and a mean gradient of up to 20 mmHg are normally seen across the aortic valve; a velocity of 3–4 m/s or a mean gradient of 20–35 mmHg may also be seen across a normally functioning aortic prosthesis but requires further evaluation. A peak velocity of up to 1.9 m/s and a mean gradient of up to 6 mmHg may be seen across the mitral prosthesis. Several mechanisms explain these Doppler gradients across structurally normal valves (Table 32.4). Higher velocities/gradients may be related to structural disease (thrombus, pannus, degenerated bioprosthesis); on the other hand, high gradients may not be manifest in patients with prosthetic dysfunction and low cardiac output state, hence the importance of using other features to diagnose valvular dysfunction (Tables 32.5, 32.6; see also Question 24 in Chapter 6). The analysis of leaflet motion and structure on TEE allows the differentiation between a dysfunctional prosthesis that requires operative correction and a structurally normal prosthesis. For instance, a high transprosthetic gradient with a normal leaflet motion corresponds to a normally functioning valve with a high velocity. Also, cinefluoroscopy is a very helpful adjunctive technique that allows analysis of the mechanical prosthesis leaflet excursion (to assess stenosis) and the prosthesis seating (to assess dehiscence and regurgitation).

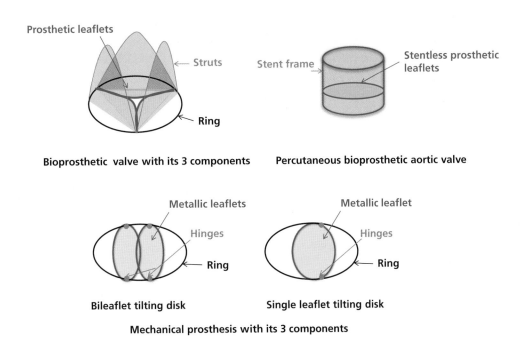

Figure 32.54 Types of prosthetic valves. Surgical bioprostheses typically have a metallic stent frame that extends from the sewing ring to each strut.

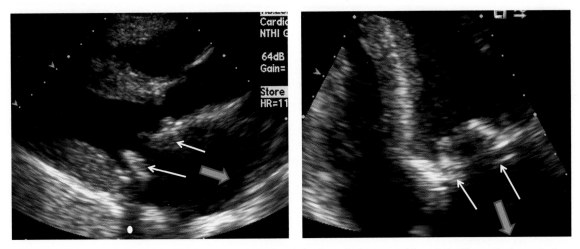

Figure 32.55 Bioprosthetic porcine valve as evidenced by the large struts/vertical columns in the center of the mitral orifice on the long-axis view and four-chamber view (two of the three struts are seen, *arrows*). The ring and the struts are hyperechogenic because of the metallic stent frame.

It may be difficult to see prosthetic valves because of the sewing ring at the annulus. This may shadow the valvular structure and the Doppler flow. Here, black shadowing is seen posteriorly, behind the struts (*dot*). Also, there is shadowing/reverberations from the valve itself in the case of a mechanical valve or a heavily calcified bioprosthetic valve, which limits visualization.

However, it is often ***possible to assess aortic prosthesis regurgitation by TTE Doppler***. This is done on parasternal long-axis and apical views, because the ventricular side is not intercepted by the valve. It is ***hard to assess mitral prosthesis regurgitation by TTE Doppler*** because the regurgitant flow and the LA are both shadowed behind the mitral valve (*thick arrow*). However, there would still be a large PISA on the ventricular side, and the increased forward E velocity can still be assessed. TEE is most helpful for mitral prosthesis assessment, because TEE looks directly at the LA.

It is possible to assess aortic or mitral prosthesis stenosis by analyzing forward flow velocities.

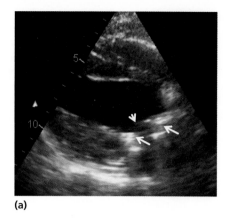

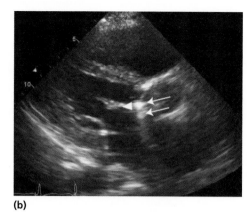

(a)   **(b)**

Figure 32.56 (a) Metallic mitral prosthesis. As in bioprostheses, a hyperechogenic metallic ring is seen (*arrows*). In metallic prostheses, thin reverberating leaflets are moving within the ring (*arrowhead*), while in bioprostheses, thick struts/columns are seen within the ring.

(b) Aortic mechanical prosthesis, with two metallic points (hinges) in the middle of the aortic orifice (*arrows*). This is a St. Jude bileaflet tilting disk valve. Evaluation of AI with color Doppler is possible, as the flow will be directed toward the LV (*arrowhead*) and not shadowed by the valve or its ring.

Table 32.4 Beside the occluder profile, four causes of pressure gradient across a prosthetic valve.

1. **Pressure recovery, particularly across a bileaflet tilting disk valve**
   The smaller central orifice in bileaflet valves may give rise to a high-velocity jet. This corresponds to a localized pressure drop that is largely recovered once the central flow reunites with flow from the two lateral orifices. Doppler recording often includes this high-velocity jet, which leads to overestimation of the gradient and thus, underestimation of EOA
2. **Patient/prosthesis mismatch**
   Prosthetic EOA is too small in relation to the patient's body size, resulting in abnormally high postoperative gradients (EOA ≤0.85 cm²/m² of BSA for aortic prosthesis, ≤ 1.2 cm²/m² for mitral prosthesis). Prosthesis may function adequately at rest but is unable to accommodate the hemodynamics of exercise
   Mostly occurs with mitral prosthesis ≤27 mm in size or aortic prosthesis ≤21 mm
3. **High flow state or severe regurgitation across the valve increases velocity and gradients**
   a. In this case, the use of the simplified Bernoulli equation ($P = 4\,V_A^2$) further overestimates gradient. Use the true Bernoulli equation ($P = 4\,[V_{prosthesis}^2 - V_{LVOT}^2]$), calculate the orifice area, or use the dimensionless index (LVOT VTI/aortic VTI) for assessment of stenosis
   b. Dynamic LVOT obstruction following aortic valve replacement: ~10% of AS patients have asymmetric septal hypertrophy (>1.5:1). Upon relief of the aortic obstruction, the afterload reduction unmasks dynamic subaortic obstruction. The obstruction is often due to obliteration of a hyperdynamic cavity, and SAM may be seen
4. **Prosthetic obstruction** (thrombus, pannus, degenerated bioprosthesis)

Because of the occluder profile, most prostheses have EOA of 1.5–3 cm² with mild gradient.
EOA, effective orifice area; VTI, velocity–time integral.

Table 32.5 Echocardiographic differentiation between a physiologically high gradient and an intrinsic aortic prosthesis obstruction.

	Normal	**Stenosis**
Peak velocity	<3 m/s	>4 m/s
TEE and cinefluoroscopy	Normal leaflet excursion and structure	Abnormal
Dimensionless index[a]	>0.30	<0.25
Contour of transaortic Doppler	Triangular, early peaking	Rounded, symmetrical
Acceleration time (AT)[b]	<100 ms	>100 ms
Effective orifice area (EOA)[c]	>1.2 cm²	<0.8 cm²

[a] Dimensionless index = LVOT VTI/aortic VTI.
[b] AT (acceleration time in milliseconds) is measured as the duration from the onset of aortic ejection to the maximal jet velocity.
[c] EOA is calculated using the continuity equation.
Adapted with permission from Zoghbi WA, et al. J Am Soc Echocardiogr 2009; 22: 975–1014.

Table 32.6 Echocardiographic differentiation between a physiologically high gradient and an intrinsic mitral prosthesis obstruction.

	Normal	Stenosis
Peak velocity	<1.9 m/s	>2.5 m/s
TEE and cinefluoroscopy	Normal leaflet excursion and structure	Abnormal
Dimensionless index[a]	>0.45	<0.4
PHT	<130 ms	>200 ms
EOA[b]	≥2 cm²	<1 cm²
PA pressure and RV function	Normal or improving	Abnormal

[a] Dimensionless index = LVOT VTI/Mitral VTI.
[b] EOA is calculated using the continuity equation (preferred to pressure half-time method).
Adapted with permission from Zoghbi WA, et al. J Am Soc Echocardiogr 2009; 22: 975–1014.

C. Prosthetic and periprosthetic valvular regurgitation

Prosthetic valves normally have mild closure backflow, which manifests as a small central jet with a tilting disk valve and two small crisscross jets with a bileaflet valve. Also, paravalvular leaks are frequently seen, especially early postoperatively (5–20%), and these are usually mild and hemodynamically insignificant. Several echocardiographic and fluoroscopic features suggest significant regurgitation. More specifically, dehiscence or rocking movement suggests paravalvular regurgitation, while immobile "stuck" strut(s) suggest valvular regurgitation. On echo-Doppler, the following features, some of which are indirect features, suggest significant regurgitation:

a. Worsening of LA or LV size or function
b. Worsening of PA pressure and RV function
c. Aortic diastolic flow reversal in the case of aortic prosthesis or large forward E velocity in the case of mitral prosthesis
d. A very large jet diameter (vena contracta)
e. Large PISA (on the apical view for the mitral valve, long-axis view for the aortic valve, cases where PISA is not hidden by shadowing)
f. Green color suggesting turbulent flow
g. Intensity and shape of the CW Doppler envelope (dense regurgitant envelope in AI or MR; steep deceleration in AI with a steep PHT)

X. Brief note on Doppler physics and echo artifacts

A. Doppler physics

The Doppler probe emits echoes at a certain frequency and captures the frequency of the reflected pulses; the change in frequency is called Doppler shift. This shift allows the calculation of the flow velocity (the flow is what modifies the emitted frequency). In PW Doppler, reflected echoes are only detected from one particular site, called the sample volume. The transducer "gate" opens for a specific period of time that corresponds to the depth of the sample volume. The transducer emits pulses and captures reflected pulses intermittently, at a specific rate called pulse repetition frequency (PRF) or sampling rate, which corresponds to the depth of the volume interrogated.

The PW must sample each reflected pulse at least twice during each cycle to appropriately measure the reflected frequency (and thus the velocity) (Figure 32.57). If the reflected frequency is more than half the sampling rate, this frequency cannot be accurately measured. The maximum frequency that can be accurately measured is half the PRF and is called the Nyquist limit (the Nyquist limit frequency has a corresponding Nyquist velocity limit). Thus, if blood flow is faster than the Nyquist velocity, its velocity cannot be appropriately sampled and measured. Deeper structures necessitate longer travel time and, thus, a lower sampling rate or Nyquist limit. As compared with superficial structures, it is harder to detect higher velocities of deeper structures, particularly if a high-frequency transducer (TEE) is used.

To measure higher velocities, increase the Nyquist limit and shift the baseline in one direction, so that velocities up to 2× Nyquist limit can be detected.

Color Doppler is a collection of PW Dopplers, as it captures multiple sample volumes along the sector interrogated, and displays a color for each sample volume. The size of the color corresponds to the size of the flow but also to its velocity in relation to the Nyquist limit; that is how the same MR volume may look more or less severe depending on the setting, flow velocity, and eccentricity. Changing the Nyquist limit or the color gain changes the perceived size of the flow.

CW Doppler continuously sends out and receives ultrasound waves, and thus does not have a Nyquist limit.

The transducer emits waves of a certain frequency (both for ultrasound and for Doppler imaging) and captures the reflected frequency of blood (Doppler) but also cardiac structures (ultrasound). A high frequency provides better axial and lateral resolution; however, the high-frequency waves get more attenuated and have reduced penetration. Therefore, TEE and vascular ultrasound transducers are high-frequency transducers (~7.5 MHz) as the imaged structures are superficial. A TTE transducer has a low frequency (~2.5–3.5 MHz). Deeper structures necessitate longer travel time and, thus, longer pulse wave duration and lower pulse frequency; the velocities of deeper structures are better resolved with a lower-frequency transducer.

B. Artifacts

While being aligned with the flow allows better assessment of velocities, being orthogonal to a structure allows a better 2D definition of this structure, a better definition of its dimension (e.g., LVOT diameter is better measured in the long-axis than the apical view), and a better assessment of myocardial thickening. It also allows a better measurement of Doppler jet diameter (e.g., vena contracta of MR or AI is best

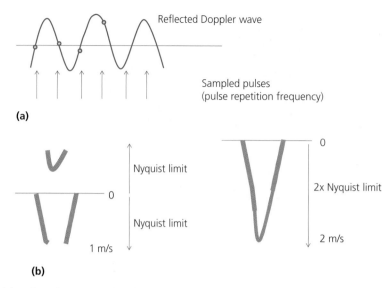

Figure 32.57 (a) Frequency of the reflected wave. On pulsed-wave Doppler, there must be two sampled pulses for every reflected wave, allowing adequate tracing of the waves (*dots*) and measurement of the frequency. One pulse per cycle does not allow appropriate delineation of the waves. **(b)** If the PW velocity exceeds the Nyquist limit (leading to aliasing), shift the baseline into one direction; this allows sampling of velocities of up to 2× Nyquist limit. The thickness of the envelope corresponds to the range of frequencies across the sample volume. Slow flow leads to a large range of velocities across the sample volume and a thick envelope (spectral broadening).

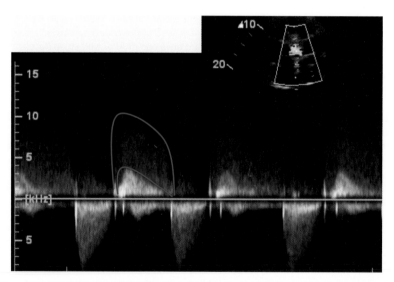

Figure 32.58 In this interrogation of the aortic valve in the apical five-chamber view, two envelopes are seen in diastole (above the baseline): AI and another, more dense envelope that corresponds to the LV inflow (E wave). Despite being in another plane, LV inflow is superimposed on the AI flow as a result of the *beam width artifact*. Similarly, **MR flow may be superimposed on AS flow, leading to overestimation of AS severity.**

measured in the parasternal long-axis view). This is due to the fact that axial resolution is superior to lateral resolution. *Moreover, lateral resolution worsens with depth, as it depends on the beam width at each level.* In fact, at a deep level, signals are reflected and backscattered from the entire slice thickness. This is called **beam width artifact** and may affect both echo and Doppler signals (Figures 32.58, 32.59). In addition, at a certain depth, strong reflectors adjacent to the image plane may appear in the image plane; this is called **side lobe artifact**. A calcified aortic valve may create the impression of calcium in the LA on the apical view; the posterior mitral annular calcium may create a band artifact in the LA.

   Range ambiguity artifact. For both echo imaging and color Doppler, the ultrasound probe samples signals from a certain depth at a determined time interval. A structure B that is at twice the depth of structure A will reach the transducer at the next sampling time for A, which results in this deep structure appearing close to the superficial structure A. This is called *range ambiguity artifact* and is seen with deep imaging.

   While reflection creates an image, refraction may create a **double image or mirror image artifact**. This may be seen on echo but also on Doppler (e.g., mirror image of MR velocity seen on the other side of the baseline; mirror image of the pulmonary artery reflects in the ascending aorta on TEE, mimicking dissection flap). This may be attenuated by reducing the gain.

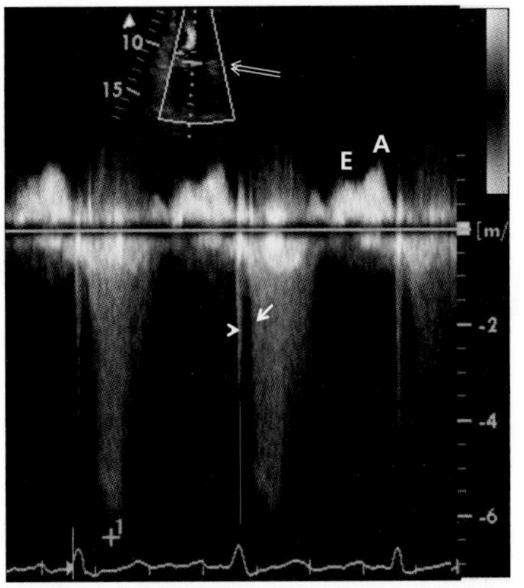

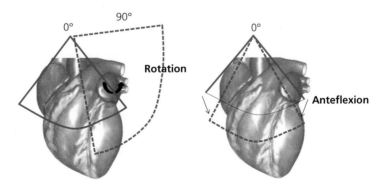

Figure 32.59 The Doppler cursor is placed across the mitral valve (*double arrow*). In diastole, E and A velocities are captured. In systole, the flow below the baseline suggests MR. However, no MR is seen on color Doppler. Also, this flow (*arrow*) does not start at the peak of R wave, nor immediately after A wave, which suggests an aortic or LVOT flow rather than a mitral flow. In fact, a narrow line corresponding to a trivial MR is seen at the peak of R wave (*arrowhead*). This flow occurs later than MR and represents the dagger shape of LVOT obstruction. It is captured on the mitral interrogation because of beam width artifact.

Reverberation and shadowing artifacts may also be seen, and these have been discussed in Section IX, *Prosthetic valves*. One form of reverberation artifact is the rib projection on the echo image, creating, for example, the impression of a "grainy" apical thrombus on the apical views. This grainy structure, however, does not follow the heart motion.

2. TRANSESOPHAGEAL ECHOCARDIOGRAPHY (TEE) VIEWS

The TEE probe and transducer can be manipulated in several planes (Figure 32.60):

- Up and down motion of the whole probe.
- Rotation from an axial horizontal plane (0°) to a vertical plane (90°).
- Clockwise or counterclockwise turn of the whole probe. Clockwise turn moves the tip towards the right-sided structures.
- Anteflexion moves the tip superiorly, while retroflexion moves the tip inferiorly. A result similar to anteflexion may be achieved by pulling the probe up.

Rather than focusing on multiple structures in one view, a stepwise focus on one structure at a time, and going through multiple views focusing on this one structure, is a reasonable approach to TEE imaging.

Figure 32.60 Illustration of angle rotation and anteflexion on TEE.

A. First step: mitral valve and left-sided chambers (see Figures 32.61–32.68)

Start with the following transesophageal views, focusing on the mitral valve and the left-sided chambers: *four-chamber view* at 0° rotation, *two-chamber view* at 60–90° rotation, and *long-axis view* at 90–120° rotation. On each view, record the image without color for structural assessment, then use color for mitral assessment. The mitral valve cusps are identified on these views.

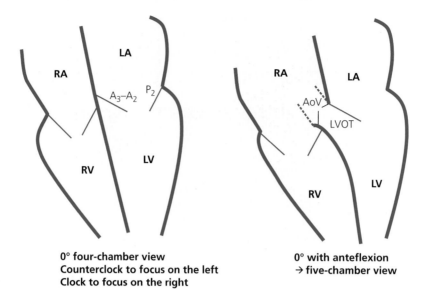

0° four-chamber view
Counterclock to focus on the left
Clock to focus on the right

0° with anteflexion
→ five-chamber view

Figure 32.61 TEE: 0° four- and five-chamber views.

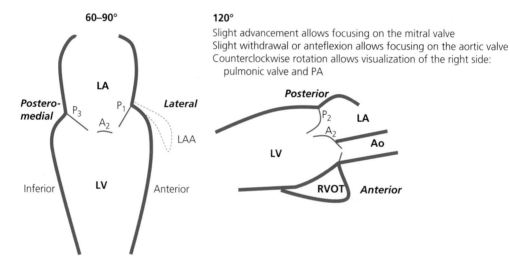

60–90°

120°
Slight advancement allows focusing on the mitral valve
Slight withdrawal or anteflexion allows focusing on the aortic valve
Counterclockwise rotation allows visualization of the right side:
   pulmonic valve and PA

Figure 32.62 TEE **two-chamber and long-axis views.** To understand the orientation, look at Figure 32.63. *The two-chamber view* looks at the intercommissural mitral plane (from the posteromedial commissure to the lateral commissure), the LAA being at the lateral side. The *three-chamber view* looks at the anterior–posterior mitral plane, at the center of the mitral valve (A_2–P_2). The posterior aspect is closest to the esophageal probe and is seen on top, while the anterior structures, aorta and RV, are away from the probe. Both these views are critical during percutaneous positioning of a Mitraclip.

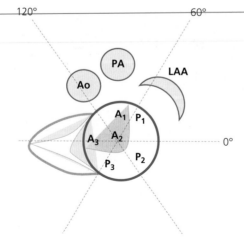

Figure 32.63 Illustration of an axial view of the mitral plane, showing the relationship of the cusps with the septum, aorta, and LAA. Also, **illustration of how various TEE rotations cut the mitral valve**. Those cuts approximate TTE cuts (0° correlates with the apical four-chamber view, 60° correlates with the apical two-chamber view, and 120° correlates with the long-axis view).

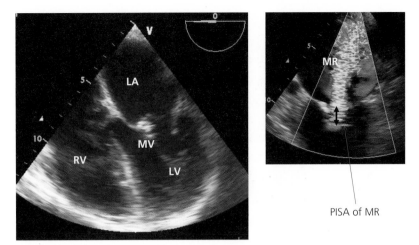

Figure 32.64 TEE **four-chamber 0° view**. Note the calcification of the mitral valve. This is a rheumatic valve with leaflet restriction not just in diastole but also in systole, the latter explaining the severe MR on Doppler. PISA of MR represents flow acceleration as the regurgitant flow comes from the LV towards the LA. PISA of MR is seen on the LV side. The *double arrow* indicates the PISA radius.

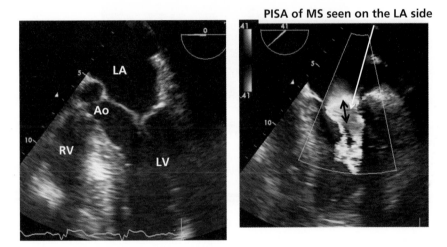

Figure 32.65 TEE **five-chamber view**. Another case of restricted leaflets from a rheumatic process. In this case, no significant MR is seen on Doppler, but significant MS is present, secondary to leaflet restriction in diastole. A large PISA of MS is seen on the LA side (*double arrow*).

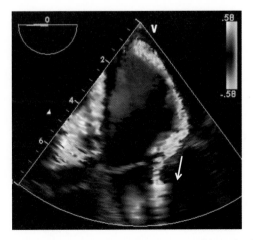

Figure 32.66 Severe eccentric MR is seen on the TEE four-chamber view, "hugging" the LA wall (Coanda effect). The posterior leaflet is tethered (direction of the *arrow*) in a patient with prior inferior infarct, resulting in a posteriorly directed jet.

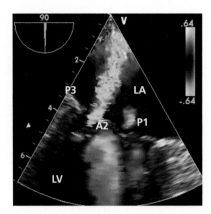

Figure 32.67 MR is seen on the 90° two-chamber view. Note that, in this view, the mitral orifice is cut at two different locations, creating two jets. One anterior cusp is hanging between two posterior cusps.

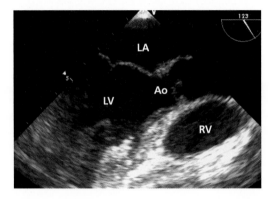

Figure 32.68 TEE **long-axis (120°) view.**

B. Second step: aortic valve evaluation (see Figure 32.69)

Go to 0° again, anteflex or pull the probe until the aortic valve is opened (*five-chamber view*). Then rotate to 30–50° while anteflexed or pulled, which allows the acquisition of the *short-axis view of the aortic valve*. Then further rotate to 120°, obtaining a *long-axis view with a focus on the aortic valve*. This is similar to the long-axis view obtained under the "First step," except that the focus is on the aortic valve. In fact, from the 120° long-axis view focused on the mitral valve, the aortic valve may be targeted by slight withdrawal or anteflexion of the probe.

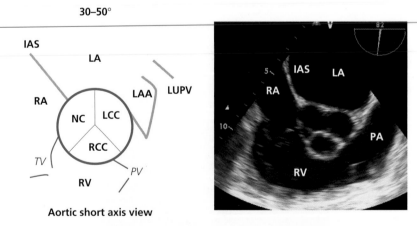

Figure 32.69 Aortic valve short-axis view. Anteflexion is necessary to see the aortic valve (at the level of the high LA). More anteflexion or slight probe withdrawal allows visualization of LAA, which is higher than the aortic valve. Note that the non-coronary cusp is the cusp in line with the interatrial septum.

   Clockwise rotation from this view allows a focus on the right side and excellent visualization of the tricuspid and pulmonic valves. LUPV, left upper pulmonary vein; LCC, left coronary cosp; NC, noncoronary cusp; PV: pulmonic valve; RCC, right coronary cusp; TV: tricuspid valve.

C. Third step: left atrial appendage (Figure 32.70)

The left atrial appendage (LAA) is best seen through a modification of the short-axis aortic view obtained under the "Second step". The LAA is slightly higher than the aortic valve, which is higher than the four-chamber view. To see the LAA, further anteflex or pull up from the aortic short-axis view. After the LAA is visualized and centered, it is inspected at multiple rotation angles (30°–90°). The LAA is a pencil-like structure, bordered laterally by a ridge sometimes called the "coumadin ridge"; the latter separates the LAA from the left upper pulmonary vein.

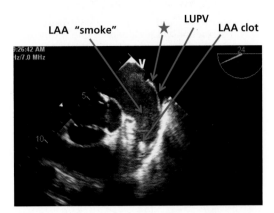

Figure 32.70 Anteflexion from the level of the short-axis view leads to the **LAA view**. A thrombus is seen at the tip of the LAA, along with spontaneous echo contrast ("smoke") in the LAA and LA. The structure identified by the *star* is the "coumadin ridge," a normal band separating the LAA from the left upper pulmonary vein (LUPV). Counterclockwise torque of the probe allows better visualization of the LUPV.

D. Fourth step: right-sided structures (see Figures 32.71, 32.72)

On any of the prior views (especially four-chamber, long-axis, and aortic short-axis views), a *clockwise torque* of the probe moves the ultrasound tip towards the right chambers and allows evaluation of the RA, RV, tricuspid and pulmonic valves.

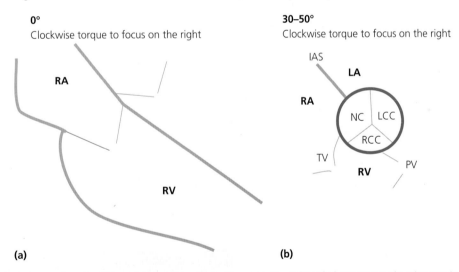

Figure 32.71 (a) Clockwise torque from the 0° four-chamber view allows a **focus on the right-sided structures**. The crista terminalis ridge may be seen by an anteflexion/retroflexion sweep of the RA.

(b) Clockwise rotation from the aortic short-axis view allows a focus on the right side and excellent visualization of RV inflow and tricuspid valve. The interatrial septum is also well visualized. The pulmonic valve may be visualized in the same plane or may require counterclockwise rotation.

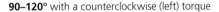
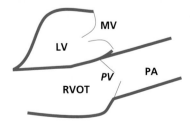

Figure 32.72 From a 90–120° LV/aortic view, torquing the TEE probe to the left, using a counterclockwise maneuver, usually allows visualization of the RVOT, pulmonic valve, and PA (whereas a torque to the right using a clockwise maneuver allows visualization of the RA/RV). *The RVOT, pulmonic valve, and PA are the only "right-sided" structures that may require counterclockwise rotation. Actually, PA and RVOT are to the left of the aorta.*

E. Fifth step: interatrial septum (see Figures 32.73–32.76)

The three best views to visualize the interatrial septum (IAS) are:

- 0° four-chamber view with a clockwise torque to the right (mitral and posterior IAS rims)
- 30–50° aortic view with a clockwise torque to the right (aortic and posterior IAS rims)
- Bicaval 90° view: from the 0° view or the aortic view torqued towards the right-sided structures, a 90° rotation allows visualization of the SVC and IVC (bicaval view) (SVC and IVC rims). The interatrial septum and the fossa ovalis, i.e., the overlap of the septum primum and secundum, are well seen. The septum primum is membranous and thin, whereas the septum secundum is muscular. In a PFO, the septum primum and secundum are not coapted and a tunnel is visualized in between. In ASD, the issue is not a lack of coaptation; rather, a defect is present in the IAS between the septum primum and septum secundum, usually >8 mm. An ostium primum ASD is characterized by an absent mitral rim, while a sinus venosus ASD is characterized by an absent SVC rim.

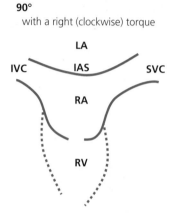

Figure 32.73 Interatrial septum (IAS) bicaval view ("Mickey Mouse" view). Try to slightly torque the probe to see the thinnest portion of the IAS, i.e., the membranous septum primum, which meets and overlaps with the septum secundum to form the fossa ovalis.

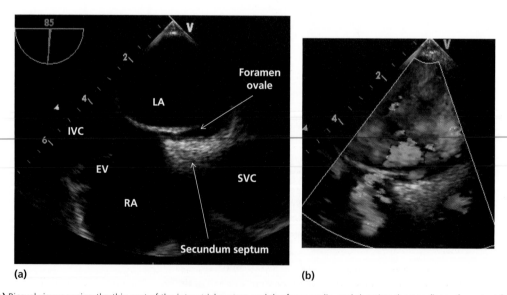

(a)   (b)

Figure 32.74 (a) Bicaval view opening the thin part of the interatrial septum and the fossa ovalis, and showing the two flaps of a patent foramen ovale. The thick, muscular flap is the septum secundum, while the thin, membranous flap is the septum primum. **(b)** Flow is seen across the foramen ovale. EV, Eustachian valve.

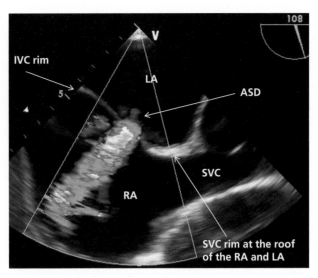

Figure 32.75 Bicaval view showing an ostium secundum ASD. ASD is a defect; in contrast, PFO is a tunnel resulting from malapposition of the primum and secundum septa, without any defect (Figure 32.74).

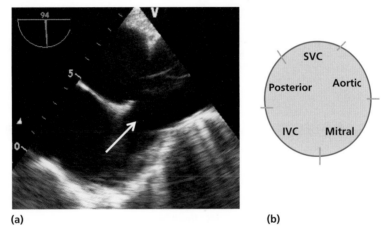

(a) **(b)**

Figure 32.76 **(a)** Bicaval view showing sinus venous ASD (*arrow*). Note the lack of any SVC rim. **(b)** Interatrial septum viewed from the side. Various rims are identified. The SVC and IVC rims are seen on the bicaval view, the aortic and posterior rims are seen on the aortic short-axis view, while the mitral rim is seen on the four-chamber view.

F. Sixth step: structures at the base of the heart (see Figures 32.77, 32.78)

Go back to the aortic short-axis view or the four-chamber view, then pull the probe up at a 0° angle. From right to left, the following structures are visualized:

Right upper pulmonary vein, SVC, aorta, PA, LAA, left upper pulmonary vein (pulmonary veins are at the extreme, aorta is more rightward than PA).

Anteflexion from this level allows the visualization of the main PA bifurcating into the right and left PA.

The left upper pulmonary vein is visualized through a left torque. The left lower pulmonary vein is visualized by advancing the transducer slightly or reducing the anteflexion. The right upper pulmonary vein (RUPV) may be visualized by clockwise torque of the probe to the right. If this is unsuccessful, two other maneuvers allow visualization of the RUPV:

- From the five-chamber view, the probe is turned to the right. The RUPV is seen next to the SVC.
- From the bicaval view (~90° view), the probe is rotated 20° or slightly turned to the right. The RUPV will appear next to the SVC.

The RUPV is the most important vein to assess, as it is involved in 90% of anomalous pulmonary venous return (an anomalous RUPV drains into the RA or SVC, while an anomalous left pulmonary vein drains into the innominate vein).

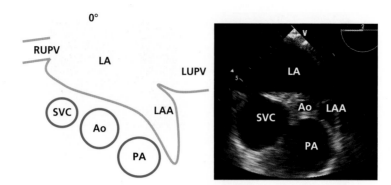

Figure 32.77 0° view at a high level, allowing visualization of structures at the base of the heart. This view shows the left upper pulmonary vein (LUPV), but may not show the right upper pulmonary vein (RUPV) well. In order to properly visualize the RUPV:

- From the five-chamber view, the probe is turned to the right. The RUPV is seen next to the SVC.

- From the bicaval view (~90° view), the probe is rotated 20° or slightly turned to the right; the RUPV will appear next to the SVC.

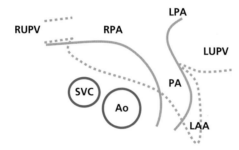

Figure 32.78 Anteflexion from Figure 32.77 shows an even higher level. The PA is seen bifurcating into left PA (LPA) and right PA (RPA).

G. Seventh step: transgastric views (see Figures 32.79–32.82)
These views are mainly useful to:

- Assess LV function and RV function, as the transesophageal views foreshorten the LV and RV, particularly the apex.
- Assess the transaortic valve gradient.
- Further evaluate the mitral and tricuspid valves.

From the 0° transesophageal view, advance the probe into the stomach then perform anteflexion to look towards the heart. This allows the acquisition of the RV/LV cross-sectional (short-axis) view. More anteflexion or slight withdrawal allows visualization of the mitral and tricuspid valves. Then, rotate the probe to 90° to acquire a two-chamber view of the left side. Clockwise rotation at 0° and 90° allows a focus on the right side.

Further advance the probe and rotate to 120°. This allows evaluation of the aortic valve and is the best TEE view for transaortic velocity measurement (the aorta is in a straight line with the Doppler signal).

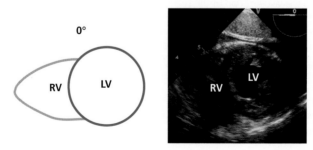

Figure 32.79 Short-axis 0° transgastric view, showing both the LV and RV.

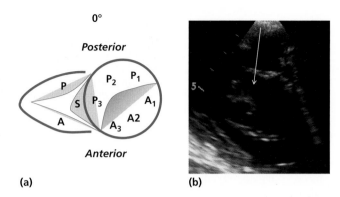

(a)

(b)

Figure 32.80 (a) Short-axis 0° transgastric view with more anteflexion than in Figure 32.79, allowing a focus on the mitral and tricuspid valves. The **ventricles/valves are seen in reverse compared with TTE, with the posterior leaflets appearing on top**. **(b)** Short-axis transgastric view, focusing on the tricuspid valve (*arrow*).

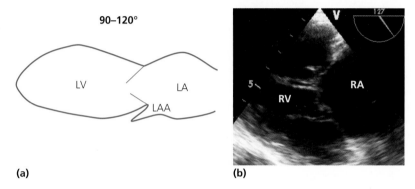

(a)

(b)

Figure 32.81 (a) Transgastric two-chamber view showing the LA–LV (90°). **(b)** Clockwise rotation from the LA–LV allows visualization of the RA–RV (right-sided two-chamber view).

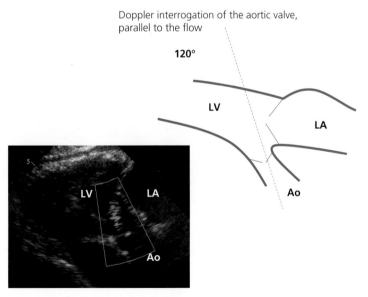

Figure 32.82 Transgastric long-axis view (120°) (deeper gastric level than Figure 32.81). This is often the only TEE view that allows measurement of the AS gradient.

H. Eighth step: aorta
(a) Ascending aorta
The ascending aorta is assessed through the transesophageal long-axis view (120°). From this view, the probe is progressively pulled up above the aortic valve, allowing visualization of the whole ascending aorta in a longitudinal plane. Also, a progressive pull from the aortic short-axis view (30°) allows visualization of the ascending aorta in an axial plane.

(b) Descending aorta

At a low transesophageal or transgastric level (0° rotation), the probe handle is flipped 180°, i.e., flipped on itself, until the circular descending aorta is seen. The descending aorta is then sequentially imaged on progressive pullback, until the longitudinal aortic arch is seen.

I. Advantages and indications of TEE

- TEE is mostly useful for: (a) determining the severity of MR, especially in acute cases or eccentric jets, and the mechanism of MR (determine if the leaflets/cusps are thickened, prolapsed or flail); (b) diagnosing mitral or aortic vegetations and the abscess complications of endocarditis; and (c) assessing mitral prostheses, and, less so, aortic prostheses.
- *TEE is complementary to TTE in native aortic valve disease, in MS, and in the assessment of tricuspid endocarditis.* For example, in *MS*, TTE is superior to TEE in defining the severity of subvalvular thickening, as the TEE best "sees" the LA rather than the LV side of the mitral valve. For *AI severity assessment*, TTE is as good as TEE; TEE is superior for defining the aortic valve structure (e.g., bicuspid, endocarditis). For *AS gradient calculation*, TTE is superior to TEE; in fact, obtaining AS gradient by TEE requires adequate transgastric views, which cannot be obtained in all patients. For *tricuspid endocarditis*, TTE and TEE may have similar diagnostic yield; however, TEE is superior in case of pacemaker leads or indwelling catheter.
- When endocarditis is suspected, perform a TTE first (TTE has a sensitivity of 60%). If TTE is negative and the clinical suspicion is not low, perform TEE.
- TEE is used to diagnose left atrial appendage thrombus before AF cardioversion.
- TEE allows the diagnosis of occult causes of stroke: PFO, atrial septal aneurysm, thoracic aorta plaques/thrombi. For PFO assessment, inject agitated saline intravenously and look for right-to-left shunting during the release phase of Valsalva, within 3–5 cardiac cycles of RA filling. If air bubbles are seen in the left chambers later than five cardiac cycles after reaching the RA, the shunt is at the pulmonary rather than the cardiac level.
- TEE is excellent for the diagnosis of aortic dissection type A or B.
- TEE may also be useful if the TTE windows are poor.

L. What is spontaneous echo contrast (SEC)?

Also called "smoke," it is seen on TEE in the left atrial appendage ± left atrium, and consists of increased blood echogenicity from red blood cell aggregation (not platelet aggregation). It is due to blood stasis and occurs under low-flow states, mainly AF. It is not a clot and is independent of the coagulation and platelet cascades, but is a strong predictor of thrombus formation and future thromboembolic events (risk of embolic events, 12% per year). SEC, per se, is not suppressed by antiplatelet or anticoagulant therapy. SEC may also occur in the absence of AF, in cases of cardiomyopathies with low flow and severely enlarged and dysfunctional LA.

Should "smoke" preclude DC cardioversion of AF? Not per se, but it should raise the suspicion of an associated thrombus. Heavy smoke and/or a severely depressed left atrial appendage emptying velocity (<25 cm/s [normal, > 40 cm/s]) may preclude DCCV if a clot cannot be definitely ruled out by TEE (i.e., look more carefully for clots in case of a heavy smoke).

M. Three-dimensional TEE of the mitral valve (see Figure 32.83)

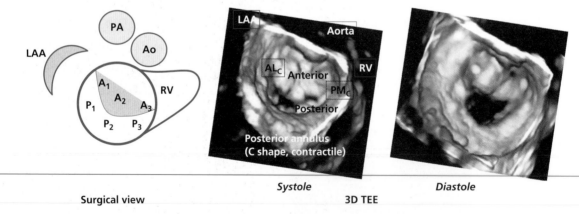

Figure 32.83 Three-dimensional TEE view of the mitral valve (en-face view). This view mimics the surgical view of the mitral valve, as the valve is inspected through the LA (left/right flip of Figure 32.63). For orientation, identify the anterior leaflet (leaflet with the convex border), the anterior annulus (flat), and the posterior annulus (C-shaped). The posterior annulus has a C shape, and is muscular and contractile. It contracts in systole and contributes to mitral valve competence, which explains how the annulus is narrower in systole than in diastole. There are two commissures: posteromedial (PM$_c$) and anterolateral (AL$_c$). Note the gap between A$_2$ and P$_2$ in systole, the source of MR.

Further reading

Nagueh SF, Appleton CP, Gillebert TC, et al. Recommendations for the evaluation of left ventricular diastolic function by echocardiography. J Am Soc Echocardiogr 2009; 22: 107–33 *(+ update in April 2016)*.

Zoghbi WA, Chambers JB, Dumesnil JG, et al. Recommendations for evaluation of prosthetic valves with echocardiography and Doppler ultrasound. J Am Soc Echocardiogr 2009; 22: 975–1014.

Lancelotti P, Moura L, Pierard LA, et al. European Association of Echocardiography recommendations for the assessment of valvular regurgitation. Eur J Echocardiogr 2010; 11: 307–32.

Lang RM, Badano LP, Mor-Avi V, et al. Recommendations for cardiac chamber quantification by echocardiography in adults. J Am Soc Echocardiogr 2015; 28: 1–39.

33 Stress Testing, Nuclear Imaging, Coronary CT Angiography

I. Indications for stress testing

Stress testing is indicated for diagnostic and, more importantly, prognostic evaluation of CAD. Its sensitivity is reduced in single-vessel CAD and in non-LAD disease.

A. Stable angina

1. Stress testing is useful for:
- The diagnostic and the prognostic assessment of patients with *intermediate CAD probability*
- The prognostic assessment of patients with *high CAD probability*

2. Stable angina is defined by three features: (1) chest pain or angina equivalent, (2) occurs with exertion or stress, and (3) resolves with rest or with NTG, within 30 seconds to 5 minutes.

3. The presence of all three features implies that angina is typical or definite. If only two features are present, angina is possible or atypical. Chest pain without any other feature is non-anginal pain. The combination of angina features, age, sex, and risk factors establishes the probability of CAD (Forrester and Duke classifications, combined in Table 33.1).

4. According to Bayes' theorem, stress testing is particularly useful in patients with an *intermediate pre-test probability* of CAD, in whom the stress test result significantly increases or reduces the probability of CAD.

If the *pre-test probability is high*, stress testing, regardless of the results, will only a have minor effect on the probability of CAD; thus, stress testing is not indicated for diagnostic purposes, but may be performed for prognostic purposes and for deciding if the patient will benefit from revascularization. Extensive ischemia warrants coronary angiography and revascularization, whereas medical therapy is an acceptable first-line option for a low- or intermediate-risk stress test.

If the *pre-test probability of CAD is low* (<15%), stress testing is often not needed. Even if the stress test is positive, the probability of CAD will only increase from <15% up to 20%, which means that the stress test is likely falsely positive. However, if judged necessary, stress ECG may be performed (class IIa).

> Stress testing of patients with low pre-test probability of CAD is the most common cause of a false-positive stress test. In fact, pre-test probability is the most important determinant of the validity of stress test results.

B. Low/intermediate-risk or low/intermediate-probability unstable angina (non-ischemic ECG, negative cardiac markers, and absence of a typical chest pain at rest or HF)

Perform stress testing at 6 hours after presentation.

C. Recent STEMI that was not urgently reperfused with PCI, whether thrombolysis was acutely administered or not

In the absence of angina recurrence or severe HF (conditions that would require a coronary angiogram), submaximal or symptom-limited stress testing may be performed at 4 days (before discharge) to see if there is any residual ischemia within or around the infarcted territory, whether reperfused or not, or in other areas.

Practical Cardiovascular Medicine, First Edition. Elias B. Hanna.
© 2017 John Wiley & Sons Ltd. Published 2017 by John Wiley & Sons Ltd.

Table 33.1 Clinical probability of CAD.

High probability of CAD (>85%)
- Typical angina in older patients (age ≥40 for men, ≥ 60 for women)
- Typical angina in patients with a combination of multiple risk factors (diabetes, smoking, hyperlipidemia, especially when all three are present)

Intermediate probability of CAD (15–85%)
- Typical angina in younger patients (age <40 for men, < 60 for women)
- Possible angina or non-anginal pain in older patients (age ≥40 for men, ≥ 60 for women) or in patients with multiple risk factors

Low probability of CAD (<15%)
- Possible angina in younger patients without a combination of multiple risk factors

---

D. Known CAD of borderline significance on the coronary angiogram (45–70% stenosis)

In this case, stress imaging may be performed *after* coronary angiography to determine if the stenosis is significant. A significant stenosis leads to ischemia in the correspondent territory on the echo or nuclear images. Alternatively, fractional flow reserve (FFR) may be performed during coronary angiography to determine whether the stenosis is significant.

II. Contraindications to all stress testing modalities

- Recent STEMI ≤ 2 days
- High-risk ACS (perform coronary angiogram)
- Active HF
- Severe AS; symptomatic HOCM
- Arrhythmias: uncontrolled AF, uncontrolled VT, second-degree Mobitz II or third-degree AV block
- HTN >180/110 mm Hg

Additional contraindication for adenosine nuclear testing: history of severe asthma or current, decompensated COPD.

Risk of death from stress testing is <1/10,000. Morbidity (MI, arrhythmias) is 5/10,000. The risk is greater when the test is performed in the early post-MI setting.

> Stress testing may be indicated after STEMI but is relatively contraindicated after NSTEMI, even a stabilized NSTEMI. In NSTEMI, the myocardial injury is small and most of the myocardium is ischemic rather than necrotic; revascularization is needed to prevent MI recurrence or progression to a large MI. Conversely, in non-reperfused STEMI, the territory may be fully infarcted already, and one has to prove ischemia by stress testing or angina recurrence before proceeding with revascularization.

> Carefully assess for AS and HOCM on physical exam, and perform an echo before stress testing if a suspicious murmur is heard. The contraindications to treadmill testing and the risks apply to pharmacological stress testing as well.

III. Stress testing modalities

Three stress testing modalities are available:

1. *Treadmill stress ECG*
2. *Treadmill stress imaging* (echo, nuclear). Echo assesses ischemia (exercise-induced hypokinesis), while ***nuclear imaging assesses the difference in coronary flow reserve*** between the area subtended by a stenosis and the areas subtended by non-obstructed coronary arteries.
3. *Pharmacological stress imaging* (echo, nuclear, MRI). Dobutamine, often with atropine, is used for stress echocardiography; adenosine is used to assess the difference in coronary flow reserve with nuclear imaging. Dobutamine may be used for nuclear imaging, but is less sensitive than adenosine in nuclear imaging. The cardiac workload is less with dobutamine than with exercise, and thus dobutamine echocardiography is also less sensitive than maximal exercise echocardiography or exercise nuclear imaging (See Appendix 1).

Since exercise achieves the highest cardiac workload and provides prognostic information independent of imaging (exercise time, symptoms, ECG response, BP response, and heart rate response), exercise stress testing is preferred to pharmacological testing. The selection of a stress test modality depends on three factors (Figure 33.1): (i) the patient's ability to walk; (ii) the presence of baseline ECG abnormalities that preclude ischemic assessment on stress ECG, mainly LBBB or resting ST-segment depression >1 mm; (iii) compelling indication for treadmill stress imaging (for its higher sensitivity and specificity), such as intermediate-to-high pre-test probability of CAD or prior revascularization.

> *In patients with LBBB or ventricular paced rhythm,* adenosine nuclear stress testing is classically the best testing modality, even if the patient is able to exercise. Exercise or dobutamine exaggerates the septal motion abnormality and the septal defect associated with LBBB, falsely suggesting ischemia (in LBBB, the septum contracts earlier with earlier interruption of diastolic blood flow than the remaining LV segments). However, exercise or dobutamine stress echo may be done and interpreted cautiously and correlates with angiographic findings; analyzing anterior and apical thickening rather than septal excursion improves the specificity.[1]

The Bruce treadmill protocol is the exercise protocol most commonly used. It consists of 3-minute stages, with an increase of speed and inclination at each stage (Table 33.2).

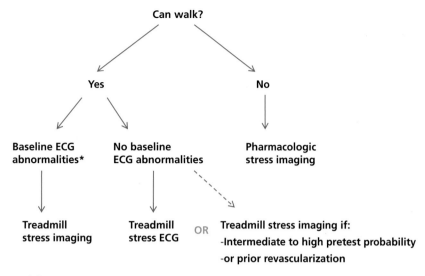

Figure 33.1 Stress testing modality.
Baseline ECG abnormalities precluding stress ECG interpretation:
- LBBB, paced rhythm, or non-specific intraventricular conduction delay ≥120 ms
- Any ST depression ≥1 mm
- LVH or digoxin therapy with any ST depression, even if <1 mm
- Pre-excitation (WPW)

These conditions will routinely have worsening of the ST depression during stress and during tachycardia, regardless of ischemia (false-positive result).
Other ECG abnormalities and clinical situations:
- RBBB or resting ST depression <1 mm ↓ specificity of stress ECG but do not preclude interpretation.
- LVH without any resting ST depression: stress ECG remains reasonably specific for ischemia.
- AF: patients may become quickly tachycardic or may not increase their heart rate enough if they are on rate-controlling medications. Exercise testing, is, however, appropriate and assesses the adequacy of rate control.
- History of PCI or CABG: stress imaging is preferred to stress ECG. Stress ECG is less sensitive in this context and cannot localize ischemia. Stress ECG is poorly sensitive for the diagnosis of single-vessel restenosis.

Table 33.2 Standard Bruce treadmill protocol.

Stage	Inclination (°)	Speed (mph)	MET
1	10	1.7	5
2	12	2.5	7
3	14	3.4	10
4	16	4.2	13
5	18	5	16

In patients who are not able to cope with the workload of a standard Bruce protocol (e.g., elderly, weak), a **modified Bruce protocol** may be performed. Stages 1, 2, and 3 of the modified Bruce protocol consist of an inclination of 0, 5, and 10° respectively, for a speed of 1.7 mph. Thus, stage 3 of the modified Bruce protocol is equivalent to stage 1 of the Bruce protocol. The energy expenditure achieved with the modified Bruce protocol is much lower than the energy expenditure of the standard Bruce protocol. A modified Bruce protocol is also called "submaximal stress testing."

The metabolic equivalent (MET) corresponds to the energy expenditure for an activity level. The reference, 1 MET, is the resting metabolic rate obtained during quiet sitting and corresponds to the consumption of 3.5 ml/kg/min of O_2. METs and O_2 consumption increase with the peak exercise achieved.

IV. Results
A. Diagnostic yield of exercise stress ECG
For the exercise stress ECG or imaging to be valid, the patient should:

1. Reach target HR, which is 85% of the maximal HR (=85% of [220 − age])
   and
   Achieve a good workload ≥6–7 METs, which means finish 5 minutes of the Bruce protocol.
2. Or attain high-risk criteria before this goal.

A sufficient workload is necessary to produce ischemia or nuclear hypoperfusion in the presence of a hemodynamically significant CAD. Otherwise, the test is less sensitive, and pharmacologic stress imaging should be performed. *Note, however, that with exercise stress imaging the sensitivity is still acceptable if the patient partially achieves the heart rate or workload goals, because stress imaging is more sensitive*

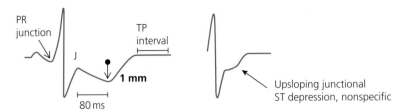

Figure 33.2 During sinus tachycardia, atrial repolarization becomes accentuated and extends over the ST segment, leading to PR depression + junctional ST depression. Referencing the ST segment to the PR junction accounts for the effect of atrial repolarization.

than stress ECG. One study suggested that even with stress ECG, a negative test at a submaximal heart rate was still predictive of a low event risk if ≥7 METs are achieved.[2]

Achieving the appropriate heart rate is even more important with dobutamine stress echocardiography than exercise stress echocardiography, as dobutamine induces less cardiac workload and thus less ischemia than exercise.

B. Positive stress ECG

A positive stress ECG is defined as descendant (downsloping) or horizontal ST depression ≥1 mm measured at 60–80 ms past the J point, during exercise or within 3 minutes of recovery in at least one lead. While ST displacement should generally be measured relative to the TP segment, PQ or PR junction is chosen as the isoelectric point during exercise (Figure 33.2). If baseline ST depression is present, the exertional worsening of ST depression, rather than the absolute ST depression during exercise, is used to assess ischemia. If baseline ST elevation is present, exertional ST depression is measured in absolute values.

The lateral precordial leads (especially V_5) are the most specific and most sensitive for exercise-induced ischemia. Isolated inferior changes are less specific and are often a false-positive result.

ST depression occurring during exercise usually persists ≥3 minutes into recovery.[3] If it does not, the ST depression is considered less specific; in particular, quick recovery of ST depression in <1 minute was predictive of a low risk of cardiac events and CAD, as low as a negative ECG result.[2]

About 10% of patients develop the diagnostic ST depression only during recovery, most typically and most specifically *during the first 3 minutes of recovery,*[3] sometimes preceded by equivocal or upsloping ST depression at peak exercise. *This recovery-only ST depression is as predictive of CAD and coronary events as ST depression that starts at peak exercise.*[4]

Upsloping ST depression or T-wave changes are non-diagnostic.

Notes
- ST depression does not localize ischemia, and often occurs in V_5 regardless whether ischemia is anterior or inferior.
- T-wave inversion is not specific. Normalization of an inverted T wave during exertion may be a true normalization of a non-specific T abnormality or an ischemic pseudo-normalization (less frequent).
- ST elevation in areas without prior Q waves indicates a local transmural myocardial ischemia, implying either a very tight stenosis or exercise-induced spasm (high-risk finding). ST elevation localizes ischemia.
  ST elevation in areas with baseline Q waves does not mean active ischemia, but indicates greater dysfunction of the infarcted myocardium (possible dyskinesis) and a worse prognosis.
- The occurrence of LBBB or RBBB does not necessarily mean ischemia; it is frequently rate-related and not specific for ischemia. Stress testing may be interrupted if one cannot be sure the wide complex rhythm is sinus (vs. VT).
- Normally, during exercise, the QRS axis becomes more vertical as the heart empties. The paradoxical occurrence of left axis or LAFB is very specific for ischemia. Also, the occurrence of a full right axis (LPFB) implies ischemia.
- Chest pain without ECG changes does not necessarily make the stress test positive. A typical and limiting angina, i.e., chest pain that starts during testing and resolves with rest or within 5 minutes of NTG, should be noted and dictates stress imaging or coronary angiography, particularly if associated with distress or diaphoresis. In fact, even with a normal ST response, a typical angina is almost as predictive of coronary events and CAD as an abnormal ST response, especially in men.[2] 10% of CAD patients have chest pain during stress testing without ST changes.

C. High-risk positive stress ECG (see Table 33.3)

In general, 40% of Duke Treadmill Score (DTS) results fall in the low-risk category (no further testing is needed), 10% fall in the high-risk category (indication for a coronary angiogram), and 50% fall in the intermediate-risk category, where stress imaging may need to be performed to further delineate the risk.[6]

DTS score is not well validated in elderly patients and in patients with a history of coronary revascularization. DTS has a strong independent prognostic value that is additional to that provided by coronary anatomy, EF, and history of CAD/MI. The original analysis that validated DTS included patients with MI (~30% of patients had prior MI) but excluded patients with prior revascularization; most patients were <65 years of age. An analysis from the GISSI trial also validated DTS in post-MI patients.

Table 33.3 High-risk stress ECG and Duke Treadmill Score (DTS).

1. Early ST depression or severe angina at stages 1 or 2 (at <6 minutes)
2. ST depression ≥2 mm, especially if more than five leads
3. ST elevation in leads without prior Q waves (→ signifies transmural ischemia, very high risk)
4. Sustained reduction of SBP >10 mmHg in comparison with the baseline, inability to increase SBP beyond the baseline with progressive exercise
5. Arrhythmias:
  • Sustained VT
  • Non-sustained VT or complex PVCs (couplets, triplets, polymorphic) associated with other ischemic signs[a]
6. Heart rate:
  • A decrease in HR of <12 bpm in the first minute of recovery is a strong predictor of cardiovascular mortality (implies lack of vagal reactivation soon after exercise)
  • Inability to achieve 85% of maximal heart rate (chronotropic incompetence) not only reduces stress test sensitivity, but also implies an increased mortality (because of autonomic dysfunction *and* an association with twice the risk of CAD and perfusion defects).[5] A similar prognostic value is found for a low chronotropic reserve index: (peak HR − resting HR)/([220-age] − resting HR) (low if <0.8, or <0.62 if on β-blockers)

Duke Treadmill Score [b]
= Exercise time on Bruce protocol − 5 × (the most severe ST depression) − 4 × (angina score)
  • Score ≥+5: Low cardiovascular risk (<1% mortality and cardiac events per year)
  • Score +4 to −10: Intermediate cardiovascular risk (1–3% mortality, 1–5% cardiac events per year)
  • Score ≤ −11: High cardiovascular risk (>3% mortality, > 5% cardiac events per year)

[a] Exercise-induced NSVT or complex PVCs portend an increased mortality in the case of underlying CAD or associated ischemic ST changes. In the absence of ischemic signs, VT may be a form of idiopathic VT initiated by exercise (e.g., RVOT VT), ARVD, or may in fact be SVT with rate-related bundle branch block. Post-exertional frequent PVCs, on the other hand, portend a stronger prognostic value than exertional PVCs, as they imply a lack of vagal reactivation soon after exercise.
[b] Exercise time is the time spent on a standard rather than modified Bruce protocol; 9 minutes on a modified Bruce protocol does not give a score of 9, but is equivalent to 3–4 minutes on a standard Bruce protocol. Angina score is 0 if no angina, 1 if non-exercise-limiting angina, 2 if exercise-limiting angina

Note: blood pressure response during exercise

Normally, SBP increases with exercise (high stroke volume) while DBP remains unchanged or decreases (vasodilatation). SBP may decrease during progressive exercise after an initial peaking from the catecholaminergic surge, but it does not decrease below baseline.

Exertional hypotension may be due to:

• Extensive ischemia.
• Cardiomyopathy: the lack of contractile reserve in systolic HF, or the lack of filling reserve in diastolic HF, prevents the increase in stroke volume. If cardiac output cannot increase and fill the dilated systemic space induced by exercise, BP decreases (BP = [CO × SVR]: if SVR ↓ but CO cannot ↑, BP ↓).
• AS or HOCM: LVOT obstruction prevents the exertional increase in stroke volume.
• Hypovolemia or antihypertensive drugs.

On the other hand, **post-exertional hypotension** is usually benign and is related to the sudden reduction of venous return and cardiac output while the systemic space is still dilated; also, the empty, hypercontractile ventricle may trigger a vasovagal response. Post-exertional hypotension may also be seen with severe AS or HOCM upon sudden cessation of activity (i.e., sudden decrease in venous return, AS and HOCM being very sensitive to preload reduction).

In hypovolemic patients, dobutamine may induce hypotension as it vasodilates without being able to increase the stroke volume (limited preload); it may also induce LVOT obstruction.

An increase in SBP to >214 mmHg, or an increase in DBP, may imply abnormal systemic vasoreactivity and a risk of future HTN.

D. Limitations of DTS and exercise stress ECG: value of stress imaging

Exercise stress ECG has a low sensitivity for CAD detection, especially in patients with single-vessel non-LAD disease. While it is more sensitive in patients with more extensive CAD, a significant proportion of these patients is still missed. In the Duke stress testing database of *symptomatic* patients, *most of whom had definite or possible angina* (two or three angina features), a low-risk DTS was still associated with a ~10% risk of left main and/or three-vessel CAD, and a ~10% risk of two-vessel or proximal LAD disease.[6] Thus, **a high-risk subgroup is concealed within the low DTS group and is often picked up by nuclear imaging.**[7–9] Also, ~12% and 55% of patients with three-vessel CAD had a low and intermediate DTS score, respectively. However, a very low-risk DTS with over 10 METs of exercise capacity (8 minutes of Bruce protocol) and no ST depression has been associated with an extremely low prevalence of moderate or severe ischemia on nuclear imaging (<2%).[10]

Importantly, the high-risk DTS had a definitive diagnostic value, with a 99% risk of significant CAD (slightly less in women), and a 75% risk of left main or three-vessel CAD.[6]

Thus, while DTS has a good prognostic value, a low-risk DTS does not exclude CAD and, *depending on the pre-test clinical probability and risk,* may conceal some high-risk subgroups. Those high-risk subgroups are often picked up by stress imaging. This explains why stress imaging may be the preferred testing modality in patients with intermediate to high pre-test probability (to avoid missing CAD, especially high-risk CAD).[8] *In patients with a low or intermediate pre-test probability, stress ECG is an appropriate and preferred test in light of its high negative predictive value in these subgroups.*[5] *Also, a very low-risk DTS of >+8, as opposed to a low-risk DTS of 5–8, is associated with a very low prevalence of moderate or severe ischemia, obviating the need for stress imaging.*[10]

Table 33.4 Sensitivity and specificity of various stress tests

Test	Sensitivity	Specificity
Stress ECG	65%	70% (lower in women)
Stress echo	75–80% (lower with dobutamine)	85%
Stress nuclear	80–85%	70% (lower in women)

For all these tests, the sensitivity is higher in left main or three-vessel CAD. Also, the prognostic value is superior to the diagnostic value.

In addition to sensitivity, stress ECG has specificity limitations, particularly in women. In *symptomatic* patients, ST depression has a good positive predictive value of ~75% in men, but only ~50% in women.[11] In fact, exertional ST depression is common in women in general, including *asymptomatic* women. In asymptomatic women, ST depression is encountered on ~5% of stress tests and does not, per se, affect the long-term prognosis, even when ST is depressed >2 mm.[12–14] This is particularly related to the lower pre-test probability, but also the higher prevalence of microvascular dysfunction in women, and a digoxin-like effect of estrogen on the ECG. Conversely, DTS and exercise parameters maintain a prognostic value in women similar to that in men. **ST depression retains a prognostic and diagnostic value in *symptomatic women with an intermediate to high pre-test probability*.**

Stress imaging has a stronger *diagnostic and prognostic value* than stress ECG. It has a higher sensitivity than stress ECG, and similar specificity (stress nuclear) or higher specificity (stress echo) (Table 33.4). It picks up the false-negative stress ECG and the significant CAD in ~20% of patients with low-risk DTS;[6–9] also, in intermediate-risk DTS, it better delineates the patient's risk as low or high.[7] On the other hand, in patients with abnormal ECG response, a normal stress imaging usually overrules the result of the stress ECG.[7] Even in patients with a markedly positive exercise ECG (≥2 mm ST depression), a normal stress echo or nuclear scan usually implies a low risk.[15–17] The following exceptions apply:
- A high-risk DTS is always high risk, regardless of imaging results.[6]
- An abnormal ST-segment or chest pain response with a normal stress imaging is usually a low-risk stress test. However, *if the patient's pre-test probability of CAD is high*, the abnormal ECG or chest pain response may dictate coronary angiography even if imaging is normal. Nuclear stress testing may miss multivessel disease because of balanced ischemia; exercise stress echo may miss an ischemic response if imaging is performed after the patient's heart rate has already declined; and dobutamine stress echo has reduced sensitivity because of its inherently lower workload. In a patient with *intermediate-to-high clinical probability of CAD*, ECG, chest pain, BP, and exercise parameters may pick up those imaging pitfalls. The assessment of both ECG and imaging responses improves the sensitivity of the study in a patient with a high pre-test probability. When both ECG and imaging are abnormal, the specificity is boosted.

In sum, a normal stress imaging or a low-risk stress ECG is associated with <1% risk of cardiac events per year for the next 2 years ("warranty period" of 2 years).[6,7,18] Within this low-risk population, a high-risk subgroup exists and is captured using pre-test clinical probability of CAD and a combination of ECG, imaging, and exercise parameters. *For all these tests, the sensitivity is higher in left main or three-vessel CAD. Also, the prognostic value is superior to the diagnostic value.*

E. Stress echocardiography
Normally, the myocardial segments become hypercontractile with stress, meaning the myocardial *thickening* and *excursion* increase with stress. An ischemic response is characterized not only by a lack of hyperkinesis, but by a paradoxical worsening of contraction in comparison to baseline: a normal myocardial segment at rest becomes hypokinetic or akinetic with stress, a hypokinetic segment becomes akinetic or dyskinetic. The change from akinesis to dyskinesis is the only deterioration that does not, by itself, imply ischemia. Also, isolated hypokinesis of the inferobasal or inferoseptal segments is frequently seen in normal individuals and is not diagnostic of ischemia.

Two other responses are taken into account but are less specific for ischemia (their value depends on the pre-test probability of CAD):

i. Lack of hypercontractile response. This may be related to ischemia, but is often related to inappropriate workload, severe HTN, underlying cardiomyopathy, imaging in early recovery after heart rate has declined, prior β-blocker therapy, or older age.

ii. Tardokinesis of a myocardial segment, meaning delayed contraction of a segment.

The following cases scenarios complicate ischemic assessment with stress echo:

i. Baseline hypokinesis: ischemia may manifest as worsening of hypokinesis or extension of hypokinesis to adjacent segments. However, this adjacent hypokinesis may be missed if the adjacent segments are tethered by the normal myocardium, or it may be overcalled if the adjacent segments are tethered by the dysfunctional myocardium. Nuclear testing is preferred in patients with baseline wall motion abnormality because of its higher sensitivity.

ii. LBBB or abnormal postoperative septal motion: the assessment of myocardial thickening, rather than excursion, of the anterior wall and apex provides appropriate diagnostic yield.[1,19]

F. Nuclear myocardial perfusion imaging (MPI), using single photon emission computed tomography (SPECT) (see also Appendices 1 and 2)

While having an excellent prognostic value, superior to stress ECG and overruling low or intermediate stress ECG results, SPECT MPI is flawed by a small but significant risk of missing multivessel disease. **The brightness of the nuclear uptake is not an absolute radioactive count, it is comparative to the pixel with the highest radioactive count:** resting segments are compared to other resting segments, while stress segments are compared to other stress segments. This means that in **diffuse balanced ischemia**, in which all the myocardium is equally ischemic (severe triple-vessel CAD), nuclear counts are equally low, which makes all pixels appear bright and the images appear normal. This rarely occurs, as one area is usually more ischemic than the others. **The more common caveat is that only one area looks ischemic, while the others look normal despite being ischemic.** Thus, nuclear testing may miss assessing the true extent of ischemia in multivessel disease. A patient with severe LAD stenosis, but more severe RCA stenosis, may appear to have only an inferior defect, because the anterior wall is less ischemic and may thus look bright.

In one study, despite angiographically severe three-vessel CAD, SPECT MPI showed no defect in 18% of patients and a single-vessel disease pattern in 36% of patients.[20] A nuclear substudy of the FAME trial found that in patients with angiographic multivessel disease, ~50% of vessels with FFR <0.80 were not identified on nuclear imaging, and 34% of patients with ischemia by FFR had a negative nuclear scan.[21] Thus, in multivessel disease, the lack of defect in one territory on nuclear imaging does not imply the lack of ischemia in that territory, and a completely normal scan is not uncommon. A high pre-test probability of CAD, chest pain during exercise testing, abnormal ECG or BP response, transient ischemic dilatation (TID), and EF on gated SPECT allow the diagnosis.

TID is the ratio of LV volume at stress compared to rest, the LV volume used being time-averaged from both systole and diastole using the non-gated perfusion images (ECG-gated LV volumes may be used with more weight provided for the systolic volume than the diastolic volume).[22,23] A post-exertional TID (ratio >1.2) proved highly specific (95%) for severe and extensive CAD, with a higher sensitivity than perfusion imaging in extensive CAD (71% vs. 33%).[22]

> While a falsely negative stress ECG is "bailed out" by stress imaging, a falsely normal nuclear scan may be bailed out by TID or by the stress ECG portion. Those situations are suspected in patients with a high pre-test probability of disease.

Nuclear imaging also has specificity issues. Soft tissue attenuation may create the impression of fixed or sometimes partially reversible defects, i.e., defects that are present at rest and worsen with stress. Classically, an inferior artifact related to diaphragmatic attenuation is seen in men, while an anterior defect related to breast attenuation is the dominant artifact in women. As the soft tissue moves between rest and stress, the attenuation artifact may vary between rest and stress and mimic a reversible defect. Alternatively, true ischemia in a territory that has an attenuation artifact may be difficult to diagnose (the change in defect severity between stress and rest may be missed).

> A fixed defect may signify any of the following:
>
> **i.** Attenuation artifact. The attenuation artifact is associated with normal wall motion on gated SPECT imaging *and* is usually mild (>50–60% nuclear uptake).
> **ii.** Myocardial scar.
> **iii.** Hibernating myocardium.
>
> Both scar and hibernation are associated with abnormal wall motion on SPECT imaging. The defect is usually mild/moderate in hibernation, vs. severe in scar (<50% nuclear uptake in scar). Thus, a fixed defect with a wall motion abnormality is not necessarily a scar, and may represent a hibernating, ischemic myocardium, especially in the absence of Q waves or akinesis, or if the defect is not severe. In one study, 75% of fixed defects without Q waves reversed with revascularization. A coronary angiogram is therefore indicated when a large, fixed defect is associated with angina, HF, or low EF. Most of those fixed defects normalize after revascularization.[24] In the COURAGE trial, rest defects improved with PCI and medical therapy, again implying hibernation.

In general, however, when it is not associated with severe symptoms or reduced EF, a fixed defect, even if real (e.g., patients with prior MI), does not imply an increased cardiac risk in comparison to a normal scan, as the fixed defect is mostly a small scar with appropriate LV compensation.[25–27]

In comparison with stress echo, nuclear imaging has the advantage of a higher sensitivity, particularly in: (i) single vessel disease; (ii) patients with underlying myocardial wall motion abnormalities; (iii) poor echo windows. Stress echo has the advantage of a higher specificity, especially in women prone to breast attenuation artifact on nuclear imaging and ST depression on stress ECG.

Note: value of the ECG during pharmacological stress testing

ST changes that occur with dobutamine should be taken into account and may imply ischemia; however, the sensitivity and specificity are less than those of the imaging part of the test. ST depression with adenosine is uncommon, because adenosine does not usually induce ischemia; however, when ST depression occurs (in ~1–2% of tests), it implies severe CAD with vasodilator-induced steal from the diseased coronary artery. Thus, ST depression induced by adenosine is insensitive but is very specific for CAD (even more so than ST depression induced by exercise) and has a strong prognostic implication.

G. Use of antianginal agents before stress testing

These agents prolong the time to onset of ST depression, increase the exercise tolerance, and may normalize the ECG or the images. Also, β-blockers prevent the heart rate from achieving the target. Thus, if possible, the last dose of β-blocker and other antianginal agents is held before stress testing.

On the other hand, stress testing may be performed under maximal medical and β-blocker therapy to assess the effectiveness of medical therapy and the prognosis under medical therapy. In fact, when treatment fails to reduce ischemia by >5%, or when residual defects involve >10% of the myocardium, the coronary event risk is high and warrants revascularization (COURAGE nuclear substudy).

In general, in patients without a history of CAD who are referred for diagnostic evaluation of a possible angina, the last dose of antianginal drug(s) is withheld before the test to increase its *diagnostic yield*. In patients with known CAD who are referred for a change in symptoms, stress testing may be performed on the current antianginal therapy to assess for residual ischemia despite medical therapy, and thus the *residual prognosis*.

A summary of high-risk stress test features and risk stratification is provided in Table 33.5. Indications to stop a stress test are provided in Table 33.6. General factors that affect the sensitivity and specificity of stress testing are provided in Table 33.7.

Table 33.5 Risk stratification with stress testing.

High risk: cardiac mortality >3%/year, cardiac events >5%/year
- DTS ≤ −11
- Reversible large and/or severe perfusion defect (summed stress score >+8, corresponding to ischemia involving >10% of the myocardium)[a]
- Fixed large or severe perfusion defect with LV dilatation/low EF
- Rest- or stress-induced LV dysfunction with EF ≤ 35%, even if the defect appears mild or moderate
- On stress echo: ischemia of ≥3 segments (out of 17), or >one coronary distribution, especially if it occurs at a low rate <120 bpm or a low dose of dobutamine (≤10 mcg/kg/min)

Intermediate risk: cardiac mortality 1–3%/year, cardiac events 1–5%/year
- DTS −10 to +4
- Summed stress score 4–8

Low-risk: cardiac mortality and cardiac events <1%/year (~0.5% with stress imaging). Warranty period ~2 years
- DTS ≥+5 (≥ +8 is very low risk)
- No perfusion defect or small perfusion defect with a summed stress score <4

---

[a]On nuclear imaging, the myocardium is divided into 20 segments. Each segment is given a score of 0 (no defect) to +4 (very severe defect, < 25% nuclear uptake) at stress. The summed stress score is obtained by adding the scores of all segments with defects. Since the maximum summed score is 80 rather than 100, the summed score is multiplied by 1.25 to obtain the percent of myocardium at risk.

Table 33.6 Indications to stop the stress test.

---

1. Achievement of high-risk criteria (severe ST ↓ ≥3 mm, ST ↑, sustained VT, ↓ SBP >10 mmHg below baseline)
2. Occurrence of some arrhythmias that do not necessarily make the test positive for ischemia but mandate interruption of the test (relative indication): ventricular triplet or NSVT, SVT or AF with a fast rate, high-degree AV block
3. Severe chest pain or chest pain accompanied by high-risk criteria
4. HTN (>250/120 mm Hg)
5. Severe dyspnea/cyanosis/ataxia

In the absence of the preceding, do not simply stop the stress test if the target heart rate is achieved; the patient needs to achieve a good workload

---

Table 33.7 Factors that reduce the sensitivity and specificity of any stress testing modality.

Reduced specificity
- *Low pre-test probability (<10–20%): this is, by far, the most common cause of a false-positive stress test*
- Abnormal baseline ECG, LVH
- Severe acute or chronic HTN can lead to ischemic signs on ECG/imaging even without CAD
- Any cardiomyopathy
- Anemia, hypokalemia, mitral valve prolapse
- AF, SVT
- Female sex (partly because of the lower pre-test probability in women, and because women more commonly have microvascular spasm)

Reduced sensitivity
- Poor workload
- Single-vessel, low-risk CAD
- Use of antianginal agents

Appendix 1. Mechanisms of various stress modalities

Exercise or dobutamine effect on ECG and echo

Exercise and dobutamine elicit ischemia by increasing myocardial demands, which translates into ST depression on ECG and hypokinesis on echo. Dobutamine increases inotropism and chronotropism, but reduces LV diastolic volume (preload); conversely, exercise increases preload, and thus, the cardiac workload is higher with exercise than with dobutamine. Hence, dobutamine is less sensitive than a maximal exercise echocardiogram.

Exercise or dobutamine effect on nuclear imaging

The increased myocardial demand elicits coronary microvascular dilatation, which increases the coronary flow by 4–5 times in normal coronary arteries. A flow-limiting coronary stenosis limits the increase in coronary flow; therefore, on nuclear perfusion imaging, areas with significant stenosis light up much less with stress than stenotic areas.

> While ECG and echo detect ischemia, nuclear imaging detects the disparities in coronary flow induced by exercise or dobutamine.

Adenosine effect on nuclear and MRI perfusion imaging

Adenosine often assesses CAD without eliciting ischemia. Adenosine vasodilates the coronary microvasculature and, similarly to exercise, increases coronary flow differentially between areas subtended by a stenosis and those that are not; areas with significant stenosis light up much less with adenosine than stenotic areas. *The same differential flow effect is detected by MRI perfusion imaging.* Since this occurs without an increase in O_2 demands, the difference in coronary flow reserve is detected on nuclear or MRI flow imaging even without inducing ischemia or ECG changes (the patient being at rest, a lack of increase of coronary flow in the stenotic artery does not translate into ischemia). This is also why adenosine echo is not a sensitive test for CAD. Adenosine may, however, induce ischemia and ECG changes by inducing a coronary steal and by reducing the perfusing pressure past a critical stenosis (the flow cannot increase enough to match the vasodilated microcirculation). This signals a worse stenosis and prognosis. Adenosine increases coronary flow at least as much as exercise, and thus adenosine nuclear imaging is at least as sensitive as exercise nuclear imaging and more sensitive than dobutamine imaging. The prognostic value of exercise nuclear imaging is, however, superior to adenosine nuclear imaging, as exercise parameters are strong prognostic markers.

Regadenoson (Lexiscan) is more selective for adenosine α_{2a} receptor and has fewer side effects, including less risk of bronchospasm. It is administered as a bolus, and has a 2–3-minute half-life.

> Depending on its severity, ischemia induces the following sequence:
>
> Impaired perfusion (seen on nuclear stress testing) → abnormal diastolic function → abnormal systolic function (seen on stress echo) → abnormal ECG (seen on stress ECG) → angina
>
> This explains the difference in sensitivity between various tests. The abnormal contractility seen on echo develops ~20 seconds after ischemia, and resolves ~25–30 seconds after resolution of ischemia. This explains why delayed echocardiographic imaging after peak exercise may miss wall motion abnormalities.

Appendix 2. Nuclear stress imaging (see Figures 33.3, 33.4, 33.5)

Nuclear stress testing is usually performed using **SPECT imaging** and SPECT tracers, but may be performed with positron emission tomography (PET) imaging and PET tracers, such as rubidium and nitrogen. **PET has a higher resolution than SPECT (less artifacts) and while the obtained images are relative perfusion images (like SPECT), PET can provide an absolute quantification of myocardial flow.** Absolute flow measurement by PET, and the calculation of stress/rest flow ratio, may circumvent the problem of balanced ischemia. Nuclear imaging has resting and stress parts. Nuclear agent injections at rest and stress can be done the same day if the patient is not obese; otherwise, a 2-day technetium test is required.

Two nuclear isotopes may be used for SPECT: technetium and thallium. The **technetium** carrier (e.g., sestamibi, Myoview) is taken up by the mitochondria of myocardial cells and does not redistribute out of the cells; technetium rather decays inside those cells, within 24 hours. A higher-dose injection during the second part of the study (i.e., stress) is therefore necessary to identify stress defects if the rest study was performed the same day.

- For 1-day technetium studies: first injected dose = 10 mCi; second injected dose, ~2 hours later = 30 mCi. A "rest–stress" or "stress–rest" sequence may be performed, but *rest–stress is preferred as it provides a true rest study* and prevents the contamination of rest images with the previously taken stress images, increasing the ability to detect reversibility. In the stress–rest sequence, a stress-induced defect may falsely persist onto the rest images and look partially fixed.
- For 2-day technetium studies: inject 30 mCi each time. A dual-isotope technique may be used: thallium at rest, then technetium at stress 4 hours later. Two-day studies are indicated for obese patients, as thallium or a 10 mCi dose of technetium may not allow good image acquisition.

Thallium is extracted by the myocardial cells, similarly to potassium, and quickly starts to redistribute out of the cells 10–15 minutes later. It has a long physical half-life (73 hours) but a short stay in the myocardium. Thallium uptake is reduced in ischemia but its redistribution becomes slower, in such a way that 3–4 hours later the nuclear concentration should be equal in ischemic and non-ischemic territories; in stress-induced ischemia, images taken 4 hours post-stress will show redistribution and reversibility of a defect that was present at stress.

A defect that is present during stress only is a reversible, ischemic defect. An infarcted, non-viable myocardium, and sometimes a hibernating or stunned myocardium, have a low nuclear uptake at stress and rest (fixed defect). A severely reduced nuclear uptake at rest, i.e., < 50% uptake in comparison to a reference region, is more likely a non-viable infarction than hibernation.

Technetium has a shorter half-life than thallium, and thus higher doses than thallium can be used. In addition, the photon energy of technetium is higher (140 keV vs. 80 keV). For these reasons, *technetium provides better-quality images with fewer artifacts, even more so in obese patients.*

Also, **nuclear SPECT gated to the ECG** may be used to compare myocardial counts in systole and diastole (myocardial brightening in systole corresponds to myocardial thickening), and to define endocardial excursion between systole and diastole. This allows EF calculation and is usually done on the post-stress images, usually with technetium studies (because technetium provides higher nuclear counts); it may be done at rest as well, for comparison of rest and stress EF and LV systolic volumes. A striking difference between echo and nuclear

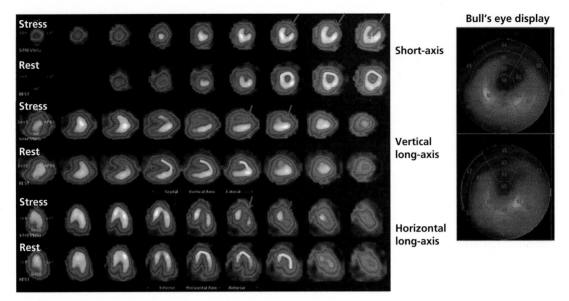

Figure 33.3 Nuclear images are displayed in three views:
- *Short-axis cuts* going from the apex to the base
- *Vertical long-axis cuts* (VLA cuts): similar to the echocardiographic apical two-chamber cuts, these cuts show the anterior and inferior walls, going septal to lateral.
- *Horizontal long-axis cuts* (HLA cuts): similar to the apical four-chamber cuts, these cuts show the septal and lateral LV walls, going anterior to inferior.

The upper images of each series are the stress images, the lower images are the rest images. A defect of the anterior wall (*arrows*) is visible on the short axis, HLA, and VLA views, extending from the base of the anterior wall to the apex. This defect is largely reversible and suggests anterior ischemia. A "bull's eye" map displays the myocardium in a two-dimensional plot, the center being the apex, the contour being the base.

Beware of attenuation artifacts: diaphragmatic attenuation of the inferior wall leading to a false, fixed inferior defect, breast attenuation of the anterior wall leading to a fixed anterior defect, and artifacts related to extracardiac tracer activity (bowel or liver uptake will look bright and will attenuate the counts of the inferior wall at stress and/or at rest). A true fixed defect should lead to regional wall motion abnormalities (infarct or hibernation). If gated SPECT does not show any wall motion abnormality, the defect is likely an attenuation artifact. Conversely, a defect that is severe (<50% nuclear uptake) is usually a true defect. Occasionally, breast attenuation may be associated with an anterior defect that is partially reversible, as the breast moves between rest and stress imaging, therefore reducing the specificity of any anterior defect in women.

Note that **the color intensity and brightness is comparative to the pixel with the highest radioactive count** (rest pixels are compared to each other; stress pixels are compared to each other, not to the rest pixels). It is not an absolute radioactive count. This means that in **diffuse balanced ischemia**, in which all the myocardium is equally ischemic, the images may look normal, as nuclear counts are equally low and all pixels appear bright. This rarely occurs, as one area is usually more ischemic than the others. **The more common caveat is that only one area looks ischemic, while the others look normal despite being ischemic.** Thus, nuclear testing may underestimate the true extent of ischemia in multivessel disease. A patient with severe LAD stenosis, but more severe RCA stenosis or inferior scar, may only have inferior defect, because the anterior wall has better nuclear uptake and thus may look bright. Looking at some extra high-risk features can compensate for this: LV dilatation on the perfusion stress images (called *transient ischemic dilatation* [TID]), which is a sign of diffuse ischemia with stress. TID index >1.15 (115%) with exercise or >1.35 with adenosine is significant. TID is not always seen even with severe ischemia, as the images are taken 15–30 minutes post-stress, giving time for the myocardium to recover its function. Another sign of severity is *lung nuclear uptake*, seen when imaging is performed 10–15 minutes post-stress, mainly with thallium; lung uptake is a sign of increased pulmonary capillary pressure with exercise, related to severe ischemia with exercise or to LV dysfunction. While the RV may be normally visualized by increasing the gain, *transient RV visualization* on stress images without gain change is a sign of severe ischemia.

assessment of EF may be due to error in gating, such as gating the cardiac cycle from R to T rather than from R to R, or a flat QRS that prevents appropriate R-to-R gating. Also, poor gating may occur when the R-to-R cycle is strikingly variable, as in AF.

With technetium, the images are taken 60 minutes after rest or adenosine stress, and 15–30 minutes after exercise stress. This waiting time allows clearance of the liver/GI uptake, this uptake being lower during exercise (less GI diversion of the cardiac output). With thallium, since it redistributes quickly, images are taken 10–15 minutes after exercise, then 4 hours later to assess the redistribution. The perfusion images are reflective of the nuclear uptake at the time of injection, not at the restful time of imaging, as the nuclear agents do not redistribute during this short period of time. However, the myocardial contractility and excursion are reflective of the myocardial function at the time of imaging (EF obtained is a post-stress EF).

If the patient is unable to walk, stress testing may be performed with adenosine or dobutamine. Adenosine (or regadenoson) testing increases coronary flow at least as much as exercise, and thus adenosine testing is at least as sensitive as treadmill nuclear imaging, and is more sensitive than dobutamine nuclear imaging. The latter should only be performed if asthma precludes adenosine use. A negative adenosine stress test result, however, has a shorter warranty period over the long term than a treadmill stress test, because exercise time, per se, has a prognostic value. Adenosine is a short-acting vasodilator administered as a 4- to 6-minute infusion (half-life 30 seconds). The nuclear agent is injected at 2–3 minutes of infusion. Adenosine vasodilates the microcirculation and increases

Short axis

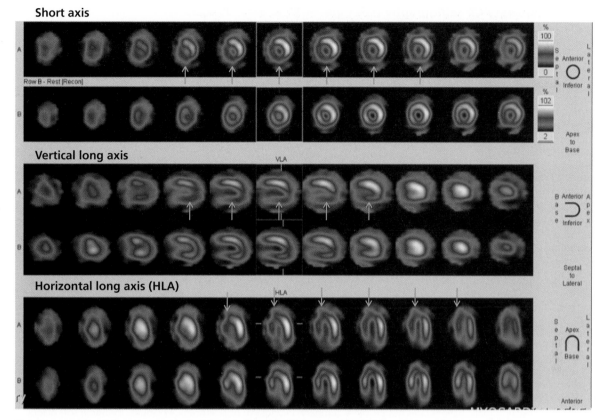

Vertical long axis

Horizontal long axis (HLA)

Figure 33.4 A severe defect (*arrows*) is noted in the inferior and septal walls at stress. This defect reverses to a large extent on the rest images. The ischemia is severe, as the defect is severe and extends into more than one coronary distribution. In fact, over 10% of the myocardium is ischemic (taking into account the extent but also the severity of the nuclear defect). No TID is noted. Severe RCA stenosis is suspected.

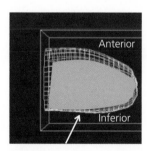

Figure 33.5 Gated SPECT myocardial excursion of the previous case (Figure 33.4). LV end-systolic volume is shown in gray, while LV end-diastolic volume is marked by the "fishnet." Note that the excursion of the inferior and apical wall is diminished (hypokinesis, *arrow*). The calculated EF is 50%.

coronary flow four to five times but cannot increase coronary flow past significant stenoses >50–70%; therefore, areas without significant stenosis will light up much more with adenosine than stenotic areas. This difference in vasoreactivity is detected even without inducing ischemia or ECG changes, as myocardial workload is not markedly increased. Caffeine is a competitive antagonist of adenosine at the receptor level and should not be used for 24 hours prior to the test. In case of bronchospasm occurring with adenosine, administer IV aminophylline.

Perform low-level treadmill exercise along with vasodilator stress testing; this reduces the common side effects of adenosine (flushing, non-specific chest pain or dyspnea, nausea) and reduces the splanchnic/GI nuclear uptake, eventually lessening artifacts and improving image quality. Also, drinking cold water before imaging may accelerate elimination of the tracer from the GI tract. When a significant GI artifact is present, stress images may be repeated a little later, providing more time for tracer clearance.

Review of the raw, moving cine images allows a better appreciation of whether a defect is an attenuation artifact or a true defect. The dark breast contour is identified over the heart, and photopenia expected behind this contour; the breast position may vary between the rest and stress studies, creating a falsely reversible defect, and this is identified on the raw cine images.[28] A defect in the anteroapical wall outside the breast contour is a true defect. A superiorly placed diaphragm may lead to inferior attenuation artifact (the superior diaphragm is identified as a linear density on the lateral heart view). GI uptake close to a defect is suspicious for GI uptake artifact. Excessive cardiac motion with its inherent artifacts may also be appreciated.

Appendix 3. Coronary CT angiography (see Figures 33.6, 33.7, 33.8, 33.9)

A. Role and indications of coronary CT angiography

Coronary CT angiography (CTA) is not a substitute for coronary angiography. It has somewhat the same indications as stress testing and is an alternative to stress testing in intermediate-probability stable angina, and low-risk or low/intermediate-probability unstable angina. It allows a safe early discharge of patients presenting to the ED with chest pain.[29] It is also useful when the stress test result is equivocal, when baseline ECG abnormalities are present, or when the patient is unable to walk.

The ideal candidate must have a very regular, normal **sinus rhythm that can be slowed to <65 bpm**, must not have frequent PVCs/PACs or AF, and must not be obese. CTA cannot adequately assess stented coronary segments <3 mm and **heavily calcified coronary arteries**. In patients with bypass grafts, CTA can assess the bypass graft bodies, but not the anastomoses with the native arteries or the native arteries distal to the anastomoses.

A normal CTA has a very high negative predictive value for significant stenosis (99%). However, the positive predictive value is more limited (70–80%), especially in the presence of heavy calcifications, such as a calcium score >400.[30] CTA does not provide any information on the functional ischemic effect of a borderline lesion and is inferior to stress testing in that regard. *It has similar prognostic value to stress testing.* A large trial randomized symptomatic outpatients with intermediate pretest clinical probability of CAD to coronary CTA versus stress testing (mostly stress imaging). An abnormal result was slightly more frequent in the CTA group (~12% vs. 8%), with relatively more true-positive findings (~75% vs. 50%).[31] *However, both strategies were associated with a low and similar rate of cardiac events at 2 years, which attests to the validity of both strategies.*

Cardiac CTA may be used to assess LV function in patients with technically limited echo. CTA is very valuable for the assessment of congenital coronary anomalies.

B. Role of CT imaging for coronary calcium scoring

CT can assess the total coronary calcium burden and the calcium burden of each coronary artery. Coronary calcium is quantified using the Agatston score. Coronary calcium correlates strongly and closely with the extent of atherosclerotic plaque burden. Coronary calcium score also strongly correlates with the long-term occurrence of coronary events.

However, calcium scores only have a weak correlation with the presence and severity of an angiographic stenosis, and thus a high calcium score in an asymptomatic patient does not dictate a coronary angiogram. Also, individual plaques, including soft plaques particularly prone to rupture and eroded plaques, may not be calcified; thus, the presence of calcium is not closely associated with the propensity of an individual plaque to rupture, and patients with ACS may not have any coronary calcium.

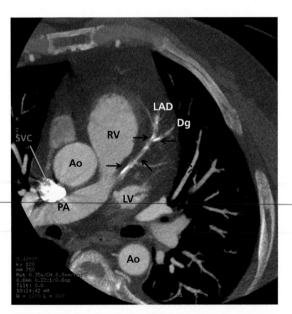

Figure 33.6 This is an axial CT view. The right ventricle is the most anterior structure, the left ventricle is posterior. The main pulmonary artery (PA) and its distal branches are visible. The ascending and descending aorta (Ao) as well as the SVC are seen. The LAD is the artery that runs between the right and left ventricles, over the septum. Left circumflex would run in the left AV groove, between the LA and LV (not seen in this image). RCA would run in the right AV groove, between RA and RV. LAD has some brightness (calcium) proximally and distally (*right-facing horizontal arrows*) and in one of its branches as well (second diagonal [Dg], *left-facing horizontal arrow*). These are calcified stenoses that seem eccentric and, when assessed in multiple views, are ~50% stenotic.

The LAD also has a soft, non-calcified stenosis in the mid segment (*oblique arrow*) between the two calcified stenoses. This stenosis looks dark, darker than contrast (soft, non-calcified stenosis). It is a severe 80% mid-LAD soft stenosis. This soft stenosis is responsible for this patient's ACS.

Always assess lesions in two views (or more if appropriate): axial, oblique, curved, sagittal, or coronal.

Reproduced with permission from Hanna EB, Quintal R, Jain N. Cardiology: Handbook for Clinicians. Arlington, VA: Scrub Hill Press, 2009.

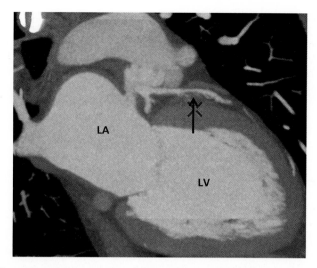

Figure 33.7 This is an oblique view of the proximal LAD (a vertical cut through the LAD plane). A soft stenosis is visible in the mid-LAD and is rated at 50% (compare the lumen proximal to the stenosis with the lumen at the level of the stenosis, *arrow*). LA and LV are also visible.Reproduced with permission from Hanna EB, Quintal R, Jain N. Cardiology: Handbook for Clinicians. Arlington, VA: Scrub Hill Press, 2009.

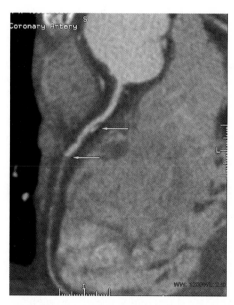

Figure 33.8 This is a curved view of the RCA. The curved view is a processed view in which the coronary artery of interest is straightened and shown in one plane. There is a proximal plaque that has calcium and a soft component as well (mixed plaque) (*top arrow*). Further down in the mid-vessel, a cutoff is seen, beyond which the opacification is severely decreased (*bottom arrow*). There must be a severe stenosis or an occlusion at this level. Coronary angiography confirmed the presence of mid-RCA occlusion.Reproduced with permission from Hanna EB, Quintal R, Jain N. Cardiology: Handbook for Clinicians. Arlington, VA: Scrub Hill Press, 2009.

Outside of acute chest pain presentations and ACS, a score of 0 makes the risk of coronary events very low and the presence of significant CAD very unlikely (very high negative predictive value). However, a high coronary calcium score only has a weak correlation with the severity of angiographic stenosis. Calcium scoring is not useful in the ACS setting: in one study, a significant proportion (~20%) of ACS patients with significant CAD had no coronary calcium.[32]

Coronary events at 5 years according to the calcium score: Score 0=< 1%; score 1–100=< 5%; score 101–300=6.5%; score >300=11%.[33]

Currently, the role and indications of CT calcium imaging are not clear. It may have a role in asymptomatic patients who are at an intermediate to high risk of coronary events according to the Framingham risk score (risk over 1% per year) to further risk-stratify and intensify medical therapy and LDL/HTN control. Coronary calcifications tend to progress over time, and the speed of progression may have a prognostic value. However, there is a measurement variability, and there are no data supporting the value of repeating calcium scoring.

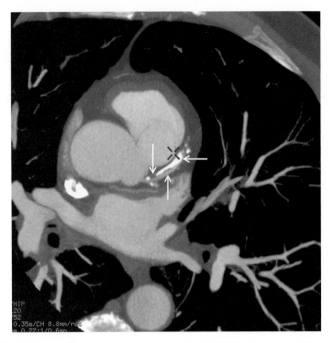

Figure 33.9 This is an axial CT view. The LAD has a soft plaque proximally (short stenosis ~50%, *down arrow*). It is followed by eccentric calcification that seems to obstruct less than 50% of the lumen (*up arrow*). Further down, this calcification seems to hide the whole vessel (*horizontal arrow*). It may simply be a rim of concentric calcium, mildly stenotic, that prevents the reader from seeing and assessing the underlying lumen, but it may also be a severe calcified stenosis. When the calcium is concentric and hides the lumen in multiple views, the significance of the underlying stenosis cannot be evaluated. ***Severe calcifications are the most important limitation to coronary CTA and significantly reduce the specificity of the test.***Reproduced with permission from Hanna EB, Quintal R, Jain N. Cardiology: Handbook for Clinicians. Arlington, VA: Scrub Hill Press, 2009.

C. Brief CTA technique

CT imaging is prone to artifacts, mostly related to the temporal resolution, the heart being a moving organ. With 64-slice CT imaging (0.6 mm thickness per slice), multiple gantry rotations are required to cover the cardiac length (~4 cm per rotation); 256-slice CT can cover the whole heart in one rotation and one cardiac cycle.

Also, during each rotation, the same cardiac structure moves within the cardiac cycle. A 64-slice CT performs a 180° rotation in ~160 ms only; in patients with slow heart rate (cardiac cycle >1 second), this corresponds to a small window of the cardiac cycle, during which the motion is limited. A dual-source CT scans an area with only 90° of rotation, thus requiring ~80 ms only. This improves the temporal resolution.

With retrospective gating, each slice is acquired multiple times at multiple phases of the cardiac cycle. Multiple gantry rotations (180 ms) and multiple acquisitions are performed over each slice, using the spiral CT technique. The table moves slowly, allowing images of the same area to overlap. The fact that each area is imaged at multiple points of the cardiac cycle allows a retrospective search for the cardiac phase during which the images have less artifacts. This reconstruction is called *multiphasic retrospective gating*.

Sequential prospective gating images each slice at one cardiac phase only, and is more sensitive to rate irregularities between the different gantry rotations. This may be less of a problem with 256-slice CT covering the whole heart in one rotation and one cycle.

D. CTA Artifacts

- Irregular heart rate may cause misalignment of adjacent slices, because adjacent slices are at different phases of the cardiac cycle for the same R–R phase (e.g., 70% of R–R corresponds to a different cardiac phase during a different cardiac cycle). This is called *step artifact*. Fast heart rate may also cause it by increasing the number of cardiac cycles acquired during the ~10 seconds of imaging, and by increasing the relative importance of slight timing variations. Respiratory motions may also cause these malalignments.
- Motion artifacts related to cardiac, coronary, or respiratory motion may occur during each cardiac cycle, leading to streaks and blurring artifacts. These artifacts are less likely to occur in the relatively quiet mid- to end-diastolic phase (~60–80% of R–R interval), and at the end-systolic phase when the coronaries are relatively stationary (~30% of R–R interval). These artifacts are increased in case of fast rate (less stationary time). Motion and step artifacts may be less pronounced at one R–R phase, hence the need to analyze the coronaries at multiple phases and the value of multiphasic reconstruction in this context.
- Increased image noise (grainy appearance) in obese patients. This may be improved by increasing the tube voltage.
- Partial volume effect or *beam hardening* is the artifact caused by an adjacent structure that has a high/bright CT attenuation (PM lead, coronary calcification). A high CT number will be assigned to the whole pixel, which will thus appear bright. This leads to overestimation of the dimension of coronary calcium.
- Poor timing of contrast injection leading to inappropriate aortic and coronary filling (the left side appears less dense than the right side of the heart).

References

1. Bouzas-Mosquera A, Peteiro J, Alvarez-Garcia N, et al. Prognostic value of exercise echocardiography in patients with left bundle branch block. JACC Cardiovasc Imaging 2009; 2: 251–9. *29% of patients with LBBB have ischemia, translating into a double mortality, ~5% per year.*

2. Christman MP, Bittencourt MS, Hulten E, et al. Yield of downstream tests after exercise treadmill testing. J Am Coll Cardiol 2014; 63: 1264–74.

3. Barlow JB. The "false positive" exercise electrocardiogram: value of time course patterns in assessment of depressed ST segments and inverted T waves. Am Heart J 1985; 110: 1328–36.

4. Lachterman B, Lehmann KG, Abrahamson D, Froelicher VF. 'Recovery only' ST-segment depression and the predictive accuracy of the exercise test. Ann Intern Med 1990; 112: 11–16.

5. Lauer MS, Francis GS, Okin PM, et al. Impaired chronotropic response to exercise stress testing as a predictor of mortality. JAMA 1999; 281: 524–9.

6. Shaw LJ, Peterson ED, Shaw LK, et al. Use of a prognostic treadmill score in identifying diagnostic coronary disease subgroups. Circulation 1998; 98: 1622–30.

Low-risk DTS/exercise test

7. Hachamovitch R, Berman DS, Kiat H, et al. Exercise myocardial perfusion SPECT in patients without known coronary artery disease: incremental prognostic value and use in risk stratification. Circulation 1996; 93: 905–14.

8. Poornima IG, Miller TD, Christian TF, et al. Utility of myocardial perfusion imaging in patients with low-risk treadmill scores. J Am Coll Cardiol 2004; 43: 194–9.

9. Bouzas-Mosquera A, Peteiro J, Álvarez-García N. Prediction of mortality and major cardiac events by exercise echocardiography in patients with normal exercise electrocardiographic testing. J Am Coll Cardiol 2009; 53: 1981–90.

10. Bourque JM, Holland BH, Watson DA, Beller GA. Achieving an exercise workload of ≥10 metabolic equivalents predicts a very low risk of inducible ischemia: does myocardial perfusion imaging have a role? J Am Coll Cardiol 2009; 54: 538–45.

ST changes in women

11. Barolsky SM, Gilbert CA, Faruqui A, et al. Differences in electrocardiographic response to exercise of women and men: a non-Bayesian factor. Circulation 1979; 60: 1021–7.

12. Gulati M, Pandey DK, Arnsdorf MF, et al. Exercise capacity and the risk of death in women: the St James Women Take Heart Project. Circulation 2003; 108: 1554–9.

13. Mora S, Redberg RF, Cui Y, et al. Ability of exercise testing to predict cardiovascular and all-cause death in asymptomatic women: a 20-year follow-up of the Lipid Research Clinics Prevalence Study. JAMA 2003; 290: 1600–7.

14. Kohli P, Gulati M. Exercise stress testing in women. Circulation 2010; 122: 2570–80.

Strongly positive stress ECG

15. Krishnan R, Lu J, Dae M, et al. Does myocardial perfusion scintigraphy demonstrate clinical usefulness in patients with markedly positive exercise tests? An assessment of the method in a high-risk subset. Am Heart J 1994; 127: 804–16.

16. Shalet BD, Kegel JG, Heo J, et al. Prognostic implications of normal exercise SPECT imaging in patients with markedly positive exercise electrocardiograms. Am J Cardiol 1993; 72: 1201–3.

17. Kobal SL, Wilkof-Segev R, Patchett MS, et al. Prognostic value of myocardial ischemic electrocardiographic response in patients with normal stress echocardiographic study. Am J Cardiol 2014; 113: 945–9.

18. Hachamovitch R, Hayes S, Friedman JD, et al. Determinants of risk and its temporal variation in patients with normal stress myocardial perfusion scans. What is the warranty period of a normal scan? J Am Coll Cardiol 2003; 41:1329–40.

19. Geleijnse ML, Vigna C, Kasprzak JD, et al. Usefulness and limitations of dobutamine–atropine stress echocardiography for the diagnosis of coronary artery disease in patients with left bundle branch block: a multicentre study. Eur Heart J 2000; 21: 1666–73.

Nuclear myocardial perfusion imaging in multivessel disease:

20. Lima RSL, Watson DD, Goode AR, et al. Incremental value of combined perfusion and function over perfusion alone by gated SPECT myocardial perfusion imaging for detection of severe three vessel coronary artery disease. J Am Coll Cardiol 2003; 42: 64–70.

21. Melikian N, De Bondt P, Tonino O, et al. Fractional flow reserve and myocardial perfusion imaging in patients with angiographic multivessel coronary artery disease. JACC Cardiovasc Interv 2010; 3: 307–14.

TID

22. Mazzanti M, Germano G, Kiat H, et al. Identification of severe and extensive coronary artery disease by automatic measurement of transient ischemic dilation of the left ventricle in dual-isotope myocardial perfusion SPECT. J Am Coll Cardiol 1996; 27: 1612–20.

23. Heston TF, Sigg DM. Quantifying transient ischemic dilation using gated SPECT. J Nucl Med 2005; 46: 1990–6. *By gated SPECT, TID is best assessed as (EDV + 5 × ESV) stress/(EDV + 5 × ESV) rest.*

Fixed defects

24. Liu P, Kiess MC. Okada RD, et al. The persistent defect on exercise thallium imaging and its fate after myocardial revascularization: Does it represent scar or ischemia? Am Heart J 1985; 110: 996–1001.

25. Gibson RS, Watson DD, Craddock GB, et al. Prediction of cardiac events after uncomplicated myocardial infarction: a prospective study comparing predischarge exercise thallium-201 scintigraphy and coronary angiography. Circulation 1983; 68: 321–36.

26. Brown KA. Prognostic value of Thallium 201 myocardial perfusion imaging A diagnostic tool comes of age. Circulation 1991; 83: 363–81.

27. Bodenheimer MM, Wackers FJT, Schwartz RG, et al. Prognostic significance of a fixed thallium defect one to six months after onset of acute myocardial infarction or unstable angina. Multicenter Myocardial Ischemia Research Group. Am J Cardiol 1994; 74: 1196–2000.

Attenuation artifacts

28. Hendel RC, Gibbons RJ, Bateman TM. Use of rotating (cine) planar projection images in the interpretation of a tomographic myocardial perfusion study. J Nucl Cardiol 1999; 6: 234–40.

CT

29. Litt HI, Gatsonis C, Snyder B, et al. CT angiography for safe discharge of patients with possible acute coronary syndromes. N Engl J Med 2012; 366: 1393–403.
30. Graham M, Cook JA, Hillis GS, et al. 64-slice computed tomography angiography in the diagnosis and assessment of coronary artery disease : systematic review and meta-analysis. Heart 2008; 94: 1386–93.
31. Douglas PS, Hoffmann U, Patel MR, et al. Outcomes of anatomical versus functional testing for coronary artery disease. N Engl J Med 2015; 372: 1291–300. *PROMISE trial*.
32. Henneman MM, Schuijf JD, Pundziute G, et al. Noninvasive evaluation with multislice computed tomography in suspected acute coronary syndrome: plaque morphology on multislice computed tomography versus coronary calcium score. J Am Coll Cardiol 2008; 52: 216–22.
33. Detrano R, Guerci AD, Carr JJ, et al. Coronary calcium as a predictor of coronary events in four racial or ethnic groups. N Engl J Med 2008; 358:1336–45.

Further reading

Gibbons R, Chatterjee K, Daley J, et al. ACC/AHA/ACP-ASIM guidelines for the management of patients with chronic stable angina: a report of the American College of Cardiology/American Heart Association Task Force on Practice Guidelines (Committee on Management of Patients With Chronic Stable Angina). J Am Coll Cardiol 1999; 33: 2092–197.

Tavel M. Stress test. In: Surawicz B, Knilans T. Chou's Electrocardiography in Clinical Practice, 5th edn. Philadelphia, PA: Saunders, 2001, pp. 208–38.

Fihn SD, Gardin JM, Abrams J, et al. 2012 ACCF/AHA/ACP/AATS/PCNA/SCAI/STS Guideline for the diagnosis and management of patients with ischemic heart disease. J Am Coll Cardiol 2012; 60: e44–164.

Part 11 CARDIAC TESTS: INVASIVE CORONARY AND CARDIAC PROCEDURES

34 Angiographic Views: Coronary Arteries and Grafts, Left Ventricle, Aorta, Coronary Anomalies, Peripheral Arteries, Carotid Arteries

I. Right coronary artery

A. Course

The right coronary artery (RCA) courses over the right AV groove, turns around and continues over the posterior AV groove, then reaches the intersection of the AV groove and the posterior interventricular groove (designated the crux), where it gives the PDA and PLB branches.

B. Branches (proximally to distally) (Figure 34.1)

1. *Conus branch* (CB) is the first RCA branch. It supplies the RVOT and has a separate ostium in 50% of individuals.

2. *Sinus node branch* (SN) originates from the RCA in 60% of individuals and from the LCx in 40%.

3. *Acute marginal branches* (AM) supply the RV (1–3 branches).

4. *Posterior descending artery* (PDA) runs on the posterior interventricular groove and supplies inferior septal branches to the inferior 25–30% of the septum (known as "inferior wall"). PDA runs parallel to the LAD, which supplies the anterior 70–75% of the septum.

5. *Posterolateral branches* (PLBs) originate from the posterior AV groove past the crux and supply the posterior wall. This part of the RCA gives rise to the AV nodal branch.

C. Segments of the RCA

- Proximal RCA: RCA before the AM branches.
- Mid-RCA: RCA around the AM branches.
- Distal RCA: RCA past the AM branches, including distal RCA at the level of the crux, PDA, and PLBs.

Practical Cardiovascular Medicine, First Edition. Elias B. Hanna.
© 2017 John Wiley & Sons Ltd. Published 2017 by John Wiley & Sons Ltd.

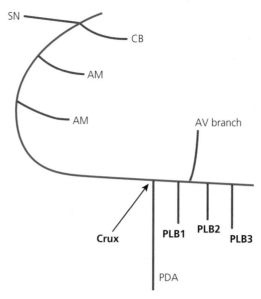

Figure 34.1 RCA course and branches. The intersection of the AV groove and the inferior septum is the crux.

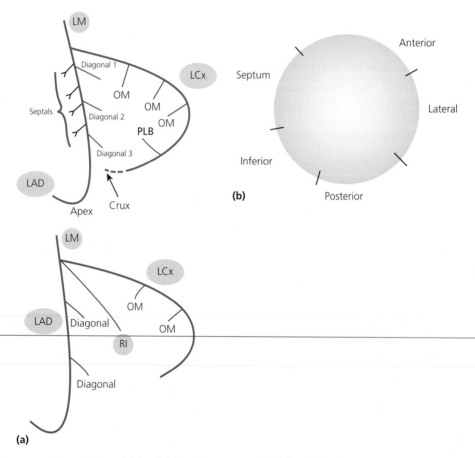

Figure 34.2 (a) Left coronary system on LAO cranial view. **(b)** LV walls on cross-sectional view of the LV.

II. Left coronary artery

A. Left main (LM) branches into the left anterior descending and left circumflex arteries

B. Left anterior descending artery (LAD) (see Figure 34.2)

1. LAD courses over the anterior interventricular groove, then reaches and frequently (80%) wraps around the apex distally. LAD gives: (i) *diagonal* (Dg) branches, usually 1–3 large diagonal branches which supply the anterior and high lateral walls; and (ii) *septal* branches which supply the anterior septum, i.e., ~70–75% of the thickness of the septum. The inferior septum is supplied by the PDA, which runs parallel to the LAD. Some patients have a dual LAD system, in which one trunk (frequently intramyocardial) gives all the septal branches and another trunk gives all the diagonal branches.

2. Segments
   - Proximal LAD=LAD proximal to the first septal branch (which is often, but not always, proximal to the first diagonal branch)
   - Mid LAD=LAD around all the major diagonal branches
   - Distal LAD=LAD distal to the major diagonal branches

C. Left circumflex coronary artery (LCx) (see Figure 34.2)

1. LCx courses over the left AV groove (like the RCA on the opposite side). It does not usually reach the crux, unless the left system is dominant.
2. Branches
   a. One to several obtuse marginal (OM) branches supply the LV free lateral wall.
   b. One or more left PLBs arise from the left AV groove before the crux. These left PLBs are adjacent to the right PLBs.
   c. PDA branch may arise from the distal LCx at the crux level in a dominant or co-dominant left system.

D. Ramus intermedius (RI) branch

Sometimes, the left main (LM) trifurcates into LAD, RI, and LCx (instead of bifurcating into LAD and LCx). RI is, in a way, a very proximal diagonal or a very proximal OM, and supplies the anterolateral wall.

Dominance refers to which artery, RCA or LCx, gives the PDA (inferior wall) and the PLB branches (posterior wall).

- RCA dominance (85% of the population): RCA gives both the PDA and the PLBs. LCx gives only the OM branches and may give some, but not all, PLBs. LCx does not reach the crux.
- Left dominance (8% of the population): LCx gives both the PDA and the PLBs. In this case, RCA is small and does not reach the crux.
- Co-dominance (7% of the population): RCA gives the PDA while LCx gives all of the PLBs and sometimes a second, parallel PDA.

At or near the crux, the dominant artery gives rise to the AV nodal branch.

In ~25% of patients with RCA dominance, there are significant anatomic variations in the origin of the PDA: double PDA, early origin of the PDA proximal to the crux, or partial supply of the PDA territory by a low AM branch that wraps around the inferior RV wall and reaches the inferior septum (*streaker branch*). Also, the inferior wall may be partially supplied by a long wraparound LAD or by OM branches that wrap around the posterior wall.

In ACS, the unstable ruptured lesion is identified as:

1. Eccentric stenosis with irregular, overhanging borders
2. Contrast staining at the lesion site after it clears from the rest of the vessel
3. Round filling defect inside the lumen, with swirling around it

The latter two features signify *thrombus* (Figure 34.3). Unlike angioscopy or OCT, coronary angiography allows thrombus visualization in only 50% of the cases.

Lesion haziness may signify (Figure 34.3):

1. Ulcerated plaque, with contrast faintly seeping inside the ruptured intima
2. Eccentric stenosis unseen on the current view (in this case, an orthogonal view may show severe stenosis)
3. Heavy calcification

III. Coronary angiography views. Recognize the angle of a view: LAO vs. RAO, cranial vs. caudal

A. Differentiate left anterior oblique (LAO) from right anterior oblique (RAO) views

Look at the spine or the central catheter in the descending aorta, then see whether the tip of the catheter is at its left (LAO) or right (RAO). For example, *in the LAO view, one "grabs" the* **catheter tip** *with the* **left hand** *while "grabbing" the central aortic catheter (or spine) with the right hand* (Figure 34.4). If the catheter tip overlaps with the central catheter or the spine, it is an anteroposterior (AP) view or a shallow-angled view.

B. Differentiate cranial from caudal views

In cranial views, the dome of the diaphragm is seen over the heart shadow (Figure 34.5).

IV. Coronary angiography views. General ideas: cranial vs. caudal views

- **Caudal views** properly assess the distal LM bifurcation, proximal LAD, and the whole LCx. The mid and distal LAD segments are usually foreshortened and overlapped with the Dg branches.
- **Cranial views** properly assess the mid and distal LAD, diagonal branches, and septal branches. Cranial views are usually good views for the ostial LM, but are often inadequate for the LM bifurcation area (distal LM and proximal LAD and LCx) (Figure 34.6).

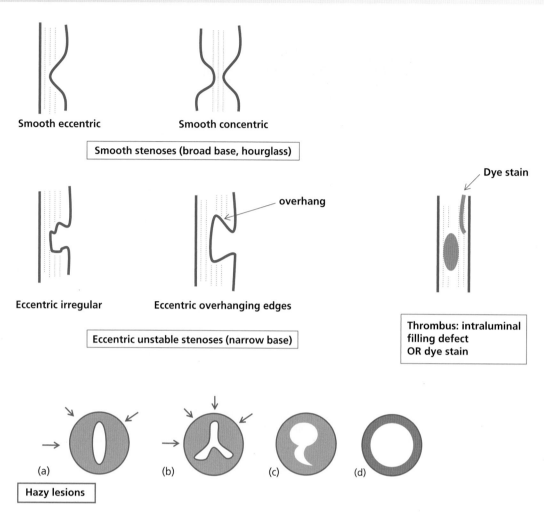

Figure 34.3 The top two rows show the difference in morphology between stable stenoses (usually smooth), unstable stenoses, and thrombus.
The bottom row shows hazy lesions. A hazy lesion could be an eccentric stenosis with no angiographic view orthogonal to the narrow lumen (**a and b**, *arrows* are angiographic angles). The narrow lumen is *white* and falsely projects as a large lumen at all angles. A hazy lesion could also be **(c)** a ruptured plaque, or **(d)** a lesion surrounded by a concentric shell of calcium. It often implies severe or unstable stenosis.

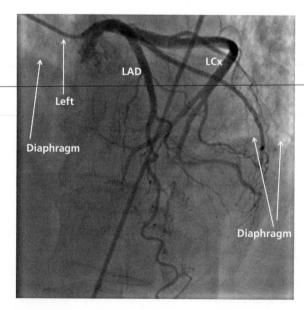

Figure 34.4 LAO view, cranial. Note the diaphragm overlapping with the heart shadow, and note the catheter tip at the left of the central aortic catheter/spine.

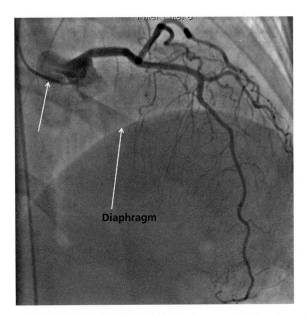

Figure 34.5 Shallow RAO view, cranial. Note the diaphragm overlapping with the heart shadow and the catheter tip slightly to the right of the central catheter in the descending aorta (the catheter tip is grabbed with the right hand, while the central catheter is grabbed with the left hand). **Also, if the ribs are looking down towards the right-hand side of the operator, the view is RAO**.

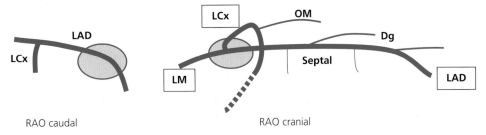

Figure 34.6 Illustration of the difference between caudal and cranial views. *Caudal* views show well the LM bifurcation into the LAD and LCx, as well as the LCx. *Cranial* views pull the LCx up and do not properly show the LM bifurcation and the proximal LAD–LCx area, but show the areas outside it (mid and distal LAD and ostial LM). The *circles* indicate the areas that are not well seen in each view.

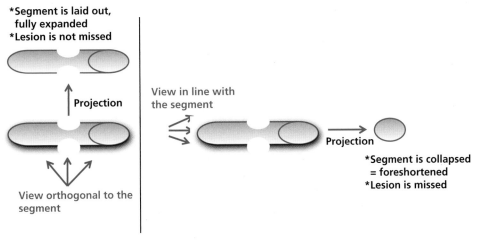

Figure 34.7 View orthogonal to a segment vs. view foreshortening a segment.

- In fact, on the **caudal views, LCx is down**, LAD is up; LAD and LCx are well separated, and their bifurcation off the LM is well visualized. On the **cranial views, LCx moves up**, along with the cranial angulation, and overlaps with the proximal LAD ± first diagonals; in addition to the overlap, the distal LM bifurcation and the proximal LAD are foreshortened. Yet, in patients with a vertical heart or a long LM, the caudal views may not open up the LM bifurcation properly; the cranial views may prove better for this purpose, particularly upon deep inspiration, which makes the heart even more vertical.

V. Coronary angiography views. General ideas: foreshortening and identifying branches

A. Foreshortening

A coronary segment is best assessed by a view orthogonal to it, i.e., a view that lays it out and fully expands it. Foreshortening implies looking at a coronary segment in line with its path, which, in two-dimensional imaging, condenses this segment and hides a stenosis by the contrast filling proximal and distal to it (Figure 34.7).

B. Arteries running on the border of the heart shadow

On any standard view, arteries that run on the border of the heart shadow, or are directed towards that border or touch it are usually diagonal or OM branches (depending on the view), **not LAD.**

VI. Left coronary views (see Figure 34.8)

A. RAO caudal (25° RAO, 25° caudal)

This is the best overall view and the **best LCx view** (Figures 34.9–34.12). In addition, it allows good assessment of the **distal LM and the proximal LAD**. The mid LAD is not well seen on this view as it is often foreshortened and overlapped with Dg branches that run above it and underneath it. The very distal apical LAD is usually well seen. If the ostial LCx overlaps with the distal LM, going more caudal will better separate the ostial LCx and the distal LM.

The RAO caudal view may be confusing when the LAD is totally occluded, in which case a large diagonal may simulate the LAD; a diagonal aims toward the heart border, whereas the LAD remains within the center of the heart shadow (Figure 34.13). In this instance, the cranial views further define whether the artery in question is LAD or Dg.

In patients with a tortuous or sharply angulated LCx, this view may foreshorten the proximal LCx, the proximal tortuosity, and even a proximal stenosis. This is reduced by deep inspiration (elongates the LCx). Also, AP caudal or LAO caudal complements this limitation of RAO caudal by showing the ostial/proximal angulation and tortuosity.

The **AP caudal view** often gives similar information to the RAO caudal view (Figure 34.14).

> LCx moves in the same direction as the image intensifier, while LAD moves in an opposite direction. When LM and proximal LCx are overlapped on RAO caudal view, going more caudal pulls LCx further down and LAD up, opening up the LM bifurcation.

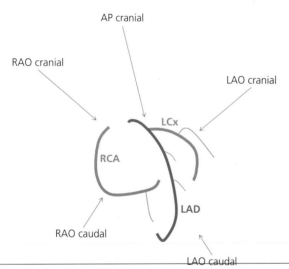

Figure 34.8 Heart in an anteroposterior view. Imagine how you look at the coronary arteries from various angles.

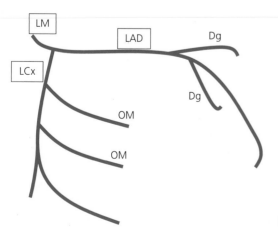

Figure 34.9 RAO caudal view (25°, 25°).

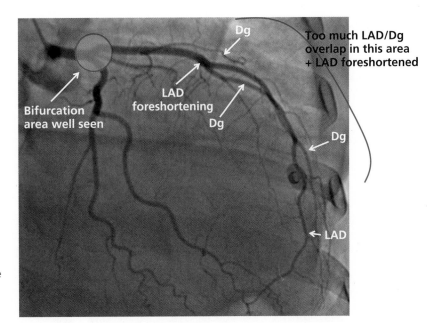

Figure 34.10 RAO caudal view. Distal LM bifurcation area is well seen; if not, the view may be angled more caudally to pull the LCx down. The mid-LAD is foreshortened and overlapped with diagonal branches. The foreshortened area looks more dense, as it is "squashed." The proximal LCx has a foreshortened area: this may be improved by imaging in deep inspiration, which straightens tortuosities.

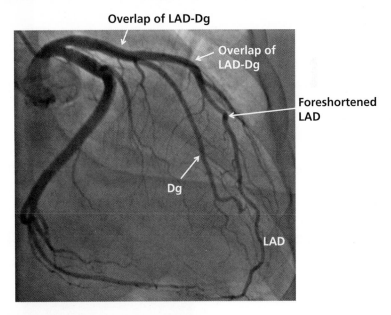

Figure 34.11 RAO caudal view. The ribs are looking down towards the right-hand side of the operator (RAO view) and the diaphragm is not seen (caudal view). Note how this view is good for the distal LM bifurcation, and how the mid-LAD overlaps with the diagonals and has some bends looking towards the X-ray detector (foreshortening).

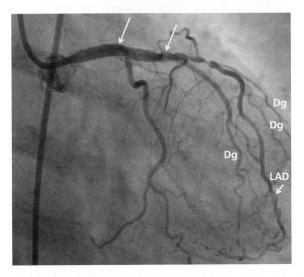

Figure 34.12 RAO caudal view in a patient with a vertical heart. Note that, in this particular case, even the LM bifurcation is not well opened. The distal LM, ostial LCx, and ostial LAD are overlapped (*left arrow*). This bifurcation may be opened by going more caudal; since the LCx follows the image intensifier, going more caudal pulls the LCx down and the LAD up, which opens up the bifurcation. In addition, the first diagonal is overlapped with the proximal/mid LAD (*right arrow*), which is expected in RAO caudal view.

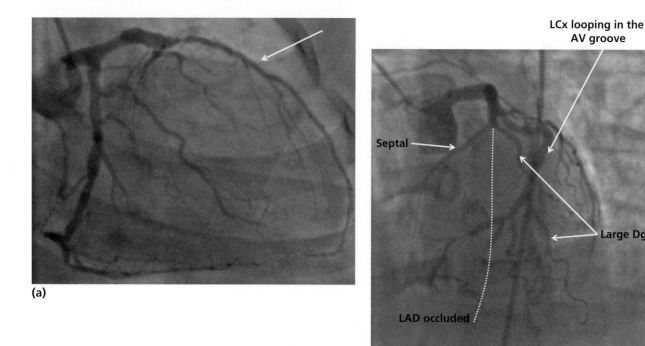

Figure 34.13 (a) RAO caudal with a large diagonal and a totally occluded LAD. The arrow points to a diagonal branch that simulates the LAD. The fact that it goes *out towards the heart border* implies that it is a diagonal branch rather than LAD, the LAD being totally occluded.

(b) LAO cranial of the same patient. LAO cranial shows the Dg going to the side, towards the heart border. No LAD is seen in the center of the heart shadow; the LAD is occluded past the diagonal and septal branches. Of note, the LAD usually runs parallel to the spine on this view (*dashed arrow*). This view confirms that the LAD is occluded when the RAO caudal view is suspicious.

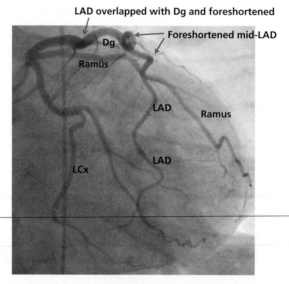

Figure 34.14 AP caudal view. Similarly to RAO caudal view, the AP caudal view shows the distal LM and the proximal LAD and LCx. The LM trifurcation is well visualized here. Note the foreshortening of the mid-LAD, wherein a large mid-LAD loop is looking towards the detector. The ramus reaches out towards the heart border, while the LAD remains inside the heart shadow.

B. LAO caudal (40° LAO, 30° caudal)

This view allows a good assessment of the **LM, proximal LAD, proximal LCx**, and proximal branches (Figure 34.15).

To obtain a good LAO caudal view, angle the image intensifier so that the tip of the catheter is positioned in the center of the cardiac silhouette. If it is not in the center of the cardiac silhouette, move the image intensifier more caudal or less LAO to obtain a good LAO caudal view, or instruct the patient to hold his breath in end-expiration, which makes the heart more horizontal.

This view looks at the heart from below and is best in patients with a horizontal heart, where the image intensifier can be almost perpendicular to the heart. This view may not properly open the LM bifurcation in patients with a vertical heart, and may be suboptimal in obese patients with a lot of soft tissue attenuation (may skip this view in those cases and rather obtain an AP caudal view). On the other hand, *in patients with a vertical heart or a long LM, cranial views may allow better delineation of the distal LM and proximal and early mid-LAD than caudal views* (Figures 34.16, 34.17, 34.18).

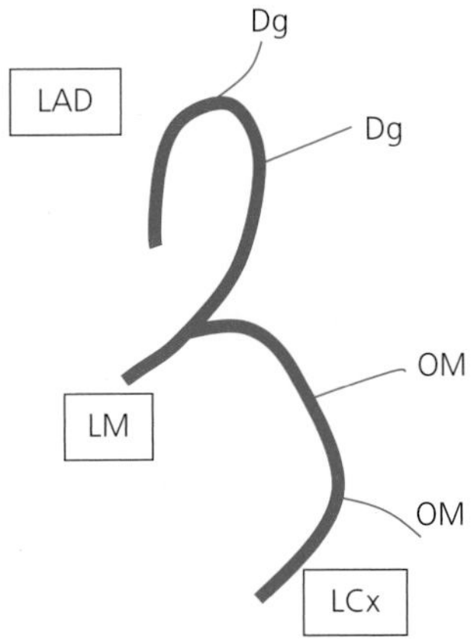

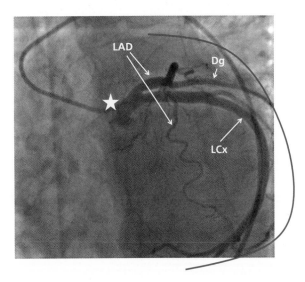

Figure 34.15 LAO caudal view (40°, 30°). Catheter tip is at the center of heart shadow. LM is at the center, LAD is up, and LCx is down. OM and Dg are in the sector between LAD and LCx.

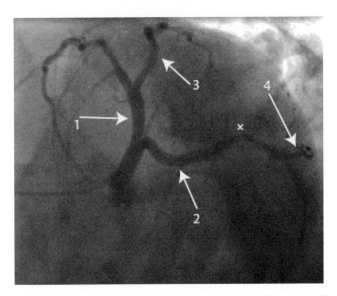

Figure 34.16 LAO caudal view of a vertical heart. The catheter tip (*star*) is not in the center of the heart shadow (delineated by the *blue line*); hence, the distal LM bifurcation is not properly opened. The view needs to be angled more caudally or less LAO to center the catheter tip, or the view needs to be taken in deep expiration to make the heart horizontal. LAO caudal is difficult to optimize in patients with a vertical heart.

Figure 34.17 LAO caudal view of a horizontal heart. Note that the catheter tip is at the center of the cardiac silhouette, and the delineation of the LM bifurcation is excellent. 1, LAD; 2, LCx; 3, diagonal; 4, OM; x, LCx stenosis.

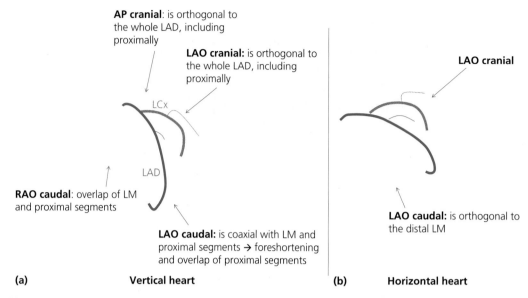

(a)   **Vertical heart**   **(b)**   **Horizontal heart**

Figure 34.18 (a) Vertical heart. LAO caudal is not orthogonal to the LM bifurcation and does not "see" it well. Cranial views, on the other hand, are orthogonal to the LM bifurcation and may allow good visualization of the distal LM/proximal LAD.

   (b) Horizontal heart. LAO cranial view is suboptimal with overlap and foreshortening of the proximal and mid LAD/LCx/Dg. LAO caudal view, on the other hand, is optimal and opens the bifurcation well. Deep inspiration makes the heart more vertical and may optimize the LAO cranial view, particularly the LM bifurcation, while imaging at end-expiration provides a better LAO caudal view.

C. AP cranial or shallow RAO cranial (5° RAO, 35° cranial)

This view allows good assessment of the ***mid and distal LAD***, as well as the diagonal and septal branches that originate from the mid and distal LAD and their points of bifurcation from the LAD. The distal LM, proximal LAD, proximal LCx, and the proximal branches are overlapped together and not well delineated (Figures 34.19, 34.20). Disease in the proximal portion of the LAD, LCx, ramus, or Dg may look like distal LM disease. Away from the LM bifurcation, the ostial LM is often well seen, as in all cranial views.

   Sometimes, however, in patients with a vertical heart or a long LM, the distal LM bifurcation is well seen, especially with deep inspiration.

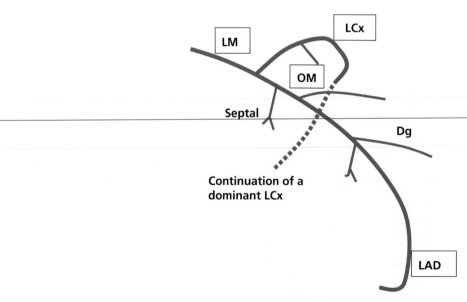

Figure 34.19 Shallow RAO cranial view (5°, 35°).

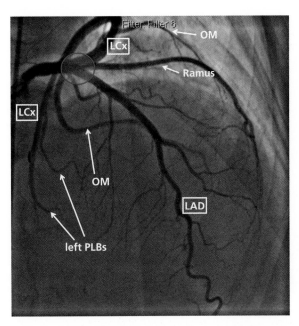

Figure 34.20 Shallow RAO cranial view. Note the overlap of the distal LM, proximal LAD, proximal LCx, and proximal ramus (*circled area*). When LCx is dominant, the distal LCx and distal OMs (left PLB branches) may be well seen on cranial views, including this view, but more so on the LAO cranial view.

D. LAO cranial (40° LAO, 30° cranial)

This view allows a good assessment of the **mid and distal LAD**, as well as the diagonal and septal branches that originate from the mid and distal LAD. The distal LM, proximal LAD, and proximal LCx are overlapped and foreshortened. The LCx is not well seen because of its overlap with the OM branches, but the mid/distal segments of the OM branches may be well seen as they run over the heart border (Figures 34.21–34.24). *Similarly to the AP cranial view, the distal LM bifurcation may be well seen without foreshortening in patients with a vertical heart or long LM, particularly with deep inspiration.*

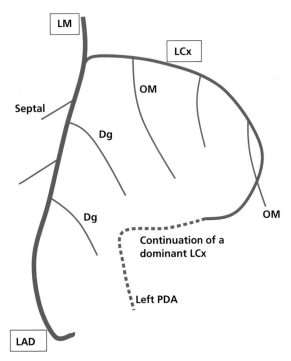

Figure 34.21 LAO cranial view (40°, 30°). The LCx and OMs run on the border of the heart shadow in this view, whereas the LAD runs over the center of the heart shadow, parallel to the spine. The diagonal and OM branches are in the sector between the LAD and LCx.

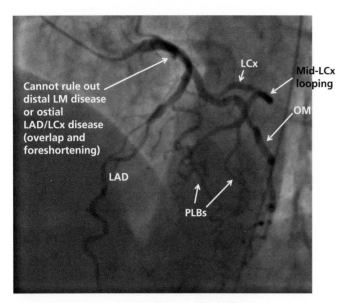

Figure 34.22 LAO cranial view. Note the overlap at the level of the distal LM.

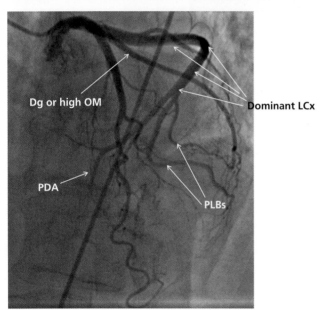

Figure 34.23 LAO cranial view showing a dominant LCx. The distal PLBs and PDA are well seen on this view. This view is the best view for the distal, dominant LCx.

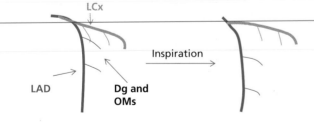

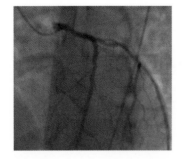
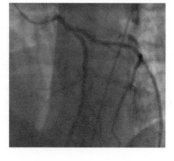

Figure 34.24 LAO cranial view. If there is too much overlap in the proximal area (*left-sided images*), move the view more cranially, as this will bring the LCx up and the LAD down. Alternatively, one may image in end-inspiration (*right-sided images*), which makes the heart more vertical and relieves the proximal overlap. **Cranial views are usually best in patients with a vertical heart.**

This is also the best view to determine whether the LCx is a dominant LCx (Figure 34.23). In such a case, the LCx is seen looping all the way down the AV groove until the crux and giving a left PDA which runs parallel to the LAD. Thus, the LAO cranial view allows a good assessment of the distal, dominant LCx as well as the left PDA, the same way it allows a good assessment of the distal RCA and right PDA.

This view is also the view that best differentiates a large Dg branch from the LAD in the case of a totally occluded LAD. Two features distinguish the LAD from an enlarged diagonal:

1. The diagonal loops to the left and reaches toward the border of the heart shadow, whereas the LAD runs parallel to the spine and loops at the apex (Figures 34.25, 34.26). Occasionally, in an enlarged LV, the apex is moved to the left and thus the LAD course may simulate a diagonal course.

2. The LAD always gives septal branches, straight parallel branches which buckle very little in systole. In contrast, the diagonal does not give any septal branch and buckles in systole.

Shallow RAO cranial may also help define a dominant LCx, and may help in the LAD/diagonal differentiation when the LAD is totally occluded.

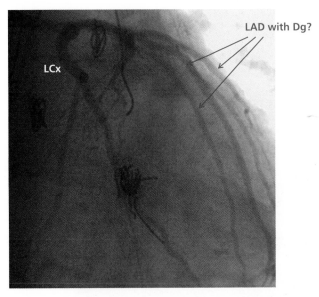

Figure 34.25 RAO caudal view. One gets the impression that the LAD is patent and is seen along with large diagonal branches. See Figure 34.26.

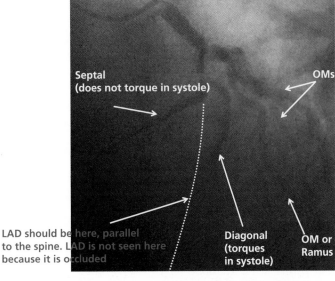

Figure 34.26 LAO cranial view of the patient from Figure 34.25. What seems like LAD on the RAO caudal view is actually a ramus or a high OM. On Figure 34.25, the outmost branch indicated by the arrow is a diagonal branch (which runs on the heart border of an RAO caudal view), while the other two branches, including the large branch that mimics LAD, are OM branches.

E. RAO cranial (30° RAO, 30° cranial)
Similarly to other cranial views, this view allows good assessment of the mid and distal LAD and the diagonal branches originating from the mid and distal LAD, as well as the ostial LM (Figures 34.27, 34.28).

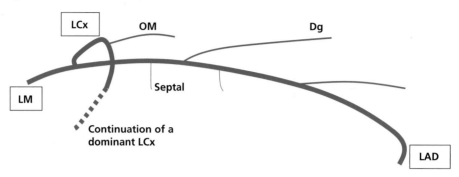

Figure 34.27 RAO cranial view (30°, 30°).

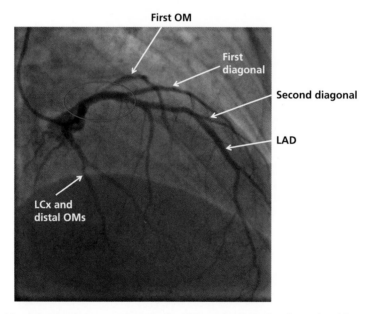

Figure 34.28 RAO cranial view. The circled area is the area where the distal LM, proximal LAD, first diagonal, and first OM overlap.

F. Other views: 90° left lateral, LAO straight, RAO straight
The 90° left lateral view is appropriate for the assessment of the very proximal and the distal LAD. It is usually inadequate for the assessment of the mid-LAD, because of LAD–diagonal overlap at the mid-LAD level. It is particularly useful **when other views do not adequately display the ostial/proximal LAD** and may be the only view that shows the ostial LAD.

   RAO straight resembles RAO caudal, and LAO straight resembles LAO cranial, with more overlap. Straight views are particularly useful during interventions in obese patients. They reduce the blurriness induced by soft tissue (caudal views) or the diaphragm (cranial views).

G. Views useful for left main assessment
In general, both cranial and caudal views are useful to assess the **ostial LM**. Also, the straight AP or shallow RAO view (5°) and the straight LAO view (30°) are often excellent additional views for ostial LM assessment. Collimation with magnification over the LM is also helpful.

   The **distal LM** is best assessed in the caudal views.

H. A minimum of two views is required for left coronary assessment
The **RAO caudal view** and **one cranial view** may be performed. The former allows the assessment of LM, LCx, and proximal and apical LAD; the latter allows the assessment of the mid and distal LAD and diagonal branches.

VII. Right coronary views

A. LAO straight

This is an **en-face view of the AV groove**. It allows good assessment of the proximal and mid RCA. The distal RCA, PDA, and PLBs are all overlapped (Figures 34.29, 34.30).

B. LAO cranial (30° LAO, 15° cranial)

This is the best RCA view. It shows the proximal and mid RCA, but also opens up the distal RCA bifurcation (Figures 34.29, 34.30).

Cranial views are important for the assessment of the distal RCA bifurcation, and one should obtain at least an LAO cranial or AP cranial view.

C. AP cranial (30° cranial)

This view allows the **best assessment of the distal RCA bifurcation** and serves as an adjunctive view when LAO cranial does not open up the bifurcation well. This view foreshortens the mid- RCA, and thus is not appropriate for mid-RCA assessment (Figure 34.31).

On the LAO straight, LAO cranial, and AP cranial views, the true RCA course has two bends (Figure 34.32). The lack of those bends signifies that the artery seen is actually a large AM branch rather than the main RCA continuing into the PDA. In this case, the main RCA is either non-dominant or occluded and does not provide a PDA. Moreover, in some anatomical variants, one large AM branch loops down to the inferior septum and provides a distal PDA. *This AM branch is called the streaker branch; it has no bend, and should not be confused with the true RCA* (Figures 34.33, 34.34).

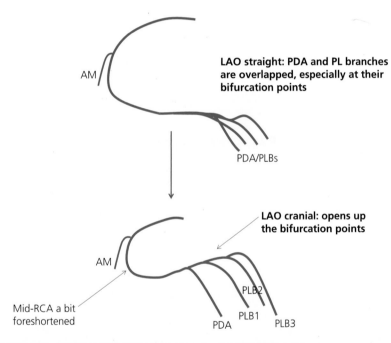

Figure 34.29 RCA views: **LAO straight vs. LAO cranial**. LAO cranial opens the distal RCA bifurcation.

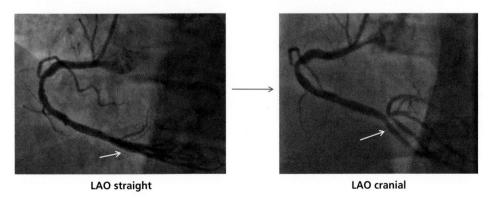

Figure 34.30 Note how the LAO cranial opens the distal RCA branches (*arrows*).

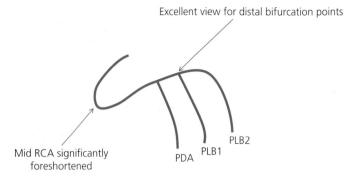

Excellent view for distal bifurcation points

Mid RCA significantly
foreshortened

PDA   PLB1   PLB2

Figure 34.31 AP cranial view. Note how the distal RCA is well laid out.

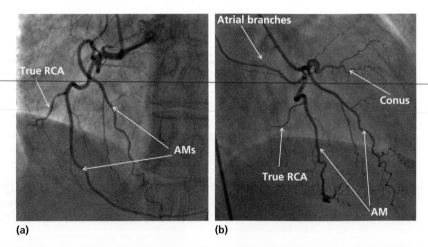

Figure 34.32 The true RCA has two distal bends on the LAO and AP cranial views (*arrows*). This is an AP cranial view.

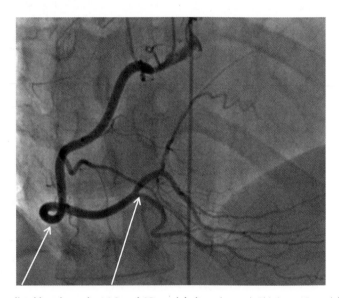

Atrial branches

True RCA

Conus

AMs

True RCA

AM

(a)   (b)

Figure 34.33 (a) LAO cranial view. It may seem that the RCA continues down and gives the PDA. In reality, the RCA finishes early in the AV groove (true RCA being the posterior-most straight branch). The branch continuing down is actually an AM branch. The lack of any bend is the clue to this interpretation. The patient either has a non-dominant RCA or an occluded mid-RCA. RAO view would confirm this interpretation. In this case, the RCA is non-dominant.

(b) RAO straight view from the same patient. The main RCA is posterior, in the AV groove. This view separates the AM branches, which go to the right, from the atrial branches, which go to the left.

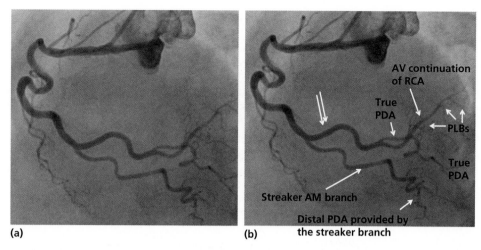

(a)   (b)

Figure 34.34 (a) LAO cranial view of the RCA. Try to identify the true RCA, PDA, and PL branches. **(b)** Same LAO cranial view with annotations. The true RCA makes a bend (*double arrow*). The branch that does not make a bend is actually a distal AM branch that loops down to the inferior septum and provides a distal PDA; this AM branch is called the streaker branch.

D. RAO straight (30° RAO)

This view looks at the AV groove from the side, and thus directly looks at the mid-RCA running in the AV groove, allowing excellent assessment of the mid-RCA. The proximal RCA is foreshortened ("looking toward us"), the distal RCA is foreshortened, and the distal RCA branches (PDA, PL) are overlapped as they run towards the apex (Figure 34.35).

This view has two additional uses: (1) if, on the LAO view, there is a question whether the artery seen is the true RCA ending into a PDA vs. a large AM branch in a patient with occluded or non-dominant RCA, the RAO view will delineate the true RCA in the AV groove. The true RCA will keep looping down towards the crux, as opposed to an AM branch, which will run to the right (Figures 34.33, 34.34); (2) during coronary interventions, this view indicates whether the guide is coaxial with the ostium ("looking toward us") and facilitates wiring of the true RCA instead of AM branches.

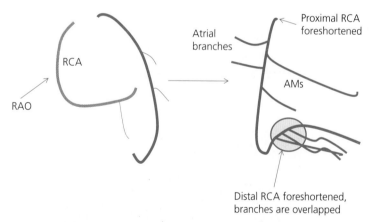

Figure 34.35 *RAO straight* (30°) looks at the AV groove from the side rather than en face, and shows the mid-RCA. It separates the ventricle from the atrium. AM branches go towards the ventricular side, while atrial branches go towards the atrial side.

E. Routine RCA views

In routine cases, image the RCA in two views: LAO cranial and RCA straight. Alternatively, one may obtain LAO straight and AP cranial views. Take at least one cranial view, sometimes two, to define distal bifurcation disease.

If the ostial RCA needs to be further assessed, two views are particularly useful: steep LAO view (50–60°) and LAO caudal view. These views are also useful during stent positioning in the ostial RCA.

VIII. Improve the angiographic view in case of vessel overlap or foreshortening: effects of changing the angulation, effects of respiration, and vertical vs. horizontal heart

A. LCx moves with the image intensifier

In case of overlap of branches that need to be set apart, remember that the LCx moves in the same direction as the image intensifier, whereas the LAD, Dg, catheter tip, and sternal wires move in the opposite direction. For example, if the image intensifier moves to a steeper LAO angle, LCx will move to the left and the catheter tip will move to the right.

Examples:

- *On LAO cranial view*:
  - ○ Steeper LAO allows more LAD–LCx separation.
  - ○ Steeper cranial allows more LAD–LCx and diagonal–LCx separation (similar to deep inspiration, Figure 34.24).
- *On RAO cranial view*:
  - ○ If the LCx overlaps with the LAD and is a bit above the LAD, move the image intensifier more cranial or take the picture during deep inspiration to lift the LCx further above the LAD; or move leftward to AP cranial view to move the LCx a bit more leftward.
  - ○ If the LCx (or OM) overlaps with the LAD and is a bit below the LAD, go less cranial.
  - ○ If the first diagonals overlap with the LAD and are a bit above the LAD, go more cranial. Moving to AP cranial also helps.

B. Effects of respiration

Expiration makes the heart horizontal, thus improving the vessel separation on the LAO caudal view but worsening the vessel overlap on the LAO cranial and RAO cranial views, i.e., the overlap of LAD, Dg, and proximal LCx/proximal OMs.

 Deep inspiration makes the heart more vertical. On a cranial view, if the LCx is overlapped with the LAD or is slightly above it, deep inspiration will push the LCx further up and the diaphragm down, allowing better exposure of the LAD (Figure 34.24). On a caudal view, if the LCx is overlapped with the LAD, deep inspiration will worsen the proximal LAD/LCx overlap. In addition, deep inspiration elongates the heart and thus straightens tortuosities, allowing better visualization of tortuous segments.

C. Vertical vs. horizontal heart

In the case of a vertical heart, LAO caudal is not orthogonal to the LM bifurcation and does not "see" it well. Cranial views, on the other hand, are orthogonal to the LAD and LCx planes and may allow good visualization of the distal LM and proximal LAD (Figure 34.18).

IX. Saphenous venous graft views

For the angiographic assessment of SVGs, obtain at least two views:

1. One straight oblique view, typically the view used to engage the graft (RAO for a left graft and LAO for a right graft). This view is useful to assess the ostium and body of the graft.

2. One angled view for the assessment of the graft anastomosis and the native vessel. For example (Figures 34.36–34.39):
   a. RAO caudal or AP caudal view for an OM graft
   b. RAO cranial, AP cranial, or LAO cranial view for a Dg or LAD graft
   c. LAO cranial ± AP cranial for an RCA graft (Figure 34.36).

If one view does not allow proper assessment of the anastomosis, obtain the second listed view. In addition, similarly to the LIMA-to-LAD, a left lateral view may be used to assess the anastomosis of the SVG-to-LAD graft.

 In many cases, it is difficult to define whether the native branch is an OM or a Dg branch, especially when the native branch is a proximal OM or Dg. The LAO cranial (or straight) often proves helpful: in this view, OM branches run on the border of the cardiac silhouette, whereas Dg branches run over the heart shadow (Figure 34.37). RAO caudal and LAO caudal may prove useful as well (Figure 34.38). ***The comparison of the graft angiogram and the native vessel angiogram obtained in the same view*** also allows the identification of the grafted branch. In addition, there are cases where one needs to identify which OM is grafted or if the grafted OM is the same OM visualized on the native angiogram (as opposed to an OM that is totally occluded and not visualized on the native angiogram). Again, comparing the graft angiogram and native vessel angiogram obtained in the same view and referencing vessels to the sternal wires will prove useful.

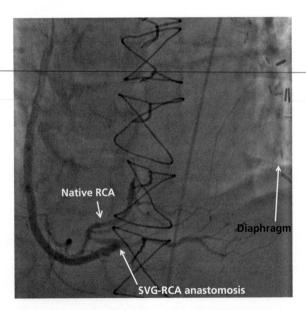

Figure 34.36 AP cranial view properly showing the SVG-to-RCA anastomosis and the native RCA.

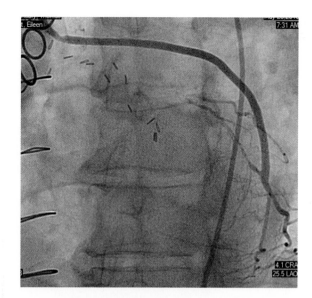

Figure 34.37 On this LAO cranial view, the grafted artery is at the left rather than right heart shadow → left coronary branch. It is running at the border of the heart, which, on LAO cranial view, implies OM branch rather than Dg.

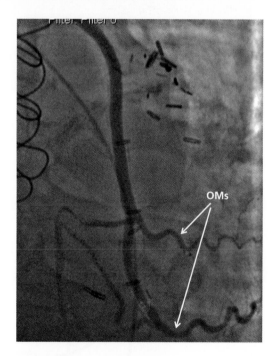

Figure 34.38 AP caudal view showing sequential SVG to OM2 and OM3. In this view, diagonal branches would be on top, running on the border of the heart shadow.

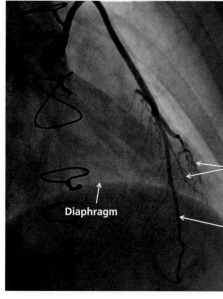

Figure 34.39 RAO cranial view (diaphragm is seen over the heart shadow, ribs are looking down towards the right). Is this SVG connected to a Dg, LAD, or OM? The anastomosed artery is not running at the border of the cardiac silhouette and is going to the apex. Thus, SVG is connected to the LAD and retrogradely fills a diagonal.

In order to identify the original target of a totally occluded SVG, see which view is orthogonal to the ostium/stump. *If the **LAO** view is orthogonal to the ostium, it is a **right**-sided graft; if the **RAO** view is orthogonal to it, it is a **left**-sided graft* (Figure 34.40). If multiple SVGs are occluded, confirm that you are engaging different ones by referencing to the sternal wires in a straight view (RAO or LAO).

Some grafts connect to two or more distal targets (Figure 34.41). A *sequential graft* (or jump graft) connects to one branch, e.g., OM1, in a side-to-side anastomosis, then continues and connects to another branch, e.g., OM2, in an end-to-side anastomosis. A *split graft* (or Y graft) consists of two grafts, A and B, with a common stem: graft A connects to one branch, e.g. OM1, and graft B comes off graft A and separately connects to another branch, e.g., diagonal. Sequential and jump grafts reduce the number of aortic anastomoses and may, in selective cases, have a lower likelihood of failure as a result of the higher flow across the graft.

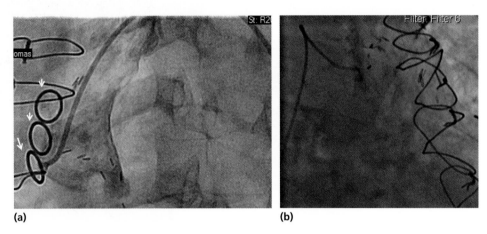

(a) (b)

Figure 34.40 **(a)** SVG to **RCA** on **LAO** view (catheter at the left of the spine). In this case, the surgeon had placed rings around the venous grafts' origins to allow identification during angiography. **(b)** SVG to a **left** coronary branch on **RAO** view (catheter tip at the *right* of the spine, ribs are looking down towards the *right*).

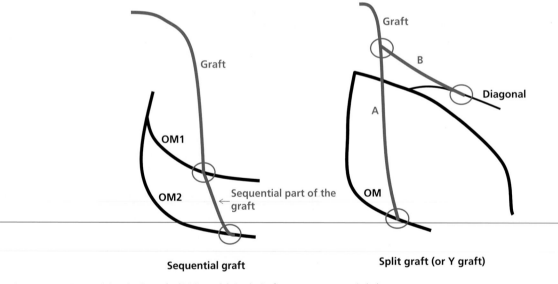

Figure 34.41 Sequential and split grafts (RAO caudal view). Graft anastomoses are circled.

X. LIMA-to-LAD or LIMA-to-diagonal views

Three views should be obtained in case of LIMA graft:

- The LIMA ostium and body are assessed in a straight view, typically the view used to engage the LIMA (e.g., RAO straight or AP view).
- The native LAD is assessed in a view that is good for the LAD, such as AP cranial or LAO cranial view.
- The LIMA-to-LAD anastomosis may be well seen on the cranial views. However, it is best assessed on a 90° lateral view, a view that is routinely obtained in all LIMA cases (Figure 34.42).

Furthermore, when redo CABG or heart surgery is contemplated in a patient with a previously placed LIMA graft, the left lateral view is very important in planning surgery as it shows how close the LIMA is to the sternum. In addition, a straight AP view will be useful to assess how far the LIMA is from the midline.

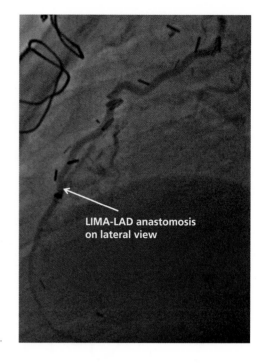

Figure 34.42 Left lateral view showing the LIMA-to-LAD anastomosis.

XI. Left ventriculography
A. RAO, LAO, and LAO cranial views
The RAO view allows the assessment of the anterior, apical and inferior walls, whereas the LAO view allows the visualization of the septal, posterolateral, and apical walls (Figure 34.43). The LAO cranial view is preferred to the straight LAO view; in fact, the straight LAO view fore-shortens the lateral wall and septal wall and overlaps the septal wall with the anterior wall, whereas the LAO cranial, by being orthogonal rather than aligned with the heart, opens up the septal and lateral walls, as well as the base (LVOT) and the LA (Figures 34.44, 34.45, 34.46).

The standard views are RAO (30°), LAO (40–60°), and LAO cranial (40–60° LAO, 20–25° cranial). The standard injection is 7–8 ml/s for a total of 20–24 ml (an enlarged LV may require a larger volume). ***The pigtail catheter should be positioned in the mid-cavity, mid-way between the base and the apex, and should be free-moving.*** A position too close to the apex induces ventricular ectopy, while a position too close to the LVOT/aorta does not fill the LV appropriately. A position too close to the base/mitral valve, particularly when the catheter feels "stuck" and not freely moving, often implies catheter impingement somewhere in the mitral apparatus (e.g. chordae). This may induce and overestimate mitral regurgitation; it may also lead to myocardial stain wherein the whole volume is injected over the impinged area, with a risk of LV perforation. In the latter situation, the catheter should be pulled out and repositioned before injection. *A pigtail multihole catheter is used rather than an end-hole catheter*, to avoid the risk of myocardial stain.

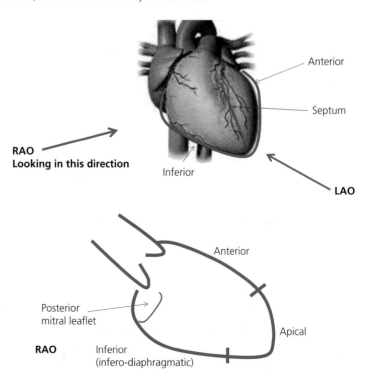

Figure 34.43 Top figure: Illustration of how the RAO and LAO views "look" at the heart. **Lower figure:** RAO view. The left ventriculogram being a two-dimensional luminogram, the anterior wall and the apex are seen, but the septum and the posterolateral wall are not seen.

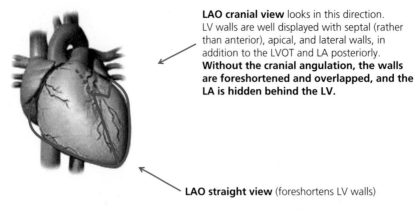

LAO cranial view looks in this direction. LV walls are well displayed with septal (rather than anterior), apical, and lateral walls, in addition to the LVOT and LA posteriorly. **Without the cranial angulation, the walls are foreshortened and overlapped, and the LA is hidden behind the LV.**

LAO straight view (foreshortens LV walls)

Figure 34.44 LAO straight vs. LAO cranial view. LAO cranial better opens the LV wall without foreshortening.

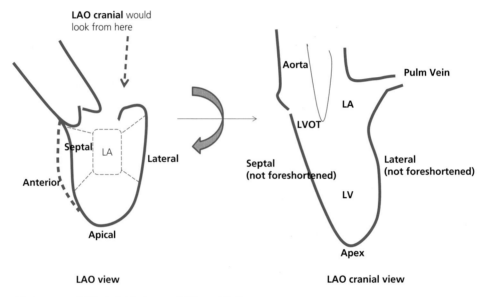

LAO cranial would look from here

Aorta

Pulm Vein

LA

LVOT

Septal   LA   Lateral

Anterior

Septal (not foreshortened)

Lateral (not foreshortened)

LV

Apical

Apex

LAO view

LAO cranial view

Figure 34.45 Left ventriculogram on **LAO straight view vs. LAO cranial view**.

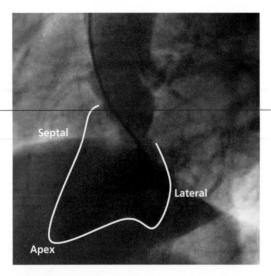

Septal

Lateral

Apex

Figure 34.46 Left ventriculogram performed in LAO straight view.

If LVEDP or PCWP >25 mmHg, ventriculography is avoided or only performed after giving nitroglycerin, using a small contrast volume.

Typically, one RAO view is performed. An LAO cranial view is additionally or alternatively performed when either of the following is suspected: (1) posterolateral MI; (2) VSD; (3) MR; (4) LVOT obstruction (e.g., HOCM, goose-neck deformity of the LVOT in primum ASD).

B. Mitral valve

The two leaflets of the mitral valve are shown in Figure 34.47. While one may get the impression of two leaflets on the RAO view, this often only shows the posterior leaflet, which engulfs the anterior leaflet by virtue of its crescentic shape.

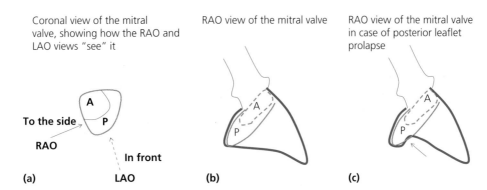

Coronal view of the mitral valve, showing how the RAO and LAO views "see" it

To the side
RAO

In front

(a)   LAO

RAO view of the mitral valve

(b)

RAO view of the mitral valve in case of posterior leaflet prolapse

(c)

Figure 34.47 **(a)** Illustration of how the RAO and LAO views look at the mitral valve. RAO looks at the mitral valve from the side (right heart side), while LAO looks from in front. **(b)** Illustration of how the mitral valve is seen on the RAO view (in gray). The anterior leaflet is not often seen on the RAO view, as it is engulfed within the crescent-shaped posterior leaflet. **(c)** In posterior prolapse, the mitral valve bulges at the base of the LV (*arrow*).

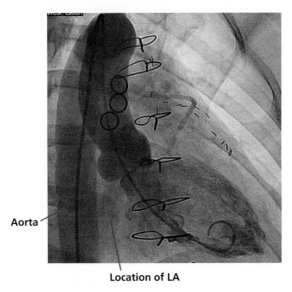

Aorta

Location of LA

Figure 34.48 RAO view of the LV. Look how the aorta overlaps with the LA. Go steeper RAO to separate the aorta from the LA.

C. Assessment of mitral regurgitation

When the severity of a regurgitation on echo-Doppler is unclear or not consistent with the clinical presentation, invasive assessment is justified. Left ventriculography and aortography are the most accurate invasive methods of mitral and aortic regurgitation assessment, respectively. In order to appropriately assess mitral regurgitation:

1. Use a 6 Fr pigtail catheter (rather than 4 Fr)
2. Inject a large bolus of contrast per second and sustain it for 4 seconds, to allow a steady-state contrast opacification of the LV and LA (e.g., 12 ml/s for a total of 48 ml). In severe MR, the large LA requires a large amount of contrast to be adequately filled and outlined.
3. Ectopy should be avoided or minimized
4. The catheter should be in the mid-cavity (LVOT placement reduces LV and LA filling)
5. Use a view that allows full visualization of the LA. In the standard 30° RAO, the LA overlaps with the descending aorta behind it, which blurs how strongly and fully the LA is opacified (Figure 34.48). Hence, it is important to go steeper on the RAO angulation (45–60° RAO) to provide a clear area between the mitral valve and the aorta (Figure 34.49). Alternatively, the LAO cranial view may be used.

To grade mitral regurgitation, the extent of LA opacification is compared to the LV opacification during the period of maximal LV filling:

1+ (mild MR): a small puff of regurgitant contrast is seen in the LA but does not fully opacify the LA.
2+ (moderate MR): LA is fully opacified, but faintly (LA < LV).
3+ (severe MR): LA is fully opacified and is as well opacified as the LV (LA = LV).
4+ (very severe MR): LA is more densely opacified than the LV (LA > LV), typically within one cardiac cycle; and/or contrast is seen refluxing in the pulmonary veins. In grades 3+ and 4+, LA is enlarged.

When LA is so large, larger than the LV, it is difficult to opacify the LA as much as the LV even when 50% of the flow is regurgitant; thus, 3+ severe MR may appear 2+.

Mitral regurgitation may also be graded using the *angiographic regurgitant fraction*. After calibration of fluoroscopic dimensions using the diameter of the pigtail loop, the LV end-diastolic and end-systolic volumes are derived from measurement of the end-diastolic and end-systolic areas. The difference between the two is the *total stroke volume*. Only part of this volume, the *forward stroke volume*, eventually reaches the systemic circulation and is measured using thermodilution cardiac output. The regurgitant fraction is equal to: *(total stroke volume – forward stroke volume)/total stroke volume* (>50% is severe).

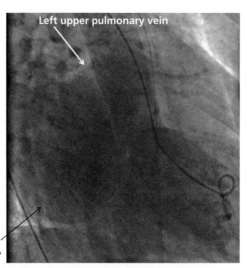

Figure 34.49 Steep RAO view shows severe MR with full delineation of the LA, which opacifies at least as much as the LV. Contrast spills back into the pulmonary vein. Thus, MR is graded 4+. LA is aneurysmal and approximates LV size.

XII. Aortography for assessment of aortic insufficiency

Aortography is best performed in the LAO view. This view is orthogonal to the aortic arch and opens the aortic arch without foreshortening and without overlap of the ascending and descending aorta. This allows assessment of the aorta along with AI, aortic dilatation being one of the most common causes or accompaniments of AI.

Aortography is performed using a 6 Fr pigtail catheter, with a large injection of 20 ml/s for 50–60 ml. The large per-second volume of 20 ml is necessary to fill the large aorta.

AI is graded similarly to MR:

1+ Small puff of regurgitant contrast is seen in the LV but does not fully opacify it.
2+ LV fills fully but is less opacified than the aorta.
3+ LV fills fully and is as opacified as the aorta.
4+ LV fills fully and is more opacified than the aorta, typically within one cardiac cycle. LV is enlarged in grades 3+ and 4+.

XIII. Coronary anomalies

Coronary artery anomalies occur in 0.3–0.9% of individuals without structural heart defects, and in 3–36% of those with structural heart defects. Among all patients undergoing coronary angiography, the most common coronary anomalies are the following:

1. Separate ostia of the LAD and LCx (0.41%).
2. Origin of the LCx from the RCA or the right sinus of Valsalva (LM only gives LAD and looks unusually long in this case) (0.37%).
3. Anterior and unusually high origin of the RCA (higher than the sinus of Valsalva) (0.18%).
4. RCA originating from the left sinus of Valsalva (0.13%).
5. Left main originating from the right sinus of Valsalva (from the RCA or from a separate ostium) (0.02%).
6. Less common anomalies: coronary artery fistula (to RV, RA, or PA usually) (0.1–0.2%); anomalous coronary artery originating from the PA.

The three most common anomalies are benign and are not, per se, associated with any hemodynamic effect. In the case of anomalous LCx origin, the LCx always courses posterior to the aorta, hence the benign nature of this anomaly.

> An anomalous LCx origin is suspected when the first left angiographic view shows an unusually long LM, this long LM being in fact the LAD, as the LCx is missing.

A. Anomalous LM or RCA origin and course

In the case of anomalous LM or RCA originating from the opposite sinus, the anomalous artery may follow one of the following four courses (Figure 34.50): (1) anterior to the PA; (2) posterior to the aorta; (3) subpulmonic, also called septal (the anomalous coronary artery dives underneath the septal LVOT then re-emerges more distally); (4) interarterial. Only the interarterial course is associated with myocardial ischemia during exercise, with a subsequent risk of VT/VF and sudden cardiac death during exercise. "Squeezing" of the coronary artery between the aorta and PA is often offered as a simplistic, yet inaccurate, explanation. When the course is interarterial, the anomalous coronary artery has a sharply angled, oblique origin, sharper than seen in the other anomalies. This sharp origin creates a slit-like ostium which gets stretched when the aorta distends during exercise, and thus it further narrows and leads to exertional ischemia. In addition, this anomalous origin is prone to spasm, torsion, or kinking, or an intramural course through the aortic wall. The interarterial course is the most common course of anomalous LM and even more so anomalous RCA (>75%). The other three anomalous courses have very rarely been associated with sudden death.

In order to define the anomalous course, **left ventriculography or aortography should be performed in an *RAO view*, and the anomalous coronary is spotted as a "dot" or an "eye" around the aorta** (the eye is a loop anterior to the aorta) (Figures 34.51, 34.52).

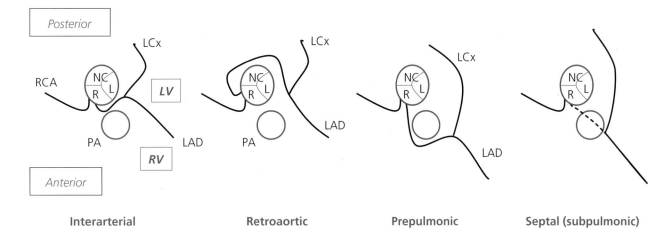

Anomalous left main originating from the right sinus

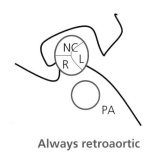

Always retroaortic

Anomalous left circumflex originating from the right sinus

Figure 34.50 Axial cuts across the aortic cusps and the PA, showing the course of anomalous left main artery and anomalous left circumflex artery originating from the right sinus.

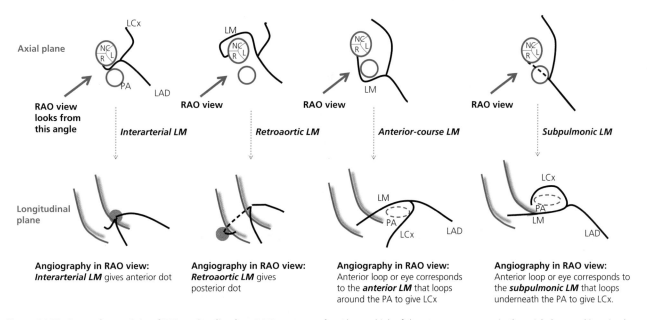

Figure 34.51 Anomalous origin of LM as visualized on RAO aortography. Always think of the coronary anatomy in the axial plane and imagine how the anomalous coronary artery projects on the RAO angle (dot vs. loop/eye). The eye of an anterior-course LM is formed by the upward loop of the LM and the downward loop of the LCx. The eye of a subpulmonic LM is formed by the downward loop of the LM and the upward loop of the LCx.

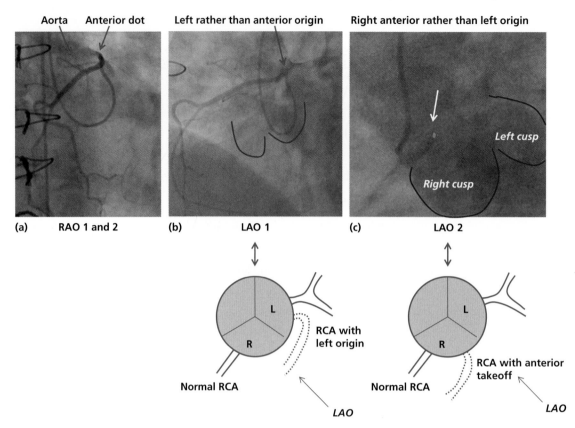

Figure 34.52 Anomalous RCA engaged with AL1. Two cases (1 and 2) are presented.

(a) *RAO view of both cases 1 and 2.* An anterior dot is seen, suggesting that the anomalous RCA has an interarterial course. However, in the particular case of RCA, this takeoff does not necessarily imply a left RCA origin and is, in fact, more commonly seen with an anterior RCA origin. Before presuming that the RCA originates from the left cusp, ensure it is not just an anterior-origin RCA by looking at a non-selective LAO 40° view with imaging of the cusps; LAO splays out the left and right cusps and distinguishes a left origin from a right anterior origin.

(b) *On LAO of case 1,* RCA is seen originating from the left cusp and the LM is seen filling next to it, implying a left-originating RCA rather than an anterior-origin RCA.

(c) *On LAO of case 2,* RCA is seen originating from the anterior surface of the right cusp (*arrow*) rather than the left cusp, implying an anterior-origin RCA.

It is most important to remember that an ***anterior dot implies interarterial course***, whereas a posterior dot (retroaortic course) or an eye/loop (subpulmonic or anterior course) are benign. These rules also apply to the anomalous RCA originating from the left sinus and to the anomalous LAD originating from the right sinus. CT or MRI are used to confirm those findings (class I).

In the particular case of the RCA, a left RCA origin should be distinguished from the benign anterior RCA origin (Figure 34.52).

The sudden death or the exertional symptoms of chest pain or syncope typically manifest before the age of 25, if ever. The risk of sudden cardiac death with anomalous LM is unclear. In autopsy series, 27–80% of patients with anomalous interarterial LM had died suddenly, and up to 30% of patients with anomalous RCA had died suddenly. However, this does not represent the absolute risk of sudden death from an anomalous coronary artery; rather, it is the relative frequency of sudden death among patients with anomalous coronary artery who happened to die and receive an autopsy (selection bias). Stress testing is insensitive for the diagnosis of ischemia or prediction of sudden death related to an anomalous coronary artery and should not be used for risk-stratifying an anomalous LM. Surgery is indicated in patients with anomalous interarterial LM, regardless of symptoms or stress testing, or anomalous interarterial RCA with documented evidence of ischemia on stress testing. Surgery may consist of coronary reimplantation, but often consists of bypass surgery to the anomalous artery, preferably using a mammary graft; since the artery is only obstructed during exercise, the mammary graft may not mature, and therefore ligation of the native artery is usually performed, the flow becoming totally dependent on the mammary graft.

B. Coronary artery fistula

A coronary artery fistula is a communication between a coronary artery and a cardiac chamber (*coronary cameral fistula*) or a vascular structure such as the PA or the coronary sinus (*coronary arteriovenous fistula*). Approximately 60% of these fistulas arise from the RCA, 30–40% from the LAD, and 5% involve both coronary arteries and terminate most commonly on the right side of the heart (most frequently **RV** [41%], then RA and PA); only 3% terminate in the LV. ***LAO view*** looks at the septum and differentiates a left-sided vs. right-sided termination; ***RAO view*** looks at the AV groove and differentiates RV termination (anterior to the AV groove), RA termination (posterior to the AV groove), and PA termination (Figure 34.43).

Acquired fistula may be seen after a penetrating trauma, PCI, RV biopsy, or cardiac surgery. The origin and course of fistulas are delineated by coronary angiography, CT, or MRI. Congenital coronary fistulas are often small and benign; they are often diagnosed in adulthood as a result of a murmur, which is typically continuous but sometimes only heard in systole. However, a fistula may have two major untoward consequences: (1) significant left-to-right shunting with O_2 step-up, pulmonary hypertension, and both right-sided and left-sided enlargement (fistula to RA or RV); (2) coronary steal, i.e., reduction in blood flow distal to the site of fistulization with myocardial ischemia. The proximal segment of the coronary artery attempts to compensate and undergoes progressive aneurismal dilatation; atherosclerosis, thrombosis, and endarteritis may develop. Small fistulas have an excellent prognosis and ~23% close spontaneously. Fistula-related complications are present in 11% of patients younger than 20 years and 35% of patients older than 20 years. Many fistulas progressively enlarge over time and insidiously lead to symptoms at a later age.

Some fistulas are simple and consist of a single origin and a single track, whereas others are complex (multiple origins or plexiform network). A large fistula (2–3× the caliber of the distal vessel) or any fistula with hemodynamic effect should be closed surgically or percutaneously; percutaneous closure is possible when a single large communication is identified (oversized coil embolization).

C. Anomalous coronary artery originating from the pulmonary artery
In this case, a coronary artery originates from the PA. This is different from coronary-to-PA fistula, wherein the coronary artery originates normally but communicates with the PA. A coronary artery originating from the PA is one of the most serious coronary anomalies and often leads to death in infancy if untreated, particularly since the coronary artery involved is often the left coronary artery. *The main issue is the low pressure in the main PA, which is more dreadful than its low oxygenation.* The low PA pressure explains why the flow in the aberrant coronary artery is directed retrogradely towards the pulmonary artery, and is derived via anastomotic vessels from the contralateral, normally arising coronary artery. Severe myocardial ischemia is therefore present. The few patients who are diagnosed in adulthood have an RCA originating from the PA, or a left coronary artery arising from the PA with a relatively small left coronary system and abundant right-to-left collaterals.

XIV. Lower extremity angiography
A. Anatomical tips (see Figures 34.53, 34.54, 34.55)

B. Technical tips
Angiography of the abdominal aorta is performed using a 4–5 Fr multihole pigtail catheter or pigtail-like catheter (e.g., OmniFlush). The catheter is positioned at the level of L1, which coincides with the level of the renal arteries. Angiography is obtained using a 10–12 ml/s injection for a total of 20–24 ml (4 Fr OmniFlush catheter allows the injection of this volume).

If bilateral iliofemoral runoff is performed using a bolus-chase technique, the contrast dose is 7–8 ml/s for 60–70 ml. The bolus fills the patient's aorta and iliac arteries, and the use of 7 ml vs. 8 ml depends on the size of these vessels. The duration of the injection depends on the patient's height; less than a 10-second injection may be done in small patients.

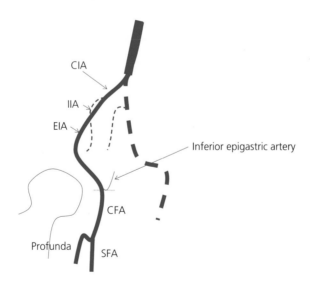

Figure 34.53 Right oblique view of the aorta, iliac and femoral arteries. Note how the iliac arteries dive posteriorly, then emerge and become superficial at the level of the inguinal ligament to form the CFA over the head of the femur. The lower loop of the inferior epigastric artery corresponds to the inguinal ligament, and thus defines the point where the deep external iliac artery emerges to the surface and becomes the CFA. A femoral stick above the loop of the inferior epigastric artery is a deep stick in the pelvic area, at a level where the artery cannot be appropriately compressed for hemostasis and where bleeding can seep through loose, non-concealing pelvic tissue.

The internal iliac artery gives gluteal branches to the thigh and deep pelvic branches, and may receive collaterals from the inferior mesenteric artery and the median sacral artery in case of common iliac occlusion. The CFA gives the *profunda femoris*, which sharply dives posteriorly and laterally in the thigh *close to the femur*, and the *SFA, which continues anteriorly and medially, away from the femur,* and is almost as anterior as the CFA early on. The CFA and profunda give circumflex branches to the hip, and the profunda gives perforating branches to the thigh throughout its course. The SFA only gives distal geniculate branches to the knee area. CFA, common femoral artery; CIA, common iliac artery; EIA, external iliac artery; IIA, internal iliac artery; SFA, superficial femoral artery.

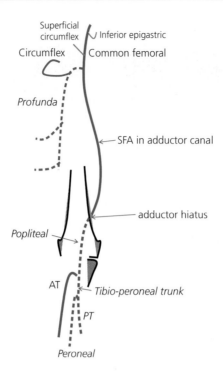

Figure 34.54 Femoropopliteal anatomy. A right lower extremity is shown. *Dashed arteries* are posterior arteries. SFA runs in the *adductor canal*, between the sartorius muscle anteriorly and the adductor muscles posteriorly. It dives posteriorly into the popliteal fossa behind the femur at the level of the *adductor hiatus*, which, in terms of fluoroscopic bony landmarks, coincides with the point at which the SFA intersects with the femur in an AP view. *SFA becomes popliteal artery at this adductor hiatus level.* Thus the popliteal artery starts much higher than the knee joint space (*dashed artery*). The popliteal artery is a posterior artery; below the knee, it gives the anterior tibial (AT) artery then continues straight in the posterior leg compartment as the tibioperoneal trunk. The AT artery is an anterior branch that emerges anteriorly by bending below the fibula head (AT genu), lies deep in the anterior leg compartment over the interosseous membrane (deeper than the anterior tibial muscle), supplies the anterior leg compartment, then emerges superficially as the dorsalis pedis artery and the lateral tarsal artery at the foot level. The tibioperoneal trunk gives rise to the posterior tibial (PT) artery and the peroneal artery, both of which supply the posterior compartment of the leg. The peroneal artery ends at the lateral malleolus and communicates with the AT through the anterior perforating branch; the PT runs to the medial malleolus and continues to the plantar foot.

Laterally to medially, the infrapopliteal vessels encountered are: AT, peroneal, then PT (distally, the peroneal becomes more lateral than the AT).

There are several anatomical variants. Some patients have a trifurcation of AT, PT, and peroneal artery (as opposed to two bifurcations). Other patients have a very high takeoff of the AT close to the knee joint.

In ~8% of patients, the AT ends early and the peroneal artery provides the dosalis pedis artery through an anterior perforating branch. In another small proportion of patients, there is no anatomical large dorsalis pedis artery at the level of the foot; the AT ramifies early on and ends as a lateral tarsal artery that supplies the foot.

Note about the femoral vein: in contrast to the groin/CFA level, where the vein is medial to the artery, the femoral vein quickly crosses over and becomes lateral to the SFA and to the popliteal artery, up until the mid-popliteal level at the knee joint level, where the vein becomes posterior to the popliteal artery. Thus, when attempting retrograde popliteal arterial access, the needle should be positioned 3–4 cm above the knee joint to enter the artery 6–7 cm above the knee joint, where the artery and veins are not overlapped.

Below the knee, every infrapopliteal artery is surrounded by two veins.

Alternatively, one may selectively engage a contralateral iliac artery using the OmniFlush or IMA catheter with the help of a slippery wire (Glidewire): (1) from a right femoral access, the OmniFlush catheter is torqued towards the left iliac, (2) the Glidewire is then advanced beyond the OmniFlush catheter tip, then torqued and advanced into the left iliac, (3) the catheter and wire are then slightly pulled until the catheter perfectly embraces the aortoiliac bifurcation; the catheter is then advanced over the wire more distally (Figure 34.56). For selective unilateral iliofemoral runoff, the contrast dose is 5 ml/s for a total of 30 ml (alternatively, as low as 4 ml/s for 20 ml may be used in short patients with small arteries) *The per-second dose is adjusted according to the diameter of the vessels (a large vessel needs a large bolus to fill it); the total duration, and thus the total dose, is adjusted according to the height of the patient.*

C. Angiographic tips

The runoffs are typically performed in AP view. In *iliac* imaging, a *contralateral* view is helpful in opening up the bifurcation of the common iliac artery into the external and internal iliac arteries and removing any overlap (20° contralateral oblique ± 20° caudal). In *femoral* imaging, a 30° *ipsilateral* view is helpful in opening up the common femoral bifurcation and identifying the ostium of the SFA; the SFA is more anterior and medial than the profunda and directed away from the femur. A more oblique view may help open the femoral bifurcation when the profunda is overlapped with the SFA on a shallow oblique view.

When the common iliac artery is occluded, collaterals develop through the contralateral internal iliac artery, the inferior mesenteric artery (which anastomoses with the internal iliac artery), or the median sacral artery. *When the external iliac artery is occluded,* collaterals

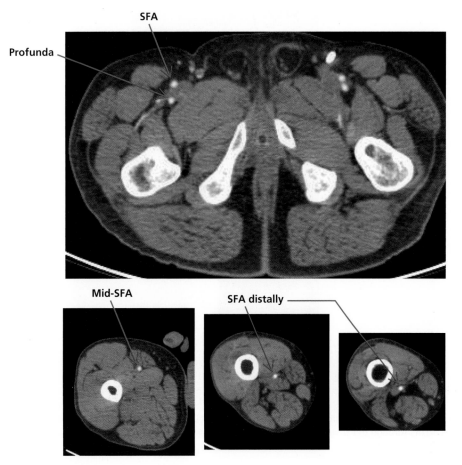

Figure 34.55 Axial CT scan images showing the SFA anatomy.
Top: note the anteroposterior relationship between SFA and profunda.
Bottom left: SFA in the adductor canal, anterior to the adductor muscles. It becomes progressively more posterior as it goes down the thigh.
Bottom right: SFA just proximal then distal to the adductor hiatus.

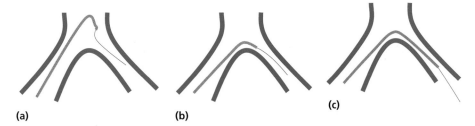

Figure 34.56 OmniFlush or IMA catheter used to selectively engage the left iliac/femoral artery through a right femoral access. **(a)** The left iliac is wired through a properly directed OmniFlush catheter, albeit not selectively engaged. A slippery wire (Glidewire) is used. **(b)** After the wire gains some distance into the left iliac, the whole system (catheter + wire) is pulled back to embrace the aortoiliac curvature, providing support for further wire and catheter advancement, as seen in **(c)**.

develop through the ipsilateral internal iliac artery but also the mammary artery (as it goes down from the chest and anastomoses with the inferior epigastric artery) (Figure 34.57). *When the SFA is occluded*, the profunda, which is rarely diseased, supplies collaterals to the popliteal artery through the geniculate branches and reconstitutes the SFA distally (Figures 34.58, 34.59).

Beware of confusing the profunda with the SFA in a case of ostial SFA occlusion. Unlike the SFA, the profunda provides branches at the thigh level. A medial profunda branch segment may still be mislabeled as proximal SFA when the true SFA is totally occluded; in this case, use a steep ipsilateral oblique view at the common femoral level to see whether this branch has a posterior course directed toward the femur (profunda), or an anterior course that curves away from the femur (SFA). A path too close to the femur on the AP or oblique view indicates that the artery is a profunda rather than SFA (Figures 34.60, 34.61).

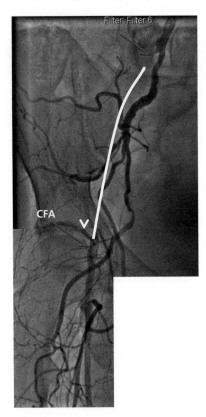

Figure 34.57 External iliac occlusion extending into the common femoral artery (CFA), with reconstitution from the internal iliac artery at the level of the CFA. **The reconstitution occurs through the *superficial circumflex artery*** (*arrowhead*), a lateral artery lower than the inferior epigastric artery. The *white line* indicates the path of the occlusion.

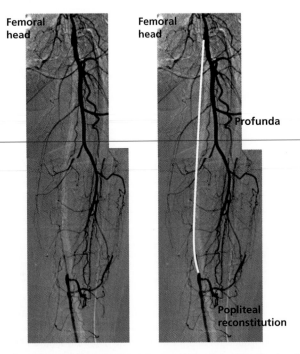

Figure 34.58 Totally occluded left SFA from the ostium to the popliteal level. It reconstitutes through profunda collaterals. The *right panel* shows the path of the occluded SFA (*white line*).

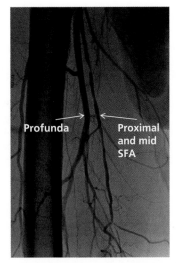

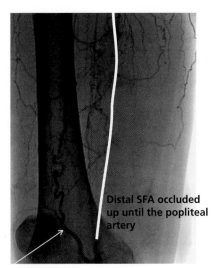

Profunda

Proximal and mid SFA

Distal SFA occluded up until the popliteal artery

Collaterals from profunda

Figure 34.59 Totally occluded right distal SFA with collaterals mostly originating from the profunda; additionally, some bridging collaterals are seen.

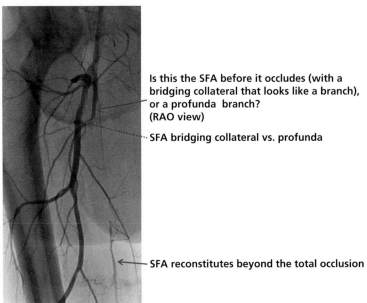

Is this the SFA before it occludes (with a bridging collateral that looks like a branch), or a profunda branch? (RAO view)

··· SFA bridging collateral vs. profunda

SFA reconstitutes beyond the total occlusion

Figure 34.60 Differentiate SFA from profunda in the case of SFA occlusion.

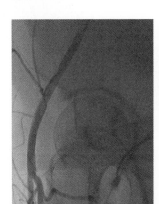

SFA

Profunda
Steep RAO view (~75°)

Figure 34.61 Same patient as Figure 34.60. An almost lateral view (*left panel*) shows that the branch in question is actually SFA not profunda, as it is anterior and directed away from the femur, whereas the profunda dives towards the femur. Successful revascularization of this SFA was performed (*right panel*).

In moderate iliac or common femoral disease disease, pressure gradients should be obtained across the stenosis. A significant pressure gradient is a peak-to-peak gradient > 20 mmHg at rest or with vasodilators (nitroglycerin). Pressure gradients may be obtained by catheter pullback; however, owing to respiratory fluctuations in arterial pressure, this method is often inadequate in assessing moderate instantaneous gradients; in addition, the catheter itself may create an obstruction and worsen the gradient, or a curved catheter may abut the arterial wall and falsely create a damped pressure past a stenosis. The best technique consists of advancing a 0.014" coronary pressure wire through a catheter and positioning it distal to the lesion, followed by simultaneous pressure measurements distal to the lesion (pressure wire transducer) and proximal to the lesion (using any catheter ≥ 5 Fr or a long 4 Fr sheath advanced close to the lesion). Alternatively, simultaneous pressure measurements may be performed using a 6 Fr sheath positioned proximal to the lesion and a straight 4 Fr catheter (e.g., Glidecath) advanced beyond the lesion. Make sure both transducers are zeroed at the same level.

XV. Carotid angiography
A. Anatomical and technical tips
Aortic arch angiography is performed in the view that opens up the aortic arch, that is, the LAO view (20 ml/s for a total of 40 ml). The aortic arch is classified as type I–III, depending on how steep it is, i.e., depending on the distance between the peak of the aortic arch and the origin of the right innominate trunk (Figure 34.62).

A true *bovine arch* is characterized by a left common carotid artery that comes off the innominate artery at least few millimeters beyond its origin, and is seen in 9% of the population. The left common carotid and innominate arteries may share a common bifurcating origin from the aortic arch; this is sometimes erroneously called bovine arch. While vertebral arteries usually originate from the subclavian arteries, the *left vertebral artery originates from the aortic arch in 5% of patients*. The aortic arch angiogram defines the arch's anatomy and any disease in the proximal portions of the four major vessels.

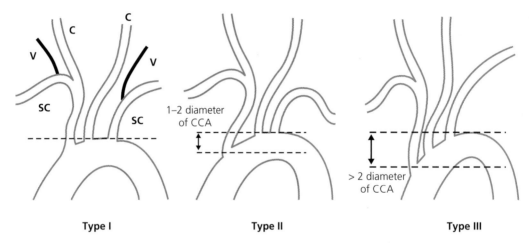

Figure 34.62 Aortic arch types I, II, and III. The distance between the top of the aortic arch and the right innominate is referenced to the diameter of the common carotid artery (CCA). C, carotid; SC, subclavian; V, vertebral. Reproduced with permission of HMP Communications from Madhwal S, Rajagopal V, Bhatt D, et al. Predictors of difficult carotid stenting as determined by aortic arch angiography. J Inv Cardiol 2008; 20: 200–4.

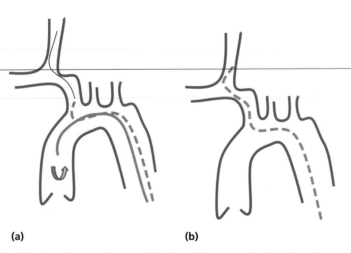

Figure 34.63 (a) On an *LAO view*, the JB1 catheter is torqued counterclockwise until it engages the right innominate trunk (goes from *solid to dashed*). Then a Wholey wire is advanced through the JB1 and torqued into the right common carotid artery; *RAO caudal view* may help open the common carotid–subclavian bifurcation. Occasionally, the wire may be going up the vertebral artery rather than the carotid artery. **(b)** The JB1 catheter is subsequently advanced over the Wholey wire to selectively engage the common carotid artery.

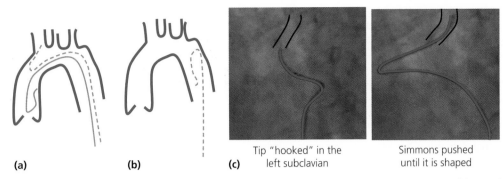

(a)   (b)   (c)   Tip "hooked" in the   Simmons pushed
                                  left subclavian   until it is shaped

Figure 34.64 Simmons catheter used to engage the innominate and carotid arteries. There are several techniques to shape it: **(a)** it may be advanced over the wire until it is shaped over the aortic valve (*solid gray*), then pulled back with a counterclockwise rotation until it engages the innominate artery (*dashed gray*). **(b)** Alternatively, the Simmons catheter can be shaped in the descending aorta then advanced to engage the vessel of interest. **(c)** The tip of Simmons may be hooked into the left subclavian artery, then pushed until it is shaped in the aortic arch; a figure of eight may be seen before full shaping of the catheter.

In aortic arch types I, II, and sometimes III, a JR4 catheter may be used to selectively engage the innominate and the left carotid arteries, in an LAO view. After being positioned in the ascending aorta, the JR4 catheter is pulled with a **counterclockwise rotation** to selectively engage the innominate artery then the left common carotid artery. On the right, after selectively engaging the innominate artery, a Wholey wire or a Glidewire is used to selectively enter the right common carotid artery, followed by advancement of the JR4 catheter over the wire (Figure 34.63). Beware of advancing the Wholey wire distally beyond the common carotid artery. Other catheters with tips longer and straighter than JR4 are preferably used (e.g., JB1 catheter, HeadHunter). RAO caudal view (20°, 20°) opens the right innominate bifurcation into the right common carotid artery and guides selective wiring of the common carotid artery.

In a type III arch, the curved catheters (Simmons or Vitek) may need to be used to engage both common carotid arteries. In a bovine arch, the curved catheters may be needed to engage the left common carotid artery (Figure 34.64). The wire is advanced until it is looped over the aortic valve, then the catheter is advanced until its base is on the aortic valve. Subsequently, the wire is removed and the catheter is allowed to take its shape in the ascending aorta over the aortic valve; the catheter is then pulled back until it engages the vessel of interest.

B. Angiographic tips

Once a common carotid artery is selectively engaged, the carotid bulb and the internal carotid artery (ICA) are positioned in the field of view; typically, the carotid bulb is located at the angle of the jaw. The carotid is then imaged in two views, using a 4–5 ml/s injection for a total of 10 ml per view: 30° ipsilateral oblique and 90° lateral view. A contralateral oblique view and an AP view may be used in case of overlap or unclear lesion severity. Note that the external carotid artery (ECA) is differentiated from the ICA by the fact that the ECA provides branches at the extracranial level, and that the ECA is actually internal to the ICA on an AP view (opposite to what the names may suggest). The ICA does not provide any branch at the cervical level. The right vertebral artery, if accidentally engaged, is distinguished from the right common carotid artery by its smooth straight course in the neck without branches and by the loop it makes at the level of C1.

The intracerebral circulation is also imaged in two views: lateral view and AP cranial view (Town view). *The first large ICA branch is the ophthalmic artery*, seen at the intracerebral level. In unilateral carotid disease, collaterals may be provided by: (i) contralateral ICA (crossover of flow from one ICA side to another through the circle of Willis may be visualized); (ii) ECA (through a communication between the superficial temporal artery and the ophthalmic artery); (iii) vertebral artery (through the circle of Willis and the posterior communicating artery). On the other hand, in a patient with severe vertebrobasilar disease, the posterior circulation may be provided by the ICA through the posterior communicating artery. Non-selective imaging of the vertebral arteries is necessary in severe carotid disease to assess the risk of an intervention.

QUESTIONS AND ANSWERS

Question 1. On RAO caudal view, in the LAD area, one artery is seen at the border of the heart shadow, another is seen over the heart shadow. Which one is the LAD?

Question 2. On RAO caudal view, in the LAD area, one large artery is seen running at the border of the heart shadow. No other large artery is seen. What is the large artery seen? And what is the likely status of the LAD?

Question 3. How would you confirm the findings of Question 2?

Question 4. On LAO caudal view, the distal LM, proximal LAD, and LCx are overlapped. Is this situation more likely to happen with a vertical or a horizontal heart? How would you open up the LM bifurcation in this case?

Question 5. Is there is a situation where a cranial view may show well the proximal LAD and even the distal LM bifurcation?

Question 6. A cranial view shows a lot of overlap in the proximal and mid-LAD area. How can the image be improved?

Question 7. A patient has an occluded proximal LAD and a large proximal diagonal branch originating before the occlusion. On LAO cranial view (or any cranial view), how would you avoid miscalling this large diagonal LAD?

Question 8. On RAO caudal view, which branches run on the border of the heart shadow? On LAO cranial view and other cranial views, which arteries run on the border of the heart shadow?

Question 9. On RAO caudal view, the proximal LCx is foreshortened and overlapped with the distal LM. How can you open the distal LM and proximal LCx?

Question 10. A patient has a borderline ostial LM stenosis on the caudal views. What other views allow good delineation of the ostial LM?

Question 11. In which case is a cranial view a valuable view for the LCx?

Question 12. What is the single best RCA view?

Question 13. What part of the RCA is not well seen on the LAO straight view?

Question 14. What are, in order, the best views for the distal RCA, i.e., the views that open the distal RCA bifurcation?

Question 15. On LAO cranial view, RCA appears to course distally in a straight line, without any bend (Figure 34.33A). What can be said of this RCA?

Question 16. Which RCA view looks at the AV grove from its side rather than en face, only allowing assessment of the mid-RCA, while foreshortening the proximal and distal RCA?

Question 17. On LAO straight view, a venous graft appears attached to an artery running on the heart border. What is the grafted artery?

Question 18. On RAO straight view, a venous graft appears to be attached to an artery running on the heart border. What is the grafted artery?

Question 19. On RAO straight view, a venous graft appears to be attached to an artery running on the lower part of the heart. What is the grafted artery?

Question 20. What three views need to be obtained for a LIMA graft?

Question 21. In order to assess MR by LV angiography, what view should be used and how much contrast should be injected?

Question 22. In order to diagnose the course of an anomalous LM (originating from the right sinus) or RCA (originating from the left sinus), aortography should be performed in what view?

Question 23. RCA appears to be originating from the left sinus. What is the other anomalous RCA origin that is sometimes confused with a left-originating RCA? Which view allows the distinction?

Answer 1. The diagonal branch runs on the border of the heart shadow. The artery that is more centered is the LAD (Figures 34.10, 34.11, 34.12).

Answer 2. The artery seen is likely a large diagonal branch. The LAD is likely occluded.

Answer 3. Obtain LAO cranial view (Figure 34.13).

Answer 4. This scenario is more likely to happen with a vertical heart. LAO caudal looks at the heart from underneath it and displays it better if it is horizontal. To open up the LM bifurcation, the LCx needs to be pulled further down and to the right. Thus, change the view to a more caudal and less leftward angle (Figures 34.16, 34.18).

Answer 5. Vertical heart.

Answer 6. The LAD moves in an opposite direction to the image intensifier. Going more cranial will push the LAD down and separate it from the LCx. Also, imaging in deep inspiration will make the heart more vertical and provide a better cranial view (less overlap) (Figure 34.24).

Answer 7. The LAD stays in the center of the heart shadow, and in the LAO cranial view, it runs parallel to the spine. Conversely, the diagonal branch takes a turn and aims towards the border of the heart shadow (Figures 34.13, 34.26). Also, the LAD gives septal branches which are characteristically straight and do not torque in systole.

Answer 8. On the *RAO caudal* view, branches running on the border of the heart shadow are diagonal branches. On the *LAO cranial* view, branches running on the border of the heart shadow are OM branches; diagonal branches loop and aim towards the heart border, but do not usually run over it. On *other cranial* views, branches running on the border of the heart shadow can be either OM or diagonal branches (Figures 34.20, 34.21, 34.28).

Answer 9. Angle the image more caudally.

Answer 10. Cranial views are good for ostial LM. Also, LAO straight and AP straight are good views for ostial LM.

Answer 11. When the LCx is dominant, the cranial views show the LCx looping proximally then continuing distally and giving left PLBs and a PDA. The distal LCx, in this case, is well seen on cranial views. If the LCx is not dominant, it is only seen looping proximally without a deep distal continuation. In fact, whenever the LCx is well seen distally beyond its loop on a cranial view, suspect a dominant LCx. On LAO cranial view, the left PDA runs parallel to the LAD.

Answer 12. LAO cranial (30° LAO, 15° cranial).

Answer 13. The distal RCA bifurcation is not well seen on LAO straight (PDA and PLBs are overlapped). LAO cranial, on the other hand, opens the distal RCA bifurcation.

Answer 14. (1) AP cranial; (2) LAO cranial.

Answer 15. This RCA is either occluded in its mid-segment or non-dominant. A dominant, patent RCA should have two distal bends on the LAO straight, LAO cranial, and AP cranial views.

Answer 16. RAO straight view (Figure 34.35).

Answer 17. OM branch (Figure 34.37). In left coronary imaging, LAO straight resembles LAO cranial.

Answer 18. Diagonal branch.

Answer 19. OM branch. In left coronary imaging, RAO straight resembles RAO caudal.

Answer 20. (i) Straight view for the LIMA body (AP or RAO usually); (ii) cranial view for the native LAD (the cranial view may also show the LIMA–LAD anastomosis); (iii) 90° left lateral view for the LIMA–LAD anastomosis.

Answer 21. MR should be assessed in an extreme RAO view (e.g., 45–60°), which allows the separation of the large LA from the descending aorta. LAO cranial may also be used. A large injection is used and sustained over 4 seconds, to allow a steady-state filling of the LV and LA (12–13 ml/s for a total of 48–52 ml).

Answer 22. RAO view, which shows the "dot" and "eye" signs.

Answer 23. Anterior RCA takeoff from the right sinus may be confused with left RCA takeoff. LAO view allows the distinction. Anterior takeoff is benign, while left takeoff may lead to ischemia (Figure 34.52).

Further reading
Anomalous coronaries

Chaitman BR, Lesperance J, Saltiel J, Bourassa MG. Clinical, angiographic, and hemodynamic findings in patients with anomalous origin of the coronary arteries. Circulation 1976; 53: 122–31.

Kimbiris D, Iskandrian AS, Segal BL, Bemis CE. Anomalous aortic origin of coronary arteries. Circulation 1978; 58: 606–15.

Lowe JE, Oldham HN, Sabiston DC. Surgical management of congenital coronary artery fistulas. Ann Surg 1981; 194: 373–80.

Serota H, Barth CW, Seuc CA, et al. Rapid identification of the course of anomalous coronary arteries in adults: the "dot and eye" method. Am J Cardiol 1990; 65: 891–8.

Yamanaka O, Hobbs RE. Coronary artery anomalies in 126,595 patients undergoing coronary angiography. Cathet Cardiovasc Diagn 1990; 21: 28–40.

Sherwood MC, Rockenmacher S, Colan SD, Geva T. Prognostic significance of clinically silent coronary artery fistulas. Am J Cardiol 1999; 83: 407–11.

35 Cardiac Catheterization Techniques, Tips, and Tricks

I. View for the engagement of the native coronary arteries: RAO vs. LAO
In order to engage a native coronary artery, a view that is orthogonal to its takeoff, i.e., LAO view, should be used (Figure 35.1).

II. Design of the Judkins and Amplatz catheters (see Figures 35.2–35.7)
In general, with any Judkins catheter, a larger arm makes the catheter point down, whereas a shorter arm makes the catheter look up.

III. Engagement of the RCA (see Figure 35.8)
Advance the **JR4 catheter** to the aortic valve, then pull slightly to free the catheter, then pull and clockwise torque 90–180° in one motion (both the pull and clockwise motions must be coordinated). If the catheter is excessively torqued (>180°), one should be prepared for a slight counterclock as the catheter engages the RCA. The torque is not transmitted to the tip unless the catheter is moved. Torquing the catheter in place does not lead to any torque transmission to the tip; then, immediately as the catheter is pulled, all the excessive torque is transmitted. The key to a successful RCA engagement is a **coordinated and simultaneous pull and torque** (90–180°). In addition, the catheter tip has a tendency to dive down when the torque gets transmitted, hence the importance of keeping a pulling tension on the catheter as the torque is transmitted.

A second technique consists of positioning the catheter 2–3 cm above the ostium, followed by a clockwise torque; the catheter will dive into the RCA ostium. A pulling tension needs to be maintained during the torque maneuver, as the catheter may dive too low upon torque transmission.

The RCA courses in the AV groove, which appears as a moving "white band" over the heart shadow. If one watches the cardiac silhouette on fluoroscopy, this white band is seen and is a clue to the course of the RCA.

An **AR catheter** is handled similarly to a JR4, except that the torque transmits to the tip more easily and the catheter has less tendency to dive down upon torque transmission. It points more downward than JR4.

Practical Cardiovascular Medicine, First Edition. Elias B. Hanna.
© 2017 John Wiley & Sons Ltd. Published 2017 by John Wiley & Sons Ltd.

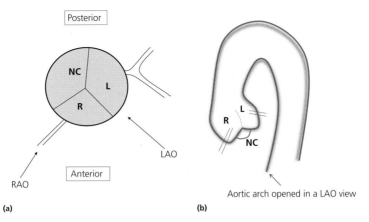

Posterior

Figure 35.1 (a) Axial cut at the level of sinuses of Valsalva. R is the right cusp, L is the left cusp, and NC is the non-coronary cusp. LAO view is orthogonal to the ostia, and therefore displays the coronary arteries in front of the operator, permitting the catheters to be torqued towards the appropriate plane. **(b)** Aortic arch opened in LAO view.

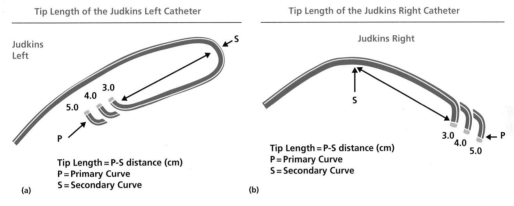

Figure 35.2 (a) Judkins left (JL) catheter. The size of the Judkins catheter is the distance between the primary and secondary curve, in cm (JL3→6). The secondary curve is what sits on the contralateral aortic wall. **(b)** Judkins right (JR) catheter. Courtesy of Mark Freed and Robert Safian, Physician's Press, Royal Oak, MI.

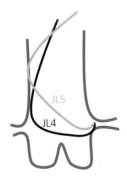

Figure 35.3 In the case of an elongated or enlarged aorta (elderly, hypertensive, or tall patient), the JL4 arm may be too short and the catheter may point up and risk dissecting the left main upon contrast injection. In addition, the secondary curve may fall down and the catheter may fold on itself. Use a larger curve (JL5, JL6) to make the catheter look down and be coaxial with the ostium.

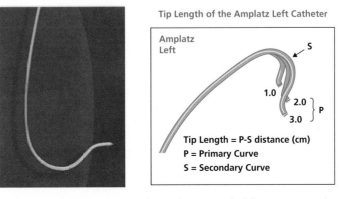

Figure 35.4 The Amplatz left (AL) catheter has a "duck" shape. AL may be used to engage the left coronary artery but also a right coronary artery with superior takeoff. Courtesy of Mark Freed and Robert Safian, Physician's Press, Royal Oak, MI.

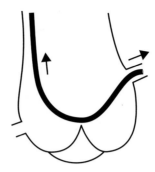

Figure 35.5 AL sits both on the back wall of the aorta and on the aortic valve (usually *contralateral cusp*), and thus provides support both from the opposite wall of the aorta and from the cusp. AL **points up**, but may point down if the AL curve is small relatively to the aorta. In addition, if the AL curve is small, the AL may not sit on the aortic valve. Reproduced with permission of Wolters Kluwer Health from Baim DS. Coronary angiography. In Grossman W, Baim DS. Grossman's Cardiac Catheterization, Angiography, and Intervention, 7th edn. Philadelphia, PA: Lippincott Williams & Wilkins, 2006, pp. 187–221.

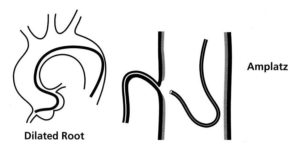

Dilated Root   **Amplatz**

Figure 35.6 AL engaging the RCA. AL looks up if the AL curve is proportionate to the aortic size; less frequently, AL looks down if its curve is small in relation to the aorta (e.g., AL1 in a dilated aortic root). Courtesy of Mark Freed and Robert Safian, Physician's Press, Royal Oak, MI.

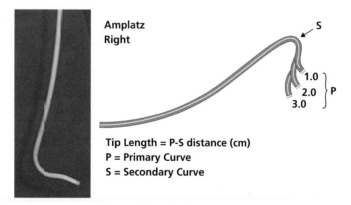

Amplatz Right

S

1.0
2.0 } P
3.0

Tip Length = P-S distance (cm)
P = Primary Curve
S = Secondary Curve

Figure 35.7 The primary-to-secondary distance distinguishes Amplatz right (AR) 1, 2, and 3. *The size of the secondary curve (S), per se, distinguishes **AR catheter from AL catheter.*** AR has a smaller curve than AL. Therefore: (1) AR does not sit on the aortic cusps or the back wall of the aorta, and does not provide support from these structures; (2) as opposed to AL, AR points down. The AR catheters represented in this illustration are **AR mod (modified AR)** catheters, the only type of AR catheters currently in use. Courtesy of Mark Freed and Robert Safian, Physician's Press, Royal Oak, MI.

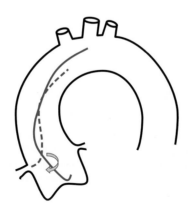

Figure 35.8 Engagement of RCA.

A *no-torque catheter* (3DRC or Williams right catheter) is, in a way, a JR4 catheter that is already torqued (Figure 35.9). All the operator has to do is advance it to the aortic valve then pull it to engage the RCA. A slight torque may be necessary if the RCA is not immediately engaged. For experienced operators, this catheter may not offer any advantage over the JR4 catheter, including no advantage in anomalous RCA takeoff. It has a short tip like JR4 and points slightly more upward than JR4.

In general, even with a JR4 catheter, less of a pulling tension is required to engage the RCA *transradially*.

The torque does not easily transmit in patients with tortuous iliac arteries and aorta, in which cases a long femoral sheath that straightens the tortuosity and lands in the aorta should be used (e.g., 23 cm or 45 cm sheath). *Also, the torque may not easily transmit in patients with a steep aortic arch, where JR4 may prove difficult to use; a catheter that requires less torque, such as AR or no-torque catheter, is preferred in these patients.*

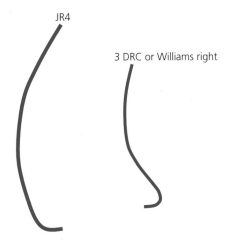

JR4

3 DRC or Williams right

Figure 35.9 The 3DRC catheter is, in a way, a JR4 that is already torqued. It simplifies JR4 engagement but does not have any major advantage over JR4 for experienced operators. It may facilitate RCA engagement when the torque does not get well transmitted, e.g., steep aortic arch.

IV. How to gauge the level of the RCA origin in relation to the aortic valve level

In some patients, one may get the impression that the RCA origin is low, very close to the aortic valve. More specifically, in an elderly patient with an elongated, almost horizontal ascending aorta, the origin of the RCA seems to be displaced downward (Figure 35.10). In fact, the distance between the aortic valve and the coronary origin is the same as in a normal aorta; however, the level of this origin is down. That is why, in those patients, one should seek the RCA origin at a level close to the aortic valve.

Once the catheter is at the outer curvature of the aorta, it is already too high, above the RCA level; it should be readvanced to the aortic valve and pulled back more slowly. Again, use the white opacity of the AV groove to help localize the RCA.

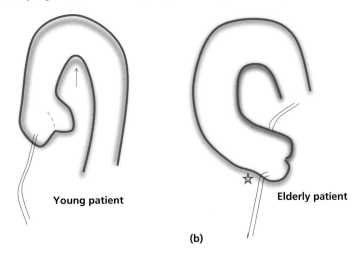

Young patient

Elderly patient

(a)

(b)

Figure 35.10 (a) Origin of the RCA in a young patient. **(b)** Origin of the RCA in an old patient with **elongated** ± dilated aorta: RCA seems to be displaced downward and is at the same level as the aortic valve.

Tip: **the way the catheter body is shaped in the ascending aorta gives an idea about the shape of the aorta. *Once the catheter reaches the outer curvature of the aorta (star), it is already too high.***

Also, the steepness of the aortic arch (*arrow*) dictates how difficult the torque transmission will be. In a steep arch, a catheter that requires less torque is preferred (AR, Williams right).

V. What is the most common cause of failure to engage the RCA? What is the next step?

The most common cause of failure to engage the RCA is an **anomalous anterior and high takeoff** (Figure 35.11). In this case, use an extreme LAO view, or better, a 90° left lateral view to be orthogonal to the origin of the RCA and attempt engaging in this view, initially using the JR4 catheter. JR4 may fail to engage the RCA because its tip is too short to reach. Alternatively, **switch to an AL0.75 or AL1 catheter**. Non-selective contrast injections help identify the level of the RCA.

   If the above two techniques fail or if the RCA is not seen during contrast injections over the right sinus of Valsalva, RCA may be origi-nating further up or from **the left sinus of Valsalva**, in which cases a larger AL is needed. For RCA originating from the left, a larger AL (1.5 or 2) may be used and aimed towards the left, or a left Judkins may be used (e.g., JL5 if JL4 is used to engage the left coronary artery).

VI. JR4 catheter engages the conus branch. What is the next step?

The RCA origin is posterior and lower than the conus origin (Figure 35.12). Thus, when the conus is engaged but not deeply so, one may continue to clockwise torque the catheter, aiming more posteriorly. If this fails, **switch to a catheter that points down in comparison to the JR4, such as JR5 or AR.**

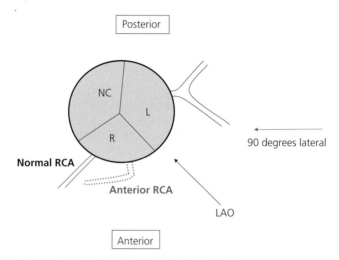

Figure 35.11 Axial cut at the level of the sinuses of Valsalva. A 90° lateral view is orthogonal to an anterior RCA and allows easier engagement. AL catheter may be necessary to reach an anterior RCA.

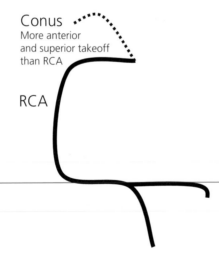

Figure 35.12 Relationship of the conus branch and RCA. If JR4 falls into the conus branch, a catheter with a more inferior takeoff, such as JR5 or AR, will successfully engage the RCA.

VII. Left coronary artery engagement: general tips

In patients with an elongated aorta (widely folding aorta) or a dilated aorta, such as tall or elderly hypertensive patients, the short arm of the JL4 catheter tends to fold on itself even before reaching the left coronary level (Figure 35.13). Even when the ostium is successfully engaged, the catheter tip **points up** in the left main artery, with a subsequent risk of left main dissection and inappropriate imaging (Figure 35.3). A catheter with a larger arm, i.e., larger primary-to-secondary-curve distance, should be used (e.g., JL5, JL6). Furthermore, in those cases, *it is important to advance the catheter over the wire until it reaches the aortic valve before taking out the wire, to prevent the catheter from "flipping" over itself.*

   If, on the other hand, the JL catheter is **pointing down** underneath the ostium, or the aorta is too narrow for the catheter, a smaller JL arm should be used.

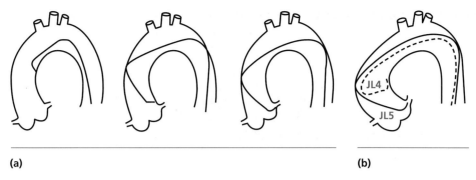

(a)   **(b)**

Figure 35.13 (a) Engagement of the left coronary artery in patients with normal-size aorta. **(b)** Engagement of the left coronary artery in patients with elongated aorta. In this case, make sure to advance the catheter all the way to the aortic valve before taking the wire out, otherwise the arm of the JL catheter may fold on itself. Reproduced with permission of Wolters Kluwer Health from Baim DS. Coronary angiography. In Grossman W, Baim DS. Grossman's Cardiac Catheterization, Angiography, and Intervention, 7th edn. Philadelphia, PA: Lippincott Williams & Wilkins, 2006, pp. 187–221.

Other technical tips (Figure 35.14)

1. **When the aorta is too wide**, the whole catheter (arm and tip) falls below the coronary origin and *points up*.
   a. If the JL4 arm is not too short, one may push the catheter against the aortic valve to reshape it, and keep pushing gently until the tip catches the ostium (step 1 in Figure 35.15). Next, the catheter is slightly pulled until it becomes more coaxial with the ostium (step 2 in Figure 35.15).
   b. One may pull up the catheter and readvance it with a **clockwise** torque. Clockwise torque makes the catheter turn up. *Asking the patient to take a deep breath may also help, as it straightens the aorta.*
   c. If (a) and (b) do not work, or if the aorta is significantly dilated/elongated, switch to a larger catheter (JL5).
2. **When the aorta is too narrow**, only the catheter tip falls below the coronary origin and *points down*.
   a. One may pull up and readvance with a clockwise torque to turn the catheter up.
   b. One may switch to a smaller catheter (JL3.5).
   Throughout all of these manipulations, the catheter body in the ascending aorta and aortic arch should be monitored. A catheter that is twisted out of its shape indicates an excessive torque that should be reversed.

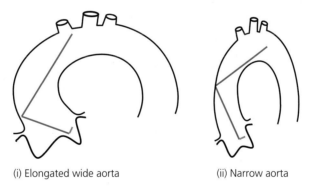

(i) Elongated wide aorta   (ii) Narrow aorta

Figure 35.14 Two scenarios wherein the JL catheter falls below the left coronary origin and does not engage by a simple pull. In **(i)**, a longer JL arm is needed (e.g., from JL4 to JL5). In **(ii)**, a shorter JL arm is needed (e.g., from JL4 to JL3.5).

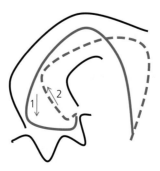

Figure 35.15 JL catheter engagement when it falls *slightly* below the left coronary ostium in a wide aorta (two steps, 1 and 2).

VIII. Management of a JL catheter that is sub-selectively engaged in the LAD or LCx

If the JL4 keeps selectively engaging the LAD in a patient with a short LM or separate ostia for the LAD and the LCx, how can the catheter be directed toward the LCx?

Unlike the JR catheter, the JL catheter has a hinge point on the aorta (secondary curve) so that clockwise rotation of the JL catheter moves it posteriorly. Thus, to move the catheter from the LAD to the LCx, which is more posterior, the catheter is typically rotated clockwise. To move the catheter from the LCx to the LAD, the catheter is rotated counterclockwise. In a patient with a large aorta, when the JL4 catheter is not resting on the aorta, the opposite maneuvers may be effective.

On the other hand, it is often more effective to **switch catheters.** Two principles allow the selection of the right catheter: (1) the LAD points up, whereas the LCx points down; (2) a larger JL catheter arm makes the catheter point down and moves the tip from the LAD to the LCx (e.g., JL5 points down in comparison to JL4, EBU4 points down in comparison to EBU3.5). Thus, in order to move the catheter from the LAD to the LCx, one may use a larger JL catheter (JL4→JL5); in order to move the catheter from the LCx to the LAD, one may use a smaller JL catheter (JL5→JL4; or JL4→JL3.5)

In addition, when the LM is short, one may use a short-arm AL catheter to selectively engage the LCx (AL1.5). A short-arm AL tends to point down (opposite of short-arm JL), and thus would selectively point towards the LCx.

IX. Specific maneuvers for the Amplatz left catheter
A. Engagement
Advance a wire until it loops over the aortic valve, then advance the AL catheter all the way over the wire onto the aortic cusp: the tip of the AL must catch the cusp of interest, while the body must sit on the contralateral cusp. Next, push the catheter up with a counterclockwise rotation in order to catch the left coronary ostium, or push with a clockwise rotation in order to catch the RCA ostium (Figure 35.16). During those manipulations, the wire is kept inside the catheter body to improve catheter pushability and torqueability; the wire is pulled out when the catheter is close to the ostium.

Once the AL catches the ostium, slightly withdraw the catheter for deeper and more coaxial engagement.

When used to engage a SVG, the same AL manipulation is performed, except that the AL catheter is not advanced all the way down to the aortic valve level. The AL is advanced to the ascending aortic level above the native coronary level. The wire is pulled and the AL tip is allowed to catch the aortic wall, then AL is pushed with a clockwise or counterclockwise rotation to catch the appropriate SVG (usually, clockwise torque is used for the left SVG).

B. Disengagement
If a well-seated AL is pulled out, the tip has a tendency to be "sucked" in deeper. Thus, in order to disengage an AL, one should push it until it prolapses out of the ostium, then clock it out (push and clock). As opposed to Judkins catheters, AL disengagement should be performed under fluoroscopy. In some cases, pushing the catheter may further advance it inside the artery; therefore, gentle maneuvering under fluoroscopy with a change in strategy may be required.

More specifically, when using a small-curve AL that is not sitting on the valve, i.e. when the tip is not looking upward, pushing the AL catheter may further advance it (Figure 35.17). Also, when an AL guide catheter is used, pushing may further advance rather than retract the catheter; this is because guide catheters are stiffer than diagnostic catheter and are less likely to flip out of the ostium with a push. Thus, when an AL guide is used, one may directly pull it under fluoroscopy, preferably over a balloon catheter.

X. If you feel that no torque is getting transmitted, what is the next step?
1. Ensure that the catheter has not been kinked as a result of excessive torquing. A kinked catheter is characterized by a severely damped or erratic pressure tracing.

2. It is likely that there is severe aortoiliac tortuosity preventing torque transmission. Under fluoroscopy, look at the shape of the catheter in the aortoiliac region to confirm, then exchange the standard short sheath (11 cm) for a long sheath that lands in the distal aorta (23 cm sheath) or better, in the thoracic aorta (45 cm sheath).

3. A very steep aortic arch may prevent torque transmission. In this case, for the RCA, use a catheter that does not require significant torquing (AR, Williams right).

XI. Appropriate guide catheters for left coronary interventions
Guide catheters have a stiffer shaft but a larger internal diameter than diagnostic catheters. Guide catheters rely on three elements for support: (1) coaxial guide alignment with the coronary takeoff; this is the most important aspect of support and is achieved not just by advancing the catheter into the ostium but by clockwise (RCA guide) or counterclockwise torque; (2) deep engagement; (3) Support from abutting the opposite aorta and/or the aortic valve (AL guides abut both the opposite aortic wall and the aortic valve, while the extra-backup guides abut the opposite aortic wall).

Guides useful for left coronary interventions (Figure 35.18)
- **Extra-backup guides** (e.g., EBU, XB, Voda). Those guides have one bend and a long tip, longer than the JL tip, which allows more coaxial and deeper support than JL. While long, the exact tip length varies with the size of the EBU; a relatively shorter tip tends to point towards the upward-looking LAD, whereas a longer tip points towards the downward-looking LCx. When the LM is long, an EBU guide with long tip is used and advanced deep into the LM, close to the ostium of the LCx, in order to reduce the non-supported distance before the sharp LM–LCx angle.
- **AL guide:** AL is particularly useful in patients with a short LM, wherein a short AL guide (AL1.5) points down towards the LCx (Figure 35.19). Outside this, AL1.5 or 2 is useful in cases that require robust support and in transradial cases. An AL guide is also useful in case of a high coronary takeoff (use AL2 or 3, depending on how high the takeoff is and how large the aorta is).
- **JL guide** does not usually provide adequate coaxial support because of the bend at its tip. It is useful for ostial LM intervention or interventions where extra support is not needed (e.g., LM is short and the LAD or LCx is neither calcified nor tortuous). The JL guide has a tip that is even shorter than the diagnostic JL tip.

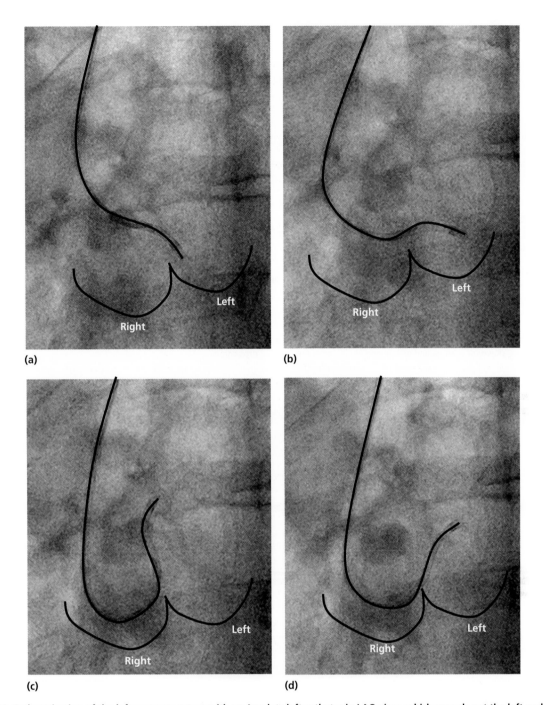

Figure 35.16 Catheterization of the left coronary artery with an Amplatz left catheter in LAO view, which spreads out the left and right coronary cusps. (a, b) The wire is sent towards the left coronary cusp, then the catheter is advanced over the wire in such a way that its tip catches the left coronary cusp, while its body aims towards the right coronary cusp. The wire is kept inside the catheter for pushability and torqueability. **(c)** After the tip catches the left cusp, the catheter is pushed with a slight counterclockwise torque until it catches the ostium. **(d)** The catheter is then pulled for more coaxial engagement.

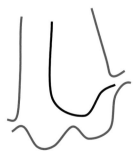

Figure 35.17 Small-arm Amplatz catheter. Pushing it may further dive it inside the left coronary artery rather than disengage it.

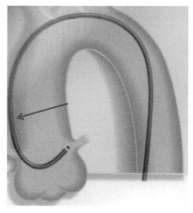
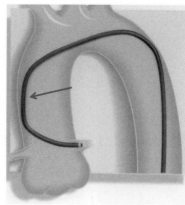
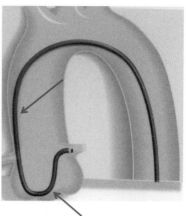

-XB 3.5 looks up
-Provides support from
the opposite
aorta (*arrow*)

XB 4.0 looks down

AL 2 with support from the
opposite aortic cusp and
the opposite aorta

Figure 35.18 Extra-backup guides and AL guide for the left coronary artery. XB with the long tip (XB4, as opposed to XB3.5) is useful for LCx intervention (looking down) or for a patient with a long LM. Courtesy of Cordis Corporation.

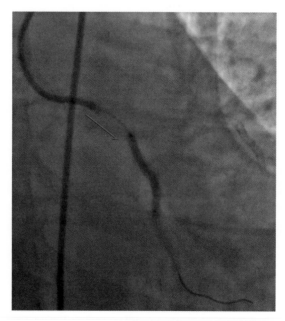

Figure 35.19 Small-arm AL guide catheter (AL1) is used to engage the LCx in a patient with a short LM. A small AL arm points down towards the LCx (*arrow*) and provides good coaxial support for a LCx intervention in a patient with a short LM.

XII. Appropriate guide catheters for RCA interventions (Figure 35.20)

A. Horizontal RCA takeoff
* JR4, hockeystick 1 or 2 (the longer tip of hockeystick 2 may allow deep engagement and extra support in complex cases).

B. Inferior RCA takeoff
* First option: multipurpose (multipurpose 2 has a longer tip than multipurpose 1).
* Other options: AR1 or 2, right coronary bypass guide (RCB), JR5 or short tip JR4. AL1 may be used if the aorta is dilated, which makes the AL1 point down.

C. Superior RCA takeoff
* AL (0.75 or 1) or XB RCA for an upwardly sharp takeoff ("shepherd crook" RCA). These guides provide extra backup support from the opposite aortic wall (Figure 35.21). They are also used in a ***highly tortuous RCA*** requiring a lot of support.
* Hockeystick 2, internal mammary (IM) guide, 3DRC, left coronary bypass guide (LCB), or JR3.5 may be effective (the shorter arm of JR3.5 points more upward than JR4). They provide support by being coaxial. Hockeystick 2 also allows support through deep intubation of its long tip.

D. High anterior RCA takeoff
* AL (0.75 or 1) or hockeystick 2.

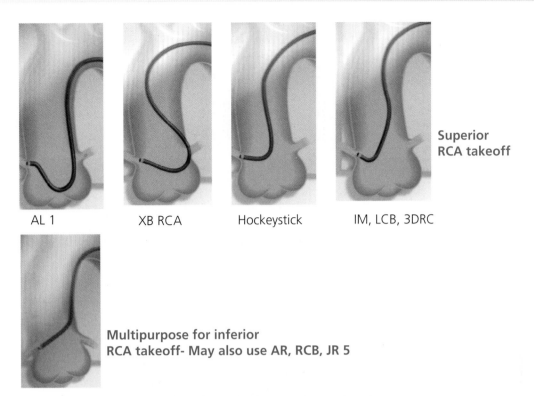

AL 1   XB RCA   Hockeystick   IM, LCB, 3DRC

**Superior
RCA takeoff**

**Multipurpose for inferior
RCA takeoff- May also use AR, RCB, JR 5**

Figure 35.20 Guide catheters for superior RCA takeoff and inferior RCA takeoff. Courtesy of Cordis Corporation.

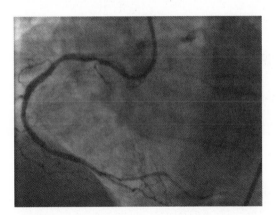

Figure 35.21 AL1 guide catheter engaging the RCA, and providing good backup support from the aortic cusp and the opposite aortic wall.

XIII. Selective engagement of SVGs: general tips
In order to engage SVGs, it is important to understand their locations and takeoffs (Figure 35.22).

a. From bottom to top, one finds SVG-to-RCA, then SVG-to-LAD or diagonals, then SVG-to-OM.

b. The SVG-to-RCA originates from the right surface of the aorta, above the RCA and almost in the same plane as the RCA (or slightly more posterior).

The SVG-to-LAD or SVG-to-diagonal branch originates from the anterior surface of the aorta.

The SVG-to-OM originates from the left posterior surface of the aorta.

c. The SVG-to-RCA has a downward takeoff, whereas the SVGs to the left coronary branches have an upward takeoff (particularly upward in the case of SVG-to-OM).

The SVG-to-RCA is best engaged in an LAO view, which is orthogonal to this SVG takeoff. SVGs to the left coronary branches are best engaged in an RAO view, which is orthogonal to the takeoff of these SVGs (Figures 35.22, 35.23) (***Right SVG → LAO; Left SVG → RAO).***

When rings are attached to the SVGs, engage each SVG in a view orthogonal to the ring, i.e., a view where the ring is seen as a straight column.

XIV. Specific torque maneuvers for engaging the SVGs
In order to engage the SVG-to-RCA, the catheter is positioned above the level of the RCA, then pulled with a counterclockwise rotation. As opposed to what may make intuitive sense, counterclockwise torquing is used to engage the SVG-to-RCA rather than clockwise torquing (this is opposite to native RCA engagement).

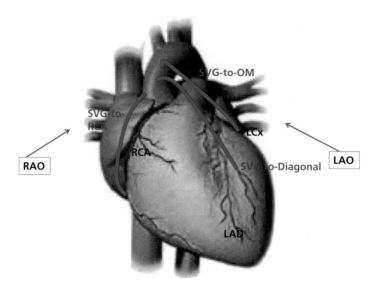

Figure 35.22 Location of SVGs:

• Down to up: SVG-to-RCA, SVG-to-LAD or diagonal, then SVG-to-OM
• Right to left: SVG-to-RCA, SVG-to-LAD or diagonal, then SVG-to-OM
• Inferior takeoff for SVG-to-RCA. Superior takeoff for SVG-to-LAD or diagonal and, more so, SVG-to-OM.
  LAO view is orthogonal to the takeoff of SVG-to-RCA, while RAO view is orthogonal to the takeoff of SVG-to-left coronary branches.

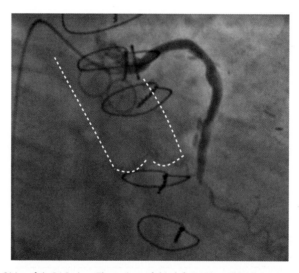

Figure 35.23 Catheter engaging SVG-to-OM graft in RAO view. The ostium of this *left SVG* is well laid out on an *RAO view*. The catheter is torqued to aim to the left border of the aorta on this view (*dashed line* is the aortic contour).

In order to engage an SVG to a left coronary branch, advance the catheter down to the aortic valve, torque it counterclockwise, then pull up and torque clockwise around the expected level of the graft.

Overall, a *counterclockwise* torque is necessary for the right SVG, and a *clockwise* torque around the graft level is necessary for the left SVG.

If, after engaging one SVG, the catheter keeps falling in this same SVG as one is trying to engage other SVGs, what should be done next?

The catheter needs to be moved out of the curvature that keeps leading it into the first SVG. The catheter should be pulled up a few centimeters above this SVG, torqued clockwise or counterclockwise about 90–180° to get out of the same curvature, then advanced to the level where the other SVG is thought to be. Appropriate torquing is then performed at this level.

For example, if the catheter keeps falling in the SVG-to-diagonal when one is trying to engage the SVG-to-OM, withdraw the catheter, torque it counterclockwise at a high level, then advance it and clockwise torque it at the expected SVG-to-OM level (above the SVG-to-diagonal level).

XV. Appropriate catheters for engaging SVGs (see Figure 35.24)

A. SVG-to-RCA
Since this graft has an inferior takeoff, a catheter pointing down is necessary for engagement:

1. A multipurpose catheter is the most appropriate catheter for this graft. It points down and has a long supportive tip that dives deeply and coaxially into the SVG.
2. AR1 and right coronary bypass (RCB) catheters are alternatives. The RCB catheter is somewhat similar to JR4, except that its short tip points down.

JR4 points slightly up and thus does not usually provide appropriate diagnostic images; the contrast may spill out and give the impression of a non-filling, occluded graft. Moreover, JR4 is certainly not an appropriate interventional guide for this SVG.

B. SVGs to the left coronary branches
JR4 is often an appropriate diagnostic catheter for the left-sided SVGs. However, since these SVGs have a superior takeoff, JR4 is not an appropriate interventional catheter. Guiding catheters pointing up are usually necessary for SVG intervention:

1. Hockeystick guide catheter, which is a catheter that has a slightly superior angle. The long-tip hockeystick 2 guide is preferred to hockeystick 1 for deep engagement and support (Figure 35.25).
2. AL1.5 or AL2 (depending on the aortic size).
3. A left coronary bypass (LCB) catheter (short-tip catheter pointing up), an internal mammary catheter, or JR4 catheter may be used for the SVG-to-LAD or diagonal, which tends to have a less superior takeoff than the SVG-to-OM. The LCB catheter is somewhat similar to JR4, except that its short tip points up.

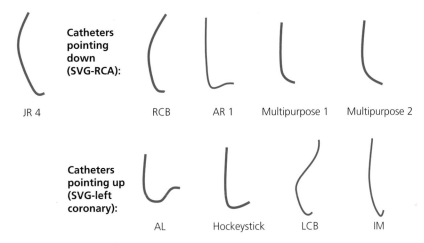

Figure 35.24 Shapes of various catheters.

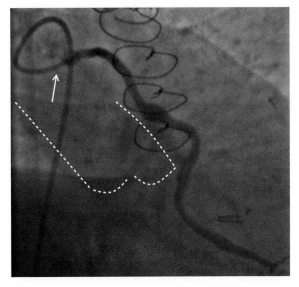

Figure 35.25 A hockeystick 2 guide catheter is used to engage the SVG-to-OM graft in an RAO view. The long arm of the hockeystick 2 points slightly upward, which proves very useful in left-sided SVG interventions (*arrow*). It allows both coaxial and backup support.

XVI. Engagement of the left internal mammary artery graft

Steps necessary to engage the left internal mammary artery (LIMA) graft (Figure 35.26):

1. Position a JR4 catheter in the aortic arch, then pull it back with a ***counterclockwise*** rotation until the left subclavian is engaged. This is performed in the LAO view, because the LAO view opens up the aortic arch and the origins of the major vessels.

2. Advance an exchange-length wire into the left subclavian artery. If the subclavian artery is very tortuous, a polymer hydrophilic wire (Glidewire) is used to maneuver through the left subclavian artery.

3. Then advance an exchange-length wire and exchange the JR4 catheter for an internal mammary (IM) catheter. Advance the latter over the wire beyond the bend of the subclavian artery.

4. An AP or RAO view may be used in order to selectively engage the LIMA. The RAO view foreshortens the subclavian but is orthogonal to the LIMA takeoff. Pull the IM catheter with a slight ***counterclockwise*** torque until it engages the LIMA. During this process, inject small puffs of contrast to identify where the LIMA originates. LIMA often originates *around the subclavian bend*, but it may originate a bit more distally or proximally before the bend. *The LIMA is between the vertebral artery and the thyrocervical trunk.* Seeing the thyrocervical trunk during a puff injection points to a need to pull the catheter slightly more.

Occasionally, if the aorta and the subclavian artery are too tortuous, leave the 0.035″ wire in the IM catheter during torque manipulations to provide more stiffness and allow more torque transmission to the catheter. Also, make sure a long 45 cm sheath is advanced in the aorta for support.

5. After obtaining the LIMA views, the catheter is disengaged and pullback pressure recorded across the ostium of the left subclavian artery. One of the most common causes of ischemia in the LIMA-to-LAD territory is left subclavian stenosis, and this should be systematically checked.

If the LIMA graft proves difficult to engage, do not persevere in the engagement attempts, as there is a risk of dissecting the LIMA ostium. Perform non-selective imaging near the LIMA ostium, with a relatively higher volume of contrast (e.g., 5 ml/s for 12 ml). In addition, inflate a blood pressure cuff across the left arm and perform the contrast injection at the peak cuff inflation. This diverts the non-selective contrast into the LIMA.

If the left subclavian artery proves difficult to engage, perform an aortic arch angiogram to analyze its takeoff. It is likely that the aortic arch is a type III arch, with the left subclavian originating more proximally than thought, proximal to the aortic arch bend.

When the LIMA needs to be engaged for interventional purposes and difficulty is encountered, a 0.014″ hydrophilic or a soft coronary wire is used to selectively enter the LIMA, then the guide is gently tracked over this wire.

The *right internal mammary artery (RIMA)* is engaged using the same steps as the LIMA, with a counterclockwise torque to enter the right innominate in an LAO view. However, an RAO caudal view may be needed to open the subclavian–carotid bifurcation and allow wiring of the subclavian. Once the IM catheter is advanced into the right subclavian, the LAO view is more appropriate to cannulate the ostium of the RIMA, and the catheter needs to be clockwise torqued rather than counterclockwise torqued.

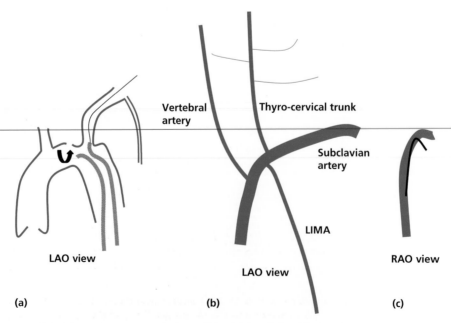

Figure 35.26 (a) Engagement of the left subclavian artery with a JR4 catheter (*counterclock*), followed by wire advancement into the left subclavian artery, then catheter exchange for an IM catheter, then engagement of the LIMA. **(b)** LIMA is between the vertebral artery and the thyrocervical trunk, at the subclavian bend. **(c)** The engaged IM catheter is shown in an RAO view, which foreshortens the subclavian artery but opens up the ostium of the LIMA.

XVII. Left ventricular catheterization

The LAO view may be used, as it displays the right and left coronary sinuses and the aortic orifice in between; it is particularly useful when a wire is used to cross the valve, to ensure that the wire does not go into the coronary arteries. After crossing the aortic valve, RAO view may be used, as it is orthogonal to the long axis of the LV and allows proper catheter positioning in the mid-LV.

In the absence of aortic stenosis, a pigtail catheter is used to access the LV (Figure 35.27). A guidewire is kept inside the pigtail catheter all the way to the tip, but not beyond the tip. This wire provides stiffness and support to the catheter, particularly when a 4 Fr pigtail catheter is used. The valve is crossed with the pigtail catheter itself: the pigtail is advanced over the aortic valve and allowed to loop (figure-of-9), then pulled back with a slight clockwise or counterclockwise torque; it may fall into the LV during this pullback. If it does not, slightly torque the catheter to direct it in a different plane, then readvance it and pull it. This maneuver is repeated, each time with a slightly different torque. *The loop has to be over the center of the valve, not eccentric over one cusp.* If the catheter repeatedly fails to fall into the LV, one may advance the wire beyond the pigtail catheter and use it to access the LV (the wire is directed through catheter torque).

If the catheter arm falls in the LV but the pigtail tip is still in the aorta, advance the wire beyond the tip. This will invariably make the whole catheter fall in the LV (Figure 35.28).

Aortic stenosis

In aortic stenosis, the left ventricle is accessed using an Amplatz left (usually AL1), multipurpose, or Judkins right catheter pointing toward the aortic valve orifice *and a straight-tip 0.035″ wire* (e.g., straight-tip, stiff-shaft Glidewire). The LAO view is used as it opens up the left and right cusps and allows one to aim at the aortic orifice in between and avoid the coronaries, as opposed to the RAO view that superimposes the left and right cusps. The catheter is torqued in a way that looks toward the aortic orifice, and the wire is advanced; the catheter is used to direct the wire in various planes. *It is often best to start with an aortic cusp injection (6 ml/s for 12 ml) to localize the exact AS jet, so that one can point the catheter/wire toward it.* Serial catheter rotations with wire readvancement are performed until the wire crosses the aortic valve. Beside torquing, the catheter may be slightly advanced and pulled to direct the wire in different planes. The key to successful crossing of a stenotic valve is to aim in the direction of the aortic orifice (Figure 35.29). The valve calcification seen on fluoroscopy is also a useful guide to the location of the aortic orifice.

To reduce the risk of stroke during these manipulations, the catheter is flushed every 2 minutes and heparin anticoagulation is provided. After crossing the valve, the Amplatz catheter is exchanged for a double-lumen pigtail catheter using a long 260 cm Amplatz superstiff wire. Amplatz wire has a soft atraumatic but non-supportive tip which should be shaped into a large pigtail curve to allow stable positioning in the LV during catheter exchanges. Simultaneous LV and aortic pressures are recorded through the double-lumen catheter. The cardiac output is simultaneously obtained through a Swan catheter that has been left in the PA, and the valve area is calculated.

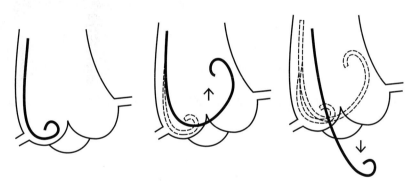

Figure 35.27 Pigtail catheter advancement. This is an LAO view, but one may use an RAO view. Advance the wire as far as the tip of the catheter to stiffen it, advance the catheter, then pull back with a slight clockwise or counterclockwise torque. Reproduced with permission of Wolters Kluwer Health from Baim DS. Coronary angiography. In Grossman W, Baim DS. Grossman's Cardiac Catheterization, Angiography, and Intervention, 7th edn. Philadelphia, PA: Lippincott Williams & Wilkins, 2006, pp. 187–221.

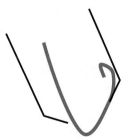

The pigtail bend is in the LV but the pigtail tip is not → advance a wire → the whole system falls all the way in.

Figure 35.28 Dealing with a situation when the pigtail bend is in the LV, but the pigtail tip is not.

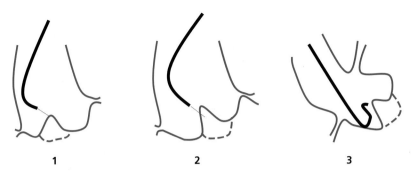

1   **2**   **3**

Figure 35.29 Various aortic root shapes, with various locations of the aortic orifice on LAO view. A different catheter is necessary in each case to direct the wire into the aortic orifice: **(1)** JR4; **(2)** Multipurpose catheter; **(3)** AL1 or 2 catheter. This aortic orifice is often indirectly localized using the aortic valve calcifications. *Moreover, an aortic cup injection (6 ml/s for 12 ml) helps localize the exact AS jet, so that one can point the catheter/wire toward it.* The aortic configuration (3), wherein the aorta is severely elongated and horizontal while the aortic valve is vertical, is commonly seen in elderly patients.

XVIII. Engagement of anomalous coronary arteries

A. Anomalous LCx originating from the right coronary sinus

This anomalous LCx always has a posterior course and an origin posterior to the RCA. It points downward. It may be engaged by: (1) further clockwise rotation of the JR4 catheter beyond the origin of the RCA; (2) use of a catheter pointing down such as AR or RCB, or, better yet, multipurpose (multipurpose being the best guide for anomalous LCx intervention).

B. Anomalous LM originating from the right sinus

Unless it takes a less common posterior course, this anomalous LM is usually anterior to the RCA, and has a downward takeoff. It is best engaged with a multipurpose catheter, AR, or a short AL (AL0.75 or 1), with a clockwise rotation from the neutral position.

C. Anomalous RCA originating from the left sinus

This RCA is usually anterior and more cephalad than the LM. It can be engaged with a large AL (e.g., AL1.5 or 2) or a long JL catheter (JL5) that is sometimes pushed and looped over the aortic valve. A JL catheter is usually successful when the RCA is close to the LM, while AL may be necessary when the RCA is anterior.

XIX. Specific tips for coronary engagement using a radial approach

A. Tips

Four important tips are critical to successful coronary engagement through a radial access (Figure 35.30):

- *The guidewire should be advanced and looped over the aortic valve. The catheter should then be advanced over the wire all the way until it touches the aortic valve below the coronary ostia.* This allows the catheter to be appropriately shaped and prevents it from sliding out of the ascending aorta (the catheter approaches the coronary ostium from below). This is not necessary in femoral manipulations, except if the aorta is large or if AL is used.
- *The catheter should not only touch the aortic valve, it should be maneuvered to specifically touch the corresponding cusp* (e.g., left coronary cusp for left coronary engagement). If the catheter does not fall swiftly into its cusp, the wire is directed toward this cusp and the catheter is then advanced over it.
- *Engagement of the coronary ostia is facilitated by leaving the guidewire within the catheter to enhance torqueability* and prevent the catheter from looping on itself. This is particularly important in the left coronary engagement and in patients with tortuous subclavian vessels or a short ascending aorta (short patients).
- A deep breath vertically elongates the aorta and the subclavian artery and attenuates the sharp catheter turn from the subclavian into the aorta, which facilitates engagement.

Also, a long sheath (25 cm) may circumvent tortuous radioulnar loops and any spastic area, improving torqueability. A long sheath limits the spasm that may occur later on, during catheter advancement or exchange through the radial artery, and is advised during interventions or when multiple catheters are exchanged.

If the wire keeps falling into the descending rather than ascending aorta, the catheter should be used to direct the wire into the ascending aorta, generally with a counterclockwise maneuver, and the patient may be asked to take a deep breath (this vertically elongates the aortic arch and the origins of the left subclavian and right innominate, creating a more vertical angle into the ascending aorta). A Glidewire may be used during these manipulations, as it more easily slips into the ascending aorta.

B. Importance of patient's height, subclavian tortuosity, right radial vs. left radial

Short patients with short and steep aortas are difficult to engage from a right radial access, as the catheter will take a sharp turn from the innominate artery into the ascending aorta, which reduces torqueability and increases the chance of catheter loop and prolapse out of the ascending aorta (Figure 35.30B). A deep breath elongates the aorta and may facilitate coronary engagement; a left Amplatz catheter advanced over the wire onto the aortic valve may prove useful (Figure 35.31).

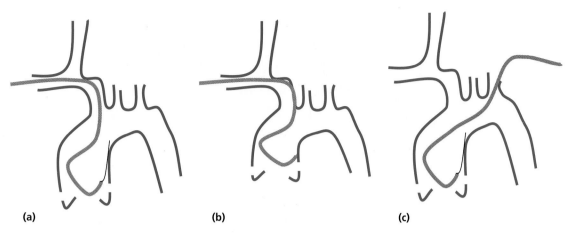

(a)   (b)   (c)

Figure 35.30 Engagement of a coronary artery through a radial approach.

(a) It is best to advance the catheter over the wire all the way down to the valve before starting the manipulations, to ensure appropriate catheter shaping and prevent the catheter from looping on itself or sliding out of the ascending aorta into the arch.

(b) A short ascending aorta translates into a sharper catheter turn into the ascending aorta, less support, and more tendency to loop and prolapse out of the ascending aorta.

(c) A left radial approach is associated with a less sharp turn at the aortic level, and thus easier catheter maneuvering and support than a right radial approach.

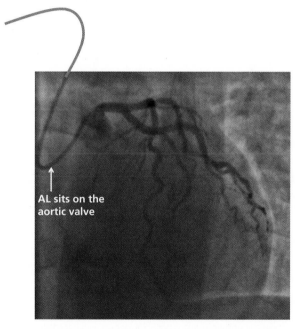

Figure 35.31 AL2 is used to engage the left coronary artery through a right radial approach in a patient with a short aorta. Amplatz left catheters may prove useful if the special radial and Judkins catheters are unsuccessful. They sit on the aortic valve and are less likely to loop and prolapse, providing good support.

In addition, severe tortuosity of the right subclavian and the right innominate–aortic arch junction is much more common than left subclavian tortuosity (10–20% vs. 5%), which further complicates the right radial approach (Figure 35.32). This is particularly common in patients with several of the following four features: short stature, old age (>75), female sex, and hypertension. *A left radial access may, thus, be preferred in patients with several of those features (e.g., old patients of short stature) or those with severe right subclavian tortuosity.* A hydrophilic Glidewire is frequently needed to cross the subclavian loops.

A catheter advanced through the left radial access follows a path close to the femoral path, with a less sharp turn at the ascending aortic level than a right radial access. The support from a left radial access is therefore generally better, and a left radial access is particularly useful in patients with short aortas (Figure 35.30C). A left radial access is more readily feasible in patients with a small body habitus, wherein the operator works from the right side of the patient and leans over to the left, similarly to using a left femoral access.

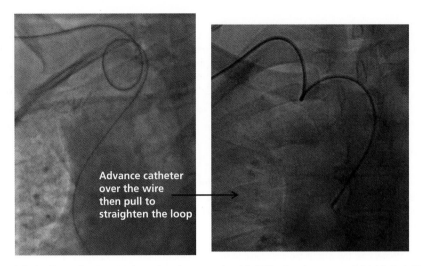

Figure 35.32 Severe right subclavian/ innominate tortuosity or loop is present in ~10–20% of patients, especially elderly (>75), short, hypertensive, and female patients. A hydrophilic 0.035″ wire (Glidewire) is used to traverse the tortuosity, ideally as the patient takes a deep breath, then advanced far into the aorta. The catheter is then advanced over the wire as far as possible. The whole system is then pulled back (right image), which allows the tortuosity to straighten.

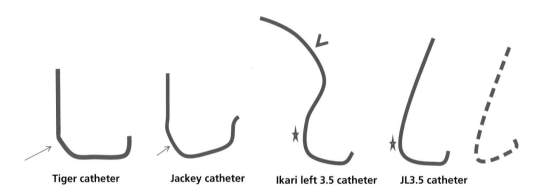

Figure 35.33 Specific radial catheters, particularly helpful for a right radial approach. Compare them to JL catheter. **(i)** *Tiger and Jackey*: note the long secondary curve that allows the catheter to rest over the contralateral aorta for support (*arrows*). Tiger's tip tends to point up, while Jackey's tip may point down. **(ii)** *Ikari left*: unlike the limited aortic contact of JL, Ikari has a long secondary curve that sits on the opposite aortic wall and provides good support (*stars*). In addition, Ikari left has a natural bend that embraces the right innominate angulation (*arrowhead*), attenuating the catheter's tendency to turn over itself (*dashed* JL catheter).

C. Judkins catheter sizes in transradial procedures; catheters for diagnostic and interventional transradial procedures

- From a *left radial approach*, no change in Judkins arm size is generally needed for right or left coronary engagement.
- From a *right radial approach*: (1) left coronary engagement usually requires a catheter that is 0.5 smaller than what would be used with the femoral or left radial approach (e.g., JL3.5, XB3 or 3.5); (2) RCA requires the same curve or a larger one (e.g., JR5).
- Special radial catheters may be used, and these are particularly useful during a right radial approach. Tiger and Jackey catheters are useful diagnostic catheters; the Tiger catheter points upward, while the Jackey catheter generally points downward (Figure 35.33).
- Amplatz left catheters may prove useful if the special radial and Judkins catheters are unsuccessful. They sit on the aortic valve and are less likely to loop and prolapse, which allows them to provide good support, particularly during interventions (Figure 35.31).
- *For diagnostic procedures*: Tiger/Jackey (for both left and right coronary arteries) or Judkins catheters are the initial catheters used.
- *For simple left coronary interventions*, a Judkins catheter or Ikari left catheter may be used.
- *For complex left coronary interventions*, the following may be used: AL catheter (AL1.5 or 2), EBU catheter, or the Ikari left catheter, which is a modified Judkins catheter designed to embrace the brachiocephalic angle and the aortic wall. *From a transradial approach, EBU and Ikari left are manipulated somewhat similarly to AL* (Figure 35.16): (i) they are initially **advanced until their tip catches the left cusp (over the wire)**; (ii) they are then **pushed against the cusp in a U fashion** until their tip points up and catches the ostium. Alternatively, Ikari left may just be pulled to engage the ostium, similarly to a Judkins catheter. *In a way, Ikari left may be maneuvered either as an EBU-like or a Judkins-like catheter.*
- *For simple RCA interventions*, JR4 or JR5 may be used.
- *For complex RCA interventions*, AR (especially the longer-tip AR2), hockeystick 2, or AL0.75 catheter may be used.

D. How to engage the RCA using the Tiger catheter that was used for left coronary engagement

After engaging the left coronary and obtaining the images with a Tiger catheter, the catheter is disengaged under fluoroscopy, then slightly pulled with a torque maneuver to get out of the left coronary plane. The catheter is then pushed down to the valve, avoiding the plane of the left coronary ostium. At this point, the catheter is pulled with a slight clock or counterclock maneuver to engage the RCA. ***It is generally easier to engage the RCA from a radial approach than from a femoral approach, and less torque is generally required***. Furthermore, the catheter is less prone to diving down. While the RCA is engaged with a clockwise rotation from a femoral approach, a clockwise or counterclockwise rotation may prove useful from a right radial approach.

XX. Damping and ventricularization of the aortic waveform upon coronary engagement

When a catheter engages a coronary artery, the pressure at its tip may damp or ventricularize. Damping is characterized by flattening of the pressure tracing with significant drop in the systolic and diastolic pressures; it indicates pressure reduction at the tip of the catheter (Figure 35.34). Ventricularization is characterized by a change in pressure from an aortic to a "ventricular-like" tracing and reflects severe ostial narrowing. The stenotic lesion restricts blood flow into the engaged artery from which the pressure is being recorded; *since coronary flow mainly occurs in diastole, the drop in pressure across the stenosis is mainly diastolic*. Ventricularization may be obvious and may manifest as a severe drop in diastolic aortic pressure and a change from a triangular to a rectangular shape. ***Subtle or early ventricularization is more common and is identified by two features:*** *(1) diastolic pressure changes from downsloping (aortic) to upsloping (ventricular); (2) A waves appear on the tracing.* Also, in addition to the drop and change in diastolic pressure, the systolic pressure usually decreases during ventricularization.

Damping that occurs before engagement of a coronary artery usually alerts to the presence of air or clot in the catheter, or to twisting of the catheter after excessive torquing. Damping upon coronary engagement has several causes: (1) severe ostial disease, with the catheter further reducing or occluding flow across the ostium and leading to reduced pressure in the coronary artery; (2) ostial spasm; (3) small coronary artery engaged with a large catheter that occludes it, particularly when a right coronary catheter selectively engages the small conus branch; (4) catheter against the arterial wall or against a plaque which damps the pressure at its tip. Ventricularization only occurs with ostial narrowing (causes [1] to [3]) and is not seen when a catheter is against the arterial wall. Since damping and ventricularization often signify occlusion of flow across the ostium, injecting contrast while damped or ventricularized replaces the remaining oxygenated blood with contrast. The latter is not quickly cleared because of reduced flow, which further reduces myocardial oxygen supply. ***Lack of contrast clearance from the coronary arteries or, worse, from the myocardium (myocardial stain) is a serious consequence of damping, which imminently leads to ischemia and ventricular fibrillation and dictates immediate catheter disengagement.*** In addition, vigorous injection while damped or ventricularized may lead to coronary dissection, since the catheter is surrounded by ostial disease or is against the vessel wall. It may also lead to embolization of thrombus or air if these were the causes of damping.

Thus, one should not inject contrast or flush with saline while damped or ventricularized, but should disengage and attempt to re-engage after taking a non-selective image to check for ostial disease, attempt to engage the right coronary if the conus branch was previously engaged, and administer sublingual nitroglycerin if ostial spasm was likely. A ***catheter with side holes*** allows contrast clearance, reduces the risk of ventricular fibrillation, and provides some coronary perfusion while the catheter is seated in the coronary artery between coronary injections; it may be useful during a coronary intervention where the guiding catheter has to remain engaged for a prolonged time. Yet, it is important to realize that a catheter with side holes only partly reduces catheter-related ischemia and does not prevent the dreaded risk of dissection. Moreover, this catheter will transmit a normal pressure recording that is partly related to the transmission of pressure from the side holes positioned in the aorta, rather than from the tip positioned at the ostium, therefore providing a false reassurance. The spilling of contrast in the aorta results in lower image quality and greater contrast use.

During a coronary intervention, ventricularization often occurs when the guiding catheter is too deeply engaged, particularly if the artery is small or has moderate ostial disease. Slight pullback or torque is appropriate. Interestingly, ***the administration of nitroglycerin may induce or worsen ventricularization early on***; the increase in flow induced by vasodilators may worsen the drop in pressure across the ostial obstruction, particularly diastolic pressure, leading to ventricularization (drop in pressure = flow × resistance). However, nitroglycerin may improve ventricularization later on, once spasm, a component of ostial obstruction, is relieved.

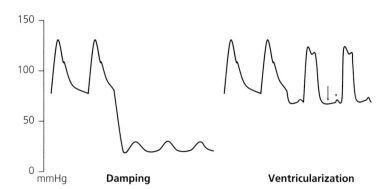

Figure 35.34 Examples of damping and ventricularization of the aortic pressure upon coronary engagement. In *ventricularization*, the diastolic pressure does not necessarily drop to levels that are as low as the left ventricular diastolic pressure, but the shape of the tracing changes from an arterial one to a ventricular one, i.e., the diastolic segment between the spikes is upsloping *(arrow)* and A wave is seen *(arrowhead)*.

XXI. Technique of right heart catheterization

1. From jugular, subclavian, brachial, or femoral venous access, the right heart catheter is advanced to the RA. At this point, the catheter is connected to the pressure transducer (through the manifold, for example) and flushed, and the RA pressure is recorded after ensuring proper zeroing at the mid-chest level.

2. The catheter is then advanced to the RV, then the PA, while the balloon at the tip of the catheter is inflated and pressures are recorded. Special handling is required when a femoral access is used. At the base of the RV (bottom part of the cardiac silhouette), the catheter is pushed, then torqued *clockwise with a slight pull* until it points superiorly and falls into the PA. *Deep inspiration and cough may assist in crossing the pulmonic valve and advancing the catheter distally.*

Alternatively, the catheter tip may be "hooked" in the ostium of a hepatic vein or directed towards the lateral RA with the balloon inflated. When advanced, it creates a loop in the RA. Once a loop is formed, further catheter push directs the tip of the loop towards the RV, then towards the RVOT and PA (Figure 35.35).

A Swan wire or a supportive 0.014" wire may be advanced beyond the catheter tip, with the balloon inflated, and used to cross the pulmonic valve into the PA. This wire is particularly helpful in patients with dilated RV. The wire also provides stiffness to the catheter and helps it track into the distal PA, preventing its prolapse into the RV. The catheter is advanced over the wire while the balloon is inflated, except in TR, where the inflated balloon may project the catheter backward, along the regurgitant flow.

3. After recording the PA pressure, the catheter is advanced with the balloon inflated until it wedges, i.e., the tip becomes immobile on fluoroscopy and one sees a change from PA pressure to PCWP on the monitor. PCWP is recorded, the balloon is then deflated and the catheter pulled back to the PA position. Avoid flushing in the PCWP position, as this may injure the pulmonary capillaries.

4. Cardiac output (CO) is measured using the thermodilution technique while the catheter is in the PA. Also, an oxygen sample is obtained from the PA (both for CO calculation using the Fick equation *and* for detecting a shunt). An oxygen sample is simultaneously obtained from the arterial sheath to calculate Fick CO.

5. The catheter is then pulled back and SVC and IVC blood samples obtained for oximetry (shunt screen). All oximetry samples should be collected within a few minutes in a calm steady state to avoid fluctuation of O_2 consumption and mixed venous O_2 saturation in the same patient. If catheterization is performed from a femoral access, the SVC is easily engaged by advancing a multipurpose catheter over a 0.035" wire into the SVC, immediately after removing the Swan catheter. The Swan catheter does not float easily into the SVC.

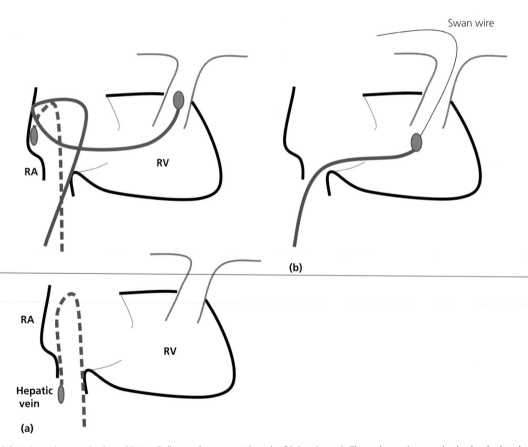

Figure 35.35 (a) Catheter loop at the *lateral RA wall* allows advancement into the PA (top image). The catheter tip may also be *hooked at the ostium of a hepatic vein* (bottom image), pushed until it loops in the RA, then released with balloon deflation. In right HF with dilated hepatic veins, the catheter tends to dive deeply into the hepatic vein (unwanted effect) rather than be "stuck" at its ostium. **(b)** Alternatively, the catheter is kept straight, and a Swan wire advanced into the PA. These techniques are especially useful in patients with dilated RV and/or TR. Remember that cough and deep inspiration also allow easier catheter tracking into the PA.

6. Left heart catheterization is performed afterward.

7. In special settings, simultaneous tracings may be necessary. During simultaneous recordings, "re-zero" both transducers simultaneously at the same level. After simultaneous recordings, switch catheter–transducer connections and ensure that the measurements and the pressure gradient remain unchanged (indirectly proving proper zeroing)

    a. When suspecting constrictive pericarditis, standard right heart catheterization is initially performed. Afterward, the LV is accessed and simultaneous LV pressure and PCWP recordings are obtained, followed by simultaneous LV and RV pressure recordings. These recordings may be repeated after a saline challenge.

    b. When assessing for aortic stenosis, right heart catheterization is performed first and the right heart catheter is left in the PA. The left ventricle is then accessed, using the technique described in Section XVII. Simultaneous LV–aortic pressure tracings are then recorded through the double-lumen catheter. CO is simultaneously obtained through the Swan catheter that was left in the PA, and the valve area is calculated.

    c. When assessing for mitral stenosis, right heart catheterization is performed first and the right heart catheter is left in the PA. The left ventricle is then accessed and simultaneous LV pressure and PCWP recordings are obtained. CO is obtained (or repeated) after pulling the right heart catheter into the PA. In order to adequately calculate valve area, make sure CO is performed close to the timing of gradient measurement. Some maneuvers may be performed if needed (e.g., handgrip, exercise), after which LV pressure, PCWP, PA pressure, and CO are evaluated again.

    d. If pulmonary hypertension is not associated with an increased PCWP, and if pulmonary arterial hypertension is suspected, a vasodilator may be infused and PA pressure, PCWP, and systemic pressure reassessed at each up-titration. During the last titration of the vasodilator, measure CO and assess RA pressure on pullback.

Note The right bundle being a slender bundle, the right heart catheter may produce a transient RBBB. In a patient with LBBB, this may lead to complete AV block. **Beware of AV block in any patient with LBBB undergoing right heart catheterization.** A temporary pacemaker should be readily available.

36 Hemodynamics

I. Right heart catheter (see Figure 36.1)

For catheterization technique, see Chapter 35, Section XXI.

II. Overview of pressure tracings: differences between atrial, ventricular, and arterial tracings (Figures 36.2, 36.3, 36.4)

III. RA pressure abnormalities

Summary of RA pressure abnormalities (Figures 36.5, 36.6, 36.7):

- **Deep X and deep Y descents:** constrictive pericarditis, restrictive cardiomyopathy, and, most frequently, severe RV failure. Deep X and deep Y descents reflect loss of atrial and ventricular compliances, wherein atrial pressure goes sharply down and then up; they may also reflect the distension of the pericardium and the functional constriction seen in severe RV dilatation.
- **Large V wave with deep Y descent:** severe TR and/or RV failure. The X that precedes the V wave may be flattened and "carried up" by the large V wave (*flat X* = systolic flow blunting).
- **Deep X and flat Y** (blunting of diastolic flow): tamponade (mnemonic: **Flat Y Tamponade** = FYT). In tamponade, not only is chamber compliance impaired, but ventricular filling is totally impeded in diastole, explaining the flat Y. Y may also be flat with sinus tachycardia.
- **Large V wave:** severe TR and/or RV failure. In severe TR, the V wave is not only tall but wide and plateaus throughout systole, approximating the RV systolic pressure; this leads to a **ventricularized** RA pressure.
- **Large A wave:** impaired RV compliance.

IV. Pulmonary capillary wedge pressure (PCWP) abnormalities

PCWP is obtained by inflating the balloon-tipped catheter in a distal PA position until it occludes the PA branch. This leads to a stagnant column of blood beyond the balloon, the pressure of which equalizes with the downstream pulmonary venous pressure and thus the LA pressure. Similarly to LA pressure, PCWP has A, X, V, and Y waves. Mean PCWP is equal to mean LA pressure. However, PCWP is delayed ~50–100 ms in comparison to LA pressure because of the delay in retrograde pressure transmission from the LA through the pulmonary vasculature; therefore, PCWP's A and V waves peak later than LA's A and V waves. In addition, PCWP has a smoother contour with less steep and deep V downslope than LA pressure, as the pressure waveform gets damped while being transmitted from the LA through the pulmonary capillaries.

Practical Cardiovascular Medicine, First Edition. Elias B. Hanna.
© 2017 John Wiley & Sons Ltd. Published 2017 by John Wiley & Sons Ltd.

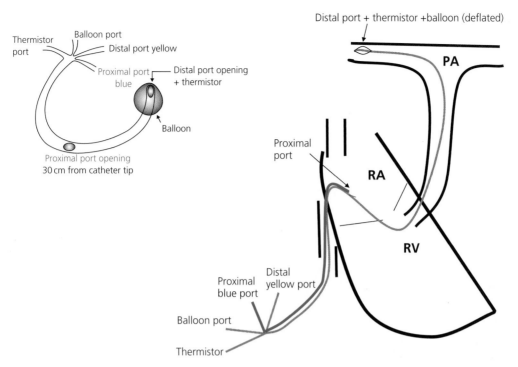

Figure 36.1 The Swan–Ganz balloon flotation catheter has four ports. (1) The ***distal yellow port*** communicates with the distal tip of the catheter; it is connected to the transducer and used to obtain pressures as the catheter is advanced through the right-sided chambers (RA → PA → PCWP). (2) The ***proximal blue port*** communicates with another lumen, 30 cm proximal to the tip. When the catheter tip is in the PA, the blue port opens in the RA; at this location, the blue port is used to inject saline into the RA and obtain cardiac output by the thermodilution technique. The blue port may also be used to record RA pressure simultaneously with PA pressure, particularly when a Swan–Ganz catheter is used for continuous monitoring in the cardiac unit. (3) The ***balloon port*** communicates with the distal balloon and allows wedging of the catheter tip (PA pressure → PCWP). (4) The ***temperature sensor port*** also communicates with the distal catheter tip; after cold saline is injected through the blue port (RA), the temperature sensor (PA) analyzes the temperature change over time and allows calculation of CO. Reproduced with permission of Demos Medical from Hanna and Glancy (2012).[1]

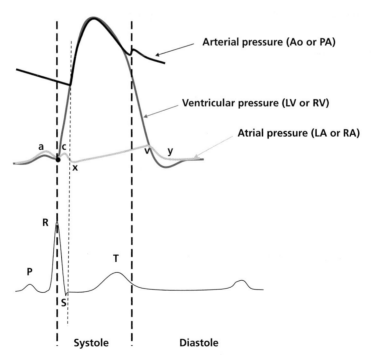

Figure 36.2 Timing of atrial, ventricular, and arterial pressures in relation to each other and to the ECG.
1. ***Atrial pressure*** has an A wave that follows the P wave, and **a V wave that peaks at or after the end of the T wave and almost intersects with the ventricular pressure descent (slightly precedes it).** Unlike the ventricular and arterial pressures, which peak during the ST–T segment, atrial pressure peaks before the ST–T segment (A wave) and after the ST–T segment (V wave).
2. ***Ventricular pressure*** increases in diastole and has an A wave.
3. ***Arterial pressure*** decreases in diastole, has no A wave, and has a dicrotic notch (the latter 3 features distinguish it from ventricular tracing).
Ventricular end-diastolic pressure (EDP) is the post-A ventricular pressure and corresponds to the peak of R wave (*black dot*).
  Reproduced with permission of Demos Medical from Hanna and Glancy (2012).[1]

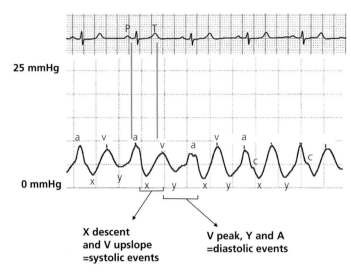

Figure 36.3 Atrial pressure tracing (RA or PCWP). A wave corresponds to atrial contraction and follows the electrocardiographic P wave. X descent corresponds to the atrial relaxation and to the downward pulling of the tricuspid annulus in early systole. V wave corresponds to atrial filling during ventricular systole while the tricuspid valve is closed. Y descent occurs in early diastole as the tricuspid valve opens and the RA rapidly empties. Thus, X descent and the upslope of V wave are systolic events (coincide with the pulse), whereas the peak of V wave, the Y descent, and the A wave are diastolic events.

V wave corresponds to atrial compliance (a large V wave implies a volume overload that overwhelms the atrial compliance). On the other hand, A wave corresponds to ventricular compliance. In normal individuals, RA pressure is characterized by A wave > V wave. LA is normally less compliant than RA, because it is constrained by pulmonary veins and it is thicker than RA, and thus LA V wave > A wave.

The C wave is a small positive deflection on the atrial tracing that sometimes interrupts the X descent; it corresponds to the brief protrusion of the tricuspid valve into the RA in early systole during isovolumic ventricular contraction.

The A wave is only seen in sinus rhythm; it is not seen in atrial fibrillation (AF). However, a C wave may be seen in AF and may mimic the A wave.
Reproduced with permission of Demos Medical from Hanna and Glancy (2012).[1]

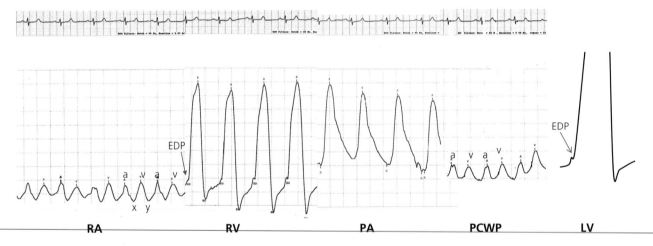

Figure 36.4 RA, RV, PA, and PCWP tracings obtained while advancing the catheter from RA to PA. LV pressure from LV catheterization is shown. In general, mean RA pressure is equal to RV diastolic pressure, and mean PCWP is equal to PA diastolic pressure and LV end-diastolic pressure. RA pressure and RV end-diastolic pressure are lower than PA diastolic pressure and PCWP, except in cases of "equalization of diastolic pressure" (tamponade, constriction, severe RV failure).
Concerning RA and PCWP pressures: note the A, X, V, Y waves and the timing of A and V waves (V peaks after ECG T wave).
Concerning PA: in contrast to the RV pressure, which increases throughout diastole (upsloping) and has A wave bump, PA pressure decreases throughout diastole (downsloping), does not have an A bump, and has a dicrotic notch. *In contrast to the RA or PCWP tracing*, the systolic PA peak occurs during the ST–T interval and the PA pressure is downsloping in diastole.
Example of normal pressures (in mmHg):
RA pressure (mean) = <u>5</u>; **RV** pressure = **25/5**; **PA** pressure = **25/12**; **PCWP** = **12**; **LV** pressure = 120/12 (LVEDP = **12**)
Reproduced with permission of Demos Medical from Hanna and Glancy (2012).[1]

A. Differential diagnosis of a large V wave

A large V wave is a V wave that is ≥ 2× the mean PCWP, or ≥ 10 mmHg larger than the mean PCWP. While classically associated with severe MR, *a large V wave implies volume overload that overwhelms the LA compliance*. Thus, V wave may not be large in severe but compensated chronic MR (e.g., asymptomatic MR patients), and may, on the other hand, be large in decompensated HF even in the absence of MR. In fact, the causes of a large V wave are: (1) severe and decompensated MR; (2) decompensated LV failure; (3) mitral stenosis; (4) VSD. In one study, ~40% of patients with a large V wave did not have significant MR, while only 40% of patients with severe MR had a large V wave.[2] A gigantic V wave, i.e., a V wave that is ≥ 2.5× the mean PCWP, or >50 mmHg, is usually secondary to MR.

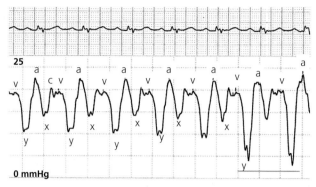

Figure 36.5 Typical deep X and deep Y descents on RA tracing, consistent with constrictive pericarditis but also with restrictive cardiomyopathy and severe RV failure. In severe RV failure, a large V wave with a flattened X descent may also be seen. V wave and Y descent become particularly prominent in inspiration (end of the tracing).

Normally, mean RA pressure declines with inspiration. A flat RA pressure without significant inspiratory drop of the mean, as in this case, is characteristic of RV failure and constriction. Only the depth of Y descent changes with inspiration. In severe RV failure, RA and RV compliances are severely overwhelmed, such that RA pressure may paradoxically rise with the inspiratory rise in preload, despite the direct transmission of negative intrathoracic pressure.

Reproduced with permission from Hanna and Glancy (2012).[1]

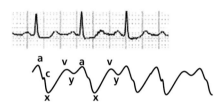

Figure 36.6 Deep X with flat Y on RA tracing, suggestive of tamponade. This may also be seen with sinus tachycardia, which shortens diastole and may thus attenuate Y descent. Reproduced with permission of Demos Medical from Hanna and Glancy (2012).[1]

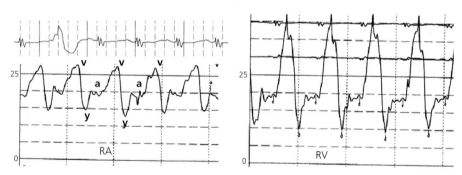

Figure 36.7 Ventricularized RA pressure in a patient with severe TR. The V wave is not only ample but wide and peaks during the ST–T segment, similarly to the RV systolic pressure. Note that Y descent is deep but X descent is flattened. Compare to RV pressure in the same patient. Reproduced with permission of Demos Medical from Hanna and Glancy (2012).[1]

B. Differentiate a large V wave from PA pressure

A large V wave may resemble PA pressure (Figures 36.8, 36.9). Five features help differentiate PCWP from PA pressure:

- V wave peaks after T wave, whereas systolic PA pressure peaks during T wave.
- V wave has a *gradual upslope and a sharp downslope*, which is opposite to the PA pressure (V wave has a more "peaked," narrow appearance).
- The segment between V waves is rather horizontal or upsloping and an A wave is usually seen, whereas on the PA pressure tracing the segment between the systolic peaks is downsloping, has a dicrotic notch, and does not have an A wave.
- Mean PCWP should be ≤ diastolic PA pressure and < mean PA pressure. *Upon balloon deflation and pullback of a wedged PA catheter, one should normally see a change in both the timing and the height of the pressure tracing corresponding to PA pressure.* The lack of a significant change (e.g., mean PCWP ≈ mean PA pressure) means that PCWP was actually a damped PA pressure. Conversely, a significant change suggests but does not confirm true wedging.
- In difficult cases, one may obtain a blood sample from the wedged catheter tip and check O_2 saturation. PCWP saturation = arterial saturation (usually >95%), whereas PA saturation = mixed venous saturation. This is the best confirmatory method of appropriate wedging, as in rare cases, A and V waves may be seen with a hybrid PA–PCWP tracing. It may, however, be difficult to withdraw blood from a wedged Swan catheter; a balloon flotation catheter with multiple distal side-holes may be used (Berman catheter).

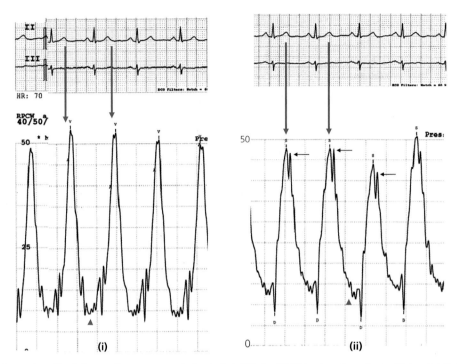

Figure 36.8 On gross inspection of both figures, they may seem similar. In fact, **(i)** is the PCWP tracing of a patient with severe MR and gigantic V waves, while **(ii)** is his PA pressure tracing. Reproduced with permission of Demos Medical from Hanna and Glancy (2012).[1]

Keys to differentiate:

1. Timing: note that in (i) the V wave peaks *after the end of the ECG T wave*, whereas in (ii) the systolic PA pressure peaks *before the end of the T wave* (*down-arrows*).
2. The segment between V waves is horizontal, whereas the segment between PA peaks, i.e., diastolic PA pressure, is downsloping (*arrowheads*).
3. PA pressure has a dicrotic notch. PA pressure has a sharp upslope and a slow downslope, which is opposite to the shape of V wave.
4. PA pressure is double-peaked. The second peak (*horizontal arrow*) corresponds to the transmission of V wave to the PA pressure. Note that V wave is almost as large as systolic PA pressure, yet the mean PCWP is certainly lower than the mean PA pressure.

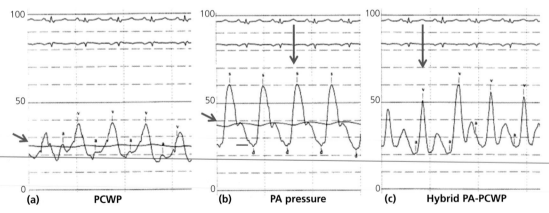

Figure 36.9 (a, b) PCWP tracing shows a large V wave of ~38 mmHg, with a mean PCWP of 26 mmHg. The mean PCWP (*left oblique arrow*) is lower than the mean PA pressure (*right oblique arrow*), and is equal to the PA diastolic pressure (*bar*), all of which is consistent with a true PCWP.

(c) Tracing C is recorded after inflation of the PA catheter balloon. It may mimic a PCWP tracing with a large V wave. However, the mean of this pressure tracing almost approximates the mean PA pressure and exceeds the PA diastolic pressure. Also, the timing does not fit with PA pressure: the presumed V waves peak as early as the PA pressure peaks, during the ECG T waves (*vertical arrows*), and have a sharp upslope, similar to the PA pressure upslope; the presumed A waves precede the ECG P waves. Thus, this is not a true PCWP tracing. The PA catheter is "underwedged," which results in a hybrid PA–PCWP waveform.

C. Case of pulmonary hypertension: differentiate PCWP from a damped PA pressure

In severe pulmonary hypertension (PH), two issues arise. *First,* in severe PH, the segmental PA branches are dilated, which makes it difficult for the catheter to occlude these branches; thus, the wedged PA waveform may be a damped PA waveform and may overestimate the true PCWP (it is a hybrid PA–PCWP waveform with arterial rather than PCWP characteristics) (Figure 36.9). *Second,* a phasic PCWP depends on appropriate retrograde transmission of LA pressure through the pulmonary vasculature without any anatomical barrier; in case of severely elevated pulmonary arteriolar or venous resistance, retrograde transmission of LA pressure is attenuated, producing a damped and flattened

PCWP that lacks distinct waves and descents. In the latter situation, mean PCWP may approximate mean LA pressure, but the waveform is flat and featureless and falsely creates or overestimates a transmitral gradient. **In sum, the PCWP of PH may be a false PCWP (damped PA waveform), or a true PCWP that is, nonetheless, featureless (damped PCWP waveform).**

Other cases where PCWP lacks A and V waves and potentially overestimates the true PCWP: (i) catheter overwedging; (ii) catheter in the upper lung zone 1, where the pulmonary capillaries are collapsed by the alveolar pressure and where PCWP reflects alveolar pressure rather than capillary pressure (this false PCWP may exceed PA diastolic pressure). In patients with elevated PCWP, it is harder for the alveolar pressure to compress the pulmonary capillaries, and thus zone 1 significantly shrinks and is unlikely to be catheterized.

> Beside the issue of PCWP–LA pressure correlation, a major pitfall of LA pressure itself is that it is not equivalent to LV preload, which is LV end-diastolic volume. Patients with a very steep LV pressure–volume relationship, such as patients with acute HF or severe diastolic HF, may have a relatively normal LV preload volume with a high LA pressure.

V. LVEDP

LV diastolic pressure slightly increases throughout diastole, and, except in AF, has an A wave that corresponds to the atrial A wave. LVEDP is located at the downslope of the A wave. In normal individuals with compliant LV, LV pressure increases only slightly after A wave, so that post-A LV pressure is not significantly higher than pre-A LV pressure. In *compensated LV dysfunction*, LV pressure is normal throughout diastole but increases only after A wave; similarly, LA pressure is overall normal and increases only after A wave, explaining why mean LA pressure better correlates with pre-A LV pressure than with LVEDP. In *decompensated LV dysfunction*, LV pressure is high throughout diastole and increases further after A wave (Figure 36.10, Table 36.1).

To identify LVEDP, search for a bump on the LV upstroke; the bump is A wave and the point that follows this bump is LVEDP (Figure 36.11). *While LVEDP varies with respiration, the most accurate LVEDP is obtained when the respiratory pressure is 0 mmHg, which, unless the patient actively exhales, corresponds to end-expiration and coincides with the highest recorded LVEDP point. This end-expiratory rule applies to all measured pressures.*

Note: Normal hemodynamic values

- RA: mean ≤ 7 mmHg
- RV: ≤ 35/8
- PA: ≤ 35/12 (mean PA pressure ≤ 20 mmHg)
- LVEDP: ≤ 16 mmHg
- PCWP: mean ≤ 12 mmHg. Note that values up to 15–18 mmHg may not lead to congestion in patients with chronic heart failure who have increased pulmonary capillary lymphatic drainage. However, except for patients with poor LV compliance, such as patients with new-onset acute heart failure or severe diastolic heart failure, PCWP of 15–18 mmHg corresponds to an unnecessary increase in LV volume preload and may be safely reduced to 12 mmHg (see Chapter 5, Figure 5.5).

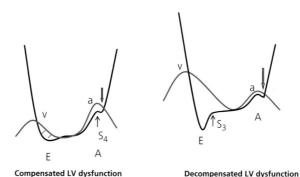

Figure 36.10 Diastolic superimposition of LA pressure (or PCWP, in *blue*) **and LV pressure** (in *black*). *Downward arrows* point to LVEDP.

In compensated LV dysfunction, LV pressure is normal before A wave but increases after A wave (LVEDP). On PCWP tracing, V wave is normal, A wave is increased, but mean PCWP is overall normal and better correlates with the pre-A LV pressure than the elevated LVEDP (PCWP < LVEDP).

In decompensated LV dysfunction, both pre-A and post-A LV pressures are elevated. On PCWP tracing, V wave is large, and mean PCWP is equal to LVEDP or larger than LVEDP, depending on how large V wave is.

Table 36.1 Correlation between LVEDP and mean PCWP.

- Normally, LVEDP ~ mean PCWP
- LVEDP > PCWP: compensated LV dysfunction, AI
- LVEDP ≈ PCWP in decompensated LV failure
- LVEDP < PCWP: MS, MR with large V wave, decompensated LV failure with large V wave
  In MS, end-diastolic PCWP is higher than LVEDP, whereas in MR or LV failure with a large V wave, end-diastolic PCWP remains equal to LVEDP, but mean PCWP is larger than LVEDP (driven by the large V wave).

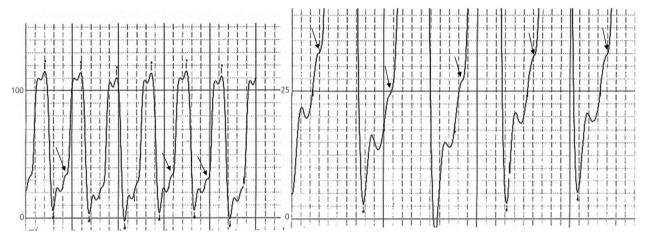

Figure 36.11 LVEDP corresponds to the bump seen on the LV upstroke (*arrows*), often coinciding with the peak of R wave on the ECG (LVEDP may be further delayed from R peak when the ACIST automatic injector system is used). This bump is LV A wave. In this figure, LV pressure steeply increases during and after A wave, leading to a pronounced A wave and a high LVEDP of 32 mmHg. **LVEDP does not correspond to the flat/plateau portion of LV diastole.** Always look for these bumps when assessing LVEDP, as long as the rhythm is sinus. Reproduced with permission of Demos Medical from Hanna and Glancy (2012).[1]

Table 36.2 Fick equation.

O_2 **consumption** (ml O_2/min)	= **Arterial O_2 delivery − venous O_2 return**
	= **CO × arterial O_2content − CO × venous O_2content**
	= **CO** (liters blood/min) × **AV difference in O_2content** (ml O_2/l blood)
⇒ **CO** (liters blood/min)	= **O_2 consumption** (ml O_2/min) divided by:
	AV difference in O_2content (ml O_2/l blood)
1. Arterial O_2 content (ml/l)	= SaO$_2$ × Hb(g/dl) × maximal capacity of 1g of Hb to carry O_2 (1.36ml O_2/g of Hb) × 10
2. Venous O_2 content (ml/l)	= SvO$_2$ × Hb × 1.36 × 10
⇒ **CO**	= **O_2 consumption (ml/min) divided by:**
	1.36 × hemoglobin × (SaO$_2$ − SvO$_2$) × 10

SaO$_2$ and SvO$_2$ are expressed as decimal fractions. ***In the absence of a left-to-right shunt, SvO$_2$ corresponds to O_2 saturation of the PA, where the venous blood achieves its best mixing from all sources*** (SVC, IVC, coronary sinus); sampling of the RA may selectively capture one of these three sources rather than their mixture. CO, cardiac output; Hb, hemoglobin; SaO$_2$, arterial O_2 saturation (transcutaneous O_2 saturation may be used instead of SaO$_2$ if an arterial sheath has not been placed); SvO$_2$, mixed venous O_2 saturation.

VI. Cardiac output and vascular resistances

The cardiac output may be measured using **three different methods**: (1) true Fick method, which is the most accurate method; (2) assumed Fick method; (3) thermodilution. The Fick equation is shown in Table 36.2.

Short of truly measuring it, O_2 consumption may be assumed to be 125 ml/min/m² of BSA or 3 ml/min/kg at rest. This assumption is subject to a large variation between individuals and within the same individual depending on the degree of wakefulness and anxiety at different times during the procedure. This assumption may be associated with discrepancies of 25% or more in comparison with the true Fick method. Thus, using 125 ml/min/m² of BSA may underestimate CO in a fully awake anxious or agitated young patient, or a septic patient with elevated O_2 consumption, and may overestimate CO in elderly patients, in heart failure patients who have reduced O_2 consumption, and in obese patients (the formula uses true body weight and surface area, which overestimates O_2 consumption of the obese). In addition, this equation is even more subject to error in patients receiving O_2 therapy, especially >30% or 2 l/min, as O_2 may increase SvO$_2$ disproportionately to SaO$_2$ and lead to overestimation of cardiac output (compared to SaO$_2$, SvO$_2$ is on a steeper portion of the O_2–hemoglobin dissociation curve, which explains the sharper rise with O_2 therapy).

Thermodilution is measured using a PA catheter that has a thermistor at its distal tip. After the catheter is positioned in the PA, 10 ml of cold (room temperature) saline is injected instantaneously through the blue RA port. The thermistor analyzes how quickly the temperature drops as blood reaches the PA and how quickly it recovers. The higher the cardiac output, the more brief and sharp the temperature change will be with a small area under the curve. The colder the injectate, and the more instantaneously it reaches the RA, the more accurate the measured cardiac output. Usually three measurements are obtained to average the slight variability of cardiac output (~10%) that occurs with various levels of wakefulness. When used for valve area calculation, the cardiac output and pressure gradient should be measured almost simultaneously to account for this variation. *This method is valid in most cases, and has <5–10% error in comparison with the true Fick method, except in TR, low cardiac output, and right-to-left or left-to-right shunt:*

- *TR:* some data suggest that thermodilution underestimates CO by ~15% in moderate or severe TR, as the cold blood keeps recirculating and elongates the thermodilution curve. However, other data suggest a good correlation between true Fick and thermodilution in TR, as TR truly reduces CO.

- *Low cardiac output <3.5 l/min* (particularly <2.5 l/min): the injectate warms up excessively as it is traveling slowly through the RA and RV, before it reaches the PA, and gives the wrong impression of a slight and brief temperature change at the tip, hence the impression of a higher CO (up to 35% higher).
- *Shunts:* right and left cardiac outputs not being equal in shunt cases, thermodilution estimates the right rather than the left cardiac output, i.e., Qp rather than Qs. But even Qp is not adequately estimated in shunts. A large left-to-right shunt considerably dilutes the injectate and prevents any meaningful temperature change at the thermistor.

Mixed venous O_2 saturation (SvO_2) provides the best assessment of the adequacy of cardiac output. Given a normal hemoglobin level and a normal arterial O_2 saturation, and in the absence of O_2 therapy, a normal SvO_2 >60% corresponds to an adequate cardiac output that matches the peripheral O_2 demands. Patients with inappropriately reduced CO increase their peripheral extraction of O_2, thus reducing SvO_2. Patients who are sedated may have a low CO that, nonetheless, matches their peripheral demands, explaining the normal SvO_2 despite the low CO. On the other hand, heart failure patients exerting themselves or patients with septic shock may have a normal or high CO that is, nonetheless, not high enough to match their peripheral demands; therefore, SvO_2 is low despite the high CO.

High-flow O_2 therapy increases O_2 delivery and raises SvO_2 disproportionately to SaO_2. SvO_2 may exceed 60% despite a low CO. SvO_2 still correlates with the appropriateness of O_2 delivery, but less so with the appropriateness of CO. *The only situation where SvO_2 is normal despite an inappropriately low cardiac output is high-flow O_2 therapy.*

In the absence of a left-to-right shunt, the oxygen saturation of the PA represents the best measurement of SvO_2, PA being the chamber where the venous blood achieves its best mixing from all sources. In the presence of a shunt, SvO_2 is O_2 saturation of the chamber just proximal to the shunt, i.e., proximal to the O_2 step-up.

The evaluation of systemic vascular resistance (SVR) is useful in assessing shock states, while the evaluation of pulmonary vascular resistance (PVR) is useful in assessing pulmonary hypertension. Vascular resistance is obtained by the general equation:

$$\text{Resistance} = \Delta \text{ pressure/CO}$$
$$\rightarrow \text{SVR (in dyn.s.cm}^{-5}) = (\text{mean systemic arterial pressure} - \text{RA pressure}) \times 80/\text{CO}$$
$$\rightarrow \text{PVR (in dyn.s.cm}^{-5}) = (\text{mean PA pressure} - \text{PCWP or LA pressure}) \times 80/\text{CO}$$
$$\rightarrow \text{PVR (in Woods units)} = (\text{mean PA pressure} - \text{PCWP or LA pressure})/\text{CO}$$

Despite a potential discrepancy, LVEDP may be used as a surrogate of LA pressure when a proper PCWP tracing cannot be obtained.

$$\text{Normal SVR} = 700-1500 \text{ in dyn.s.cm}^{-5}; \text{ normal PVR} < 2.5 \text{ Wood units}$$

VII. Shunt evaluation
A. Left-to-right shunt
Normally, $SvO_2 = O_2$ saturation of PA

$$\approx O_2 \text{ saturation of RV} \approx O_2 \text{ saturation of RA}$$

$$\approx \text{average } O_2 \text{ saturation of SVC and IVC} \left(= [3 \times SVC + 1 \times IVC] / 4 \right)$$

O_2 saturation of the SVC is normally lower than O_2 saturation of the IVC by a few percentage points (~5%); the renal O_2 extraction being relatively low, the renal venous O_2 saturation is high and increases the IVC O_2 saturation (above-diaphragm IVC). Mixed venous blood is a mixture of IVC (~55%), SVC (~45%), and coronary sinus blood (~5%). While the IVC flow is normally higher than the SVC flow (55% vs. 45% of cardiac output), mixed venous O_2 saturation more closely approximates SVC O_2 saturation than IVC O_2 saturation as a result of the very low O_2 saturation of the coronary sinus return (~30–40%). Note also that, *in shock states,* blood is directed away from the splanchnic system and IVC O_2 saturation may become lower than SVC O_2 saturation.

A significant left-to-right shunt is characterized by an O_2 step-up of ≥7% between chambers. More specifically, O_2 step-up of 8% between SVC and RA, 6% between RA and PA, or 5% between RV and PA identifies a left-to-right shunt with a high sensitivity and specificity. During a routine right heart catheterization, two blood samples are typically acquired (PA and SVC). If a significant shunt is detected on this screen (8% between SVC and PA), a full oximetry run with sampling of all cardiac chambers needs to be performed. O_2 saturation of the RA is most subject to false measurement, depending on whether the sample is obtained close to the stream of the SVC, IVC, or coronary sinus. If the RA saturation is low on one sample only, it is likely that this sample was obtained close to the coronary sinus and represents a normal finding (e.g., 55% on one RA sample, while the remaining RA samples and the PA sample are 65%). Thus, try to collect multiple RA samples to avoid this sampling artifact, and preferably sample the RA at the mid-lateral level, with the catheter looking towards the border of the RA silhouette.

B. Right-to-left shunt
Arterial O_2 saturation ≥95% on ambient air rules out significant right-to-left shunt. Arterial O_2 saturation <95% may be secondary to a right-to-left shunt or, more commonly, lung disease or sedation. A right-to-left shunt is presumed present when arterial O_2 saturation is <95% and does not resolve with O_2 therapy and with taking a few deep breaths. In this case, pulmonary venous O_2 saturation (PV O_2) is considered 98% and the reduced arterial O_2 saturation is considered an O_2 step-down from shunting. On the other hand, if right-to-left shunt is deemed absent, PV O_2 is considered equal to the low arterial O_2 saturation.

Alternatively, if ASD or PFO is present, one may access the left upper pulmonary vein and directly measure PV O_2 and any potential O_2 step-down.

C. Calculation of shunt flow ratios

In the absence of shunting, the pulmonary (right heart) blood flow is equal to the systemic (left heart) blood flow. A left-to-right shunt increases the pulmonary blood flow, which becomes equal to the sum of the systemic blood flow plus the shunt flow. The *net shunt flow ratio* is equal to:

$$\text{Pulmonary blood flow (Qp) / systemic blood flow (Qs)}$$

→ Using the Fick equation for flow:

$$\text{Qp} = O_2 \text{ consumption (ml/min) divided by}$$
$$1.36 \times \text{hemoglobin} \times (\text{PV } O_2 - \text{PA } O_2) \times 10$$

$$\text{Qs} = O_2 \text{ consumption divided by}$$
$$1.36 \times \text{hemoglobin} \times (\text{SA } O_2 - \text{MV } O_2) \times 10$$

$$\text{Qp/Qs} = (\text{SA } O_2 - \text{MV } O_2) \text{ divided by}$$
$$(\text{PV } O_2 - \text{PA } O_2)$$

where SA O_2 is systemic arterial O_2 saturation, MV O_2 is mixed venous O_2 saturation obtained in the right-sided chamber just proximal to the O_2 step-up, PV O_2 is pulmonary venous O_2 saturation, and PA O_2 is pulmonary arterial O_2 saturation (Figure 36.12).

A Qp/Qs ratio of <1.5 signifies that the net left-to-right shunt is small. Qp/Qs of 1.5–2 and >2 signify intermediate and large left-to-right shunts, respectively, and are indications to repair the defect. Qp/Qs <1.0 signifies a net right-to-left shunt, i.e., reversal of a left-to-right shunt and typically contraindicates closure of the shunt.

> Qp/Qs corresponds to the net shunt ratio. The patient may have large left-to-right and right-to-left shunts (bidirectional shunt) with hypoxemia and pulmonary hypertension, but a small Qp/Qs ratio as the ratio assesses the net shunting into the predominant direction, e.g., left-to-right. In the latter case, Qp/Qs underestimates the severity of shunting, which may be better assessed by echo or by the calculation of the absolute left-to-right and right-to-left shunts (see Appendix 1).

Other pitfalls of Qp/Qs

- The simplified Qp/Qs equation is not accurate in ***patients receiving O_2 therapy*** with FiO_2 >30%. O_2 therapy increases the contribution of free O_2 to the overall blood O_2 content, especially blood O_2 content of the pulmonary veins, where O_2 partial pressure is highest. The high left-sided O_2 content that gets shunted strikingly increases the right-sided O_2 saturation at the shunt level, which is on a steep portion of the O_2 saturation–hemoglobin curve. O_2 step-up and Qp/Qs will be exaggerated.
- ***High systemic CO*** causes SvO_2 to be higher than normal and lessens interchamber variability and O_2 step-up. A higher SvO_2 is on a flatter portion of the O_2 saturation–hemoglobin curve, so that a lot more O_2 is needed to increase O_2 saturation at the shunt level. If SVC O_2 is 85%, a 2:1 shunt is necessary to have an O_2 step-up of only 5-7%. In other words, ***in the case of high cardiac output and high SVC O_2, a smaller O_2 step-up implies a larger shunt.*** Anemia, on the other hand, directly reduces SvO_2 but also increases CO and, overall, does not affect the degree of O_2 step-up.

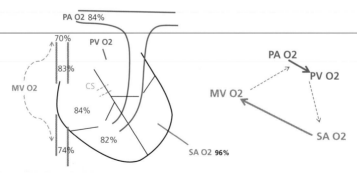

Figure 36.12 O_2 saturation at various levels. Note that MV O_2 and SA O_2 used as numerator in the Qp/Qs equation correspond to the "extreme" chambers (connected by *gray arrow*), while PA O_2 and PV O_2 used as denominator correspond to the in-between chambers (connected by *blue arrow*).

There is an O_2 step-up of ≥8% between the SVC and the PA. The O_2 step-up occurs at the level of the low SVC, signifying a possible sinus venosus ASD.

MV O_2 = (3 × high SVC + 1 × IVC)/4 = (3 × 70 + 74)/4 = 71

Qp/Qs = (SA O_2 − MV O_2)/(PV O_2 − PA O_2) = (96 − 71)/(96 − 84) = 2.1

In the absence of right-to-left shunt, PV O_2 = SA O_2. SA O_2 >95% on ambient air rules out any significant right-to-left shunt. For simplification, one may use SVC O_2 saturation (in this case, high SVC) as an estimation of MV O_2. Reproduced with permission of Demos Medical from Hanna and Glancy (2012).[1]

VIII. Valvular disorders: overview of pressure gradients and valve area calculation

(A more detailed discussion of the hemodynamics of valvular stenosis and regurgitation is provided in Chapter 6.)

A. Transaortic pressure gradient

Aortic stenosis (AS) is assessed by simultaneously recording the LV and aortic pressures. Simultaneous recordings may be obtained by using a 6 Fr or 7 Fr double-lumen pigtail catheter, with one lumen communicating with the aorta and one lumen in the LV. Each lumen is connected to a transducer, and it is critical to calibrate and zero both transducers simultaneously at the same level and ensure none of the tracings is damped (aortic tracing has a dicrotic notch, LV tracing has an early diastolic dip and mid-systolic spiking). Moreover, it is important that the LV catheter is placed in the LV body, not in the LVOT. In fact, patients with AS may have a small subaortic gradient in addition to the transaortic gradient, which is part of the AS anatomy. Placing the catheter in the LVOT may underestimate the transaortic gradient by up to 30 mmHg. In addition, the LV catheter with side holes must be fully inside the LV, without aortic contamination; if a few side holes are in the aorta, the peak LV pressure will be falsely reduced, and thus the gradient will be reduced.

Alternatively, the transaortic pressure gradient may be obtained by catheter pullback across the aortic valve. This is followed by superimposition of the non-simultaneous tracings and calculation of the peak-to-peak and mean gradients. This method is useful in routine cardiac catheterization when AS is unsuspected and serves to rule out significant AS. In fact, in the absence of a gradient upon pullback, or if the peak-to-peak gradient is <15 mmHg, severe AS is almost excluded. In the assessment of severe AS, the pullback technique is less accurate than the simultaneous method. The pullback method is not reliable in AF, where significant beat-to-beat variability in pressure mandates simultaneous recordings.

The transaortic pressure gradient may also be measured by obtaining simultaneous LV and femoral arterial pressure recording. A 4 Fr catheter is used to measure LV pressure while the side arm of a 6 Fr sheath is used to measure the femoral pressure (the sheath should be significantly larger than the catheter inside it to allow adequate measurement of the femoral pressure). This technique has two shortcomings: (i) the femoral arterial tracing is delayed in comparison to the aortic tracing; (ii) due to a phenomenon of reflected pressure waves and systolic amplification in the periphery, the systolic femoral pressure is higher than the systolic aortic pressure, sometimes considerably higher (by 20–50 mmHg), particularly in young patients or in those with concomitant aortic insufficiency. Thus, the superimposition of the femoral and aortic peak pressures should be verified upon pullback. A long sheath (e.g., 65 cm) that lands in the thoracic aorta may be used to circumvent this pitfall.

Illustrations of transaortic pressure gradient are shown in Figures 36.13 and 36.14. A discussion of low-gradient AS with low EF, low-gradient AS with normal EF, and pressure recovery phenomenon are discussed in Chapter 6, Section 4 (*Aortic stenosis*).

B. Transmitral pressure gradient

Simultaneous LA–LV pressures should be obtained, and ideally LA pressure should be directly accessed through a trans-septal puncture. In practice, PCWP is often used as a surrogate of LA pressure, and PCWP–LV simultaneous recordings are often used to assess MS (Figure 36.15). There are three pitfalls in using PCWP, all of which lead to the overestimation of transmitral gradient:

i. PCWP tracing is delayed by 50–150 ms in comparison to LA pressure tracing.
ii. PCWP is more damped than LA pressure with less deep and steep Y descent.
iii. The obtained PCWP may not be a true PCWP and may rather be a damped PA pressure (hybrid PA–PCWP), as described in Section IV.

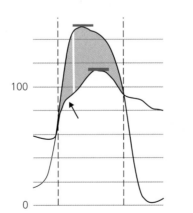
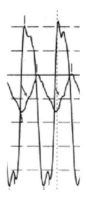

Figure 36.13 Aortic stenosis. *Peak-to-peak gradient* is the difference between the two *peaks (blue bars)*, **peak instantaneous gradient** is the largest difference between the two *curves (white vertical line)*, and **mean gradient** is the integration of all gradients *(gray area)*. LV pressure peaks early and the aortic pressure peaks late, which is the opposite of what is found in HOCM.

Note the **anacrotic notch** beyond which the aortic upstroke is slowed *(arrows)*. The aortic upstroke starts normally then is sharply impeded after the valve stops opening, creating this bend called an anacrotic notch. The aortic pressure has a *slow upstroke after the anacrotic notch and peaks late* (**pulsus tardus**). Also, the pulse pressure is reduced because of reduced stroke volume (**pulsus parvus**). In elderly patients with reduced arterial compliance, the pulse pressure may not be reduced and the anacrotic notch may be absent.

The mean gradient usually approximates the peak-to-peak gradient and is about 65% of the peak instantaneous gradient. In severe AS with severely delayed aortic upstroke, the mean gradient area may end up being larger than the peak-to-peak gradient.

Note that, in AS, the aortic pressure upstroke is less steep than the LV pressure upstroke; if the LV and aortic upstrokes are superimposed, suspect subaortic obstruction or error in zeroing creating a false gradient (e.g., the LV and aortic transducers are zeroed at two different levels).

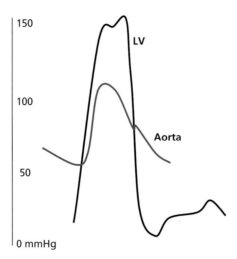

Figure 36.14 This simultaneous LV–aortic pressure recording simulates severe AS. However, the upstrokes of both tracings are parallel, which is unusual in AS, wherein the aortic upstroke is less steep than the LV upstroke and peaks late. This is a hint to an error in zeroing; in fact, the two transducers were zeroed at different levels. When performing simultaneous pressure recordings, one should re-zero both transducers at the same level and, after the initial recordings, swap transducers to verify that the gradient remains unchanged. Also, upon catheter pullback from the LV, verify that both pressures superimpose in the aorta and that the pullback gradient is similar to the simultaneous gradient. Reproduced with permission of Demos Medical from Hanna and Glancy (2012).[1]

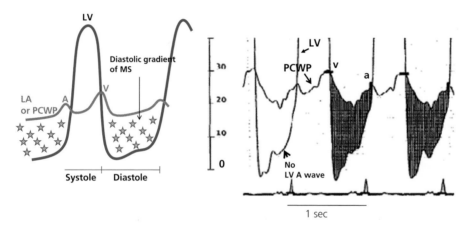

Figure 36.15 Two examples of mitral stenosis with a diastolic pressure gradient between PCWP and LV at a heart rate of 60 bpm (*dark filled areas*). Due to the phase delay of PCWP, the tracing of PCWP has been shifted to the left so that the *peak of V wave is bisected by the LV downslope.* ***There is no LA–LV diastasis, i.e., LA pressure remains higher than LV pressure throughout diastole, despite a heart rate of 60 bpm, signifying severe MS.*** LA A wave is pronounced but LV A wave is reduced because of ventricular underfilling (this is similar to the lack of S_4 in MS).

   In mild or moderate MS (valve area >1.5 cm²), diastasis is reached at end-diastole. However, diastasis may not be reached if the patient is tachycardic (tachycardia converts a mild anatomic MS into a severe hemodynamic MS). Reproduced with permission of Demos Medical from Hanna and Glancy (2012).[1]

To correct for the phase delay, one may shift the PCWP leftward until the peak of V wave is bisected by the LV downstroke (or slightly precedes it). Two situations particularly exaggerate the PCWP pitfalls and affect its use as a surrogate of LA pressure in MS:

i. Large V wave, where the "spread-out," slow V downslope of PCWP creates a false gradient, not seen with the sharp V downslope of LA pressure.

ii. Pulmonary hypertension: pulmonary hypertension makes it difficult to wedge the PA and obtain a true PCWP. Even when PCWP is obtained, it is usually a damped, flat tracing that falsely suggests a high PCWP–LV gradient.

A proper PCWP that is appropriately damped without a large V wave is usually a satisfactory substitute for LA pressure, with overestimation of the transmitral gradient by only 2 mmHg according to some investigators.

   Typically, severe MS is characterized by the following three hemodynamic findings:

- LV and LA pressures do not equalize at the end of diastole (diastasis is not reached), even when the heart rate is controlled at 60–75 bpm and even after a pause of 1 second.
- Mean transmitral gradient ≥ 5 mmHg at a heart rate < 75–80 bpm.
- LA A wave may be prominent yet LV A wave is discrepantly absent (LV underfilling).

When mitral valve area is 1–1.5 cm² but the heart rate is slow (≤ 60 bpm) and the cardiac output is low, diastasis may be reached at the very end of diastole and the gradient may decline to 5 mmHg.

On the other hand, when the mitral valve area is >1.5 cm² but tachycardia (or heart rate >80 bpm), high-output state (e.g., anemia), or concomitant MR is present, diastasis may not be reached and the gradient may be >5–10 mmHg, as **the gradient is highly dependent on cardiac output and heart rate.**

Patients with elevated LA pressure and ample V wave, such as patients with severe MR, have an early diastolic pressure gradient between LA and LV, but, as opposed to severe MS, LA and LV pressures equalize at mid-diastole (diastasis) and there is no LA–LV end-diastolic gradient.

C. Transvalvular gradients in tachycardia and AF

Transaortic AS gradient is reduced in inappropriate tachycardia or short R–R interval, from the reduced stroke volume, and is increased after a PVC or a long R–R interval. Tachycardia may, however, be associated with an increase in transaortic gradient if inotropism and cardiac output are increased, since an increase in cardiac output strikingly increases transvalvular gradients. Try to control the rate before assessing AS, and average the gradient from 5–10 beats.

Changes in R–R cycle affect diastolic time much more than systolic time. Thus, transmitral MS gradient may strikingly increase after a short R–R cycle (opposite of AS), as the diastolic time allowed for LA emptying is reduced and the per-second diastolic flow increases. *The increased gradient during tachycardia is relevant to the decision making and approximates MS gradient on stress testing* (gradient is actually higher during exercise testing than during the short R–R cycles of AF, because exercise not only increases heart rate but increases stroke volume and the overall cardiac output). *It is always important to comment on heart rate in any MS study, as tachycardia can convert an anatomically mild MS into a physiologically severe MS with a high gradient.*

D. Valve area calculation

According to Gorlin, the valve orifice area is equal to:

$$\text{Flow across the valve} / (\text{constant} \times \sqrt{\text{pressure gradient}})$$

Flow across the valve is not continuous. In fact, the cardiac output expressed in liters per minute crosses the valve during the intermittent time it is open, i.e., in less than a minute. Therefore, the per-second flow rate across the valve is actually larger than the cardiac output. For the mitral and tricuspid valves, if the cardiac output is 5 liters/minute and if the diastolic duration is 35 seconds per minute, the flow across the mitral and tricuspid valves is actually 5 liters per 35 seconds, or 0.14 liters/second; thus, the flow across the valve is equal to the cardiac output divided by the diastolic filling time expressed in seconds per minute.

The diastolic filling time is the diastolic filling period (DFP) per each beat (expressed in seconds) multiplied by the heart rate, or the diastolic filling time of all beats occurring in a 10-second period multiplied by 6 (Figure 36.16).

Thus, mitral valve area =

$$\frac{\text{CO (liters/minute)} \times 1000 / \text{diastolic filling time (seconds/minute)}}{37.7 \times \sqrt{\text{mean transmitral gradient}}}$$

$$\frac{\text{CO} \times 1000 / (\text{DFP [seconds/beat]} \times \text{HR [beats/minute]})}{37.7 \times \sqrt{\text{mean transmitral gradient}}}$$

For the aortic and pulmonic valves, the diastolic filling time and the diastolic filling period per beat are replaced by the systolic ejection time (expressed in seconds per minute) and the systolic ejection period per beat (SEP).

Thus, aortic valve area =

$$\frac{\text{CO} \times 1000 / \text{systolic ejection time (seconds/minute)}}{44.3 \times \sqrt{\text{mean transaortic gradient}}}$$

$$\frac{\text{CO} \times 1000 / (\text{SEP [seconds/beat]} \times \text{HR [beats/minute]})}{44.3 \times \sqrt{\text{mean transaortic gradient}}}$$

A simpler equation (Hakki formula) has been validated for both mitral and aortic valves:

$$\text{Valve area} = \text{CO} / \sqrt{\text{gradient}}$$

In Hakki's equation, mean gradient is used for the mitral valve, while mean gradient or peak-to-peak gradient is used for the aortic valve. This formula is not well tested in patients with bradycardia (<40 bpm), tachycardia (>100 bpm), or atrial fibrillation.

These equations show that for a fixed valvular area, gradient is dependent on the square of the CO. Thus, a twofold increase in CO almost translates into a fourfold increase in gradient, while a low CO translates into a low gradient even if the stenosis is severe.

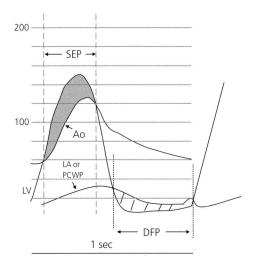

Figure 36.16 LV, aortic (Ao) and PCWP tracing in a patient with AS (LV–Ao gradient, *gray area*) and MS (PCWP–LV gradient in diastole, *dashed area*). Illustration of how to obtain SEP and DFP. Reproduced with permission of Demos Medical from Hanna and Glancy (2012).[1]

Calculation of valvular area in atrial fibrillation
In atrial fibrillation, average the mean valvular gradient over 10 beats. Then measure the systolic ejection time (or diastolic filling time) spent in a 10-second period throughout all the beats contained in these 10 seconds, and multiply this time by 6 to obtain the systolic ejection time in seconds/minute. Then apply Gorlin's equation.

Calculation of valvular area in the case of coexisting regurgitation of the same valve
In the case of severe regurgitation of the same valve being evaluated for stenosis, CO obtained by Fick or thermodilution cannot be used in Gorlin's or Hakki's equation. The latter CO is the net flow that reaches the systemic circulation, whereas at the level of the valve the flow is a summation of the net systemic flow and the backward regurgitant flow. Using the smaller net CO in Gorlin's equation *falsely decreases the valve area*. In this case, the angiographic CO ([LV diastolic volume – LV systolic volume] × HR) may be used, as it integrates all the ejected flow, including the flow that ultimately goes backward. Also, knowing that in severe regurgitation the regurgitant flow is usually at least as large as the net forward flow, the total flow across the valve is at least twice the CO; therefore twice the CO may be used in Gorlin's equation instead of CO. This allows a rough and conservative estimate of the valve area, as the regurgitant flow may be larger than the forward flow, and therefore the true valve area may even be larger than the corrected calculation.

A regurgitation affecting a valve other than the valve of interest does not impact upon valvular area calculation using Gorlin's equation but may lead to a low CO and a lower gradient across the valve of interest.

E. Five findings suggestive of severe aortic insufficiency (AI) (Figures 36.17, 36.18)
1. Widened pulse pressure is seen with chronic severe AI (enlarged LV with a large stroke volume). This is a very sensitive finding in chronic AI, but not specific (may be seen in non-compliant aorta).
2. Dicrotic notch is absent. This is particularly true when the aorta is non-compliant, as in acute AI or AI of the elderly; the dicrotic notch may persist in chronic AI of young patients.
3. LVEDP sharply rises while aortic diastolic pressure sharply falls → LV pressure and aortic pressure approximate in end-diastole. This is seen with acute or decompensated AI.
4. Peripheral systolic amplification of arterial pressure is more exaggerated in AI.
5. LVEDP exceeds not only mean PCWP but end-diastolic PCWP. This leads to early mitral closure on echo and is a sign of acute or decompensated AI.

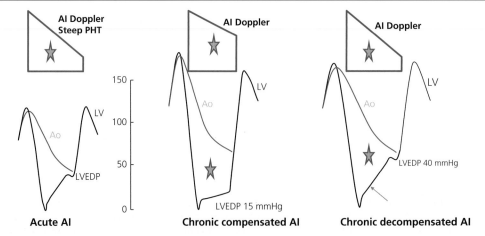

Figure 36.17 LV–aortic pressure tracings in acute AI and chronic AI. Chronic decompensated AI has all five AI features. In acute and decompensated AI, the steep diastolic approximation of LV and aortic pressures (triangle, *star*) translate into a similarly steep AI Doppler. Conversely, in compensated AI, LV and aortic pressures do not approximate in end-diastole.

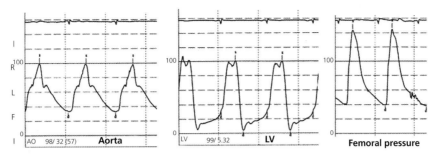

Figure 36.18 On the aortic tracing, the aortic pressure drops precipitously in diastole, while the LV pressure sharply rises. LVEDP approximates aortic end-diastolic pressure. This suggests acute or decompensated AI. The fact that systolic aortic pressure is low implies either acute AI or chronic end-stage AI (with reduced EF and total stroke volume). The *dicrotic notch* may persist in chronic AI with compliant aorta. An *anacrotic notch* is noted here; anacrotic notch may be seen in AI even when the associated AS is not severe; because of the high flow crossing it, the aortic valve may become functionally obstructive. Unlike in severe AS, this anacrotic notch is high on the aortic upstroke and the aortic upstroke remains sharp rather than "tardus."

   Note that the femoral pressure is much larger than the aortic pressure. This is the peripheral systolic amplification that is exaggerated in AI.

IX. Dynamic LVOT obstruction
(See also Chapter 7.)

   In the presence of a gradient between the LV and the aorta, and if LVOT obstruction is suspected, use an end-hole catheter, rather than a multihole catheter, and slowly pull back across the LVOT to localize the site of pressure drop. Once the site of pressure drop is localized, a double-lumen pigtail catheter may be used for simultaneous LV–aortic pressure recording and exact gradient determination. Unlike the fixed obstruction of AS, dynamic LVOT obstruction worsens throughout systole as the LV cavity becomes smaller. Thus, dynamic LVOT obstruction is worse in late systole and is characterized by four features (Figures 36.19–36.22):

1. Early and sharp aortic upstroke (spike), followed by a pressure drop (plateau)
2. Late LV peak with a late LV–aortic gradient
3. Brockenbrough phenomenon after a pause
4. Gradient is dynamic with maneuvers

This dynamic LVOT obstruction may be secondary to HOCM or to a hypercontractile small LV cavity in a hypovolemic patient with a degree of hypertensive hypertrophy ("hypertensive obstructive cardiomyopathy").

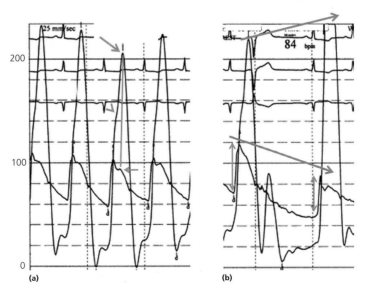

(a)   (b)

Figure 36.19 Dynamic LVOT obstruction.

   (a) The LVOT obstruction worsens throughout systole as the LV becomes smaller, which explains why the aortic pressure drops and plateaus after an early peak (spike-and-dome appearance, *horizontal arrow*), and why LV pressure peaks in late systole (*upper arrow*) and has a narrow, dagger shape. The LV pressure has a bend that corresponds to the point of worsened obstruction (*arrowhead*). The LV–aortic pressure gradient is a late gradient (*vertical line*); this is similar to the Doppler finding of a late-peaking dagger-shaped velocity across the LV. As opposed to AS, the peak-to-peak gradient approximates the peak instantaneous gradient in HOCM.

   (b) The behavior of LV and aortic pressures after a premature beat helps corroborate the diagnosis. Following a pause, the increased myocardial contractility worsens the dynamic LV obstruction. Thus, while the LV pressure and the pressure gradient increase, the stroke volume decreases, which reduces the aortic pulse pressure (*double arrows*) (= Brockenbrough sign). In AS, the obstruction is fixed and thus the increased contractility after a premature beat leads to increased stroke volume, and, consequently, an increase in the transaortic gradient (as per Gorlin's equation, the transaortic gradient increases with increased flow across the valve). As opposed to HOCM, the aortic pulse pressure increases as well.

   Reproduced with permission of Demos Medical from Hanna and Glancy (2012).[1]

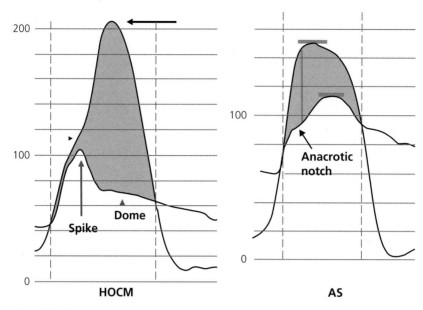

Figure 36.20 Contrast LV–aortic tracings in HOCM vs. AS. In HOCM, the aortic pressure peaks early while the LV pressure and the gradient peak late, after a bend (*arrowhead*). In AS, the LV pressure peaks early while the aortic pressure peaks late, after an anacrotic notch. Reproduced with permission of Demos Medical from Hanna and Glancy (2012).[1]

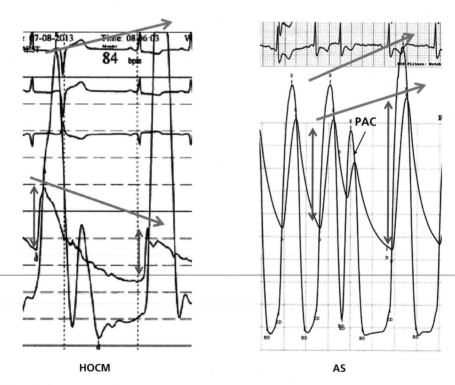

Figure 36.21 Brockenbrough phenomenon after a premature beat in HOCM. Note the increased pressure gradient but reduced aortic pulse pressure (*double arrows*) after a pause in HOCM, vs. the increased pressure gradient but also increased aortic systolic and pulse pressure in AS. The *arrows* indicate the change in LV pressure vs. aortic pressure. The pressure gradient increases much more markedly with HOCM than with AS after this pause. Also, because of the increased obstruction, *the spike-and-dome morphology becomes more apparent after a pause.*

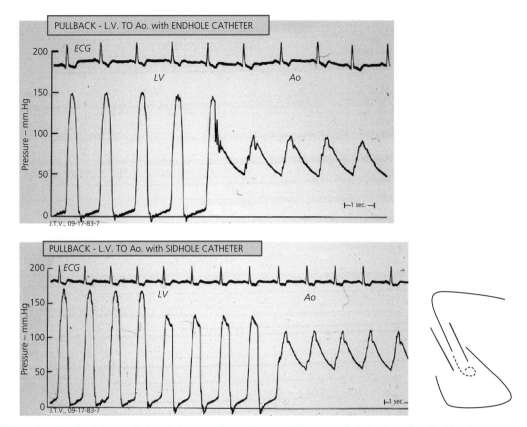

Figure 36.22 LV–aortic pullback using an endhole catheter in a patient with severe AS (*upper tracing*). A pullback from the LV to the aorta using a catheter with side holes contaminates the LVOT pressure with aortic pressure and creates the impression of a drop in pressure across the LVOT rather than the aortic valve (*lower tracing*).

Conversely, in a patient with LVOT obstruction, the LVOT catheter may transmit the aortic pressure rather than the LVOT pressure, as holes are spread across both the LVOT and the aorta, which may create the impression of an aortic rather than an LVOT drop in pressure.

This illustrates the importance of an end-hole catheter in localizing the site of obstruction during a pullback maneuver. Once the obstruction is localized, a multihole LV catheter (e.g., double-lumen pigtail) may be used for simultaneous pressure recordings, as in Figure 36.21.

Reproduced with permission of Demos Medical from Hanna and Glancy (2012).[1]

X. Pericardial disorders: tamponade and constrictive pericarditis (see Figures 36.23, 36.24)
(See Chapter 17.)

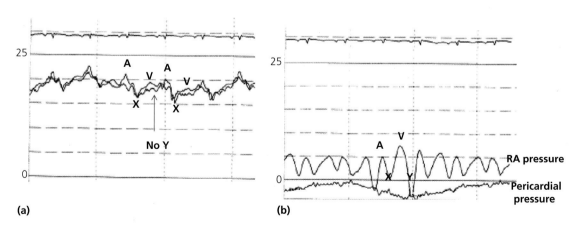

(a)   (b)

Figure 36.23 (a) Simultaneous pericardial and RA pressures are recorded in **tamponade**, before pericardiocentesis. **The RA and pericardial pressures are elevated and equalized** (~20 mmHg); this defines tamponade. The two tracings are actually superimposed. Furthermore, X descent is seen, but Y descent is flat (mnemonic: **Flat Y Tamponade = FYT**). V wave almost continues straight into A wave. **(b)** Post-pericardiocentesis, pericardial pressure becomes normal (negative pressure ≤ 0 mmHg). RA pressure is normal with clear V wave and Y descent. Had the pericardial pressure or RA pressure not normalized, and had these pressures remained equal, effusive–constrictive pericarditis would have been suggested.

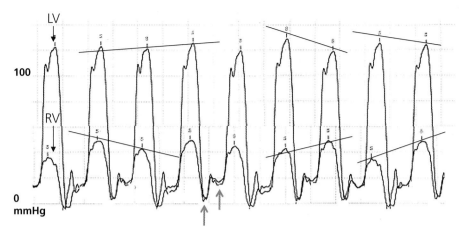

Figure 36.24 Simultaneous RV–LV pressure recording. This recording is the most important recording in assessing the presence of constrictive pericarditis. It shows the following:

1. **Diastolic dip–plateau pattern of RV and LV tracings** (dip = *lower vertical gray arrow*, plateau = *upper vertical gray arrow*). It is not specific for constrictive pericarditis and, similarly to the deep X and deep Y on RA tracing, may be seen in decompensated systolic or diastolic ventricular failure with severe loss of compliance, including restrictive cardiomyopathy.
2. **Equalization of end-diastolic pressures of RV and LV**, mainly seen in inspiration (LV pressure > RV pressure at other times). Equalization of RV and LV end-diastolic pressures may be seen in RV failure as well, except that RV supersedes LV pressures at times.
3. While (1) and (2) correspond to the analysis of diastolic RV and LV pressures, the third feature corresponds to the analysis of systolic RV and LV pressures. **Discordance of peaks**, wherein the systolic peaks of RV and LV move in opposite directions, is very specific for constrictive pericarditis. This contrasts with restrictive cardiomyopathy or decompensated ventricular failure, wherein the peaks are concordant. There is discordance on this recording, as RV peak increases when LV peak decreases. The two *black lines* illustrate this concept.

Reproduced with permission of Demos Medical from Hanna and Glancy (2012).[1]

XI. Exercise hemodynamics

In patients with unexplained exertional dyspnea, a Swan catheter may be placed and exercise performed on a supine cycle ergometer mounted on the catheterization table. Invasive PA pressure, PCWP, and CO are measured during exercise. This may unveil occult LV diastolic dysfunction as a cause of the patient's dyspnea. On the bicycle, the work is started at 25 watts (W), and increased by ~25 W every 2 minutes (mild exercise ~50 W, heart rate 110 bpm; moderate exercise ~100 W, heart rate 130 bpm; maximal exercise ~150–200 W). At each stage, the patient must pedal at 60–80 rpm to achieve the estimated work.

During exercise, venous return increases and stroke volume increases as a result of the increased preload (Frank–Starling mechanism) and the inotropic reserve. Normally, in early exercise, LV end-diastolic volume increases (preload increases) while end-systolic volume decreases (EF increases). At high levels of tachycardia, as diastole shortens, the rising LV end-diastolic volume plateaus or even declines, while stroke volume continues to rise from the reduction of end-systolic volume.

Even in normal individuals, PCWP and PA pressure increase to some extent with exercise, and PCWP frequently exceeds 15 mmHg. PA pressure increases as a result of the increased cardiac output (similarly to the exertional rise of systemic arterial pressure). The normal values of exertional PA pressure and PCWP are shown in Table 36.3.[3]

Whether in normal individuals or in those with LV diastolic dysfunction, most of the rise of PCWP (≥80%) already occurs at a low level of exercise (at 1.5 minutes of 25 W).[4] In diastolic dysfunction, PCWP will rise sharply early on, then continue the rise, but the early rise already gives a good idea of the final response. In fact, in diastolic dysfunction, PCWP already rises with passive leg elevation, before cycling (~40% of the eventual rise).[4] Two studies found that PCWP adjusted to the workload in W/kg provides a more accurate assessment of diastolic function (normal PCWP is <25 mmHg/W/kg).[5,6] PCWP returns to baseline value quickly, within 1 minute of recovery, as the preload sharply declines.

HF, including HFpEF, is characterized by an excessive rise of PCWP and PA pressure, beyond the numbers in Table 36.3, and a blunted rise of cardiac output. In fact, the capacity to increase LV diastolic volume is limited (limited preload reserve with limited capacity to use the Frank–Starling mechanism), and the capacity to reduce LV systolic volume is limited (limited contractile reserve). This translates into a limited stroke volume reserve and a back-up rise in pressure. More specifically, in one study, the stroke volume index did not significantly rise in HFpEF patients (rose <20%, stroke volume index remained ~40 ml/m² vs. > 60 ml/m² in controls).[5] Also, there is a limited chronotropic response in HFpEF. *Because cardiac output cannot match the rising O_2 consumption, PA O_2 saturation declines with exercise.*

Other modalities of stress testing may be employed to unveil occult LV diastolic dysfunction and elicit a rise of PCWP and PA pressure (CO blunting cannot be properly assessed with these modalities): (1) 45° passive leg raising using a wedge or a supine bike (increases venous return); (2) adenosine infusion (adenosine is an arterial but not a venous dilator; thus, it increases venous return and may increase PCWP); (3) leg positive pressure, which consists of inflating BP cuffs at 90 mmHg around both legs for few minutes (increases venous return);[7] (4) sustained handgrip isometric exercise using a dynamometer, for 3 minutes (causes a reflex increase in BP, heart rate, and CO); (5) atrial pacing up to 85% of the maximal age-predicted heart rate. As opposed to exercise, pacing is associated with a reduction of LV preload and a reduction of stroke volume and LVEDP during the pacing phase, even in patients with CAD or LV dysfunction. Yet, in the latter patients, pacing increases diastolic stiffness, therefore increasing LVEDP shortly after termination of pacing, once preload reincreases. It also increases PCWP during pacing by reducing LA emptying.

Table 36.3 Normal exertional values of PCWP, PA pressure, and cardiac output, according to age.

Patients <50 years of age
- Mean PCWP <18–20 mmHg
- Systolic PA pressure <40 mmHg; mean PA pressure <30 mmHg

Patients ≥50 years of age
- Mean PCWP <25 mmHg
- Systolic PA pressure <50–55 mmHg; mean PA pressure <40 mmHg

In all patients, at peak exercise
- Cardiac output usually increases to >10 l/min, and cardiac index increases to >6 l/min/m² (even at low workloads)
- In relative terms, cardiac index more than doubles and stroke volume index increases 25–40%
- PA O₂ saturation does not decline significantly

At rest, PCWP and PA pressure are measured at end-expiration, where the respiratory pressure is 0. However, during exercise, the end-expiratory pressure is a positive pressure (active exhalation), and thus the most representative exercise pressures average the inspiratory and expiratory numbers. However, some studies have used the above pressure cutoffs in end-expiration.[4]

Appendix 1. Advanced hemodynamic calculation: a case of shunt with pulmonary hypertension

Case scenario
The following O₂ saturations are obtained (Figure 36.25):

> Right circulation: SVC 58%, IVC 66%, RA 68%, PA 73%
> Left circulation: pulmonary vein (PV) 93%, aorta 85%

The following pressures are obtained:

> PA pressure = 75/21, mean 43 mmHg; PCWP = 16 mmHg; RA pressure = 13 mmHg; aortic pressure = 130/77 mmHg; hemoglobin (Hb) = 14 g/dl; body surface area (BSA) = 2.1 m²

What is the direction of the shunt? Should this shunt be closed?

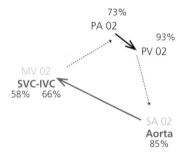

Figure 36.25 The numerator of the Qp/Qs is in blue (extreme chambers), while the denominator is in black (between chambers).

Answer
There is a significant O₂ step-up at the level of the RA, indicating a left-to-right shunt across an ASD (>8% O₂ step-up between SVC and PA, PA having the best mixture of shunted blood). There is a significant O₂ step-down between the PV and the aortic level, indicating a right-to-left shunt with hypoxemia. Thus, this patient has a bidirectional shunt with severe pulmonary hypertension, worrisome for Eisenmenger syndrome.

$$\text{MV O}_2 = (3\ \text{SVC} + 1\ \text{IVC})/4 = 60\%$$
$$\text{Qp/Qs} = (\text{SA O}_2 - \text{MV O}_2)/(\text{PV O}_2 - \text{PA O}_2) = (85 - 60)/(93 - 73) = 1.25\ \text{(Figure 36.25)}$$

A Qp/Qs ratio in the 1–1.5 range does not imply that the shunt flow is small. Since the oximetry suggests significant bidirectional shunting, the patient may very well have large left-to-right and right-to-left shunts, the net shunt being slightly left-to-right. One must calculate the absolute Qp and Qs and the absolute shunt flow in each direction to address the true severity of the shunt in each direction, rather than solely rely on Qp/Qs.

$$\text{Qp} = \text{O}_2 \text{ consumption}/(\text{Hb} \times 1.36 \times [\text{PV O}_2 - \text{PA O}_2] \times 10)$$
$$= (125\ \text{ml/min/m}^2 \times \text{BSA})/(14 \times 1.36\ [0.93 - 0.73] \times 10) = 6.9\ \text{l/min}$$
$$\text{Qs} = \text{O}_2 \text{ consumption}/(\text{Hb} \times 1.36 \times [\text{SA O}_2 - \text{MV O}_2] \times 10)$$
$$= 5.5\ \text{l/min}$$

Q effective = theoretical right- and left-sided flow had there not been any shunt, in which case SA O₂ = PV O₂ and PA O₂ = MV O₂
$$= \text{O}_2 \text{ consumption}/(\text{Hb} \times 1.36 \times [\text{PV O}_2 - \text{MV O}_2] \times 10)$$
$$= (125\ \text{ml/min/m}^2 \times \text{BSA})/(14 \times 1.36 \times [0.93 - 0.60] \times 10)$$
$$= 4.2\ \text{l/min}$$

Left-to right shunt=Qp – Q effective=2.7 l/min
Right-to-left shunt=Qs – Q effective=1.3 l/min

Thus, there is a large left-to-right shunt (40% of Qp), and moderate right-to-left shunt. To appreciate the severity of this left-to-right shunt, **remember that in patients with isolated left-to-right shunt, a Qp/Qs of 1.5 corresponds to a shunt flow that is 33% of Qp (Qp=1.5 units, Qs=1 unit, and the shunt flow=0.5 unit). A Qp/Qs of 2 corresponds to a shunt flow that is 50% of Qp (Qp=2, shunt=1, Qs=1).**

 Thus, from the standpoint of left-to-right flow, the patient qualifies for ASD closure. One must additionally determine if the severe pulmonary hypertension is due to an Eisenmenger process or is simply due to the increased flow across the pulmonary arteries without much of an increase in PVR. For this purpose, one must measure PVR and see if PVR is >6 Wood units or >2/3 SVR, in which case a vasoreactivity testing is indicated to rule out Eisenmenger syndrome.

PVR=(mean PA pressure – PCWP)/Qp=(43 – 16)/6.9=4 Wood units.
SVR=(mean aortic pressure – RA pressure)/Qs=(95 – 13)/5.5=15 Wood units

Note that Qp, rather than the cardiac output obtained by thermodilution, should be used to calculate PVR. The patient's PVR is only mildly elevated and is much lower than SVR, suggesting that the pulmonary hypertension is mainly related to the increased flow. This patient is, therefore, a candidate for shunt closure.

QUESTIONS AND ANSWERS: Additional hemodynamic cases

Question 1. The following oximetry run is obtained:
IVC 77%, high SVC 84%, low SVC 90%
High RA 88%, mid-RA 85%, low RA 78%, RV 84%, PA 86%
Left upper pulmonary vein 99%, aorta 96%
Is there a significant shunt? Calculate Qp/Qs.

Question 2. A simultaneous LV–LA recording is shown (Figure 36.26). What does it suggest?

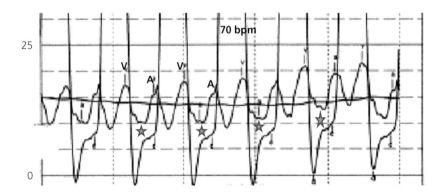

Figure 36.26

Question 3. The patient in Question 2 underwent mitral valvuloplasty. Which chambers are represented on this simultaneous recording (Figure 36.27)? Is there any residual MS? What else is suggested on this recording?

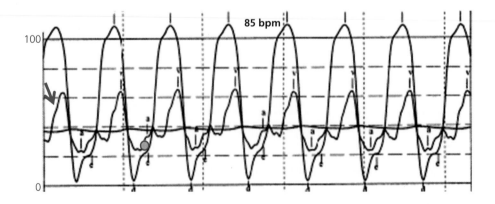

Figure 36.27

Question 4. What do these aortic and PA tracings suggest (Figure 36.28)?

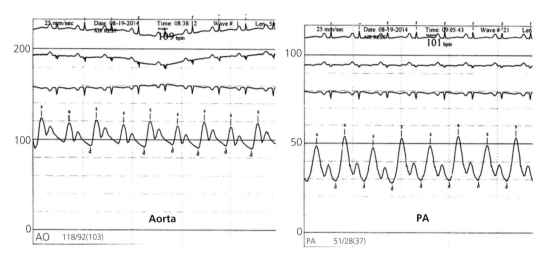

Figure 36.28

Question 5. A 69-year-old hypertensive, obese woman (BMI 35) with sleep apnea presents with dyspnea on exertion. Echo shows normal EF with mild LVH and grade 1 diastolic dysfunction. Pulmonary function testing is normal. A right heart catheterization is performed. Hemodynamics at rest: RA pressure 5 mmHg, PA 42/20 mmHg (mean 27 mmHg), PCWP 10 mmHg (with a prominent A wave of 14 mmHg > V wave). Cardiac output is 6.7 l/min with cardiac index 3.4 l/min/m². Stroke volume index = cardiac index/heart rate = 40 ml/min/m² (heart rate 85 bpm). Arterial O_2 saturation is 95% (ambient air), PA O_2 saturation is 75%. What is the diagnosis?
A. Mild pulmonary hypertension related to sleep apnea
B. HFpEF
C. Exercise hemodynamics are required to establish a diagnosis

Question 6. Exercise hemodynamics were performed on the patient in Question 5, using a supine bicycle. Hemodynamic parameters were measured upon leg raising, before cycling, then upon cycling (25 W to 150 W). Hemodynamics with leg raising, before cycling: PA pressure 55/28 mmHg, PCWP 15 mmHg (V = A = 22 mmHg).

Hemodynamics with peak exercise (150 W, 140 bpm): PA pressure 75/35 mmHg, mean 48 mmHg; PCWP 27 mmHg, prominent V = 36 mmHg; cardiac output by thermodilution = 12 l/min, with cardiac index 6 l/min/m²; stroke volume index = 42 ml/min/m²; arterial O_2 saturation 85%, PA O_2 saturation 42%.

At 2 minutes post-recovery, arterial saturation went up to 98%, PA saturation was 81%. Which of the following statements is (are) correct?
A. PA pressure and PCWP rose excessively with exercise, implying HFpEF (the cutoff for abnormal exertional PCWP is 25 mmHg, the cutoff for abnormal exertional systolic PA pressure is 55 mmHg)
B. The cardiac output rose with exercise but not enough, as manifested by the low PA O_2 saturation
C. The stroke volume rose <20–25%, implying a limited preload reserve
D. The pressure–volume relationshsip of the LV is steep
E. Exertional PA O_2 saturation is low because of the inappropriate cardiac output but also the low arterial O_2 saturation
F. Low arterial O_2 is partly due to the high exertional PCWP and reduced O_2 diffusion, but mostly due to lack of appropriate rise in ventilation (obesity-hypoventilation)

Answer 1. There is a step-up at the level of the low SVC, suggesting a shunt at this level, likely a sinus venosus ASD. Furthermore, the IVC O_2 being normally higher than the SVC O_2 (outside shock), even the high SVC sample is contaminated by a spillover of the left-to-right shunt. Thus, IVC O_2 is the best representation of the mixed venous O_2 in this case, rather than the average of IVC O_2 and high SVC O_2.

Note that the RA saturation is highly variable, depending on whether it is sampled next to the IVC (78%), SVC (88%), or in between (85%). The best mixture of all venous return is achieved at the PA level. Overall, the 9% O_2 step-up between the IVC and the PA suggests significant left-to-right shunt.

The left upper pulmonary venous O_2 is 99%, while aortic O_2 is 96%. Should pulmonary venous O_2 (PV O_2) be considered 99% in the Qp/Qs calculation? In the absence of right-to-left shunt and when aortic O_2 is >95%, PV O_2 is considered equal to aortic O_2, 96% in this case rather than 99%. The sampling of one out of four pulmonary veins may be affected by sampling contamination (not here) or by a better function of one lung quadrant.

Thus: Qp/Qs = (aortic O_2 – IVC O_2)/(PV O_2 – PA O_2) = (96 – 77)/(96 – 86) = 1.9.

Answer 2. Note the lack of LV–LA diastasis in end-diastole despite a heart rate of 70 bpm, implying severe MS (the diastolic gradient is marked by the *star*). Also, a mean gradient >5 mmHg at a heart rate <80 bpm suggests severe MS. The large V wave and the large A wave on the LA tracing are consistent with severe MS. MS often leads to prominent V and A waves; at an early stage A wave may be most prominent, at a late stage V wave may be most prominent. Note the lack of LV A wave despite the prominence of LA A wave: this is characteristic of MS, where the large LA A wave can barely fill the LV through the stenotic mitral valve.

Answer 3. Figure 36.27 is a simultaneous LV–LA (or LV–PCWP) recording. The large V wave may mimic PA pressure. Distinguish this LA tracing from PA tracing using the following:

1. The tracing is upsloping in diastole and has an A wave, implying LA pressure rather than PA.
2. Timing: the pressure peak occurs after the LV pressure plateau (rather than simultaneous with it), implying that it is not PA pressure. Rather, it almost intersects with the LV descent, implying it is a V wave.
3. The pressure peak has a gradual upslope and a sharper downslope, implying a V wave.

V wave has become gigantic after valvuloplasty (~65 mmHg), definitely implying acute MR. A lack of diastasis is seen in diastole (*blue dot*). However, at this particular time, MS is likely mild, the diastolic gradient and the hemodynamic severity being exaggerated by the high transmitral flow initiated by MR and the faster heart rate.

Answer 4. Note the following three findings:

1. A very narrow aortic pressure: narrow in *height* (pulse pressure <25% of systolic pressure) and narrow in *width* in systole. This implies a low stroke volume/cardiac output. Clinically, a narrow pulse pressure is the best correlate of a low stroke volume. Invasively, the systolic area of the waveform correlates with the stroke volume.
2. The waveform morphology and height vary alternately between beats. This is called pulsus alternans and implies a low cardiac output. Differentiate this from pulsus paradoxus, wherein the pulse varies cyclically (with respiration), rather than alternately.
3. The dicrotic notch is very prominent on both the PA and aortic waveforms. In fact, the aortic and PA pulses are called dicrotic pulses. A prominent dicrotic notch results from severe peripheral vasoconstriction (conversely, the dicrotic notch is attenuated in cases of peripheral vasodilatation and extensive peripheral runoff). In a way, it also implies a low cardiac output.

In sum, this patient has severe low-output systolic HF. His PA saturation is very low at 40% and he has sinus tachycardia, further confirming the low-output state.

Answer 5. C. The prominent A wave on PCWP tracing is a hint to the presence of LV dysfunction, albeit a compensated LV dysfunction (mean PCWP is normal, but post-A PCWP and LVEDP may be abnormal). In decompensated LV dysfunction, V wave becomes prominent, much more so than A wave (Figure 36.10).

Answer 6. All are correct. The cardiac output did not rise enough and the stroke volume almost did not rise at all. The LV cavity is small and stiff and is unable to dilate and accept the increased venous return (limited preload reserve). It is unable to use the Frank-Starling mechanism, wherein a higher preload would raise the stroke volume. It does not accept preload, which backs up in the pulmonary circulation. Filling pressures rise despite a lack of change of preload, a sign of a steep LV pressure–volume relationship in diastole. Note that some abnormalities already manifest with leg raising, before exercise.

References

1. Hanna EB, Glancy DL. Practical Cardiovascular Hemodynamics. New York, NY: Demos Medical, 2012.
2. Fuchs RM, Heuser RR, Yin FCP, Brinker JA. Limitations of pulmonary wedge V waves in diagnosing mitral regurgitation. Am J Cardiol 1982; 49: 849–54.
3. Kovacs G, Berghold A, Scheidl S, Olschewski H. Pulmonary artery pressure during rest and exercise in healthy subjects: a systematic review. Eur Resp J 2009; 34: 888–94.
4. Borlaug BA, Nishimura RA, Sorajja P, et al. Exercise hemodynamics enhance the early diagnosis of heart failure with preserved ejection fraction. Circ Heart Fail 2010; 3: 588–95.
5. Maeder MT, Thompson BR, Brunner-La Roca HP, Kaye DM. Hemodynamic basis of exercise limitation in patients with heart failure and normal ejection fraction. J Am Coll Cardiol 2010; 56: 855–63.
6. Dorfs S, Zeh W, Hochholzer W, et al. Pulmonary capillary wedge pressure during exercise and long-term mortality in patients with suspected heart failure with preserved ejection fraction. Eur Heart J 2014; 35: 3103–12.
7. Yamada H, Kusunose K, Nishio S, et al. Pre-load stress echocardiography for predicting the prognosis in mild heart failure. JACC Cardiovasc Imaging 2014; 7: 641–9.

37 Intracoronary Imaging

1. INTRAVASCULAR ULTRASOUND (IVUS)

I. Image basics

The arterial wall has three layers: (1) intima, typically white (echodense); (2) media, a thin black band; (3) adventitia, a thick, white, onion-skin external layer. The lumen is black (echolucent). In normal vessels, the intima is very thin, thinner than the media. In atheromatous arteries, the intima is essentially composed of atheroma, and its thickness corresponds to the plaque thickness; the media undergoes atrophy and becomes thinner than the intima. **When one is looking at an IVUS image, the first step is to find the black band inside the arterial wall. This black band is the media; inside it are the intima and the lumen** (Figures 37.1, 37.2).

Because of a blood stasis artifact, the lumen may look white and "foggy" and the lumen–intima boundary may be blurry, making luminal measurement difficult. In addition, the "foggy" lumen may be confused with a thrombus or with an echolucent intima, e.g., lipid-rich intima or intima with a necrotic core, falsely suggesting unstable disease. In order to improve blood stasis artifact, flush the coronary artery with contrast or saline whenever there is luminal blurriness (Figure 37.3). One may also use the color signal feature available with the Volcano system, wherein blood echogenicity is assigned a red color.

Vascular structures seen in the surroundings of the imaged artery may be arterial branches (e.g., septal, diagonal branches) or coronary veins. If, upon pullback, the structure enters the intima and joins the main vessel, the structure is a branch. Otherwise, it is a vein. Arterial branches are useful landmarks that identify the disease location and correlate it with angiography (Figures 37.4, 37.5, 37.6). Also, in the case of dissection, if the wire position is in question (true lumen vs. false lumen), seeing branches that join the lumen confirms the true luminal position of the wire.

In the presence of atherosclerosis, the media undergoes expansion in such a way that the luminal area remains normal. This is called **positive remodeling** or the Glagov phenomenon (Figures 37.7, 37.8). When the plaque area occupies more than 40% of the total vessel area (external elastic membrane area), luminal narrowing is seen. However, ~10–20% of atherosclerotic vessels undergo **negative remodeling**, wherein the media constricts and further narrows the lumen beyond what is expected from atherosclerosis. Thus, *luminal narrowing depends on the amount of atherosclerosis but also the type and extent of remodeling*.

Practical Cardiovascular Medicine, First Edition. Elias B. Hanna.
© 2017 John Wiley & Sons Ltd. Published 2017 by John Wiley & Sons Ltd.

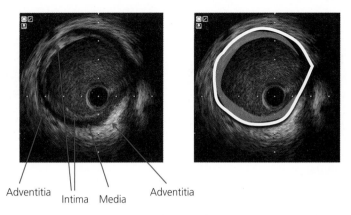

Adventitia Intima Media Adventitia

Figure 37.1 The left image is duplicated on the right with blue shading highlighting the intima and a white line highlighting the media.

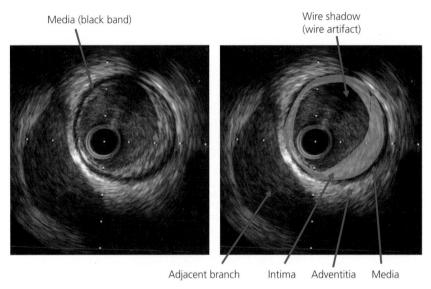

Media (black band)

Wire shadow
(wire artifact)

Adjacent branch   Intima   Adventitia   Media

Figure 37.2 The left image is duplicated on the right with blue shading highlighting the intima. A wire artifact is seen as a black shadow. An adjacent vessel is seen. The imaged vessel is the proximal LAD and the adjacent vessel is the ramus.

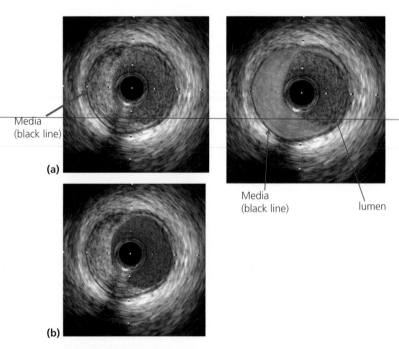

Media
(black line)

(a)

Media
(black line)

lumen

(b)

Figure 37.3 (a) Intima is marked in blue in the right-hand image. Note that the lumen is hazy, and one cannot definitely rule out echolucent (dark) plaque within this lumen. **(b)** After flushing the lumen, its boundaries become sharper, which makes luminal and intimal calculations easier and rules out echolucent plaque or intraluminal thrombus.

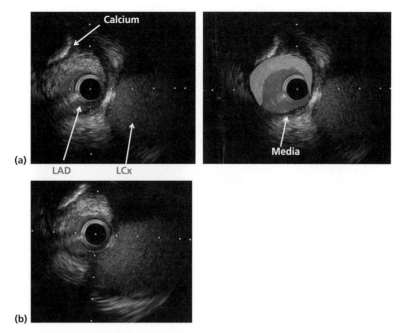

Figure 37.4 **(a)** Ostial LAD with LCx adjacent to it. The blue shading marks the intima, the gray shading marks the lumen. The black line surrounding the intima is the media. Always start by identifying the media, then identify the intima and lumen. **(b)** The severe LAD disease with constrictive remodeling extends until the very ostium, just as the LCx meets the LAD. The LAD lumen is narrow as a result of atherosclerosis but also as a result of vessel constriction. In fact, the media-to-media diameter of this ostial LAD (external elastic membrane [EEM] diameter) is only 3 mm (the distance between two dots being 1 mm)

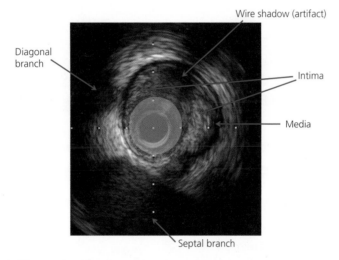

Figure 37.5 Diseased LAD at the level of first septal and first diagonal branches.

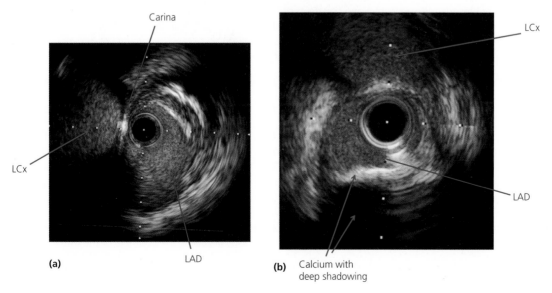

Figure 37.6 (a, b) Two IVUS images of a left main bifurcating into LAD and LCx. In (b), note that the ostial LAD is heavily calcified with a luminal area of 4 mm².

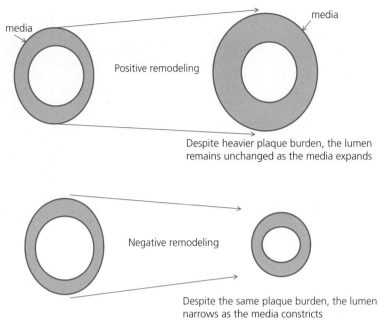

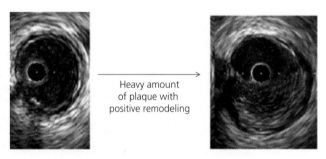

Figure 37.7 Positive and negative remodeling.

Figure 37.8 Example of positive remodeling (EEM area has expanded to accommodate atherosclerosis). Remodeling index = EEM area at the level of the lesion (right)/EEM area at the level of the reference (left).

II. Plaque types

IVUS identifies three types of plaques, i.e., three types of intima:

- *Echolucent, soft intima* is less echogenic (less white) than the adventitia. A soft plaque may be hard to differentiate from a foggy lumen.
- *Echodense, fibrous intima* is as bright as or brighter than the adventitia. Most atherosclerotic lesions are fibrous.
- *Calcified intima* is brighter than the adventitia and has deep shadowing (Figures 37.4, 37.6). The calcium is quantified by the arc it encompasses (e.g., 90°, 180°) and its depth. Superficial calcium is defined as calcium in the top half of the intima and is particularly adverse to stent expansion.

In addition, one should look for signs of plaque instability (Figures 37.9–37.12):

a. *A ruptured or ulcerated plaque* is a plaque that has been split. It contains a cavity that communicates with the lumen, with a variable amount of overlying, ruptured fibrous cap.
b. *A dark, echolucent area* within a plaque represents a soft lipid-rich component, a necrotic core, intra-plaque hemorrhage, or an intra-intimal thrombus.
c. *A thrombus* is an intraluminal or intra-intimal echolucent mass having a layered or lobulated appearance (± speckled texture). It is sometimes hard to differentiate from soft echolucent plaque or necrotic or lipid-rich areas. Also, blood stasis artifact may hide a thrombus or create the impression of a thrombus. When in doubt, flush the coronary artery to clear blood stasis.

In addition, heavy atheroma with positive remodeling is often seen in ACS and is a marker of instability. While positive remodeling reduces the severity of coronary stenosis, it is a marker of heavy atherosclerosis and plaque progression, frequently through prior plaque ruptures, and is thus a negative prognostic marker.

When measuring the luminal area in a ruptured/ulcerated plaque, exclude the ulcerated area, as it is not true lumen. The lesion may not look severe on angiography because the ruptured cavity fills with contrast, concealing the tightness of the true lumen.

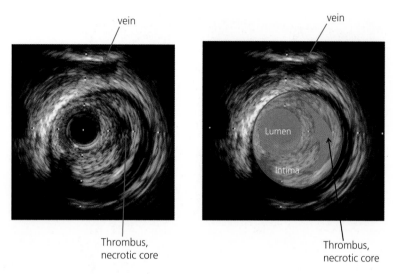

Figure 37.9 Lesion with necrotic core. Intima and necrotic core are highlighted in the right-hand image.

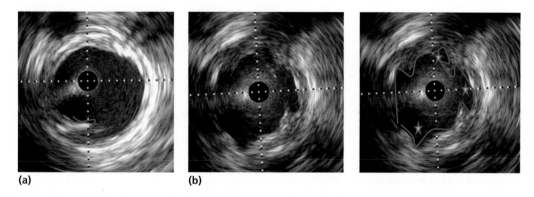

Figure 37.10 Ulcerated lesions. **(a)** Ulcer demarcated at 6 o'clock. **(b)** Stenosis with multiple ulcers demarcated at 12, 3, and a little after 6 o'clock (*stars* in right-hand image). The blue line delineates the intima–lumen boundary.

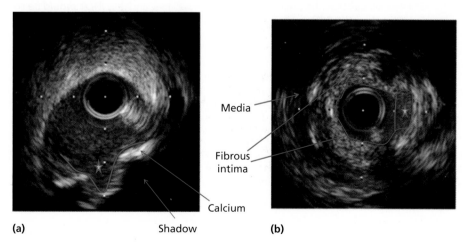

Figure 37.11 Further examples of ulcers. **(a)** LAD ulcer at 6 o'clock (*star*). Also, a superficial calcified arc of 45° is seen with deep shadowing. **(b)** Crater/ulcer at 3 o'clock (*star*). Lumen area measures ~2.5 mm² , excluding the crater (using the imaginary interrupted line).

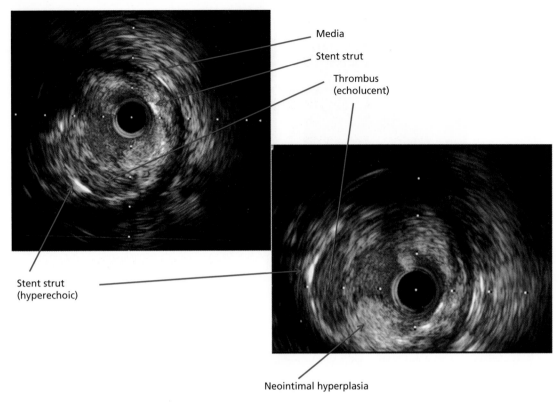

Media

Stent strut

Thrombus
(echolucent)

Stent strut
(hyperechoic)

Neointimal hyperplasia

Figure 37.12 Stent thrombosis and neointimal hyperplasia.

III. Basic IVUS measurements

The following are basic IVUS measurements (Figure 37.13):

a. *External elastic membrane (EEM)* cross-sectional area (CSA), also called total vessel CSA: EEM corresponds to the outer boundary of the media. This is the boundary between the black band (media) and the outer adventitia.

b. *Lumen CSA* at the level of the stenosis (*minimal luminal area [MLA]*): this is the most important measurement and the one correlating the most with outcomes.

c. *Intima + media CSA* = atheroma CSA = EEM area minus lumen area.

d. *Area of stenosis*: contrary to a common misconception, the area of stenosis does not reference the stenosis to the EEM area. As a result of positive remodeling, the EEM area is larger than the original non-diseased vessel area, and thus **MLA should be compared to the most normal surrounding lumen rather than the EEM area.** The reference lumen is the most normal-looking lumen, i.e., the largest lumen with the smallest plaque burden within 10 mm of the lesion. One may average the proximal and distal references.

Conversely, referencing the plaque to the EEM area is called *plaque burden* or *percent cross-sectional narrowing* and is dependent on the amount of atheroma.

e. In patients with a stent, the *stent area* is the area bounded by the stent struts, while the neointimal hyperplasia area is equal to stent area minus lumen area (Figures 37.14, 37.15). **The stent should be sized to the reference lumen area, not the EEM area.** The stent should be sized to 100% of the distal reference or 90% of the average proximal and distal references. Sizing the stent to the EEM area results in stent oversizing with a risk of perforation or edge dissection. An undersized stent is a stent with an area that is less than the reference lumen area. A stent is underexpanded when (Figure 37.14):

* It is appropriately sized but the minimal stent area (MSA) (i.e., the stent area in the tightest spot) is less than the reference lumen area.
* The diameter of the stent is less than the nominal stent diameter (e.g., a 3 mm stent is only expanded to 2.5 mm).
* It is asymmetric with a minimal-to-maximal stent diameter <0.7.

Underexpansion is typically focal in calcified or fibrotic spots.

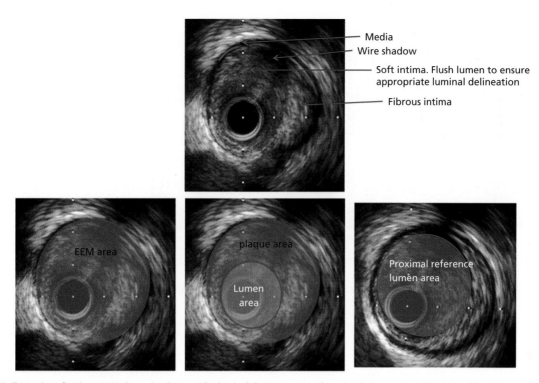

Figure 37.13 Illustration of various IVUS-determined areas. The luminal diameter across the stenosis is ~2 mm, with a minimal luminal area (MLA) of 3.5 mm² (1 mm grid). The EEM diameter is 4 mm, with EEM area (total vessel area) of ~12.5 mm². The proximal reference lumen diameter is 3 mm, with a proximal reference lumen area of 7 mm².

The area of stenosis is MLA in reference to the reference lumen area, not vessel area. Thus, the area of stenosis is equal to (reference lumen − stenotic lumen)/reference lumen = (7 − 3.5)/7 = 50%.

The plaque burden is: plaque area/EEM area = (EEM area − stenotic lumen)/EEM area = (12.5−3.5)/12.5 = 72%.

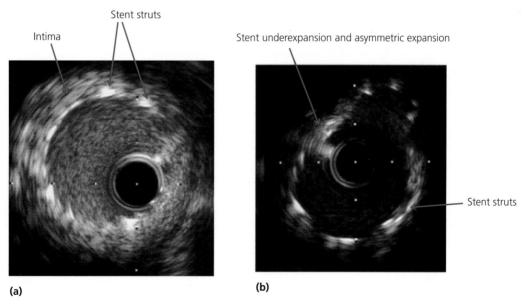

Figure 37.14 Stents. **(a)** Ostial LM stent with intima seen underneath the struts. **(b)** Stent underexpansion and asymmetric expansion. The minimal stent diameter is 2.5 mm, while its maximal diameter is 4 mm.

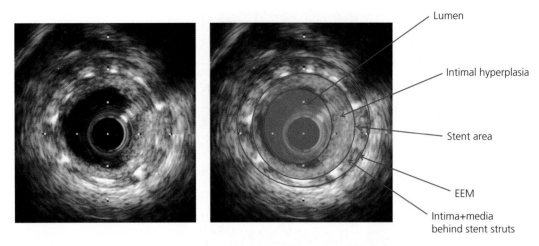

Figure 37.15 Stent with neointimal hyperplasia. In-stent restenosis percent is equal to neointimal hyperplasia area/stent area.

IV. Interpretation of how a severe stenosis may look mild angiographically, yet severe by IVUS; significance of lesion haziness (see Figure 37.16)

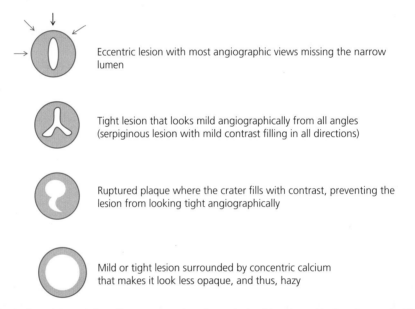

Eccentric lesion with most angiographic views missing the narrow lumen

Tight lesion that looks mild angiographically from all angles (serpiginous lesion with mild contrast filling in all directions)

Ruptured plaque where the crater fills with contrast, preventing the lesion from looking tight angiographically

Mild or tight lesion surrounded by concentric calcium that makes it look less opaque, and thus, hazy

Figure 37.16 Causes of lesion haziness. Interpretation of how a severe stenosis may look mild angiographically, yet severe by IVUS.

V. Endpoints of stenting

The endpoints of stenting are:

1. Full apposition to the vessel wall, i.e., no gaps between the stent and the underlying intima (Figure 37.17).
2. Good expansion with a minimal stent area that is 100% of the smallest reference lumen area or >80–90% of the average reference lumen area (i.e., average of the proximal and distal reference areas).
3. Good expansion with a minimal stent area that matches the nominal stent diameter (e.g., a 3 mm stent should have a 7 mm² area).
Stent underexpansion is a predictor of stent thrombosis and restenosis, much more so than stent malapposition.
4. Symmetric stent expansion with minimal/maximal stent diameter ≥0.7
5. No edge dissections that are deep (extend to the media), circumferential (>1 quadrant), long (>5 mm), or associated with MLA <4 mm². The latter edge dissections require additional edge stenting. Also, edge disease or plaque shift with MLA <4 mm² increases the risk of future events and may necessitate stenting.

VI. Assessment of lesion significance by IVUS

Several studies have tried to associate ischemia with a single minimal luminal area cutoff by IVUS. MLA <3 mm² for non-left main arteries had a good correlation with FFR <0.75 in one study, whereas MLA <4 mm² had a good correlation with ischemia determined by coronary vascular reserve in another study.[1,2] More recently, cutoffs of 2.4 mm² for any epicardial vessel, 3 mm² for the proximal LAD, and 2.75 mm² for the mid-LAD were found to have the best correlation with FFR ≤0.80.[3,4]

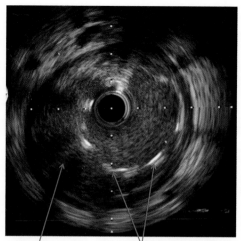

Left main lumen   Ostial LAD stent with one strut hanging in LM

Figure 37.17 The stent is well expanded in the ostial LAD with one strut hanging in the left main (standard ostial stenting technique). Had this been a left main stent, a major stent malapposition would have been diagnosed (stent not touching the vessel wall).

However, the use of a single anatomical cutoff clearly has issues: a 4 mm² MLA may limit flow in a large proximal vessel but not in a distal small vessel. In fact, the area of a normal 2.5 mm vessel is 4.9 mm²; thus a stenosis with MLA 4 mm² corresponds to a 28% area of stenosis and should not be considered functionally significant. Even in a 3 mm vessel (7.12 mm² area), a 4 mm² MLA corresponds to a 44% area of stenosis, unlikely to be significant.[5] Furthermore, the drop in flow across a lesion correlates with length as well as diameter, i.e., a focal 4 mm² stenosis may not be significant. Deferral based on IVUS MLA >4 mm² is appropriate and associated with excellent clinical outcomes; however, the decision to treat a lesion with MLA <4 mm² is less appropriate.[6] An intermediate lesion is better assessed functionally, while IVUS is still useful for lesion assessment in ACS. IVUS is useful before lesion stenting for sizing and for evaluation of some unstable morphological features (e.g., plaque rupture, circumferential calcifications that dictate rotational atherectomy), and is useful after stenting to assess stent expansion, apposition, and distal edge dissections.

VII. Assessment of left main by IVUS
See Chapter 38, Section XI.

2. OPTICAL COHERENCE TOMOGRAPHY (OCT)

OCT uses infrared light. An optical beam is directed at the tissue, and the small portion of light that reflects from subsurface tissues is collected. Since it uses light, OCT has a much higher resolution than ultrasound/IVUS, an almost microscopic resolution (10 micrometers with OCT vs. 150 micrometers with IVUS).

On OCT, the intima is yellow, the media is dark lucent, and the adventitia is often not visualized (when visualized, adventitia is dark red). The morphology of various lesion types is shown in Figures 37.18 and 37.19.
Advantages of OCT include:

1. Greater definition of the lumen boundaries than IVUS, allowing a more accurate calculation of lumen CSA. Also, it allows better assessment of stent expansion and the apposition of the stent to the intima.
2. Visualization of the thin fibrous cap and diagnosis of cap rupture. A thin cap is defined as a cap thinner than 65 micrometers. Most plaque ruptures (80%) occur over a thin-cap fibroatheroma.
3. Better assessment of plaque composition than IVUS (lipid-rich plaque vs. fibrous plaque). OCT is as good as IVUS for the assessment of calcifications.
4. Better visualization of thrombus than IVUS (Figure 37.19).
5. Better visualization of stent edge dissections (Figure 37.20). While edge dissections are seen by angiography in 5% of stenting procedures, they are seen by IVUS and OCT in 10% and 30% of stenting procedures, respectively. However, small edge dissections (<1 quadrant, <5 mm in length, not extending to the media, and associated with MLA >4 mm²) do not need to be stented.

Disadvantages of OCT include:

1. Poor tissue depth penetration of 1–2.5 mm, as opposed to 10 mm with IVUS. Thus, OCT may not visualize the full depth of the intima and may not be able to measure the plaque burden.
2. Requires a blood-free medium for imaging. OCT imaging is performed quickly in order to allow imaging during a single contrast injection (e.g., 4 ml/s for 16 ml). Blood that has not cleared from some areas may lead to swirls or to speckle artifacts that simulate thrombi. This also implies that OCT cannot be used to assess the ostial left main or the ostial RCA, as the guide catheter has to be appropriately engaged beyond the ostium to allow coronary contrast filling, which prevents the imaging of that ostium.
3. The imaging depth is lower than with IVUS. OCT penetrates ~3.5–4 cm of the blood-free medium, which means that OCT is suboptimal for large vessel imaging.

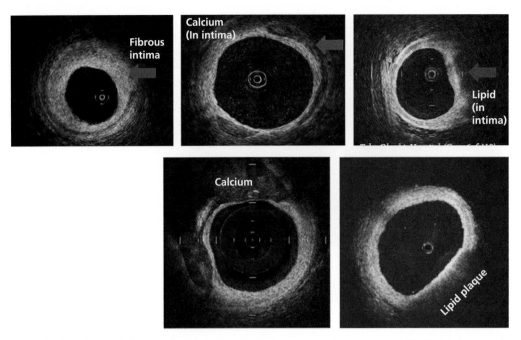

Figure 37.18 OCT. *Fibrotic plaque* is characterized by being bright (high signal). As opposed to IVUS, *calcium* on OCT is dark (low signal) and is well demarcated with low attenuation of light, allowing deeper imaging. *Lipid plaque* is also dark but attenuates light more than calcium, which explains the loose edges and the shadowing; it is homogeneous. Courtesy of St. Jude Medical.

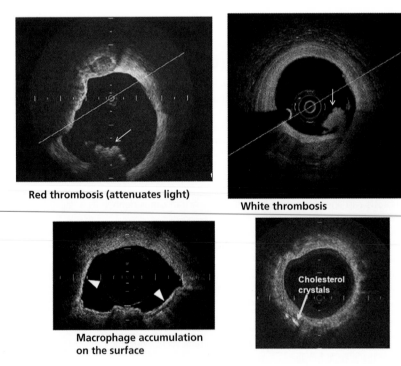

Figure 37.19 Thrombus, macrophage accumulation, and cholesterol crystals imaged by OCT. Macrophage accumulation appears as a bright line on the surface of the plaque and is associated with shadowing. Macrophages usually accumulate superficially within the fibrous cap, and are a sign of instability. In fact, macrophages are the cells that rupture the cap. Cholesterol crystals look like bright dots. Courtesy of St. Jude Medical.

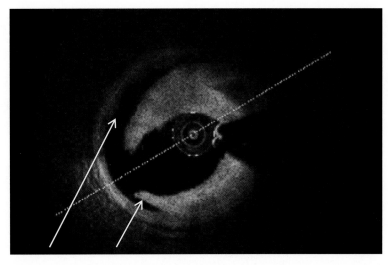

Figure 37.20 Stent edge dissection. Arrows show the dissection planes. The dissection is deep (reaches the media between 10 and 12 o'clock) and extends more than 1 quadrant. This dissection is thus clinically significant.Courtesy of St. Jude Medical.

References

IVUS

1. Takagi A, Tsurumi Y, Ishii, et al. Clinical potential of intravascular ultrasound for physiological assessment of coronary stenosis. Relationship between quantitative ultrasound tomography and pressure-derived fractional flow reserve. Circulation 1999; 100: 250–5.
2. Abizaid A, Mintz GS, Pichard AD, et al. Clinical, intravascular ultrasound, and quantitative angiographic determinants of the coronary flow reserve before and after percutaneous transluminal coronary angioplasty. Am J Cardiol 1998; 82: 423–8.
3. Kang SJ, Lee JY, Ahn JM, et al. Validation of intravascular ultrasound-derived parameters with fractional flow reserve for assessment of coronary stenosis severity. Circ Cardiovasc Interv 2011; 4: 65–71.
4. Koo BK, Yang HM, Doh JH, et al. Optimal intravascular ultrasound criteria and their accuracy for defining the functional significance of intermediate coronary stenoses of different locations. JACC Cardiovasc Interv 2011; 4: 803–11.
5. Kern MJ. Coronary physiology in the cath lab: beyond the basics. Cardiol Clin 2011; 29: 237–67.
6. Abizaid A, Mintz G, Mehran R, et al. Long-term follow-up after percutaneous transluminal coronary angioplasty was not performed based on intravascular ultrasound findings: importance of lumen dimensions. Circulation 1999; 100: 256–61.

Further reading

OCT

Jang IK, Bouma BE, Kang DH, et al. Visualization of coronary atherosclerotic plaques in patients using optical coherence tomography: comparison with intravascular ultrasound. J Am Coll Cardiol 2002; 39: 604–9.
Jang IK. Optical coherence tomography or intravascular ultrasound? JACC Cardiovasc Interv 2011; 4: 492–4.
Suh WM, Seto AH, Margey RJ, Cruz-Gonzalez I, Jang IK. Intravascular detection of the vulnerable plaque. Circ Cardiovasc Imaging 2011; 4: 169–78.
Bezerra HG, Costa MA, Guagliumi G, Rollins AM, Simon DI. Intracoronary optical coherence tomography: a comprehensive review. JACC Cardiovasc Interv 2009; 2: 1035–46.

38 Percutaneous Coronary Interventions and Complications, Intra-Aortic Balloon Pump, Ventricular Assist Devices, and Fractional Flow Reserve

I. Major coronary interventional devices
A. Balloon angioplasty
1. Mechanisms of action
Angioplasty expands the external elastic membrane of the stenotic segment, creating a larger total vessel area that compensates for the intimal plaque; this is similar to the positive remodeling phenomenon (Figure 38.1). Some axial plaque redistribution, proximally and distally, may also reduce the stenosis, at the expense of creating edge stenoses.

2. Pitfalls
a. Angioplasty fractures the intimal plaque, allowing it to yield for vessel expansion. **Dissection** of the intima (coronary plaque) is, thus, a normal finding with angioplasty, and the dissection planes may extend deep into the media (true dissection). In heavily fibrotic or calcified stenoses, dissections are necessary to allow the plaque to yield and prevent early recoil. Dissections are angiographically seen after ~30% of balloon angioplasties. Mild and shallow dissections (angiographic type A or B dissections) are not associated with worsened long-term outcomes; to the contrary, the well-expanded, fractured vessel may be associated with less long-term constriction/restenosis. However, a severe dissection may obstruct the lumen and impair flow. Also, dissection may lead to abrupt vessel closure within minutes to 24 hours after angioplasty; this occurs in 5–10% of angioplasties and is treated with bailout stenting.

b. **Elastic recoil** is the immediate vessel constriction that occurs after angioplasty. After the vessel appropriately yields to balloon inflation, it may quickly constrict upon balloon deflation (within 10 minutes). More prolonged inflation of the vessel with an appropriately sized balloon (sized 1:1 to the reference luminal diameter) at a high pressure reduces this phenomenon.

c. **High risk of restenosis** (~40%). Restenosis starts beyond the first month and is mainly due to **negative remodeling**, which is a form of late vessel constriction (as opposed to elastic recoil, a form of early vessel constriction).

3. Compliant vs. non-compliant balloons
Non-compliant balloons do not expand much beyond their nominal size even at high pressures (<10% overexpansion), allowing one to exert high pressure across a calcified, unyielding lesion without balloon overexpansion across the soft spots.

4. Balloon angioplasty with a balloon that is scored with blades (cutting balloon) or wires (Angiosculpt) allows the plaque to yield more easily, at lower inflation pressures. Theoretically, this increases the success of angioplasty and may be associated with less severe dissections. Also, a scored balloon is less likely to slip during balloon inflation. Standard, non-scored balloons tend to slip when inflated across a heavily fibrotic stenosis ("watermelon seeding"). Using longer balloons, slower inflation, and scored balloons reduces this phenomenon.

Practical Cardiovascular Medicine, First Edition. Elias B. Hanna.
© 2017 John Wiley & Sons Ltd. Published 2017 by John Wiley & Sons Ltd.

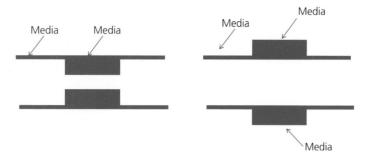

Figure 38.1 Main mechanism of action of balloon angioplasty. Angioplasty pushes the plaque and its media out, making the media larger at the treatment site. In order for this to happen, the plaque has to yield; frequently, it fractures, sometimes deeply into the media (dissection).

5. Cases where plain balloon angioplasty is sometimes performed, without stenting

- Vessels <2.0 mm
- Bifurcation lesions, in which a diseased side branch is dilated while the main branch is stented
- Treatment of DES restenosis

B. Bare-metal stents (BMSs)

A stent addresses all three balloon angioplasty pitfalls. It covers and seals the dissection planes or, at least, prevents them from expanding and promoting abrupt vessel closure. It has enough radial strength to prevent early (elastic recoil) and late (restenosis) vessel constriction. Stenting improves the immediate and late PCI result, but is not without its own pitfalls:

i. Stent thrombosis: while preventing abrupt vessel closure, stenting is associated with a risk of stent thrombosis, mainly in the first month. This risk is 0.5–1% in patients receiving dual antiplatelet therapy (DAT) with aspirin and clopidogrel, and 5–10% in patients receiving single antiplatelet therapy with aspirin.

ii. In-stent restenosis (ISR): restenosis is reduced to 20–25% with stenting. Overall, stenting *eliminates the late negative remodeling* seen after plain angioplasty, *but increases the degree of neointimal hyperplasia*, which starts 1 month after stenting and progresses for up to 6–8 months. The rate of clinical restenosis after BMS, i.e., angina recurrence, is ~15%.

Note on technical aspects

The stent is mounted on a compliant balloon and is apposed to the vessel wall through balloon inflation. Prior to advancing a stent, lesion pre-dilatation with a slightly undersized balloon breaks the fibrosis and calcium, which allows stent delivery and expansion. Sometimes, "direct stenting" not preceded by balloon angioplasty may be performed. Factors favoring successful direct stenting are: absence of calcium at the target or other coronary vessels, absence of severe proximal tortuosity, non-critical stenosis, and age <70 years.

The stent is usually deployed at a pressure ≤14 atm to prevent edge overinflation by the compliant stent balloon and the risk of edge dissection. After stent deployment, stent dilatation may be performed with a shorter non-compliant balloon placed within the stent and inflated at a higher pressure (15–18 atm) to ensure proper stent expansion.

C. Drug-eluting stents (DESs)

(*First-generation DESs:* sirolimus [Cypher] and paclitaxel [Taxus, Ion]; *second-generation DESs:* everolimus [Xience V, Promus, Synergy], zotaralimus [Resolute]).

A DES consists of a stent platform similar to a BMS, with two additional components: a drug, and a polymer that controls the local drug delivery over 3–6 months. The drug inhibits cell proliferation and thus neointimal hyperplasia, with a restenosis rate of <5–10%. On the other hand, by delaying stent strut coverage, the risk of stent thrombosis persists beyond the first month. With the first-generation DESs, this risk of stent thrombosis remained significant for the first 12 months and mandated DAT for 12 months. The second-generation DESs are associated with a dramatic reduction in the risk of stent thrombosis and target vessel MI (vs. first-generation DESs); the risk of stent thrombosis is very low even after clopidogrel interruption at 3–6 months.

The risk of stent thrombosis with DES is similar to BMS, as long as clopidogrel is used for the proper duration. The proper duration of dual antiplatelet therapy with second-generation DES is: (i) 6 months in the setting of stable CAD PCI, with a possible reduction to 3 months if needed (class IIb); (ii) 12 months in the setting of ACS, with a possible reduction to 6 months if needed (class IIb).

While DES does not clearly reduce mortality or MI in comparison to BMS, it dramatically reduces restenosis and repeat revascularizations. DES is superior to BMS in all subsets of patients, but is *particularly superior and indicated in the following cases*:

a. One of *five features* indicative of a high risk of restenosis: diabetes, long lesions >20 mm, small vessel <3 mm, bifurcation stenting, chronic total occlusion (CTO).
b. In-stent restenosis.
c. Proximal LAD, left main, or multivessel disease, where restenosis is more consequential.

In complex lesions with several of those features, the restenosis rate remains high even with DES, ≥ 10%, with an even higher rate of target vessel revascularization related to disease progression outside the stented area.

On the other hand, since DES mandates longer antiplatelet therapy, it used to be less favored in the following situations:

- Patients at a high bleeding risk (e.g., anemia, recent major bleed)
- Planned surgery in the next 6 months
- Requirement for chronic warfarin therapy

However, since second-generation DES appear as safe as BMS, the above situations are no longer considered more problematic for DES than BMS. Note that 1–6 months of triple therapy followed by long-term clopidogrel+warfarin therapy is acceptable with second-generation DES (ESC guidelines consider 1 month of triple therapy acceptable in high-bleeding-risk patients).

D. Rotational atherectomy (Rotablator) and orbital atherectomy

The atherectomy devices consist of a burr mounted over a catheter. As opposed to angioplasty, which expands the media without affecting plaque volume, atherectomy acts by removing plaque; it cuts the atheroma into small microparticles that are subsequently eliminated by the reticuloendothelial system. Those microparticles are typically very small, smaller than the red blood cells, and thus do not usually plug the microcirculation, as long as each atherectomy pass is limited to <30 seconds and vasodilators are used between passes. The Rotablator achieves better immediate results than angioplasty but is associated with a similar rate of late restenosis; the heat injury initiates both negative remodeling and neointimal hyperplasia. Atherectomy is useful in heavily calcified lesions that do not yield with high-pressure balloon angioplasty, meaning that the balloon never fully expands across the lesion. The lack of full balloon expansion is different from the more common elastic recoil, wherein the balloon expands but the vessel quickly collapses back. **A stent should never be used for an unyielding lesion**, i.e., a lesion where the balloon does not fully expand, as the stent will fail to appropriately expand and a catastrophic stent thrombosis may occur.

After balloon angioplasty fails to expand a lesion, the patient is brought back 4–6 weeks later for rotational atherectomy. It is not performed in a patient with dissection planes soon after angioplasty, as a major vessel perforation may be created by atherectomy.

E. Aspiration thrombectomy

As an adjunct to balloon and stenting, aspiration thrombectomy catheters (suction catheters: Export, Pronto catheters) can be used to aspirate thrombi.

Aspiration thrombectomy catheters have been mainly studied at a large scale in acute STEMI. Initial data suggested that they improve microcirculatory and cellular perfusion (TAPAS trial). However, large trials (TASTE and TOTAL) did not show any clinical benefit from the systematic use of thrombectomy and there was a small stroke hazard. The selective use of thrombectomy in STEMI patients with a large thrombus burden may still be justified.

The Angiojet rheolytic thrombectomy catheter may be used for a heavy thrombus burden, especially in acute STEMI that results from SVG occlusion. It is mostly valuable in lower extremity acute limb ischemia, often as an adjunct to local thrombolysis.

Wires with a distal basket, called *distal embolic protection devices*, are mainly useful during PCI of venous grafts. They have not shown a benefit in acute MI: native coronary arteries have numerous side branches, such that a distal basket will prevent embolization into the distal vessel but will favor embolization into side branches, some of which are large. Also, placement of the distal protection may increase the time to reperfusion and may create arterial injury per se (especially if the basket moves during device manipulations).

II. Stent thrombosis, restenosis, and neoatherosclerosis

A. Thrombosis

Stent thrombosis usually occurs within 1 month of stent placement but can occur later with DES or BMS. It is prevented with dual antiplatelet therapy (DAT) and adequate stent expansion. Stent thrombosis typically leads to STEMI, the prognosis of which is much worse than that of spontaneously occurring STEMI (high clot burden), with a 15–45% risk of mortality.

Timing of stent thrombosis: acute (within 24 hours), subacute (between 1 and 30 days), late (between 1 and 12 months), and very late (>12 months). Late and very late stent thromboses are rare, but may be seen with DES or BMS, especially if both antiplatelet agents are discontinued. The risk of late stent thrombosis is probably similar with second-generation DES and BMS(0.2–0.4% per year) (DAPT trial). After the first month, stent thrombosis usually occurs ≥ 7 days after clopidogrel discontinuation, implying that brief clopidogrel interruption for non-cardiac surgery may be safe.

There are three categories of risk factors for stent thrombosis (Table 38.1).

Table 38.1 Risk factors for stent thrombosis.

---

a. Mechanical
Stent underexpansion, stent malapposition, edge dissection, edge plaque shift (especially if the plaque is necrotic and active)

b. Pharmacological
Acutely, a delayed loading of ADP receptor antagonist is a risk factor for acute thrombosis. Non-compliance with the recommended duration of DAT is the most important risk factor for subacute and late stent thrombosis. Clopidogrel non-responsiveness increases the risk of stent thrombosis, which remains low, in absolute terms, in stable CAD PCI. The latter is rarely a standalone factor in stent thrombosis

c. Underlying patient and lesion
- ACS presentation, particularly STEMI, is by far the most important predictor of stent thrombosis in this category
- Other factors: diabetes, renal failure, small vessel, long lesion, poor runoff and bifurcation PCI (especially dual stenting)

B. Restenosis

1. Mechanisms

a. *After plain balloon angioplasty*, two processes lead to restenosis:
- Negative arterial remodeling (arterial constriction).
- Neointimal hyperplasia.

Both processes start beyond 1 month (1–6 months). As opposed to stenting, the main mechanism of restenosis after angioplasty is negative remodeling, which peaks earlier than neointimal hyperplasia.

b. *After stenting*:
- Stent underexpansion (suboptimal stent deployment).
- Focal or diffuse in-stent neointimal hyperplasia. *Neointimal hyperplasia* refers to smooth muscle cell and macrophage migration from deep in the vessel wall (media) to the surface of the struts. This is followed by cellular proliferation and production of extracellular matrix (fibrosis). Restenosis leads to a "fibrotic" narrowing of the stent lumen, different from thrombosis, and different from atherosclerosis.

  When the stent is underexpanded, even a mild degree of neointimal hyperplasia may lead to significant restenosis. Underexpansion is a common factor in restenosis, especially DES restenosis, where neointimal hyperplasia is milder than with BMS. This makes stent underexpansion a major factor in >50% of DES restenoses.

2. Neointimal hyperplasia

Neointimal hyperplasia starts to develop 1 month after angioplasty or stent placement, peaks at 3–6 months, and does not progress beyond 6–8 months with BMS or 12 months with DES. After DES, neointimal hyperplasia is milder but also more delayed than after BMS. Either way, neointimal hyperplasia does not usually progress beyond those timelines. However, progression of atherosclerosis in the nearby segments and neoatherosclerosis inside the stented segment may occur beyond those timelines (even more so with SVG stenting).

3. Patterns of restenosis

Restenosis may be focal (42% of cases of BMS restenosis), diffuse (21%), proliferative (extends beyond stent margins; 30%), or totally occlusive (7%). With DES, restenosis is often focal, sometimes purely at the edges, in relation to uncovered edge disease, progressive edge disease, or neointimal hyperplasia and negative remodeling at the edges. High-pressure inflation of the compliant stent balloon may also induce edge injury and restenosis.

4. Clinical presentation

Restenosis usually leads to recurrence of stable angina, but it may lead to MI presentation in ~10% of patients (usually NSTEMI). Therefore, while it is less catastrophic than stent thrombosis, restenosis is not benign.

5. Treatment

Restenosis is treated with balloon angioplasty if the main problem is technical (i.e., the stent is underexpanded) or if the in-stent restenosis is focal. Focal restenosis has good outcomes with balloon angioplasty and a recurrent restenosis rate of ~20%. A cutting balloon may also be used. Conversely, diffuse in-stent restenosis and edge restenosis are treated with DES placement within the previously placed BMS or DES (DES stent "sandwich"). Alternatively, a drug-coated balloon may be used (available in Europe). *IVUS* helps determine the mechanism and guide the treatment of in-stent restenosis.

Sandwich DES stenting for DES restenosis is associated with a ~15–20% risk of recurrent restenosis. Placing a heterogeneous sandwich DES, i.e., a different type of DES within the restenosed DES, is not clearly superior to a homogeneous sandwich DES.

C. Neoatherosclerosis

Beyond 1 year, atherosclerosis starts to grow over the stent neointima; this is referred to as neoatherosclerosis. As opposed to neointimal hyperplasia, neoatherosclerosis is characterized by a lipid-laden plaque with foamy macrophages and a fibrous cap. It tends to appear earlier and more frequently with DES (30–50% at 1–2 years) than BMS (16% at 5 years). It explains *late restenosis* and partly explains the *very late stent thrombosis* seen with both types of stents.

D. Mechanisms of recurrent target vessel disease after stenting (Table 38.2)

Table 38.2 Recurrent target vessel disease/angina after stenting.

---

1. First 1–2 months
- *Mechanical issues* leading to subacute stent thrombosis (acute severe presentation) or residual stenosis (insidious presentation): stent underexpansion, edge disease or edge dissection, failure to cover the entire target lesion

2. 1–12 months
- *Stent restenosis*
- *Late stent thrombosis* from stent underexpansion[a]
- *Disease progression* outside the stented area, especially at the edges (more so in ACS)

3. Over 1 year
- *Neoatherosclerosis*
- *Late presentation of neointimal hyperplasia*
- *Disease progression* outside the stented area

---

[a] Also, necrotic plaque protrusion through the stent (more so in ACS) may predispose to restenosis or thrombosis.

III. Peri-PCI antithrombotic therapy (see Table 38.3)

Table 38.3 Peri-PCI antithrombotic therapy.

Stable CAD PCI

Planned PCI

1. Aspirin 325 mg >2 h before PCI if aspirin-naïve (otherwise, aspirin 81 mg the day of the procedure)

2. Clopidogrel 600 mg ≥ 2 h, 300 mg ≥ 24 h, or 75 mg ≥ 7 days before PCI

3. GPI: no benefit in elective PCI preloaded with clopidogrel (except for bailout)

4. UFH or bivalirudin:

   Bivalirudin ↓ bleeding in comparison to UFH or UFH + GPI, with similar anti-ischemic benefit

   Dose of UFH: 70–100 units/kg to a goal ACT 250–300 s if GPI is not used

   50–70 units/kg to a goal ACT 200–250 s if GPI is used

Ad-hoc PCI

- Preloading all patients undergoing coronary angiography with clopidogrel, for the possibility of PCI, has not been shown to be superior to in-lab loading in stable CAD. Thus, clopidogrel 600 mg is administered during the procedure, once a decision is made to proceed with PCI

- GPI is not routinely indicated, regardless of whether UFH or bivalirudin is used. GPI is only considered for bailout

---

NSTE–ACS

Antiplatelet therapy

1. Aspirin 325 mg on admission, then 81 mg daily

2. Clopidogrel 300 mg or ticagrelor 180 mg on admission of all NSTE–ACS patients

   May withhold in a subgroup of patients with a high probability of needing CABG

3. Upstream GPI *is not indicated*, even if an ADP receptor antagonist is not started on admission

4. After coronary angiography, if PCI is to be performed:

   - Add 300 mg of clopidogrel if 300 mg has already been given

   or load with 600 mg of clopidogrel in the cath lab if no clopidogrel has been given

   or load with prasugrel 60 mg in the cath lab (even if clopidogrel has been given)

   or load with ticagrelor 180 mg in the cath lab (even if clopidogrel has been given)

   - GPI if troponin (+) *and* no clopidogrel or ticagrelor preload

   or if PCI complications (bailout use of GPI)

   - GPI on top of prasugrel or ticagrelor: unclear benefit?

Anticoagulant therapy

UFH pre-catheterization and during PCI

or UFH pre-catheterization and switch to bivalirudin during PCI

or Fondaparinux 2.5 mg SQ QD pre-catheterization with standard-dose UFH or bivalirudin during PCI

or Enoxaparin pre-catheterization. If the patient received 1 mg/kg SQ enoxaparin within 8 h of PCI and has already received two doses of enoxaparin, no additional anticoagulation is needed during PCI. If enoxaparin was given 8–12 h ago or only one SQ dose was given, add 0.3 mg/kg IV bolus during PCI

Avoid switching between UFH and enoxaparin. The switch to bivalirudin is, however, appropriate and does not attenuate the bleeding reduction seen with bivalirudin

---

STEMI

1. Aspirin 325 mg in the emergency room

2. Clopidogrel 600 mg, prasugrel 60 mg, or ticagrelor 180 mg *upstream* in the emergency room

3. No upstream GPI before PCI regardless of PCI delay (if PCI delay, give fibrinolytics rather than GPI)

4. Upstream UFH (60 units/kg, up to 4000 units)

5. During PCI:

   - May use UFH or bivalirudin

   - GPI is used if: (i) clopidogrel or ticagrelor not preloaded in emergency room, or (ii) high thrombus burden

---

GPI: glycoprotein IIb-IIIa inhibitors

IV. Complex lesion subsets

A. Multivessel PCI

According to clinical trials, multivessel PCI compares favorably with CABG if the stenoses are technically amenable to PCI. The presence of a chronic total occlusion or one or more technically difficult lesions or long lesions (angiographic SYNTAX score ≥ 23) should favor CABG, especially because CABG provides a more complete revascularization. Diabetes favors CABG as well, as CABG provides lower rate of repeat revascularization and better survival compared with PCI in diabetes.

B. Long lesions and diffuse disease (multiple lesions in series)

Normally, the stent should be implanted from normal reference to normal reference if possible (starting 2 mm before and 2 mm after the lesion); this will avoid edge dissections and edge plaque shift. In case of diffuse disease with tandem lesions in series, the most severe lesions are stented (spot stenting), while the intermediate ones may be left untreated. FFR may be used to guide PCI in diffuse disease: stent the areas where the pressure drop is largest, as assessed by FFR pullback tracing. FFR may be reassessed after stenting each lesion. If possible, the distal lesion should be stented first, followed by the proximal lesion; this obviates the need to cross the proximal stent with the distal stent.

While DES length does not increase restenosis rate as strongly as BMS length, very long stenting ("full metal jacket"), even with DES, is associated with a high risk of restenosis and is preferably avoided. Furthermore, long stenting may compromise future placement of bypass grafts and is preferably avoided, especially in the LAD.

C. Bifurcation lesions

Side branch (SB) narrowing may occur after main branch (MB) PCI. This is related to plaque shift (snowplow phenomenon). The likelihood of this depends on the degree of ostial SB narrowing. When the ostium of the SB has >50% stenosis (= true bifurcation lesion), there is a risk of SB occlusion with MB stenting (14–35%). Bifurcation stenoses are approached as follows:

- Double wiring, i.e., wiring of both SB and MB, is indicated when the SB is large (>2–2.5 mm) *and* has significant disease. Occasionally, if the supplied territory is very large, SB is wired even in the absence of significant disease.
- Pre-dilate SB if it is significantly diseased at baseline or after MB dilatation.
- Avoid planned dual stenting (NORDIC, BBC-1, and CACTUS trials), except when SB is very large with diffuse (not just ostial) disease.
- Post-dilate SB *only if* occlusion, impaired flow, or ± severe narrowing (>90%) develops (NORDIC 3 trial).
- Stent SB only in case of suboptimal balloon angioplasty result, i.e., one of the following four features: SB occlusion, poor flow, dissection, or ± severe residual stenosis (>90%) in a large SB. SB is more readily post-dilated or provisionally stented when it is large (e.g., LCx in distal left main stenting). After dual stenting, final kissing balloon inflation is necessary to resolve MB stent distortion.

FFR studies have shown that SB narrowing that occurs after stenting is often functionally non-significant. The narrowing is partly due to a benign geometric kinking of SB when MB is straightened by the stent. In addition, ***provisional rather than planned stenting is associated with a lower periprocedural MI and similar long-term outcomes***. Stent-induced occlusion of a large branch may result in significant myocardial ischemia/necrosis, though in most patients the long-term prognosis is good and many initially occluded SBs are patent on follow-up.

D. Chronic total occlusion (CTO)

CTO implies a total coronary occlusion that is >3 months old. An occlusion may develop progressively over time and lead to an insidious, chronic angina presentation. It may also develop or progress acutely/subacutely leading to STEMI or NSTEMI; when this acute occlusion is not treated early on, it enters the category of CTO 3 months later. Well-developed collaterals may provide flow equivalent to a 50–90% stenosis, which helps maintain myocardial viability and prevents resting myocardial ischemia. When the coronary occlusion develops progressively rather than abruptly, the myocardial function may be normal at rest or depressed, but not infarcted (hibernating rather than necrotic myocardium). Hibernation is distinguished from infarction by the persistence of angina, lack of Q waves, lack of echocardiographic thinning, and the presence of ischemia on stress testing.

CTO PCI is indicated in symptomatic patients who have a large ischemic burden on stress testing, especially if symptoms or ischemia are refractory to medical therapy. PCI reduces angina and reduces the need for CABG. On the other hand, opening an occlusion that was associated with a large transmural infarct (STEMI or Q-wave MI), and a myocardium that is now akinetic and minimally ischemic, is not beneficial and is not indicated (OAT trial). The success rate of CTO PCI can exceed 80% when using a hybrid algorithm, with mortality rates of 0–2% (see Appendix, Question 7). Restenosis rate is markedly reduced with DES (~10%).

Five main features predict failure of the antegrade approach to CTO PCI:

- Heavy calcification across the CTO.
- Sharp angle/tortuosity >45° within the CTO site.
- Presence of a side branch at the occlusion point without any stump (the wire will preferentially go into the side branch).
- Long CTO >2–3 cm.
- Presence of a network of thin bridging collaterals around the occlusion (caput medusa). These are sometimes hard to distinguish from intralesional microchannels, which, to the contrary, predict a high success rate. CTO with antegrade, microchannel flow is called functional CTO; the vessel continues to opacify past the CTO in an antegrade fashion.

Polymer-coated wires may be used in a functional CTO to slide through the microchannels. Otherwise, drilling wires with progressively heavier tips are used, with the support of a catheter advanced to the occlusion site. Double arterial access with engagement of the contralateral coronary is usually necessary. Contralateral injections allow collateral retrograde filling of the index vessel and thus proper visualization of the wire progression. Antegrade vessel opacification usually ceases once the wire and catheter are advanced to the CTO site, making contralateral guidance critical in most cases.

V. Sheath management

If heparin is used during PCI, the sheath is removed when ACT <170 seconds (~2–3 hours after PCI).

If bivalirudin is used, the sheath is removed 1.5 hours after the infusion is discontinued, the half-life being 25 minutes in patients with normal renal function; wait 2–3 hours in advanced renal failure (GFR <30 ml/min), where the half-life is ~1 hour.

If enoxaparin is used, remove the sheath 6–8 hours after the last SQ dose of enoxaparin.

General duration of manual pressure over the femoral artery: 10 minutes if a 4 Fr sheath is used and 5 more minutes for each higher French size. 4–6 Fr sheaths are usually used for diagnostic coronary angiography; ≥ 5 Fr sheaths are used for PCI.

In general, the patient is maintained flat in bed 4 hours after 4 Fr sheath removal, and 6 hours after 6 Fr sheath removal. A vascular closure device may be used (polyethylene glycol [Mynx], collagen [Angio-Seal], or suture-based device [Perclose]). When a closure device is used, the sheath is pulled out immediately after PCI, even while anticoagulation with heparin or bivalirudin is therapeutic; prolonged occlusive manual compression is not needed and the patient can ambulate 2–4 hours later. ***However, while convenient, closure devices do not reduce local vascular and bleeding complications***. They may, in fact, increase local vascular complications (small risk of arterial occlusion). It is safe to restick the same artery immediately after Mynx or Perclose closure. It is preferred to wait 3 months after Angio-Seal deployment, but, if needed, a restick may be performed 24 hours after deployment, 1 cm proximal to the initial stick.

If a radial access is used, heparin is given regardless of PCI to prevent radial occlusion (UFH 5000 units or 50 units/kg). If an intervention is planned, a therapeutic dose of bivalirudin may be given instead of UFH. The sheath is removed at the end of the procedure and hemostasis achieved with the use of an inflatable transradial band. *Patent hemostasis* should be used, meaning that the transradial band is only inflated with enough volume to stop the bleeding, not more (the transradial band is only inflated 1 ml of air beyond the occlusive volume); and pulse oximetry should continue to show a waveform even with ulnar occlusion. The band is kept untouched for 30 min then deflated progressively (~3 ml every 15 min).

Patients are generally hospitalized for 1 day after PCI, during which they are monitored for access complications, contrast nephropathy, and periprocedural MI. Low-risk patients without major comorbidities (HF, renal failure) undergoing a non-complex PCI through a radial access may be discharged on the day of the procedure.

VI. Post-PCI mortality and coronary complications

A. Mortality

Mortality after diagnostic angiography is ~0.1%, but this increases significantly in **severe AS** or **left main disease** (up to 0.5%), where any transient arrhythmia or hypotension, sometimes induced by sedation, may initiate an irreversible, vicious circle of myocardial ischemia and further hypotension. Also, in left main disease, the catheter abutting a left main plaque may create a left main dissection.

Mortality after PCI is <1% (~0.5%). Complications and mortality after PCI are related to both the patient and the lesion characteristics:

a. *Patient characteristics:* ACS presentation, unstable hemodynamics/emergent case, severe HF or severe LV dysfunction, older age, CKD
b. *Lesion characteristics:* severe calcifications, tortuosity, multivessel CAD, CTO, degenerated venous graft (especially left venous graft, where guide support is difficult)
Patient characteristics are a stronger determinant of complications than lesion characteristics.

B. Coronary dissection

A coronary dissection is seen after 30% of balloon angioplasties. It may also occur at the edges of a stent, when overinflation of the stent's balloon damages the edges. The frequency of stent edge dissection is 5% angiographically, 10% by IVUS, and 30% by OCT (the latter frequently detects some small and clinically insignificant dissections). Coronary dissection is more common in diffuse or calcified disease. Coronary dissection may also result from wire manipulations or from a deep-seated guiding catheter. Dissections typically propagate distally (antegradely).

1. Angiographic types of coronary dissection

- Type A: luminal haziness that does not persist after dye clearance.
- Type B: parallel tract or double lumen seen during dye injection, does not persist after dye clearance.
- Type C: extraluminal dye stain that persists after dye clearance (different from thrombus, where the stain is intraluminal). It looks angiographically similar to a type 1, localized perforation.
- Type D: spiral luminal filling defect that *significantly narrows* the true lumen. Flow may be slow but completely fills the artery.
- Type E: luminal filling defect with incomplete distal flow.
- Type F: total occlusion.

2. Treatment

When occurring after plain balloon angioplasty, types A and B dissections are often benign and do not affect outcomes; they may be treated with prolonged low-pressure balloon dilatation (balloon sized 1:1 to the vessel). After stenting, any angiographic edge dissection (except possibly type A) is worrisome as it increases the risk of stent thrombosis and warrants intracoronary imaging or further stenting. On IVUS or OCT, superficial dissections that do not reach the media, extend to less than one quadrant, and are <5 mm in length are benign. Edge dissections are frequently seen on OCT and do not necessarily warrant further stenting if they have benign features.

Whether with angioplasty or stenting, angiographic dissections types C through F carry an increased risk of thrombosis and vessel closure and are treated with further stenting. Stent distally to stop the propagation of the dissection, then proximally to seal the source of dissection; when the dissection extends very distally in a spiral fashion, it may not be possible to stent distally and one may only stent the proximal entry point to stop the expansion of the false lumen and collapse it. When the guide dissects the ostial left main or RCA and leads to hemodynamic compromise, proximal stenting may need to be performed first to relieve the extent of ischemia. In small or severely tortuous vessels where stenting is not possible, perform prolonged low-pressure balloon inflation with a well-sized balloon (not undersized).

Since type C dissection may, in fact, be a localized perforation that manifests 24–48 hours later, the patient needs to be carefully monitored and an echo needs to be obtained ± repeated 24 hours later, looking for hemopericardium.

3. Intramural hematoma is a bleeding inside the media that displaces the internal elastic membrane inward without a dissection entry or exit point. On IVUS, it appears like a deep medial dissection without superficial extension. Angiographically, it may simulate a dissection or may appear smooth, ***simulating a refractory spasm***. It is usually treated with further stenting at a low pressure.

C. Periprocedural MI

Two types of periprocedural MI may be seen:

a. Q-wave transmural MI occurs in ~1% of PCIs. It is often the result of abrupt vessel closure, thrombus formation, or occlusion of a major side branch.
b. Non-Q-wave MI is usually due to either:
  i. Distal microembolization, microvascular spasm, and microcellular reperfusion injury in a successfully opened vessel. A sluggish flow in spite of a patent epicardial artery (TIMI 2 flow or less) is called *no reflow*.
  ii. Loss of small side branches.
  iii. Transient procedural complications, such as thrombus or flow-limiting dissection.

No reflow is reduced with the use of IIb–IIIa inhibitors, and with the use of filter devices during venous graft interventions. Once it occurs, it is treated with intracoronary adenosine, verapamil, or nitroprusside.

Before saying that the patient has "no reflow," always make sure there is no mechanical obstruction or dissection (angiographically or on IVUS).

According to the 2012 ACC universal MI definition, periprocedural non-Q-wave MI is defined by an increase in troponin I to >5× the upper limit of normal, along with: (1) prolonged chest pain, or (2) ischemic ST changes or new Q waves, or (3) new wall motion abnormality, or (4) angiographic evidence of procedural, flow-limiting complications. However, as opposed to the more recognized prognostic value of post-PCI CK-MB elevation (>3–10× normal), the degree of troponin rise used in the 2012 definition does not clearly carry an independent negative prognostic value. Therefore, an expert consensus document has suggested the use of CK-MB elevation ≥ 10× normal or troponin I elevation ≥ 70× normal to define periprocedural MI. Lesser degrees of CK-MB elevations, as well as isolated troponin elevation post-PCI, are of questionable prognostic value.

The above definition applies for patients with normal baseline biomarkers. If the biomarker values are elevated but stable or falling, periprocedural MI is diagnosed by ≥ 50% reincrease of a previously downward trending troponin or CK-MB value. In patients who present with elevated biomarkers that are on the rise and who undergo PCI within 24 hours of presentation, periprocedural MI is defined by the occurrence of procedural thrombotic/occlusive complications, prolonged ischemic symptoms ≥ 30 minutes, new ischemic ST abnormalities, or Q waves after PCI, along with an increase of the next troponin I or CK-MB by at least 50% (this is the definition used in trials, e.g., ACUITY, EARLY ACS, CHAMPION Phoenix trials).

The increase in biomarkers reflects a more extensive and unstable atherosclerotic burden that predisposes to future ischemic events. The latter is likely the main reason for survival impairment, rather than the minor injury induced by PCI. This explains why the unadjusted increase in mortality with periprocedural MI is more striking than the adjusted increase in mortality, and that only marked biomarker rise post-PCI carries an independent prognostic value.

Note that *spontaneous NSTEMI carries a much stronger independent prognostic value than periprocedural MI*, despite less biomarker elevation (3× higher mortality, according to ACUITY trial data). In fact, in NSTEMI, the adverse outcome is related not only to the minor myocardial injury but to the ruptured, active plaques that carry a high risk of a large infarction, which is not the case in controlled periprocedural MI.

Periprocedural MI occurs in 5–10% of PCI cases and the incidence is reduced with the current antiplatelet regimens. Most periprocedural MIs are clinically silent. Cardiac markers should be checked 12–24 hours after all complicated PCIs and in patients with ischemic symptoms during or after PCI. Cardiac markers may also be checked routinely, 12–24 hours after any PCI (class IIa recommendation).

Chest pain is relatively common after PCI (~30%) and should be immediately evaluated with an ECG. A mild pain may simply be secondary to the continuous stretch of the treated vessel segment by the deployed stent. On the other hand, pain may be related to distal microembolization, coronary spasm, coronary dissection, or loss of small side branches, and may be associated with periprocedural MI.

Pain is initially treated with nitroglycerin. If pain is severe and persistent or associated with new ST-segment abnormalities or hemodynamic changes, coronary angiography is repeated and PCI performed urgently if needed (coronary thrombosis, dissection, large side branch occlusion). *An increase in cardiac markers is an adverse prognostic marker that does not dictate, per se, a repeat coronary angiography.*

Chest pain that occurs during PCI has similar causes. In addition, guide catheter dissection of the left main or ostial RCA should be considered and carefully assessed by angiography.

Differential diagnosis of post-PCI hypotension
- Access site complications: hematoma, retroperitoneal bleed
- Coronary perforation with tamponade
- Acute stent thrombosis or occlusive edge dissection → diagnosis by ECG
- Left main or RCA dissection (induced by the guiding catheter) → diagnosis by ECG
- Vagal shock from pain or sheath removal
- Excessive use of sedatives or antihypertensives in a hypovolemic patient

D. Coronary perforation
1. Causes of coronary perforation
A coronary perforation may be secondary to:

a. Wire tip tearing the distal end of a branch, especially when a polymer wire is inadvertently advanced too deeply. Wire perforations are usually limited, type 1 or 2 perforations.
b. Balloon or stent inflation, in which case the perforation is a large, type 2 or 3 perforation. This is more common with an oversized balloon, especially in a calcified vessel.
c. Rotablator perforation, usually the largest perforation.

2. Classification and management of coronary perforations

- **Concealed perforation (type 1)** manifests as an extraluminal stain. It requires no specific treatment except monitoring. Both type 1 perforation and type C dissection manifest as an extraluminal stain and may be indistinguishable angiographically. In the former, the stain is periadventitial, whereas in the latter, the stain is in the media.
- **Limited perforation (type 2)** manifests as a myocardial or epicardial blush/stain without jetting. It can usually be managed with prolonged balloon inflation (≥5 min) at the perforation site or just proximal to it. An echo is performed and repeated 24 hours later.
- **Freeflowing, jet-like dye streaming (type 3)**. The streaming may be pericardial, leading to immediate tamponade, or ventricular, better tolerated hemodynamically.

  Two procedures are to be immediately and concomitantly performed in case of a type 3 perforation, and this may require two physicians: (i) pericardiocentesis, and (ii) prolonged balloon inflation proximal to the perforation site. Afterwards, a second femoral access (7 or 8 Fr) is obtained and a second guiding catheter is used to double-engage and double-wire the perforated coronary artery. A Graftmaster covered stent is advanced through the second guiding catheter while the balloon is still inflated through the first guiding catheter, the balloon being only briefly deflated to advance the covered stent to the perforation site. Even short periods of balloon deflation may lead to hemodynamic compromise; thus, the double-guide technique obviates the need for a prolonged interval without an inflated balloon while the covered stent is advanced. Emergent surgery may be required if the perforation fails to seal with balloon inflation and a covered stent cannot be used.

A non-sealing perforation of a branch or distal vessel, which is usually a wire-induced perforation, may be treated by distal thrombin injection. *Thrombin* is injected through the lumen of an over-the-wire balloon catheter, the balloon being positioned distally and appropriately inflated to prevent any leak of thrombin into the proximal vessel. Contrast injection through the inflated balloon is performed first to ensure it is well sealed. Also, through a selective microcatheter positioned very distally in the branch, one may embolize *small coils* or small *fat particles* harvested from the femoral access site (cut into pieces <1 mm and mixed with saline).

Anticoagulation is not immediately reversed during the above maneuvers (e.g., prolonged balloon inflation), as this may lead to extensive coronary thrombosis.

> Note that a stain/blush that does not clear (type 2 perforation) implies a degree of sealing of the perforation and is, thus, less threatening than a blush that quickly flows and clears.

VII. Femoral access complications

All femoral bleeding complications are increased with PCI (vs. diagnostic catheterization), female sex, higher anticoagulant dose, GPI therapy, and HTN.

A. Groin hematoma

A large hematoma is a hematoma that is associated with a significant drop in hemoglobin, a requirement for transfusion, or hemodynamic compromise. In addition, it may lead to nerve compression and neurological symptoms (femoral or lateral cutaneous nerve).

B. Retroperitoneal hematoma (~0.7% of PCIs)

While the common femoral artery is a superficial compressible artery, the external iliac artery dives deep in the loose pelvis and is not compressible, even at its distal part. Thus, an iliac stick, i.e., a high stick above the inguinal ligament, has a 5× higher risk of a free-flowing, deep bleed called retroperitoneal bleed. Retroperitoneal bleed may, however, occur with a lower stick. It may also be due to inadvertent puncturing or cannulation of a small branch during access, such as the inferior epigastric artery.

Such a bleed should be immediately considered in a patient with flank or back pain, unexplained bradycardia or vagal shock, or unexplained tachycardia or hypotension that does not quickly and sustainably improve with fluid administration and atropine (if appropriate), and without a large superficial hematoma. After initial quick fluid resuscitation, the patient with persistent, unexplained hypotension is urgently taken back to the cath lab and a contralateral access obtained. Iliac angiography is obtained and, if contrast extravasation is seen, a prolonged balloon inflation is performed. This may be followed by placement of a covered stent across the perforation if it is iliac. If the perforation is common femoral, stenting is better avoided and prolonged balloon inflation alone, very short stenting, or surgical correction may be performed. If the perforation results from the puncture of a small branch, this branch may be wired then coiled; alternatively, an over-the-wire balloon may be advanced into it, followed by thrombin injection through the balloon lumen.

> When retroperitoneal hematoma is suspected with any degree of hemodynamic compromise, iliac angiography through a contralateral access is urgent. **CT scan is not necessary to confirm the diagnosis in a persistently hypotensive patient, nor should the diagnosis rely on a drop in hemoglobin level**. The patient may fall into a progressive irreversible shock with unnecessary delay. A CT scan is justified only in a hemodynamically stable, non-tachycardic, comfortable patient who has an unexplained drop of a routinely checked hemoglobin, sometimes preceded by a transient hypotension that has quickly stabilized. This patient likely had a self-limited retroperitoneal bleed that spontaneously clotted. CT scan serves to confirm the diagnosis in this particular case.

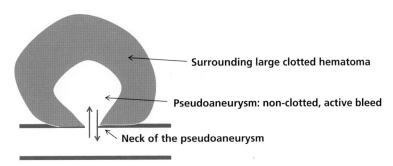

Figure 38.2 A pseudoaneurysm is characterized by a non-clotted active bleed and may be surrounded by a clotted, larger area of hematoma. A to-and-fro flow is seen from the arterial lumen.

C. Femoral pseudoaneurysm

A pseudoaneurysm is an expansile collection of blood that has two features differentiating it from a hematoma: (i) it is not clotted, and (ii) it remains in communication with the arterial lumen, i.e., there is active bleeding (Figure 38.2). In contrast, a hematoma is clotted blood without active bleeding. A pseudoaneurysm must be distinguished from a hematoma (exam, ultrasound), as it is an active bleed that will continue to expand.

A hematoma may initiate intrinsic fibrinolysis, which may dissolve the clot that initially plugs the arteriotomy site; thus, *a hematoma may evolve into a pseudoaneurysm.*

A bruit is heard on exam and a pulsatile mass is felt. The diagnosis is made by ultrasound Doppler, which shows a mass that communicates with the femoral artery through a *to-and-fro, high turbulence mosaic flow.*

The risk is higher with a low superficial femoral or profunda stick, as those arteries are not supported by bony structures and are difficult to compress; the profunda, in particular, dives posteriorly and deeply into the thigh, immediately upon takeoff, making it particularly prone to uncontrollable bleed or pseudoaneurysm.

A pseudoaneurysm that is <3.5 cm with a small neck (less than a few millimetres) is treated with ultrasound-guided prolonged compression (45 minutes) or ultrasound-guided thrombin injection. A large pseudoaneurysm >3.5 cm, a pseudoaneurysm with a large neck, or a pseudoaneurysm that fails thrombin therapy is corrected surgically.

D. Arteriovenous fistula

The risk is increased when the access is low, at the superficial femoral or profunda level, or when a venous sheath is used along with the arterial sheath. Below the femoral bifurcation, the femoral veins cross over to become anterior then lateral to the arteries, rather than medial, and risk getting punctured on the way to the arterial access.

A continuous femoral bruit is heard. At least one-third of fistulas close within 1 year, mostly within 4 months. The remaining fistulas tend to remain stable without complications on 1-year follow-up, as these fistulas are usually small.

Monitoring is usually the first line of therapy, with serial clinical and ultrasound follow-ups every 3 months. Surgical correction is indicated in the case of progressive growth or complications (limb ischemia, DVT, HF). The shunt flow across the fistula being much less than 30% of the cardiac output (Qp/Qs << 1.5) and less than a dialysis AV fistula flow, most AV fistulae (90%) are asymptomatic and do not require repair.

E. Limb ischemia

Limb ischemia may be related to impairment of flow by the sheath itself in patients with a small or diseased femoral artery. Also, the sheath may further impair the already reduced baseline flow of any severe PAD. If limb ischemia is not promptly corrected by sheath removal, a femoral dissection, thrombus, or distal embolization should be suspected. Heparin is administered and a femoral ultrasound is urgently performed, followed by urgent vascular surgery (for exploration and thrombectomy) or percutaneous intervention through a contralateral access.

> *Retrograde iliac dissection* may occur with wire advancement. Being retrograde, it is generally benign and seals with the antegrade flow.

VIII. Renal, stroke, and atheroembolic complications

A. Contrast nephropathy (increase in creatinine >0.5 mg/dl *or* > 25%)

The incidence is ~3–5%, but is higher in the case of a pre-existing renal failure, HF (or worse, shock), dehydration, or diabetes with renal failure (diabetes alone is not a risk factor). A high contrast load (>3× the GFR in ml/min) or multiple contrast studies within 72 hours are major risk factors. In patients with pre-existing moderate renal failure, the risk is ~25%. In patients with a baseline creatinine >4–5 mg/dl, the risk is >50%. In the absence of risk factors, the risk is <2%. The risk of severe renal failure requiring dialysis or irreversible renal failure is, however, ~5× lower. Most contrast nephropathies eventually improve and renal function returns to baseline. However, 18% are left with some irreversible impairment of renal function.

Creatinine starts to rise 24–48 hours after PCI, peaks at 3–5 days, and improves at 1 week. Creatinine often declines the day after the procedure because of dilution/hydration; a slight rise in creatinine at 24 hours may be an early sign of contrast nephropathy.

Prevention of contrast nephropathy:

- Hydration with normal saline (better than 0.45% saline), ***in the absence of HF***: 100 ml/h for a few hours before the procedure and 12 hours after the procedure. *In HF with clinical or hemodynamic congestion, hydration aggravates volume overload and may potentially worsen the risk of renal impairment.*
- Bicarbonate drip has not shown superiority to saline hydration.
- Use the smallest amount of contrast (30 ml for a diagnostic coronary angiogram, if possible; total contrast <2–3× GFR for PCI).

B. Stroke

Periprocedural incidence: 0.07% after routine diagnostic cardiac catheterization, up to 1% after crossing the aortic valve in severe AS, up to 0.4% after PCI.

Ischemic stroke is related to atheroembolization of aortic plaques (as the catheters scrape the aorta), embolization of thrombi formed on the wires/catheters, or embolization of an LV thrombus. This risk increases with age, peripheral arterial disease, or venous graft interventions. Patients with prior CABG generally have heavy aortic atherosclerosis; in addition, difficult left venous graft engagement and retrograde embolization during ostial venous graft intervention may lead to stroke.

Hemorrhagic stroke is rare and may be related to anticoagulation.

C. Cholesterol atheroembolization

Atheroembolization may occur in patients with severe aortic or iliac atherosclerosis, who slough off cholesterol debris during the procedure. This may lead to distal cyanosis (blue toes), livedo reticularis, subacute progressive renal failure (occurring >1 week later, with eosinophiluria), and mesenteric ischemia.

IX. Intra-aortic balloon pump (IABP) or intra-aortic balloon counterpulsation

A. Overview of IABP

An IABP is a balloon mounted on a catheter, inserted through a femoral artery (7–8 Fr sheath). It is placed just distal to the left subclavian artery (at the level of the *tracheal carina* fluoroscopically) and extends proximal to the renal arteries. It has two lumens: (i) a helium gas line connected to the balloon, and (ii) a central arterial lumen attached to the arterial monitor (Figure 38.3). Newer IABP catheters have a fiberoptic tip that allows arterial pressure monitoring without the need for the arterial lumen; the arterial port may be capped in this case. In the absence of a fiberoptic tip, thrombosis of the arterial lumen prevents monitoring of the arterial waveform and may dictate balloon removal, or the use of a suboptimal radial line for monitoring.

The IABP inflates in early diastole, just at the dicrotic notch. It deflates at end-diastole, just at the isovolumic contraction phase before the aortic upslope: this creates a negative pressure in the aorta that "sucks" flow from the LV, thus reducing afterload and myocardial wall stress. This increases cardiac output by ~20%, up to 0.5–1 liters/minute, and decreases LV filling pressure and PCWP by ~20%. Furthermore, the reduction in afterload decreases myocardial O_2 demands, which reduces myocardial ischemia.

Note that an IABP reduces systolic and end-diastolic BP, but creates a third component to BP, called *augmented BP*, that is higher than the unassisted systolic BP (Figures 38.4, 38.5, 38.6).

Assisted systolic and end-diastolic pressures are reduced in comparison to the corresponding unassisted pressures.

The end-diastolic pressure should generally be reduced by ~10–15 mmHg in comparison to the baseline end-diastolic pressure to ensure proper support. The mean arterial pressure increases, and more importantly cardiac output and tissue perfusion increase even if the mean arterial pressure is unchanged. Systemic pressure is not a parameter by which the efficacy of IABP should be gauged. The organs below the balloon level are not adversely affected, because they still receive the enhanced cardiac output during systole.

B. Effect of IABP on coronary flow

IABP inflation in diastole increases aortic diastolic pressure. In addition, IABP reduces LVEDP. Thus, IABP improves the gradient that drives coronary flow (aortic diastolic pressure minus LVEDP), which improves coronary flow in low-output states with non-obstructed coronary arteries. In the case of a critical coronary stenosis, coronary flow increases upstream of the stenosis but does not increase distal to the critical stenosis, even in shock. In fact, one landmark study by Kern et al. positioned a Doppler wire past critical coronary stenoses and demonstrated that ***IABP does not increase coronary flow velocity, a surrogate of flow, in a coronary artery beyond a critical stenosis*** (flow-limiting stenosis). Once the stenosis is treated with angioplasty, IABP increases distal coronary flow in comparison to no IABP augmentation. Another study demonstrated that coronary pressure is not increased by IABP distally to a severe stenosis (>70–80% stenosis). ***Thus, IABP improves myocardial ischemia distal to a severe stenosis through the reduction in O_2 demands rather than through an increase in coronary flow or pressure.*** Only when a non-obstructed artery supplies large collaterals (grade 2 or 3) to the occluded site can IABP increase flow distal to the coronary occlusion. Conversely, after PCI, IABP consistently increases coronary flow and plays a great role in relieving ischemia related to microvascular obstruction and no reflow, and thus in relieving persistent ST elevation.

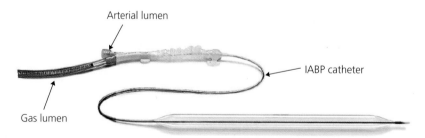

Figure 38.3 IABP catheter connected to two lumens: arterial lumen and gas lumen. Courtesy of Maquet.

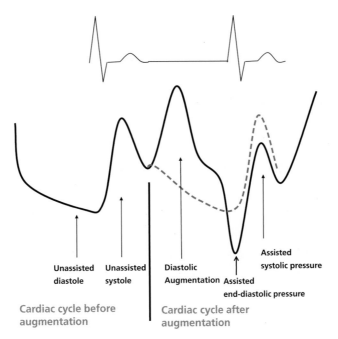

Figure 38.4 Unassisted and assisted aortic pressure. Balloon inflation occurs at the dicrotic notch, which corresponds to the end of T wave on the ECG (***end of T inflation***); balloon deflation occurs at the isovolumic contraction, which corresponds to the peak of R wave (***R-wave autodeflation***). The timing of balloon deflation is fine-tuned **until the dicrotic notch is concealed within the balloon inflation and until the nadir diastolic pressure is 10–15 mmHg lower than the unassisted diastole.** Note that the assisted end-diastolic pressure is lower than the unassisted end-diastolic pressure, the assisted systolic pressure is lower than the unassisted systolic pressure, and the augmented pressure is higher than the systolic pressure. The *blue tracing* corresponds to the aortic tracing had there not been balloon augmentation. Compare the diastolic and systolic pressures before and after augmentation.

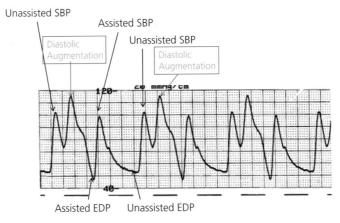

Figure 38.5 1:2 IABP inflation. Note that in a 1:2 or 1:3 mode, the SBP that immediately precedes augmentation is actually the unassisted SBP. **The two pressures to the left of augmentation are the unassisted pressures, while the pressures to the right are the assisted pressures.** EDP, end-diastolic pressure. Courtesy of Maquet.

C. Triggering and timing

The IABP is often timed and triggered to the surface ECG. It inflates at the end of T wave, which corresponds to the dicrotic notch and beginning of diastole, and deflates at the peak of R wave, which corresponds to the beginning of the isovolumic contraction (Figures 38.4, 38.5, 38.6). The device can be triggered every beat/every QRS (1:1 inflation) or every other beat/QRS (1:2, 1:3). Timing is adjusted to achieve the optimal waveform and is best done under 1:2 or 1:3 pumping mode, so that arterial tracings from consecutive beats with and without assistance can be compared. Adjustment of timing is rarely necessary with the current IABP systems, as these systems look at the aortic pressure and automatically fine-tune the timing to achieve the best arterial waveform.

The arterial waveform can also be used for triggering and timing but should not be used in irregular rhythm, as the balloon may remain inflated between cardiac cycles. Ventricular pacing spikes may be used for timing of patients who are 100% ventricular-paced

Arterial pressure waveform

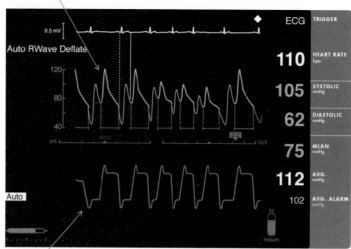

Balloon inflation waveform

Figure 38.6 IABP monitor showing the ECG, the arterial pressure waveform, and the balloon inflation waveform. The IABP is inflating in a 1:1 mode. Note that the IABP deflates at the peak of R wave (*top dashed line*, corresponds to the downslope of the balloon inflation waveform), and inflates at the end of T wave (*solid line*). Note that during shorter R–R intervals there is less augmentation in pressure (less helium delivered to the balloon). Courtesy of Maquet.

Table 38.4 Causes of lack of appropriate pressure augmentation.

---

1. a. **Late inflation or early deflation** (leads to suboptimal increase in coronary perfusion and suboptimal sucking effect).
   b. **Late balloon deflation or early inflation** (balloon inflated in systole increases afterload).
   c. **With these dysfunctional timings**, one of the dips on the tracing in Figure 38.4 widens or gets effaced. Changing the timing corrects this.
2. **Shock state that is not cardiogenic** in nature, such as hypovolemic shock or septic shock. In septic shock, afterload is already reduced and IABP does not further increase stroke volume.
3. **Tachycardia >120 bpm** reduces diastolic time, and thus reduces balloon filling and inflation during this brief time. The reduced diastolic time during each cardiac cycle is the main issue, rather than a limited ability to circulate gas at high rates; switching to 1:2 does not necessarily help.
4. **Balloon kinking** may lead to poor augmentation or poor deflation. Check the catheter and tubing for a visible kink, ensure the balloon has fully exited the sheath and get an X-ray, and position the patient flat, as bending the groin area may kink the catheter.
5. **Gas leak due to loose connections or balloon leak/rupture**. The latter may result from inflation against calcified aortic plaques and may lead to clotting inside the balloon and balloon entrapment. The blue, balloon inflation waveform is abbreviated and **blood is seen coming out of the gas lumen**. IABP should be placed on standby and **removed quickly** (<30 min), to prevent balloon clotting and entrapment.

---

and who do not have a good-amplitude QRS. In fact, even in patients who are paced, it is preferred to use the ECG for timing. If the arterial lumen is thrombosed, a radial line may be used to monitor the arterial waveform but not to adjust the timing, as balloon inflation and deflation are seen relatively later on the radial waveform than on the aortic waveform. The radial waveform may be connected to the IABP console.

D. Troubleshooting and lack of appropriate augmentation (Table 38.4)
If there is no pressure augmentation and the helium balloon inflation waveform is flat or abbreviated, consider gas leak (check tubing connections, check for blood in the gas lumen). Also, consider catheter kink and ensure that the balloon is fully out of the sheath.

A **helium balloon inflation waveform that is overexpanding** suggests impaired balloon deflation (catheter is kinked or balloon is partially in the sheath).

E. Indications for IABP
1. Cardiogenic shock due to acute ischemia/infarction: IABP is used in conjunction with PCI, is placed before or after PCI, and kept until the patient stabilizes (IABP used as a bridge to recovery). Outside shock, IABP is also useful in patients with a large STEMI who have persistent ischemia or ST elevation after primary PCI (IABP improves microvascular no reflow).
2. Mechanical complications related to MI (ventricular septal rupture, papillary muscle rupture): IABP is used as a bridge to surgical treatment.
3. Patients with low EF undergoing multivessel or left main PCI. In patients with extensive multivessel disease and EF <30% undergoing PCI, planned IABP placement was associated with a significant reduction in 4-year mortality compared with no IABP or bailout IABP (BCIS-1 trial). IABP did not reduce the short-term mortality. Rather, the mortality benefit emerged beyond several months of follow-up and was significant at 51 months.
4. Coronary complications occurring during PCI and leading to ischemia/shock: IABP as a bridge to recovery.

5. Prophylactically, pre- and post-cardiac surgery in the following high-risk cases: severe LV dysfunction, ongoing ischemia, high-grade left main stenosis, decompensated AS.

IABP may also be placed post-cardiac surgery for cardiogenic shock.

6. Refractory ischemic arrhythmias: IABP is placed during revascularization, or after revascularization if these arrhythmias persist.

IABP is a temporizing measure, a bridge to a more definitive therapy (CABG, PCI). It is also a supportive measure pending an expected recovery after a complicated PCI or CABG with transient ischemia and stunning.

F. Contraindications

IABP is contraindicated in moderate or severe AI and in HOCM (since intracavitary obstruction increases with afterload reduction). Severe peripheral arterial disease is a relative contraindication. Rather than being due to the balloon itself, *limb ischemia is related to the sheath* occluding flow to the ipsilateral limb. The use of a sheathless IABP limits limb ischemia, but sheathless insertion is contraindicated in severely obese patients because of the risk of subcutaneous catheter kink. Ipsilateral iliac angioplasty should be performed before IABP insertion in patients with iliac disease.

G. Care and follow-up

- Daily chest X-rays are performed to check the catheter position. If needed, the catheter may be manipulated and repositioned through the sheath.
- IV therapeutic doses of heparin (goal PTT 46–70 s) are provided to: (i) prevent limb ischemia from the large sheath, (ii) prevent thrombosis over the balloon.
- Daily CBC, as IABP may lead to hemolytic anemia and mild thrombocytopenia. *Severe thrombocytopenia is not* secondary to IABP.
- The IABP is weaned off when the patient is stable, usually 24–48 hours after placement, and after appropriate therapy of the underlying cardiac condition. The patient must be:
  - Stable from the hemodynamic standpoint, i.e., have a stable systemic pressure and peripheral perfusion with or without small doses of inotropes/vasopressors, and preferably with the support of vasodilators that will simulate the IABP effect, if the blood pressure allows (nitroprusside, nitroglycerin).
  - Stable from the ischemic standpoint.
- When the patient is ready to be weaned off, IABP inflation is changed from 1:1 to 1:2 then 1:3 over the course of one to several hours to ensure tolerability. If the patient tolerates weaning, IABP may be removed. Heparin is held for ~2 hours and 1:1 pumping is resumed during these hours to prevent balloon clotting. The pump is shut off and IABP removed when ACT <160 s or PTT <50 s.

X. Percutaneous LV assist device: Impella and TandemHeart
A. Impella or transvalvular LV assist device

Impella is the prototype transvalvular LV assist device. It is a microaxial rotatory pump that expels blood from the LV to the aorta. The flow is continuous rather than pulsatile. Impella 2.5 can provide up to 2.5 l/min of flow support and is inserted percutaneously through the femoral artery; the pump segment diameter is 12 Fr while the catheter is 9 Fr and can be left in place for up to 5 days (Figures 38.7, 38.8). Impella CP can provide up to 4 l/min of support and is also inserted percutaneously (14 Fr pump). Impella 5.0 can provide up to 5 l/min of support and is inserted surgically (21 Fr). In addition to increasing cardiac output, ***Impella reduces the end-diastolic volume (preload) and the end-systolic volume (wall tension or afterload), which reduces O$_2$ demands***. The reduction in end-diastolic pressure also improves subendocardial perfusion and microcirculatory flow.

Impella reduces afterload differently from IABP: the former reduces LV volume (flow device) while the latter reduces aortic resistance (pressure device). However, the two devices should not be combined. The diastolic augmentation of IABP increases the diastolic afterload of Impella, which is a continuous pump, and counteracts the Impella flow in diastole. This drastically reduces the diastolic and overall Impella flow. Besides, significant hemolysis may occur as the Impella pumps against an inflated balloon.

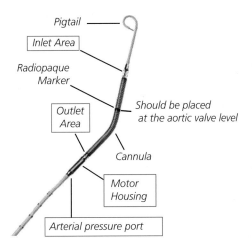

Figure 38.7 Impella 2.5 assist device. Blood is pulled from the LV through the *inlet area* and pumped into the ascending aorta through the *outlet area*. The *motor* is above the outlet area and purging prevents it from being contaminated with blood. The *arterial pressure port* is above the motor. The catheter bend is positioned across the aortic valve. Courtesy of Abiomed.

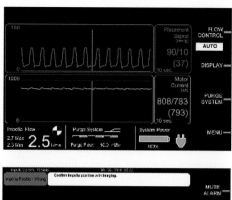

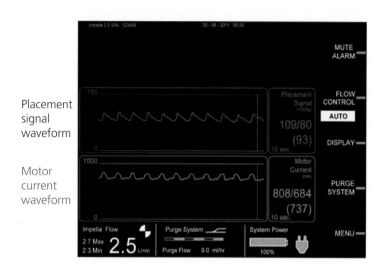

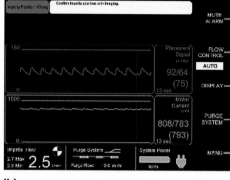

(a)   **(b)**

Figure 38.8 (a) The Impella console shows two waveforms: the aortic waveform (*on top*) captured by the arterial port above the motor, and the motor current waveform (*bottom*). The Impella flow is an estimate derived from the motor current. While the pump is continuous, the current and flow are higher in systole than diastole because of the higher delta pressure between the LV and the aorta.

(b) There are two situations wherein the motor current waveform becomes flat (but not necessarily low): the inflow and outflow ports are both in the LV or both in the aorta. If they are both in the LV, the aortic port may show a ventricular waveform (*top*) but may also show an arterial waveform (*bottom*), as the aortic pressure port, which is upstream of the inflow and outflow, may still be in the aorta.

If the LV is underfilled and gets sucked by Impella, the flow will be lower than the programmed flow and the motor current may dampen and decline. Courtesy of Abiomed.

Impella provides a constant axial flow, and, as opposed to IABP, there is no need for ECG or pressure waveform synchronization. The arterial pressure increases but the pulse pressure narrows since part of the cardiac output is provided by this non-pulsatile pump. **The more Impella contributes to the cardiac output, the less pulsatile the blood flow is.** For example, during coronary balloon inflation in high-risk coronary intervention, the pulse pressure is severely reduced and the aortic pressure may become a flat pressure line provided by Impella.

With IABP, the absolute increase in cardiac output depends on the baseline cardiac output; thus, in the sickest patients with severe heart failure and limited cardiac reserve, cardiac output may only increase by 0.2 liters/minute, which necessitates the adjunctive use of inotropic agents. The benefit of IABP in this context is mainly seen in terms of reducing myocardial ischemia. Impella 2.5, on the other hand, increases cardiac output by 2.5 l/min in the most severe cases of heart failure. For example, if an Impella is applied to a patient with a cardiac output of 5 l/min, the preload reduction reduces the native stroke volume and cardiac output to 4 l/min, but Impella provides 2.5 l/min of extra flow, making the new cardiac output 6.5 l/min, i.e., providing a total increase in cardiac output of 1.5 l/min. If Impella is applied to a patient with a cardiac output of 2 l/min, the unloading of the LV reduces the native cardiac output to 1.6 l/min, but Impella provides 2.5 l/min of extra flow, making the new cardiac output 4.1 l/min, i.e., providing a total increase in cardiac output of 2.1 l/min. Also, **the more depressed the aortic pressure (low afterload), the higher the flow provided by the Impella pump in both systole and diastole.** Thus, **Impella further improves cardiac output in severe LV failure while unloading the LV and reducing O$_2$ demands.** The patient is less likely to require inotropic agents with Impella than with IABP support. It is important to maintain adequate preload during Impella therapy, as a low preload reduces the benefit from Impella and its potential to increase the overall cardiac output. It is also important to maintain a low arterial afterload (mean BP <90 mmHg), as the axial Impella pumping is impeded by a high upstream, aortic pressure. In light of its superior flow, Impella CP is generally used in cardiogenic shock, while Impella 2.5 is used to support PCI.

In an animal study of cardiogenic shock, *Impella improved coronary flow in unobstructed coronary arteries by up to ~45%*, significantly more than IABP (~15%) (Sauren et al.). Impella improves coronary flow through the increase in mean arterial pressure but also through the reduction of LVEDP and microvascular resistance. Moreover, **Impella unloads the LV and reduces O$_2$ demands more dramatically than IABP.**

PROTECT II was a randomized, multicenter trial comparing the Impella system with IABP in patients requiring hemodynamic support during non-emergent, high-risk PCI (unprotected left main PCI and LVEF <35% or three-vessel PCI and LVEF <30%). The mean SYNTAX score was high at 30. In the per-protocol analysis, Impella patients had fewer major adverse events at 90 days than the IABP patients (40.8% vs. 51.4%; $p = 0.029$), despite a more frequent use of rotational atherectomy.

Impella contraindications

Impella is contraindicated in moderate or severe AS (aortic valve area <1.5 cm^2), as the Impella catheter may worsen the aortic obstruction. It is also contraindicated in moderate or severe AI, and in the presence of LV thrombus. Severe peripheral arterial disease is a relative contraindication.

B. TandemHeart LV assist device

TandemHeart is a left atrial-to-iliac artery bypass. It consists of an extracorporeal centrifugal pump that withdraws blood from the left atrium via a 21 Fr trans-septal cannula and pumps it into the iliac artery (15–17 Fr cannula) at a continuous flow rate of up to 3.5 l/min (15 Fr outflow cannula) or 5 l/min (17 Fr outflow cannula). The iliac flow retrogradely supplies the systemic circulation. The left atrial cannula is inserted trans-septally through the femoral vein. The maximum output depends on the diameter of the outflow cannula. In order to prevent limb ischemia from the large arterial cannula, a sheath is placed antegradely in the femoral artery and connected in a Y fashion with the iliac cannula. Similarly to Impella, this percutaneous LVAD unloads the LV and improves subendocardial perfusion, with a potential for more cardiac output increase than Impella 2.5. While Impella directly unloads the LV, TandemHeart indirectly unloads the LV, and it is therefore less effective in reducing afterload and less effective in reducing O$_2$ consumption. Thus, while both devices provide good hemodynamic support and myocardial ischemic protection, Impella 2.5 is likely more suited for high-risk PCI or MI, where ischemic protection is the primary concern, whereas TandemHeart is likely more suited for cardiogenic shock, where hemodynamic support is the primary concern. The availability of Impella CP, which provides both ischemic protection and large flow rate, has lessened the need for TandemHeart.

XI. Extracorporeal membrane oxygenation (ECMO)

Peripheral venoarterial ECMO consists of a femoral venous cannula (~23 Fr), a femoral arterial cannula (~17 Fr), an extracorporeal pump (non-pulsatile), and an oxygenator. ECMO drains unoxygenated blood from the IVC and returns oxygenated blood through the femoral artery. In the absence of any forward cardiac output, blood will retrogradely flow from the femoral artery towards the upper body. Peripheral ECMO provides a cardiopulmonary bypass wherein oxygenation and flow are *almost* fully provided by the machine (see below why peripheral ECMO should not provide *full* support). ECMO provides flow at ~4–5 l/min. ECMO is particularly useful in:

1. Patients with witnessed cardiac arrest who had an immediate start of cardiopulmonary resuscitation, yet a lack of return of spontaneous circulation in >10 minutes. *ECMO may be placed at the bedside in a patient with cardiac arrest and ongoing chest compressions, using groin access.*

2. Patients with profound cardiogenic shock and biventricular failure, where LV support alone with Impella may not be enough. This may apply to patients with MI or severe myocarditis.

Femoral–femoral ECMO has several caveats that explain why some intrinsic LV output should be maintained:

1. The LV continues to receive venous return from the bronchial and thebesian veins, and thus may overdistend in the absence of some intrinsic LV function. ECMO increases pressure afterload and may make it harder for the intrinsic LV to open the aortic valve and decompress. LV overdistension may lead to coronary compression, irreversible myocardial injury, pulmonary edema, and hemorrhage. The LV needs to be monitored by echo and vented if necessary: this is performed using adjunctive IABP, Impella, or inotropes. In a patient with cardiac arrest, ongoing chest compressions should be continued to vent the LV. An LA cannula may also be inserted through a trans-septal puncture to vent the left heart. While ECMO flow is non-pulsatile, the maintenance of intrinsic LV function leads to a perceptible pulse on the arterial waveform. An 80% ECMO flow and 20% LV flow is desired.

2. While necessary, the preservation of LV pumping means that the upper body is partly supplied by the LV rather than the ECMO. Competition between ECMO flow (coming from the lower body) and intrinsic LV flow may lead to deoxygenation of the upper body. This is monitored by checking the arterial O$_2$ saturation of the right radial artery (furthest away from ECMO flow).

After a few days, ECMO is weaned off by progressively reducing its flow to 1.5 liters/minute while monitoring systemic pressure and LV function by echo. Before removal, the cannulae are clamped for 15 minutes to ensure hemodynamic stability. Vasopressors may need to be up-titrated during the weaning process. Pulmonary edema may worsen as venous return increases.

As an alternative to ECMO in patients with biventricular failure and shock requiring temporary support, an ***extracorporeal biventricular assist device*** may be used (CentriMag BiVAD). The cannulae of the right assist device are surgically placed in the RA and PA, while the cannulae of the left assist device are surgically placed in the LV (or LA) and the aorta. The pump, and the optional oxygenator, are outside the body. BiVAD is less expeditious but more effective than ECMO, and may be used for 30 days (as opposed to a few days only for ECMO).

Veno–venous ECMO drains blood from a femoral venous access and returns it into a jugular access. It is used in patients with preserved circulation but severe respiratory failure, such as acute respiratory distress syndrome. It has shown a mortality reduction during the H1N1 epidemic.

XII. Fractional flow reserve (FFR)

A. FFR concept and application

FFR is measured using a 0.014" coronary pressure wire which has a micromanometer 3 cm from its floppy tip (at the junction of the radiopaque distal tip and the radiolucent part of the wire). This wire is advanced into the coronary artery and measures pressure distal to the stenosis (Pd). This pressure is compared to the aortic pressure (Pa) obtained through the guiding catheter. In a simplistic way, FFR compares pressure distal to the stenosis to pressure in the aorta (Pd/Pa) under maximal hyperemia. However, FFR actually aims to evaluate the ratio of maximal myocardial flow in the presence of a stenosis to the theoretical maximal myocardial flow had there not been a stenosis. Since myocardial flow = microvascular flow = pressure/ microvascular resistance, maximal microcirculatory vasodilatation needs to be achieved in order to make pressure correlate linearly with flow (Figure 38.9). In a patient with a significant stenosis, flow may be normal at rest but

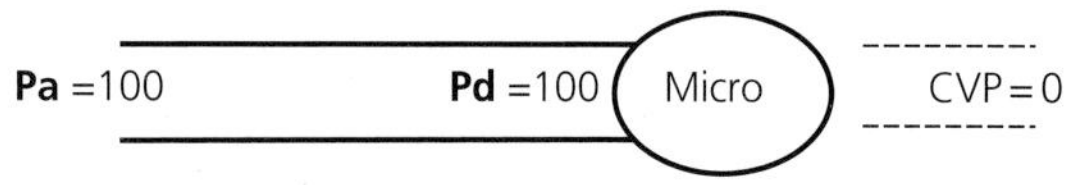

Pa =100   Pd =100 Micro   CVP = 0

Myocardial flow in the absence of stenosis= Flow 1= (Pa-CVP)/microvascular resistance

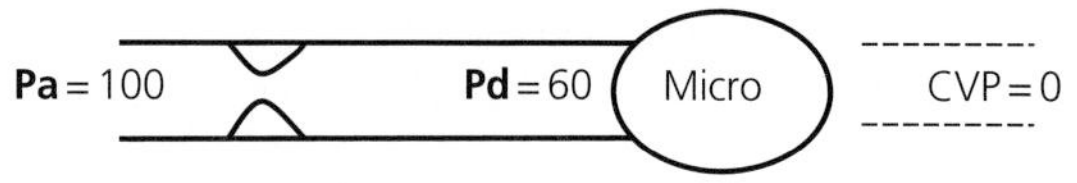

Pa = 100   Pd = 60 Micro   CVP = 0

Myocardial flow in the presence of stenosis= Flow 2=(Pd-CVP)/microvascular resistance

FFR= $\dfrac{\text{Flow 2}}{\text{Flow 1}}$

$= \dfrac{\text{(Pd-CVP)/microvascular resistance}}{\text{(Pa-CVP)/microvascular resistance}}$

During maximal hyperemia, microvascular resistance is low and equal in both conditions (in the absence of microcirculatory impairment or in the presence of microcirculatory impairment that is steady over time)

→ Flow and pressure are linearly related

→ FFR= (Pd-CVP)/ (Pa-CVP)~ Pd/Pa

Figure 38.9 Concept of FFR. FFR evaluates the ratio of maximal myocardial flow in the presence of a stenosis to the theoretical maximal myocardial flow had there not been a stenosis. Reproduced with permission of Demos Medical from Hanna EB. Fractional flow reserve. In: Hanna EB, Glancy DL. Practical Cardiovascular Hemodynamics. New York, NY: Demos Medical, 2012, p. 193.

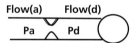

Flow(a)   Flow(d)

Pa   Pd

(Pa-Pd)= Flow(a) /resistance across the stenosis

If flow(a) ↑→ More drop in pressure past the stenosis

At maximal hyperemia, flow(a) ↑ and thus Pd further drops.
Since Pd linearly correlates with flow(d) at maximal hyperemia, this further drop in Pd represents a further drop in flow(d) at maximal hyperemia

Figure 38.10 The drop in pressure and thus the drop in flow across a stenosis is dependent on the proximal flow, which depends on the amount of viable myocardium supplied by the artery. Thus, for the same stenosis severity (e.g., 80%), a proximal left anterior descending artery stenosis is more likely to be significant than a small diagonal stenosis (e.g., FFR 0.65 in the former and FFR 0.90 in the latter).

Also, for the same stenosis severity, length increases the significance of a stenosis. According to the Poiseuille law, resistance across a stenosis correlates with (viscosity × length)/radius[4].

Reproduced with permission of Demos Medical from Hanna EB. Fractional flow reserve. In: Hanna EB, Glancy DL. Practical Cardiovascular Hemodynamics. New York, NY: Demos Medical, 2012, p. 194.

does not increase enough with maximal vasodilatation; thus, vasodilatation allows the calculation of the maximum achievable flow ratio (corresponding to exertional flow).

The drop in flow across a stenosis corresponds to the severity of luminal narrowing, the length of stenosis, the extent of viable myocardium supplied by the artery, and the presence of collaterals (Figure 38.10). A 75% mid-LAD lesion supplying a normal anterior wall is more likely to be significant than a 75% small diagonal stenosis or 75% mid-LAD stenosis supplying an infarcted anterior wall.

The preferred hyperemic stimulus is intravenous adenosine administered through a central venous line or a large antecubital vein. The FFR number obtained before adenosine administration is simply a drop in pressure across a stenosis and does not correspond to a drop in flow; "baseline FFR" or "pre-adenosine FFR" are inappropriate descriptions, "baseline pressure ratio" being the appropriate characterization of the ratio obtained before adenosine administration. After adenosine infusion, the myocardial flow increases because of microcirculatory dilatation, the pressure further drops across the lesion (Figure 38.10), and, more importantly, this additional pressure drop correlates with an actual flow drop, i.e., FFR.

Systemic hemodynamics such as heart rate or blood pressure or stable microvascular dysfunction do not affect the drop in myocardial flow secondary to a coronary stenosis, and therefore FFR remains accurate in these circumstances. Moreover, FFR takes into account the contribution of collateral flow: a lesion is more likely to be significant if the artery provides collaterals. FFR <0.75 is hemodynamically

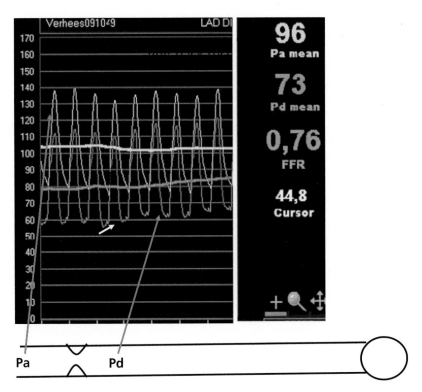

Figure 38.11 The upper tracing illustrates Pa, the pressure at the guide catheter tip, while the lower tracing illustrates Pd, the pressure obtained through the wire sensor. When the lesion is significant with FFR <0.80, the distal pressure takes a ventricularized morphology, wherein the pressure is horizontal or upsloping in diastole (*white arrow*), sometimes with A wave. Reproduced with permission of Demos Medical from Hanna EB. Fractional flow reserve. In: Hanna EB, Glancy DL. Practical Cardiovascular Hemodynamics. New York, NY: Demos Medical, 2012, p. 196.

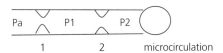

Figure 38.12 Serial stenoses. The calculation of local FFR across each stenosis under maximal hyperemia, i.e., P_1/Pa and P_2/P_1, underestimates the true severity of each lesion; had there not been another lesion, the local flow across each lesion would be higher and the pressure drop across each lesion would be higher than estimated by the local FFR. In fact, P_1 does not have a linear correlation with the myocardial flow past lesion 1, as the presence of lesion 2 prevents maximal hyperemia past lesion 1, and thus, P_1/Pa and P_2/P_1 are not true FFR values. P_2, the summation of pressure drop across both stenoses, linearly correlates with myocardial flow past lesion 2, and P_2/Pa is an adequate estimate of myocardial flow drop across all lesions.

Reproduced with permission of Demos Medical from Hanna EB. Fractional flow reserve. In: Hanna EB, Glancy DL. Practical Cardiovascular Hemodynamics. New York, NY: Demos Medical, 2012, p. 197.

significant and accurately identifies ischemia on non-invasive stress testing with 100% specificity, whereas FFR >0.80 has a sensitivity of >90% for excluding ischemia. When FFR is between 0.75 and 0.80, ischemia is generally present but clinical variables are necessary to guide revascularization.

Also, *when FFR is <0.80, the distal coronary pressure becomes ventricularized and loses its dicrotic notch* (Figure 38.11). In fact, blood flows in the left coronary artery predominantly during diastole. If a stenosis is present, the diastolic drop in pressure is larger than the systolic drop in pressure (drop in pressure across a stenosis = flow/ resistance → larger diastolic flow translates into a larger diastolic pressure drop). Therefore, the shape of the pressure curve recorded by the wire is different from the aortic pressure curve, with a flat or ventricularized diastole. During hyperemia, diastolic blood flow increases with a lesser increase in systolic flow, further accentuating the ventricularized shape of the distal pressure signal. FFR <0.80 without distal pressure ventricularization suggests an error in zeroing or error in equalization of both transducers at the aortic level. Pull back the wire to the tip of the guide and verify appropriate equalization.

B. Special situation: serial stenoses (Figure 38.12)

Place the wire distal to all lesions and assess the summation FFR. If FFR ≤0.80, perform a wire pullback maneuver under steady-state hyperemia (intravenous adenosine infusion) and assess the local pressure drop, i.e., flow drop, across each lesion. Treat the lesion with the highest focal drop, then reassess FFR to see if the remaining lesion is focally significant. After treating one of the lesions, the flow increases, which leads to further pressure drop across the other lesion, and as a result the true FFR across this other lesion will be lower than initially expected.

C. Special situation: diffuse disease

If FFR ≤0.80 but pressure pullback reveals a gradual decline in pressure without a focal drop, the patient may not be served by revascularization. This may be seen in patients with mild or moderate diffuse disease and small coronary arteries. In fact, 8% of arteries with mild diffuse coronary atherosclerosis and without a focal stenosis have a graded continuous fall in pressure along the arterial length with FFR <0.75, explaining myocardial ischemia and angina without angiographically obstructive disease.

D. Special situation: ostial disease

If the guiding catheter is too deeply engaged in a patient with ostial disease, the pressure at its tip corresponds not to the aortic pressure but to the pressure distal to the lesion. In this case, both the guiding catheter tip and the pressure wire sensor are distal to the stenosis. The guiding pressure (false Pa) and the sensor pressure (Pd) correlate closely and the FFR is falsely increased.

Thus, while the guide may be temporarily engaged during wiring, it must be disengaged when FFR measurements are obtained. Damping or ventricularization of the guide pressure upon engagement, if present, may be used to confirm engagement then to confirm disengagement as damping resolves.

On the other hand, when assessing a coronary lesion in a patient who has moderate ostial disease or a small ostium that damps upon guide engagement, deep guide seating creates an ostial obstruction and prevents maximal hyperemic flow, and thus maximal pressure drop at the level of the lesion (serial stenoses concept). *FFR at the level of the lesion is, again, falsely increased. Guide pressure (Pa) ventricularization at rest or with hyperemia is a hint to this phenomenon.* The guide needs to be withdrawn in the aorta during FFR measurement.

E. Artery supplying an old infarcted myocardium: value of FFR in assessing residual ischemia and viability

When part of the territory supplied by a coronary artery is infarcted, this territory receives reduced myocardial flow, and thus the maximal achievable flow across this myocardial territory is reduced. Also, as opposed to a viable myocardium, the hyperemic response of a chronically infarcted myocardium is impaired. Thus, suppose that a patient with no history of anterior myocardial infarction has a 70% mid-LAD stenosis and FFR 0.70. If that same patient with the same LAD stenosis has a history of myocardial infarction with necrosis of three-quarters of the supplied territory, FFR may end up being ~0.85, and *there may not be a significant difference between the resting and hyperemic pressure ratio (impaired microcirculation)*. It has been shown that patients who are positive for residual ischemia after myocardial infarction, as assessed by nuclear imaging, have lower values of FFR compared to patients without residual ischemia. In the infarcted territory, FFR <0.75 identifies residual ischemia that is completely reversible with stenting with a specificity of 100% and a sensitivity of 87%. In another study, FFR ≤0.71 had an 88% positive predictive value for significant myocardial recovery after revascularization.

F. FFR vs. nuclear perfusion imaging in multivessel disease

Myocardial perfusion imaging (MPI) techniques are based on the concept of relative flow reserve (i.e., comparison of hyperemic flow in a stenotic artery vs. hyperemic flow in a non-stenotic artery) and require the presence of at least one normal vascular bed to demonstrate ischemia. In one study, despite angiographically severe three-vessel coronary artery disease, myocardial perfusion imaging showed no defect in 18% of patients and a single-vessel disease pattern in 36% of patients.

A nuclear substudy of the FAME trial found that in patients with angiographic multivessel disease, ~50% of vessels with FFR <0.80 were not identified on nuclear imaging, and *34% of patients with ischemia by FFR had a negative nuclear scan*.

H. Left main disease: FFR and IVUS

The assessment of left main lesion severity by angiography is subject to large inter- and intra-observer variability, particularly for 30–60% stenoses. In left main disease, several prospective studies have shown that deferral of coronary artery bypass grafting (CABG) based on FFR >0.80 is associated with good long-term outcomes, similar to the outcomes of patients with left main FFR ≤0.80 who receive CABG.

IVUS may be used to guide left main revascularization. However, various studies have provided various cutoffs for what should be considered significant left main disease. While one retrospective study found that the lack of revascularization of a stenotic left main artery with a minimal lumen area <7.5 mm² was associated with poor outcomes, other studies have found different cutoffs, such as a minimal lumen area <6 mm², or a minimal lumen diameter <2.5 mm. The functional significance also depends on the patient's original left main diameter and the presence of branch vessel disease (LAD or LCx disease). Additionally, the lack of coaxiality and the potential oblique luminal distortion may overestimate the minimal luminal area. Hence, IVUS of the LM should be performed from two different angles, one through an LAD wire and the other through an LCx wire.

FFR seems to provide a more uniform and reproducible assessment of the significance of left main disease, but FFR has limitations as well: the frequent presence of concomitant lesions in the LAD, LCx, or both interferes with an isolated evaluation of the left main lesion. *Left main FFR is falsely increased in the presence of severe LAD or LCx disease (serial stenoses concept)*; this is particularly important in patients with proximal LCx disease and no LAD disease, in whom the referral to CABG is based on left main disease. One study has shown that *if the composite FFR of the LM plus the downstream LAD or LCx disease is ≥0.65, the isolated LM FFR is adequately approximated by placing the pressor sensor between the LM and the downstream disease*. If the summation FFR is <0.65, the intermediate wire placement will overestimate the true, isolated LM FFR (by an average of ~0.08). Both FFR and IVUS modalities may be needed in left main assessment.

QUESTIONS AND ANSWERS

Question 1. Which of the following is *untrue*?
A. Thrombosis mostly occurs the first month after stent implantation
B. In-stent restenosis mostly occurs 1–12 months after stent implantation
C. Neoatherosclerosis occurs >1 year after stent implantation
D. Risk factors for stent thrombosis are twofold: mechanical or pharmacological issues

Question 2. A patient has 90% mid-LAD stenosis at a bifurcation with a large diagonal branch. The diagonal branch also has 90% stenosis. What is the best PCI strategy?
A. Wire both LAD and diagonal, dilate the LAD, then dilate the diagonal, then stent the LAD while jailing the diagonal wire. Redilate the diagonal only if it has impaired flow post-stenting. No need to stent the diagonal
B. Plan for an upfront two-stent technique using crush or culotte technique

Question 3. After mid-LAD stenting, a spiral dissection is seen at the edge and is spiraling down distally to the apical LAD, impairing flow across the artery. The patient has chest pain. What type of dissection is this?

Question 4. The dissection of Question 3 becomes subtotally occlusive. What is the next step?
A. Stent distally
B. Stent proximally, at the edge of the stent

Question 5. A patient has an 80% mid-LCx stenosis. The reference vessel diameter is ~3 mm. The lesion is treated with a 3 mm compliant balloon at a high pressure of 19 atm, but the balloon never fully expands and the lesion does not yield. What is the next step?
A. Dilate the lesion with 3 mm non-compliant balloon
B. Dilate the lesion with 2.75 mm non-compliant balloon
C. Use rotablation
D. Use cutting balloon
E. Stent the lesion

Question 6. In patients with multivessel CAD involving the LAD or the left main, PCI is an alternative to CABG when:
A. SYNTAX score is ≤22 without diabetes
B. SYNTAX score is <32 without diabetes
C. SYNTAX score is ≤22 regardless of diabetes

Question 7. A patient has CTO of the mid-RCA that is ~5 cm long with heavy calcium. It reconstitutes distally before the bifurcation, through LAD septal collaterals. There is a cap at the occlusion site and the distal reconstitution has a 2.5 mm caliber. What is the first recanalization strategy?
A. Antegrade recanalization with polymer wire escalation
B. Antegrade recanalization with heavy-tip wire escalation
C. Antegrade recanalization with subintimal tracking followed by reentry
D. Retrograde recanalization through the septal collaterals

Question 8. A patient underwent an uneventful PCI of the mid-RCA through a femoral access. The femoral access is closed using a closure device. One hour after the procedure, the patient is noted to be diaphoretic and hypotensive (BP 90/65), with a rise in pulse (from baseline 60 to 90 bpm). On exam, his access site is soft without hematoma. He does not complain of chest pain and ECG is unremarkable. Hypotension does not improve with a quick fluid bolus. What is the next step?
A. Continue fluid administration and check hemoglobin
B. Continue fluid administration, check hemoglobin, and obtain a stat CT scan of the abdomen
C. Take the patient urgently to the catheterization laboratory, perform contralateral femoral access, and obtain iliofemoral angiography

Question 9. Concerning differences between groin hematoma and pseudoaneurysm, which of the following is *untrue*?
A. Hematoma is a clotted blood collection, wherein the bleeding has already stopped (no communication with the lumen)
B. Pseudoaneurysm is a non-clotted blood collection that continues to communicate with the true lumen through the arteriotomy (the arteriotomy is the neck of the pseudoaneurysm)
C. Pseudoaneurysm consists of active bleeding into the blood collection
D. On ultrasound, a hematoma is characterized by a to-and-fro, high-turbulence mosaic flow
E. A hematoma may evolve into a pseudoaneurysm through intrinsic thrombolysis

Question 10. A patient undergoes mid-RCA stenting. At the end of the procedure, it is noted that the ostium of the RCA has been dissected by the guiding catheter. The dissection extends into the right coronary cusp. What is the next step?
A. Refer to cardiac surgery (aortic dissection)
B. Stent the ostium of the RCA and treat the cusp dissection conservatively with clinical and CT monitoring

Question 11. A mid-RCA stenosis has been treated over a polymer wire. The polymer wire has been inadvertently advanced into a small PDA branch. At the end of the procedure, it is noted that the polymer wire tip has perforated the small PDA branch. There is a small myocardial blush in the septum at the level of the branch. This blush only slowly clears. What type of perforation is this?

Question 12. How should the perforation of Question 11 be managed?
A. Prolonged balloon inflation distally (~3–5 minutes), close to the level of the perforated branch
B. Rewire the small branch and advance a balloon catheter into it. Afterwards, remove the wire, inflate the balloon, and inject thrombin, coil, or fat particles into the excluded branch
C. Reverse anticoagulation
D. A then B

Question 13. A patient has a proximal LAD stenosis and a mid-LAD stenosis. A pressure wire is placed between the two stenoses. The FFR number is 0.85. Which of the following statements are true (multiple options)?
A. This number is an adequate representation of the significance of the proximal LAD stenosis

B. Had there not been a mid-LAD stenosis, the FFR number at this level would be >0.85

C. Had there not been a mid-LAD stenosis, the FFR number at this level would be <0.85

D. 0.85 is not a true FFR across the proximal stenosis, as the mid-LAD stenosis prevents the achievement of maximal hyperemia across this proximal stenosis

Question 14. A patient has mid-LAD stenosis of 70%. A pressure wire is advanced in the LAD for FFR. The patient has a small left main with mild ostial disease, which makes the guiding catheter obstruct the ostium and leads to ventricularization of the guiding catheter pressure during engagement. The FFR measured across the LAD while the catheter is engaged is 0.82 (under maximal hyperemia). How will this FFR number change if the catheter is disengaged?

A. FFR will rise (e.g., 0.87), as the guiding catheter was creating additional ostial obstruction

B. FFR will drop (e.g., 0.75)

Question 15. On Figure 38.5, during 1:2 IABP balloon augmentation, identify the assisted systolic and diastolic pressures, as well as the unassisted pressures.

Answer 1. D. Risk factors for stent thrombosis are threefold: mechanical, pharmacological, and patient/lesion characteristics.

Answer 2. A. Provisional stenting is preferred to a two-stent strategy. In a true bifurcation, the diagonal is dilated before LAD stenting, to reduce the risk of post-stent occlusion. After LAD stenting, the diagonal is only dilated if flow is impaired (NORDIC 3), or, possibly, if it is left with a stenosis >90% (BBC-1 and NORDIC-IV trials).

Answer 3. Type D dissection.

Answer 4. B. Generally, the dissection is initially stented distally to prevent further propagation, then proximally. However, in cases where the dissection extends too far distally or the distal extent cannot be properly assessed, it is reasonable to stent proximally to collapse the false lumen and block its expansion. This may also be done in unstable patients.

Answer 5. C. A lesion that does not fully yield during balloon inflation should not be stented. The lack of full balloon expansion is different from the more common elastic recoil, wherein the balloon expands but the vessel quickly collapses back. A stent treats elastic recoil and dissections that occur after balloon angioplasty, but will not be able to expand a lesion that does not yield to balloon angioplasty. The stent will fail to appropriately expand and a catastrophic stent thrombosis may occur. Rotablation should be used in this case, usually 4–6 weeks after balloon angioplasty attempt. Balloon angioplasty may have created dissection planes, which contraindicate the immediate use of rotablation, hence the waiting period. The pressure of balloon angioplasty is what makes the lesion yield, not the type of balloon. A non-compliant balloon allows high inflation pressure without much of a growth in balloon size and is safer to use for high pressure inflation >14 atm (i.e., a 3 mm balloon stays close to 3 mm in size). However, the yielding power of high pressure, 19 atm in this case, is the same with either balloon.

Answer 6. A. This is based on the SYNTAX and FREEDOM trials. If SYNTAX score is >22 or diabetes is present, CABG is associated with a mortality reduction in comparison to PCI. Otherwise, there is no clear mortality difference between CABG and PCI.

Answer 7. C. The "hybrid CTO algorithm" has been developed to allow quick recanalization of difficult CTOs:

1st step: does the CTO have: (i) a clear proximal cap, and (ii) a robust distal reconstitution target away from a bifurcation point? If so, antegrade recanalization should be attempted.

2nd step: if, in addition, the CTO is <20 mm, especially without calcification or angulation at the CTO level, antegrade recanalization may be performed through the true intima using wire escalation technique. If several adverse features are present, subintimal wiring with a knuckled polymer wire may be performed, followed by distal reentry.

3rd step: in the absence of a clear proximal cap or a robust distal target that provides space for antegrade reentry, retrograde recanalization may be performed.

Answer 8. C. The patient has unexplained hypotension, without major groin hematoma and without suspicion of any cardiac issue (MI, tamponade). The top diagnosis is retroperitoneal hematoma. CT scan should not be performed in an unstable patient as the patient may quickly go into a full-blown shock during the waiting time. A quick bedside echo may be performed before taking the patient to the lab, to rule out tamponade from coronary perforation.

Answer 9. D. A pseudoaneurysm is characterized by to-and-fro flow.

Answer 10. B. Retrograde cusp dissection is generally benign and heals spontaneously. It does not require aortic surgery. CT scan may be performed and repeated to ensure the dissection does not antegradely extend into the ascending, tubular aorta, in which case surgery may be needed. Surgery is particularly indicated when the dissection extends >4 cm in the ascending aorta. Ostial coronary dissection induced by a guide is a major coronary dissection that readily progresses to occlusion. The coronary ostium should be treated with stenting.

Answer 11. Type 2 perforation.

Answer 12. D. If, after prolonged inflation, myocardial blush continues to be seen during contrast injections, distal fat, coil or thrombin injection is the next therapy. Reversing anticoagulation is not initially necessary, and may lead to extensive thrombus formation during prolonged balloon inflation.

Answer 13. C and D. Local FFR across each stenosis is not a true FFR and is a higher number than the true FFR, as maximal flow cannot be achieved across each stenosis, and thus maximal pressure drop cannot be achieved. Only the summation FFR, obtained by placing the wire past all stenoses, is an adequate representation of the significance of the overall disease. The true local FFR across the proximal stenosis may be obtained after treating the mid-LAD stenosis.

Answer 14. B. When the guiding catheter creates an ostial obstruction, it prevents maximal hyperemic flow and thus maximal pressure drop at the level of the lesion (serial stenoses concept). FFR at the level of the lesion is, thus, falsely increased. Guide pressure (Pa) ventricularization at rest or with hyperemia is a hint to this phenomenon. The guide needs to be withdrawn in the aorta during FFR measurement, allowing a proper drop of the FFR number.

Answer 15. In 1:2 mode, the assisted pressures are the two pressures that immediately follow augmentation, while the *unassisted* pressures are the two pressures that immediately precede augmentation (*to the left* of it). The systolic pressure over which the balloon inflates is actually an unassisted pressure. The assisted systolic and diastolic pressures are lower than the unassisted systolic and diastolic pressures, respectively.

Further reading

Periprocedural MI

Prasad A, Gersh BJ, Bertrand ME, et al. Prognostic significance of periprocedural versus spontaneously occurring myocardial infarction after percutaneous coronary intervention in patients with acute coronary syndromes. An analysis from the ACUITY trial. J Am Coll Cardiol 2009; 54: 477–86.

Thygesen K, Alpert JS, Jaffe AS, et al. Third universal definition of myocardial infarction. ESC/ACCF/AHA/WHF expert consensus. Circulation 2012; 126: 220–35.

Moussa ID, Klein LW, Shah B, et al. Consideration of a new definition of clinically relevant myocardial infarction after coronary revascularization. J Am Coll Cardiol 2013; 62: 1563–70.

BMS, DES, DES restenosis and thrombosis, neoatherosclerosis, thrombectomy

Hochman JS, Lamas GA, Buller CE, et al. Coronary intervention for persistent occlusion after myocardial infarction. N Engl J Med 2006; 355: 2395–407. *OAT trial.*

Tu JV, Bowen J, Chiu M, et al. Effectiveness and safety of drug-eluting stents in Ontario. N Engl J Med 2007; 357: 1393–402.

Mauri L, Silbaugh TS, Wolf RE, et al. Long-term clinical outcomes after drug-eluting and bare-metal stenting in Massachusetts. Circulation 2008; 118: 1817–27.

Aminian A, Kabir T, Eeckhout E. Treatment of drug-eluting stent restenosis: an emerging challenge. Catheter Cardiovasc Interv 2009; 74: 108–16.

Nakazawa G, Otsuka F, Nakano M, et al. The pathology of neoatherosclerosis in human coronary implants. J Am Coll Cardiol 2011; 57: 1314–22.

Stone GW, Maehara A, Witzenbichler B, et al. Intracoronary abciximab and aspiration thrombectomy in patients with large anterior myocardial infarction: the INFUSE-AMI randomized trial. JAMA 2012; 307: 1817–26.

Jolly SS, Cairns JA, Yusuf S, et al. Randomized trial of primary PCI with or without routine manual thrombectomy. N Engl J Med 2015; 372: 1389–98. *TOTAL trial. In contrast to the TAPAS trial, the TASTE and TOTAL trials did not show any clinical benefit of the routine use of thrombectomy.*

Antithrombotic data

Steinhubl SR, Berger PB, Mann JT 3rd, et al. Early and sustained dual oral antiplatelet therapy following percutaneous coronary intervention: a randomized controlled trial. JAMA 2002; 288: 2411–20. *CREDO trial.*

Ferguson JJ, Califf RM, Antman EM, et al. Enoxaparin vs unfractionated heparin in high-risk patients with non-ST-segment elevation acute coronary syndromes managed with an intended early invasive strategy: primary results of the SYNERGY randomized trial. JAMA 2004; 292: 45–54.

Kastrati A, Mehilli J, Schühlen H, et al. A clinical trial of abciximab in elective percutaneous coronary intervention after pretreatment with clopidogrel. N Engl J Med 2004; 350: 232–8. *ISAR REACT trial,*

Stone GW, McLaurin BT, Cox DA, et al. Bivalirudin for patients with acute coronary syndromes. N Engl J Med 2006; 355: 2203–16. *ACUITY trial.*

Levine GN, Bates ER, Blankenship JC, et al. 2011 ACCF/AHA/SCAI guideline for percutaneous coronary revascularization. J Am Coll Cardiol 2011; 58: e44–122.

Periprocedural MI

Prasad A, Gersh BJ, Bertrand ME, et al. Prognostic significance of periprocedural versus spontaneously occurring myocardial infarction after percutaneous coronary intervention in patients with acute coronary syndromes. An analysis from the ACUITY trial. J Am Coll Cardiol 2009; 54: 477–86.

Thygesen K, Alpert JS, Jaffe AS, et al. Third universal definition of myocardial infarction. ESC/ACCF/AHA/ WHF expert consensus. Circulation 2012; 126: 220–35.

Moussa ID, Klein LW, Shah B, et al. Consideration of a new definition of clinically relevant myocardial infarction after coronary revascularization. J Am Coll Cardiol 2013; 62: 1563–70.

Access complications

Kelm M, Serings SM, Jax T, et al. Incidence and clinical outcome of iatrogenic femoral arteriovenous fistulas: Implications for risk stratification and treatment. J Am Coll Cardiol 2002; 40: 292–7.

Farouque HM, Tremmel JA, Raissi Shabari F, et al. Risk factors for the development of retroperitoneal hematoma after percutaneous coronary intervention in the era of glycoprotein IIb/IIIa inhibitors and vascular closure devices. J Am Coll Cardiol 2005; 45: 363–8.

IABP, Impella

Flynn MS, Kern MJ, Donohue TJ, et al. Alterations of coronary collateral blood flow velocity during intraaortic balloon pumping. Am J Cardiol 1993; 71: 1451–5. *Coronary collateral velocity is measured upon balloon inflation over the antegrade wire; the only flow perceived is the retrograde collateral flow. The patient with grade 2 collaterals had improvement of retrograde flow with IABP (this was not the case in patients without obvious angiographic collaterals).*

Kern MJ, Aguirre F, Bach R, et al. Augmentation of coronary blood flow by intra-aortic balloon pumping in patients after coronary angioplasty. Circulation 1993; 87: 500–11.

Sauren LD, Accord RE, Hamzeh K, et al. Combined Impella and intra-aortic balloon pump support to improve both ventricular unloading and coronary blood flow for myocardial recovery: an experimental study. Artif Organs 2007; 31: 839–42.

Yoshitani H, Akasaka T, Kaji S, et al. Effects of IABP on coronary pressure in patients stenotic coronary arteries. Am Heart J 2007; 154: 725–31.

Weber DM, Raess DH, Henriques JPS, Siess T. Principles of Impella cardiac support. Card Interv Today 2009 Aug–Sep; (Suppl): 9–16.

Naidu SS. Novel percutaneous cardiac assist devices: the science of and indications for hemodynamic support. Circulation 2011; 123: 533–43.

Perera D, Stables R, Clayton T, et al. Long-term mortality data from the balloon pump-assisted coronary intervention study (BCIS-1): a randomized, controlled trial of elective balloon counterpulsation during high-risk percutaneous coronary intervention. Circulation 2013; 127: 207–12.

ECMO

Davies A, Jones D, Bailey M, et al. Extracorporeal membrane oxygenation for 2009 influenza A (H1N1) acute respiratory distress syndrome. JAMA 2009; 302: 1888–95.

Kulkarni T, Sharma NS, Diaz-Guzman E. Extracorporeal membrane oxygenation in adults: a practical guide for internists. Cleve Clin J Med 2016; 83: 373–84.

FFR

Pijls NH, van Son JA, Kirkeeide RL, De Bruyne B, Gould KL. Experimental basis of determining maximum coronary, myocardial, and collateral blood flow by pressure measurements for assessing functional stenosis severity before and after percutaneous transluminal coronary angioplasty. Circulation 1993; 87: 1354–67.

Abizaid AS, Mintz GS, Abizaid A, et al. One-year follow-up after intravascular ultrasound assessment of moderate left main coronary artery disease in patients with ambiguous angiograms. J Am Coll Cardiol 1999; 34: 707–15.

Pijls NH, De Bruyne B, Bech GJ, et al. Coronary pressure measurement to assess the hemodynamic significance of serial stenoses within one coronary artery: validation in humans. Circulation 2000; 102: 2371–7.

De Bruyne B, Hersbach F, Pijls NH, et al. Abnormal epicardial coronary resistance in patients with diffuse atherosclerosis but "normal" coronary angiography. Circulation 2001; 104: 2401–6.

De Bruyne B, Pijls NH, Bartunek J, et al. Fractional flow reserve in patients with prior myocardial infarction. Circulation 2001; 104: 157–62.

Fassa AA, Wagatsuma K, Higano ST, et al. Intravascular ultrasound-guided treatment for angiographically indeterminate left main coronary artery disease: a long-term follow-up study. J Am Coll Cardiol 2005; 45: 204–11.

Hamilos M, Muller O, Cuisset T, et al. Long-term clinical outcome after fractional flow reserve-guided treatment in patients with angiographically equivocal left main coronary artery stenosis. Circulation 2009; 120: 1505–12.

Melikian N, De Bondt P, Tonino O, et al. Fractional flow reserve and myocardial perfusion imaging in patients with angiographic multivessel coronary artery disease. JACC Cardiovasc Interv 2010; 3: 307–14.

Sharif F, Trana C, Muller O, De Buyne B. Practical tips and tricks for the measurement of fractional flow reserve. Catheter Cardiovasc Interv 2010; 76: 978–85.

Hanna EB. Fractional flow reserve. In: Hanna EB, Glancy DL. Practical Cardiovascular Hemodynamics. New York, NY: Demos Medical, 2012, pp. 193–207.

Index

Note: Page numbers followed by '*f*' refer to Figures; those followed by a '*t*' refer to Tables

Practical Cardiovascular Medicine, First Edition. Elias B. Hanna.
© 2017 John Wiley & Sons Ltd. Published 2017 by John Wiley & Sons Ltd.